Emergency
Care and Transportation of the Sick and Injured

American Academy of Orthopaedic Surgeons

Editors:

Bruce D. Browner, MD, FAAOS

Andrew N. Pollak, MD, EMT-P, FAAOS

Carol L. Gupton, BSEMS, NREMT-P

JONES AND BARTLETT PUBLISHERS

Sudbury, Massachusetts

BOSTON   TORONTO   LONDON   SINGAPORE

American Academy of Orthopaedic Surgeons

Jones and Bartlett Publishers

40 Tall Pine Drive
Sudbury, MA 01776
978-443-5000
www.emtb.com
www.jbpub.com

Jones and Bartlett Publishers Canada
2406 Nikanna Road
Mississauga, ON L5C 2W6 CANADA

Jones and Bartlett Publishers International
Barb House, Barb Mews
London W6 7PA UK

Production Credits

Chief Executive Officer: Clayton E. Jones
Chief Operating Officer: Donald W. Jones, Jr.
V.P., Managing Editor: Judith H. Hauck
V.P., Manufacturing and Inventory Control: Therese Bräuer
V.P., Production and Design: Anne Spencer
Emergency Care Acquisitions Editor: Kimberly Brophy
Emergency Care Associate Editors: Carol Brewer and Jennifer Reed
Senior Marketing Manager Emergency Care: Alisha Barry
Senior Production Editor: Linda S. DeBruyn
Web Product Manager: Adam Alboyadjian
IT Manager: Nicole Healey
Design Manager: Kristin Ohlin
Production Services Manager: Philip Regan
Design and Composition: Studio Montage
Cover Photograph: © 2000 Bruce Ayres/Stone
Text Printing and Binding: The Courier Company
Cover Printing: Lehigh Press

This textbook is intended solely as a guide to the appropriate procedures to be employed when rendering emergency care to the sick and injured. It is not intended as a statement of the standards of care required in any particular situation, because circumstances and the patient's physical condition can vary widely from one emergency to another. Nor is it intended that this textbook shall in any way advise emergency personnel concerning legal authority to perform the activities or procedures discussed. Such local determinations should be made only with the aid of legal counsel.

Notice: The patients described in "You Are the EMT" and "Assessment in Action" throughout this text are fictitious.

Library of Congress Cataloging-in-Publication Data

Emergency care and transportation of the sick and injured / editors Andrew N. Pollak, Carol Gupton; American Academy of Orthopaedic Surgeons.— 8th ed.
    p. cm.
Includes index.
    ISBN 0-7637-1666-9
    1. Medical emergencies. 2. Transport of sick and wounded. I. Pollak, Andrew N.
    II. Gupton, Carol L. III. American Academy of Orthopaedic Surgeons.
RC86.7.A43 2001
616.02'5—dc21

                    2001052032

ISBN 0-7637-2046-1 (hard cover)

Additional credits appear on page 986 which constitutes a continuation of the copyright page.

Printed in the United States of America
05 04 03 02   10 9 8 7 6 5 4 3 2

Brief Contents

Contents

Section 1 Preparing to be an EMT-B

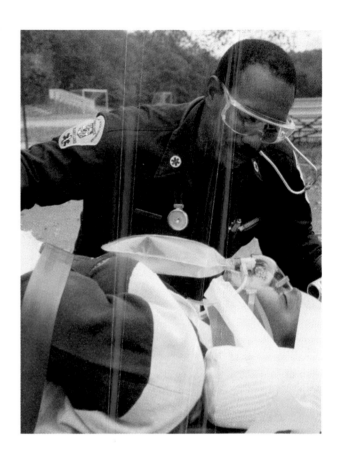

3 Medical, Legal, and Ethical Issues 64

Section 2 Airway

Section 3 Patient Assessment

contents

Section 4 Medical Emergencies

contents

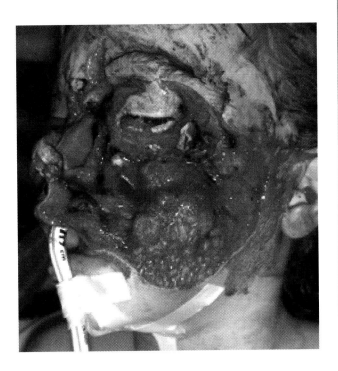

contents

Section 5 Trauma

contents

24 Soft-Tissue Injuries 562

25 Eye Injuries 586

26 Face and Throat Injuries 600

contents

contents

Section 6 Special Populations

Section 7 Operations

Section 8 Enrichment

EMT-B Skill Drills

Technology Resources

A key component in our program, interactivities and simulations help students become great EMT-Bs.

www.emtb.com

Anatomy Review— interactive anatomical figure labeling.

Web Links— present current information including trends in health care, the EMS community, and new equipment.

Online Outlook— activities further reinforce and expand on topics covered in each chapter.

Online Chapter Pretests— prepare students for training with instant results, feedback on incorrect answers, and page references.

Online Review Manual— prepare for regional, state, and national exams with this handy review manual providing instant results, feedback, and page references.

Distance Learning—

The Eighth Edition is now available with two distance learning options, Blackboard and WebCT.

Providing complete web-based course management solutions, both Blackboard and WebCT offer the ability to:

- Integrate PowerPoint presentations from the Instructor's ToolKit CD-ROM and eLearning interactivities and resources from www.emtb.com.

- Generate customized exams using the Instructor's TestBank. Exams taken online can be graded in real-time and can provide as much or as little feedback as desired.

- Participate in online forums and real-time chats, post announcements, and communicate easily with an entire class via e-mail.

- Upload course syllabi, additional course material, and course assignments.

preview

Interactivities

9-1-1 Scenarios—
actual 9-1-1 calls and questions
to prepare EMT-Bs for the field.

Videos: Skills in Action—
watch an experienced provider
perform critical skills.

Interactive Simulations—
experiment with EMT-B
skills in the safety of a virtual
environment.

Assessment in Action—
challenge students' problem-
solving abilities using scenarios
and get feedback.

Interactive Ready for Review—
test comprehension of chapter
material.

Vocabulary Explorer

Interactive Online Glossary—
expand students' medical
vocabulary, complete with
sound and images.

Animated FlashCards—
review vital vocabulary
and key concepts.

preview

Chapter Resources

TECHNOLOGY

www.emtb.com

- Online Chapter Pretest
- Interactivities
- Vocabulary Explorer
- Anatomy Review
- Web Links
- Online Review Manual
- Distance Learning

Chapter FEATURES

- Skill Drills
- Vital Vocabulary
- Pediatric Needs
- Geriatric Needs
- EMT-B Safety
- EMT-B Tips
- Documentation Tips
- Remember
- Prep Kit

Navigation Toolbar
Found at the beginning of each chapter, the navigation toolbar will guide you through the technology resources and text features available for that chapter.

You Are the EMT
Each chapter opens with a case study that will stimulate classroom discussion, capture students' attention, and provides an overview of the chapter. Additional case studies and challenging questions are included in the end-of-chapter Prep Kit.

preview

You are the EMT

While waiting for a light to change, you and your partner hear the unmistakable sound of gunshots. Moments later, dispatch sends you to the Jacks or Better pub for a shooting.

Penetrating trauma can produce injuries ranging from minor soft-tissue wounds to fatalities, either of which can present with little visible outward signs indicating the severity of the injury. This chapter will provide information on the methods recommended to control bleeding along with helping you answer the following questions:

1. Why does internal bleeding often go unnoticed until the patient "crashes"?

2. Under what circumstances might the rarely used tourniquet be the best choice for bleeding control?

Bleeding

After managing the airway, recognizing bleeding and understanding how it affects the body are perhaps the most important skills you will learn as an EMT-B. Bleeding can be external and obvious or internal and hidden. Either way, it is potentially dangerous, causing first weakness and, if left uncontrolled, eventually shock and death. The most common cause of shock after trauma is bleeding.

The purpose of this chapter is to help you understand how the cardiovascular system reacts to blood loss. The chapter begins with a brief review of the anatomy and function of the cardiovascular system. It then describes the signs, symptoms, and emergency medical care of both external and internal bleeding. The chapter concludes with a discussion on the relationship between bleeding and hypovolemic shock.

Anatomy and Physiology of the Cardiovascular System

The cardiovascular system circulates blood to all of the body's cells and tissues, delivering oxygen and nutrients and carrying away metabolic waste products ▶ Figure 22-1 . Certain parts of the body, such as the brain, spinal cord, and heart, require a constant flow of blood to live. The cells in these organs cannot tolerate a lack of blood for more than a few minutes. Other organs, such as the lungs and kidneys, can survive for short periods of time without adequate blood flow. After that, their cells begin to die. This can lead to a permanent loss of function or, if enough cells die, death.

The cardiovascular system, the main system responsible for supplying and maintaining adequate blood

- The pump (the heart)
- A container (the blood vessels that reach every cell in the body)
- The fluid (blood and body fluids)

The Heart

The heart is a hollow muscular organ about the size of a clenched fist. It is an involuntary muscle that is under the control of the autonomic nervous system, but it has its own regulatory system. Thus, it can function even if the nervous system shuts down.

The heart is always working; all other organs depend on it to provide a rich blood supply. For this reason, it has a number of special features that other muscles do not. First, because the heart can tolerate a serious interruption of its blood supply for only a few seconds, its blood supply is as rich and well distributed as possible ▶ Figure 22-2 . Second, the heart works as two paired pumps ▶ Figure 22-2 . Each side of the heart has an upper chamber (atrium) and a lower chamber (ventricle), both of which pump blood. Blood leaves each chamber of a normal heart through a one-way valve, which keeps the blood moving in the proper direction by preventing a backflow.

The right side of the heart receives oxygen-poor (deoxygenated) blood from the veins of the body. Blood enters into the right atrium from the vena cava, then fills the right ventricle. After the right ventricle contracts, blood flows into the pulmonary artery and the pulmonary circulation. The now oxygen-rich (oxygenated) blood returns to the left side of the heart from the lungs through the pulmonary veins. Blood enters the left atrium, then passes into the left ventricle. This side of

Documentation Tips

Documentation Tips provide advice on how to document patient care and highlight situations where documentation is especially crucial.

EMT-B Tips

EMT-B Tips provide advice from masters of the trade.

EMT-B Safety

Safety Tips are included to reinforce safety concerns for both the EMT-B and the patient.

preview

Chapter Resources

Remember
Remember boxes contain key points from the chapter to help students retain important information.

Remember

General Steps in Administering Medication

1. Obtain an order from medical control.
2. Verify the proper medication and prescription.
3. Verify the form, dose, and route of the medication.
4. Check the expiration date and condition of the medication.
5. Reassess the vital signs, especially heart rate and blood pressure, at least every 5 minutes or as the patient's condition changes.
6. Document.

But what if the same patient is also having chest pain "just like my other heart attack"? In that case, you may be able to apply the oxygen, but you may have to call medical control or follow standing orders before helping to administer the patient's nitroglycerin spray. Knowing and understanding the local protocols under which you will be working are absolutely essential.

In addition to getting approval to administer a medication, you must verify the online order, which means that you should restate the name of the medication, the dose to be given, and the route of administration to medical control. Verifying the order will help to reduce the chance of a miscommunication leading to the administration of an inappropriate medication.

Next, you must reconfirm that the patient can tolerate the medication. For example, suppose that you have received and verified the order to give one sublingual nitroglycerin tablet to a patient with a cardiac condition. While you were getting the order, however, the patient began to sweat more and became less responsive. A repeat blood pressure reading is 80/60 mm Hg. Using your knowledge about nitroglycerin, you would decide not to give the medication. Instead, you would notify medical control of the changes in the patient's condition and seek further orders.

Pediatric Needs

Children are not small adults, especially when it comes to the administration of medications. The approach to this population differs from that of the adult. First the dosages will be different. Sometimes they are smaller; sometimes, however, they can be larger. This has to do with the way that children metabolize medications. Most of the assisted medications will be smaller doses. Let's look at epinephrine, for example. The dose for the adult is 0.3 to 0.5 mg and the child will be given 0.2 to 0.3 mg. The approach to the injection is also different, the injection for an adult will be in the lateral thigh and the child will be in the medial thigh. Location of the injection has to do with the development of blood vessels and muscle mass in the thigh. So to avoid hitting a blood vessel, to ensure the larger spectrum of the muscle, and to ensure proper distribution of the medication, it is important to use the medial thigh in the infant and small child. When administering an MDI to children, they may not have the coordination needed to use an inhaler. It will be easier if a spacer device is added to the inhaler to ensure the child receives the full benefit of the medicine. The last and most important issue around medication administration in children is the affective side. Children are not cognitively or emotionally the same as adults. Therefore it may require you a little more time and effort to explain each procedure. It is also in your best interest to tell the child the truth. It is very important to gain the trust of the child in the short time you have to bond with him or her.

Skill Drill 7-4 Inserting an Oral Airway With a 90° Rotation

Depress the tongue so the tongue remains forward.

Insert the oral airway sideways from the corner of the mouth, until the flange reaches the teeth.

Rotate the oral airway at a 90° angle. Remove the tongue blade as you exert gentle backward pressure on the oral airway, until it rests securely in place against the lips and teeth.

If you encounter difficulty while inserting the oral airway, an alternative method may be used by following these steps ▲ **Skill Drill 7-4**

1. **Use a tongue blade** to depress the tongue, ensuring that the tongue remains forward (**Step 1**).
2. **Insert the oral airway sideways** from the corner of the mouth, until the flange reaches the teeth (**Step 2**).
3. **Rotate the oral airway** at a 90° angle, removing the tongue blade as you exert gentle backward pressure on the oral airway, until it rests securely in place against the lips and teeth (**Step 3**).

In some instances, a patient may become responsive and regain the gag reflex after you have inserted an oral airway. If this occurs, gently remove the airway by pulling it out, following the normal curvature of the mouth and throat. Be prepared for the patient to vomit.

Have suction available, and log roll the patient onto his or her side to allow any fluids to drain out.

Nasopharyngeal Airways

A **nasopharyngeal (nasal or trumpet) airway** is usually used with a patient who has an intact gag reflex and is not able to maintain an airway ▶ **Figure 7-15**. Patients with an altered mental status or those who have just had a seizure may also benefit from this type of airway. If a patient has sustained severe trauma to the head or face, you should consult medical control before inserting a nasopharyngeal airway. Extreme care must be used with such trauma patients. If the airway is accidentally pushed through the hole caused by a fracture of the base of the skull, it may penetrate through the cranium and into the brain.

This type of airway is usually better tolerated by patients who have an intact gag reflex. It is not as likely as the oropharyngeal airway to cause vomiting. You should coat the airway well with a water-soluble lubricant before it is inserted. Be aware that slight bleeding may occur even when the airway is inserted properly. However, you should never force the airway into place. Follow these steps to ensure correct placement of the nasopharyngeal airway ▶ **Skill Drill 7-5**

1. **Before inserting the airway**, be sure you have selected the proper size. Measure from the tip of the patient's nose to the earlobe.

Pediatric Needs

In children, the alternative method of inserting an oral airway, using a tongue blade to hold the tongue down while inserting the airway, is the only acceptable method. Because the airways of children are undeveloped, rotating an oropharyngeal airway in the posterior pharynx may cause damage. For more discussion on pediatric airways, see Chapter 32.

Pediatric Needs and Geriatric Needs

Pediatric Needs and Geriatric Needs highlight specific concerns and procedures for special populations.

Geriatric Needs

Geriatric patients often take many medications. They might also save medications left over from prior medical conditions. Make every effort to identify which medications are current and what conditions they are being used to treat. Ask family members to help distinguish current from outdated medications, or look at the expiration dates on the medication labels. Take either a list of the current medications or the drugs themselves with you to the emergency department.

Elderly patients can become confused about their medication regimen. Uncertainty as to whether or not they missed a dose may cause the patients to repeat the medication, possibly leading to an overdose. If you think an overdose has occurred, contact medical control.

Remember, medications can interact with each other, creating potentially harmful conditions for the patient. Even though a medication may be indicated for a special condition, it might be contraindicated in the presence of another medication. For example, if the patient is taking the heart medication propranolol (Inderal) and has an acute episode of shortness of breath, any asthma remedy might be rendered ineffective by the heart medication.

The new medication sildenafil (Viagra) can have potentially fatal interactions with common heart medications. Ask a patient who has been prescribed nitroglycerin if he has used Viagra within the previous 24 hours. Report this to medical control.

While medications do help people to recover from acute conditions and adjust to chronic diseases, they can pose serious problems for the geriatric patient. You should distinguish current from prior medications, suspect accidental or intentional overdoses, and be prepared for potentially lethal medication interactions. Document all findings and inform medical control.

Documentation Tips

When documenting a medication, the proper form includes the name of the medication, dose and route, and vital signs before and after administration. For instance:

10:30 am—VS: P 88, R 18, BP 128/68—nitro, 0.4 mg SL

10:35 am—VS: P 80, R 18, BP 124/60

Epinephrine has the following characteristics:

- Secreted naturally by adrenal glands
- Decreases muscle tone of bronchiole tree
- Dilates passages in lungs
- Constricts blood vessels
- Increases heart rate and blood pressure

ADMINISTERING EPINEPHRINE BY METERED-DOSE INHALER. Asthma, also known as "reactive airway disease," can be a life-threatening condition. Therefore, some patients use epinephrine inhalers to relieve bronchial spasms quickly. The trade names of some of these inhalers include Primatene Mist, Bronitin Mist, Bronkaid Mist, and Medihaler-Epi. Since epinephrine tends to increase heart rate and blood pressure, most patients with asthma also use certain chemical cousins of epinephrine that produce fewer side effects. Metaproterenol (Alupent or Metaprel) and albuterol (Proventil or Ventolin) both work more on the bronchial spasms and less on the cardiovascular system.

ADMINISTERING EPINEPHRINE BY INJECTION. Patients who know that they are allergic to insect stings often carry epinephrine for SC or IM injections, just in case they are stung. In these individuals, insect venom causes the body to release histamine, which lowers blood pressure by relaxing the small blood vessels and allowing them to leak. The release of histamine may also cause wheezing from bronchial spasms and swelling of the airway tissues (edema), which make it difficult for the patient to breathe. Epinephrine acts as a specific antidote to histamine, countering both of these harmful effects. It constricts the blood vessels, allowing blood pressure to rise and reducing the swelling. In the lungs, it has the opposite effect: it dilates these passages, so the flow of air is less restricted. You can also expect the patient's heart rate to increase after administration of epinephrine.

You may be trained to administer SC and IM injections of epinephrine, depending on local protocol

exercise or when the patient becomes suddenly scared. Because epinephrine is secreted by the adrenal glands, it is also known as adrenaline. Epinephrine has different effects on different body tissues and is used as a medication in several forms. Generally, **epinephrine** will increase heart rate and blood pressure and decrease the muscle tone of the bronchiole tree. Therefore, it can ease breathing problems caused by the bronchiole spasms that are common in asthma and allergic reactions. In a person who is close to anaphylactic shock as a result of an allergic reaction, epinephrine may also help to maintain the patient's blood pressure.

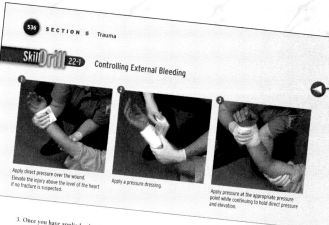

536 SECTION 5 Trauma

Skill Drill 22-1 Controlling External Bleeding

① Apply direct pressure over the wound. Elevate the injury above the level of the heart if no fracture is suspected.

② Apply a pressure dressing.

③ Apply pressure at the appropriate pressure point while continuing to hold direct pressure and elevation.

3. **Once you have applied a dressing and controlled the bleeding,** you can create a pressure dressing to maintain the pressure by firmly wrapping a sterile, self-adhering roller bandage around the entire wound. Use 4" × 4" or 4" × 8" sterile gauze pads for small wounds, and sterile universal dressings for larger wounds. If sterile gauze pads are not immediately available, use a clean handkerchief, sanitary napkin, or clean cloth. If no material is available, use your gloved hand to continue to provide the necessary pressure.

Cover the entire dressing, above and below the wound. Stretch the bandage tight enough to control bleeding but not so tight as to decrease blood flow to the extremity. You should still be able to palpate a distal pulse on the injured extremity after applying the pressure dressing. If bleeding continues, the dressing is probably not tight enough. Do not remove a dressing until a physician has evaluated the patient. Instead, apply additional manual pressure through the dressing. Then add more gauze pads over the first dressing, and secure them both with a second, tighter, roller bandage.

Bleeding will almost always stop when the pressure of the dressing exceeds arterial pressure. On those rare occasions when direct pressure fails to stop bleeding from a large gaping wound, you may need to pack the wound with sterile gauze pads, in addition to direct hand pressure. Applying ice may help control bleeding and reduce the pain **(Step 2)**.

4. **If a wound continues to bleed** despite use of direct pressure, elevate the extremity and try placing additional pressure over a proximal **pressure point**, or pulse point. A pressure point is a spot where a blood vessel lies near a bone. This technique is also useful if you have no material on hand to use for a dressing. Because a wound usually draws blood from more than one major artery, proximal compression of a major artery rarely stops bleeding completely, but it helps to slow the loss of blood. You must be thoroughly familiar with the location of the pulse points for this to work ▶ **Figure 22-9 (Step 3)**.

SPECIAL TECHNIQUES. Much of the bleeding associated with broken bones occurs because the sharp ends of the bones cut muscles and other tissues. As long as a fracture remains unstable, the bone ends will move and continue to injure partially clotted vessels. Therefore, stabilizing a fracture and decreasing movement is a high priority in the prompt control of bleeding. Often, simple splints will quickly control bleeding associated with a fracture ▶ **Figure 22-10** . If not, you may need to use another splinting device.

Skill Drills
Skill Drills provide written step-by-step explanations and visual summaries of important skills and procedures.

---

742 SECTION 6 Special Populations

Figure 32-7 Any number of objects can obstruct a child's airway. Some of the more common ones include batteries, coins, toys, buttons, and candy.

TWO-RESCUER BVM VENTILATION. This procedure is similar to one-rescuer ventilation except that it requires two rescuers, one to hold the mask to the patient's face and maintain the patient's head position, the other to ventilate the patient. This technique is usually more effective in maintaining a tight seal.

Airway Obstruction

Children, especially those younger than 5 years, can (and do) obstruct their airway with any object that they can fit into their mouth: hot dogs, balloons, grapes, or coins ◀ **Figure 32-7** . In cases of trauma, a child's teeth may have been dislodged into the airway. Blood, vomit-us, or other secretions can also cause partial or complete obstruction.

Another source of airway obstructions are infections, including pneumonia, croup, and epiglottitis ▶ **Figure 32-8** . **Croup** is an infection of the airway below the level of the vocal cords, usually caused by a virus. **Epiglottitis** is an infection of the soft tissue in the area above the vocal cords. Infection should be considered as a possible cause of airway obstruction if a child has congestion, fever, drooling, and cold symptoms. Such children must be taken immediately to the emergency department. Without special equipment and training, attempts to clear an airway that is blocked by infection can worsen the obstruction.

Signs and Symptoms

Obstruction by a foreign object may involve the upper or the lower airway. Signs and symptoms that are frequently associated with an upper airway obstruction include decreased or absent breath sounds and stridor. **Stridor** has been described as a high-pitched noise heard mainly on inspiration and is usually caused by swelling of the area surrounding the vocal cords or upper airway obstruction. In children with croup, it resembles the bark of a seal.

Figure 32-8 Epiglottitis is an infection that can cause airway obstruction in children.

Signs and symptoms of a lower airway obstruction include **wheezing**, a whistling sound caused by air traveling through narrowed air passages within the bronchioles, and/or rales. **Rales** are caused by the flow of air through liquid, present in the air pouches and smaller airways in the lungs. They produce a crackling sound like that of blowing bubbles through a straw in a glass filled with liquid. The best way to auscultate breath sounds in a child is to listen on both sides of the chest at the level of the armpit ▶ **Figure 32-9** .

Emergency Medical Care

Treatment of the child with an airway obstruction depends on whether or not the patient is unconscious and whether the obstruction is partial or complete.

If the child is conscious and you know for sure that there is a foreign body in the airway—that is, if someone actually saw the object go into the child's mouth—encourage the child to cough to clear the airway. Abdominal thrusts are also recommended to

Vital Vocabulary
Vital Vocabulary is easily identified and defines key terms students must know in the field. A comprehensive list follows each chapter, and Vocabulary Explorer on www.emtb.com provides interactivities.

Chapter Resources

Prep Kit
End-of-chapter activities reinforce important concepts and improve students' comprehension. Additional instructor support and answers to all activities are contained in the **Instructor's Resource Kit**.

Ready for Review
thoroughly summarizes chapter content. An interactive Ready for Review is provided on www.emtb.com to help students prepare for exams.

Assessment in Action
promotes critical thinking through the use of case studies and provides you with discussion points for your classroom presentation.

Prep Kit

Ready for Review

Medications come in seven different forms: tablets and capsules, solutions and suspensions, metered-dose inhalers, topical medications, transdermal medications, gels, and gases. They may be administered through nine different routes: intravenous, intramuscular, or subcutaneous injection; orally; sublingually; intraosseously, transcutaneously; by inhalation; and by rectum. In all but the intravenous injection route, the medication is absorbed into the bloodstream through various body tissues. These routes of administration often determine the speed with which the medication takes effect.

Three medications are typically carried on the EMS unit: oxygen, oral glucose, and activated charcoal. There are three additional medications that the EMT-B may help the patient self-administer: metered dose inhaler medications, nitroglycerin, and epinephrine. Remember, though, that these may differ depending on local protocol. The administration of any medication requires approval by medical control, either through direct orders given on-line or standing orders that are part of the local protocols.

There are five steps to follow in administering medications, four of which occur before you give the medication: Obtain an order from medical control, verify the proper medication, verify the dose and route, and check the expiration date of the medication. The fifth step is to accurately document the patient's history, assessment, treatment, and response.

Vital Vocabulary

absorption The process by which medications travel through body tissues until they reach the bloodstream.

action The therapeutic effect of a medication on the body.

activated charcoal An oral medication that binds and adsorbs ingested toxins in the gastrointestinal tract, for treatment of some poisonings and medication overdoses. Charcoal ground into a very fine powder that provides the greatest possible surface area for binding medications that have been taken by mouth; it is carried on the EMS unit.

adsorption To bind or stick to a surface.

contraindication Situations in which a medication should not be given because it would not help or may actually harm a patient.

dose The amount of medication given on the basis of the patient's size and age.

epinephrine Medication that increases heart rate and blood pressure but also eases breathing problems by decreasing muscle tone of the bronchiole tree; the EMT-B may be allowed to help the patient self-administer the medication.

gel A semi-liquid substance that is administered orally through capsules or plastic tubes.

generic name The original chemical name of a medication (in contrast to one of its "trade names"); not capitalized.

hypoglycemia An abnormally low blood glucose level.

indication A therapeutic use for a specific medication.

inhalation Breathing into the lungs; a medication delivery route.

intramuscular (IM) injection Injection into a muscle; a medication delivery route.

intraosseous (IO) Into the bone; a medication delivery route.

intravenous (IV) injection Injection directly into a vein; a medication delivery route.

metered-dose inhaler (MDI) A miniature spray canister through which droplets or particles of medication may be inhaled.

nitroglycerin Medication that increases cardiac perfusion by blood flow by causing arteries to dilate; the EMT-B may be allowed to help the patient self-administer the medication.

oral By mouth; a medication delivery route.

oral glucose A simple sugar that is readily absorbed by the bloodstream; it is carried on the EMS unit.

over-the-counter (OTC) medications Medications that may be purchased directly by a patient without a prescription.

oxygen A gas that all cells need in order to metabolize; the heart and brain, especially, cannot function without oxygen.

per os (PO) Through the mouth; a medication delivery route; same as oral.

per rectum (PR) Through the rectum; a medication delivery route.

pharmacology The study of the properties and effects of medications.

prescription medications Medications that are distributed to patients only by pharmacists according to a physician's order.

side effects Any effects of a medication other than the desired ones.

solution A liquid mixture that cannot be separated by filtering or allowing the mixture to stand.

sublingual (SL) Under the tongue; a medication delivery route.

suspension A mixture of ground particles that are distributed evenly throughout a liquid but do not dissolve.

subcutaneous (SC) injection Injection into the tissue between the skin and muscle; a medication delivery route.

topical medications Lotions, creams, and ointments that are applied to the surface of the skin and affect only that area; a medication delivery route.

trade name The brand name that a manufacturer gives a medication; capitalized.

transcutaneous Through the skin; a medication delivery route.

transdermal medications Medications that are designed to be absorbed through the skin (transcutaneously).

Assessment in Action

You have been waiting for the new jump-kits when they finally arrived. Your service has decided to carry activated charcoal and glucose gel in the new kit. In addition to the protocols, your crew has also decided to carry cards on the patient-assisted medications inside the kits.

It is your job to put those cards together. The cards will include information on activated charcoal and glucose gel as well as epinephrine, nitroglycerin, and metered-dose inhalers.

1. The cards will include all information necessary for any EMT to appropriately administer these medications. Which of the following lists give complete information for any medication?
   A. Actions, dose, route of administration, indications, contraindications, and side effects
   B. Dose, indications, contraindications, generic name and prescription name
   C. Indications, contraindications, generic name, side effects, and the local pharmacy
   D. Generic name, trade names, side effects, route of administration, and your medical director's name

2. Appropriate information to include on an information card about activated charcoal includes administration. A good way to administer activated charcoal is to:
   A. pour it in a glass to drink.
   B. sip it through a straw.
   C. chew it as a tablet.
   D. administer it under the tongue.

3. The appropriate method to administer the patient-assisted medication called epinephrine is to:
   A. administer it under the tongue.
   B. chew it as a tablet.
   C. inject it between the skin and muscle.
   D. swallow it as a liquid.

4. Another patient-assisted medication is a metered dose inhaler. Information on the card will include instructions to:
   A. shake well before administering.
   B. refrigerate prior to using.
   C. administer under the tongue.
   D. turn the device upside down.

5. The medication that is used most commonly in the form of a gas outside the hospital environment is:
   A. nitroglycerin.   B. metered-dose inhaler.
   C. oxygen.   D. carbon dioxide.

6. One of the contraindications for oral glucose is the patient who:
   A. is a diabetic.   B. cannot swallow.
   C. has a digestive problem. D. is having chest pain.

7. The other name for epinephrine is:
   A. metaproterenol.   B. albuterol.
   C. nitroglycerin.   D. adrenaline.

Challenging Questions

8. Why are "spacers" used?

9. Why does nitroglycerin have a tendency to lower blood pressure?

Points to Ponder

You are dispatched to an "unconscious patient" to find a middle-aged man, wide-awake, sitting in a living room chair. He is complaining that someone called you and that he does not need any help. He explains that he "just got dizzy and passed-out for a second." As you continue your assessment, the only notable finding is that the patient's blood pressure is quite elevated. The patient states that he only takes his blood pressure medicine when his headaches get too bad. In further questioning, he explains that he is supposed to take one tablet twice a day, but it affects his "manhood." You remember from your pharmacology lecture that some blood pressure medication make the patient unable to achieve an erection. He also states that his headaches have been occurring for about three days. Your patient tells you that he "don't need to see no damned doctor" and refuses transport. What are the potential risks for this patient if he does not take his blood pressure medication as prescribed? How would you counsel him and what would you say? How will you deal with him if he becomes more talkative about his "sex life?"

Issues Education and Counseling, Refusal of Treatment.

Online Outlook

A medication may have many different names, which may be a bit confusing for you at first. To learn more about trade names and generic names of medications, complete Exercise 10 at the www.emtb.com.

Vital Vocabulary
provides key terms and definitions from the chapter.

Points to Ponder
tackles cultural, social, ethical, and legal issues through case studies.

Online Outlook
guides exploration of topics online, where additional activities reinforce and expand on important information from the chapter.

Patient Assessment Flowchart

The Patient Assessment Flowchart provides a quick visual reference for the entire patient assessment process.

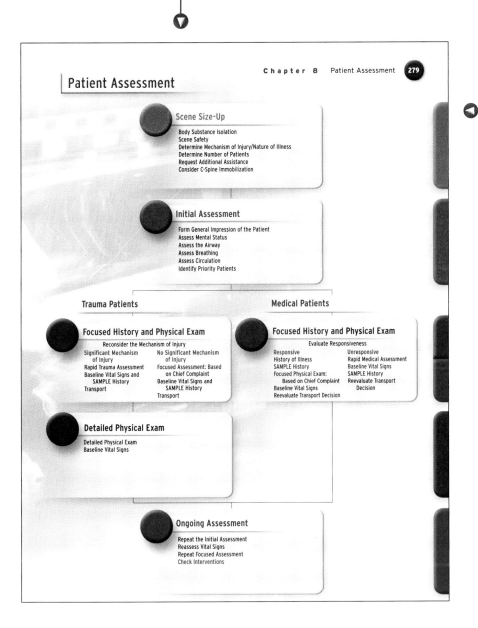

Divided into six sections, the patient assessment flowchart is color-coded to the chapter content for easy reference. The flowchart is repeated at the beginning of each section to show students "at a glance" where they are in the patient assessment process.

preview

Instructor Resources

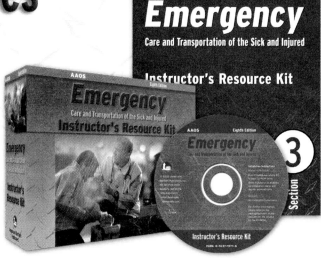

Instructor's ToolKit CD-ROM

ISBN: 0-7637-1972-2

Preparing for class is easy with the resources found on this CD-ROM, including:

PowerPoint Presentations, providing you with a powerful way to make presentations that are educational and engaging to your students. The slides can be edited and modified to meet your needs.

Lecture Outlines, providing you with complete, ready-to-use lesson plans that outline all of the topics covered in the text. The lesson plans can be modified and customized to fit your course.

Image Bank, providing you with a selection of the most important images found in the textbook. You can use them to incorporate more images into the PowerPoint presentations, make handouts, or enlarge a specific image for further discussion.

Instructor's Resource Kit

ISBN: 0-7637- 2044-5 * 8-Volumes

ISBN: 0-7637-1971-4 * CD-ROM

The Instructor's Resource Kit is your guide to the entire teaching and learning system. Available as either a series of self-contained booklets, one for each section of the text, or on one handy CD-ROM, this indispensable kit contains:

Detailed lesson plans that are keyed to the PowerPoint presentations with sample lectures, lesson quizzes, and teaching strategies.

Teaching tips and ideas to enhance presentations.

Answers to all end-of-chapter student questions found in the text.

Instructor's TestBank

ISBN: 0-7637-1948-X * Print

ISBN: 0-7637-1949-8 * CD-ROM

Following the EMT-Basic National Standard Curriculum, this TestBank provides you with:

- more than 1,500 multiple-choice and scenario-based questions
- pages reference to the *Eighth Edition*

With the TestBank on CD-ROM, you can originate tailor-made tests quickly and easily by selecting, editing, organizing, and printing a test along with an answer key.

Instructor's Slide Set on CD-ROM

ISBN: 0-7637-2042-9

This easy-to-use CD-ROM will assist you in emphasizing key points and stimulating classroom discussion through realistic examples, chapter-by-chapter. Over 1,200 electronic images are sure to grab the viewer's attention.

Trauma Slide Set on CD-ROM

ISBN: 0-7637-2048-8

Bring the "real world" to your classroom discussion with approximately 100 real-life trauma images.

Instructor's Slide Set

ISBN: 0-7637-0934-4

Provides 1,200 35mm slides.

Instructor's Upgrade Slide Set

ISBN: 0-7637-1942-0

This Upgrade Slide Set was created for users of the Slide Set for *Emergency Care and Transportation of the Sick and Injured*, Seventh Edition. It was designed for instructors who would like to upgrade easily and cost effectively.

You are the EMT Video Series

ISBN: 0-7637-1025-3 * 10 videos

These videos capture real-life scenes from the street and are enriched with thought-provoking questions. Use these videos for initial training to identify correct and incorrect procedures. Each video comes with a booklet that will help you guide class discussions. Videos run approximately 25-30 minutes.

The EMS Call—ISBN: 0-7637-1014-8

The Well-Being of the EMT—ISBN: 0-7637-1016-4

Lifting and Moving—ISBN: 0-7637-1017-2

Airway Management—ISBN: 0-7637-1019-9

Patient Assessment—ISBN: 0-7637-1018-0

Communication—ISBN: 0-7637-1071-7

Managing the Geriatric Patient— ISBN: 0-7637-1022-9

Trauma Management and Spinal Immobilization—ISBN: 0-7637-1020-2

Pediatric Emergencies I—ISBN: 0-7637-1021-0

Pediatric Emergencies II—ISBN: 0-7637-1015-6

Student Resources

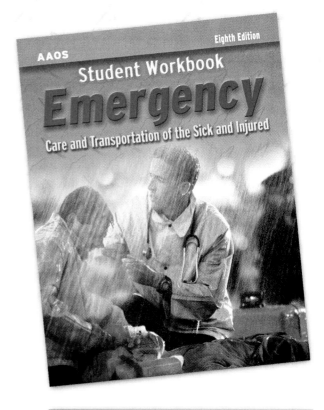

Student Workbook

ISBN: 0-7637-1943-9

This resource is designed to encourage critical thinking and aid comprehension of the course material through:

- case studies and corresponding questions
- figure labeling exercises
- crossword puzzles
- matching, fill-in-the-blank, short answer, and multiple-choice questions
- skill drill activities

Review Manual

ISBN: 0-7637-1945-5 * Print

ISBN: 0-7637-1947-1 * CD-ROM

ISBN: 0-7637-1946-3 * Online at www.emtb.com

This Review Manual has been designed to prepare students to sit for exams by including the same type of scenario-based and multiple-choice questions that they are likely to see on classroom and national examinations. The manual is available in print, on CD-ROM, and Online. It provides answers to all questions with brief explanations and page references.

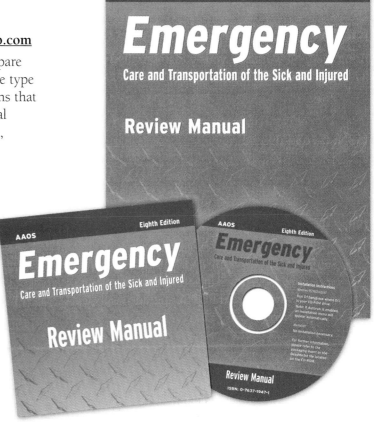

EMT-B Mobile Field Guide

ISBN: 0-7637-1944-7

This essential resource is packaged with each copy of *Emergency Care and Transportation of the Sick and Injured*, Eighth Edition. It provides instant, portable access to the *EMT-B Field Guide* on your PalmPilot™, eBook Reader, Windows CE™ based handheld device, or Windows PC.

The Field Guide provides the vital emergency information needed by prehospital personnel. It's a great resource for fast review of important step-by-step procedures, offering just the right amount of information to guide actions and reactions in the field.

The EMT-B Field Guide

ISBN: 0-7637-0880-1

This handy reference covers basic information from patient management tips to guidelines on helping a patient use medication. A few special features include a prescription medication reference and documentation tips. *The EMT-B Field Guide* is pocket-sized, spiral-bound, and water resistant for ready-reference in the field.

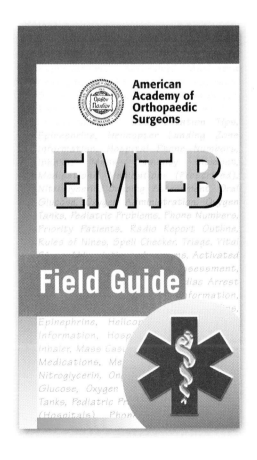

preview

Acknowledgments

Editors

Bruce D. Browner, MD, FAAOS

Dr. Browner is a senior member of the orthopaedic trauma community in the United States. He has been active at both the national and international levels in clinical program and technology development, education, research, and health policy. Prior to his orthopaedic residency, he completed a fellowship at the Shock Trauma Research Unit at Albany Medical College. Upon completion of his training, he spent four years on the faculty of the Maryland Shock Trauma Center. He subsequently spent 10 years at the University of Texas Medical School in Houston and Hermann Hospital where he served as Director of the Division of Orthopaedic Surgery and Chief of the Orthopaedic Service. Eight and one half years ago, he assumed his current position in Connecticut. Dr. Browner has served on the Board of Directors, and the Committees on Injuries, Health Care Finance, and International Affairs of the American Academy of Orthopaedic Surgeons. He is currently Chairman of the Advisory Council for Orthopaedic Surgery, member of the Health Policy Steering and International Committees, and a senior member of the Committee on Trauma of the American College of Surgeons. He has also been appointed the Founding Chairman of Trauma Committee by Societe International de Chirgurgie Orthopedique et de Traumatologie (S.I.C.O.T.). Dr. Browner was a founding member and past President of the Orthopaedic Trauma Association. He is the senior editor of *Skeletal Trauma*, the leading textbook on fractures and dislocations in the world. He was the Chairman of the Editorial Panel for the Seventh Edition of *Emergency Care and Transportation of the Sick and Injured*. He is a member of the International Steering Committee for the Bone and Joint Decade: 2000–2010, and is currently involved in an international effort to control the global road traffic injury epidemic.

Gray-Gossling Professor and Chairman
Department of Orthopaedic Surgery
University of Connecticut Health Center
Farmington, CT

Director of Orthopaedic Department
Hartford Hospital
Hartford, CT

Andrew N. Pollak, MD, EMT-P, FAAOS

Dr. Pollak has been active in EMS activities since 1980 when he started as a volunteer firefighter and first responder. During his career he has served as an EMT-A, an EMT-Paramedic, and as a flight physician with a hospital-based aeromedical ambulance service. He is currently an Attending Orthopaedic Trauma Surgeon at the R Adams Cowley Shock Trauma Center in Baltimore, Maryland. He remains active in EMS as Fire Surgeon for the Baltimore County Fire Department and as an educator and administrator. He is the director of the hospital-based rapid response field unit known as the Shock Trauma Go Team.

Associate Professor and Acting Chairman
Department of Orthopaedic Surgery
University of Maryland School of Medicine

Attending Orthopaedic Traumatologist
R Adams Cowley Shock Trauma Center
Baltimore, MD

Carol L. Gupton, NREMT-P

Carol Gupton has been involved in EMS since 1985 and has been a paramedic for 10 years. She is currently an EMS Instructor for the Omaha Fire Department. Her experience includes a faculty appointment with Creighton University's paramedic program and 5 years of service as a paramedic and EMS advisor for the La Vista Volunteer Fire Department. She is the Nebraska PHTLS state coordinator and co-chair of the Midlands EMS Protocol Committee and has authored several chapters in EMS textbooks. She received her Bachelor's of Science in EMS from Creighton University in 1994 and has been certified as a nationally registered paramedic since 1991. Carol has been actively teaching all levels of EMS including First Responders, EMT-B, Paramedic, AMLS, and PEPP, for 15 years.

Bachelor of Science, EMS
EMS Instructor
Omaha Fire Department
Prehospital Provider Education, Inc.
Omaha, NE

acknowledgments

Reviewers (continued)

Rockey Johnson
Kentucky State Fire and Rescue/
    STAT Care
Louisville, KY

Bob Lovelace, BF, EMT-P, I/C
Huron Valley Ambulance
Plymouth, MI

Don Lundy, BS, NREMT-P
Charleston County EMS
Charleston, SC

David M. Magnino
California Highway Patrol Academy
West Sacramento, CA

Bonnie Maynard
Nashville Fire Department
Nashville, TN

Jeff McDonald, EMT-P
Tarrant County College – Northeast
Hurst, TX

Michael E. Murphy, RN, CEN, EMT-P
Rockland Paramedic Services
Nanuet, NY

Michael Panté, NREMT-P
Robert Wood Johnson
    University Hospital
New Brunswick, NJ

Jeff Pollakoff, EMT-P
UCLA Center for Prehospital Care
Los Angeles, CA

Monte Posner, MSW, EMT-B, CIC
TIMER
Staten Island, NY

Richard Prentiss
Miami-Dade Community College
Miami, FL

Tom Raithby, EMT-2
Fairfield, New Brunswick
Canada

Robb Rehberg, MS, ATC, NREMT
Montclair State University
Upper Montclair, NJ

Michael Reilly
Community Medical Center
Toms River, NJ

Gina Riggs, NREMT-P
Kiamichi Technology Center
Poteau, OK

Jose Salazar, MPH, NREMT-P
Loudoun County Fire & Rescue
Leesburg, VA

Paul Schifando
LA County Fire Department
Los Angeles, CA

William H. Seifarth, MS, NREMT-P
Maryland Institute for Emergency
    Medical Services Systems
Baltimore, MD

Vince Shaffer
Medix School
Kennesaw, GA

Gary L. Shirley
Mississippi Gulf Coast
    Community College
Gulfport, MS

James Stefka
East Texas Medical Center
Brownsboro, TX

Jim Stevens
St. Louis Community College
Dayton, OH

Gail Stewart
Florida Association of Professional
    EMTs and Paramedics
Tallahassee, FL

Denise Tiedeman, EMT-B
Tidewater Community College
Virginia Beach, VA

John Todaro, REMT-P, RN
Florida College of
    Emergency Physicians
Orlando, FL

Ed Travers, BSN, RN, CEN, EMT-P
Massachusetts Bay
    Community College
Burlington, MA

Ariel Villarreal
Broward Community College
Pembroke Pines, FL

James E. Walker, Jr., EMT-B
Northeastern University
Burlington, MA

Willy Wright, EMT-P
Staten Island EMS
Staten Island, NY

The American Academy of
Orthopaedic Surgeons would like
to acknowledge the following
individuals for their contributions
to previous editions of *Emergency
Care and Transportation of the
Sick and Injured.*

Ken Beers, MS
Monroe Community College
Rochester, NY

Stephen M. Belkoff, PhD, EMT-P
University of Maryland
Baltimore, MD

Scott S. Bourn, RN, MSN, EMT-P
Beth-El College of Nursing and Health
    Sciences University of Colorado
Colorado Springs, CO

Kenneth J. Bouvier, NREMT-I
EMS Education
New Orleans, LA

Kevin S. Brame, MA
Orange County Fire Authority
Orange, CA

Andrew Burgess, MD
R Adams Cowley Shock
    Trauma Center
Baltimore, MD

**Alexander M. Butman, BA, DSC,
    REMT-P**
Emergency Training Institute
Fairlawn, OH

Jack Campbell, MD
Truman Medical Center-West
Kansas City, MO

Greg P. Carlson, NREMT-P
Wisconsin Indianhead
    Technical College
New Richmond, WI

Eduardo E. Castro, MD
Massachusetts General Hospital
Boston, MA

Paul Coffey
Massachusetts Department of
    Public Health
Boston, MA

**John "Chip" Coleman, SSgt, USAF,
    NREMT-P**
USAF School of Healthcare Sceinces
Sheppard AFB, TX

Alasdair K.T. Conn, MD
Massachusetts General Hospital
Boston, MA

Holly Frost Davis, BS, NREMT-P
Northern Virginia Community College
Annandale, VA

Kim Dickerson, EMT-P, RN
Edison Community College
Fort Myers, FL

Suzanne Goodrich, RN-MSN
UCI Medical Center
Orange, CA

Larry G. Gosdin, RN, BA, EMT-P
Emergency Medical Services Program
Gadsden, AL

Donald Graesser, PhD
Bergen County EMS Training Center
Paramus, NJ

Jack T. Grandey, NREMT-P
Wilderness EMS Institute
Pittsburgh, PA

Jaime S. Greene, BA, EMT-B
School District of Palm Beach County
West Palm Beach, FL

Fred Harchelroad, MD, FAAEM, FACMT
Allegheny University of the
Health Sciences
Pittsburgh, PA

Deborah Parkman Henderson, PhD, RN
Harbor-UCLA Medical Center
Torrance, CA

Lenworth M. Jacobs, MD, MPH, FACS
University of Connecticut School
of Medicine
Hartford Hospital
Hartford, CT

Rickard L. Judd, PhD, EMSI
Central Connecticut State University
New Britain, CT

Barbara L. Klingensmith, BA, MS, NREMT-P
Edison Community College
Fort Myers, FL

Rebecca Layman, EMT-B
R Adams Cowley Shock
Trauma Center
Baltimore, MD

L. Scott Levin, MD
Duke University Center
Durham, NC

Scott A. McConnell, BA, EMT-P
Lima Technical College
Lima, OH

Michael G. Miller, NREMT-P
West Suburban Hospital
Oak Park, IL

Anthony J. Misner, BA, EMT-P
Yosemite Community
Education Center
Oakhurst, CA

Robert G. Nixon, BA, EMT-P
Lifecare Medical Training
Walnut Creek, CA

Hilary C. Onyiuke, MD
Hartford Hospital
Hartford, CT

Craig B. Ordway, MD
State University of New York
Stony Brook, NY

Paul E. Pepe, MD, MPH, FACEP, FCCM
Allegheny University of the
Health Sciences
Pittsburgh, PA

Edward L. Pesanti, MD
University of Connecticut
Health Center
Farmington, CT

Jonathan Politis, BA, NREMT-P
Town of Colonie
Latham, NY

Pamela Poore, RN
Little Company of Mary
Emergency Department
Torrance, CA

Linda Quan, MD
Children's Hospital Regional
Medical Center
Seattle, WA

John Rinard, BBA, EMT-P
Texas Tech University Health
Science Center
Lubbock, TX

Fredrick H. (Ted) Rogers, NREMT-P
St. Petersburg Junior College
St. Petersburg, FL

Vincent M. Santoro, MD
Hartford Hospital
Hartford, CT

Michael Sayre, MD
University of Cincinnati
Cincinnati, OH

Dave Schottke, RN, REMT-P, MPH
Washington D.C.

James S. Seidel, MD, PhD
Harbor-UCLA Medical Center
Torrance, CA

Sandra Stinson, RN, NREMT-P, I/C
Southwest Mississippi Regional
Medical Center
McComb, MS

Samuel J. Stratton, MD
Harbor-UCLA Medical Center
Torrance, CA

Vincent P. Tamariz, MD
Harbor-UCLA Medical Center
Torrance, CA

J.J. Tepas III, MD
University of Florida Health Science
Center-Jacksonville
Jacksonville, FL

Stephen H. Thomas, MD
Massachusetts General Hospital
Boston, MA

Donna Tidwell, BS, RN, EMT-P
Columbia State Community College
Columbia, TN

John M. Watson, MD
Hartford Hospital
Hartford, CT

Brian S. Zachariah, MD
University of Texas, Southwestern
Dallas, TX

Preparing to be an EMT-B

Section 1

Introduction to Emergency Medical Care

Objectives

Cognitive

1. Define Emergency Medical Services (EMS) systems (p 4).
2. Differentiate the roles and responsibilities of the EMT-B from other prehospital care providers (p 5).
3. Describe the roles and responsibilities related to personal safety (p 14).
4. Discuss the roles and responsibilities of the EMT-B towards the safety of the crew, the patient, and bystanders (p 14).
5. Define quality improvement and discuss the EMT-B's role in the process (p 11).
6. Define medical direction and discuss the EMT-B's role in the process (p 10).
7. State the specific statutes and regulations in your state regarding the EMS system (p 12).

Affective

8. Assess areas of personal attitude and conduct of the EMT-B (p 14).
9. Characterize the various methods used to access the EMS system in your community (p 10).

Psychomotor

None

www.emtb.com

Online Chapter Pretest
Interactivities
Vocabulary Explorer
Anatomy Review
Web Links
Online Review Manual
Distance Learning

Skill Drills
Vital Vocabulary
Pediatric Needs
Geriatric Needs
EMT-B Safety
EMT-B Tips
Documentation Tips
Remember
Prep Kit

Rarely does a day pass that people do not hear the sound of a siren as an ambulance responds to someone's call for help. This chapter represents the starting point for your initial training and education as an EMT-Basic as you learn how to meet the needs of those who call 9-1-1.

This chapter will help to introduce you to the exciting profession of EMS (Emergency Medical Services). It will also help you answer the following questions:

1. How would you define a "real emergency?"

2. In the overall scheme of prehospital medicine, what are the primary roles and responsibilities of an EMT-B?

Introduction to Emergency Medical Care

This book has been designed to serve as the text and primary resource for the emergency medical technician basic (EMT-Basic) course. This chapter describes the content and objectives of the EMT-Basic course. It also discusses what will be expected of you during the course and what other requirements you will have to meet to be licensed or certified as an EMT-Basic in most states. The differences between basic first aid training, a Department of Transportation (DOT) First Responder training course, and the training for the EMT-Basic, EMT-Intermediate, and EMT-Paramedic are described.

Emergency medical services (EMS) is a system. The key components of this system and how they influence and affect the EMT-Basic and his or her delivery of emergency care are carefully discussed. Next, the administration, medical direction, quality control, and regulation of EMS services are presented. The chapter ends with a detailed discussion of the roles and responsibilities of the EMT-Basic as a health care professional.

Course Description

You are about to enter an exciting field. **Emergency medical services (EMS)** consists of a team of health care professionals who, in each area or jurisdiction, are responsible for and provide prehospital emergency care and transportation to the sick and injured (▶ Figure 1-1). Each emergency medical service is part of a local or regional EMS system that provides the many varied prehospital and hospital components required for the delivery of proper emergency medical care. The standards for prehospital emergency care and the individuals who provide it are governed by the laws in each state and are typically regulated by a state office of EMS.

The individuals who provide the emergency care in the field are trained and, except for licensed physicians, must be state-licensed or certified **emergency medical technicians (EMTs)**. EMTs are categorized into three training and licensure levels: EMT-Basic, EMT-Intermediate, and EMT-Paramedic. An **EMT-Basic** (EMT-B) has training in basic emergency care skills, including automated external defibrillation, use of definitive airway adjuncts, and assisting patients with certain medications. An **EMT-Intermediate** (EMT-I) has advanced training in specific aspects of advanced life support, such as intravenous (IV) therapy and cardiac monitoring. An **EMT-Paramedic** (EMT-P) has extensive training in advanced life support, including IV therapy, pharmacology, cardiac monitoring, and other advanced assessment and treatment skills.

Although the specific training and licensure requirements vary from one state to another, the training that is

Figure 1-1 As an EMT-B, you will be part of a larger team that responds to a variety of calls and provides a wide range of prehospital emergency care.

required in almost every state follows or exceeds the guidelines that are recommended in the current US DOT (Department of Transportation) National Standard Curriculum for each EMT level.

After you have successfully completed the Basic Life Support/Cardiopulmonary Resuscitation (BLS/CPR) course for health care providers and met the other prerequisites, you are ready to take the EMT-B course. Like any introductory course, the EMT-B course covers a great deal of information and introduces many skills. Everything you learn in the course will be important to your ability to provide high-quality emergency care once you are licensed and ready to practice. In addition, the knowledge, understanding, and skills that you acquire in the EMT-B course will serve as a foundation for the additional knowledge and training that you will receive in future years.

This textbook covers the material and skills that are identified in the US DOT 1994 EMT-Basic National Standard Curriculum and in the 1994 National EMS Education and Practice Blueprint. In addition to the required core content, it includes additional information that will help you to understand and apply the material and skills that are included in the EMT-B level. Your instructor will furnish you with reading assignments. It is important that you complete the assigned reading before each class.

In class, the instructor will review the key parts of the reading assignment and clarify and expand on them. He or she will also answer any questions that you have and will clarify any points that you or others find confusing ▶ Figure 1-2 . Unless you have carefully read the assignment and made notes before coming to class, you will not fully understand or benefit from the classroom presentation and discussions. You will also need to take additional notes during class ▶ Table 1-1 .

The EMT-B course will include four types of learning activities:

1. **Reading assignments** from the textbook and presentations and discussions held in class will provide you with the necessary knowledge base.
2. **Step-by-step demonstrations** will teach you hands-on skills that you then need to practice repeatedly in supervised small group workshops.
3. **Summary skills sheets** will help you to memorize the sequence of steps in complex skills that contain a large number of steps or variations so that you can perform the skill with no errors or omissions.
4. **Case presentations and scenarios** used in class will help you learn how to apply the knowledge and skills acquired in class situations like those you will find in the field.

EMT-B Training: Focus and Requirements

EMT-B training is divided into three main categories. The first and most important category focuses on the care of life-threatening or potentially life-threatening conditions. To deal with these, you will learn how to do the following:

- Size up the scene and situation
- Ensure that the scene is safe
- Perform an initial assessment of the patient
- Obtain a history of this episode and a pertinent past medical history
- Identify life-threatening injuries or conditions
- Establish and maintain an open airway
- Provide adequate ventilation
- Manage conditions that prevent proper ventilation

Figure 1-2 In the classroom, you will learn both didactic and practical skills to prepare you for various types of calls.

TABLE 1-1 Study Tips for Using This Textbook

- **Complete each assignment** diligently and carefully.
- **Read the textbook** like a textbook, not like a newspaper, magazine, or novel.
- **Read each chapter** several times and underline key points. Take notes!
- **Ask your instructor** to clarify any questions you note in your reading or in class.
- **Take additional notes** when the assigned material is expanded upon in class.
- **Remember:** The only absurd question is the one that a student has and fails to ask.

- Provide high-flow supplemental oxygen
- Perform cardiopulmonary resuscitation (CPR)
- Perform automated or semiautomated external defibrillation (AED)
- Control external bleeding
- Recognize and treat shock
- Care for patients in an acute life-threatening medical emergency
- Assist patients in taking certain medications that they carry and that their physician has pre-scribed for an acute episode
- Identify and rapidly prepare, or "package," patients (by positioning, covering, and securing them) for rapid initiation of transport when necessary

The second category of training covers conditions that, although not life-threatening, are key components of emergency care or are necessary to prevent further harm before the patient is moved. You will learn to do the following:

- Identify patients for whom spinal precautions should be taken and immobilize them properly
- Dress and bandage wounds
- Splint injured extremities
- Care for burns
- Care for cases of poisoning
- Deliver a baby
- Assess and care for a newborn
- Manage patients with behavioral or psychological problems
- Cope with the psychological stresses on patients, families, your fellow EMT-Bs, and yourself

The third category covers important issues that are related to your ability to provide emergency care. You will develop the following related skills:

- Understanding the role and responsibilities of the EMT-B
- Following your service's protocols and orders from medical direction
- Understanding ethical and medicolegal problems
- Emergency vehicle and defensive driving
- Using equipment carried on the ambulance
- Checking and stocking the ambulance
- Communicating with patients and others at the scene

- Using the radio and communicating with the dispatcher
- Giving a precise patient radio report and obtain-ing direct medical direction
- Giving a full verbal report when transferring the patient's care at the hospital
- Preparing proper documentation and completing the patient care report
- Working with other responders at a crash scene
- Cooperating with operations at special rescue, mass-casualty, and hazardous materials incidents

Certification Requirements

To be recognized and perform as an EMT-B, you must meet certain training and other requirements. The spe-cific requirements differ from state to state. You should ask your instructor or contact your state EMS office to find out about the requirements in your state. Generally, the criteria will include the following:

- High school diploma or equivalent
- Proof of immunization against certain communi-cable diseases
- Valid driver's license
- Successful completion of a recognized health care provider's BLS/CPR course
- Successful completion of a state-approved EMT-B course
- Successful completion of a state-recognized written certification examination
- Successful completion of a state-recognized practical certification examination
- Demonstrating that you can meet the mental and physical criteria necessary to be able to safely and properly perform all the tasks and functions described in the defined role of an EMT-B
- Compliance with other state and local provisions

The **Americans with Disabilities Act (ADA)** of 1990 protects individuals who have a disability from being denied access to programs and services that are provided by state or local governments and prohibits employers from failing to provide full and equal employ-ment to the disabled. To obtain further information about the ADA and employment as an EMT-B, you should con-tact your state EMS office.

In most states, individuals who have been convicted of driving while under the influence of alcohol or other drugs, or have been convicted of certain felonies, may be denied certification as an EMT-B.

States may exclude from certification persons with a history of a health problem that could make their performance of EMT-B tasks dangerous to themselves or others.

Overview of the Emergency Medical Services System

HISTORY OF EMS. As an EMT-B, you will be joining a long tradition of people who have provided emergency medical care to their fellow human beings. With the early use of motor vehicles in warfare, volunteer ambulance squads were organized and went overseas to provide care for the wounded in World War I. In World War II, the military trained special corpsmen to provide care in the field and bring the casualties to aid stations staffed by nurses and physicians. In the Korean conflict, this evolved to the field medic and rapid helicopter evacuation to nearby Mobile Army Surgical Hospital units, where immediate surgical intervention was provided. Many advances in the immediate care of trauma patients resulted from the casualty experiences in the Korean and Vietnam conflicts.

Unfortunately, emergency care of the injured and ill at home had not progressed to a similar level. As late as the early 1960s, emergency ambulance service and care across the United States varied widely. In some places, it was provided by well-trained advanced first aid squads that had well-equipped modern ambulances. In a few urban areas, it was provided by hospital-based ambulance services that were staffed with interns and early forms of medics. In many places, the only emergency care and ambulance service was provided by the local funeral home using a hearse that could be converted to carry a cot and serve as an ambulance. In other places, the police or fire department used a station wagon that carried a cot and a first aid kit. In most cases, both of these were staffed by a driver and an attendant who had some basic first aid training. In the few areas where a commercial ambulance was available to transport the ill, it was usually similarly staffed and served primarily as a means to transport the patient to the hospital.

Many communities had no formal provision for prehospital emergency care or transportation. Injured persons were given basic first aid by police or fire personnel at the scene and were transported to the hospital in a police or fire officer's car. Customarily, patients with an acute illness were transported to the hospital by a relative or neighbor and were met by their family physician or an on-call hospital physician, who assessed them and then summoned any specialists and operating room staff

> As an EMT-B, you will be joining a long tradition of people who have provided emergency medical care to their fellow human beings.

that were needed. Except in large urban centers, most hospitals did not have the staffed emergency departments to which we are accustomed today.

EMS as we know it today had its origins in 1966 with the publication of *Accidental Death and Disability: The Neglected Disease of Modern Society.* This report, prepared jointly by the Committees on Trauma and Shock of the National Academy of Sciences/National Research Council, revealed to the public and Congress the serious inadequacy of prehospital emergency care and transportation in many areas. A number of key items were recommended in the report, some of which follow:

- Development of national courses of instruction for prehospital emergency care and transportation by fire, police, rescue, and ambulance personnel
- Development of nationally accepted textbooks and training aids for these courses
- Development of federal guidelines for the design of ambulances and the equipment they carry
- Development and adoption of general policies and regulations pertaining to ambulance services and qualification and supervision of ambulance personnel in each state
- Adoption by each municipality (or district or county) of means to supply the necessary proper prehospital emergency care and transport within its jurisdiction
- Establishment of hospital emergency departments with staffing by physicians, nurses, and other personnel who are trained in resuscitation and the immediate care of the seriously injured and ill

As a result, Congress mandated that two federal agencies address these issues. The National Highway Traffic Safety Administration (NHTSA) of the DOT, through the Highway Safety Act of 1966, and the Department of Health and Human Services, through the Emergency Medical Act of 1973, created funding sources and programs to develop improved systems of prehospital emergency care.

In the early 1970s, the DOT developed and published the first National Standard Curriculum to serve as the guideline for the training of EMTs. To support the EMT course, the American Academy of Orthopaedic Surgeons prepared and published the first EMT text-book—*Emergency Care and Transportation of the Sick and Injured*—in 1971. The textbook you are reading is the eighth edition of that publication. Through the 1970s, following the recommended guidelines, each state developed the necessary legislation, and the EMS system was developed throughout the United States. During the same period, emergency medicine became a recognized medical specialty, and the fully staffed emergency departments that we know today became the accepted standard of care.

In the late 1970s and early 1980s, the DOT developed a recommended National Standard Curriculum for the training of paramedics and identified a part of the course to serve as training for basic EMTs.

By 1980, EMS had been established throughout the nation. The system was based on the following two key changes:

- The introduction of legislation that made it the responsibility of each municipality, township, or county to provide proper prehospital emergency care and transportation within its boundaries
- The establishment of recognized and regulated standards for the training of ambulance personnel and equipment required on each ambulance

These changes ensured that, regardless of where an individual became hurt or acutely ill, he or she would receive timely, proper emergency care and transport to the hospital. During the 1980s, many areas enhanced the EMT National Standard Curriculum by adding EMTs with higher levels of training who could provide key components of **advanced life support (ALS)** care (advanced lifesaving procedures). The availability of paramedics (EMT-Ps) and ALS on calls that require or benefit from advanced care has grown steadily in recent years. In addition, with the evolution in training and technology, the EMT-B and EMT-I can now perform a number of important advanced skills in the field that were formerly reserved for the EMT-P.

The way EMS systems work may differ depending on the geographic area and population served. Regardless of the area, however, the NHTSA is available to evaluate EMS systems, based on the following 10 criteria in their Technical Assistance Program Assessment Standards:

1. Regulation and policy
2. Resource management
3. Human resources and training
4. Transportation equipment and system
5. Medical and support facilities
6. Communications system
7. Public information and education
8. Medical direction
9. Trauma system and development
10. Evaluation

Levels of Training

Public Basic Life Support and Immediate Aid

With the development of EMS and increased awareness of the need for immediate emergency care, millions of laypeople have been trained in BLS/CPR. In addition to CPR, many individuals have taken short basic first aid courses that include control of bleeding and other simple skills that may be required to provide immediate essential care. These courses are designed to train individuals so that those in the workplace, teachers, coaches, baby-sitters, and the like, can provide the necessary critical care in the minutes before EMTs or other responders arrive at the scene.

In addition, many individuals, such as those who regularly accompany groups on camping trips or are in other situations in which the arrival of EMS may be delayed because of remote location, are trained in advanced first aid. This course includes basic life support and the essential additional care and packaging that may be necessary until the help of rescuers and EMTs can be obtained at a remote location.

First Responders

Because the presence of a person who is trained and able to initiate basic life support and other urgent care cannot be ensured, the EMS system includes immediate care by **first responders**, such as law enforcement officers, fire fighters, park rangers, ski patrollers, or other organized rescuers who often arrive at the scene before the ambulance and EMTs (**▶ Figure 1-3**). The DOT has established a First Responder Curriculum to provide these individuals with the training necessary to initiate immediate care and then assist the EMTs on their arrival. The course focuses on providing immediate basic life support and urgent care with limited equipment. It also familiarizes the student with the additional procedures, equipment, and packaging techniques that EMTs may use and with which the first responder may be called upon to assist.

Just as it is essential for the first responder to do enough for the patient, it is also essential for the first responder not to try to do too much. One of the most serious dangers to patients is improper removal from a vehicle or crash scene. Permanent paralysis and other injuries have been caused by these well-intentioned but potentially dangerous actions.

First responders are trained by using the DOT First Responder Curriculum, which includes training in basic life support. First responders can provide basic life support before the ambulance arrives by assessing the injury or illness, providing air to the lungs and blood to the brain, and controlling bleeding, all of which can be done with little or no equipment.

EMT-Basic

The EMT-B course requires a minimum of 110 hours (more in some states) and includes the essential knowledge and skills required to provide basic emergency care in the field. The course serves as the foundation on which additional knowledge and skills are built in advanced EMT training. On arrival at the scene, you and the other EMTs who have responded with the ambulance should assume responsibility for the assessment and care of the patient, followed by proper packaging

and transport of the patient to the emergency department. With the publication and adoption of the US DOT 1994 EMT-Basic National Standard Curriculum, selected ALS skills have been added to this level. These skills include automated external defibrillation, use of airway adjuncts (▼ **Figure 1-4**), and assisting patients with the use of their physician-prescribed medications, such as nitroglycerin, epinephrine, and metered-dose inhalers.

EMT-Intermediate

The EMT-Intermediate (EMT-I) course and training are designed to add knowledge and skills in specific aspects of ALS to individuals who have been trained and have experience in providing emergency care as an EMT-B. These additional skills include IV therapy, interpretation of cardiac rhythms and defibrillation, orotracheal intubation, and, in many states, the knowledge and skills necessary to administer medications.

EMT-Paramedic

The EMT-Paramedic (EMT-P) has completed an extensive course of training that significantly increases knowledge and mastery of basic skills and covers a wide range of ALS skills (▼ **Figure 1-5**). These skills include the following:

- Electrocardiogram monitoring and interpretation of cardiac rhythms
- Advanced cardiac life support (ACLS) protocols and skills
- Manual defibrillation and external cardiac pacing

Figure 1-3   First responders, such as law enforcement officers, are trained to provide immediate basic life support until EMTs arrive on the scene.

Figure 1-4   EMT-Bs are trained to use airway adjuncts.

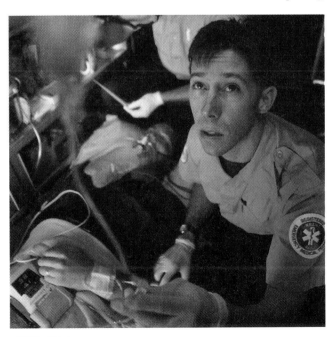

Figure 1-5   Advanced training covers a wide range of ALS skills.

- Orotracheal and nasotracheal intubation
- Needle cricothyroidotomy
- Needle decompression for tension pneumothorax
- IV therapy
- Advanced pharmacology: drug calculations and medication administration (IV, IV infusion, IO, ET, and injections)

Components of the EMS System

Access

Easy access to help needed in an emergency is essential. In most of the country, an emergency communications center that dispatches fire, police, rescue, and EMS units can be reached by dialing 9-1-1. At the communication center, trained dispatchers obtain the necessary information from the caller and, following dispatch protocols, dispatch the ambulance crew and other equipment and responders that may be needed (▼ Figure 1-6).

In an enhanced 9-1-1 system, the address of the telephone from which the call is made is displayed on a screen. The connection is frozen until the dispatcher releases it so that if the caller is unable to speak, his or her location remains displayed. Most emergency communications centers also include special equipment so that individuals with speech or hearing disabilities can communicate with the dispatcher via a keyboard and printed messages. In some areas, rather than 9-1-1, a different special published emergency number may be used to call for EMS. Training the public in how to summon an EMS unit is an important part of the public education responsibility of each EMS service.

Figure 1-6 Trained dispatchers obtain information about the call and then send responders to the scene as needed.

In many municipalities, EMS is a part of the fire department. In others, it is a part of the police department or is an independent public safety service. In some areas, a contractor may provide either the basic EMS or ALS service. In some areas, ALS is provided by paramedics who are based at a hospital or who may cover a number of towns in a region.

Administration and Policy

Each EMS service operates in a designated **primary service area (PSA)** in which it is responsible for the provision of prehospital emergency care and the transportation of the sick and injured to the hospital.

EMS services are usually administered by a senior EMS official. Daily operations and overall direction of the service is provided by an appointed chief executive officer and several other officers who serve under him or her. When the EMS service is a part of a fire or police department, the department chief will usually delegate the responsibility for directing EMS to an assistant chief or other officer whose sole responsibility is to manage the EMS activities of the department. To provide clear guidelines, most services have written operating procedures and policies. When you join a service, you will be expected to learn and follow them.

The chief executive of the service is in charge of both the necessary administrative tasks (eg, scheduling, personnel, budgets, purchasing, vehicle maintenance) and the daily operations of the ambulances and crews. Except for medical matters, he or she operates as the chief (similar to a fire chief or police chief) of EMS for the service and the PSA that it covers.

Medical Direction and Control

Each EMS system has a physician **medical director** who authorizes the EMTs in the service to provide medical care in the field. The appropriate care for each injury, condition, or illness that you will encounter in the field is determined by the medical director and is described in a set of written standing orders, or protocols. **Medical control** is either off-line (indirect) or online (direct), as authorized by the medical director. Standing orders are a type of indirect medical direction. Each EMT must know and follow the protocols developed by his or her medical director.

The service's protocols will also identify an EMS physician who can be reached by radio or telephone for medical control during a call (► Figure 1-7). This is a type of direct online medical control. On some calls, once the squad has initiated any immediate urgent care and gives its radio report, the online medical control physician may either confirm or modify the proposed treatment plan or may prescribe any additional special orders that the EMT-Bs are to follow for that patient. The point at which the EMT-Bs should give their radio report or obtain online medical direction will vary.

The medical director provides the ongoing working liaison between the medical community, hospitals, and the EMTs in the service. If treatment problems arise or different procedures should be considered, these are referred to the medical director for his or her decision and action. To ensure that the proper training standards are met, the medical director determines and approves the continuing education and training that are required of each EMT in the service and approves any that individuals obtain elsewhere.

Quality Control and Improvement

The medical director is responsible for maintaining <u>quality control</u>, ensuring that all staff members who are involved in caring for patients meet appropriate medical care standards on each call. To provide the necessary quality control, the medical director and other involved staff review patient care reports.

<u>Continuous quality improvement (CQI)</u> is a circular system of continuous internal and external reviews and audits of all aspects of an EMS call. To provide CQI, periodic run review meetings are held in which all those who are involved in patient care review the run reports and then discuss any areas of care that appear to need change or improvement. Positive feedback is also discussed. If a problem appears to be repeated by a single EMT or crew, the medical director will discuss the details with the individuals involved and, if necessary, assign remedial training or some other

> Each EMS system has a physician medical director who authorizes the EMTs in the service to provide medical care in the field.

development activity. The medical director is also responsible for ensuring that appropriate continuing education and training are available.

Information and skills in emergency medical care change constantly. You need refresher training or continuing education as new modalities of care, equipment, and understanding of critical illnesses and trauma develop. Equally, when you have not used a particular procedure for some time, skill decay may occur. Therefore, your medical director might establish a CQI process to correct the deficit. For example, an emergency department physician noted that despite their assessments, many EMT-Bs were missing a high number of closed long bone fractures, resulting in poor prehospital care. A subsequent audit of calls led to a review and retraining session for assessment and care of fractures. This same process can apply to CPR or any other type of skill that you do not use often. Ensuring that your skills and knowledge are current is one of the ongoing commitments of being an EMT.

Other Physician Input

EMS is an extension of the emergency medical care provided in the emergency department by physicians and the other specialists who provide definitive care in the hospital. Besides the direction that the medical director and direct online medical control physicians provide, your training and practices are based on input from many specialty professional associations at the national, state, and local levels.

As an EMT-B, you are part of the professional continuum of care provided to patients who often have life-threatening conditions. Physicians are at the top of the professional continuum pyramid. Many physician experts from the specialties of emergency medicine, traumatology, orthopaedics, cardiology, anesthesiology, radiology, and other medical disciplines participate in the ongoing work of EMS. The efforts of these groups—often through professional associations such as the American Academy of Orthopaedic Surgeons, the American College of Emergency Physicians, the American College of Surgeons, and the National

Figure 1-7 Online or direct medical control is provided by a physician.

Association of EMS Physicians—include research, the establishment of standards for quality assurance, continuing education, and publications.

Regulation

Although each EMS system, medical director, and training program has vast latitude, their training, protocols, and practices must conform with the EMS legislation, rules, regulations, and guidelines adopted by each respective state. The state EMS office is responsible for authorizing, auditing, and regulating all EMS services, training institutions, courses, instructors, and providers within the state. In most states, the state EMS office obtains input from an advisory committee made up of representatives of the services, service medical directors, medical associations, hospitals, training programs, instructors' associations, EMT associations, and the public in that state.

Equipment

As an EMT-B, you will use a wide range of different emergency equipment. During the EMT-B course, you will be introduced to, and learn how to use, a variety of the different appliances and devices that you may need to use on a call. You will also learn when the use of each is indicated and when it is contraindicated because it will not be of benefit or may cause harm. Although the use of different models and brands of a given device will follow the same generic principles and methods, some variation and peculiarities exist from one model to another. When you join a service, you should check each key piece of equipment before going on duty to ensure that it is in its assigned place, that it is working properly, and that you are familiar with the specific model carried on your ambulance.

The Ambulance

Each EMT-B may be called upon to drive the ambulance. Therefore, you must familiarize yourself with the roads in your PSA or sector. Before going on duty, you should check all the equipment and supplies and communication equipment that the ambulance carries and make sure that it is fully fueled, that it has sufficient oil and other key fluids, and that the tires are in good condition and properly inflated (► **Figure 1-8**). You should also test each of the driver's controls and each built-in unit and control in the patient compartment. If you have not driven the specific ambulance before, it is a good idea to take it out and become familiar with it before you respond to a call. Maintenance and safe driving of the ambulance are discussed in detail in Chapter 35.

Transport to Specialty Centers

In addition to hospital emergency departments, many EMS systems include specialty centers that focus on specific types of care (eg, trauma, burns, poison, or psychiatric conditions) or specific types of patients (eg, children). Specialty centers require in-house staffs of surgeons and other specialists; other facilities must page operating teams, surgeons, or other specialists from outside the hospital. Typically, only a few hospitals in a region are designated as specialty centers. Transport time to a specialty center may be slightly longer than that to an emergency department, but patients will receive definitive care more quickly at a specialty center. You must know the location of the centers in your area and when, according to your protocol, you must transport the patient directly to one. Sometimes, air medical transport will be necessary. Local, regional, and state protocols will guide your decision in these instances.

Interfacility Transports

Many EMS services provide interfacility transportation for nonambulatory patients or patients with both acute and chronic medical conditions requiring medical monitoring. This may include transferring patients to and from hospitals, skilled nursing facilities, board and care homes, or even their home residence.

During ambulance transportation, the health and well-being of the patient is the EMT's responsibility. The EMT should obtain the patient's medical history, chief complaint, and latest vital signs and provide an ongoing patient assessment. In certain circumstances, depending on local protocols, a nurse, physician, respiratory therapist, or medical team will accompany the patient. This is especially true when the patient requires care that extends beyond the EMT-B's "scope of practice."

Figure 1-8 Making sure the ambulance is fueled is part of an EMT-B's responsibility.

Working with Hospital Staff

You should become familiar with the hospital by observing hospital equipment and how it is used, the functions of staff members, and the policies and procedures in all emergency areas of the hospital. You will also learn about advances in emergency care and how to interact with hospital personnel ▶ **Figure 1-9** . This experience will help you to understand how your care influences the patient's recovery and will emphasize the importance and benefits of proper prehospital care. It will also show you the consequences of delay, inadequate care, or poor judgment.

Physicians, nurses, and other medical professionals are not likely be in the field with you to provide personal, on-the-spot instructions. However, you may consult with appropriate medical staff using the radio through established medical control procedures.

In the emergency department, hospital staff may train you by showing you assessment and treatment techniques on patients. A physician or nurse may serve as an instructor for medical subjects in your training program. Through these experiences, you will become more comfortable using medical terms, interpreting patient signs and symptoms, and developing patient management skills.

Hospital staff are usually willing to help you improve your skills and efficiency throughout your career. Some physicians and nurses may have completed the EMT curriculum as part of their formal medical training. The best patient care occurs when all emergency care providers have a close rapport. This allows you and hospital staff the opportunity to discuss mutual problems and to benefit from each other's experiences.

Working with Public Safety Agencies

Some public safety workers have EMS training. As an EMT-B, you must become familiar with all the roles and responsibilities of these agencies. Personnel from certain agencies are better prepared than you to perform certain functions. For example, employees of a utility company are better equipped to control downed power lines than you or your partner. Law enforcement personnel are better able to handle violent scenes and traffic control, while you and your partner are better able to provide emergency medical care. If you work together and recognize that each person has special talent and a job to do at the scene, effective scene and patient management will result. Remember that the best, most efficient patient care is achieved through cooperation among agencies.

Figure 1-9 As an EMT-B, you will interact with hospital staff.

Training

Your training will be conducted by many knowledgeable EMS educators. In most states, the instructors who are responsible for coordinating and teaching the EMT-B course and continuing education courses are approved and certified by the state EMS office or agency. To be certified in some states, an instructor must have extensive medical and educational training and teach for a designated period while being observed and supervised by an experienced instructor.

Most ALS training is provided in either a college or hospital setting. In most states, educational programs that provide ALS training must be approved by the state and have their own medical director. In these courses, many of the lectures and small group sessions will be presented by the medical director or other physicians and nurses. In clinical sessions in which supervised practice is obtained in the emergency department or other in-hospital settings, students are also supervised directly by physicians and other medical staff.

The quality of care that you will provide depends on your ability and the quality of your training. Therefore, your instructor and the many others who developed and participated in your training program are key members of the emergency care team.

Providing a Coordinated Continuum of Care

The emergency care of patients occurs in three progressive phases:

1. **The first phase** consists of patient assessment, initial prehospital care, proper packaging, and safe transport to the hospital.

2. **In the second phase,** the patient receives continued assessment and stabilization in the hospital emergency department.

3. **In the third phase,** the patient receives the necessary definitive specialized care.

These three phases must be provided in a coordinated continuum of care to maximize survival and reduce patient suffering and lasting adverse effects. The EMS system is designed to produce such a coordinated effort among the local EMS services, emergency department staff, and the medical staff who provide definitive care.

Roles and Responsibilities of the EMT-B

As an EMT-B, you will be the first health care professional to assess and treat the patient; as such, you have certain roles and responsibilities (▼ **Table 1-2**). Often, patient outcomes are determined by the care that you provide in the field and your identification of patients who need prompt transport.

Professional Attributes

As an EMT-B, whether you are paid or a volunteer, you are a health care professional. Part of your responsibility is to make sure that patient care is given a high priority without endangering your own safety or the safety of others. Another part of the responsibility to yourself, other EMTs, the patient, and other health care professionals is to maintain a professional appearance and manner at all times. Your attitude and behavior must reflect that you are knowledgeable and sincerely dedicated to serving anyone who is injured or in an acute medical emergency.

TABLE 1-2 Roles and Responsibilities of the EMT-B

- Ensuring your own safety and the safety of your fellow EMT-Bs, the patient, and others at the scene
- Locating and safely driving to the scene
- Sizing up the scene and situation
- Rapidly assessing the patient's gross neurologic, respiratory, and circulatory status
- Providing any essential immediate intervention
- Performing a thorough, accurate patient assessment
- Obtaining an expanded SAMPLE history
- Reaching a clinical impression and providing prompt, efficient, prioritized patient care based on your assessment
- Communicating effectively with the patient and advising him or her of any procedures you will perform
- Properly interacting and communicating with fire, rescue, and law enforcement responders at the scene
- Identifying patients who require rapid packaging, and initiating transport without delay

- Identifying patients who do not need emergency care and will benefit from further detailed assessment and care before they are moved and transported
- Properly packaging the patient
- Safely lifting and moving the patient to the ambulance and loading the patient into it
- Providing safe, appropriate transport to the hospital emergency department or other designated facility
- Giving the necessary radio report to the medical control center or receiving hospital emergency department
- Providing any additional assessment or treatment while en route
- Monitoring the patient and checking vital signs while en route
- Documenting all findings and care on the patient care report
- Unloading the patient safely and, after giving a proper verbal report, transferring the patient's care to the emergency department staff
- Safeguarding the patient's rights

As a professional, you must take pride in your appearance, grooming, and hygiene (▼ **Figure 1-10**). A professional appearance and manner help to build confidence and ease the patient's anxiety. You will be expected to perform under pressure with composure and self-confidence. Patients and families who are under stress need to be treated with understanding, respect, and compassion.

Most patients will treat you with respect and appreciation, but some will not. Some patients are uncooperative, demanding, unpleasant, ungrateful, and verbally abusive. You must be nonjudgmental and overcome your instincts to react poorly to such behavior. Remember that when individuals are hurt, ill, under stress, frightened, despondent, under the influence of alcohol or drugs, or feel threatened, they will often react with inappropriate behavior, even toward those who are trying to help and care for them. Every patient, regardless of his or her attitude, is entitled to compassion, respect, and the best care that you can provide.

Most individuals in this country can obtain proper routine medical care when they are ill and are surrounded by relatives and friends who will help to take care of them. However, when you are called to a home for a medical problem that is clearly not an emergency, remember that for some individuals, calling an ambulance and being transported to the emergency department is the only way to obtain medical care.

As a new EMT-B, you will be given a lot of advice and training from the more experienced EMT-Bs with whom you serve. Some may voice a callous disregard for some types of patients. You should not be influenced by the unprofessional attitude of these individuals, regardless of how experienced or skilled they appear.

As a health care professional and an extension of physician care, you are bound by patient confidentiality. You should not discuss your findings or any disclosures made by the patient with anyone but those who are treating the patient or, as required by law, the police or other social agencies. When discussing a call with others, you should be careful to avoid any information that might disclose the name or identity of patients you have treated. Be careful not to gossip about calls and patients with others, even in your own home.

Continuing Education

Once you no longer have the structured learning environment that is provided in your initial training course, you must assume the responsibility for directing your own study and learning. As an EMT-B, you will be required to attend a certain number of hours of continuing education approved for EMT-Bs each year to maintain, update, and expand your knowledge and skills. In many services, the required hours are provided by the training officer and medical director. In addition, most EMS education programs and hospitals offer a number of regular continuing education opportunities in each region. You may also attend state and national EMS conferences to help keep you up-to-date about local, state, and national issues affecting EMS. Since there are many levels of certification, you should ensure that the continuing education you receive is approved for the EMT-B. Whether you take advantage of these opportunities depends on you. Whether you decide to remain an EMT-B or achieve a higher level of training and certification, the key to being a good EMT and providing high-quality care is your commitment to continual learning and ever-increasing knowledge and skills.

EMTs possess special knowledge and skills that are directed to the care of patients in emergency situations. The authority that is delegated to you to care for patients is a very special one. Maintaining your knowledge and skills is a substantial responsibility. Knowledge and skills that are learned in any profession decay and weaken when they are not used on a continual basis. Consider CPR. If you have not used these skills since your original training, it is likely that you will perform CPR in a way that is less than desirable. Continuing education and refresher courses are one way by which you can maintain your skills and knowledge.

Figure 1-10 **A.** A professional appearance and manner help to build confidence and ease patient anxiety. **B.** An unprofessional appearance may promote distrust.

Prep Kit

Ready for Review

EMS is the system that provides the emergency medical care that is needed by people who have been injured or have an acute medical emergency. When the dispatcher at the 9-1-1 emergency communications center receives a call for emergency care, he or she dispatches to the scene the designated EMS ambulance squad and any fire, rescue, or police units that may be needed. The EMS ambulance is staffed by EMTs who have been trained to the EMT-Basic, EMT-Intermediate, or EMT-Paramedic level according to recommended national standards and have been certified/licensed by the state. After the EMTs size up the scene and assess the patient, they provide the emergency care that is indicated by their findings and ordered by their medical director in the service's standing order protocols or the physician who is providing online medical direction. The EMTs then package the patient and provide transport to the nearby hospital or designated specialized care facility (eg, trauma center, pediatric hospital) for further evaluation and stabilization in the emergency department and, after admission, definitive surgical or medical care.

The EMT-B course that you are now taking will present the information and skills that you will need to pass the required examinations for licensure certification and start as an EMT-B in the field. This course will provide you with the training that you need to function as an EMT-B and will serve as the essential foundation upon which you can advance your training and expertise.

The following are the essential keys to being a good EMT-B:

- Compassion and motivation to reduce suffering, pain, and death in those who are injured or acutely ill
- Desire to provide each patient with the best possible care
- Commitment to obtain the knowledge and skills that this requires
- The drive to continually increase your knowledge, skills, and ability

Once you have successfully completed this course and have been certified as an EMT-B, you will enter the next key phase of your training. When you join an EMS service, your first task will be to learn the medical protocols and operating procedures of the squad. You will also have to learn where each piece of equipment is kept on the ambulance and become familiar with how the equipment works. From your experience and the guidance provided by your crew chief and the other experienced EMT-Bs you work with, you will gain increased mastery of the skills that you learned in the course and learn how to apply your knowledge and skills in the diverse situations that are actually encountered in the field.

Once you have completed the course, you must assume responsibility for directing your own study through continuing education provided by your service's training officer and medical director or through other opportunities available to you. Your commitment to continuing learning is the key to being a good EMT.

Vital Vocabulary

advanced life support (ALS) Advanced lifesaving procedures, some of which are now being provided by the EMT-B.

Americans with Disabilities Act (ADA) Comprehensive legislation that is designed to protect individuals with disabilities against discrimination.

continuous quality improvement (CQI) A system of internal and external reviews and audits of all aspects of an EMS system.

emergency medical services (EMS) A multidisciplinary system that represents the combined efforts of several professionals and agencies to provide prehospital emergency care to the sick and injured.

emergency medical technician (EMT) An EMS professional who is trained and licensed by the state to provide emergency medical care in the field.

EMT-Basic An EMT who has training in basic emergency care skills, including automated external defibrillation, use of a definitive airway adjunct, and assisting patients with certain medications.

EMT-Intermediate An EMT who has training in specific aspects of advanced life support, such as IV (intravenous) therapy, interpretation of cardiac rhythms and defibrillation, and orotracheal intubation.

EMT-Paramedic An EMT who has extensive training in advanced life support, including IV (intravenous) therapy, pharmacology, cardiac monitoring, and other advanced assessment and treatment skills.

first responder The first trained individual, such as a police officer, fire fighter, or other rescuer, to arrive at the scene of an emergency to provide initial medical assistance.

medical control Physician instructions that are given directly by radio (online/direct) or indirectly by protocol/guidelines (off-line/indirect), as authorized by the medical director of the service program.

medical director The physician who authorizes or delegates to the EMT the authority to perform medical care in the field.

primary service area (PSA) The designated area in which the EMS service is responsible for the provision of prehospital emergency care and transportation to the hospital.

quality control The responsibility of the medical director to ensure that the appropriate medical care standards are met by EMT-Bs on each call.

Assessment in Action

You are on your way to becoming an EMT-B, the backbone of the EMS system. In this course, you will learn new terms, theories, and techniques. These fundamental concepts and principles serve as the very foundation of patient care skills.

To help you develop critical thinking skills, expanded scenarios called **Assessment in Action** appear at the end of each chapter. These scenarios are followed by discussion and multiple-choice questions that are designed to stimulate discussion with your classmates or your instructor. These discussions, along with the rest of your course work, will help you to develop the skills that you need to become a successful EMT-B.

1. Which of the following is NOT considered one of the roles and responsibilities of an EMT-B?
   A. Ensuring your own safety during an emergency response
   B. Treating only patients who are able to pay for your services
   C. Providing safe transport of patients in your care to the hospital
   D. Providing quality patient care based on your assessment findings

2. What aspect of EMS is most likely to contribute to reducing permanent injury and disability to the general population?
   A. Health care insurance for all Americans
   B. Rapid access to EMS using 9-1-1 systems
   C. Increased Medicare reimbursement for hospitals
   D. Smaller, faster, and more fuel-efficient ambulances

3. Which of the following is NOT an attribute of a professional EMT-B?
   A. Having total recall of local EMS protocols
   B. Meeting continuing education requirements
   C. Maintaining a neat, clean personal appearance
   D. Placing personal needs before the patient's needs

4. Continuous quality improvement in EMS is best described as:
   A. a local concept with little practical importance except to attorneys and legislators.
   B. a government mandate that ensures that each state receives the same amount of tax-based funding.
   C. an ongoing system of audits and reviews that ensures that the public receives the highest standard of patient care.
   D. a philosophy that suggests that only young, healthy individuals be employed in EMS to reduce on-the-job injuries.

5. The medical director of an EMS provider agency is NOT responsible for:
   A. reviewing run reports to ensure compliance with protocols.
   B. developing and implementing protocols or standing orders.
   C. providing online medical direction during emergency calls.
   D. deciding which patients will be reimbursed for insurance claims.

Points to Ponder

You recently passed the EMT class and have been working as many shifts as you can with your response agency. You have a night off and are enjoying an evening "on the town." You have been to dinner and are headed to a movie when you notice a man sitting on the ground and leaning against an office building. He is holding his head and staring at the ground. He is wearing a suit and looks as though he may have just come out of the building. You slow down to take a closer look and the person with you tells you to keep driving, that you have worked enough lately. You are not in uniform and do not have any equipment with you. Would you stop and check on this person? When off-duty, are you functioning as an EMT? What legal protections do you have when you are off-duty?

Issues Duty to Act, Identification of EMTs, Scene Safety, Burnout, Role When Not On-duty, Legal Liability.

Online Outlook

The National Highway Traffic Safety Administration's (NHTSA) mission is to save lives, prevent injuries, and reduce traffic-related health care costs and other economic costs. Learn more about the NHTSA's involvement in EMS by completing Exercise 1 at www.emtb.com.

www.emtb.com

The Well-Being of the EMT-B

Objectives

Cognitive

1. List possible emotional reactions that the EMT-B may experience when faced with trauma, illness, death, and dying (p 20).
2. Discuss the possible reactions that a family member may exhibit when confronted with death and dying (p 22).
3. State the steps in the EMT-B's approach to the family confronted with death and dying (p 23).
4. State the possible reactions that the family of the EMT-B may exhibit due to their outside involvement in EMS (p 23).
5. Recognize the signs and symptoms of critical incident stress (p 29).
6. State possible steps that the EMT-B may take to help reduce/alleviate stress (p 30).
7. Explain the need to determine scene safety (p 37).
8. Describe the various ways by which communicable diseases can be transmitted from one person to another (p 38).*
9. Discuss the importance of body substance isolation (BSI) (p 38).
10. Define the term "universal precautions" and describe when it is appropriate to use such measures (p 38).*
11. Describe the steps the EMT-B should take for personal protection from airborne and bloodborne pathogens (p 43).
12. Identify appropriate task-specific personal protective equipment (p 43).*
13. Identify possible occupational diseases and methods of risk assessment (p 46).
14. Identify the role of a testing and immunization program in protecting the EMT-B from communicable diseases (p 45).*
15. Identify the benefits of an exposure control plan (p 43).*
16. Identify how the following diseases are transmitted and discuss the steps to take to prevent and/or deal with an exposure to each: hepatitis, meningitis, tuberculosis, HIV/AIDS (p 46).*
17. List the mechanisms of disease transmission (p 39).*
18. List the components of postexposure management and reporting (p 50).*
19. Discuss the importance of obtaining a patient's history and assessment findings to identify possible communicable diseases (p 50).*
20. List the personal protective equipment necessary for each of the following situations (p 51):
    - Hazardous materials
    - Rescue operations
    - Violent scenes
    - Crime scenes
    - Exposure to bloodborne pathogens
    - Exposure to airborne pathogens

    * These are noncurriculum objectives.

Affective

21. Explain the rationale for serving as an advocate for the use of appropriate protective equipment (p 37).
22. Explain the duty to care for patients with communicable diseases (p 46).*

Psychomotor

23. Given a scenario with potential infectious exposure, the EMT-B will use appropriate personal protective equipment. At the completion of the scenario, the EMT-B will properly remove and discard the protective garments (p 41).
24. Given the above scenario, the EMT-B will complete disinfection/cleaning and all reporting documentation (p 51).

TECHNOLOGY

www.emtb.com

- Online Chapter Pretest
- Interactivities
- Vocabulary Explorer
- Anatomy Review
- Web Links
- Online Review Manual
- Distance Learning

Chapter FEATURES

- Skill Drills
- Vital Vocabulary
- Pediatric Needs
- Geriatric Needs
- EMT-B Safety
- EMT-B Tips
- Documentation Tips
- Remember
- Prep Kit

You are the EMT

You are returning to quarters after participating in an unsuccessful resuscitation attempt on an elderly woman when your partner suddenly starts sobbing.

Unfortunately, many of the victims of out-of-hospital cardiac arrests do not survive. These calls, along with others, take their emotional toll on new and seasoned providers alike. This chapter focuses on providing you with the knowledge and insights you will need to keep yourself emotionally and physically healthy as you do the often-stressful work of an EMT-B. It will also help you answer the following questions:

1. What are the common emotional reactions that you may expect to encounter from either patients or possibly other providers during times of *extreme* stress?

2. Why is the concept of scene safety so important to the well-being of prehospital caregivers?

The Well-Being of the EMT-B

There is an ancient proverb, "Physician, heal thyself." As providers of health care, doctors need to look after themselves—in all respects—so that they can minister to others. An ill physician is in no position to render care as he or she was trained to do. That dictum applies to all health care providers and goes well beyond just physical issues. In caring for the critically ill and injured, there are many factors and situations that can interfere with the EMT-B's ability to treat the patient.

The personal health, safety, and well-being of all EMT-Bs are vital to an EMS operation. As a part of your training, you will learn how to recognize possible hazards and protect yourself from them. These hazards vary greatly, ranging from personal neglect to environmental and human-made threats to your health and safety. You will also learn about the mental and physical stress that you must cope with as a result of caring for the sick and injured. Death and dying challenge you to deal with the realities of human weaknesses and the emotions of the survivors.

It is important to remain calm to perform effectively when you are confronted with horrifying events, life-threatening illness, or injury. A special kind of self-control is needed to respond efficiently and effectively to the suffering of others. This self-control is developed through the following:

• Proper training

• Ongoing experience in dealing with all types of physical and mental distress

• A dedication to serve humanity

Emotional Aspects of Emergency Care

At times, even the most experienced health care providers have difficulty overcoming personal reactions and proceeding without hesitation. Patients need to be removed from life-threatening situations. Life support measures need to be given to patients who are severely injured. You may also be called upon to recover human remains from highway accidents, aircraft disasters, or explosions **▼ Figure 2-1** . In all of these situations, you must be calm and act responsibly as a member of the emergency medical care team. You must also realize that even though your personal emotions must be kept under control, these are normal feelings. Every EMT-B who must deal with such situations has these feelings. The struggle to remain calm in the face of horrible circumstances contributes to the emotional stress of the job.

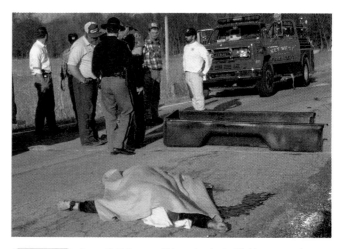

Figure 2-1 As an EMT-B, you will have to deal with the removal of bodies.

Death and Dying

Today, life expectancy has dramatically increased; nearly two-thirds of all deaths occur among those age 65 and older. Sixty percent of all deaths today are attributed to heart disease. From the age of 1 to the age of 34, trauma is the leading cause of death. Death today is likely to occur either quite suddenly or after a prolonged terminal illness. The environment of death has changed since our nation's earlier days; it no longer occurs in the home setting. The setting of death is somewhere else—in the hospital, a hospice, or a convalescent home, at the workplace, or on the highway. For this reason, we are less familiar with death than our ancestors were. We tend to deny death in America. Illness can be much more drawn-out and much more removed from daily life. Life support systems and impersonal care remove the whole experience of death from most people's awareness. The mobility of families also makes it less likely that there will be extended family support when death does occur.

Death was once both an expected and accepted fact in earlier American history. Life expectancy was brief (compared to today's), mortality rates (the ratio of number of deaths to a given population size) were high, and childbirth was hazardous, often resulting in the death of both the mother and the baby. Hardships of the times, both natural and human-made, were great. Children and adults died of disease, injuries, and the traumas of war. Most people had experienced the death of someone close to them. There were no funeral homes; mourning occurred at home in the family setting. The presence of a dead body was a natural event.

No matter what the frequency of response to emergency calls, death is something that every EMT-B will sometimes face. For some of you, it may be infrequent. Others, in urban settings, may see death many times in responding to motor vehicle crashes, drug overdoses, suicides, or homicides. Some EMT firefighters may have to deal with the mass-casualty incident of an airplane crash or a hazardous materials accident. In all these cases, coming to grips with your thoughts, understandings, and adjustment to death is not only important personally, but also a function of delivering emergency medical care.

Physical Signs of Death

Determination of the cause of death is the medical responsibility of a physician. There are both definitive and presumptive signs of death. In many states, death is defined as the absence of circulatory and respiratory function. Many states have also adopted "brain death" provisions; these provisions refer to irreversible cessation of all functions of the brain and brain stem. Questions often arise as to whether to begin basic life support. In the absence of physician orders such as do not resuscitate (DNR) orders, the general rule is: If the body is still warm and intact, initiate emergency medical care. An exception to this rule is cold temperature (hypothermia) emergencies. Hypothermia is a general cooling of the body in which the internal body temperature becomes abnormally low: 95°F (35°C). It is considered a serious condition and is often fatal. At 86°F (30°C), the brain can survive without perfusion for about 10 minutes. When the core temperature drops to 82.4°F (28°C), the patient is in grave danger; however, individuals have survived a hypothermia accident with a temperature of 64.4°F (18°C). In cases of hypothermia, the patient should not be considered dead until he or she is warm and dead.

PRESUMPTIVE SIGNS OF DEATH. Most medicolegal authorities will consider the presumptive signs of death that are listed in (▼ **Table 2-1**) adequate, particularly when they follow a severe trauma or occur at the end stages of long-term illness such as cancer or other prolonged diseases. These signs would not be adequate in cases of sudden death due to hypothermia, acute poisoning, or cardiac arrest. Usually, in these cases, some combination of the signs is needed to declare death, not just one of them alone.

TABLE 2-1 Presumptive Signs of Death

- Unresponsiveness to painful stimuli
- Lack of a pulse or heartbeat
- Absence of breath sounds
- No deep tendon or corneal reflexes
- Absence of eye movement
- No systolic blood pressure
- Profound cyanosis
- Lowered or decreased body temperature

DEFINITIVE SIGNS OF DEATH. Definitive or conclusive signs of death that are obvious and clear to even non-medical persons include the following:

- Obvious mortal damage, such as a body in parts (decapitation)

- **Dependent lividity**: blood settling to the lowest point of the body, causing discoloration of the skin.

- **Rigor mortis**, the stiffening of body muscles caused by chemical changes within muscle tissue. It develops first in the face and jaw, gradually extending downward until the body is in full rigor. The rate of onset is affected by the body's ability to lose heat to its surroundings. A thin body loses heat faster than a fat body. A body on a tile floor loses heat faster than a body wrapped up in a blanket in a bed. Rigor mortis occurs sometime between 2 and 12 hours after death.

- **Putrefaction** (decomposition of body tissues). Depending on temperature conditions, this occurs sometime between 40 and 96 hours after death.

Medical Examiner Cases

Involvement of the medical examiner, or the coroner in some states, depends on the nature and scene of the death. In most states, when trauma is a factor or the death involves suspected criminal or unusual situations such as hanging or poisoning, the medical examiner must be notified (▼ **Figure 2-2**). When the medical examiner or coroner assumes responsibility of the scene, that responsibility supersedes all others at the scene, including the family's. The following are considered the medical examiner's cases:

- When the person is dead on arrival (DOA)

- Death without previous medical care or when the physician is unable to state the cause of death

- Suicide (self-destruction)

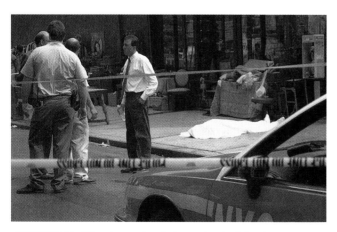

Figure 2-2 When trauma is a factor or the death involves a suspected criminal situation, the medical examiner is required.

> ## Remember
>
> **Definitive Signs of Death**
>
> - Obvious mortal damage
> - Dependent lividity
> - Rigor mortis
> - Putrefaction

- Violent death

- Poisoning, known or suspected

- Death resulting from accidents

- Suspicion of a criminal act

If emergency medical care has been initiated, keep thorough notes of what was done or found. These records may be important during a subsequent investigation.

The Grieving Process

The death of a human being is one of the most difficult events for another human being to accept. If the survivor is a relative or close friend of the deceased, it is even more difficult. Emotional responses to the loss of a loved one or friend are appropriate and should be expected. In fact, it is expected that you will feel emotional about the death of a patient. Feelings and emotions are part of the grieving process. All of us experience these feelings after a stressful situation that causes us personal pain.

In 1969, Dr. Elisabeth Kubler-Ross published research revealing that people go through several stages of grieving. The stages of grieving are as follows:

1. **Denial.** Refusal to accept diagnosis or care, unrealistic demands for miracles, or persistent failure to understand why there is no improvement.

2. **Anger, hostility.** Projection of bad news onto the environment and commonly in all directions, at times almost at random. The person lashes out. Someone must be blamed, and those who are responsible must be punished. This is usually an ugly phase.

3. **Bargaining.** An attempt to secure a prize for good behavior or promise to change lifestyle. "I promise to be a 'perfect patient' if only I can live until 'x' event."

4. **Depression.** Open expression of grief, internalized anger, hopelessness, the desire to die. It rarely involves suicidal threats, complete withdrawal, or giving up long before the illness seems terminal. The patient is usually silent.

TABLE 2-2 Responding to Grief

Don't Say...	Try Instead...
Give it time. Things will get better.	I'm sorry.
You should not question God's will.	It is okay to be angry.
You have to get on with your life.	It must be hard to accept.
You have to keep on going.	That must be painful for you.
You can always have another child.	Tell me how you are feeling.
You're not the only one who suffers.	Let's spend some time together.
The living must go on.	If you want to cry, it's okay.
I know how you feel.	People really cared for…

5. **Acceptance.** The simple "yes." Acceptance grows out of a person's conviction that all has been done and the person is ready to die.

Stages may follow one another or occur simultanously. They may last different amounts of time.

Even though the event (death) has not yet happened, the patient knows that it will happen. The patient has no control over this process. The patient will die whether or not he or she is ready to die. Furthermore, being ready to die does not mean that the patient will be happy about dying. You may encounter situations in which the patient is close to death, and you may need to provide reassurance and emotional care.

What Can the EMT-B Do?

Do helpful things, and make simple suggestions. Ask whether there is anything that you can do that will be of help, such as calling a relative or religious advisor. Provide gentle and caring support. Reinforcing the reality of the situation is important. This can be accomplished by merely saying to a grieving person, "I am so sorry for your loss." It is not important that you have a well-rehearsed script, for it is not likely that your exact words or consolations will be remembered. Being yourself and sincere are important.

Some statements tend to be trite, and some suggest a kind of silver lining behind the clouds. Although they may be intended to make the person feel better about a situation, they also can be viewed as an attempt to diminish the person's grief. The grieving person needs to grieve. Statements like these can also indicate our inability to comprehend the profound sadness of grief because we have not experienced that kind of loss.

Attempts to take grief away too quickly are not good. If you do not know how the person really feels, you should not say so. People may be offended by responses that give advice or explanations about the death ▲ **Table 2-2** . Statements such as "Oh, you shouldn't feel that way" are judgmental. If you judge what the grieving person is feeling, it is likely that he or she will stop talking with you. There is no reason why grieving people should not feel what they are feeling. Remember anger is a stage of grieving. The anger may be directed at you. The anger seems irrational to everyone but the person grieving. A professional attitude is a necessity.

Statements and comments that suggest action on your part are generally helpful. These statements imply a sense of understanding; they focus on the grieving person's feelings. It is not necessary to go into an extensive discussion. All you need to do is be sincere and say, "I am so sorry. I just want you to know that I am thinking about you." What people really appreciate is somebody who will listen to them. Simply ask, "Would you like to talk about how or what you are now feeling?" Then accept the response.

Dealing with the Patient and Family Members

There is no right or wrong way to grieve. Each person will experience grief and respond to it in his or her own way. Family members may express rage, anger, and despair. Many people will be rational and cooperative. Their concerns will usually be relieved by your calm, efficient manner. Your actions and words, even a simple touch, can communicate caring. While you must treat all patients with respect and dignity, use special care with dying patients and their families. Be concerned about their privacy and their wishes, and let them know that you take their concerns seriously. However, it is best to be honest with patients and their families; do not give them false hope.

Initial Care of the Dying, Critically Ill, or Injured Patient

Individuals who are in the process of dying as a result of trauma, an acute medical emergency, or a terminal disease will feel threatened. That threat may be related to their concern about survival. These concerns may involve feelings of helplessness, disability, pain, and separation. They are related to the individual's sense of self and understanding of death (▼ Table 2-3).

ANXIETY. Anxiety is a response to the anticipation of danger. The source of the anxiety is often unknown; but in the case of seriously injured or ill patients, the source is usually recognizable. What may increase the anxiety are the unknowns of the current situation. Patients may ask the following:

- What will happen to me?
- What are you doing?
- Will I make it?
- What will my disabilities be?

Patients who are anxious may have the following signs and symptoms:

- Upset
- Sweaty and cool (diaphoretic)
- Rapid breathing (hyperventilating)
- Fast pulse (tachycardic)
- Restless
- Tense
- Fearful
- Shaky (tremulous)

TABLE 2-3   Concerns of the Dying, Critically Ill, or Injured Patient

- Anxiety
- Pain and fear
- Anger and hostility
- Depression
- Dependency
- Guilt
- Mental health problems
- Receiving unrelated bad news

For the anxious patient, time seems to be extended; seconds seem like minutes, and minutes seem like hours.

PAIN AND FEAR. Pain and fear are very closely interrelated. Pain often is associated with illness or trauma. Fear is generally thought of in relation to the oncoming pain and the outcome of the damage. It is often helpful to encourage patients to express their pains and fears, since expression of them begins the process of adjustment to the pain and acceptance of the emergency medical care that may be necessary. Some individuals have difficulty in openly admitting their fear. The fear may be expressed as bad dreams, withdrawal, tension, restlessness, "butterflies" in the stomach, or nervousness. In some cases, it may be expressed as anger.

ANGER AND HOSTILITY. Anger may be expressed by very demanding and complaining behavior. Often, this may be related to the fear and anxiety of the emergency medical care that is being given. Sometimes, the fear is so acute that the patient may want to express anger toward you or others but is unable to do so because of the dependency factor. If you find that you are the target of the patient's anger, make sure that you are safe; do not take the anger or insults personally. Be tolerant, and do not become defensive.

The anger may also be expressed physically, and you may be the target of the displaced aggression. If the patient or a relative becomes so emotionally upset that you are physically assaulted or you believe that this could happen, back out of the situation. Such hostility must be contained. If emergency medical care is not possible under these circumstances, law enforcement intervention is required.

DEPRESSION. Almost all dying patients feel some degree of depression because of internalized anger and other factors. Some patients may have many dissatisfactions and regrets about their lives; others may be wrapped up in concerns about financial, legal, social, or family problems. The patient should be encouraged to express his or her feelings. Assisting the patient and his or her family in resolving unsettled matters may decrease feelings of depression.

DEPENDENCY. When emergency medical care is given to any individual, a sense of dependency develops. Individuals who are placed in this position often feel helpless and may become resentful. The resentfulness may arouse feelings of inferiority, shame, or weakness.

GUILT. Many patients who are dying, their families, or the caregivers of those patients may feel guilty over what has happened to them. Occasionally family members and/or long-term caregivers may feel a degree of relief when an extended illness is finally over. That relief may later turn into guilt. Most of the time, however, no one can explain these feelings. The magnitude of the guilt may be very great. Sometimes, feelings of guilt can result in a delay in seeking emergency medical care.

MENTAL HEALTH PROBLEMS. Mental health problems such as disorientation, confusion, or delusions may develop in the dying patient. In these instances, the patient may display behavior inconsistent with normal patterns of thinking, feeling, or acting. Common characteristics of such behavior may include the following:

- Loss of contact with reality
- Distortion of perception
- Regression
- Diminished control of basic impulses and desires
- Abnormal mental content, including delusions and hallucinations

In some long-term situations, generalized personality deterioration may occur.

RECEIVING UNRELATED BAD NEWS. A patient who is in critical condition or is dying may not want to hear of unrelated bad news, such as the death of someone close to them. Such news may depress the patient or cause the patient to give up hope.

Caring for Critically Ill and Injured Patients

Patients need to know who you are and what you are doing. Let the patient know that you are attending to his or her immediate needs and that these are your primary concerns at this moment (▼ **Figure 2-3**). As soon as possible, explain to the patient what is going on. Confusion, anxiety, and other feelings of helplessness will be decreased if you keep the patient informed from the start.

Avoid Sad and Grim Comments

EMT-Bs, other safety personnel, family, and bystanders must avoid grim comments about a patient's condition. Remarks such as "This is a bad one" or "The leg is badly damaged, and I think he will lose it" are inappropriate. These remarks may upset or increase anxiety in the patient and compromise possible recovery outcomes. This is especially true for the patient who may be able to hear but not to respond.

Orient the Patient

You should expect a patient to be disoriented in an emergency situation. The aura of the emergency situation—lights, sirens, smells, and strangers—is intense. The impact and effect of injuries or acute illness may cause the patient to be confused or unsettled. It is important to orient the patient to his or her surroundings (▼ **Figure 2-4**). Use brief, concise statements such as "Mr. Smith, you have had an accident, and I am

Figure 2-3   Let the patient know immediately that you are there to help.

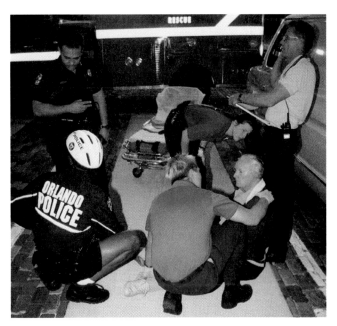

Figure 2-4   The aura of an emergency situation can be confusing and frightening to the patient. Make sure you explain to the patient what has happened.

now splinting your arm. I am John Foxworth of the New Britain EMS; I will be caring for you."

Be Honest

In approaching any patient, you must decide how much each patient is able to understand and accept. You should be honest without additionally shocking the patient or giving information that is unnecessary or that may not be understood. Simply explain what you are doing, and allow the patient to be part of the care being given; this can relieve feelings of helplessness as well as some of the fear.

Acknowledge the Seriousness of the Condition

There may be occasions when a patient may refuse emergency medical care and insist that you do nothing or leave him or her alone. In these cases, it is important to impress on the patient the seriousness of the condition without causing undue alarm. Saying, "Everything will be okay," when it is obvious that it is not, is not being truthful. Generally, seriously ill or injured patients know that they are in trouble.

Allow for Hope

In trauma and acute medical conditions, patients may ask whether they are going to die. You may feel at a loss for words. You may also know, on the basis of past experience or in view of the seriousness of the present situation, that the prognosis is poor. But it is not up to you to tell the patient that he or she is dying. Statements such as "I don't know if you are going to die; let's fight this one out together" or "I am not going to give up on you, so do not give up on yourself" are helpful. These statements transmit a sense of trust and hope, and they let the patient know that you are doing everything possible to save his or her life. If there is the slightest chance of hope remaining, you want that message transmitted in your attitude and in the statements you make to the patient.

Locate and Notify Family Members

Many patients will be concerned and ask you to notify their family or others close to them. The patient may or may not be able to assist you in doing this. You should see to it that an appropriate and responsible person makes an effort to locate the desired persons. Assuring the patient that someone is going to do this may be a significant part of the patient's care.

Injured and Critically Ill Children

Injured and critically ill children who have life-threatening conditions should be cared for as any patient would be, insofar as an assessment of airway, breathing, and circulation (ABC) and immediate life threats are concerned. Due regard should be given to variations in height, weight, and size in providing emergency medical care. Because of the increased excitement and extraordinary nature of the emergency scene for a child, it is important that a relative or responsible adult accompany the child, to relieve anxiety and assist in care as appropriate.

Dealing with the Death of a Child

The death of a child is a tragic and dreaded event. It is not unusual to think about the fact that the dead or dying child has a lot more to do and should have many more years to live. In our society, we assume that only old people are supposed to die. Children die less frequently now than they did in earlier times, so most people are unprepared for what they will feel when a child dies. You may think about your own children and those whom you know: nephews, nieces, grandchildren, and children of close friends. And you may think, "Why should this child, who is only 5 years old, die?"

Answering the difficult questions of your own mortality will be of help when dealing with the death of a child. But, still, the death of a child will not be an easy subject to talk about. This will be especially so for the family. And as an EMT-B involved in a call that involves the death of a child, you will also likely experience stress.

One of your responsibilities may be to help the family through the initial period after the death. As an EMT-B, until more definitive and professional help can be available, you may be in the best position to help the family begin to cope with their loss. How a family initially deals with the death of a child will affect its stability and endurance. You can help a family through its initial period of grief and alert the family to the follow-up counseling and support services that are available.

Helping the Family

If the child is dead, acknowledging the fact of the death is important. This should be done in a private place, even if that is inside an ambulance. Often, the parents cannot believe that the death is real, even if they have been preparing for it, as in the case of a terminal illness such as leukemia. Reactions vary, but shock, disbelief, and denial are common. Some parents show little emotion at the initial news.

If it is possible and appropriate, find a place where the mother and father can hold the child. This is important in the parents' grieving process; it helps to lessen the sense of disbelief and makes the death real. Even if the parents do not ask to see the child, you should tell them that they may. Your decision in permitting the parents to see the child may need some discretion. For example, in the case of a traumatic death in which there is significant disfigurement, that decision might have to be delayed. The delay may involve having support services available or contacting the family physician or others who can help the parents through this difficult situation. This may involve preparing the parents for what they will see and the changes brought on by rigor mortis, asphyxiation, and so forth.

Sometimes, you do not need to say much. In fact, silence can sometimes be more comforting than words. You can express your own sorrow. Do not overload grieving parents with a lot of information; at this point, they cannot handle it. Nonverbal communication, such as holding a hand or touching a shoulder, may also be valuable. Let the family's actions be your guide about what is appropriate. It is important that parents be encouraged to talk about their feelings.

Stressful Situations

Many situations, such as mass-casualty scenes, serious automobile crashes, excavation cave-ins, house fires, infant and child trauma, amputations, abuse of an infant/child/spouse/elderly person, and death of a coworker or other public safety personnel, will be stressful for everyone involved. During these situations, you must exercise extreme care in both your words and your actions. Be careful to present a professional demeanor in words and actions at the scene. Words that do not seem important, or that are said jokingly, may hurt someone. Conversations at the scene must be professional. You should not say, "Everything will be all right," or "There is nothing to worry about." A person who is trapped in a wrecked car, hurting from head to foot and worrying about a loved one, knows that all is not well. What will reassure the patient is your calm and caring approach to the emergency situation. Briefly explain your plan of action to assist the patient in the crisis. Inform the patient that you need his or her help and the assistance of family members or bystanders to carry out the plan of action.

How a patient reacts to injury or illness may be influenced by certain personality traits. Some patients may become highly emotional over what may seem to be a minor problem. Others may show little or no

emotion, even after serious injury or illness. Many other factors influence how a patient reacts to the stress of an EMS incident. Among these factors are the following:

- Socioeconomic background
- Fear of medical personnel
- Alcohol or substance abuse
- History of chronic disease
- Mental disorders
- Reaction to medication
- Age
- Nutritional status
- Feelings of guilt

You are not expected to always know why a patient is having an unusual emotional response. However, you can quickly and calmly assess the actions of the patient, family members, and bystanders. This assessment will help you to gain the confidence and cooperation of everyone at the scene. In addition, you should use a professional tone of voice and show courtesy, along with sincere concern and efficient action. These simple considerations will go far to relieve worry, fear, and insecurity. Calm reassurance will inspire confidence and cooperation. Compassion is important, but you must be careful. Your professional judgment takes priority over compassion. For example, suppose a screaming child with no obvious life-threatening injuries is covered with another patient's blood. This frightened child appeals to your compassion and thus gets your attention. In the meantime, an unconscious, nonbreathing adult nearby could die from lack of care.

Patients must be given the opportunity to express their fears and concerns. You can easily relieve many of these concerns at the scene. Usually, patients are concerned about the safety or well-being of others who are involved in the accident and about the damage or loss of personal property. Your responses must be discreet and diplomatic, giving reassurance when appropriate. If a loved one has been killed or critically injured, you should wait, if possible, until clergy or emergency department staff can give the patient the news. They can then provide the psychological support the patient may need.

Some patients, especially children and the elderly, may be terrified or feel rejected when separated from family members by the uniformed EMS provider team. Other patients may not want family members to share their stress, see their injury, or witness their pain.

Figure 2-5 Children may be frightened when separated from family members.

It is usually best if parents go with their children and relatives accompany elderly patients (▲ **Figure 2-5**).

Religious customs or needs of the patient must also be respected. Some people will cling to religious medals or charms, especially if any attempt is made to remove them. Others will express a strong desire for religious counsel, baptism, or last rites if death is near. You must try to accommodate these requests. Some people have religious convictions that strongly oppose the use of drugs, blood, and blood products. If you obtain such information, it is imperative that you report it to the next level of care.

In the event of a death, you must handle the body with respect and dignity. It must be exposed as little as possible. Learn your local regulations and protocols about moving the body or changing its position, especially if you are at a possible crime scene. Even in these situations, cardiopulmonary resuscitation (CPR) and appropriate treatment must be given unless there are obvious signs of death.

Uncertain Situations

There will be times when you are unsure whether a true medical emergency exists. If you are unsure, contact medical control about the need to transport. If you cannot reach medical control, it is always best to transport the patient. For both ethical and medicolegal reasons, a physician must examine all patients who are transported and judge the degree of medical need.

You must also realize that the most minor symptoms may be early signs of severe illness or injury. Symptoms of many illnesses can be similar to those of substance abuse, hysteria, or other conditions. You must accept the patient's complaints and provide appropriate care until you are able to transfer care of the patient to a higher level (eg, paramedic, nurse, or physician). Your local protocols will direct your actions in these uncertain situations. When in doubt, err on the side of caution, and acquire the patient's consent and transport to the medical facility.

Stress Warning Signs and the Work Environment

EMS is a high-stress job. Understanding the causes of stress and knowing how to deal with them are critical to your job performance, health, and interpersonal relationships. To prevent stress from affecting your life negatively, you need to understand what stress is, its physiologic effects, what you can do to minimize these effects, and how to deal with stress on an emotional level.

Stress is the impact of stressors on your physical and mental well-being. Stressors include emotional, physical, and environmental situations or conditions that may cause a variety of physiologic, physical, and psychologic responses. The body's response to stress begins with an alarm response, followed by a stage of reaction and resistance, and then recovery or, if the stress is prolonged, exhaustion. This three-stage response is referred to as the **general adaptation syndrome**.

The physiologic responses involve the interaction of the endocrine and nervous systems, resulting in chemical and physical responses. This is commonly known as the *fight-or-flight response*. Positive stress, such as exercise, as well as negative forms of stress, such as shift work, long hours, or the frustration of losing a patient, all have the same physiologic manifestations. These include the following:

- Increased respirations and heart rate
- Increased blood pressure
- Dilated venous vessels near the skin surface (causes cool, clammy skin)
- Dilated pupils
- Tensed muscles
- Increased blood glucose levels
- Perspiration
- Decreased blood flow to the gastrointestinal tract

Stress may also have physical symptoms such as fatigue, changes in appetite, gastrointestinal problems, or headaches. Stress may cause insomnia or hypersomnia, irritability, inability to concentrate, and hyperactivity or underactivity. Additionally, stress may manifest itself in psychologic reactions such as fear, dull or nonresponsive behavior, depression, oversensitivity, anger, irritability, and frustration. Often, today's fast-paced lifestyles compound these effects by not allowing a person to rest and recover after periods of stress. Prolonged or excessive stress has been proven to be a strong contributor to heart disease, hypertension, cancer, alcoholism, and depression.

Many people are subject to cumulative stress, whereby insignificant stressors accumulate to a larger stress-related problem. In the emergency services environment (EMS, police, firefighters), stressors may also be sudden and more severe. Some events are unusually stressful or emotional, even by emergency services standards. These acute severe stressors result in what is referred to as critical incident stress. Events that can trigger critical incident stress include the following:

- Mass-casualty incidents

- Serious injury or traumatic death of a child

- Crash with injuries, caused by an emergency services provider while responding to or from a call

- Death or serious injury of a coworker in the line of duty

Posttraumatic stress disorder (PTSD) may develop after a person has experienced a psychologically distressing event. It is characterized by re-experiencing the event and overresponding to stimuli that recall the event. PTSD is sometimes referred to as "Vietnam veteran's disease" because of its classification as a mental disorder following the Vietnam conflict. Stressful events in EMS are sometimes psychologically overwhelming. Some of the symptoms include depression, startle reactions, flashback phenomena, and dissociative episodes (eg, amnesia of the event).

An emergency services provider need not suffer through the emotional aftermath of these difficult situations. A process called **critical incident stress management (CISM)** was developed to address this need (▶ **Figure 2-6**). This process confronts the responses to critical incidents and defuses them, directing the emergency services personnel toward physical and emotional equilibrium. CISM can occur formally, as a debriefing for those who were on scene. A trained CISM team of peers and mental health professionals may facilitate this. Additionally, CISM can occur at an ongoing scene in the following circumstances:

EMT-B Safety

Coworkers often notice a change in behavior or attitude before a supervisor does. This is especially true in EMS, where close relationships develop between people who work together and share rooms, meals, and social interaction. This may allow you to help someone before job performance is negatively affected.

- When personnel are assessed for signs and symptoms of distress while resting

- Before re-entering the scene

- During a scene demobilization in which personnel are educated about the signs of critical incident stress and given a buffer period to collect themselves before leaving

The most common form of CISM is peer defusing, when a group informally discusses events that they experienced together.

Stress and Nutrition

Anyone can respond to a sudden physical stress for a short time. If stress is prolonged, especially if physical action is not a permitted response, the body can quickly be drained of its reserves. This can leave it depleted of key nutrients, weakened, and more susceptible to illness.

Your body's three sources of fuel—carbohydrates, fat, and protein—are consumed in increased quantities

Figure 2-6   Critical incident stress management plays an important role in helping providers to relieve stress.

during stress, particularly if physical activity is involved. The quickest source of energy is glucose, taken from stored glycogen in the liver. However, this supply will last less than a day. Protein, drawn primarily from muscle, is a long-term source of glucose. Tissues can use fat for energy. The body also conserves water during periods of stress. To do so, it retains sodium by exchanging and losing potassium from the kidneys. Other nutrients that are susceptible to depletion are the vitamins and minerals that are not stored by the body in substantial quantities. These include water-soluble B and C vitamins and most minerals.

As EMS providers, we do not have control of what stressors we will face on any given day. Consequently, stress in one form or another is an unavoidable part of our lives. As one would study for a test, dress properly for a day of snow skiing, or train for a sporting event, we should physically prepare our bodies for stress. Physical conditioning and proper nutrition are the two variables over which we have absolute control. Muscles will grow and retain protein only with sufficient activity. Bones will not passively accumulate calcium. In response to the physical stress of exercise, bones store calcium and become denser and stronger. Regular,

well-balanced meals are essential to provide the nutrients that are necessary to keep your body fueled (▼ **Figure 2-7**). Vitamin-mineral preparations that provide a balanced mix of all the nutrients may be necessary to supplement a less than perfectly balanced diet.

Stress Management

There are many methods of handling stress. Some are positive and healthy; others are harmful or destructive. Americans consume more than 20 tons of aspirin per day, and doctors prescribe muscle relaxers, tranquilizers, and sedatives more than 90 million times per year to patients in the United States. Although these medications have legitimate uses, they do nothing to combat the stress that may cause the medical problems described previously.

The term "stress management" refers to the tactics that have been shown to alleviate or eliminate stress reactions. These may involve changing a few habits, changing your attitude, and perseverance (▶ **Table 2-4**).

A clue to the management of stress comes from the fact that it is not the event itself but the individual's reaction to it that determines how much it will strain the body's resources. Remember that stress is defined as

Key

⬤ Fat (naturally occurring and added)

▾ Sugars (added)

These symbols show fats, oils and added sugars in foods.

FATS, OILS & SWEETS
Use sparingly

MILK, YOGURT & CHEESE GROUP
2-3 servings

MEAT, POULTRY, FISH, DRY BEANS, EGGS & NUTS GROUP
2-3 servings

VEGETABLE GROUP
3-5 servings

FRUIT GROUP
2-4 servings

BREAD, CEREAL, RICE & PASTA GROUP
6-11 servings

Figure 2-7 A healthy diet is illustrated by the USDA Food Guide Pyramid.

TABLE 2-4 Strategies to Manage Stress

Change or eliminate stressors.

Change partners to avoid a negative or hostile personality.

Change work hours.

Cut back on overtime.

Change your attitude about the stressor.

Stop wasting your energy complaining or worrying about things that you cannot change, such as:

- Skid row alcoholics
- Abused children
- Nursing home transfers
- Cleaning contaminated EMS units

Try to adopt a more relaxed, philosophical outlook.

Expand your social support system apart from your coworkers.

Sustain friends and interests outside emergency services.

Minimize the physical response to stress by employing various techniques, including:

- A deep breath to settle an anger response
- Periodic stretching
- Slow, deep breathing
- Regular physical exercise
- Progressive muscle relaxation

anything that you perceive as a threat to your equilibrium. Stress is an undeniable and unavoidable part of our everyday life. By understanding how it affects you physiologically, physically, and psychologically, you can more successfully manage it.

Supporting patients in emergency situations is difficult. It is stressful for them but also for you. You are vulnerable to all the stresses that go with your profession. It is critical that you recognize the signs of stress so that it does not interfere with your work or life away from work, including your family life. The signs and symptoms of chronic stress may not be obvious at first. Rather, they may be subtle and not present all the time ▶ Table 2-5 .

The following sections provide some suggestions for how to cope better with stress. Some of them may be useful in helping you to prevent problems from developing. Others may help you to solve problems, should they develop.

LIFESTYLE CHANGES. Your well-being is of primary importance to effective EMS operations. The effectiveness and efficiency with which you do your job depend on your ability to stay in shape and avoid the risk of personal injury. **Burnout** is a condition of chronic fatigue and frustration that results from mounting stress over time. To avoid burnout, you need to be in good physical and mental health. Be aware of the potential hazards in rescue and emergency medical care. You must also learn how to avoid or prevent personal injury or illness.

TABLE 2-5 Warning Signs of Stress

Irritability toward coworkers, family, and friends

Inability to concentrate

Difficulty sleeping, increased sleeping, or nightmares

Anxiety

Indecisiveness

Guilt

Loss of appetite (gastrointestinal disturbances)

Loss of interest in sexual activities

Isolation

Loss of interest in work

Increased use of alcohol

Recreational drug use

NUTRITION. To perform efficiently, you must eat nutritious food. Food is the fuel that makes the body run. The physical exertion and stress that are a part of your job require a high energy output. If you do not have a ready source of fuel, your performance may be less than satisfactory. This can be dangerous for you, your partner, and your patient. Therefore, it is important for you to learn about and follow the rules of good nutrition.

Candy and soft drinks contain sugar. These foods are quickly absorbed and converted to fuel by the body. But simple sugars also stimulate the body's production of insulin, which reduces blood glucose levels. For some people, eating a lot of sugar can actually result in lower energy levels.

Complex carbohydrates rank next to simple sugars in their ability to produce energy. Complex carbohydrates such as pasta, rice, and vegetables are among the safest, most reliable sources for long-term energy production. However, some carbohydrates take hours to be converted into usable body fuel.

Fats are also easily converted to energy, but eating too much fat can lead to obesity, cardiac disease, and other long-term health problems. The proteins in meat, fish, chicken, beans, and cheese take several hours to convert to energy.

Carry an individual supply of high-energy food to help you maintain your energy levels ▼ Figure 2-8 . Try eating several small meals throughout the day to keep your energy resources at constant high levels. Remember, however, that overeating may reduce your physical and mental performance. After a large meal, the blood that is needed for the digestive process is not available for other activities.

You must also make sure that you maintain an adequate fluid intake ▼ Figure 2-9 . Hydration is important for proper functioning. Fluids can be easily replenished by drinking any nonalcoholic, noncaffeinated fluid. Water is generally the best fluid available. The body absorbs it faster than any other fluid. Avoid fluids that contain high levels of sugar. These can actually slow the rate of fluid absorption by the body. They can also cause abdominal discomfort. One indication of adequate hydration is frequent urination. Infrequent urination or urine that has a deep yellow color indicates dehydration.

EXERCISE AND RELAXATION. A regular program of exercise will enhance the benefits of maintaining good nutrition and adequate hydration. When you are in good physical condition, you can handle job stress more easily. A regular program of exercise will increase your strength and endurance ▶ Figure 2-10 . You may wish to practice relaxation techniques, meditation, and visual imagery.

BALANCING WORK, FAMILY, AND HEALTH. As an EMT-B, you will often be called to assist the sick and injured any time of the day or night. Unfortunately, there is no rhyme or reason to the timing of illness, injury, or interfacility transfer. Volunteer EMT-Bs may often be called away from family or friends during social activities. Shift workers may be required to be apart from loved ones for long periods of time. You should never let the job interfere excessively with your own needs. Find a balance between work and family; you owe it to yourself and to them. It is important to make sure that you have the time that you need to relax with family and friends.

It is also important to realize that coworkers, family, and friends often may not understand the stress caused by responding to EMS calls. As a result of a "bad call," you might not feel like going out to a movie or attending a family event that has been planned for some time. In these situations, help from a critical incident stress debriefing team or information sessions conducted by the EMS unit's employee assistance program may assist you in resolving these problems.

Figure 2-8　Carry a supply of high-energy food with you so that you can maintain your energy levels.

Figure 2-9　Maintain an adequate fluid intake by drinking plenty of water or other nonalcoholic, caffeine-free fluid.

When possible, rotate your schedule to give yourself time off. If your EMS system allows you to move from station to station, rotate to reduce or vary your call volume. Take vacations to provide for your good health so that you will be able to respond the next time you are needed. If at any point you feel that the stress of work is more than you can handle, seek help. You may want to discuss your stress informally with your family or coworkers. Help from more experienced team members can be invaluable. You may also wish to get help from peer counselors or other professionals. Seeking this help does not make you weak in the eyes of others. Rather, it shows that you are in control of your life.

Critical Incident Stress Debriefing

You may be called to a situation so horrible that you find it difficult to respond as you were trained. You may have an immediate or delayed negative response to the incident. Do not be ashamed of such feelings; almost all responders have had the same reaction at one time or another. If you feel overwhelmed, step back and call additional resources. Sometimes, simply knowing that help is on the way can help you to overcome your fear or anxiety and enable you to respond to the situation. Remember that if you have these feelings from time to time, your partner and other members of the team may have them, too. Keep an eye on other members of your team. Confirm that they are under control and act appropriately during a major disaster.

After a stressful run or a disaster, there may be an emotional letdown. This letdown is often overlooked. However, it may be more important to deal with than the initial contact response. Critical incident stress debriefing is a way to deal with this emotional letdown phase. A critical incident is any event that causes

anxiety and mental stress to emergency workers. **Critical incident stress debriefing (CISD)** is a program in which severely stressful job-related incidents are discussed. These discussions are conducted in strict confidence with other emergency workers who are trained in CISD (▼ **Figure 2-11**). The purpose of CISD is to relieve personal and group anxieties and stress. Never be ashamed to report your feelings, because such a debriefing can be vital to your emotional well-being. It should not be dismissed as trivial or nonessential.

CISD teams consist of peer counselors and mental health professionals who help you to deal with critical incident stress. Usually, CISD meetings are held within 24 to 72 hours of a major incident. CISD meetings may also have to be repeated at a later time. A CISD meeting is not an investigation or an interrogation. It is an opportunity to discuss your feelings, fears, and reactions to the event. All information that is discussed in the meeting should remain confidential. The CISD leaders and mental health professionals will help you by listening and then offering suggestions on how to overcome the stress. CISD is designed to accelerate the normal recovery process following a critical incident. These meetings are helpful to all rescuers who are involved in an incident, whether or not they think they were stressed. A CISD meeting provides a means to quickly vent feelings in a nonthreatening atmosphere.

CISD programs are located throughout the United States. CISD teams usually can be located by calling telephone directory assistance in your area and asking for CISD. The International Critical Incident Stress Foundation, Inc. has an emergency access number: (410) 313-2473. For general information, call (410) 750-9600, or contact the foundation by e-mail at icisf@erols.com.

Figure 2-10 A regular program of exercise will increase strength and endurance.

Figure 2-11 CISD sessions are conducted in strict confidence with other emergency workers who are trained in CISD.

A comprehensive CISM system includes the following 10 components:

- Preincident stress education
- On-scene peer support
- One-on-one support
- Disaster support services
- Defusings
- CISD
- Follow-up services
- Spouse and family support
- Community outreach programs
- Other health and welfare programs, such as wellness

Workplace Issues

As our society continues to grow more and more culturally diverse, some groups that may have been satisfied in the past to accept and participate in American cultural traditions may seek instead to assert, preserve, and nurture their differences. As our society grows more culturally diverse, so do EMS workplaces. There will be challenges as these changes continue to occur. With the greater involvement of people of different backgrounds, EMS has the opportunity to serve people with more sensitivity to cultural variances.

Cultural Diversity on the Job

Each individual is different, and you should communicate with coworkers and patients in a way that is sensitive to everyone's needs (▶ **Figure 2-12**). Look at cultural diversity as a resource, and make the most of the differences among people in EMS, thus allowing them to provide optimum patient care. As the public safety workplace becomes more culturally diverse, changes may occur that could be considered disruptive. It is possible to build the strength of your workgroup through the use of diversity.

For many years, EMS and public safety have been dominated by white males, though to a lesser extent than police and fire departments because of the traditional involvement of female nurses in EMS. This trend continues to decline; more women and minorities are working in public safety. The proactive EMT-B understands the benefits of using cultural diversity to improve patient care and expects to work alongside workers with different backgrounds and to accept their differences.

As an arm of public safety, EMS has not been in existence for as long as law enforcement and fire depart-

ments. Therefore, there may be less resistance to cultural diversity in EMS than in the other areas of public safety. Depending on your work experience, you may or may not have worked with people of varying backgrounds, attitudes, beliefs, and values.

Compared with traditional workplaces, EMS might seem like chaos. People who work in an office or manufacturing facility can reasonably expect to go to work every day, see the same people, and perform basically the same tasks. In EMS and public safety work, you are exposed to people in crisis. This exposure brings out the traits and qualities that your partners and coworkers use to manage their stress. Coworkers in traditional workplaces may not be willing to show this side of themselves to others. Debriefing after the call will help in this process.

Cultural diversity in EMS allows EMT-Bs to enjoy the benefits of accentuating the skills of a broad range of people. When you accept coworkers as individuals, the need to fit them into rigid roles is eliminated. To be more sensitive to cultural diversity issues, you must first be aware of your own cultural background. Ask yourself, "What are my own issues relative to race, color, religion, and ethnicity?" Since culture is not restricted to different nationalities, you should also consider age, handicap, gender, sexual orientation, marital status, work experience, and education.

In sports, you play to your team's strengths. For example, in football, offensive lines have a fast side and a strong side, and they run plays toward either side depending on the situation. As part of an effective EMS team, you can make it part of your team culture to play to your group's strengths. This may be difficult to do;

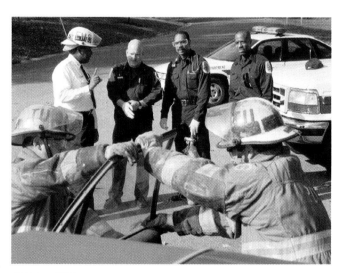

Figure 2-12 Communicate with coworkers in a way that is sensitive and respectful of individual differences.

but once you begin the process, the benefits in terms of improved patient care are immeasurable.

Your Effectiveness as an EMT-B

To be an effective EMT-B, you need to discover the diverse cultural needs of your coworkers, as well as those of your patients and their families. Although it is unrealistic to expect EMT-Bs to become cross-cultural experts with knowledge about all ethnicities, you should learn how to relate effectively.

Teamwork is essential in public safety and EMS. In order to work effectively as a team, you need to communicate to deal with cultural diversity issues.

As a health care professional, you should try to be a role model for new EMT-Bs by showing them the value of diversity. If you are working with a coworker or patient from a particular cultural group, be careful about any opinion you may have formed about that group. Do not assume that there is a language barrier, and do not appear patronizing by saying, "Some of my best friends are...." There are legitimate differences in how various cultures respond to stress. For example, you should be prepared to accept that people of different cultures might respond differently to the death of a loved one.

When you are working with patients or calling the hospital on the radio, other EMT-Bs may be sensitive to how you treat patients from their cultural group. Therefore, when referring to patients, you should use the appropriate terminology. Avoid using terms such as "cripple," "deformed," "deaf," "dumb," "crazy," and "retard" when referring to patients. Instead, use the term "disabled," and describe the specific disability.

You might want to consider taking multilingual training classes. This will not only be useful in communicating with your coworkers; it will also help to improve communication with your patients and sensitize you to the cultural richness of the people who are using the language.

Even the perception of discrimination can weaken morale and motivation and negatively affect the goal of EMS. Therefore, to achieve the benefits of cultural diversity in the EMS workplace, EMT-Bs must understand how to communicate effectively with coworkers from various backgrounds.

Avoiding Sexual Harassment

The number of sexual harassment lawsuits skyrocketed in the 1990s because of increased media attention to the problem. Furthermore, guilty verdicts encouraged others to bring suit concerning conduct that once would have gone unchallenged.

Sexual harassment is any unwelcome sexual advance, unwelcome request for sexual favors, or other unwelcome verbal or physical conduct of a sexual nature when submitting is a condition of employment, submitting or rejecting is a basis for an employment decision, or such conduct substantially interferes with performance and/or creates a hostile or offensive work environment.

Supreme Court Justice Clarence Thomas's confirmation hearings brought sexual harassment to the nation's attention. These hearings raised our awareness of sexual harassment, how it occurs, its impact on victims, and why victims might not report the behavior. The Tailhook incident that resulted in the resignations of two top US Navy officers also helped to increase our awareness.

There are two types of sexual harassment: quid pro quo (the harasser requests sexual favors in exchange for something else, such as a promotion) and hostile work environment (jokes, touching, leering requests for a date, talking about body parts). Seventy percent of sexual harassment today is considered hostile work environment. Remember, it does not matter what the intent or who the harasser was. What matters are the other person's perception and what impact that behavior had on that person. For many years, it was not uncommon to walk into a fire station and see sexually suggestive posters, calendars, or cartoons and to hear sexual jokes or comments. This situation is changing because more women are working in EMS and public safety and because of high-profile events such as the ones mentioned previously.

Because EMT-Bs and other public safety professionals depend on each other for their safety, it is especially important to try to develop nonadversarial relationships with coworkers. Most EMS facilities and fire stations make arrangements for different bunkrooms for men and women. If this is not the case at your facility, you should discuss this with your supervisor and talk openly with coworkers of the opposite gender to allow for their privacy.

If you are concerned about a particular behavior, it may be helpful to ask yourself these questions: "Would I do or say this in front of my spouse, significant other, or parents?" "Would I want my family members to be exposed to this behavior?" "Would I want my behavior videotaped and shown on the evening news?"

If you have been harassed, you should report it to your supervisor immediately and keep notes of what happened and what was said. You should confront the harasser if you feel comfortable doing so; however, this may not be for everyone. If you are asked for a date, say, "I'm not interested." If remarks or touching offends you, say, "Please don't say/do that to me; it offends me."

Substance Abuse

In the past, part of the fire service ritual was to go back to the fire station after the fire, clean and maintain the equipment, and discuss the call. At some locations, having a few beers was not uncommon. EMS today is very different from the ambulance service in which one of your parents may have participated years ago.

Drug and alcohol use in the workplace causes an increase in accidents and tension among workers, but most important, it can lead to poor treatment decisions. EMS personnel who abuse substances such as alcohol or marijuana are more likely to have problems with their work habits and their drivers' licenses may be revoked as a result. They may be absent from work more often than other workers. If the abuse has occurred within hours before the start of their shift, their ability to render emergency medical care may be lessened because of mental or physical impairment. Because of the seriousness of substance abuse, many EMS systems now require their personnel to undergo periodic random tests for illegal drug use. Since public safety workers depend so much on coworkers for their own safety, it is even more important that ways be found to manage this problem.

As an EMT-B, you will witness firsthand the tremendous effects of violence, trauma, and disease. Beyond CISD, members of the public safety community have a way of covering for each other. It is important to understand that the problem behavior will usually get worse before it gets better. Unfortunately, the stereotypical image of the alcoholic or addict lying in the gutter in an urban part of town often blinds EMS personnel to the existence of a coworker's drug or alcohol problem. Not all people with a substance abuse problem fit the stereotype.

As a member of the EMS team, you are responsible for responding to the community's emergency medical needs. Hazards in the EMS workplace are many. If you or one of the members of your team has an alcohol or other drug problem, these risks increase. Furthermore, drug use that occurs off the job does not necessarily decrease the risk. While varying state to state, a drug-alcohol-related arrest may result in the revocation of some or all driving privileges and even loss of EMT certification. Because of the tremendous risk potential, it is critical that EMT-Bs seek help or find a way to confront their partner or coworker even though there will be great pressure to allow the behavior to continue.

EMT-B Safety

Substance abuse does not just reduce an EMS responder's ability to provide patient care. It also compromises the safety of that responder and other members of the team. Ignoring a substance abuse problem puts you and those you work with at increased risk.

Addicts and alcoholics develop great skill at covering their behavior; you might even decide not to bother your coworker because you feel that he or she has caught too many tough calls lately and needs to blow off some steam. Do not let this happen. You have to find a way to confront someone who has a substance abuse problem. Because of the tremendous hazard to patients, the public, and other team members, you have a legitimate right to confront coworkers with drug and alcohol problems.

When confronting a coworker with a potential drug or alcohol problem, make it clear to the worker that if the problem is personal, it is the worker's responsibility to take care of it. You have the power to assist this person. In many workplaces, coworkers are often in a position to notice a change in a coworker's behavior or attitude before a supervisor does. This is even more the case in EMS because of the close relationship that develops between people who work in the ambulance for so many hours and share rooms, meals, and social interaction while waiting for the next call. This may allow you to help someone before his or her job performance is negatively affected.

To help reduce the potential for drug and alcohol use in the EMS workplace, EMT-Bs can learn about alcohol and other drugs. Beyond following company policy, EMT-Bs can agree among themselves what constitutes unacceptable behavior. The best time to confront these issues is usually after a call. Management sets the tone on these issues, but senior EMT-Bs can also emphasize to new EMT-Bs that drug and alcohol abuse will not be tolerated.

In a manufacturing or office environment, supervisors refer employees with problems to employee assistance programs (EAPs). EMS operations might not lend themselves easily to EAPs. Operations may be geographically spread out with minimal supervision and irregular work hours. Calls may range from a relatively simple 5-minute call to complex mass-casualty incidents that last several hours. Your partners may change regularly. And since you depend so much on each other for your safety, there will be pressure not to rock the boat. You are not

> One of the
> fundamental tools of the EMT-B
> is communication.

"turning someone in." You may be saving his or her life. Your coworker may be a great EMT-B, but if this person has unresolved substance abuse issues, the risk to fellow EMT-Bs and patients is just too great. If a substance abuse-related incident occurs during a call, it may dramatically increase the workload for other emergency responders when they respond to assist you. Early intervention is the best bet to ensure a safe, alcohol- and drug-free workplace.

Scene Safety and Personal Protection

The personal safety of all those involved in an emergency situation is very important. In fact, it is so important that the steps you take to preserve personal safety must become automatic. A second accident at the scene or an injury to you or your partner creates more problems, delays emergency medical care for patients, increases the burden on the other EMT-Bs, and may result in unnecessary injury or death.

   You should begin protecting yourself as soon as you are dispatched. Before you leave for the scene, begin preparing yourself both mentally and physically. Make sure you wear seat belts and shoulder harnesses en route to the scene. Wear seat belts and shoulder harnesses at all times unless patient care makes it impossible ▶ **Figure 2-13** . Many EMS units have mandatory seat belt policies for the driver at all times, for all EMT-Bs during transit to the scene, and for anyone who is riding with a patient.

   Protecting yourself at the scene is also very important. A second accident may damage the ambulance and may result in injury to you, your partner, or additional injury to the patient. The scene must be well marked ▶ **Figure 2-14** . If law enforcement has not already done so, you should make sure that proper warning devices are placed at a sufficient distance from the scene. This will alert motorists coming from both directions that a crash has occurred. You should park the ambulance at a safe but convenient distance from the scene. Before attempting to access patients who are trapped in a vehicle, check the vehicle's stability. Then take any necessary measures to secure it. Do not rock or push on

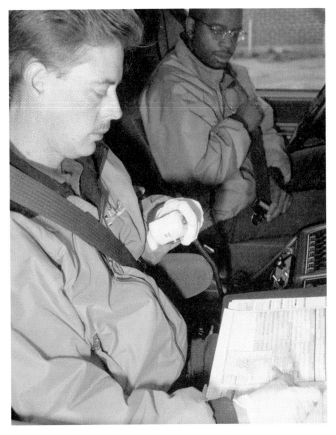

Figure 2-13   Wear seat belts and shoulder harnesses en route to the scene.

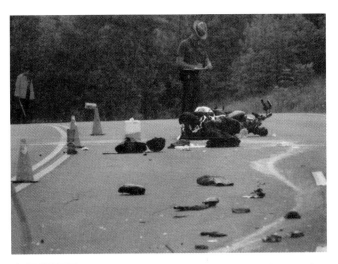

Figure 2-14   Make sure the crash scene is well marked to prevent a second crash that may damage the ambulance or result in injury to you, your partner, or the patient.

a vehicle to find out whether it will move. This can overturn the vehicle or send it crashing into a ditch.

   When working at night, you must have plenty of light. Poor lighting increases the risk of further injury to both you and the patient. It also results in poor

Figure 2-15 Wear reflective emblems or clothing to help make you more visible at night and improve your safety in the dark.

emergency medical care. Reflective emblems or clothing helps to make you more visible at night and decreases your risk of injury (▲ **Figure 2-15**).

Communicable Diseases

As an EMT-B, you will be called upon to treat and transport patients with a variety of communicable or infectious diseases. Most of these diseases are much harder to catch than is commonly believed. In addition, there are many immunizations, protective techniques, and devices that can minimize the health care provider's risk of infection. When these protective measures are used, the risk of the health care provider contracting a serious communicable disease is negligible.

Routes of Transmission

While all infections result from an abnormal invasion of body spaces and tissues by germs, different germs use different means of attack. We refer to these as the mechanisms of transmission. **Transmission** is the way an infectious agent is spread. There are four basic mechanisms: direct transmission, vehicle-borne, vector-borne, and airborne (▶ **Table 2-6**). In this context, "vehicle" means an inanimate object, while "vector" means a living object.

Risk Reduction and Prevention

Universal Precautions and Body Substance Isolation

The **Occupational Safety and Health Administration (OSHA)** develops and publishes guidelines concerning reducing risk in the workplace. It is also responsible for enforcing these guidelines. OSHA requires all EMT-Bs

to be trained in the handling of bloodborne pathogens and in approaching the patient who may have a communicable or infectious disease. Training must also be provided for issues including blood and body fluid precautions, secretion precautions, and contamination precautions.

Because health care workers are exposed to so many different kinds of infections, the Centers for Disease Control and Prevention (CDC) developed a set of **universal precautions** for health care workers to use in treating patients. These protective measures are designed to prevent workers from coming into direct contact with germs carried by patients. **Direct contact** is the exposure or transmission of a communicable disease from one person to another by physical touching. Gonorrhea is an example of a disease transmitted by direct contact, usually sexual. **Exposure** is contact with blood, body fluids, tissues, or airborne droplets by direct or indirect contact. **Indirect contact** is exposure or transmission of a disease from one person to another by contact with a contaminated object. Common colds are probably spread in this way.

The goal of universal precautions is to interrupt the transmission of germs by decreasing the chance that you will come into contact with them. Universal precautions are not universal in the sense that they will help to pro-

TABLE 2-6   Mechanisms of Transmission of Infectious Diseases

In this table (Data taken from Benenson AS (ed): *Control of Communicable Diseases in Man,* 15th ed, Washington, DC, American Public Health Association, 1990), the routes of transmission and some examples are outlined. Remember, while some germs frequently cause disease after transmission, transmission to a susceptible host is much more likely to cause asymptomatic infection and colonization.

Route	Descriptions	Source	Examples
UNIVERSAL PRECAUTIONS			
Direct	Contact, directly either with the person or with droplets sprayed (eg, by sneezing, coughing contact)	Ordinary contact	Measles, mumps, chickenpox, bacterial meningitis, influenza, diphtheria, herpes simplex
		Sexual contact	Syphilis, gonorrhea, HIV infection, hepatitis B, herpes simplex
Indirect Vehicle-borne	Spread by inanimate objects (eg, food, needles, clothing, transfused blood)	Food or water	Hepatitis A, B, C, salmonella, *Shigella*, poliomyelitis
		Blood	HIV infection
		Other	Measles, tetanus
Vector-borne Mechanical	Simple carriage by insects. The vector simply carries the germs.	Houseflies	*Shigella*
Biological	Transmission by insect in which the germ lives and grows	Ticks	Lyme disease, Rocky Mountain spotted fever
		Mosquitoes	Malaria, equine encephalitis
AIRBORNE DISEASE PRECAUTIONS			
Airborne Droplet nuclei	Residues after partial evaporation of droplets. Germs may remain viable, and the droplets may remain suspended for long periods		*Mycobacterium tuberculosis,* chickenpox
Dust	Small particles of dust from the soil may carry fungal spores and remain airborne for long periods.		*Histoplasma, Coccidioides, Mycobacterium-avium intracellulare*

tect you against all infectious diseases. Instead, the word "universal" is meant to remind you to apply precautions in all situations in which you have direct patient contact. It is impossible to tell whether an individual is free from a communicable disease, even if he or she appears healthy. Therefore, you should always take precautions.

You can also reduce your risk of exposure by following **body substance isolation (BSI)** precautions. BSI is the preferred infection control concept for fire and EMS personnel. BSI differs from universal precautions in that it is designed to approach all body fluids as being potentially infectious. However, in observing universal precautions, you assume that only blood and certain body fluids pose a risk for transmission of hepatitis B and human immunodeficiency virus. In 1988, the CDC removed many body fluids, such as sweat, tears, saliva, urine, feces, vomitus, nasal secretions, and sputum, from the risk category unless these fluids contain visible blood. However, in the dark, you may not be able to see any blood. Therefore, EMS follows the BSI concept rather than relying on universal precautions.

Modes of transmission for infectious diseases include the following:

- Blood or fluid splash
- Surface contamination
- Needlestick exposure
- Oral contamination due to lack of or improper handwashing

PROPER HANDWASHING. Proper handwashing is perhaps one of the simplest yet most effective ways to control disease transmission. You should always wash your hands before and after contact with a patient, regardless of whether you wear gloves. The longer the germs remain with you, the greater their chance of getting through your barriers. Although soap and water are not protective in all cases, in certain cases their use provides excellent protection against further transmission from your skin to others.

If no running water is available, you may use waterless handwashing substitutes (▼ **Figure 2-16**). If you use a waterless substitute in the field, make sure that you wash your hands once you arrive at the hospital. The proper procedure for handwashing is as follows:

1. Use soap and warm water.

2. Rub your hands together for at least 10 to 15 seconds to work up a lather.

3. Rinse your hands, and dry them with a paper towel.

4. Use the paper towel to turn off the faucet.

GLOVES AND EYE PROTECTION. Gloves and eye protection are the minimum standard for all patient care if there is any possibility for exposure to blood or body fluids. Both vinyl and latex gloves provide adequate protection. Your department may prefer one type of glove over the other, or you may choose yourself. You should evaluate each situation and choose the glove that works best. (Some individuals are allergic to latex. If you suspect that you are allergic, consult your supervisor for options.) Vinyl gloves may be best for routine procedures, and latex gloves may be best for invasive procedures. Never use vinyl or latex gloves for cleaning. Change latex gloves if they have been exposed to motor oil, gasoline, or any petroleum-based product. Do not use petroleum jelly with latex gloves. Wear double gloves if there is substantial bleeding. You may also wear double gloves if you will be exposed to large volumes of other body fluids. Be sure to change gloves as you move from patient to patient. For cleaning and disinfecting the unit, you should use heavy-duty utility gloves (▼ **Figure 2-17**). *You should never use lightweight latex or vinyl gloves for cleaning.*

Removing used latex or vinyl gloves requires a methodical technique to avoid contaminating yourself with the materials from which the gloves have protected you (▶ **Skill Drill 2-1**).

1. **Begin by partially removing one glove.** With the other gloved hand, pinch the first glove at the wrist—being certain to touch only the outside of the first glove—and start to roll it back off the hand, inside out. Leave the exterior of the fingers on that first glove exposed **(Step 1)**.

Figure 2-16 Use a waterless handwashing solution if there is no running water available. Be sure to wash your hands with soap once you arrive at the hospital.

Figure 2-17 Use heavy-duty utility gloves to clean the unit. You should never use lightweight latex or vinyl gloves for cleaning.

Skill Drill 2-1   Proper Glove Removal Technique

1 Partially remove the first glove by pinching at the wrist. Be careful to touch only the outside of the glove.

2 Remove the second glove by pinching the exterior with the partially gloved hand.

3 Pull the second glove inside out toward the fingertips.

4 Grasp both gloves with your free hand touching only the clean, interior sufaces.

2. **Use the still-gloved fingers** of the first hand to pinch the wrist of the second glove and begin to pull it off, rolling it inside-out toward the fingertips as you did with the first glove **(Step 2)**.

3. **Continue pulling the second glove off** until you can pull the second hand free **(Step 3)**.

4. **With your now-ungloved second hand,** grasp the exposed inside of the first glove and pull it free of your first hand and over the now-loose second glove. Be sure that you touch only clean, interior surfaces with your ungloved hand **(Step 4)**.

Gloves are the most common type of **personal protective equipment (PPE)**. In many EMS rescue operations, you must also protect your hands and wrists from injury. You may wear puncture-proof leather gloves, with latex gloves underneath. This combination will allow you free use of your hands with added protection from blood and body fluids. Remember that latex or vinyl gloves are considered medical waste and must be disposed of properly. Leather gloves must be treated as contaminated material until they can be properly decontaminated.

Eye protection is important in case blood splatters toward your eyes ▶ **Figure 2-18** . If this is a possibility, wearing goggles is your best protection. However, you need not wear goggles if you wear prescription glasses. Prescription glasses are acceptable as eye protection, but you must add removable side shields when on duty.

GOWNS AND MASKS. Occasionally, you may need to wear a mask and gown. A mask and gown provide protection from extensive blood splatter. Gowns may be worn in situations such as field delivery of a baby or major trauma. However, wearing a gown may not be practical in many situations. In fact, in some instances, a gown may pose a risk for injury. Your department will likely have a policy regarding gowns. Be sure you know your local policy. There are times when a change of uniform is preferred because trying to clean off contaminants is difficult and sometimes impossible without professional cleaning and disinfection or disposing of the uniform entirely.

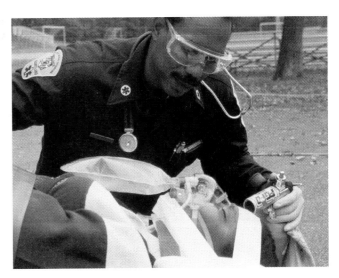

Figure 2-18 Wear eye protection to prevent blood splatter into your eyes.

MASKS, RESPIRATORS, AND BARRIER DEVICES. The use of masks is a complex issue, especially in light of OSHA and CDC requirements regarding protection from tuberculosis. You should wear a standard surgical mask if blood or body fluid spatter is a possibility. If you suspect that a patient has an airborne disease, you should place a surgical mask on the patient. However, if you suspect that the patient has tuberculosis, place a surgical mask on the patient and a High-Efficiency Particulate Air (HEPA) respirator on yourself (▼ **Figure 2-19**). However, if the patient needs oxygen, place the patient on a nonrebreathing mask with an oxygen flow rate of 10 to 15 L/min instead of a surgical mask. Do not place an HEPA respirator on the patient; it is unnecessary and uncomfortable. A simple surgical mask will reduce the risk of transmission of germs from the patient into the air. Use of an HEPA respirator should comply with OSHA standards, which state that facial hair, such as long sideburns or a mustache, will prevent a proper fit.

Although there are no documented cases of disease transmission to rescuers as a result of performing unprotected mouth-to-mouth resuscitation on a patient with an infection, you should use a pocket mask or bag-valve-mask (BVM) device (▼ **Figure 2-20**). Mouth-to-mouth resuscitation is rarely necessary in a work situation.

Remember that the outside surfaces of these items are considered contaminated after they have been exposed to the patient. You must make sure that gloves, masks, gowns, and all other items that have been exposed to infectious processes or blood are properly disposed of according to local guidelines. If you are stuck by a needle, get blood in your eye, or have any body fluid contact with the patient, report the incident to your supervisor immediately.

PROPER DISPOSAL OF SHARPS. Be careful when handling needles, scalpels, and other sharp items. The spread of HIV and hepatitis in the health care setting can usually be traced to careless handling of sharps.

- Do not recap, break, or bend needles. Even the most careful individuals may stick themselves accidentally.

- Dispose of all sharp items that have been in contact with human secretions in approved closed, rigid containers (▼ **Figure 2-21**).

Employer Responsibilities

Your employer cannot guarantee a 100% risk-free environment. Taking the risk of exposure to or acquisition of a communicable disease is a part of your job. You have a right to know about diseases that may pose a risk to you. Remember, though, that your risk for

Figure 2-19 Wear a HEPA respirator if you treat a patient whom you suspect has tuberculosis.

Figure 2-20 Barrier devices such as a pocket mask are necessary when providing artificial ventilations.

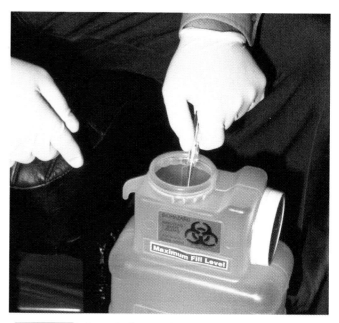

Figure 2-21 Properly dispose of sharps in a closed, rigid, marked container.

infection is not high; however, OSHA regulations, especially for private and federal agencies, require that all employees be offered a workplace environment that *reduces* the risk for exposure. Note that in some states that have their own OSHA plans, state and municipal employees must also be covered.

In addition to OSHA guidelines, other national guidelines and standards, including those from the CDC and NFPA Infection Control Standard 1581, address reducing the risk for exposure to bloodborne **pathogens** (disease-causing organisms) and airborne diseases. The standards set by these agencies set a standard of care for all fire and EMS personnel and apply whether you are a full-time paid employee or a volunteer.

PERSONAL PROTECTIVE EQUIPMENT. Personal protective equipment (PPE) is equipment that blocks entry of an organism into the body. OSHA requires that the following PPE be made available to you:

- Vinyl and latex gloves
- Heavy-duty gloves for cleaning
- Protective eyewear
- Masks (including a HEPA respirator)
- Cover gowns
- Devices for respiratory assistance

The proper PPE for each task is selected according to the way in which a communicable disease is transmitted. For example, transmission of an airborne disease can be blocked by a mask. Blood spatter into the eye can be prevented by wearing eye protection.

Wear protective eyewear whenever there is a possibility that blood or another body fluid will splatter into your eyes. If you wear prescription eyeglasses, you can add removable side shields to your glasses while you are on duty.

Because some cover gowns are not practical in the field, your department will decide whether your uniform will serve as PPE. If so, the department's exposure control plan should outline how and where contaminated uniforms are to be laundered.

The recommendations for PPE use should be followed; however, OSHA recognizes that there are times when these procedures cannot be performed. There is an "exception" statement in the OSHA regulation that states that when you believe that taking the time to use PPE will delay delivery of care to the patient or will pose a risk to your personal safety, you may choose not to use PPE. Risk to personal safety refers to the likelihood of being attacked by a person or an animal, not to concern

over acquiring a communicable disease. If you choose not to use PPE, you will have to justify this action, as an inquiry will follow.

Exposure Control Plan

Another way to reduce risk of exposure is by following your department's **exposure control plan**, which is a comprehensive plan that incorporates CDC guidelines, OSHA regulations, NFPA Infection Control Standard 1581, and other applicable state and local regulations ▶ **Table 2-7**.

Immunity

Even if germs do reach you, they may not infect you. For example, you may be immune, or resistant, to those particular germs. Immunity is a major factor in determining which hosts become ill from which germs ▶ **Table 2-8**. One way to gain immunity from many diseases today is to be immunized, or vaccinated, against them. Vaccinations have almost eliminated some childhood diseases, such as measles and polio.

Another way in which the body becomes immune to a disease is to recover from an infection from that germ. Afterward, the body recognizes and repels that germ when it shows up again. Once exposed, healthy individuals will develop lifelong immunity to many common pathogens. For example, a person who contracts and becomes infected with the hepatitis A virus may be ill for several weeks, but because an immunity will develop, will not have to worry about getting the illness again. Sometimes, however, the immunity is only partial. Partial immunity protects against new infections. But germs that remain in the body from the first illness may still be able to cause the same disease again when the body is stressed or has some impairment in its immune system. For example, tuberculosis can cause a mild, unnoticeable infection before the body builds up a partial immunity. If the infection is never treated, the infection may be reactivated when immunity is weakened; however, such individuals are protected against a new infection from another person.

Humans seem unable to mount an effective immune response to some infections, such as **HIV infection**, which is infection with the human immunodeficiency virus that can progress to acquired immunodeficiency syndrome (AIDS).

Although hepatitis A immunization is not required by OSHA, you may wish to be vaccinated as a preventive measure. Hepatitis A vaccination is not necessary if you have had hepatitis A in the past. All these vaccines are effective and rarely cause side effects. Many communi-

TABLE 2-7 Components of an Exposure Control Plan

Determination of Exposure	• Determines who is at risk for ongoing contact with blood and other body fluids • Creates a list of tasks that pose a risk for contact with blood or other body fluids • Includes personal protective equipment (PPE) required by OSHA
Education and Training	• Explains why a qualified individual is required to answer questions about communicable diseases and infection control, rather than relying on packaged training materials • Includes availability of an instructor able to train EMTs regarding bloodborne and airborne pathogens, such as hepatitis B and C, HIV, syphilis, and tuberculosis • Ensures that the instructor provides appropriate education, which is the best means for correcting many myths surrounding these issues
Hepatitis B Vaccine Program	• Spells out the vaccine offered, its safety and efficacy, record keeping, and tracking • Addresses the need for postvaccine antibody titers to identify individuals who do not respond to the initial three-dose vaccination series
Personal Protective Equipment (PPE)	• Lists the PPE offered and why it was selected • Lists how much equipment is available and where to obtain additional PPE • States when each type of PPE is to be used for each risk procedure
Cleaning and Disinfection Practices	• Describes how to care for and maintain vehicles and equipment • Identifies where and when cleaning should be performed, how it is to be done, what PPE is to be used, and what cleaning solution is to be used • Addresses medical waste collection, storage, and disposal
Tuberculin Skin Testing/Fit Testing	• Addresses how often employees should undergo skin testing • Addresses how often fit testing should be done to determine the proper size mask to protect the EMT from tuberculosis • Addresses all issues dealing with HEPA respirator masks
Postexposure Management	• Identifies whom to notify when exposure may have occurred, forms to be filled out, where to go for treatment, and what treatment is to be given
Compliance Monitoring	• Addresses how the service or department evaluates employee compliance with each aspect of the plan • Ensures that employees understand what they are to do and why it is important • States that noncompliance should be documented • Indicates what disciplinary action should be taken in the face of continued noncompliance
Record Keeping	• Outlines all records that will be kept, how confidentiality will be maintained, and how records can be assessed and by whom

TABLE 2-8 Immunity to Infectious Diseases

Type of Immunity	Characteristics	Examples	Comments
Lifelong	The illness will not recur	Measles Mumps Polio Rubella Hepatitis A Hepatitis B	Infection or vaccination provides long-term immunity to new infection. A live vaccine is required for measles only.
Partial	The person who has recovered from a first infection is unlikely to get a new infection from another person but may develop illness from germs that lie dormant from the initial infection.	Chickenpox Tuberculosis	Infection provides lifelong immunity to the patient from acquiring a new infection, but the original illness may recur, or it may recur in a different way. In the case of chickenpox, which is caused by the herpes zoster virus, an infection may recur years later in the form of shingles.
None	Exposure confers no protection from reinfection. The infection may wear down the patient's resistance.	Gonorrhea Syphilis HIV infection	No vaccine is available. Repeated infections are common. For example, there is effective immediate treatment for gonorrhea, and the germs may be eradicated; however, reinfection is likely if the high-risk practices (eg, unprotected sex) continue. For syphilis and HIV infection, the lack of immunity allows the germs to continue to cause damage within the host.

ties require you to show proof that you are up to date with their immunizations.

Remember, germs that cause no symptoms in one person may cause serious illness in another.

Immunizations

As an EMT-B, you are at risk for acquiring an infectious or communicable disease. Using basic protective measures can minimize the risk. You are responsible for protecting yourself.

Prevention begins by maintaining your personal health. Annual health examinations should be required for all EMS personnel. A history of all your childhood infectious diseases should be recorded and kept on file. Childhood infectious diseases include chickenpox,

mumps, measles, rubella, and whooping cough. If you have not had one of these diseases, you must be immunized.

The CDC and OSHA have developed requirements for protection from bloodborne pathogens such as hepatitis B and human immunodeficiency viruses. An immunization program should be in place in your EMS system. Immunizations should be kept up to date and recorded in your file. Recommended immunizations include the following:

- Tetanus-diphtheria boosters (every 10 years)
- Measles, mumps, rubella (MMR) vaccine
- Influenza vaccine (yearly)
- Hepatitis B vaccine

You should also have a skin test for tuberculosis before you begin working as an EMT-B. The purpose of the test is to identify anyone who has been exposed to tuberculosis in the past. Testing should be repeated every year.

If you know that you will be transporting a patient who has a communicable disease, you have a definite advantage. This is when your health record will be valuable. If you have already had the disease or been vaccinated, you are not at risk. However, you will not always know whether a patient has a communicable disease. Therefore, you should always follow BSI precautions if there is the possibility of exposure to blood or other body fluids.

Duty to Care

You cannot deny care to a patient who you suspect has a communicable disease, even if you believe that the patient poses a risk to your safety. To deny care to such a patient is considered to be abandonment, which is legally and ethically a serious matter that can result in both civil and criminal actions against you. It can also be considered a breach of duty (a situation in which the EMT-B does not act within an expected and reasonable standard of care). In addition to breach of duty, if the following factors are present, you may be considered negligent in your duties:

- Duty (acting reasonably in a way that a person with similar training would act)
- Damages (physically or psychologically harming a patient)
- Cause (reasonable cause and effect—having a duty and abusing it and harming another individual)

Denying care to a patient who you suspect has a communicable disease can also be considered discrimination according to the Americans with Disabilities Act (ADA), especially when a public department or agency such as EMS is involved.

You must understand the disease process and the factors necessary to put you at risk because your response to them sometimes has legal consequences.

Some Diseases of Special Concern

HIV Infection

Exposure to the virus that causes AIDS is the most feared infection risk for EMTs. It is this prospect that led to the development of universal precautions and BSI precautions. There is no vaccine to protect against

HIV infection, and despite great progress in drug treatments, AIDS is still fatal. Fortunately, it is not easily transmitted in your work setting. For example, it is far less contagious than hepatitis B. HIV infection is a potential hazard only when deposited on a mucous membrane or directly into the bloodstream. Therefore, assuming that there is no sexual contact with a patient, your real risk of infection is limited to exposure to an infected patient's blood. Exposure can take place in the following ways:

- The patient's blood is splashed or sprayed into your eyes, nose, or mouth or into an open sore or cut, however tiny; even a microscopic opening in the skin is an invitation for infection with a virus.
- You have blood from the infected patient on your hands and then touch your own eyes, nose, mouth, or an open sore or cut.
- A needle used to inject the patient breaks your skin. The risk to you from a single injection, even with a hollow-bore needle, is small, probably less than 1 in 1,000. However, this is by far the most dangerous form of exposure.
- Broken glass at a motor vehicle crash or other incident may penetrate your glove (and skin), which may have already been covered with blood from an infected patient.

Many patients who are infected with HIV do not show any symptoms. This is why the government requires health care workers to wear certain types of gloves any time they are likely to come into contact with secretions or blood from any patient. You should always put on the proper type of gloves before leaving the ambulance to care for a patient. In addition, you must take great care in handling and disposing of needles and scalpels so that others are not inadvertently exposed to them. Finally, you should cover any open wounds that you have whenever you are on the job.

If you have any reason to think that a patient's blood or secretions may have entered your system, especially through inoculation of a patient's blood, you should seek medical advice as soon as possible. If you know that the patient is infected with HIV, your physician may suggest immediate treatment to try to prevent you from becoming infected. However, if the patient seems an unlikely candidate for HIV infection, your physician may recommend that both you and the patient be tested before you undergo therapy. As scientists learn more about HIV infection, testing and treatment recommendations change. So it is important that you immediately see your doctor (or your program's designated doctor) any time you are potentially exposed to a communicable disease. Know the policy for your system and consider now what you would do in the event of exposure.

Hepatitis

The term **hepatitis** refers to an inflammation (and often infection) of the liver. Hepatitis causes fever, loss of appetite, jaundice, and fatigue. It can be caused by a number of different viruses and toxins. There is no sure way to tell which patients with hepatitis have a contagious form of the disease and which do not.
▶ **Table 2-9** shows the characteristics of different types of hepatitis, from which you can assess your risk of exposure. Hepatitis A can be transmitted only from a patient who has an acute infection, while hepatitis B and hepatitis C can also be transmitted from long-term carriers who have no signs of illness. A **carrier** is a person (or animal) in whom an infectious organism has taken up permanent residence and who may or may not cause any active disease. Carriers may never know that they harbor the organism; however, they can infect other individuals.

Hepatitis A is transmitted orally through oral or fecal contamination. This means that, generally, you must eat or drink something that is contaminated with the virus. **Contamination** is the presence of an infectious organism on or in an object. The organisms that cause hepatitis B and C are transmitted through vehicles other than food or water. For example, these organisms may enter the body through a transfusion or needlestick with infected blood, which puts health care workers at high risk for contracting hepatitis B, the more contagious and virulent form. **Virulence** is the strength or ability of a pathogen to produce disease. Hepatitis B is far more contagious than HIV. For this reason, vaccination with hepatitis B vaccine is highly recommended for EMTs. Unfortunately, not everyone who is vaccinated develops immediate immunity to the virus. Sometimes, but not always, an additional dose will provide immunity. You should be tested after vaccination (titer) to determine your immune status.

If you are stuck with a needle or injured in some other way while caring for a patient who might have hepatitis, see your doctor immediately.

Meningitis

Meningitis is an inflammation of the meningeal coverings of the brain and spinal cord. Patients with meningitis will have signs and symptoms such as fever,

You cannot withhold care from a patient who you suspect has a communicable disease.

headache, stiff neck, and altered mental status. It is an uncommon but very frightening infectious disease. Meningitis can be caused by viruses or bacteria, most of which are not contagious. However, one form, meningococcus meningitis, is highly contagious. The meningococcal bacterium colonizes the human nose and throat and only rarely causes an acute infection. When it does, it can be lethal. Patients with this kind of infection often have red blotches on their skin; however, many patients with forms of meningitis that are not contagious also have red blotches.

Because only laboratory tests can sort out the different forms of meningitis, you should use universal precautions and follow BSI precautions with any patient who is suspected of having meningitis. Gloves and a mask will go a long way to prevent the patient's secretions from getting into your nose and mouth. Again, the risk of infection is small, even if the organism is transmitted. For this reason, vaccines, which are available for most types of meningococcus, are rarely used. There are no effective treatments for the disease.

After treating a patient with meningitis, you should contact your employer health representative.

Tuberculosis

Most patients who are infected with *Mycobacterium tuberculosis* (the tubercle bacillus) are well most of the time. If the disease involves the bone or kidneys, the patient is only slightly contagious. In the United States, however, **tuberculosis** is a chronic bacterial disease that usually strikes the lungs. Disease that occurs shortly after infection is called primary tuberculosis. Except in infants, this infection is not usually serious. After the primary infection, the tubercle bacillus is rendered dormant by the patient's immune system. However, even after decades of lying dormant, this germ can reactivate. Reactive tuberculosis is common and can be much more difficult to treat, especially because an increasing number of tuberculosis strains have grown resistant to most antibiotics.

Although tuberculosis is often hard to distinguish from other diseases, patients who pose the highest risk almost invariably have a cough. Therefore, for your safety, you should consider respiratory tuberculosis to be the only contagious form, as it is the only one that is spread by airborne transmission. The droplets that are produced by coughing are not the real problem. The real problem is the droplet nuclei, which are what remains of droplets after excess water has evaporated. These particles are tiny enough to be totally invisible and can remain suspended in the air for a long time. In fact, as long as they are shielded from ultraviolet light, they can remain alive for decades. So you may be at risk by simply entering a closed room that the patient actually left long ago. Particles of that size of droplet nuclei are not stopped by routine surgical masks. Inhaled, they are carried directly to the alveoli of the lungs, where the bacteria may begin to grow.

Why is tuberculosis not more common than it is?

After all, absolute protection from infection with the tubercle bacillus does not exist. Everyone who breathes is at risk. And the vaccine for tuberculosis, called BCG, is only rarely used in the United States. Under normal circumstances, however, the mechanism of transmission used by *M. tuberculosis* is not very efficient. Infected air is easily diluted with uninfected air. And *M. tuberculosis* is one of those germs that typically causes no illness in a new host. In fact, many patients with tuberculosis do not even transmit the infection to family members. In crowded environments with poor ventilation, however, the disease spreads relatively easily.

If you are exposed to a patient who is found to have pulmonary tuberculosis, you will be given a tuberculin skin test. This simple skin test determines whether a person has been infected with *M. tuberculosis*. A positive result means that infection has occurred; it does not mean that the person has active tuberculosis. It takes at least 6 weeks for the bacteria to show up in the labora-

TABLE 2-9 Characteristics of Hepatitis

Type	Route of Infection	Incubation Period *(time before clinical signs and symptoms appear but infection may still be transmitted)*	Acute Disease *(when patient usually appears sick)*
Viral (infectious)			
Hepatitis A	Fecal-oral, infected food	2 to 6 weeks	Early symptoms of all viral hepatitis include loss of appetite, vomiting, fever, fatigue, sore throat, cough, and muscle and joint pain.
Hepatitis B	Blood, saliva, urine, sexual contact, breast milk	4 to 12 weeks	Several weeks later, jaundice (yellow eyes and skin) and right upper quadrant abdominal pain develop.
Hepatitis C	Blood, sexual contact	2 to 10 weeks	
Hepatitis D	Blood, sexual contact	4 to 12 weeks	
Toxin-Induced Medication, Drugs, Alcohol	Inhalation, skin exposure, oral ingestion, exposure or IV administration	Within hour to days following exposure	Severity of disease depends on amount of agent absorbed and duration of exposure.

tory test. So if you have the test within a few weeks of the exposure and results are positive, this means that you had already acquired the infection from somebody else. You will probably never identify the source. Most transmissions occur silently. This is why health care workers have tuberculin skin tests regularly. If the infection is found before the individual becomes ill, preventive therapy is almost 100% effective. Usually, a daily dose of isoniazid will cure the patient.

Other Diseases of Concern

SYPHILIS. Although syphilis is commonly thought of as a sexually transmitted disease, it is also a bloodborne disease. There is a small risk for transmission through a contaminated needlestick injury or direct blood-to-blood contact.

Geriatric Needs

Everyone has defenses against getting sick, but the aging process can pose a threat to our natural defense mechanisms against invading microorganisms. Our physical defenses weaken or are eliminated as we age. The skin's thinning and loss of supportive collagen, along with a reduction in the number of blood vessels, can allow bacteria or viruses to enter the body with less resistance. The respiratory system cannot trap and eliminate bacteria or viruses in the airways as it once did. Finally, the gastrointestinal system allows an easier entry for bacteria or viruses through the intestines. Not only do our physical barriers to entry weaken, but our immune system deteriorates, and invading organisms are not as easily identified as abnormal. Infectious agents can take hold in the elderly patient much more easily because of reduced defenses.

When transporting an elderly patient, protect the patient from the environment, since extremes in heat or cold can further reduce the body's defenses. If you have a cold or the flu, use respiratory precautions, including a face mask for yourself so that the patient does not get exposed to the viruses. If your patient has a cold or the flu, protect yourself. However, remember that your defense system is probably much stronger than that of the patient.

Chronic Infection (patient may no longer have signs of the relevant illness)	Vaccine Available?	Treatment	Comments
Chronic condition does not exist.	Yes	None	Mild illness; approximately 2% of patients die. After acute infection, has patient life-long immunity.
Chronic infection affects up to 10% of patients; up to 90% of newborns who have the disease.	Yes	Yes, but poor	Up to 30% of patients may become chronic carriers. Patients are asymptomatic and without signs of liver disease, but they may infect others. Approximately 1% to 2% of patients die.
Chronic infection affects 90% of patients.	No	Yes, but poor	Cirrhosis of the liver develops in 50% of patients with chronic hepatitis C; chronic infection increases the risk of cancer of the liver.
Chronic infection is very common.	No	None	Occurs only in patients with active hepatitis B infection. Fulminant disease may develop in 20% of patients.
Some chemicals may initiate an inflammatory response that continues to cause liver damage long after the chemical is out of the body.	No	Stop exposure. In patients with overdose of acetaminophen, certain drugs may subdue liver injury if given early enough.	This type of hepatitis is not contagious. Patients with toxin-induced hepatitis may have liver damage, such as jaundice. Not every exposure to a toxin will cause liver damage.

WHOOPING COUGH. Whooping cough, also called pertussis, is an airborne disease caused by bacteria that mostly affects children younger than 6 years. Signs and symptoms include fever and a "whoop" sound that occurs when the patient tries to inhale after a coughing attack.

The best way to prevent exposure is to try to place a mask on the patient and on yourself.

NEWLY RECOGNIZED DISEASES. Newly recognized diseases, such as those caused by Hantavirus or enteropathogenic *Escherichia coli,* are being reported. These diseases are not transmitted from person to person. They are not communicable diseases and do not pose a risk to you during patient care.

Multiple antibiotic-resistant organisms have recently been the subject of media scrutiny. These organisms should be viewed as no more or less contagious than other less resistant organisms of the same type. The same precautions apply.

General Postexposure Management

In many instances, you will not know that a patient has an airborne or bloodborne disease, and you could be exposed without knowing it. The Ryan White Law requires that the hospital notify your department's **designated officer**, the individual in the department who is charged with the responsibility of managing exposures and infection control issues, within 48 hours of the time the hospital identifies the patient's disease (▼ **Figure 2-22**). In the event of possible exposure, there should be a protocol in place to obtain information from your local hospital or other medical resource. You

Figure 2-22 The Ryan White Law requires that the hospital notify your designated officer within 48 hours of the time the hospital identifies the patient's disease.

Documentation Tips

The ability of your EMS service to support you in case of exposure to a communicable disease depends on your understanding of how exposure can occur and your immediate report of exposure to potentially infectious materials. Make notes right away to ensure that you remember all pertinent information, and report immediately after the response following your service's guidelines.

should be screened and given information about the necessity of medical follow-up. Treatment depends on the disease. Your designated officer will assist you with the necessary information.

If you experience a needlestick injury or some other unprotected exposure to blood, you must notify your department's designated officer as soon as possible and complete an incident report. The designated officer can contact the hospital for information; the hospital has 48 hours to report back to the designated officer. Depending on your state laws and whether it is possible, patient testing should be done, followed by baseline testing on you.

Because there are many diseases for which there are no outward signs of infection, your protection lies in the use of PPE and/or prompt reporting of exposure. Be familiar with the postexposure protocols outlined in your department's exposure control plan.

Establishing an Infection Control Routine

Infection control, procedures to reduce infection in patients and health care personnel, should be an important part of your daily routine. Take the following steps in dealing with potential exposure situations:

1. **En route to the scene,** make sure that all equipment is out and available.

2. **Upon arrival,** make sure the scene is safe to enter, then do a quick visual assessment of the patient, noting whether any blood is present.

3. **Select the proper PPE** according to the tasks you are likely to perform.

4. **Change gloves and wash hands** between patients; do not unnecessarily delay treatment for use of PPE thereby potentially putting patients at risk. Remove gloves and other gear after contact with the patient, unless you are in the patient compartment. *Remember that good handwashing is always necessary.*

5. **Limit the number of people** who are involved in patient care if there are multiple injuries and a substantial amount of blood at the scene.

6. **If you or your partner are exposed** while providing care, try to relieve one another as soon as possible so that you can seek care. Notify the designated officer and report the incident. This will also help to maintain confidentiality.

Be sure to routinely clean the ambulance after each run and on a daily basis. Cleaning is an essential part of the prevention and control of communicable diseases and will remove surface organisms that may remain in the unit.

You should clean your unit as quickly as possible so that it can be returned to service. Address the high-contact areas, including surfaces that were in direct contact with the patient's blood or body fluids or surfaces that you touched while caring for the patient after having contact with the patient's blood or body fluids.

Whenever possible, cleaning should be done at the hospital. If you clean the unit back at the station, make sure you have a designated area with good ventilation and a floor drain.

Bag any medical waste and dispose of it in a red bag at the hospital whenever possible. Any contaminated equipment that is left with the patient at the hospital should be cleaned by hospital staff or bagged for transport and cleaning at the station.

You can use a bleach and water solution at a 1:10 dilution to clean the unit. A hospital-approved disinfectant that is effective against *M. tuberculosis* can also be used. Use the cleaning solution in a bucket or pistol-handled spray container. Do not use alcohol or aerosol spray products to clean the unit.

Remove contaminated linen, and place it into an appropriate bag for handling. Each hospital may have a different system for handling contaminated linen; you should learn hospital protocols (▼ **Figure 2-23**).

Learn the regulations defining medical waste in your area. The disposal of infectious waste, such as needles, sharps, and heavily soiled dressings, may vary from hospital to hospital and from state to state.

Scene Hazards

In the course of your career, you will be exposed to many hazards. Some situations will be life-threatening. In these cases, you must be properly protected, or you must avoid the hazard completely.

Hazardous materials

Your safety is the most important consideration at a hazardous materials incident. Upon your arrival, you should first try to read labels and identification numbers. All hazardous materials should be marked with safety placards, though this is not always done. These placards are marked with colored diamond-shaped labels (▼ **Figure 2-24**). Although it is important for you to obtain information from the placards, you should never approach any object marked with a placard.

Figure 2-23 Contaminated linen should be bagged appropriately and disposed of according to your local protocols.

Figure 2-24 Hazardous materials safety placards are marked with colored diamond-shaped labels.

It is useful to carry binoculars in the ambulance so that you can read placards from a safe distance. A specially trained and equipped hazardous materials team will be called to handle disposal of materials and removal of patients. You should not begin caring for patients until they have been moved away from the scene or the scene is safe for you to enter.

The DOT's *Emergency Response Guidebook* is an important resource (▼ **Figure 2-25**). It lists most hazardous materials and the proper procedures for scene control and emergency care of patients. Several similar resources are available. Some state and local government agencies may also have information about the hazardous materials in their areas. A copy of the guidebook and other information relevant to your area should be available in your unit or at the dispatch center. Thus, you should be able to begin proper emergency management as soon as the hazardous material is identified. Again, do not go into an area and risk exposure to yourself. Do not enter the area unless you are absolutely sure that no hazardous spill has occurred.

Hazardous materials are classified according to toxicity levels, which dictate the level of protection required. The toxicity levels—0, 1, 2, 3, 4—measure

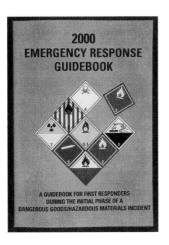

Figure 2-25 The DOT's *Emergency Response Guidebook* lists many hazardous materials and the proper procedures for scene control and emergency care of patients.

the risk the substance poses to an individual. The higher the number, the greater is the toxicity and the greater is the protection needed (▼ **Table 2-10**). It is important to remember that you are at great risk in hazardous materials situations. Do not enter the scene unless it is safe.

Electricity

Electrical shock can be produced by human-made sources (power lines) or natural sources (lightning). No matter what the source, you must evaluate the risk to you and to the patient before you begin patient care.

POWER LINES. The amount of current that is involved greatly affects the level of risk for injury. Your local power company can help you by providing training to evaluate the risks in electrical emergencies. Its staff can also teach you how to deal with power lines once the risks have been established. *You should not touch downed power lines.* Dealing with power lines is beyond the scope of EMT-B training. However, you should mark off a danger zone around the downed lines.

Energized, or "live" power lines, especially high-voltage lines, behave in unpredictable ways. You need in-depth training to be able to handle the equipment that is used in an electrical emergency. The equipment also has specific storage needs and requires careful cleaning. Dirt or other contaminants can make this equipment useless or dangerous.

At the scene of a motor vehicle crash, above-ground and below-grade power lines may become hazards. Disrupted overhead wires are usually a visible hazard. You must be careful even if you do not see sparks coming from the lines. Visible sparks are not always present in charged wires. The area around downed power lines is always a danger zone. This danger zone extends well beyond the immediate accident scene.

Use the utility poles as landmarks for establishing the perimeter of the danger zone. The danger zone must be

TABLE 2-10 Toxicity Levels of Hazardous Materials*		
Level	**Hazard**	**Protection Needed**
0	Little to no hazard	None
1	Slightly hazardous	Self-contained breathing apparatus only (level C suit)
2	Slightly hazardous	Self-contained breathing apparatus only (level C suit)
3	Extremely hazardous	Full protection, with no exposed skin (level A or B suit)
4	Minimal exposure causes death	Special HazMat gear (level A suit)

* For more information on classification of hazardous materials, see page 850.

EMT-B Safety

Experienced EMT-Bs are aware of the potential hazards that may be present when responding to the scene. At times, these situations may be dangerous to you and your crew. The best protection when hazards are present is early recognition that a hazard may exist.

EMT-B Tips

Recognize the warning signs before a lightning strike. You may feel a tingling sensation on your skin, or your hair may stand on end. Move immediately to a low-lying area. If caught in an open area, make yourself the smallest possible target.

a restricted area. Only emergency personnel, equipment, and vehicles are allowed inside this area.

If you must enter this type of situation, be sure to wear the proper protective equipment according to the type of incident. A helmet and turnout gear ▼ **Figure 2-26** are typically called for, though you cannot count on turnouts for complete protection from electrical hazards. Other protective equipment may be needed. The Protective Clothing section covers turnouts and helmets in more depth.

LIGHTNING. Lightning is a complex natural phenomenon. You are unwise to think that "lightning never strikes in the same place twice." If the right conditions remain, a repeat strike in the same area can occur.

Lightning is a threat in two ways: through a direct hit and through ground current. After the lightning bolt strikes, the current drains along the earth, following the most conductive pathway. To avoid being injured by a ground current, stay away from drainage ditches, moist areas, small depressions, and wet ropes. If you are involved in a rescue operation, you may need to delay

it until the storm has passed. Recognize the warning signs just before a lightning strike. As your surroundings become charged, you may feel a slight tingling sensation on your skin, or your hair may even stand on end. In this situation, a strike may be imminent. Move immediately to the lowest possible area.

If you are caught in an open area, try to make yourself the smallest possible target for a direct hit or for ground current. To keep from being hit by the initial strike, stay away from projections from the ground, such as a single tree. Drop all equipment, particularly metal objects that project above your body. Avoid fences and other metal objects. These can transmit current from the initial strike over a long distance. Position yourself in a low crouch. This position exposes only your feet to the ground current. If you sit, both your feet and your buttocks are exposed. Place an object made of nonconductive material, such as a blanket, under your feet. Get inside a car or your unit, if possible, as vehicles will protect you from lightning.

Fire

You will often be called to the scene of a fire. Therefore, you should understand some basic information about fire, if you do not know it already. There are five common hazards in a fire:

1. Smoke

2. Oxygen deficiency

3. High ambient temperatures

4. Toxic gases

5. Building collapse

Smoke is made up of particles of tar and carbon. These particles irritate the respiratory system on contact. Most smoke particles are trapped in the upper respiratory system, but many smaller particles enter the lungs. Some smoke particles not only irritate the airway, but also may be deadly. You must be trained in the use of appropriate airway protection, such as a

Figure 2-26 Wear a helmet made of a certified electrical nonconductor material, making sure that the chin strap is fastened securely.

Figure 2-27 You should be trained in the use of self-contained breathing apparatus and have it available if you may be working near fire scenes.

self-contained breathing apparatus or a disposable short-term device, and have it available at all fire scenes ▲ **Figure 2-27** .

Fire consumes oxygen. Particularly in a closed space, such as a room, fire may consume most of the available oxygen. This will make breathing difficult for anyone in that space. The high ambient temperatures in a fire can result in thermal burns and damage to the respiratory system. Breathing air that is heated above 120°F (49°C) can damage the respiratory system.

A typical building fire emits a number of toxic gases, including carbon monoxide and carbon dioxide. Carbon monoxide is a colorless, odorless gas that is responsible for more fire deaths each year than any other by-product of combustion. Carbon monoxide combines with the hemoglobin in your red blood cells about 200 times more rapidly than oxygen does. It blocks the ability of the hemoglobin to transport oxygen to your body tissues. Carbon dioxide is also a colorless, odorless gas. Exposure causes increased respirations, dizziness, and sweating. Breathing concentrations of carbon dioxide above 10% to 12% will result in death within a few minutes.

During and after a fire, there is always a possibility that all or part of the burned structure will collapse. Often, there are no warning signs. Therefore, you should never run into a burning building. Your hasty entry into a burning structure may result in serious injury and possibly death. Once inside the burning building, you are subject to an uncontrolled, hostile environment. Fires are not selective about their victims. You must be extremely cautious whenever you are near a burning structure or one in which a fire has just been

put out. Trained firefighters will be at the scene. Follow their instructions at the scene of any fire.

Fuel and fuel systems of vehicles that have been involved in crashes are also a hazard. Although this rarely happens, any leaking car fuel may ignite under the right conditions. If you see or smell a fuel leak, or if people are trapped in the vehicle, you must coordinate appropriate fire protection.

Make sure that you are properly protected if there is or has been a fire in the vehicle. Wear appropriate respiratory protection and thermal protection, as the smoke from a vehicle fire contains many toxic by-products. The use of appropriate protective gear at a crash scene can reduce your risk of injury. Avoid using oxygen in or near a vehicle that is smoking, smoldering, or leaking fuel.

Protective Clothing: Preventing Injury

Wearing protective clothing and other appropriate gear is critical to your personal safety. Become familiar with the protective equipment that is available to you. Then you will know what clothing and gear are needed for the job. You will also be able to adapt or change items as the situation and environment change. Remember that protective clothing and gear are safe only when they are in good condition. It is your responsibility to inspect your clothing and gear. Learn to recognize how wear and tear can make your equipment unsafe. Be sure to inspect equipment before you use it, even if you must do so at the scene.

Clothing that is worn for rescue must be appropriate for the activity and the environmental conditions in which the activity will take place. For example, bunker gear that is worn for firefighting may be too restrictive for working in a confined space. In every situation involving blood and/or other body fluids, be sure to follow BSI precautions. You must protect yourself and the patient by wearing gloves and eye protection, as well as any additional protective clothing that may be needed.

Cold Weather Clothing

When dressing for cold weather, you should wear several layers of clothing. Multiple layers provide much better protection than a single thick cover. You have more flexibility to control your body temperature by adding or removing a layer. Cold weather protection should consist of at least the following three layers:

1. **A thin inner layer** (sometimes called the transport layer) next to your skin. This layer pulls moisture away from your skin, keeping you dry and warm. Underwear made of polypropylene or polyester material works well.

2. **A thermal middle layer** of bulkier material for insulation. Wool has been the material of choice for warmth, but newer materials, such as polyester pile, are also commonly used.

3. **An outer layer** that will resist chilling winds and wet conditions, such as rain, sleet, or snow. The two top layers should have zippers to allow you to vent some body heat if you become too warm.

When choosing clothing to protect yourself from the weather, pay attention to the type of material used. Cotton should be avoided in cold, wet environments. Cotton tends to absorb moisture, causing chilling from wetness. For example, if you wear cotton trousers and walk through wet grass, the cotton soaks up the moisture from the grass. This will chill you in cold weather. However, cotton is appropriate in warm, dry weather because it absorbs moisture and pulls heat away from the body.

As an outer layer in cold weather, you might consider plastic-coated nylon, as it provides good waterproof protection. However, it can also hold in body heat and perspiration, which makes you wet both inside and out. Newer, less airtight materials allow perspiration and some heat to escape while the material retains its water resistance. Avoid flammable or meltable synthetic material anytime there is any possibility of fire.

Turnout Gear

Turnout or bunker gear is a fire service term for protective clothing designed for use in structural firefighting environments ▶ **Figure 2-28** . Turnout gear provides head-to-toe protection. It uses different layers of fabric or other material to provide protection from the heat of fire, to reduce trauma from impact or cuts, and to keep water away from the body. Like most protective clothing, turnout gear adds weight and reduces range of motion to some degree.

The exterior fabrics provide increased protection from cuts and abrasions. They also act as a barrier to high external temperatures. In cold weather, an insulated thermal inner layer of material that helps to retain body heat is recommended.

Turnout gear or a bunker jacket provides minimal protection from electrical shock. But it does protect you from heat, fire, possible flashover, and flying sparks. The front opening of the jacket should be fastened, and the jacket should be worn with the collar up and closed in front to protect your neck and upper chest. Proper fit is important so that you can move freely.

Gloves

Firefighting gloves will provide the best protection from heat, cold, and cuts ▶ **Figure 2-29** . Yet these gloves

Figure 2-28   Turnout or bunker gear provides complete head-to-toe protection.

Figure 2-29   Firefighting gloves protect your hands and wrists from heat, cold, and injury.

Figure 2-30 A helmet with side impact protection and a chin strap will not dislodge if struck by an object.

Figure 2-31 Boots should cover and protect your ankles, keeping out stones, debris, and snow. Steel-toed boots are preferred.

reduce manual dexterity. In addition, firefighting gloves will not protect you from electrical hazards. In rescue situations, you must be able to use your hands freely to operate rescue tools, provide patient care, and perform other duties. Puncture-proof leather gloves, with latex gloves underneath, will permit free use of your hands with added protection from both injury and body fluids. The Communicable Diseases section in this chapter discusses the use of latex gloves for infectious exposure prevention.

Helmets

You should wear a helmet any time you are working in a fall zone. A fall zone is an area where you are likely to encounter falling objects. The helmet should provide top and side impact protection. It should also have a secure chin strap (▲ **Figure 2-30**). Objects will often fall one after another. If the strap is not secure, the first falling object may knock off your helmet. This leaves your head unprotected as the remaining objects fall.

Construction-type helmets are not well suited for rescue situations. They offer minimal impact protection and have inadequate chin straps. Modern fire helmets offer impact protection. However, the projecting brim at the back of the neck may get in your way in a rescue situation. In cold weather, you can lose a good bit of body heat if you are not wearing a hat or helmet. An insulated hat made from wool or a synthetic material can be pulled down over the face and the base of the skull to reduce heat loss in extremely cold weather.

In situations that may involve electrical hazard, you should always wear a helmet with chin strap and face shield (Figure 2-26). The shell of the helmet should be

made of a certified electrical nonconductor. The chin strap should not stretch. In fact, it should fasten securely so that the helmet stays in place if you are knocked down or a power line hits your head. You should also be able to lock the face shield on the helmet. This will protect your face and eyes from power lines and flying sparks. A standard fire turnout helmet should meet all of these needs.

Boots

Boots should protect your feet. They should be water resistant, fit well, and be flexible so that you can walk long distances comfortably. If you will be working out-doors, you should choose boots that cover and protect your ankles, keeping out stones, debris, and snow. Steel-toed boots are preferred (▲ **Figure 2-31**). In cold weather, your boots must also protect you from the cold. Leather is one of the best materials for boots. However, other materials, such as Gore-Tex water-repellent fabric, are also very good. The soles of your boots must provide traction. Lug-type soles may grip well in snow, but they become very slippery when caked with mud.

The fit of boots and shoes is extremely important, because a minor annoyance can develop into a disabling injury. You may develop painful blisters if your feet slip around inside your boots. However, make sure you have enough room to wiggle your toes.

Boots should be puncture-resistant, protect the toes, and provide foot support. It may be difficult to obtain a good fit with firefighting boots; shoe inserts or sock lay-ering may be needed for a comfortable fit. Make sure the tops of your boots are sealed off to keep rain, snow, glass, or other materials from getting into your boots.

Socks will keep your feet warm and provide some cushioning for you as you walk. In cold weather, two pairs of socks are generally preferable to one thick pair. A thin sock next to the foot helps to wick perspiration away to a thicker, outer sock. This tends to keep your feet warmer, drier, and generally more comfortable. When you purchase new shoes or boots, keep these points in mind.

Eye Protection

The human eye is very fragile, and permanent loss of sight can occur from very minor injuries. You need to protect your eyes from blood and other body fluids, foreign objects, plants, insects, and debris from extrication. You may wear eyeglasses with side shields during routine patient care. (The Communicable Diseases section in this chapter covers eye protection against splattering body fluids.)

However, when tools are being used during extrication, you should wear a face shield or goggles. In these instances, prescription eyeglasses do not provide adequate protection. In snow or white sand, particularly at higher altitudes, you must protect your eyes from ultraviolet exposure. Specially designed glasses or goggles can provide this. In addition, your eye protection must be adaptable to the weather and the physical demands of the task. It is critical that you have clear vision at all times.

Ear Protection

Exposure to loud noises for long periods of time can cause permanent hearing loss. Certain equipment, such as helicopters, some extrication tools, and sirens, produces high levels of noise. Wearing soft foam industrial-type earplugs usually provides adequate protection.

Skin Protection

Your skin needs protection against sunburn while you are working outdoors. Long-term exposure to the sun increases the possibility of skin cancer. It might be considered simply an annoyance, but sunburn is a type of thermal burn. In reflective areas such as sand, water, and snow, your risk of sunburn increases. Protect your skin by applying a sunscreen with a minimum rating of SPF 15.

Body Armor

Though policy for most EMT-Bs directs them simply to avoid situations that may involve gunshots,

EMS responders in some areas do wear body armor (bulletproof vests) for personal protection. Several types of body armor are available. They range from extremely lightweight and flexible to heavy and bulky. The lighter vests do not stop large-caliber bullets. However, they offer more flexibility and are preferred by most law enforcement personnel. Lighter vests are commonly worn under a uniform shirt or jacket. The larger, heavier vests are worn on the outside of your uniform.

Violent Situations

The safety of you and your team is of primary concern. Civil disturbances, domestic disputes, and crime scenes, especially those involving gangs, can create many hazards for EMS personnel. Large gatherings of hostile or potentially hostile people are also dangerous. Several agencies will respond to large civil disturbances. In these instances, it is important for you to know who is in command and will be issuing orders ▼ **Figure 2-32** . However, you and your partner may be on your own when a group of people seems to grow larger and become increasingly hostile. In these cases, you should call law enforcement immediately if they are not already. You may need to wait for law enforcement to arrive before you can begin treatment.

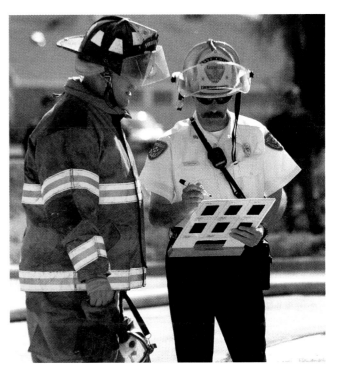

Figure 2-32 Several agencies may respond to large disturbances. It is important for you to know who is in command and will be issuing orders.

In some areas, EMS personnel wear body armor (bulletproof vests) if a scene has the potential to become violent.

Remember that you and your partner must be protected from the dangers at the scene before you can provide patient care. Law enforcement must make sure the scene is safe before you and your partner enter. A crime scene often poses potential problems for EMS personnel. If the perpetrator is still somewhere on the scene, this person could reappear and threaten you and your partner or attempt to further injure the patient you are treating. Bystanders who are trying to be helpful may interfere with your emergency medical care. Family members may be very distraught and not understand what you are doing when you attempt to splint an injured extremity and the patient cries out that what you are doing hurts. Be sure that you have adequate assistance from the appropriate public safety agency in these cases.

Sometimes EMT-Bs will be at a scene where a dangerous situation is underway, such as a hostage situation or riot. In these instances, it may be necessary for EMS personnel to be protected from projectiles such as bullets, bottles, and rocks. Law enforcement personnel will ordinarily provide for concealment or cover of personnel who are involved in the response to the incident. **Cover** and concealment involve the tactical use of an impenetrable barrier for protection. EMT-Bs should not be placed in a position that will endanger their lives or safety during such incidents.

Remember that your personal safety is of the utmost importance. You must thoroughly understand the risks of each environment you enter. Whenever you are in doubt about your safety, do not put yourself at risk. Never enter an unstable environment, such as a shooting, a brawl, a hostage situation, or a riot. Therefore, as part of your scene size-up, evaluate the scene for the potential for violence. If it is a possibility, call for additional resources. Failure to do so may put you and your partner at serious risk. Rely on the advice of law enforcement personnel, as they have more experience and expertise in handling these situations.

It is also important for you to remember that if you believe that an event is a crime scene, you must attempt to maintain the chain of evidence. Briefly, make sure that you do not disturb the scene unless it is absolutely necessary in caring for the patient.

Behavioral Emergencies

Although Chapter 19 goes into greater depth about behavioral emergencies, consider these questions as you evaluate the patient in terms of a behavioral or psychiatric emergency that may lead to a violent patient reaction:

- How does this patient relate to you?

- Are your questions answered appropriately?

- Is the patient withdrawn or detached?

- Is the patient hostile or friendly? Overly friendly?

- Does the patient understand why you are there?

- How is the patient dressed? Is the dress appropriate for the time of the year and occasion? Are the clothes clean? Dirty?

- Are the patient's movements coordinated or jerky and awkward? Is there hyperactivity? What kind?

- Are the patient's movements purposeful, for example, in putting his or her clothes on? Are the actions aimless, such as sitting and rocking back and forth in a chair?

- Has the patient harmed herself or himself? Is there damage to the surroundings?

- Does the patient present as physically rigid, or is there waxy flexibility?

- Does the patient appear relaxed, stiff, or guarded?

- What are the patient's facial expressions? Are they bland or flat, or are they expressive? Does the patient show joy, fear, or anger to appropriate stimuli? If so, to what degree?

- Are the patient's vocabulary and expressions what you would expect under the circumstances? Are they consistent with the patient's social and educational background?

It might not be possible for you to gather all of the information that these questions suggest. Sometimes, a patient who is experiencing a behavioral emergency will not respond at all. In those cases, the patient's facial expressions, pulse and respirations, tears, sweating, and blushing may be significant indicators of his or her emotional state.

The following principal determinants of violence, though not intended to be all-inclusive, are of value for the EMT-B:

- **Past history.** Has this patient previously exhibited hostile, overly aggressive, or violent behavior? This information should be solicited by EMS personnel at the scene or requested from law enforcement personnel, family, previous EMS records, or hospital information.

- **Posture.** How is this person sitting or standing? Does the patient appear to be tense, rigid, or sitting on the edge of the bed, chair, or wherever he or she is positioned? The observation of increased tension by physical posture is often a warning signal for hostility.

- **Vocal activity.** What is the nature of the speech the patient is using? Loud, obscene, erratic, and bizarre speech patterns usually indicate emotional distress. The patient who is conversing in quiet, ordered speech is not as likely to strike out against others as is the patient who is yelling and screaming.

- **Physical activity.** Perhaps one of the most demonstrative factors to look for is the motor activity of a person who is undergoing a behavioral crisis. The patient who is pacing, cannot sit still, or is displaying protection of his or her boundaries of personal space needs careful watching. Agitation is a prognostic sign to be observed with great care and scrutiny.

Other factors to take into consideration for potential violence include the following:

- Poor impulse control

- The behavior triad of truancy, fighting, and uncontrollable temper

- Instability of family structure, inability to keep a steady job

- Tattoos, such as those with gang identification or statements like "born to kill" or "born to lose"

- Substance abuse

- Functional disorder (If the patient says that he or she is hearing voices that say to kill, believe it!)

- Depression, which accounts for 20% of violent attacks

Prep Kit

Ready for Review

EMT-Bs will encounter death, dying patients, and the families and friends of those who have died. Death will be no stranger in the work of EMS personnel. Therefore, coming to grips with death and dying and understanding the concerns of the dying patient, assisting a family following the death of a loved one, and dealing with one's own feelings about death are both personally and professionally important.

When signs of stress such as fatigue, anxiety, anger, feelings of hopelessness, worthlessness, or guilt, and other such indicators manifest themselves, behavioral problems can develop. Recognizing the signs of stress is important for all EMT-Bs. CISD efforts, among other programs of support, are important in identifying potentially serious mental health problems, such as posttraumatic stress disorder, that can result from dealing with the overwhelming stress that sometimes develops in critical situations such as the death of patients. Posttraumatic stress disorder is a syndrome with onset following a traumatic, usually life-threatening event.

As an EMT-B, you will arrive at scenes where potential danger to yourself is easily apparent. Every patient encounter should be considered to be potentially dangerous. Therefore, it is essential that you take all available precautions to minimize exposure and risk. Potential risks include scene hazards and infectious and communicable diseases.

Infectious diseases can be transmitted in one of four ways: direct transmission, vehicle-borne, vector-borne, and airborne. Even if you are exposed to an infectious disease, your risk of becoming ill is small. Whether or not an acute infection occurs depends on several factors, including the amount and type of infectious organism and your resistance to that infection. Most germs colonize the human body without causing any disease at all.

You can take several steps to protect yourself against exposure to infectious diseases, including keeping up to date with recommended vaccinations, using universal precautions and following BSI precautions at all times, and handling all needles and other sharp objects with great care. Sharp items should be disposed of in closed, rigid containers. Because it is often impossible to tell which patients have infectious diseases, you should avoid direct contact with the blood and body fluids of all patients. Use special caution if you have any open sores or cuts, no matter how small. If you think you may have been exposed to an infectious disease, see your physician (or your employer's designated physician) immediately.

Four infectious diseases of special concern are HIV infection, hepatitis B, meningitis, and tuberculosis. Of these, only meningitis and tuberculosis are transmitted through the air. The tubercle bacillus can remain dormant for decades without causing disease.

Because medical therapy is almost always effective if you have not already become ill, you should get a tuberculosis test on a regular basis. Hepatitis B is by far the most common threat to health care workers. It is highly contagious and usually transmitted by needlestick. Vaccination with hepatitis B vaccine is highly recommended. Meningitis is very rare; your risk of disease, even if you acquire this infection, is very small. Using a mask and gloves will go a long way to protect you against meningitis.

You should know what to do if you are exposed to an airborne or bloodborne disease. Your department's designated officer will be able to help you follow the protocol set up in your area.

Infection control should be an important part of your daily routine. Be sure to follow the proper steps when dealing with potential exposure situations.

In the course of your career, you will be exposed to many hazards. Some situations will be life-threatening. In these cases you must be properly protected, or you must avoid the situation completely.

Scene hazards include potential exposure to hazardous materials, electricity, and fire. At a hazardous materials incident, your safety is the most important consideration. Never approach an object labeled with a hazardous materials placard. Use binoculars to read the placards from a safe distance. Do not begin caring for patients until they have been moved away from the scene by the hazardous materials team or the scene has been made safe for you to enter.

Electrical shock can be produced by power lines or by lightning. If you encounter a downed power line, *do not touch it*. Mark off a danger zone around the downed lines and contact the power company. To protect yourself from lightning, recognize the warning signs just before a lightning strike. Move immediately to the lowest area possible. If you are in an open area, make yourself the smallest target by dropping all equipment and getting into a low crouch. If possible, get inside a car or your unit.

There are five common hazards in a fire: smoke, oxygen deficiency, high ambient temperatures, toxic gases, and building collapse. You must be trained in the use of appropriate airway protection and have it available at all scenes. Do not rush into a burning building to care for a patient. The building could collapse at any time. Follow the instructions of the trained firefighters at the scene.

Violent situations such as civil disturbances, domestic disputes, and crime scenes can create many hazards for EMS personnel. Whenever you are in doubt about your safety do not put yourself at risk. If you see the potential for violence during a scene size-up, call for additional resources. Rely on the advice of law enforcement. Remember, your personal safety is of the utmost importance.

www.emtb.com

Vital Vocabulary

body substance isolation (BSI) An infection control concept and practice that assumes that all body fluids are potentially infectious.

burnout A condition of chronic fatigue and frustration that results from mounting stress over time.

carrier An animal or person who may transmit an infectious disease but may not display any symptoms of it.

communicable disease Any disease that can be spread from person to person, or from animal to person.

contagious An infectious disease that is capable of being transmitted from one person to another.

contamination The presence of infectious organisms on or in objects such as dressings, water, food, needles, wounds, or a patient's body.

cover The tactical use of an impenetrable barrier to conceal EMS personnel and protect them from projectiles (eg, bullets, bottles, rocks).

critical incident stress debriefing (CISD) A confidential group discussion of a severely stressful incident that usually occurs within 24 to 72 hours of the incident.

critical incident stress management (CISM) A process that confronts the responses to critical incidents and defuses them, directing the emergency services personnel toward physical and emotional equilibrium.

dependent lividity Blood settling to the lowest point of the body, causing discoloration of the skin.

designated officer The individual in the department who is charged with the responsibility of managing exposures and infection control issues.

direct contact Exposure or transmission of a communicable disease from one person to another by physical touching.

exposure A situation in which a person has had contact with blood, body fluids, tissues, or airborne particles in a manner that suggests that disease transmission may occur.

exposure control plan A comprehensive plan that helps employees to reduce their risk of exposure to or acquisition of communicable diseases.

general adaptation syndrome The body's three-stage response to stress. First, stress causes the body to trigger an alarm response, followed by a stage of reaction and resistance, and then recovery, or if the stress is prolonged, exhaustion.

hepatitis An infection of the liver, usually caused by a virus, that causes fever, loss of appetite, jaundice, fatigue, and altered liver function.

HIV infection Infection with the human immunodeficiency virus (HIV) that can progress to acquired immunodeficiency syndrome (AIDS).

host The organism or individual that is attacked by the infecting agent.

indirect contact Exposure or transmission of disease from one person to another by contact with a contaminated object.

infection The abnormal invasion of a host or host tissues by organisms such as bacteria, viruses, or parasites, with or without signs or symptoms of disease.

infection control Procedures to reduce transmission of infection among patients and health care personnel.

infectious disease A disease that is caused by infection, in contrast to one caused by faulty genes, metabolic or hormonal disturbances, emotional trauma, or another cause.

meningitis An inflammation of the meningeal coverings of the brain; it is usually caused by a virus or a bacterium.

Occupational Safety and Health Administration (OSHA) The federal regulatory compliance agency that develops, publishes, and enforces guidelines concerning safety in the workplace.

pathogen A microorganism that is capable of causing disease in a susceptible host.

personal protective equipment (PPE) Protective equipment that OSHA requires to be made available to the EMT. In the case of infection risk, PPE blocks entry of an organism into the body.

posttraumatic stress disorder (PTSD) A delayed stress reaction to a prior incident. This delayed reaction is the result of one or more unresolved issues concerning the incident that might have been alleviated with the use of critical incident stress management.

putrefaction Decomposition of body tissues.

rigor mortis Stiffening of the body, is a definitive sign of death.

transmission The way in which an infectious agent is spread: contact, airborne, by vehicles, or by vectors.

tuberculosis A chronic bacterial disease, caused by *Mycobacterium tuberculosis*, that usually affects the lungs but can also affect other organs such as the brain or kidneys.

universal precautions Protective measures that have traditionally been developed by the Centers for Disease Control and Prevention (CDC) for use in dealing with objects, blood, body fluids, or other potential exposure risks of communicable disease.

virulence The strength or ability of a pathogen to produce disease.

www.emtb.com

Assessment in Action

You and your partner are dispatched to a "Medical Emergency, nature unknown" at a small apartment complex in town. When you arrive, you see that law enforcement is already there, trying to manage the six or seven neighbors who have gathered outside a first-floor apartment.

After applying BSI, you enter the apartment to find a 31-year-old woman lying on the sofa. There are pills from a half-dozen bottles scattered on the carpet. From the doorway you see no chest rise and fall. You note that there is blood-tinged, foamy saliva in her mouth. She is unresponsive. While attempting to clear her airway, you note that her jaw and neck are stiff. There is no breathing, no pulse, and her skin is cool and dry. You find dependent lividity in her earlobes, neck, arms, and legs. Your partner notes her arms are stiff also. As you turn to the police officer and tell him that this patient has definitive signs of death, an older woman enters the room and starts yelling at you, accusing you of taking too long to arrive and questioning your ability as caregivers. You learn that this person is the patient's mother.

1. What BSI would be most appropriate in this situation?
   A. Gloves and mask
   B. Mask and goggles
   C. Gloves and goggles
   D. Mask and gown

2. The most effective way to prevent disease transmission is to:
   A. wear gloves.
   B. wear goggles.
   C. wash your hands.
   D. become immunized.

3. Of the signs of death exhibited in this situation, which indicate that CPR would be futile?
   A. Unresponsiveness
   B. Cool, dry skin
   C. Absence of breathing and pulse
   D. Stiffness in her jaw and neck

4. Usually dependent lividity is sufficient to confirm death. However, in this situation dependent lividity is not reliable. What are the other situations?
   A. Hypothermia
   B. Bilateral amputations
   C. Excessive bleeding
   D. Cardiac arrest

5. The patient's mother appears to be in what stage of coping with her daughter's unexpected death?
   A. Denial
   B. Anger
   C. Bargaining
   D. Acceptance

6. The most appropriate way to respond to the mother is to:
   A. ignore her.
   B. become defensive.
   C. be tolerant and empathetic.
   D. let the police handle her.

7. The patient's boyfriend arrives on the scene and says, "If only we hadn't had a fight last night, things would have been different." The patient's boyfriend is in what stage of coping with her death?
   A. Denial
   B. Anger
   C. Bargaining
   D. Acceptance

8. Approximately 1 month later you find yourself dreaming about this call. Thoughts of this call even come up when you are watching TV. Is there anything significant about these events?
   A. No, but it's a sign you have been working too hard. Go out on the town and unwind with your friends.
   B. Yes, this is a serious sign of mental stress and you should resign from your job and find another occupation.
   C. No, these reactions are expected and will go away if you isolate yourself from things that remind you of it.
   D. Yes, these reactions are signs of PTSD and you may need to diffuse with a professional.

9. A situation forcing you to deal with the death of loved ones and their families can be stressful in itself. What are some concrete methods to help prevent susceptibility to physical illness during stressful times?
   A. Keep your mind on your work
   B. Go out with the guys on a regular basis
   C. Watch your diet and exercise regularly
   D. Volunteer for as much extra work as you can

Challenging Questions

1. Why would lividity be unreliable if it occurs in a patient suffering from an overdose or poisoning?

2. In this situation, what would be appropriate empathetic responses to give to the mother?

3. Stress is known to strain body resources, even if it is "good" stress. What part of stress is so bad for our physical body?

Points to Ponder

You have been with a response agency for just over a year and they are sending you to an EMT-Intermediate class. You are still covering shifts and studying for your intermediate class in your spare time. On top of that, you have a bad cold and are taking over-the-counter medications to help with the congestion and body aches. Because of illness and vacations the agency is short-handed and you are on your second of back-to-back shifts. Between lack of sleep and the cold medications, you are very tired and even starting to hallucinate. It is about 2:00 in the morning and you have six more hours to go on your shift. You are so tired that you do not think you should be driving and trade with your partner. You are headed to the hospital with a middle-aged male experiencing difficulty breathing and are having a difficult time focusing on the patient care. What would you do? Should you finish your shift?

Issues Burnout, Well-Being of the EMT-B, Patient Care Standards, Safety.

Online Outlook

As a part of training you will begin to recognize and protect yourself from possible hazards. Nevertheless, injury and death to EMTs sometimes occur. Visit the National EMS Memorial Service Web Site and complete Exercise 2 at **www.emtb.com**.

Medical, Legal, and Ethical Issues

Cognitive

1. Define the EMT-B's scope of practice (p 66).
2. Discuss the importance of do not resuscitate (DNR) orders [advance directives] and local or state provisions regarding EMS application (p 72).
3. Define consent and discuss the methods of obtaining consent (p 69).
4. Differentiate between expressed and implied consent (p 69).
5. Explain the role of consent of minors in providing care (p 70).
6. Discuss the implications for the EMT-B in patient refusal of transport (p 71).
7. Discuss the issues of abandonment, negligence, and battery and their implications for the EMT-B (p 68).
8. State the conditions necessary for the EMT-B to have a duty to act (p 68).
9. Explain the importance, necessity, and legality of patient confidentiality (p 73).
10. Discuss the considerations of the EMT-B in issues of organ retrieval (p 75).
11. Differentiate the actions that an EMT-B should take to assist in the preservation of a crime scene (p 74).
12. State the conditions that require an EMT-B to notify local law enforcement officials (p 71).

Affective

13. Explain the role of EMS and the EMT-B regarding patients with DNR orders (p 72).
14. Explain the rationale for the needs, benefits, and usage of advance directives (p 72).
15. Explain the rationale for the concept of varying degrees of DNR (p 72).

Psychomotor

None

3

TECHNOLOGY

www.emtb.com

- Online Chapter Pretest
- Interactivities
- Vocabulary Explorer
- Anatomy Review
- Web Links
- Online Review Manual
- Distance Learning

Chapter FEATURES

- Skill Drills
- Vital Vocabulary
- Pediatric Needs
- Geriatric Needs
- EMT-B Safety
- EMT-B Tips
- Documentation Tips
- Remember
- Prep Kit

You are the EMT

While working at a two-car collision site, you see another provider take several $20 bills out of an open purse and put them in his pocket. What should you do?

Unfortunately, ethical and moral quandaries confront EMS providers routinely. How you handle them, to a large degree, will determine what type of health care professional you are. This chapter will present the basic legal concepts associated with prehospital medicine along with various ethical considerations. It will also help you answer the following questions:

1. Why is adhering to the principles of patient confidentiality an essential component of quality prehospital care?

2. What is the difference between informed and implied consent, and why is obtaining patient consent so important?

Medical, Legal, and Ethical Issues

A basic principle of emergency care is to do no further harm. Any health care provider who acts in good faith and according to an appropriate standard of care usually avoids legal exposure. Providing emergency medical care in an organized system is a recent phenomenon. **Emergency medical care**, or immediate care or treatment, is often provided by an EMT, who may be the first link in the chain of prehospital care. As the scope and nature of emergency medical care become more complex and widely available, litigation involving participants in EMS systems will no doubt increase. Providing competent emergency medical care that conforms with the standard of care taught to you will help you to avoid both civil and criminal actions. Consider the following situations:

- You are transporting a patient, and while the stretcher is being loaded into the ambulance, your partner slips, the stretcher crashes to the ground, and the patient is injured.

- You are about to begin treating a child, and the father commands you to stop.

What should you do? Even when emergency medical care is properly rendered, there are times when you may be sued by a patient who seeks to obtain relief, often in the form of a monetary award, for pain and suffering. Or administrative action, such as suspension of your state license or EMT-B certificate, may be brought against you for failure to abide by the regulations of your state EMS agency. For this reason, you must understand the various legal aspects of emergency medical care.

You must also consider ethical issues. As an EMT-B, should you stop and treat patients who were involved in an automobile crash while you are en route to another emergency call? Should you begin CPR on a patient who, according to the family, has terminal cancer? Should patient information be released to a patient's attorney on the telephone?

Scope of Practice

The scope of practice, which is most commonly defined by state law, outlines the care you are able to provide for the patient. Your medical director further defines the scope of practice by developing protocols and standing orders. The medical director gives you the legal authorization to provide patient care through telephone or radio communication (online) or standing orders and protocols (off-line) (▶ **Figure 3-1**).

You and other EMS personnel have a responsibility to provide proper, consistent patient care and to report problems, such as possible liability or exposure to airborne or bloodborne pathogens or infectious disease, to your medical director immediately.

Standards of Care

The law requires you to act or behave toward other individuals in a certain, definable way, regardless of the activity involved. Under given circumstances, you have a duty either to act or not. Generally speaking, you must be concerned about the safety and welfare of others when your behavior or activities have the potential for causing others injury or harm (▶ **Figure 3-2**). The manner in which you must act or behave is called a **standard of care**.

Standard of care is established in many ways, among them local custom, statutes, ordinances, administrative regulations, and case law. In addition, professional or institutional standards have a bearing on determining the adequacy of your conduct.

Standards Imposed by Local Custom

The standard of care is how a reasonably prudent person with similar training and experience would act under similar circumstances, with similar equipment, and in the same place. For example, the conduct of an EMT-B who is employed by an ambulance service is to be judged in comparison with the expected conduct of other EMT-Bs from comparable ambulance services. These standards are often based on locally accepted protocols.

As an EMT-B, you will not be held to the same standard of care as physicians or other more highly trained individuals would. In addition, your conduct must be judged in the light of the given emergency situation, taking into consideration the following factors:

- General confusion at the scene of the emergency
- The needs of other patients
- The type of equipment available

In this context, an **emergency** is a serious situation, such as injury or illness, that arises suddenly, threatens the life or welfare of a person or group of people, and requires immediate intervention (▼ **Figure 3-3**).

The prevailing custom of the community is an important element in determining the standard of emergency care required.

Standards Imposed by Law

In addition to local customs, standards of emergency medical care may be imposed by statutes, ordinances, administrative regulation, or case law. In many jurisdictions, violating one of these standards is said to create *presumptive negligence*. Therefore, you must become familiar with the particular legal standards that may exist in your state. In many states, this may take the form of treatment protocols published by a state agency.

Professional or Institutional Standards

In addition to standards imposed by law, professional or institutional standards may be admitted as evidence in determining the adequacy of an EMT's conduct. Professional standards include recommendations published by organizations and societies that are involved in emergency medical care. Institutional standards

Figure 3-1 Online medical direction is often communicated via radio.

Figure 3-2 Act or behave toward others in a way that shows your concern about their safety and welfare.

Figure 3-3 An emergency is a serious situation that arises suddenly, threatens the life or welfare of one or more individuals, and requires immediate intervention.

include specific rules and procedures of the EMS service, ambulance service, or organization to which you are attached.

Two notes of caution: First, you must be familiar with the standards of your organization. Second, if you are involved in formulating standards for a particular agency, they should be reasonable and realistic so that they do not impose an unreasonable burden on EMTs. Providing the best emergency medical care should be every EMT's goal, but it is not realistic to have institutional standards that *demand* the best care.

Many standards of care may be imposed on you. State health department regulations usually govern the scope and level of training. Court decisions have resulted in case law defining standards of care. Professional standards are also imposed, such as the American Heart Association's standard for basic life support (BLS) and cardiopulmonary resuscitation (CPR) (▼ Figure 3-4).

Ordinary care is a minimum standard of care. In general, it is expected that anyone who offers assistance will exercise reasonable care and act prudently. If you act reasonably, according to the accepted standard, the risk of civil suit is small. If you apply the standard practices you have been trained to use, you can likely avoid liability. For example, various organizations have defined standards for performing CPR. If you deviate from these standards, you may be liable for civil and possibly criminal prosecution. In addition, state regulatory agencies that oversee EMS operations can sanction EMS personnel for deviating from the standard of care.

Standards Imposed by States

MEDICAL PRACTICES ACT. EMS personnel are exempt from the licensure requirements of the Medical Practices

Figure 3-4 Many standards of care are imposed on you, such as those for performing CPR.

Act in most states because an EMT-B is regarded as a nonmedical professional. The practice of medicine is defined as the diagnosis and treatment of disease or illness. EMT-Bs and others in the prehospital care chain assess the need for life support and begin care. Therefore, the standard of care must be maintained within the scope of your state's provisions and licensing requirements.

CERTIFICATION. Some states provide certification or licensure of individuals who perform emergency medical care. **Certification** is the process by which an individual, institution, or program is evaluated and recognized as meeting certain predetermined standards to ensure safe and ethical patient care. Once certified, you are obliged to conform to the standards that are generally recognized nationally by various registry groups and provide an important link in nationwide EMS. You must ensure that your certification or licensure remains current; skill levels must be kept up to date.

Some organizations have recently changed their concept of certification. The American Heart Association, for example, now acknowledges only one's successful completion of a CPR course. Certification has specific legal meaning and is generally restricted to licensing agencies.

Duty to Act

Duty to act is an individual's responsibility to provide patient care. Responsibility comes from either statute or function. A bystander is under no obligation to assist a stranger in distress; there is no duty to act. There may be a duty to act in certain instances, including the following:

- You are charged with emergency medical response.

- Your service or department's policy states that you must assist in any emergency.

Once your ambulance responds to a call or treatment is begun, you have a legal duty to act. If you are off duty and come upon a crash, you are not legally obligated to stop and assist patients. However, you do have a moral and ethical duty to act because of your special training and expertise.

Negligence

Negligence is the failure to provide the same care that a person with similar training would provide. It is deviation from the accepted standard of care that may result in further injury to the patient. Determination of negligence is based on the following four factors:

1. **Duty.** It is the EMT-B's responsibility to act reasonably within the standards of his or her training.

2. **Breach of duty.** There is a breach of duty when the EMT-B does not act within an expected and reasonable standard of care.

3. **Damages.** There are damages when a patient is physically or psychologically harmed in some noticeable way.

4. **Cause.** There must be a reasonable cause and effect. An example is dropping the patient during lifting, causing a fracture of the patient's leg. If a person has a duty and abuses it, causing harm to another individual, the EMT-B, the agency and/or medical director may be sued for negligence.

All four elements must be present for the legal doctrine of negligence to apply.

Abandonment

Abandonment is the unilateral termination of care by the EMT-B without the patient's consent and without making any provisions for continuing care by a medical professional with skills at the same or a higher level. For the EMT-B, once care is started, you have assumed a duty that must not stop until an equally competent person assumes responsibility. Not performing that duty exposes the patient to harm and is a basis for a negligence suit. Abandonment is legally and ethically a serious matter that can result in both civil and criminal actions against an EMT.

For example, suppose you arrive at the scene of a single-car accident and begin care of two injured patients. A passerby tells you of a two-car accident farther down the road in which five people are injured. You turn care of the two injured patients from the first accident over to the passerby and leave to go to the other accident. Abandonment has occurred because you did not turn care of the patients over to a person with the same or a higher level of skill than yours. Consider the following general questions when you are faced with making a decision such as this one:

- What problems may develop from your actions?

- Are you neglecting your duty to your patient?

- Are you abandoning the patient if you leave the scene?

> **Under most circumstances, consent is required from every conscious, mentally competent adult before care can be started.**

- Are you violating a standard of care?

- Are you acting prudently?

Consent

Under most circumstances, consent is required from every conscious, mentally competent adult before care can be started. A person receiving care must give permission, or **consent**, for treatment. If a person is in control of his or her actions, even though injured, and refuses care, you may not care for the patient. In fact, doing so may be grounds for both criminal and civil action such as assault and battery. Consent can be actual or implied and can involve the care of a minor or a mentally incompetent patient.

Expressed Consent

Expressed consent (or actual consent) is the type of consent in which the patient expressly authorizes you to provide care or transport. It must be **informed consent**, which means that the patient has been told of the potential risks, benefits, and alternatives to treatment and has given consent to treatment. The legal basis for this doctrine rests on the assumption that the patient has a right to determine what is to be done with his or her body. The patient must be of legal age and able to make a rational decision.

A patient might agree to certain emergency medical care but not to other care. For example, a patient might agree to be removed from a car but refuse further care. An injured person might agree to emergency care at home but refuse to be transported to a medical facility. Informed consent is valid if given orally; however, it may be difficult to prove. Having the patient sign a consent form does not eliminate your responsibility to fully inform the patient.

Implied Consent

When a person is unconscious and unable to give consent or when a serious threat to life exists, the law assumes that the patient would consent to care and transport to a medical facility (▼ Figure 3-5). This is called **implied consent**. Implied consent is limited to true emergency situations and is appropriate when the patient is unconscious, delusional, unresponsive as a result of drug or alcohol use, or otherwise physically unable to give expressed consent. However, many things may be unclear about what represents a "serious threat to life." Legal proceedings would likely revolve around that question. This becomes a medicolegal judgment, which should be supported by the EMT-B's best efforts to obtain consent. **Medicolegal** is a term that relates to medical jurisprudence (law) or forensic medicine. In most instances, the law allows the spouse, a close relative, or next of kin to give consent for an injured person who is unable to give consent. Refusal of your offer to render emergency care also may be implied. For example, a patient's action in pulling his or her arm from your splint may be an indication of refusal of consent.

Minors and Consent

Because a minor might not have the wisdom, maturity, or judgment to give valid consent, the law requires that a parent or legal guardian give consent for treatment or transport (▼ Figure 3-6). However, in some states, a minor can give valid consent to receive medical care, depending on the minor's age and maturity. Many states also allow emancipated, married, or pregnant minors to be treated as adults for the purposes of consenting to medical treatment. You should obtain consent from a parent or legal guardian whenever possible; however, if a true emergency exists and the parent or legal guardian is not available, the consent to treat the

minor is implied, just as with an adult. You must never withhold lifesaving care.

Mentally Incompetent Adults

Assisting patients who are mentally ill, in behavioral (psychological) crisis, under the influence of drugs or alcohol, or developmentally delayed is complicated. An adult patient who is mentally incompetent is not able to give informed consent. From a legal perspective, this situation is similar to those involving minors. Consent for emergency care should be obtained from someone who is legally responsible, such as a guardian or conservator. In many cases, however, such permission will not be readily obtainable. Many states have protective custody statutes allowing such a person to be taken, under law enforcement authority, to a medical facility. Know the provisions in your area. Remember that when a true emergency exists, you can assume that implied consent exists.

Forcible Restraint

Forcible restraint is the act of physically preventing an individual from treating any mental or physical action. Forcible restraint of a mentally disturbed individual may be required before emergency care can be rendered. If you believe that a patient will injure himself, herself, or others, you can legally restrain the patient. However, you must consult medical control, online or off-line dependent on local protocol, for authorization to restrain or contact law enforcement personnel who have authority to restrain people. In some states, only a law enforcement officer may forcibly restrain an individual (▶ Figure 3-7). You should be clearly informed

Figure 3-5 When a serious threat to life exists and the patient is unconscious or otherwise unable to give consent, the law assumes that the patient would give consent to care and transport to the hospital.

Figure 3-6 The law requires that a parent or legal guardian give consent for treatment or transport of a minor. However, you must never withhold lifesaving care.

about local laws. Restraint without authority exposes you to civil and criminal penalties. Restraint may be used only in circumstances of risk to yourself or others.

Your service should have clearly defined protocols to deal with situations involving restraint. After restraints are applied, they must not be removed en route even if the patient promises to behave.

Remember that if the patient is conscious and the situation is not urgent, consent is required. Adults who appear to be in control of their senses cannot be forced to submit to either care or transportation.

Assault and Battery

<u>Assault</u> is defined as unlawfully placing a person in fear of immediate bodily harm without the person's consent. <u>Battery</u> is unlawfully touching a person; this includes providing emergency care without consent. Serious legal problems may arise in situations in which a patient has not given consent for treatment. Battery could be considered if you apply a splint to a suspected fracture of the lower leg or use an Epi-Pen on a patient without the patient's consent. The patient may have grounds to sue you for assault, battery, or both. To protect yourself from these charges, make sure that you obtain expressed consent or that the situation allows

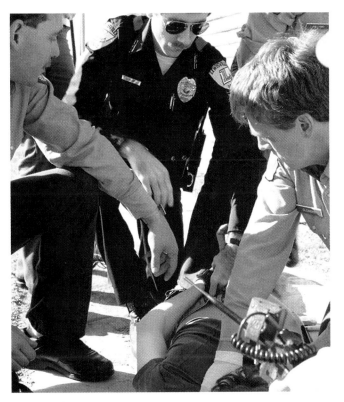

Figure 3-7 Be sure that you know the local laws about forcible restraint of a patient. In some states, only a law enforcement officer has the authority to restrain a patient.

for implied consent. Consult your medical director if you have questions or doubt about a specific situation.

The Right to Refuse Treatment

Mentally competent adults have the right to refuse treatment or withdraw from treatment at any time. However, these patients present you with a dilemma. Should you provide care against their will and risk being accused of battery? Should you leave them alone? If you leave patients alone, you risk being accused of negligence or abandonment if their condition becomes worse.

If a patient refuses treatment or transport, you must make sure that he or she understands, or is informed about, the potential risks, benefits, treatments, and alternatives to treatment. You must also fully inform the patient about the consequences of refusing treatment and encourage the patient to ask questions. Remember that competent adults who refuse specific kinds of treatment for religious reasons generally have a legal right to do so.

When a patient refuses treatment, you must assess whether the patient's mental condition is impaired. If the patient refusing treatment is delusional or confused, you cannot assume that the refusal is an informed refusal. When in doubt, it is always best to proceed with treatment. This is the best course of action because providing treatment is a much more defensible position than failing to treat a patient. Failure to treat a patient can be considered negligence.

You may also be faced with a situation in which a parent refuses to permit treatment of an ill or injured child. In this situation, you must consider the emotional impact of the emergency on the parent's judgment. In this and virtually all cases of refusal, you can usually resolve the situation with patience and calm persuasion. You may also need the help of others, such as law enforcement officials.

There will be times when you are not able to persuade the patient, guardian, conservator, or parent of a minor or mentally incompetent patient to proceed with treatment. In this case, you must obtain the signature of the individual who is refusing treatment on an official release form that acknowledges refusal. You must be sure to document any assessment findings and emergency care that you provided. You must also obtain a signature from a witness to the refusal. You should then keep the refusal with the run report and the patient care report. In addition to the release form itself, you should write a note about the refusal on the patient care report. If the patient refuses to sign the release form, the best you can do is inform your medical director and thoroughly document the situation

Documentation Tips

When a patient, parent, or guardian refuses treatment or transport, protect yourself with both a thorough patient care report and an official refusal form. Have the patient or other refusing party sign the form, document in the patient care report what you have done to ensure an informed refusal, and note the involvement of medical control in the situation. Be sure to submit the refusal form with your patient care report.

and the refusal. Report to medical control, and/or follow your local protocols with regard to this situation.

Good Samaritan Laws and Immunity

Most states have adopted **Good Samaritan laws**, which are based on the common law principle that when you reasonably help another person, you should not be liable for errors and omissions that are made in giving good faith emergency care. However, Good Samaritan laws do not protect you from a lawsuit. Only a few statutory provisions provide immunity from a lawsuit, and those usually are reserved for governments. Good Samaritan laws provide an affirmative defense if you are sued for rendering care, but they do not protect you from liability or for failure to provide proper care, nor do they pertain to acts outside the scope of care. These laws do not protect anyone from wanton, gross, or willful negligence (eg, the failure to exercise due care).

Another group of laws grants immunity from liability to official emergency medical care providers, such as EMT-Bs. These laws, which vary from state to state, do not provide immunity when injury or damage is caused by gross negligence or willful conduct.

Most states have also adopted specific laws granting special privileges to EMS personnel, authorizing them to perform certain medical procedures. Many states also grant partial immunity to EMTs and physicians and nurses who give emergency instructions to EMS personnel via radio or other forms of communication. Consult your medical director for more information about the laws in your area.

Advance Directives

Occasionally, you and your partner may respond to a call in which a patient is dying from an illness. When you arrive at the scene, you may find that family members present do not want you to try to resuscitate the patient. Without valid written documentation from a physician, such as an advance directive or a do not resuscitate (DNR) order (also known as a "Do Not Attempt Resuscitation" order), this type of request places you in a very difficult position. An **advance directive** is a written document that specifies medical treatment for a competent patient, should he or she become unable to make decisions. In this situation, a **competent** patient is able to make rational decisions about his or her well-being. An advance directive is also commonly called a living will. DNR orders give you permission *not* to attempt resuscitation. Although laws can differ from state to state, generally speaking, to be valid, **DNR orders** must meet the following requirements:

- Clearly state the patient's medical problem(s)
- Be signed by the patient or legal guardian
- Be signed by one or more physicians
- Be dated in the preceding 12 months

However, even in the presence of such a DNR order, you are still obligated to provide supportive measures (oxygen, pain relief, and comfort) to a patient who has not arrested, whenever possible. Each ambulance service, in consultation with its medical director and legal counsel, must develop a protocol to follow in these circumstances.

Because of terminal nursing home placement and hospice and home health programs, you may be faced with this situation often. Specific guidelines vary from state to state, but the following four statements may be considered general guidelines:

1. **Patients have the right to refuse treatment,** including resuscitative efforts, provided that they are able to communicate their wishes.

2. **A written order from a physician is required** for DNR orders to be valid in a health care facility.

3. **You should periodically review** state and local protocols and legislation regarding advance directives.

4. **When you are in doubt** or the written orders are not present, resuscitate.

Ethical Responsibilities

In addition to legal duties, EMTs have certain ethical responsibilities as health care providers. These responsibilites are to themselves, their coworkers, the public, and the patient. Ethics are related to action, conduct, motive, or character and how they relate to the EMT's responsibilities. From an EMS standpoint, ethics are associated with what the profession of EMS providers deems right or fitting conduct. Treating a patient ethically means doing so in a manner that conforms to professional standards of conduct.

How can you make sure that you are acting ethically, especially with all the decisions you have to make in the field ▼ Table 3-1 ?

You must meet your legal and ethical responsibilities while caring for your patients' physical and emotional needs. Patient needs vary depending on the situation.

An unquestionable responsibility is honest reporting. Absolute honesty in reporting is essential. You must provide a complete account of the events and the details of all patient care and professional duties. Accurate records are also important for quality improvement activities.

Confidentiality

Communication between you and the patient is considered confidential and generally cannot be disclosed without permission from the patient or a court order. Confidential information includes the patient history, assessment findings, and treatment provided. You cannot disclose information regarding a patient's diagnosis, treatment, or mental or physical condition without consent; if you do, you may find yourself liable for breach of confidentiality.

In certain situations, you may release confidential information to designated individuals. In most states, records may be released when a legal subpoena is presented or the patient signs a written release. The patient must be mentally competent and fully understand the nature of the release.

> Except under certain, specific circumstances you cannot disclose patient information without consent.

Another means for disclosing information is with an automatic release, which does not require a written form. This type of release allows you to share information with other health care providers so that they may continue the patient's care.

In many states, you do not need a written release to report information about cases of rape or abuse to proper authorities. Third-party payment billing forms may also be completed without written consent.

Records and Reports

Society, through its government, has formulated a policy to protect individuals with health regulations and statutes. Because certain individuals are in a position to observe and gather information about diseases, injuries, and emergency events, an obligation to compile such information and report it to certain agencies may be imposed. Even if there is no such requirement, you should compile a complete and accurate record of all incidents in which you come into contact with sick or injured patients. Most medical and legal experts believe that a complete and accurate record of an

TABLE 3-1 Ethical Decision Making

1. Consider all options available to you and the consequence of each option.

2. What decisions have been made regarding a similar situation? Is this a type of problem that reflects a rule or policy? Can an existing policy or rule be applied? *This uses the concept of "precedence."*

3. How would this action affect you if you were in your patient's or patient's family's place? *This is a form of the "Golden Rule."*

4. Would you feel comfortable having all prehospital care providers apply this action in all similar circumstances? *This is an application of Kant's "Categorical Imperative."*

5. Can you supply a good justification for your action to:
   - Your peers
   - The public
   - Your supervisor

6. How will the consequences of your decision derive the greatest benefit in view of all the alternatives? *This is the test of "utility."*

emergency medical incident is an important safeguard against legal complications. The absence of a record or a substantially incomplete record may mean that you have to testify about the events, your findings, and your actions relying on memory alone, which can prove to be wholly inadequate and embarrassing in the face of aggressive cross-examination.

The courts consider the following two rules of thumb regarding reports and records:

- **If an action or procedure** is not recorded on the written report, it was not performed.

- **An incomplete or untidy report** is evidence of incomplete or inexpert emergency medical care.

You can avoid both of these potentially dangerous presumptions by compiling and maintaining accurate reports and records of all events and patients.

Patient care reports also help the EMS system evaluate individual and service provider performance. These reports are an integral part of most quality assurance programs.

Special Reporting Requirements

Abuse of Children, the Elderly, and Others

All states and the District of Columbia have enacted laws to protect abused children, and some have added other protected groups such as the elderly and "at-risk" adults. Most states have a reporting obligation for certain individuals, ranging from physicians to any person. You must be aware of the requirements of law in your state. Such statutes frequently grant immunity from liability for libel, slander, or defamation of character to the individual who is obligated to report, even if the reports are subsequently shown to be unfounded, as long as the reports are made in good faith.

Injury During the Commission of a Felony

Many states have laws requiring the reporting of any injury that is likely to have occurred during the commission of a crime, such as gunshot wounds, knife wounds, or poisonings. Again, you must be familiar with the legal requirements of your state.

Drug-Related Injuries

In some instances, drug-related injuries must be reported. These requirements may affect the EMT-B. However, it should be stressed that the US Supreme Court has held that drug addiction, in contrast to drug possession or sale, is an illness and not a crime. Hence, an injury as a result of a drug overdose may not be within the definition of an injury resulting from a crime.

EMT-B Tips

When taking a history from a patient you suspect has been abused, you may get more accurate information if your partner interviews the parents or other caregivers separately. Abused patients are usually reluctant to speak openly in front of their abusers.

Some states, by statute, specifically establish confidentiality and excuse certain specified individuals from reporting drug cases, either to a government agency or to a minor's parents, if, in the opinion of those individuals, withholding reporting is necessary for the proper treatment of the patient. Once again, you must be familiar with the legal requirements of your state.

Childbirth

Many states require that anyone who attends at a live birth in any place other than a licensed medical facility report the birth. As before, you must be familiar with state requirements.

Other Reporting Requirements

Other reporting requirements may include attempted suicides, dog bites, certain communicable diseases, assaults, and rapes.

Most EMS agencies require that all exposures to infectious diseases be reported. You may be asked to transport certain patients in restraints, which may also need to be reported. Each of these situations can present significant legal problems. You should learn your local protocols regarding these situations.

Scene of a Crime

If there is evidence at an emergency scene that a crime may have been committed, you must notify the dispatcher immediately so that law enforcement authorities can be informed. Such circumstances should not stop you from providing necessary emergency medical care to the patient; however, your safety is a priority, so you must ensure that the scene is safe to enter. At times, you may have to transport the patient to the hospital before the authorities arrive. While emergency medical care is being provided, you must be careful not to disturb the scene of the crime any more than absolutely necessary. Notes and drawings should be made of the position of the patient and of the presence and position of any weapon or other objects that may be valuable to the investigating officers. If possible, do not cut through holes in clothing from weapon or gunshot wounds. You should confer periodically with local authorities and be aware of their wishes as to any actions you should take at the scene of the crime. It is best if these guidelines can be established by protocol.

The Deceased

In most states, EMTs do not have the authority to pronounce a patient dead. If there is any chance that life exists or that the patient can be resuscitated, you must make every effort to save the patient at the scene and during transport. However, at times death is obvious, such as in the following circumstances:

- Rigor mortis (stiffening of the body) has set in.
- Mortal injury, such as decapitation.
- Dependent lividity (discoloration of the body as a result of pooling of the blood) is present ▼ Figure 3-8 .
- The body is decomposed.

In such instances, there is no urgent reason to move the body. The only immediate action that is required of you is to cover the body and prevent its disturbance. Local protocol will determine your ultimate action in these instances.

Special Situations

Organ Donors

You may be called to a scene involving a potential organ donor. An individual who has expressed a wish to donate organs is a potential organ donor. Consent to organ donation is voluntary and knowing. Consent is evidenced by either a donor card or a driver's license

indicating that the individual wishes to be a donor ▼ Figure 3-9 . You may need to consult with medical control when faced with this situation.

You should treat a potential organ donor in the same way that you would any other patient needing treatment. The fact that a patient is a possible donor does not mean that you should not use all means necessary to keep that patient alive. Organs that are often donated, such as a kidney, heart, or liver, need oxygen at all times; you must give the possible donor oxygen, or the organs will be damaged and become useless.

Remember that your priority is to save the patient's life. You may encounter potential organ donor situations at a multiple-casualty incident. The potential organ donor should be triaged with other patients and assigned a category; the potential organ donor may have to have a lower priority than other less severely injured patients.

Be sure to learn what the specific protocols are in your area regarding these situations.

Medical Identification Insignia

Many patients will carry important medical identification and information, often in the form of a bracelet, necklace, or card that will identify whether the patient has allergies, diabetes, epilepsy, or some other serious condition ▼ Figure 3-10 . This information is helpful to you in assessing and treating the patient.

Figure 3-9 The patient may be carrying a donor card or driver's license indicating that he or she wishes to be an organ donor.

Figure 3-10 The patient may be carrying a medical identification card or wearing a bracelet or necklace that may indicate a serious medical condition.

Figure 3-8 Dependent lividity is an obvious sign of death caused by discoloration of the body from pooling of the blood to the lower parts of the body.

Prep Kit

Ready for Review

As the scope of emergency medical care becomes more complex and widely available, litigation involving participants in emergency medical services will increase.

The scope of practice outlines the care you are able to provide to the patient and is most commonly defined by law; the medical director further defines the scope of practice. The standard of care is the manner in which you must act or behave when treating sick or injured patients. Some standards are imposed by local custom, the law, and institutions.

A duty to act is the responsibility of an individual to provide patient care. If you are off duty or out of your jurisdiction, you may not have a legal duty to act; however, you do have a moral and ethical duty to act because of your training and expertise.

Negligence is the failure to provide the same care that a person of similar training would provide. Determination of negligence is based on duty, breach of duty, damages, and cause.

Abandonment is the termination of care without the patient's consent and without making provisions for the transfer of care to a medical professional with skills at the same or a higher level than yours. Abandonment is legally and ethically a very serious act.

You must receive consent from a patient before beginning care. A conscious adult patient who can make a rational decision will be able to give you expressed consent. Expressed consent must also be informed consent. When a patient is unconscious and unable to give consent, the law assumes implied consent. You should try to obtain consent from a parent or guardian of a minor whenever possible. You should never withhold lifesaving care.

Assault is defined as unlawfully placing a person in fear of immediate harm without the person's consent. Battery is unlawfully touching a person; this includes providing emergency care without consent. To protect yourself from these charges, be sure to obtain expressed consent whenever possible.

Mentally competent patients have the right to refuse treatment. In these instances, be sure to have the patient sign a refusal form, and make sure your department keeps a copy.

Many states have adopted Good Samaritan laws and other laws that provide immunity to EMS personnel, provided that injury to the patient was not the result of gross negligence or willful misconduct on the part of the EMT-B.

An advance directive is a written document that specifies medical treatment in case a mentally competent patient becomes unable to make decisions. DNR orders give you permission to not attempt resuscitation in the event of cardiac arrest. Your ambulance service should have protocols in place to follow when you are faced with an advance directive or DNR orders.

Communication between you and the patient is confidential and should not be disclosed without permission from the patient or a court order.

Records and reports are important; make sure that you compile a complete and accurate record of each incident where you come into contact with sick or injured patients. You may need to testify some day and the courts consider an action or procedure that was not recorded on the written report as not having been performed, and an incomplete or untidy report is considered evidence of incomplete or inexpert medical care.

You should know what the special reporting requirements are involving abuse of children, the elderly, and others; injuries related to crimes; drug-related injuries; and childbirth. Be sure to note whether patients are carrying some type of medical identification information. If you fail to take this information into account, you may cause harm to the patient.

Vital Vocabulary

abandonment Unilateral termination of care by the EMT-B without the patient's consent and without making provisions for transferring care to another medical professional with skills at the same level or higher.

advance directive Written documentation that specifies medical treatment for a competent patient should the patient become unable to make decisions; also called a living will.

assault Unlawfully placing a patient in fear of bodily harm.

battery Touching a patient or providing emergency care without consent.

certification A process in which a person, an institution, or a program is evaluated and recognized as meeting certain predetermined standards to provide safe and ethical care.

competent Able to make rational decisions about personal well-being.

consent Permission to render care.

DNR (Do Not Resuscitate) orders Written documentation giving permission to medical personnel not to attempt resuscitation in the event of cardiac arrest.

duty to act A medicolegal term relating to certain personnel who either by statute or by function have a responsibility to provide care.

emergency A serious situation, such as injury or illness, that threatens the life or welfare of a person or group of people and requires immediate intervention.

emergency medical care Immediate care or treatment.

expressed consent A type of consent in which a patient gives express authorization for provision of care or transport.

forcible restraint The act of physically preventing an individual from treating any physical action.

Good Samaritan laws Statutory provisions enacted by many states to protect citizens from liability for errors and omissions in giving good faith emergency medical care, unless there is wanton, gross, or willful negligence.

implied consent Type of consent in which a patient who is unable to give consent is given treatment under the legal assumption that he or she would want treatment.

informed consent Permission for treatment given by a competent patient after the potential risks, benefits, and alternatives to treatment have been explained.

medicolegal A term relating to medical jurisprudence (law) or forensic medicine.

negligence Failure to provide the same care that a person with similar training would provide.

standard of care Written, accepted levels of emergency care expected by reason of training and profession; written by legal or professional organizations so that patients are not exposed to unreasonable risk or harm.

Assessment in Action

You are dispatched to a "woman with difficulty breathing" at a farm. About 10 minutes later, you pull up in front of a small farmhouse.

You ring the doorbell and knock loudly several times but there is no response, so you decide to find out whether the door is open. It is, so you tentatively enter and shout, "We are here with an ambulance, did somebody call us? Is anybody home?" You enter the house and see an elderly woman lying in the middle of the floor. Your partner starts to assess her level of consciousness.

1. Which of the following regarding duty to act is true?
   A. You have been sent to her home, therefore you have a duty to act.
   B. Once you have established that she needs resuscitation, you have a duty to act.
   C. The duty to act is a personal choice so you can choose to treat or not.
   D. Because you are an EMT-B you have a legal duty to act.

2. Under what type of consent can you treat this patient and attempt resuscitation?
   A. Undue   C. Referred
   B. Informed   D. Implied

3. This patient had been asleep and, upon awakening, was alert and oriented to person, place, and time, but stated that she didn't wish to go to the hospital. After completion of an initial assessment, what would be the most appropriate course of action?
   A. Inform her of the possible consequences and have her sign a refusal form.
   B. Threaten legal action if she chooses not to go.
   C. Secure her to the stretcher and then transport her to the hospital.
   D. Call law enforcement so they can place her under protective custody.

4. You have established unresponsiveness, pulselessness, and apnea, and are beginning resuscitation procedures when a young man rushes into the room stating, "Don't do that, she doesn't want CPR!" What should you do?
   A. Continue treatment because you have already started, and transport.
   B. Immediately stop what you are doing and ask who he is.

C. Ask if there is any written documentation such as a DNR or advance directive.
D. Stop your procedures and have him sign a refusal of care form.

5. If, during your assessment, you had found regular respirations and a weak pulse and the relative produced a DNR order, what would be appropriate measures to take?
   A. Document the presence of DNR orders and have the relative sign the refusal of care.
   B. Continue all treatment because DNR orders are not legal outside a hospital.
   C. There is no further action to take; you may leave.
   D. Provide supportive care and transport with the DNR orders.

6. After you have completed this call and are back at the station, you receive a phone call from a man who identifies himself as this patient's son. He is asking what happened to his mother and what you did at the scene. What would be an appropriate response?
   A. Describe for him, in objective terms, what was done at the scene and offer to get a copy of the report for him.
   B. Tell him he must come down in person to receive that information, since you have no way of verifying who he is over the phone.
   C. Tell him he must call back when your report is complete, and talk to both you and your commanding officer.
   D. Tell him you are not allowed to give out that information and refer him to the family members who were present at the scene.

Challenging Question

7. You are called to the scene of a 50-year-old man who injured his leg. He was assessed, had no complaints other than his leg, and a splint was applied. Vital signs were within normal limits. There was no change in his status en route to the hospital. While he was in the emergency department, the patient suffered a cardiac arrest and died. The family sued the ambulance, the hospital, and the physician. From this information, were the four factors of negligence met?

Points to Ponder

You have been working with the same partner for about six months. As you are talking he tells you that he is having some financial problems and is going to apply for a second job at the hospital. You also find out that his wife is pregnant. She is not able to work so they have lost her income and have increased expenses with the baby and her medical bills. About a week later you are securing an elderly patient to the stretcher while your partner is gathering the patient's medications from the nightstand. You happen to look just as your partner is putting an antique pocket watch into his pocket. You have never seen him with a pocket watch and suspect that it may be the patient's. What would you do? Would you ask your partner about it? Would you report it to your supervisor? What if your partner admitted

stealing it but refused to give it back and said he would deny taking it?

Issues Ethics in EMS, Communication with your Partner, Partner Relationships.

Online Outlook

When you arrive at the scene of a terminally ill patient, you may find that family members present do not want you to try to resuscitate the patient. This places you in a very difficult situation. Learn more about this by completing Exercise 3 at www.emtb.com.

www.emtb.com

The Human Body

TECHNOLOGY

www.emtb.com

Online Chapter Pretest
Interactivities
Vocabulary Explorer
Anatomy Review
Web Links
Online Review Manual
Distance Learning

Chapter FEATURES

Skill Drills
Vital Vocabulary
Pediatric Needs
Geriatric Needs
EMT-B Safety
EMT-B Tips
Documentation Tips
Remember
Prep Kit

You are the EMT

Your rescue squad is sent to a local tavern where you find one of the patrons down on the front steps after having been shot three times in the chest and abdomen. As you cover the wounds, you wonder what internal organs have been damaged in the attack, and to what extent.

This chapter provides essential information about the basic workings of the human body and will also help you answer the following questions:

1. How does each body system respond when another body system is damaged from illness or injury?

2. Why is it necessary for an EMT-B to have a fundamental working understanding of medical terminology?

The Human Body

A working knowledge of human anatomy is important for you as an EMT-B. Even though you will not make diagnoses, you can help hospital personnel by communicating information using the correct medical terms. All EMT-Bs must be familiar with the language of topographic anatomy. By using the proper medical terms, you will be able to communicate correct information with the least possible confusion.

Using topographic anatomy is actually like using a road map. The terms that are introduced in this chapter will help you to identify the topographic (ie, on the surface) landmarks of the body. These landmarks are used as guides to locate the internal structures that lie under them. These terms also refer to the names of the major regions of the body and the way in which the locations of these regions are described in relation to one another.

Topographic Anatomy

The surface of the body has many definite visible features that serve as guides or landmarks to the structures that lie beneath them. You must be able to identify the superficial landmarks of the body—its **topographic anatomy**—to perform an accurate assessment. Understanding the terminology is also important so that you can describe patient findings correctly to your team, ALS providers, and hospital personnel.

Learning the terms that are introduced in this chapter will make your job as an EMT-B easier, since you will be able to correctly identify structures as you complete and report your assessment findings. Hospital personnel will use these terms to ask you questions about a patient. Therefore, you must learn what these terms mean and how to use them.

The terms that are used to describe the topographic anatomy are applied to the body when it is in the **anatomic position**. This is a position of reference in which the patient stands facing you, arms at the side, with the palms of the hands forward.

The Planes of the Body

The anatomic planes of the body are imaginary straight lines that divide the body (▶ **Table 4-1**). These planes help you to identify the location of internal structures and understand the relationships between and among the organs.

ANTERIOR AND POSTERIOR. **Anterior** refers to the front surface of the body, the side facing you in the anatomic position. **Posterior** refers to the back surface of the patient, or the side away from you.

MIDLINE. An imaginary vertical line drawn from the middle of the forehead through the nose and the umbilicus (navel) to the floor is called the **midline** of the body. This imaginary line divides the body into two halves that are mirror images. The nose, chin, umbilicus (navel), and spine are examples of midline structures.

MIDCLAVICULAR LINE. The **midclavicular line** is an imaginary line drawn vertically through the middle portion of the clavicle and parallel to the midline. For example, the nipples of the breasts are in the midclavicular line on either side of the body.

MIDAXILLARY LINE. The **midaxillary line** is an imaginary vertical line drawn through the middle of the axilla (armpit) parallel to the midline. This line is also in the middle of the anterior and posterior surfaces of the body.

Directional Terms

In this section, terms that indicate direction are introduced. These terms indicate distance and direction from the midline (▼ Figure 4-1), (▼ Table 4-2).

RIGHT AND LEFT. The terms "right" and "left" refer to the patient's right and left sides, not to your right and left sides.

SUPERIOR AND INFERIOR. The **superior** part of the body, or any body part, is the portion nearer to the head.

The part nearer to the feet is the **inferior** portion. These terms are also used to describe the relationship of one structure to another. For example, the nose is superior to the mouth and inferior to the forehead.

LATERAL AND MEDIAL. Parts of the body that lie farther from the midline are called **lateral** (outer) structures. The parts that lie closer to the midline are called **medial** (inner) structures. For example, the knee has medial (inner) and lateral (outer) aspects.

PROXIMAL AND DISTAL. The terms "proximal" and "distal" are used to describe the relationship of any two structures on an extremity. **Proximal** describes structures that are closer to the trunk. **Distal** describes structures that are farther from the trunk or nearer to the free end of the extremity. For example, the elbow is distal to the shoulder and proximal to the wrist and hand.

TABLE 4-1 Anatomic Planes of the Body

Term	Definition
Anterior	Front
Posterior	Back
Midline	Line drawn through nose and umbilicus
Midclavicular	In the middle of the clavicle, parallel to the midline
Midaxillary	In the middle of the armpit, parallel to the midline

TABLE 4-2 Directional Terms

Term	Definition
Right	The patient's right
Left	The patient's left
Lateral	Farther from midline
Medial	Closer to midline
Superior	Closer to the head, higher
Inferior	Farther from the head, lower
Proximal	Closer to the midline (in an extremity, closer to the trunk)
Distal	Farther from the midline (in an extremity, closer to the free end)
Dorsal	Toward the spine
Ventral	Toward the abdomen
Palmar	The front region of the hand
Plantar	The bottom of the foot

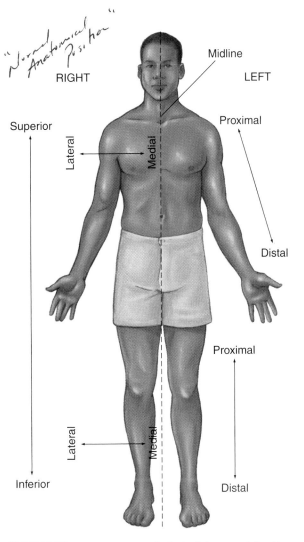

Figure 4-1 Directional terms indicate distance and direction from the midline.

SUPERFICIAL AND DEEP. **Superficial** means closer to or on the skin. **Deep** means farther inside the body and away from the skin.

VENTRAL AND DORSAL. **Ventral** refers to the anterior surface of the body. **Dorsal** refers to the posterior surface of the body, including the back of the hand.

PALMAR AND PLANTAR. The front region of the hand is referred to as the palm or **palmar** surface. The bottom of the foot is referred to as the **plantar** surface.

APEX. The **apex (plural: apices)** is the tip or the top-most portion of a structure. For example, the tips of the shoulders are the apices of the shoulder. The most superior portions of the lungs are the apices of the lungs. The exception to this is the heart.

Other Directional Terms

Many structures of the body occur bilaterally. A **bilateral** structure is a body part that appears on both sides of the midline. For example, the eyes, ears, hands, and feet are bilateral structures. This is also true for structures inside the body, such as the lungs and kidneys. Structures that appear on only one side of the body

> The surface of the body has many definite visible features that serve as guides or landmarks to the structures that lie beneath them.

are said to occur unilaterally. For example, the spleen is on the left side of the body only, and the liver is on the right side.

As part of the assessment process, you will palpate the abdomen and report your findings. Therefore, it is important that you be able to describe the exact location of areas of the abdomen. The way to describe the sections of the abdominal cavity is by **quadrants**. Imagine two lines intersecting at the umbilicus, dividing the abdomen into four equal areas ▼ **Figure 4-2** . These are referred to as the right upper quadrant (RUQ), left upper quadrant (LUQ), right lower quadrant (RLQ), and left lower quadrant (LLQ). Remember that here, too, right and left refer to the patient's right and left, not yours.

It is important to learn all of these terms and concepts so that you can describe the location of any injury or assessment findings. When you use these terms properly, any other medical personnel who care for the patient will know immediately where to look and what to expect.

Anatomic Positions

You will use these terms to describe the position of the patient as you find him or her or as you are to eventually transport the patient to the emergency department ▶ **Figure 4-3** .

PRONE AND SUPINE. These terms describe the position of the body. The body is in the **prone position** when lying face down; the body is in the **supine position** when lying face up.

FOWLER'S POSITION. A patient who is sitting up with the knees bent is in **Fowler's position**.

TRENDELENBURG'S POSITION. In **Trendelenburg's position**, the body is supine with the head lower than the feet.

SHOCK POSITION. In the **shock position**, or modified Trendelenburg's position, the head and **torso** (the trunk without the head and limbs) are supine, and the lower extremities are elevated 6″ to 12″. This helps to increase blood flow to the brain.

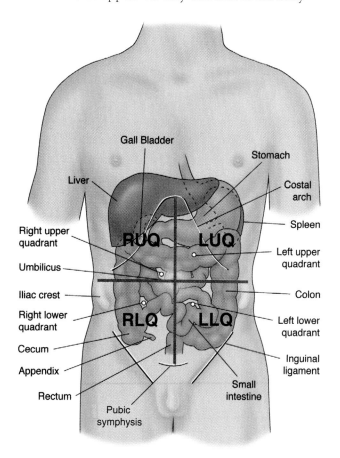

Gall Bladder
Stomach
Liver
Costal arch
Spleen
Right upper quadrant
RUQ **LUQ**
Left upper quadrant
Umbilicus
Iliac crest
Colon
Right lower quadrant
RLQ **LLQ**
Left lower quadrant
Cecum
Appendix
Inguinal ligament
Rectum
Small intestine
Pubic symphysis

Figure 4-2 The abdomen is divided into quadrants.

Figure 4-3 **A.** Prone. **B.** Supine. **C.** Shock position (modified Trendelenburg's position). **D.** Fowler's position.

The Skeletal System

The **skeleton** gives us our recognizable human form and protects our vital internal organs (▶ **Figure 4-4**). The brain lies within the skull. The heart, lungs, and great vessels are protected by the thorax, which is part of the torso. Much of the liver and spleen is protected by the lower ribs. The spinal cord is contained within and protected by a bony spinal canal formed by the vertebrae.

The 206 bones of the skeleton provide a framework for the attachment of muscles. The skeleton is also designed to allow motion of the body. Bones come into contact with one another at joints where, with the help of muscles, the body is able to bend and move.

The Skull

The **cranium** is composed of a number of thick bones that fuse together to form a shell above the eyes and ears that holds and protects the brain (▼ **Figure 4-5**). The brain connects to the spinal cord through a large opening at the base of the skull (the **foramen magnum**). The spinal cord is composed of virtually all the nerves that carry messages between the brain and the rest of the body.

The most posterior portion of the cranium is called the **occiput**. On each side of the cranium, the lateral portions are called the

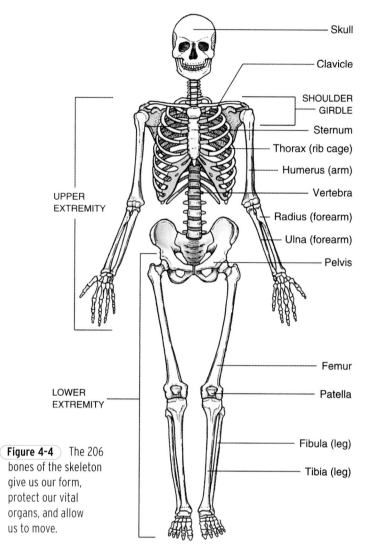

Figure 4-4 The 206 bones of the skeleton give us our form, protect our vital organs, and allow us to move.

Labels: Skull, Clavicle, SHOULDER GIRDLE, Sternum, Thorax (rib cage), Humerus (arm), Vertebra, Radius (forearm), Ulna (forearm), Pelvis, Femur, Patella, Fibula (leg), Tibia (leg), UPPER EXTREMITY, LOWER EXTREMITY

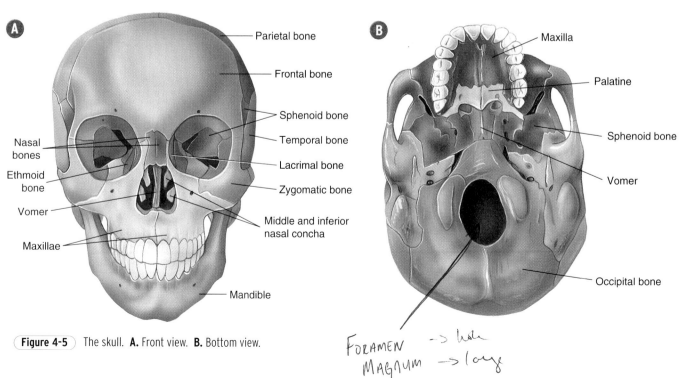

Figure 4-5 The skull. **A.** Front view. **B.** Bottom view.

A. Labels: Parietal bone, Frontal bone, Sphenoid bone, Temporal bone, Lacrimal bone, Zygomatic bone, Middle and inferior nasal concha, Mandible, Nasal bones, Ethmoid bone, Vomer, Maxillae

B. Labels: Maxilla, Palatine, Sphenoid bone, Vomer, Occipital bone

FORAMEN → hole
MAGNUM → large

temples or **temporal regions**. Between the temporal regions and the occiput lie the **parietal regions**. The forehead is called the frontal region. Just anterior to the ear, in the temporal region, you can feel the pulse of the superficial temporal artery. The thick skin covering the cranium and usually bearing hair is called the **scalp**.

The face is composed of the eyes, ears, nose, mouth, and cheeks. Six bones—the nasal bone, the two **maxillae** (upper jawbones), the two **zygomas** (cheek bones), and the **mandible** (lower jawbone)— are the major bones of the face.

The **orbit** (eye socket) is made up of two facial bones: the maxilla and the zygoma. The orbit also includes the frontal bone of the cranium. Together, these bones form a solid bony rim that protrudes around the eye to protect it. If you look at the face from the side, you can see that the eyeball sits back within the orbit. The nasal bone is very short, because most of the nose is made of flexible cartilage. In fact, only the proximal one third of the nose, the bridge, is formed by bone. Unlike the nose, the exposed portion of the ear is made up entirely of cartilage that is covered by skin. The external, visible part of the ear is called the **pinna**. The ear lobes are the fleshy parts at the bottom of each ear. About 1″ posterior to the external opening of the ear is a prominent bony mass at the base of the skull called the **mastoid process**.

The maxilla contains the upper teeth and forms the hard palate (roof of the mouth). The mandible is the only movable facial bone that has a joint (**temporomandibular joint**) where it meets with the temporal bone of the cranium just in front of each ear.

The Neck

The neck contains many important structures. It is supported by the cervical spine, or the first seven vertebrae in the spinal column (C1 through C7). The spinal cord exits from the foramen magnum and lies within the spinal canal formed by the vertebrae. The upper part of the esophagus and the **trachea** (windpipe) lie in the midline of the neck. The carotid arteries may be found on either side of the trachea, along with the jugular veins and several nerves.

Several useful landmarks can be palpated and seen in the neck (▼ **Figure 4-6**). The most obvious is the firm prominence in the center of the anterior surface commonly known as the **Adam's apple**. Specifically, this prominence is the upper part of the **thyroid cartilage**. It is more prominent in men than in women. The other, lower portion is the **cricoid cartilage**, a firm ridge of cartilage inferior to the thyroid cartilage, which is somewhat more difficult to palpate. Between the thyroid cartilage and the cricoid cartilage in the midline of the neck is a soft depression, the **cricothyroid membrane**. This is a thin sheet of connective tissue (**fascia**) that joins the two cartilages. The cricothyroid membrane is covered at this point only by skin.

Inferior to the larynx, several additional firm ridges are palpable in the anterior midline. These ridges are the cartilage rings of the trachea. The trachea connects the larynx with the main air passages of the lungs (the bronchi). On either side of the lower larynx and the upper trachea lies the thyroid gland. Unless it is enlarged, this gland is usually not palpable.

Pulsations of the carotid arteries are easily palpable in a groove about half an inch lateral to the larynx. Lying immediately adjacent to these arteries, but not palpable, are the internal jugular veins and several important nerves. Lateral to these vessels and nerves lie the **sternocleidomastoid muscles**, which allow movement of the head. These muscles originate from the mastoid process of the cranium and insert into the medial border of each collarbone and the **sternum** (breastbone) at the base of the neck.

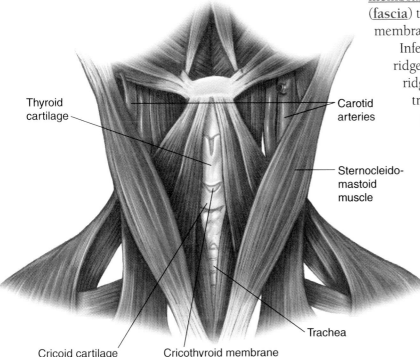

Thyroid cartilage

Carotid arteries

Sternocleidomastoid muscle

Trachea

Cricoid cartilage

Cricothyroid membrane

Figure 4-6   The principal structures of the neck include the trachea, along with many blood vessels, muscles, and nerves.

A series of bony prominences lie posteriorly, in the midline of the neck. They are the spines of the cervical vertebrae. The lower cervical spines are more prominent than the upper ones, and they are more easily palpable when the neck is flexed. At the base of the neck posteriorly, the most prominent spine is the seventh cervical vertebra (▼ **Figure 4-7**).

The Spinal Column

The spinal column is the central supporting structure of the body and is composed of 33 bones, each called a vertebra. The <u>vertebrae</u> are named according to the section of the spine in which they lie and are numbered from top to bottom (▼ **Figure 4-8**). From the top down, the spine is divided into five sections:

- <u>Cervical spine</u>. The first seven vertebrae (C1 through C7), which lie in the neck, form the cervical spine. The skull rests on the first cervical vertebra (the atlas) and articulates with it.

- <u>Thoracic spine</u>. The next 12 vertebrae make up the thoracic spine. One pair of ribs is attached to each of the thoracic vertebrae.

- <u>Lumbar spine</u>. The next five vertebrae form the lumbar or dorsal spine.

- <u>Sacrum</u>. The five sacral vertebrae are fused together to form one bone called the sacrum. The sacrum is joined to the iliac bones of the pelvis with strong ligaments at the sacroiliac joints to form the pelvis.

- <u>Coccyx</u>. The last four vertebrae form the coccyx or tailbone.

The <u>spinal cord</u> is an extension of the brain, composed of virtually all the nerves that carry messages between the brain and the rest of the body. It exits through a large hole in the base of the skull called the foramen magnum and is contained within and protected by the vertebrae of the spinal column. The spinal column is virtually surrounded by muscles. However, the posterior spinous process of each vertebra can be felt as it lies just under the skin in the midline of the back. The most prominent and most easily palpable spinous process is that of the seventh cervical vertebra at the base of the neck.

The anterior part of each vertebra consists of a round, solid block of bone called the body. The posterior part of each vertebra forms a bony arch. This series of arches from one vertebra to the next forms a tunnel that runs the length of the spine called the spinal canal. The bones of the spinal canal encase and protect the spinal cord (▶ **Figure 4-9**). Nerves branch from the spinal cord and exit from the spinal canal between each two vertebrae to form the motor and sensory nerves of the body.

The vertebrae are connected by ligaments, and between each two vertebrae is a cushion called the intervertebral disk. These ligaments and disks allow

Figure 4-7 The most prominent of the cervical vertebrae is the spine of C7.

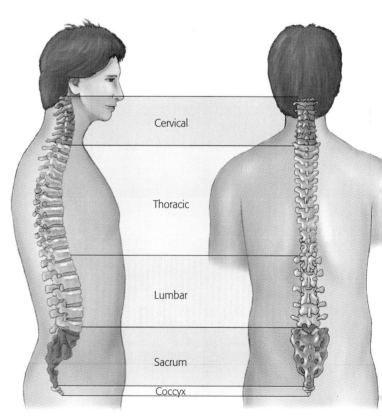

Cervical

Thoracic

Lumbar

Sacrum

Coccyx

Figure 4-8 The spinal column is composed of 33 bones divided into five sections.

some motion so that the trunk can bend forward and back. However, they also limit motion of the vertebrae so that the spinal cord will not be injured. An injury to the spine may damage part of the spinal cord and its nerves that may not be protected by the vertebrae.

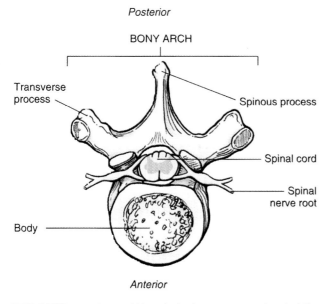

Figure 4-9   The bones of the spinal column encase and protect the spinal cord.

Therefore, until the injury is stabilized, you must use extreme caution in caring for the patient to prevent injury to the spinal cord.

The Thorax

The **thorax** (chest) is the cavity that contains the heart, lungs, esophagus, and great vessels (the aorta and two venae cavae). It is formed by the 12 thoracic vertebrae (T1 through T12) and their 12 pairs of ribs. The **clavicle** (collarbone) overlies the superior boundaries of the thorax in front and articulates posteriorly with the **scapula** (shoulder blade), which lies in the muscular tissue of the thoracic wall. The inferior boundary of the thorax is the diaphragm, which separates the thorax from the abdomen.

ANTERIOR ASPECTS. The dimensions of the thorax are defined by the **thoracic cage** (bony rib cage) and its attachments (▼ **Figure 4-10A**). Anteriorly, in the midline of the chest is the sternum. The superior border of the sternum forms the easily palpable jugular notch. The sternum has three components: the manubrium, the body, and the xiphoid process. The upper quarter of the sternum is called the **manubrium**. The body comprises the rest of the sternum except for a narrow, cartilaginous tip inferiorly, which is called the

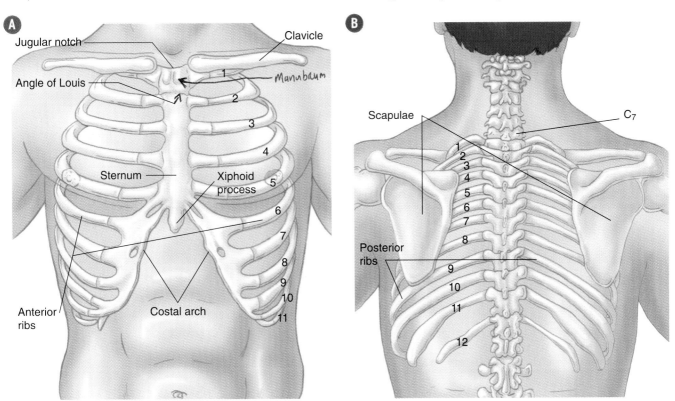

Figure 4-10   **A.** The anterior aspect of the thorax includes the following bony landmarks: the clavicle, the sternum, the xiphoid process, the angle of Louis, and the anterior ribs. **B.** The posterior aspect of the thorax includes the following bony landmarks: the scapulae, the thoracic vertebrae, and the posterior ribs.

<u>xiphoid process</u>. The junction of the manubrium and the body forms a very prominent ridge on the sternum, called the angle of Louis. The **angle of Louis** lies at the level where the second rib is attached to the sternum; it provides a constant and reliable bony landmark on the anterior chest wall.

In the midline of the upper back, the spines of the 12 thoracic vertebrae can be palpated. Twelve ribs on each side form small joints with their respective thoracic vertebrae and extend around to the front to create the walls of the thoracic cage. The upper five ribs connect to the sternum through a short bridge of cartilage. The sixth through tenth ribs insert into the costal arch. The **costal arch** is a bridge of cartilage that connects the ends of the sixth through tenth ribs with the lower portion of the sternum. The eleventh and twelfth ribs are called **floating ribs**, because they do not attach to the sternum through the costal arch. The costal arch is easily palpable and represents the boundary between the lower border of the thorax and the upper border of the abdomen.

POSTERIOR ASPECTS. On the posterior chest wall, the scapulae overlie the thoracic wall and are surrounded by large muscles (◄ **Figure 4-10B**). When the patient is standing or sitting erect, the two scapulae should lie at approximately the same level, with their inferior tips at about the level of the seventh thoracic vertebra. In the lower part of the thorax on each side, an angle called the **costovertebral angle** is formed by the junction of the spine and the tenth rib. The kidneys lie deep to (beneath) the back muscles in the costovertebral angle.

DIAPHRAGM. The **diaphragm** is a muscular dome that forms the inferior boundary of the thorax, separating the chest from the abdominal cavity (▼ **Figure 4-11**). Its contraction, along with that of the chest wall muscles, assists with allowing air to be drawn into the lungs. Anteriorly, it attaches to the costal arch; posteriorly, it attaches to the **lumbar vertebrae**. The diaphragm cannot be seen or palpated.

ORGANS AND VASCULAR STRUCTURES. Within the thoracic cage, the largest structures are the heart and lungs (▼ **Figure 4-12**). The heart lies immediately under the sternum. It extends from the second to the sixth ribs anteriorly and from the fifth to the eighth thoracic vertebrae posteriorly. The inferior border of the heart extends into the left side of the chest. Diseased hearts may be larger or smaller. The major blood vessels that travel to and from the heart also lie in the chest cavity. On the right side of the spinal column, the superior and inferior venae cavae carry blood to the heart.

Just beneath the manubrium of the sternum, the arch of the aorta and the pulmonary artery exit the heart. The arch of the aorta passes to the left and

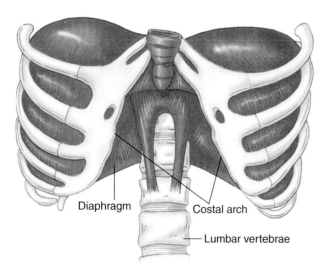

Figure 4-11   The diaphragm forms the undersurface of the thorax, separating the chest from the abdominal cavity.

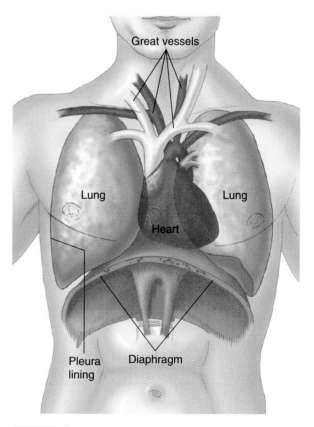

Figure 4-12   The anterior aspect of the thorax shows the relative positions of the principal organs beneath the surface.

lies along the left side of the spinal column as it descends into the abdomen. The esophagus lies behind the great vessels and directly on the anterior aspect of the spinal column as it passes through the chest into the abdominal cavity.

All space within the chest that is not occupied by the heart, great vessels, and esophagus is occupied by the lungs. Anteriorly, the lungs extend down to the surface of the diaphragm at the level of the xiphoid process. Posteriorly, the lungs extend farther inferiorly to the surface of the diaphragm at the level of the twelfth thoracic vertebra.

ANATOMIC LANDMARKS. The major palpable landmarks in the chest are obviously the ribs. Most of them can be easily felt except for the first, which is hidden under and behind the clavicle. Between each rib is the "intercostal space." These spaces can be located by palpating the jugular notch and moving lateral (the first intercostal space). Counting the successive spaces between the ribs gives us the second, third, etc. Both clavicles and the sternum can be easily palpated. The jugular notch is the top portion of the sternum. Lateral to that is the first intercostal space. Inferiorly, the costal arch is readily palpable on both sides of the anterior chest wall. In the midline, the tip of the xiphoid process is a tender and easily palpated landmark.

The major palpable landmarks in the chest are obviously the ribs.

The Abdomen

The **abdomen** is the second major body cavity; it contains the major organs of digestion and excretion. The diaphragm separates the thoracic cavity from the abdominal cavity. Anteriorly and posteriorly, thick muscular abdominal walls create the boundaries of this space. Inferiorly, the abdomen is separated from the pelvis by an imaginary plane that extends from the pubic symphysis through the sacrum (▼ Figure 4-13). Many organs lie in both the abdomen and the pelvis, depending on the posture of the patient.

The simplest and most common method of describing the portions of the abdomen is by quadrants, the four equal areas formed by two imaginary lines that intersect at right angles at the umbilicus. On the anterior abdominal wall, the quadrants thus formed are the right upper,

Figure 4-13 The boundaries of the abdomen are the anterior and posterior abdominal cavity walls, the diaphragm, and an imaginary plane from the pubic symphysis to the sacrum. **A.** Anterior view. **B.** Lateral view.

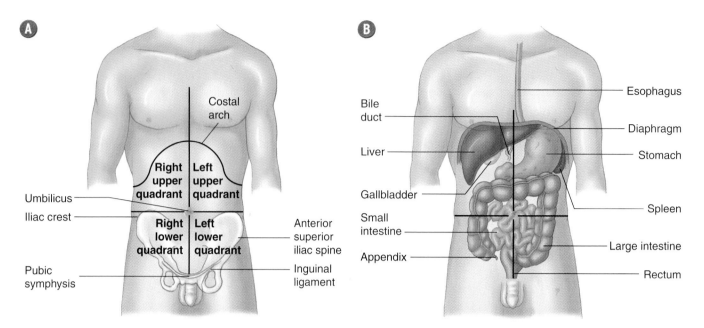

Figure 4-14 **A.** In the abdomen, quadrants are the easiest system for identifying areas. Major bony landmarks are also shown.
B. Many of the organs in the abdomen lie in more than one quadrant.

right lower, left upper, and left lower ▲ **Figure 4-14**. The terms "right quadrant" and "left quadrant" refer to the patient's right and left as you face them, not to your right and left sides. Pain or injury in a given quadrant usually arises from or involves the organs that lie in that quadrant. This simple means of designation will allow you to identify injured or diseased organs that require emergency attention.

ORGANS AND VASCULAR STRUCTURES. In the right upper quadrant (RUQ), the major organs are the liver, the gallbladder, and a portion of the colon. Most of the liver lies in this quadrant, almost entirely under the protection of the eighth to twelfth ribs. The liver fills the entire anteroposterior depth of the abdomen in this quadrant. Therefore, injuries in this area are frequently associated with injuries of the liver.

In the left upper quadrant (LUQ), the principal organs are the stomach, the spleen, and a portion of the colon. The spleen is almost entirely under the protection of the left rib cage, whereas the stomach may sag well down into the left lower quadrant when full. The spleen lies in the lateral and posterior portion of this quadrant, under the diaphragm and immediately in front of the ninth to eleventh ribs. The spleen is frequently injured, especially when these ribs are fractured.

The right lower quadrant (RLQ) contains two portions of the large intestine: the **cecum**, the first portion into which the small intestine (ileum) opens, and the ascending colon. The **appendix** is a small

tubular structure that is attached to the lower border of the cecum. Appendicitis is the most frequent cause of tenderness and pain in this region. In the left lower quadrant (LLQ) lie the descending and the sigmoid portions of the colon.

Several organs lie in more than one quadrant. The small intestine, for instance, occupies the central part of the abdomen around the umbilicus, and parts of it lie in all four quadrants. The pancreas lies just behind the abdominal cavity on the posterior abdominal wall in both upper quadrants. The large intestine also traverses the abdomen, beginning in the RLQ and ending in the LLQ as it passes through all four quadrants. The urinary bladder lies just behind the pubic symphysis in the middle of the abdomen and therefore lies in both lower quadrants and also in the pelvis.

The kidneys are called **retroperitoneal** organs because they lie behind the abdominal cavity ▶ **Figure 4-15**. They are above the level of the umbilicus, extending from the eleventh rib to the third lumbar vertebra on each side. They are approximately 5″ long and lie just anterior to the costovertebral angle.

ANATOMIC LANDMARKS. The chief landmarks in the abdomen are the costal arch, the umbilicus, the anterior superior iliac spines, the iliac crest, and the pubic symphysis. The costal arch, as was noted earlier, is the fused cartilages of the sixth through the tenth ribs. It forms the superior arching boundary of the abdomen. The umbilicus, a constant structure, is in the same

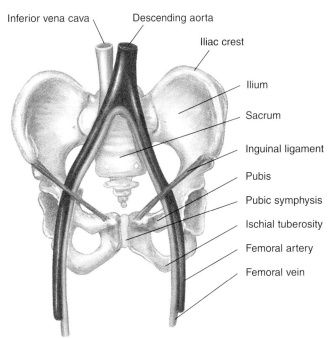

Figure 4-15 The major organs of the retroperitoneal space lie behind the abdominal cavity, above the level of the umbilicus, and extend from the eleventh rib to the third lumbar vertebra. Note that the bladder, inferior vena cava, and aorta also lie in this plane.

Figure 4-16 The pelvis is a closed bony ring that consists of the sacrum, ilium, and ischium.

horizontal plane as the fourth lumbar vertebra and the superior edge of the iliac crest, the rim of the pelvic bone. The **anterior superior iliac spines** are the bony prominences of the pelvis (ilium) at the front on each side of the lower abdomen just below the plane of the umbilicus. In the midline in the lowermost portion of the abdomen is another hard bony prominence, the **pubic symphysis**. Between the lateral edge of the pubic symphysis and the anterior superior spine on each side, you can palpate the tough **inguinal ligament**, which stretches between these two structures. Below the ligament lie the femoral vessels.

Posteriorly, you do not usually refer to abdominal quadrants. The posterior portion of the iliac crest can be palpated, as can the spines of the five lumbar vertebrae (Ll through L5) in the midline.

The Pelvis

The pelvis is a closed bony ring that consists of three bones: the sacrum and the two pelvic bones (▲ **Figure 4-16**). Much like the skull, each pelvic bone is formed by the fusion of three separate bones. These three bones are called the **ilium**, the **ischium**, and the **pubis**. These bones meet at three joints: the two posterior sacroiliac joints and the anterior midline pubic symphysis. All three joints allow very little

motion, as they are firmly held together by strong ligaments. On the lateral side of each pelvic bone—where the three component bones join—is the socket for the hip joint. This depression, in which the femoral head fits very snugly, is called the **acetabulum**.

The pelvic cavity is bounded superiorly by an imaginary plane that runs from the pubic symphysis to the top of the sacrum. Its lateral walls are formed by the inner borders of the pelvic bone, and its inferior boundary is the pelvic outlet, a layer of muscles with openings for the gastrointestinal tract (the rectum), the female reproductive system (the vagina), and the urinary tract (the urethra). In addition, the pelvis contains the final portions of the gastrointestinal tract (the rectosigmoid colon), the female reproductive organs, and the urinary bladder.

ANTERIOR ASPECTS. The prominent anterior bony landmarks of the pelvis are the pubic symphysis in the midline and the anterior superior iliac spines. The inguinal ligament attaches to these two bony prominences and can be palpated in a thin person. Just distal to the midpoint of the inguinal ligament, the femoral artery can be palpated as it enters the thigh. From the anterior superior iliac spine, the ilium extends laterally and posteriorly to form the rim of the pelvis. This bony ridge is called the **iliac crest**, or wing of the pelvis.

POSTERIOR ASPECTS. Posteriorly, the pelvis appears flat, and in the middle third, the firm bony sacrum can be palpated. Just lateral to the sacrum on either side is a joint with the iliac portion of the pelvic bone (the sacroiliac joint). In the sitting position, a bony prominence is easily felt below the middle of each buttock. These prominences are the ischial tuberosities. The sciatic nerve, which is the major nerve to the lower extremity, lies just lateral to the tuberosity as it enters the thigh.

The Lower Extremity

The main parts of the lower extremity are the thigh, the leg, and the foot (▼ **Figure 4-17**). Three joints connect the parts of the lower extremity: the hip, the knee, and the ankle. The joint between the thigh and pelvis is called the hip. The joint between the thigh and the leg is the knee. The joint between the leg and the foot is the ankle.

Pelvis (hip bone)
HIP
Femur
THIGH
Patella (knee cap)
KNEE
Fibula
LEG
Tibia (shin bone)
ANKLE
Tarsals (ankle)
FOOT
Metatarsals
Phalanges

Figure 4-17 The principal parts of the lower extremity include the thigh, leg, and foot. The principal parts of the leg include the tibia and fibula.

THIGH. On the proximal lateral side of the thigh, just below the hip joint, is a bony prominence called the **greater trochanter**. This prominence is sometimes called the "hip bone." During patient assessment, you should always compare the position of the greater trochanter with that on the opposite side as a guide to injury or deformity of the hip.

The **femur** (thigh bone) is the longest and one of the strongest bones in the body. The **femoral head** (at the top of the femur) forms the hip joint with the acetabulum of the pelvis. This ball-and-socket joint allows for flexion, extension, and motion toward (**adduction**) and away (**abduction**) from the midline. It also allows for internal and external rotation of the entire lower extremity. The shaft of the femur is surrounded by large muscles (the quadriceps in front and the hamstrings in back). Just above the knee, the medial and lateral femoral condyles can be palpated.

KNEE. Between the thigh and the leg is the largest joint in the body: the knee. The knee is essentially a hinge joint, allowing only flexion and extension between the distal femur and the proximal tibia. Adduction, abduction, and rotation of the knee are resisted by complex ligaments that are quite susceptible to injury. Anterior to the knee is a specialized bone called the **patella** (kneecap). It lies within the tendon of the quadriceps muscle and protects the front of the knee from injury.

LEG. The leg lies between the knee and the ankle joint and is composed of the **tibia** and the fibula. The tibia (shin bone) is the larger bone and lies in the front of the leg. You can palpate the entire length of the tibia on the anterior surface of the leg just under the skin. The fibula lies on the lateral side of the leg. You can palpate the head of the fibula on the lateral aspect of the knee joint. Its distal end forms the lateral malleolus of the ankle joint.

ANKLE AND FOOT. The ankle is a hinge joint that allows flexion and extension of the foot on the leg (▶ **Figure 4-18**). The end of the tibia forms the medial malleolus, and the end of the fibula forms the lateral malleolus. These two bony prominences form the socket of the ankle joint. Both are surface landmarks of the ankle joint and are easily palpated. The foot contains seven tarsal bones. The talus is one of the largest; the calcaneus, which forms the prominence of the heel, is the other large tarsal bone. The Achilles tendon inserts into the back of the calcaneus. Five metatarsal bones form the substance of the foot. The five toes are formed by 14 phalanges—two in the great toe and three in each of the smaller toes.

The Upper Extremity

The upper extremity extends from the shoulder girdle to the fingertips and is composed of the arm, elbow, forearm, wrist, hand, and fingers. The arm extends from the shoulder to the elbow.

SHOULDER GIRDLE. The proximal portion of the upper extremity is called the **shoulder girdle** and consists of three bones: the clavicle, the scapula, and the humerus (▼ Figure 4-19). The shoulder girdle is where the upper extremity attaches to the trunk. The upper extremity can move through a wide range of motion, allowing the hand to be placed in almost any position. This motion occurs at three joints within the shoulder girdle: the sternoclavicular joint, the acromioclavicular (A/C) joint, and the glenohumeral joint. Only slight motion occurs normally at the sternoclavicular and A/C joints. The ball-and-socket arrangement of the glenohumeral joint allows great freedom of motion in almost any direction.

The clavicle is a long, slender bone that lies just under the skin and provides support for the upper extremity. The clavicle is palpable through its entire length from the sternum to its attachment to the scapula. Its medial end is attached by very strong ligaments to the manubrium of the sternum to form the sternoclavicular joint. Its lateral end forms a joint with the acromion process of the scapula to create the A/C joint.

The scapula is a large, flat, triangular bone that overlies the posterior wall of the thorax and is surrounded by large muscles. Because of these muscles, only small parts of this bone are palpable. The scapula has two specially named regions that form joints with the clavicle and the humerus. The acromion process in the front forms part of the A/C joint. The glenoid fossa joins with the humeral head to form the glenohumeral joint. The spine and medial border of the scapula can be seen and palpated posteriorly. The acromion process forms the rounded edge of the shoulder girdle. You can feel this if you slowly move your finger along the clavicle and across the A/C joint.

ARM. The supporting bone of the arm is the **humerus**. Its long, straight shaft serves as an effective lever for heavy lifting. As in the thigh, there are few bony landmarks in the arm because it is covered by large muscles: the **biceps** in the front and the **triceps** in the back. The head of the humerus is covered by muscles that form the rounded prominence of the shoulder girdle laterally. The distal end articulates with both the radius and ulna at the elbow joint (▶ Figure 4-20).

The humerus joins with the radius and ulna to form the elbow, which is a relatively simple hinge joint. You can easily see and feel three prominences on the back of the elbow: the medial and lateral condyles of the humerus and the olecranon process of the ulna.

FOREARM. The forearm is composed of the radius and the ulna. The **ulna** is larger in the proximal forearm, and the **radius** is larger in the distal forearm.

Figure 4-18 The surface landmarks of the foot and ankle include the medial malleolus, the calcaneus, and the phalanges.

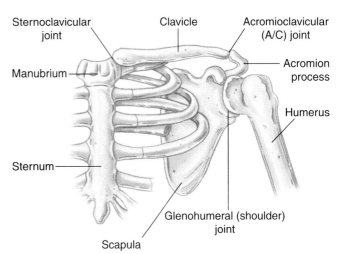

Figure 4-19 The bones of the shoulder girdle include the clavicle, the scapula, and the humerus.

The olecranon process of the ulna forms most of the elbow joint. The entire ulnar shaft from the tip of the olecranon process distally can be palpated, because it lies just under the skin on the back of the forearm. The radius is covered by muscles and cannot be palpated except in the lower third of the forearm, where it enlarges to form a major portion of the wrist joint. The radius rotates about the ulna, which allows the palm of the hand to turn up or down. At the wrist, the ends of the radius and ulna (the styloid processes) lie directly under the skin and can be easily palpated. The radial styloid is slightly longer than the ulnar styloid. The radius lies on the lateral, or thumb, side of the forearm, and the ulna is on the medial or little finger side.

WRIST AND HAND. The wrist is a modified ball-and-socket joint formed by the ends of the radius and ulna and several small wrist bones (▼ **Figure 4-21**). There are eight bones in the wrist, called carpal bones. Extending from the carpal bones are five metacarpals, which serve as a base for each of the five fingers or digits. The **carpometacarpal joint** (thumb joint) is a modified ball-and-socket joint that allows the thumb to rotate as well as to flex and extend. The other joints in the hand are simple hinge joints. In the thumb, there are two

bones beyond the metacarpal: the proximal and distal phalanges. The remaining four digits of the hand are named in order: the index, middle, ring, and little finger. Each of these contains three phalanges.

Joints

Wherever two bones come in contact, a **joint (articulation)** is formed. A joint consists of the ends of the bones that make up the joint and the surrounding connecting and supporting tissue (▶ **Figure 4-22**). Most joints in the body are named by combining the names of the two bones that form that joint. For example, the sternoclavicular joint is the articulation between the sternum and the clavicle. Most joints allow motion—for example, the knee, hip, or elbow—whereas some bones fuse with one another at joints to form a solid, immobile, bony structure. For instance, the skull is composed of several bones that fuse as a child grows. An infant, whose skull bones are not yet fused, has fontanels (soft spots) between the bones. The fontanels close as the bones fuse together when the infant's skull reaches the adult size. Some joints have slight, limited motion in which the bone ends are held together by fibrous tissue. Such a joint is called a symphysis.

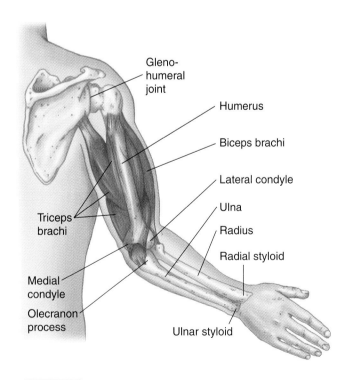

Figure 4-20 The principal bones in the arm and forearm include the humerus, the radius, and the ulna.

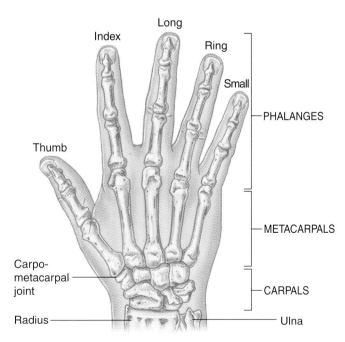

Figure 4-21 The principal bones in the wrist and hand include the carpals, the metacarpals, and the phalanges.

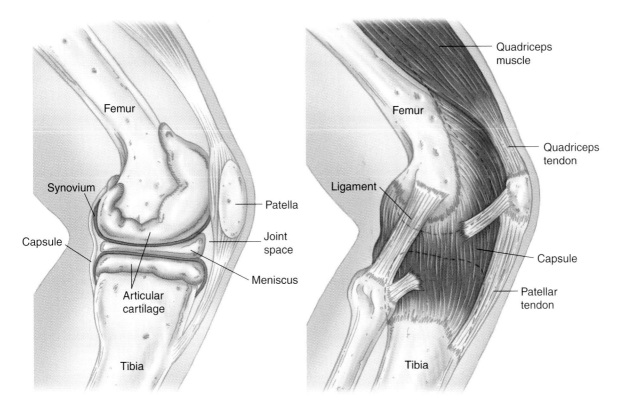

Figure 4-22   A joint consists of bone ends, the fibrous joint capsule, and ligaments. The degree to which a joint can move is determined by how the ligaments hold the bone ends and by the configuration of the bones themselves.

The bone ends of a joint are held together by a fibrous sac with a synovial lining, called the **joint capsule**. At certain points around the circumference of the joint, the capsule is lax and thin so that motion can occur. In other areas, it is quite thick and resists stretching or bending. These bands of tough, thick tissue are called **ligaments**. A joint such as the sacroiliac joint that is virtually surrounded by tough, thick ligaments will have little motion, whereas a joint such as the shoulder, with few ligaments, will be free to move in almost any direction (and will, as a result, be more prone to dislocation).

The degree of freedom of motion of a joint is determined by the extent to which the ligaments hold the bone ends together and also by the configuration of the bone ends themselves. The shoulder joint is a **ball-and-socket joint**, which allows rotation as well as bending (►**Figure 4-23**). The finger joints and the knee are **hinge joints**, with motion restricted to one plane (► **Figure 4-24**). They can only **flex** (bend) and **extend** (straighten). Rotation is not possible because of the shape of the joint surfaces and the strong restraining ligaments on both sides of the joint. Thus, although the amount of motion varies from joint to joint, all joints have a definite limit beyond which motion cannot

occur. When a joint is forced beyond this limit, damage to some structure must occur. Either the bones that form the joint will break, or the supporting capsule and ligaments will be disrupted.

The Musculoskeletal System

The human body is a well-designed system whose form, upright posture, and movement are provided by the **musculoskeletal system.** As its combination form suggests, the term musculoskeletal refers to the bones and voluntary muscles of the body. The musculoskeletal system also protects the vital internal organs of the body.

Figure 4-23   The shoulder is a ball-and-socket joint.

Figure 4-24   The knee joints are hinge joints, which allow motion in only one plane.

Muscles are a form of tissue that allows body movement. Although there are more than 600 muscles in the musculoskeletal system, they are generally divided into three types: skeletal, smooth, and cardiac ▼ Figure 4-25 .

Skeletal Muscle

<u>Skeletal muscle</u>, so named because it attaches to the bones of the skeleton, forms the major muscle mass of the body. It is also called <u>voluntary muscle</u>, because all skeletal muscle is under direct voluntary control of the brain and can be stimulated to contract or relax at will. Skeletal muscle is also called <u>striated muscle</u>, because when viewed under the microscope, it has characteristic stripes (striations). All body movement results from skeletal muscle contraction or relaxation. Usually, a specific motion is the result of several muscles contracting and relaxing simultaneously.

All skeletal muscles are supplied with arteries, veins, and nerves ▼ Figure 4-26 . Arterial blood brings oxygen

and nutrients to the muscle, and the veins carry away the waste products of muscular contraction (carbon dioxide and water). Muscles cannot function without this ongoing supply of oxygen and nutrients and removal of waste products. Muscle cramps result when insufficient oxygen or food is carried to the muscle or when acidic waste products accumulate and are not carried away.

Skeletal muscle is under the direct control of the nervous system and responds to a command from the brain to move a specific body part. Specific nerves pass directly from the brain to the spinal cord. There, they connect with other nerves that exit from the spinal cord and pass to each skeletal muscle. Electrical impulses are carried from the cells in the brain and spinal cord along the peripheral nerves to each muscle, signaling it to contract. When this normal nerve supply is lost through injury to the brain, spinal cord, or peripheral nerves, the voluntary control of the muscle is lost, and the muscle becomes paralyzed.

Most skeletal muscles attach directly to bone by tough, ropelike cords of fibrous tissue called tendons, which continue the fascia that covers all skeletal muscles. The fascia is much like the skin of a sausage in that it encases the muscle tissue. At either end of the muscle,

Cardiac muscle

Skeletal muscle

Smooth muscle

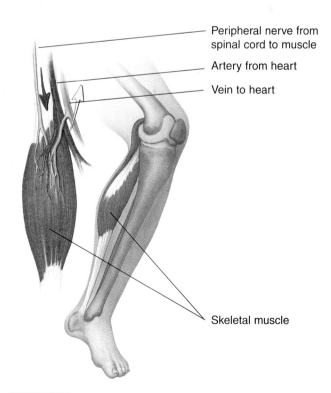

Peripheral nerve from spinal cord to muscle

Artery from heart

Vein to heart

Skeletal muscle

Figure 4-25 The three types of muscles are skeletal, smooth, and cardiac.

Figure 4-26 All skeletal muscles are supplied with arteries, veins, and nerves.

the fascia extends beyond the muscle to attach to a bone. This musculotendinous unit crosses a joint and is responsible for the motion of that joint. The proximal point of attachment of the musculotendinous unit is its origin, and the distal bony attachment is called the insertion of the muscle. When a muscle contracts, a line of force is created between the origin and the insertion, which pulls the points of origin and insertion closer together (▼ **Figure 4-27**). This motion occurs at the joint between the two bones.

Smooth Muscle

<u>Smooth muscle</u> carries out much of the automatic work of the body; therefore, it is also called **involuntary muscle**. Smooth muscle is found in the walls of most tubular structures of the body, such as the gastro-intestinal tract, the urinary system, the blood vessels, and the bronchi of the lungs. Contraction and relax-ation of smooth muscle propel or control the flow of the contents of these structures along their course. For example, the rhythmic contraction and relaxation

of the smooth muscles of the wall of the intestine propel ingested food through it, and smooth muscle in the walls of a blood vessel can alter the diameter of the vessel to control the amount of blood flowing through it (▼ **Figure 4-28**).

Smooth muscle responds only to primitive stimuli such as stretching, heat, or the need to relieve waste. An individual cannot exert any voluntary control over this type of muscle.

Cardiac Muscle

The heart is a large muscle composed of a pair of pumps of unequal force: one of lower pressure and one of higher pressure. The heart must function contin-uously from birth to death. It is a specially adapted involuntary muscle with a very rich blood supply and its own electrical system, which makes it different from both skeletal and smooth muscle. Another difference is that cardiac muscle has the property of "automaticity," which means that the heart muscle can set its own rhythm and rate without influence from the brain. This property is unique to heart muscle. Cardiac muscle can tolerate an interruption of its blood supply for only a few seconds. It requires a continuous supply of oxygen and glucose for normal function. Because of its special structure and function, cardiac muscle is placed in a separate category.

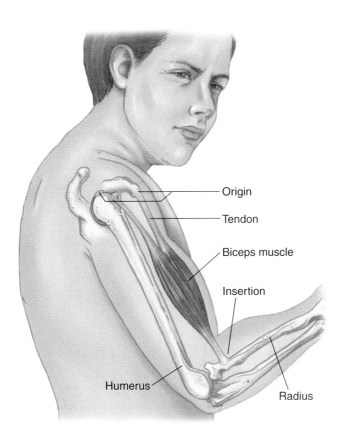

Figure 4-27   The biceps muscle causes the elbow to bend when it contracts. Note the points of tendon origin and insertion. As the muscle contracts and shortens, these points are pulled closer together, with motion occurring at the elbow joint.

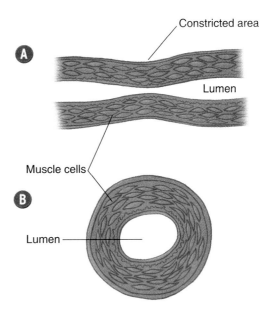

Figure 4-28   **A.** Smooth muscle lines the walls of the tubular struc-tures of the body. **B.** Contraction of the muscles narrows the diam-eter of the structure, and relaxation allows the diameter to increase in size.

The Respiratory System

The **respiratory system** consists of all the structures of the body that contribute to respiration, or the process of breathing (▼ **Figure 4-29**). It includes the nose, mouth, throat, larynx, trachea, and bronchi, which are all air passages or airways. The system also includes the lungs, where oxygen is passed into the blood and where carbon dioxide is removed from the blood to be exhaled. Finally, the respiratory system includes the diaphragm, the muscles of the chest wall, and the accessory muscles of breathing, which permit normal respiratory movement. In this text, the term "airway" usually refers to the upper airway or the passage above the larynx (voice box).

The function of the respiratory system is to provide the body with oxygen and eliminate carbon dioxide. The exchange of oxygen and carbon dioxide takes place in the lungs and in the tissues. It is a complicated process that occurs automatically unless the airways or the lungs become diseased or damaged.

The Upper Airway

The structures of the upper airway are located anteriorly and at the midline. The upper airway includes the nose, mouth, and throat. The nose and mouth lead to the oropharynx (throat). The nostrils lead to the **nasopharynx** (above the roof of the mouth, or soft palate), and the mouth leads to the oropharynx. The lining of the nasopharynx gives off watery secretions and helps to moisten the air as we breathe. Air enters through the mouth more rapidly and directly. As a result, it is less moist than air that enters through the nose.

Two passageways are located at the bottom of the pharynx: the esophagus behind and the trachea (windpipe) in front. Food and liquids enter the pharynx and pass into the esophagus, which carries them to the stomach. Air and other gases enter the trachea and go to the lungs.

Protecting the opening of the trachea is a thin, leaf-shaped valve called the **epiglottis.** This valve allows air to pass into the trachea but prevents food or liquid from entering the airway under normal circumstances.

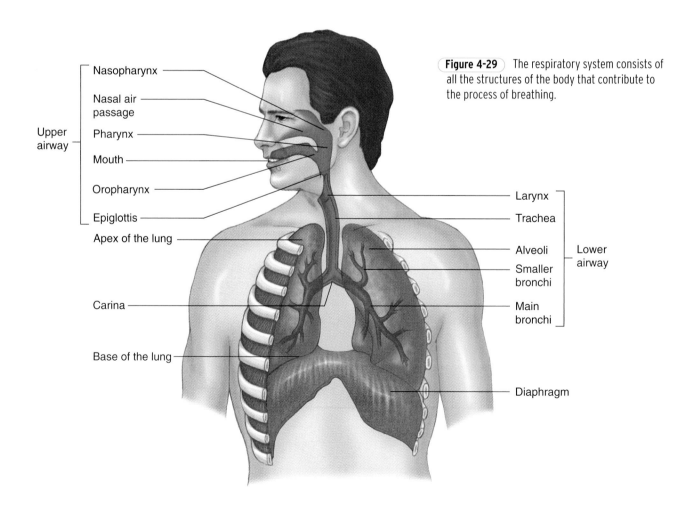

Figure 4-29 The respiratory system consists of all the structures of the body that contribute to the process of breathing.

Air moves past the epiglottis into the larynx and the trachea.

The Lower Airway

The first part of the lower airway is the larynx, a rather complex arrangement of tiny bones, cartilage, muscles, and the two vocal cords. The larynx does not tolerate any foreign solid or liquid material. A violent episode of coughing and spasm of the vocal cords will result from contact with solids or liquids.

The Adam's apple, or thyroid cartilage, is easily seen in the middle of the front of the neck. The thyroid cartilage is actually the anterior part of the larynx. Tiny muscles open and close the vocal cords and control tension on them. Sounds are created as air is forced past the vocal cords, making them vibrate. These vibrations make the sound. The pitch of the sound changes as the cords open and close. You can feel the vibrations if you place your fingers lightly on the larynx as you speak or sing. The vibrations of air are shaped by the tongue and muscles of the mouth to form understandable sounds. Immediately below the thyroid cartilage is the palpable cricoid cartilage.

Between these two prominences lies the cricothyroid membrane, which can be felt as a depression in the midline of the neck just inferior to the thyroid cartilage. Below the cricoid cartilage is the trachea. The trachea is approximately 5″ long and is a semirigid, enclosed air tube made up of rings of cartilage that are open in the back. This enables food to pass through the esophagus, which lies right behind the trachea. The rings of cartilage keep the trachea from collapsing when air moves into and out of the lungs. The trachea ends at the carina and divides into smaller tubes. These tubes are the right and left main bronchi, which enter the lungs. Each main bronchus immediately branches within the lung into smaller and smaller airways. Within the right lung, three major bronchi are formed. Within the left, there are only two. Each bronchus supplies air to one lobe of the lung.

Lungs

The two lungs are held in place within the chest by the trachea, the arteries and veins that run to and from the heart, and the pulmonary ligaments. Each lung is divided into lobes. The right lung has three lobes: the upper, middle, and lower lobes. The left lung has an upper lobe and a lower lobe. Each lobe is divided further into segments. Also within each lung, the main bronchi divide until they end in very fine airways called bronchioles. The bronchioles end in about 700 million tiny grapelike sacs called **alveoli** (▼ **Figure 4-30**).

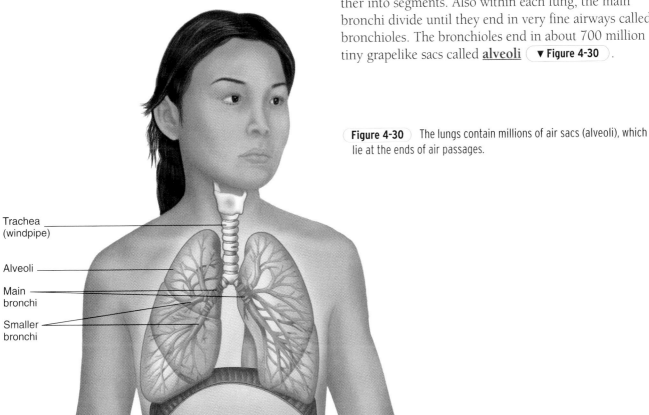

(**Figure 4-30**)   The lungs contain millions of air sacs (alveoli), which lie at the ends of air passages.

Trachea (windpipe)

Alveoli

Main bronchi

Smaller bronchi

The exchange of oxygen and carbon dioxide occurs within these alveoli. The walls of the alveoli contain a network of tiny blood vessels (pulmonary capillaries) that carry the carbon dioxide from the body to the lungs and the oxygen from the lungs to the body.

The lungs cannot expand and contract themselves because they have no muscle. There is, however, a very definite mechanism to ensure that they follow the motion of the chest wall and expand or contract with it. Covering each lung is a layer of very smooth, glistening tissue called **pleura** (▼ Figure 4-31). Another layer of pleura lines the inside of the chest cavity. The two layers are called parietal pleura (lining the chest wall) and visceral pleura (covering the lungs).

Between the parietal pleura and the visceral pleura is the **pleural space**, called a "potential" space rather than an actual space in the usual sense because normally these layers are in close contact everywhere. In fact, the layers are sealed tightly against one another by a thin film of fluid. When the chest wall expands, the lung is pulled with it and made to expand by the force exerted through these closely applied pleural surfaces. Normally, the pleural space is quite small and contains only the thin film of pleural fluid as each lung entirely fills its chest cavity.

Diaphragm

The diaphragm is unique because it has characteristics of both voluntary (skeletal) and involuntary (smooth) muscle. It is a dome-shaped muscle that divides the thorax from the abdomen and is pierced by the great vessels and the esophagus (▼ Figure 4-32). Under the microscope, it has striations like skeletal muscle. Also, it is attached to the costal arch and the lumbar vertebrae like other skeletal muscles. Thus, in many ways, it looks like a voluntary muscle; however, we do not have complete voluntary control over its function. It acts like a voluntary muscle whenever we take a deep breath, cough, or hold our breath. We control these variations in the way we breathe.

However, unlike other skeletal or voluntary muscles, the diaphragm performs an automatic function. Breathing continues while we sleep and at all other times. Even though we can hold our breath or temporarily breathe faster or slower, we cannot continue these variations in breathing pattern indefinitely. Ultimately, when the concentration of carbon dioxide is close to being disturbed, automatic regulation of breathing resumes. Therefore, although the diaphragm looks like voluntary skeletal muscle and is attached to the skeleton, it behaves, for the most part, like an involuntary muscle.

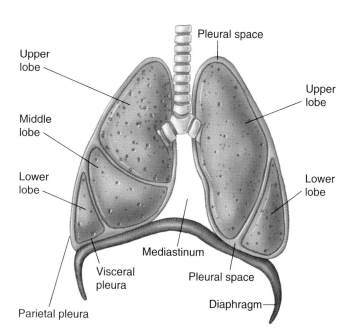

Figure 4-31 The pleura lining the chest wall and covering the lungs is an essential part of the breathing mechanism. The pleural space is not an actual space until blood or air leaks into it, causing the pleural surfaces to separate.

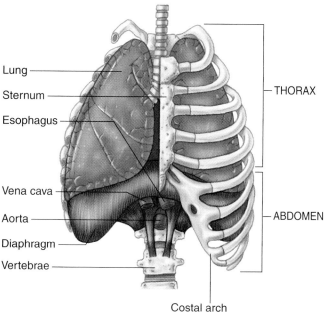

Figure 4-32 The dome-shaped diaphragm divides the thorax from the abdomen. It is pierced by the great vessels and the esophagus.

blood from the left ventricle through the body and back to the right atrium. In the systemic circulation, as blood passes through the tissues and organs, it gives up oxygen and nutrients and absorbs cellular wastes and carbon dioxide. The cellular wastes are eliminated in passages through the liver and the kidneys. The pulmonary circulation, the circuit in the lungs, carries oxygen-poor blood from the right ventricle through the lungs and back to the left atrium. In the pulmonary circulation, as blood passes through the lungs, it is refreshed with oxygen and gives up carbon dioxide.

Heart

The **heart** is a hollow muscular organ approximately the size of an adult's clenched fist. It is made of a unique, adapted tissue called cardiac muscle or **myocardium** and actually works as two paired pumps, the one on the left side being more muscular. A wall called the septum divides the heart down the middle into right and left sides. Each side of the heart is divided again into an upper chamber (**atrium**) and a lower chamber (**ventricle**).

The heart is an involuntary muscle. As such, it is under the control of the autonomic nervous system. However, it has its own electrical system and continues to function even without its central nervous system control. It is distinct from skeletal or smooth muscle in its requirement for a continuous supply of oxygen and nutrients.

The heart must function continuously from birth to death and has developed special adaptations to meet the needs of this continuous function. It can tolerate a serious interruption of its own blood supply for only a very few seconds before the signs of a heart attack develop. Thus, its blood supply is as rich and well distributed as possible.

HOW THE HEART WORKS. The heart receives the first blood distribution from the aorta. The two main coronary arteries have their openings immediately above the aortic valve at the beginning of the aorta where the pressures are highest ◄ **Figure 4-37** .

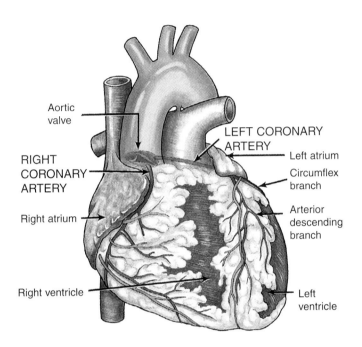

Figure 4-37   The two main coronary arteries supply the heart with blood.

Figure 4-38   **A.** The right side, or lower pressure side, of the heart pumps blood from the body to the lungs.   **B.** The left side, or higher pressure side, of the heart pumps oxygen-rich blood to all parts of the body.

The right side of the heart receives blood from the veins of the body (◀ **Figure 4-38A**). The blood enters from the superior and inferior venae cavae into the right atrium, then fills the right ventricle passing through a valve that closes to prevent backflow after the right atrial muscle contracts. Contraction of the right ventricle causes blood to flow into the pulmonary artery and the pulmonary circulation.

The left side receives oxygenated blood from the lungs through the pulmonary veins into the left atrium where it passes through a valve into the left ventricle (◀ **Figure 4-38B**). Contraction of this most muscular of the pumping chambers pumps the blood into the aorta and then to the arteries of the body.

The exit of each of the four heart chambers is governed by a one-way valve. The valves prevent the backflow of blood and keep it moving through the circulatory system in the proper direction. When a valve controlling the filling of a heart chamber is open, the other valve allowing it to empty is shut and vice versa. Normally, blood moves in only one direction through the entire system.

When a ventricle contracts, the valve to the artery opens, and the valve between the ventricle and atrium closes. Blood is forced from the ventricle out into the pulmonary artery or aorta. At the end of contraction, the ventricle relaxes. Backpressure causes the valve to the artery to close, and the entry valve to the ventricle opens as the ventricle relaxes. Blood then flows from the atrium into the ventricle. When the ventricle is stimulated to contract, the cycle is repeated.

NORMAL HEARTBEAT. In the normal adult, the heartbeat may range from 50 to 180 beats/min, depending on the level of activity. A very well-conditioned athlete may have a normal resting **heart rate** (**pulse**) of 50 to 60 beats/ min. During vigorous physical activity, the heart rate may rise normally to as fast as 180 beats/ min. The usual adult resting heart rate is between 60 and 100 beats/min (▶ **Table 4-4**). At each beat, 70 to 80 mL of blood is ejected from the adult heart. In one minute, the entire blood volume of 5 to 6 L is circulated through all the vessels.

ELECTRICAL CONDUCTION SYSTEM. A network of specialized tissue that is capable of conducting electrical current runs throughout the heart (▼ **Figure 4-39**). The flow of electrical current through this network causes smooth, coordinated contractions of the heart. These contractions produce the pumping action of the heart. Each mechanical contraction of the heart is associated with two electrical processes. The first is depolarization, during which the electrical charges on the surface of the muscle cell change from positive to negative. The second is repolarization, during which the heart returns to its resting state and the positive charge is restored to the surface.

When the heart is working normally, the electrical impulse begins high in the atria at the sinoatrial (SA)

TABLE 4-4 Normal Heart Rates	
Adults	60 to 100 beats/min
Children	80 to 100 beats/min
Toddlers	100 to 120 beats/min
Newborns	120 to 140 beats/min

(**Figure 4-39**) Electrical current flows through the heart to produce its pumping action.

SINOATRIAL (SA) NODE (pacemaker)

Internodal bundles

ATRIOVENTRICULAR (AV) NODE

Purkinje fibers

Interatrial bundle

Purkinje fibers

Right and left branches of AV bundle

AV-node 40 to 60 beats per minute

node, then travels to the atrioventricular (AV) node, and moves through the Purkinje fibers to the ventricles. This movement produces a smooth flow of electricity through the heart, which depolarizes the muscle and produces a coordinated pumping contraction. The heart's electrical system becomes disturbed if part of the heart is oxygen deficient, is injured, or dies. As a result, the heart may not continue to beat properly. Blood pressure decreases, and a patient may lose consciousness.

Arteries

The arteries carry blood from the heart to all body tissues ▶ **Figure 4-40** . They branch into smaller arteries and then into arterioles. The arterioles, in turn, branch into smaller vessels until they connect to the vast network of capillaries. The walls of an artery are made of fine, circular muscle tissue. Some arteries even have elastic tissue.

Arteries contract to accommodate loss of blood volume and also to increase blood pressure. Blood is supplied to tissues as they need it. For example, the digestive system is supplied with more blood after you eat a meal. The leg muscles are more heavily supplied when jogging. Some tissues need a constant blood supply, especially the heart, the kidneys, and the brain. Other tissues, such as the muscles in the extremities, the skin, and intestines, can function with less blood when at rest.

The **aorta** is the principal artery leaving the left side of the heart; it carries freshly oxygenated blood to the body. This blood vessel is found just in front of the spine in the chest and abdominal cavities. The aorta has many branches that supply the heart, head, neck, arms, and abdominal and thoracic organs before it ends in the lower abdomen. It divides at the level of the umbilicus into the two common iliac arteries that lead to the lower extremities. All of the aorta's branches ultimately become arterioles leading into the body's capillary network.

The **pulmonary artery** begins at the right side of the heart and carries oxygen-poor blood to the lungs. It divides into finer and finer branches until it meets with the pulmonary capillary system located in the thin walls of the alveoli. These arteries are the only ones in the body that carry oxygen-poor blood.

Figure 4-40 The principal arteries supply blood to a vast network of smaller arteries and arterioles, which nourish the tissue cells via the capillaries. Venules deliver oxygen-poor blood to the veins that return blood to the heart.

The **carotid artery** is the major artery that supplies blood to the head and brain. The carotid arteries are located on both sides of the neck. You can easily feel the carotid pulse if you place your fingers at the anterior lateral part of the neck. Since the carotid artery is rather close to the heart, you can feel its pulse even after the pulse in the distal extremities is too weak to feel.

The **femoral artery** is the major artery that supplies blood to the lower extremities. It is palpable in the groin. It divides at the level of the knee and supplies blood to the leg. At the ankle, two of these branches are palpable. You can feel a pulse at the **posterior tibial artery**, which is behind the medial prominence of the ankle (medial malleolus). You can also feel a pulse at the **dorsalis pedis artery** on the anterior surface of the foot (dorsum of the foot).

The **brachial artery** is the major vessel in the upper extremity that supplies blood to the arm. It divides into two major branches just below the elbow. This is the artery that is used in assessing blood pressure with a blood pressure cuff and stethoscope.

The **radial artery** is the major artery in the forearm and is palpable at the wrist on the thumb side (radial side). The **ulnar artery** is also palpable at the wrist on the opposite side (ulnar side, at the base of the fifth finger), although its pulse is not as strong. Both of these arteries supply blood to the hand.

Arteries branch into smaller arteries and then into arterioles. **Arterioles** are the smallest branches of an artery leading to the vast network of capillaries.

Capillaries

In the body, there are billions of cells and billions of capillaries. **Capillary vessels** are fine end-divisions of the arterial system that allow contact between cells of the body tissues and the plasma and the red blood cells. At this level, each individual cell of the body lives. Oxygen and other nutrients pass from blood cells and plasma in the capillaries to the individual tissue cells through the very thin wall of the capillary. Carbon dioxide and other metabolic waste products pass in a reverse direction from the tissue cells to the blood to be carried away. Blood in arteries is characteristically bright red, because its hemoglobin is rich in oxygen. Blood in the veins is dark bluish red, because it has passed through a capillary bed and given up its oxygen to the cells. Capillaries connect directly at one end with the flow-regulating arterioles and at the other with the venules.

Veins

Oxygen-poor blood from the capillary system next moves to the venules, which are the smallest branches of the veins (Figure 4-40). The veins then return blood to the heart.

Once blood passes through the network of capillaries and moves through the venules, it returns to the heart via a network of larger and larger veins (see Figure 4-40). Veins have much thinner walls than arteries and are generally larger in diameter. The veins becomes larger and larger and ultimately form two major vessels. These major vessels, part of the great vessels, are located in the midline, just to the left of the spine, and channel blood from the body and collect it just before it enters the heart.

The **superior vena cava** carries blood returning from the head, neck, shoulders, and upper extremities. Blood from the abdomen, pelvis, and lower extremities passes through the **inferior vena cava**. The superior and inferior venae join at the right atrium of the heart. The right ventricle receives blood from the right atrium and pumps it through the pulmonary arteries into the lungs.

The **pulmonary veins** carry oxygen-rich blood from the lungs to the left atrium. The oxygenated blood from the lungs enters the four pulmonary veins that unite at the left atrium. It then passes to the left ventricle and is pumped to the body again.

Components of Blood

Blood is a complex, thick, red fluid composed of plasma, red blood cells called erythrocytes, white blood cells called leukocytes, and platelets (▶ **Figure 4-41**).

- **Plasma** is a sticky, yellow fluid that carries the blood cells and nutrients. It also transports cellular waste material to the organs of excretion. It contains most of the compounds needed to produce a blood clot.

- The iron-containing hemoglobin molecules in **red blood cells** (erythrocytes) give color to the blood and carry oxygen.

- **White blood cells** (leukocytes) play a role in the body's immune defense mechanisms against infection.

- **Platelets** are tiny, disk-shaped elements that are much smaller than the cells. They are essential in the initial formation of a blood clot, the mechanism that stops bleeding.

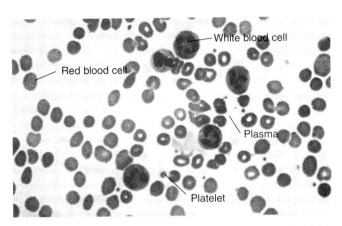

Figure 4-41   The components of blood include red blood cells, white blood cells, platelets, and plasma.

Blood under pressure will gush or spurt intermittently from an artery and is bright red. From a vein, it will flow in a steady stream and is dark bluish-red. From capillaries, it will ooze at many tiny individual points. Clotting normally takes from 6 to 10 minutes.

Physiology of the Circulatory System

The **pulse**, which is palpated most easily at the neck, wrist, or groin, is created by the forceful pumping of blood out the left ventricle and into the major arteries. It is present throughout the entire arterial system. It can be felt most easily where the larger arteries are near the skin. The central pulses are the carotid artery pulse, which can be felt at the upper portion of the neck, »and the femoral artery pulse, which is felt in the groin. The peripheral pulses are the radial artery pulse, which is felt at the wrist at the base of the thumb; the brachial artery pulse, which is felt on the medial aspect of the arm, midway between the elbow and shoulder; the posterior artery pulse, which is felt posterior to the medial malleolus; and the dorsalis pedis artery pulse, which is felt on the top of the foot ▶ **Figure 4-42** .

Blood pressure is the pressure that the blood exerts against the walls of the arteries as it passes through them. When the cardiac muscle of the left ventricle contracts, it pumps blood from the ventricle into the aorta. This muscular contraction phase is called **systole**. When the muscle of the ventricle relaxes, the ventricle fills with blood. This phase is called **diastole**. The pulsed forceful ejection of blood from the left ventricle of the heart into the aorta is transmitted through the arteries as a pulsatile pressure wave. This pressure wave keeps the blood moving through the body. The high and low points of the wave can be measured with a sphygmomanometer (blood pressure cuff) and are expressed numerically

in millimeters of mercury (mm Hg). The high point is called the systolic blood pressure (measured as the heart muscle is contracting). The low point is called the diastolic blood pressure (measured when the heart muscle is in its relaxation phase).

The average adult has approximately 6 L of blood in the vascular system. Children have less, 2 to 3 L, depending on their age and size. Infants have only about 300 mL. The loss of an amount of blood that may be negligible for an adult could be fatal for an infant.

NORMAL CIRCULATION IN ADULTS. In all healthy people, the circulatory system is automatically adjusted and readjusted constantly so that 100% of the capacity of the arteries, veins, and capillaries holds 100% of the blood at that moment. Never are all the vessels fully dilated or constricted. The size of arteries and veins is controlled by the nervous system, according to the amount of blood that is available and many other factors to keep blood pressure normal at all times. Under the condition of normal pressure, with a system that can hold just 100% of the blood available, all parts of the system will have adequate blood supply all of the time.

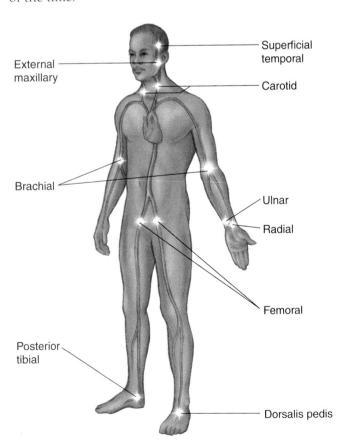

Figure 4-42   The central and peripheral pulses can be felt where the large arteries are near the skin.

<u>Perfusion</u> is the circulation of blood within an organ or tissue in adequate amounts to meet the cells' current needs. Blood enters an organ or tissue through the arteries and leaves it through the veins (▼ Figure 4-43). Loss of normal blood pressure is an indication that the blood is no longer circulating efficiently to every organ in the body. There are many reasons for loss of blood pressure. The result in each case is the same: Organs, tissues, and cells are no longer adequately perfused or supplied with oxygen and food, and wastes can accumulate. Under these conditions, cells, tissues, and whole organs may die. The state of inadequate circulation, when it involves the entire body, is called shock or hypoperfusion.

INADEQUATE CIRCULATION IN ADULTS. When a patient loses a small amount of blood, the arteries, veins, and heart automatically adjust to the smaller new volume. The adjustment occurs in an effort to maintain adequate pressure throughout the circulatory system and thereby maintain circulation for every organ. The adjustment occurs very rapidly after the loss, usually within minutes. Specifically, the vessels constrict to

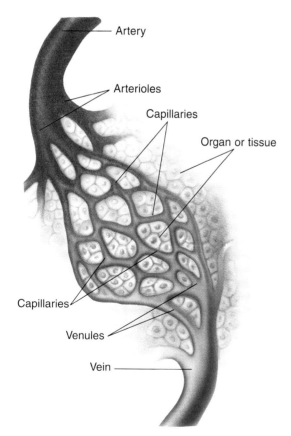

Figure 4-43 Blood enters an organ or tissue through the arteries and leaves through the veins. This process, called perfusion, provides adequate blood flow to the tissues to meet the cell's needs.

provide a smaller bed for the reduced volume of blood to fill. And the heart pumps more rapidly to circulate the remaining blood more efficiently. As the blood pressure falls, the pulse increases to attempt to keep the cardiac output constant at 5 to 6 L per minute. If the loss of blood is too great, the adjustment fails, and the patient goes into shock.

The Nervous System

The <u>nervous system</u> controls virtually all activities of the body, both voluntary and involuntary. The <u>somatic nervous system</u> is the part of the nervous system that regulates activities over which there is voluntary control. Such activities include walking, talking, and writing. The <u>autonomic nervous system</u> controls the many body functions that occur without voluntary control. These activities include body functions such as digestion, dilation and constriction of blood vessels, sweating, and all other involuntary actions that are necessary for basic body functions. Anatomically, the nervous system is divided into two parts: the central nervous system and the peripheral nervous system. Thus, the nervous system as a whole can be divided anatomically into the central and peripheral nervous systems, and functionally into somatic (voluntary) and autonomic (involuntary) components.

The Central Nervous System

The <u>central nervous system (CNS)</u> is made up of the brain and the spinal cord. From a practical point of view, the central nervous system can be considered the part of the nervous system that is covered and protected by bones. The brain is covered by the skull, and the spinal cord is covered by the spinal column. The major parts of most nerve cells (the nucleus and the cell body) lie within the central nervous system.

BRAIN. The <u>brain</u> is the controlling organ of the body. It is the center of consciousness. It is responsible for all our voluntary body activities, the perception of our surroundings, and the control of our reactions to the environment. In addition, the brain enables us to experience all the fine shadings of thought and feeling that make us individuals. The brain is subdivided into several areas, all of which have specific functions. Three major subdivisions of the brain are the cerebrum, the cerebellum, and the brain stem (▶ Figure 4-44).

The <u>cerebrum</u>, which is the largest part of the brain and is sometimes called the "gray matter," makes up

CEREBRUM

BRAINSTEM

CEREBELLUM

(handwritten annotations: "Major Motor", "function to live", "Fine motor control for cerebrum")

Figure 4-44 The brain lies well protected within the skull. Its principal subdivisions are the cerebrum, the cerebellum, and the brain stem.

about three fourths of the volume of the brain and is itself composed of four lobes: frontal, parietal, temporal, and occipital. The cerebrum on one side of the brain controls activities on the opposite side of the body. Each lobe of the cerebrum is responsible for a specific function. For example, one group of brain cells in the frontal lobe is responsible for the activity of all the voluntary muscles of the body. Brain cells in this area generate impulses that are sent along nerve fibers that extend from each cell into the spinal cord. Another area in the parietal lobe has cells that receive sensory impulses from the peripheral nerves of the body. Other parts of the cerebrum are responsible for other body functions. For instance, the occipital region, on the back of the cerebrum, receives visual impulses for the eyes; other areas control hearing, balance, and speech. Still other parts of the cerebrum are responsible for emotions and other characteristics of an individual's personality.

The **cerebellum**, which is located underneath the great mass of cerebral tissue, is sometimes called the "little brain." The major function of this area is to coordinate the various activities of the brain, particularly body movements. Without the cerebellum, very specialized muscular activities such as writing or sewing would be impossible.

The **brain stem** is so called because the brain appears to be sitting on this portion of the central nervous system as a plant sits on its stem. The brain stem is the most primitive part of the central nervous system. It lies deep within the cranium and is the best-protected part of the central nervous system. The brain stem is the controlling center for virtually all body functions that are absolutely necessary for life. Cells in this part of the brain control cardiac, respiratory, and other basic body functions.

The brain has many other anatomic areas, all of which have specific and important functions. The brain receives a vast amount of information from the environment, sorts it all out, and directs the body to respond appropriately. Many of the responses involve voluntary muscle action; others are automatic and involuntary.

SPINAL CORD. The spinal cord is the other major portion of the central nervous system ▶ **Figure 4-45** . Like the brain, the spinal cord contains nerve cell bodies, but the major portion of the spinal cord is made up of nerve fibers that extend from the cells of the brain. These nerve fibers transmit information to and from the brain. All the fibers join together just below the brain stem to form the spinal cord. The spinal cord exits through a large opening at the base of the skull called the foramen magnum. It is encased within the spinal canal down to the level of the second lumbar vertebra. The spinal canal is created by the vertebrae, stacked one on another. Each vertebra surrounds the cord, and together the vertebrae form the bony spinal canal.

The principal function of the spinal cord is to transmit messages between the brain and the body. These messages are passed along the nerve fibers as electrical impulses, just as messages are passed along a telephone cable. The nerve fibers are arranged in specific bundles within the spinal cord to carry the messages from one specific area of the body to the brain and back.

The Peripheral Nervous System

Many of the cells in the central nervous system have long fibers that extend from the cell body out through openings in the bony covering of the spinal canal to form a cable of nerve fibers that link the central nervous system to the various organs of the body. These cables of nerve fibers make up the **peripheral**

> The nervous system controls virtually all activities of the body, both voluntary and involuntary.

nervous system. The three major types of nerves are sensory nerves, motor nerves, and connecting nerves. **Sensory nerves** carry information from the body to the central nervous system. **Motor nerves** carry information from the central nervous system to the muscles of the body. **Connecting nerves** do just what their name implies: They connect the sensory and motor nerves.

The peripheral nervous system is composed of 31 pairs of peripheral nerves called spinal nerves and 12 pairs called cranial nerves. At each vertebral level from the first cervical to the fifth sacral, on each side of the spinal cord, a spinal nerve exits the spinal cord and passes through an opening in the bony canal. This spinal nerve is composed of nerve fibers from nerve cells that originate within the spinal cord. The nerve fibers conduct sensory impulses from the skin and other organs to the spinal cord. They also conduct motor impulses from the spinal cord to the muscles that are present in that segment of the body. For example, between the seventh and eighth ribs, the spinal nerve carries sensory fibers from the skin between those two ribs and also has motor nerve fibers to innervate the intercostal muscle between the seventh and eighth ribs. This specific arrangement of nerve fibers becomes more complex and confusing in both the cervical and lumbar regions because of the large number of muscles in the arms and legs that must be supplied with nerve fibers. The spinal nerves combine to form a complex nerve network (called a plexus) in these two areas: the brachial plexus for the upper extremity and the lumbosacral plexus for the lower extremity.

The 12 pairs of peripheral nerves that exit the brain through holes in the skull are called the cranial nerves. For the most part, they are very specialized nerves that provide specific functions. For example, the facial (seventh cranial) nerves send motor impulses to many of the facial muscles.

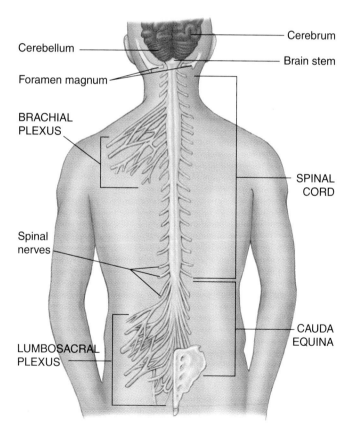

Figure 4-45 The spinal cord is a continuation of the brain stem. It exits the skull at the foramen magnum and extends down to the level of the second lumbar vertebra.

SENSORY NERVES. Sensory nerves of the body are quite complex. There are many different types of sensory cells in the nervous system. One type forms the retina of the eye; others are responsible for the hearing and balancing mechanisms in the ear. Other sensory cells are located within the skin, muscles, joints, lungs, and other organs of the body. When a sensory cell is stimulated, it transmits its own special message to the brain. There are special sensory nerves to detect heat, cold, position, motion, pressure, pain, balance, light, taste, and smell, as well as other sensations. Specialized nerve endings are adapted for each cell so that it perceives only one type of sensation and it transmits only that message.

The sensory impulses constantly provide information to the brain about what the different parts of our body are doing in relation to our surroundings. Thus, the brain is continuously made aware of its surroundings. The cranial nerves supply sensations directly to the brain. Visual sensations (what we see) reach the brain directly by way of the optic nerve (the second cranial nerve) in each eye. The nerve endings for the optic nerve lie in the retina of the eye. The nerve endings are stimulated by light, and the impulses are carried along the nerve that passes through a hole in the back of the eye socket and carries impulses to the occipital portion of the brain.

When sensory nerve endings in the extremities are stimulated, the impulses are transmitted along a peripheral nerve to the spinal cord. The cell body of the peripheral nerve lies in the spinal cord. The impulse is then transmitted from that cell body to another nerve ending in the spinal cord. The impulse is then sent up the spinal cord to the sensory area in the parietal lobe of the brain, where the sensory information can be interpreted and acted on by the brain.

MOTOR NERVES. Each muscle in the body has its own motor nerve. The cell body for each motor nerve lies in the spinal cord, and a fiber from the cell body extends as part of the peripheral nerve to its specific muscle. Electrical impulses that are produced by the cell body in the spinal cord are transmitted along the motor nerve to the muscle and cause it to contract. The cell body in the spinal cord is stimulated by an impulse produced in the motor strip of the cerebral cortex. This impulse is transmitted along the spinal cord to the cell body of the motor nerve.

CONNECTING NERVES. Within the brain and the spinal cord are cells with short fibers that connect the sensory nerves with the motor nerves. In the spinal cord, they connect the sensory and motor nerves directly,

Documentation Tips

Using correct anatomical terminology in your patient care report improves patient care by making the report more useful to hospital personnel and enhances your professional image as an EMT-B.

bypassing the brain. These connecting nerves allow sensory and motor impulses to be transmitted from one nerve to another within the central nervous system.

The connecting nerves in the spinal cord complete a reflex arc between the sensory and motor nerves of the limbs. An irritating stimulus to the sensory nerve, such as heat, will be transmitted from the sensory nerve along the connecting nerve directly to the motor nerve. This will stimulate the sensory nerve. The muscle responds promptly, withdrawing the limb from the irritating stimulus even before this information can be transmitted to the brain. When a physician taps your knee with a rubber hammer, he or she is testing to see whether your reflex arc is intact.

The Skin

The skin, the largest single organ in the body, serves three major functions: to protect the body in the environment, to regulate the temperature of the body, and to transmit information from the environment to the brain.

The protective functions of the skin are numerous. Over 70% of the body is composed of water. The water contains a delicate balance of chemical substances in solution. The skin is watertight and serves to keep this balanced internal solution intact. The skin also protects the body from the invasion of infectious organisms: bacteria, viruses, and fungi. These organisms are everywhere and are routinely found lying on the skin surface and deep in its grooves and glands. However, they never penetrate the skin unless it is broken by injury; thus, the skin provides a constant protection against outside invaders.

The energy of the body is derived from **metabolism** (chemical reactions) that must take place within a very narrow temperature range. If the body temperature is too low, these reactions cannot proceed, metabolism ceases, and the body dies. If the temperature becomes too high, the rate of metabolism increases. Dangerously high temperatures producing too high a metabolic rate can result in permanent tissue damage and death.

Functions of the Skin

The major organ for regulation of body temperature is the skin. Blood vessels in the skin constrict when the body is in a cold environment and dilate when the body is in a warm environment. In a cold environment, constriction of the blood vessels shunts the blood away from the skin to decrease the amount of heat radiated from the body surface. When the outside environment is hot, the vessels in the skin dilate, the skin becomes flushed or red, and heat radiates from the body surface.

Also, in the hot environment, sweat is secreted to the skin surface from the sweat glands. Evaporation of the sweat requires energy. This energy, as body heat, is taken from the body during the evaporation process, which causes the body temperature to fall. Sweating alone will not reduce body temperature; evaporation of the sweat must also occur.

Information from the environment is carried to the brain through a rich supply of sensory nerves that originate in the skin. Nerve endings that lie in the skin are adapted to perceive and transmit information about heat, cold, external pressure, pain, and the position of the body in space. The skin thus recognizes any changes in the environment. The skin also reacts to pressure, pain, and pleasurable stimuli.

Anatomy of the Skin

The skin is divided into two parts: the superficial epidermis, which is composed of several layers of cells, and the deeper dermis, which contains the specialized skin structures. Below the skin lies the subcutaneous tissue layer (▼ **Figure 4-46**). The cells of the epidermis are sealed to form a watertight protective covering for the body.

The **epidermis** is actually composed of several layers of cells. At the base of the epidermis is the germinal layer, which continuously produces new cells that gradually rise to the surface. On the way to the surface, these cells die and form the watertight covering. The epidermal cells are held together securely by an oily substance called sebum, which is secreted by the **sebaceous glands** of the dermis. The outermost cells of the epidermis are constantly rubbed away and then replaced by new cells produced by the germinal

EPIDERMIS

DERMIS

SUBCUTANEOUS TISSUE

Hair

Pore

Germinal layer of epidermis

Sebaceous gland

Nerve (sensory)

Sweat gland

Hair follicle

Blood vessel

Subcutaneous fat

Muscle fascia

Muscle

Figure 4-46   The skin has two principal layers: the epidermis and the dermis. Below the skin is a layer of subcutaneous tissue.

layer. The deeper cells in the germinal layer also contain pigment granules that (along with the blood vessels lying in the dermis) produce skin color.

The epidermis varies in thickness in different areas of the body. On the soles of the feet, the back, and the scalp, it is quite thick, but in some areas of the body, the epidermis is only two or three cell layers thick. The watertight seal provided by the epidermis prevents the invasion of bacteria and other organisms.

The deeper part of skin, the **dermis**, is separated from the epidermis by the layer of germinal cells. Within the dermis lie many of the special structures of the skin: sweat glands, sebaceous (oil) glands, hair follicles, blood vessels, and specialized nerve endings.

Sweat glands produce sweat for cooling the body. The sweat is discharged onto the surface of the skin through small pores, or ducts, that pass through the epidermis onto the skin surface. The sebaceous glands produce sebum, the oily material that seals the surface epidermal cells. The sebaceous glands lie next to hair follicles and secrete sebum along the hair follicle to the skin surface. In addition to providing waterproofing for the skin, sebum keeps the skin supple so that it does not crack.

Hair follicles are the small organs that produce hair. There is one follicle for each hair connected with a sebaceous gland and also with a tiny muscle. The muscle pulls the hair into an erect position when the individual is cold or frightened. All hair grows continuously and is either cut off or worn away by clothing.

Blood vessels provide nutrients and oxygen to the skin. The blood vessels lie in the dermis. Small branches extend up to the germinal layer. There are no blood vessels in the epidermis. A complex array of nerve endings also lie in the dermis. These specialized nerve endings are sensitive to environmental stimuli; they respond to these stimuli and send impulses along the nerves to the brain.

Beneath the skin, immediately under the dermis and attached to it, lies the **subcutaneous tissue**. The subcutaneous tissue is composed largely of fat. The fat serves as an insulator for the body and as a reservoir to store energy. The amount of subcutaneous tissue varies greatly from individual to individual. Beneath the subcutaneous tissue lie the muscles and the skeleton.

The skin covers all of the external surface of the body. The various orifices (openings to the body)—including the mouth, nose, anus, and vagina—are not covered by skin. Orifices are lined with mucous membranes.

Mucous membranes are quite similar to skin in that they provide a protective barrier against bacterial invasion. Mucous membranes differ from skin in that they secrete **mucus**, a watery substance that lubricates the openings. Thus, mucous membranes are moist, whereas the skin is dry. A mucous membrane lines the entire gastrointestinal tract from the mouth to the anus.

The Endocrine System

The brain controls the body through both the nervous system and the endocrine system. The **endocrine system** is a complex message and control system that integrates many body functions. It releases substances called hormones, either by target organs or into the bloodstream ▼ **Figure 4-47** . Adrenaline and insulin are examples of hormones. Each endocrine gland produces one or more hormones. Each hormone has a specific effect on some organ, tissue, or process ▶ **Table 4-5** . The brain controls the release of hormones by the endocrine glands with other (stimulating or inhibiting) hormones. The final effect influences the endocrine glands and the brain. As a result, we have a tightly controlled system with primary and secondary feedback

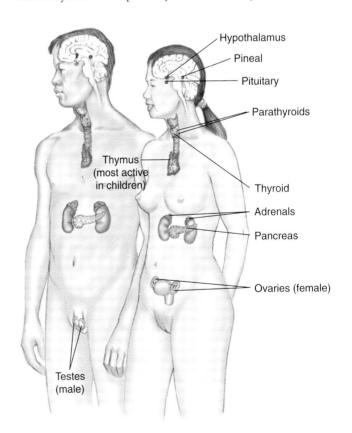

Figure 4-47 The endocrine system controls the release of hormones in the body.

loops to keep body systems in balance (▶ Figure 4-48). For example, when we are frightened, the brain stimulates the adrenal gland through a hormone to release adrenaline (epinephrine). Release of adrenaline increases our blood pressure and heart rate. The resulting increase in blood pressure and heart rate decreases the amount of hormone released by the adrenal gland. The brain then reduces the amount of stimulation to the adrenal gland. Thus, a new steady state is achieved at heightened levels of alertness. Insulin is another hormone that is intimately involved in the control of the blood glucose and metabolism of food.

Excesses or deficiencies in hormones cause various diseases. With endocrine diseases, specific body functions are increased, decreased, or absent. Diabetes mellitus is a common problem. Because production of the hormone insulin is deficient, the body is unable to use glucose normally. This disease also damages the small blood vessels in the body. The tissue damage that results is as much a part of diabetes as is the difficulty in regulating the amount of glucose in the blood.

The Digestive System

The digestive system is composed of the gastrointestinal tract (stomach and intestines), mouth, salivary glands, pharynx, esophagus, liver, gallbladder, pancreas, rectum, and anus. The function of this system is **digestion**:

the processing of food that nourishes the individual cells of the body.

How Digestion Works

Digestion of food, from the time it is taken into the mouth until essential compounds are extracted and delivered by the circulatory system to nourish all of the cells in the body, is a complicated chemical process. In succession, different secretions, primarily enzymes, are added to the food by the salivary glands, the stomach, the liver, the pancreas, and the small intestine to convert the food into basic sugars, fatty acids, and amino acids. These basic products of digestion are carried across the wall of the intestine and transported through the portal vein to the liver. In the liver, the products are processed further and then stored or transported to the heart through veins draining the liver. The heart then pumps the blood with these nutrients throughout the arteries and then to the capillaries, where the nutrients pass through the capillary walls to nourish the body's individual cells.

In normal routine activity, without any food or fluid ingestion at all, between 8 to 10 L of fluid are secreted daily into the gastrointestinal tract. This fluid comes from the salivary glands, stomach, liver, pancreas, and small intestine. In a normal adult, about 7% of the body weight is delivered as fluid daily to the gastrointestinal tract. If significant vomiting or diarrhea occurs for more

TABLE 4-5 **Endocrine Glands**			
Gland	**Location**	**Function**	**Hormones Produced**
Adrenal	Kidneys	Regulate salt, sugar, and sexual function	Adrenaline (epinephrine) and others
Ovary	Female pelvis (2 glands)	Regulate sexual function, characteristics, and reproduction	Estrogen and others
Pancreas	Retroperitoneal space	Regulate glucose metabolism and other functions	Insulin and others
Parathyroid	Neck (behind and beside the thyroid) (3–5 glands)	Regulate serum calcium	Parathormone
Pituitary	Base of skull	Regulate all other endocrine glands	Multiple, very important hormones
Testes	Male scrotum (2 glands)	Regulate sexual function, characteristics, and reproduction	Testosterone and others
Thyroid	Neck (over the larynx)	Regulate metabolism	Thyroxine and others

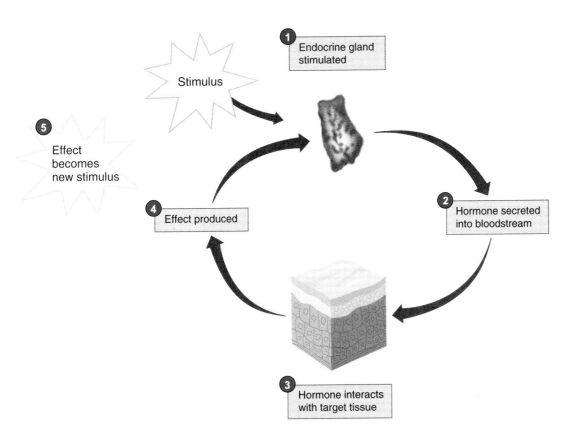

1 Endocrine gland stimulated

Stimulus

5 Effect becomes new stimulus

4 Effect produced

2 Hormone secreted into bloodstream

3 Hormone interacts with target tissue

Figure 4-48 The endocrine system is tightly controlled with primary and secondary feedback loops to keep body systems in balance.

than 2 or 3 days, the patient will lose a very substantial portion of body composition and become severely ill.

Anatomy of the Digestive System

MOUTH. The mouth consists of the lips, cheeks, gums, teeth, and tongue. A mucous membrane lines the mouth. The roof of the mouth is formed by the hard and soft palates. The hard palate is a bony plate lying anteriorly; the soft palate is a fold of mucous membrane and muscle that extends posteriorly from the hard palate into the throat. The soft palate is designed to hold food that is being chewed within the mouth and to help initiate swallowing.

SALIVARY GLANDS. There are two **salivary glands** located under the tongue, one on each side of the lower jaw, and one inside each cheek. They produce nearly 1.5 L of saliva daily. Saliva is approximately 98% water. The remaining 2% is composed of mucus, salts, and organic compounds. Saliva serves as a binder for the chewed food that is being swallowed and as a lubricant within the mouth.

OROPHARYNX. The **oropharynx** is a tubular structure about 5″ long that extends vertically from the back of the mouth to the esophagus and trachea. An automatic movement of the pharynx during swallowing lifts the larynx to permit the epiglottis to close over it so that liquids and solids are moved into the esophagus and away from the trachea.

ESOPHAGUS. The **esophagus** is a collapsible tube about 10″ long that extends from the end of the pharynx to the stomach and lies just anterior to the spinal column in the chest. Contractions of the muscle in the wall of the esophagus propel food through it to the stomach. Liquids will pass with very little assistance.

STOMACH. The stomach is located in the left upper quadrant of the abdominal cavity, largely protected by the lower left ribs. Muscular contractions in the wall of the stomach and gastric juice, which contains much mucus, convert ingested food to a thoroughly mixed semi-solid mass. The stomach produces approximately 1.5 L of gastric juice daily for this process. The principal function of the stomach is to receive food in large quantities intermittently, store it, and provide for its movement into the small bowel in regular, small amounts. In 1 to 3 hours, the semi-solid food mass derived from one meal is propelled by muscular contraction into the duodenum, the first part of the small intestine.

PANCREAS. The **pancreas**, a flat, solid organ, lies below and behind the liver and stomach and behind the peritoneum. It is firmly fixed in position, deep within the abdomen, and is not easily damaged. It contains two kinds of glands. One set of glands secretes nearly 2 L of pancreatic juice daily. This juice contains many enzymes that aid in the digestion of fat, starch, and protein. Pancreatic juice flows directly into the duodenum through the pancreatic ducts. The other gland is the islets of Langerhans, which produces insulin. Insulin regulates the amount of glucose in the blood.

LIVER. The **liver** is a large, solid organ that takes up most of the area immediately beneath the diaphragm in the right upper quadrant. It is the largest solid organ in the abdomen and has several functions. Poisonous substances produced by digestion are brought to the liver and rendered harmless. Factors that are necessary for blood clotting and for the production of normal plasma are formed here. Between 0.5 and 1 L of bile is made by the liver daily to assist in the normal digestion of fat. The liver is the principal organ for the storage of sugar or starch for immediate use by the body for energy. It also produces many of the factors that aid in the proper regulation of immune responses. Anatomically, the liver is a large mass of blood vessels and cells, packed tightly together. It is fragile and, because of its size, relatively easily injured. Blood flow in the liver is high, because all of the blood that is pumped to the gastrointestinal tract passes into the liver, through the portal vein, before it returns to the heart. In addition, the liver has a generous arterial blood supply of its own. Ordinarily, approximately 25% of the cardiac output of blood (1.5 L) passes through the liver each minute.

BILE DUCTS. The liver is connected to the intestine by the **bile ducts**. The **gallbladder** is an outpouching from the bile ducts that serves as a reservoir and concentrating organ for bile produced in the liver. Together, the bile ducts and gallbladder form the biliary system. The gallbladder discharges stored and concentrated bile into the duodenum through the common bile duct. The presence of food in the duodenum triggers a contraction of the gallbladder

to empty it. The gallbladder usually contains about 60 to 90 mL of bile.

SMALL INTESTINE. The **small intestine** is the major hollow organ of the abdomen. The cells lining the small intestine produce enzymes and mucus to aid in digestion. Enzymes from the pancreas and the small intestine carry out the final processes of digestion. More than 90% of the products of digestion (amino acids, fatty acids, and simple sugars), together with water, ingested vitamins, and minerals are absorbed across the wall of the lower end of the small intestine into veins to be transported to the liver. The small intestine is composed of the duodenum, the jejunum, and the ileum. The duodenum, which is about 12″ long, is the part of the small intestine that receives food from the stomach. Here, food is mixed with secretions from the pancreas and liver for further digestion. Bile, produced by the liver and stored in the gallbladder, is emptied as needed into the duodenum. It is greenish black, but through changes during digestion, it gives feces its typical brown color. Its major function is in the digestion of fat. The jejunum and ileum together measure more than 20′ on average to make up the rest of the small intestine.

LARGE INTESTINE. The **large intestine**, another major hollow organ, consists of the cecum, the colon, and the rectum. About 5′ long, it encircles the outer border of the abdomen around the small bowel. The major function of the colon, the portion of the large intestine that extends from the cecum to the rectum, is to absorb the final 5% to 10% of digested food and water from the intestine to form solid stool, which is stored in the rectum and passed out of the body through the anus.

APPENDIX. The appendix is a tube 3″ to 4″ long that opens into the cecum (the first part of the large intestine) in the right lower quadrant of the abdomen. It may easily become obstructed and, as a result, inflamed and infected. Appendicitis, which is the term for this inflammation, is one of the major causes of severe abdominal distress. The appendix has no known function.

RECTUM. The lowermost end of the colon is the **rectum**. It is a large, hollow organ that is adapted to store quantities of feces until it is expelled. At its terminal end is the anus, a 2″ canal lined with skin. The rectum and anus are supplied with a complex series of circular muscles called sphincters that control, both voluntarily and automatically, the escape of liquids, gases, and solids from the digestive tract.

The Urinary System

The **urinary system** controls the discharge of certain waste materials filtered from the blood by the kidneys. In the urinary system, the kidneys are solid organs; the ureters, bladder, and urethra are hollow organs **▼ Figure 4-49** . Ordinarily, we consider the urinary and genital systems together, because they share many organs.

The body has two **kidneys** that lie on the posterior muscular wall of the abdomen behind the peritoneum in the retroperitoneal space. These organs rid the blood of toxic waste products and control its balance of water and salt. Blood flow in the kidneys is high. Nearly 20% of the output of blood from the heart passes through the kidneys each minute. Large vessels attach the kidneys directly to the aorta and the inferior

> Ordinarily, the urinary and genital systems are considered together because they share many organs.

vena cava. Waste products and water are constantly filtered from the blood to form urine. The kidneys continuously concentrate this filtered urine by reabsorbing the water as it passes through a system of specialized tubes within them. The tubes finally unite to form the **renal pelvis**, a cone-shaped collecting area that connects the ureter and the kidney. Normally, each kidney drains its urine into one ureter through which the urine passes to the bladder.

A **ureter** passes from the renal pelvis of each kidney along the surface of the posterior abdominal wall behind the peritoneum to drain into the urinary bladder. The ureters are small (0.2″ in diameter), hollow, muscular tubes. **Peristalsis**, a wave-like contraction of smooth muscle, occurs in these tubes to move the urine to the bladder.

The **urinary bladder** is located immediately behind the pubic symphysis in the pelvic cavity and is composed of smooth muscle with a specialized lining membrane. The two ureters enter posteriorly at its base on either side. The bladder empties to the outside of the body through the **urethra**. In the male, the urethra passes from the anterior base of the bladder through the penis. In the female, the urethra opens at the front of the vagina. The normal adult forms 1.5 to 2 L of urine every day. This waste is extracted and concentrated from the 1,500 L of blood that circulate through the kidneys daily.

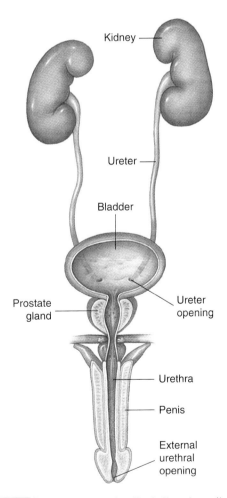

Kidney

Ureter

Bladder

Prostate gland

Ureter opening

Urethra

Penis

External urethral opening

Figure 4-49 The urinary system lies in the retroperitoneal space behind the organs of the digestive system. The urinary system in males and females includes the kidneys, ureters, urinary bladder, and urethra. This diagram shows the male urinary system.

The Genital System

The **genital system** controls the reproductive processes by which life is created. The male genitalia, except for the prostate gland and the seminal vesicles, lie outside the pelvic cavity. The female genitalia are contained entirely within the pelvis. The male and female reproductive organs have certain similarities and, of course, basic differences. They allow the production of sperm and egg cells and appropriate hormones and the act of sexual intercourse and reproduction.

FRONT VIEW

- Ureter
- Urinary bladder
- Ductus deferens
- Seminal vesicle
- Prostate gland
- Bulbourethral gland
- Corpus cavernosa
- Urethra
- Epididymis
- Testis
- Penis
- Glans penis

SIDE VIEW

- Pubic bone
- Prostate gland
- Urethra
- Corpus cavernosum
- Scrotum

Figure 4-50 The male reproductive system consists of the testicles, vasa deferentia, seminal vesicles, prostate gland, urethra, and penis.

The Male Reproductive System and Organs

The male reproductive system consists of the testicles, vasa deferentia, seminal vesicles, prostate gland, urethra, and penis ▲ **Figure 4-50** . Each **testicle** contains specialized cells and ducts; some of these produce male hormones, and others develop sperm. The hormones are absorbed directly into the bloodstream from the testicles. The **vasa deferentia (or vas deferens)** are ducts that travel from the testicles up beneath the skin of the abdominal wall for a short distance. They then pass through an opening into the abdominal cavity and into the prostate gland to connect with the urethra. The vasa deferentia carry the sperm from the testicles to the urethra. The **seminal vesicles** are small storage sacs for sperm and seminal fluid. The vesicles also empty into the urethra, at the prostate.

Semen, also called seminal fluid, contains sperm cells that are carried up each vas from each testicle to be mixed with fluid from the seminal vesicles and prostate gland. The **prostate gland** surrounds the urethra where it emerges from the urinary bladder. Fluids from the prostate gland and from the seminal vesicles mix during sexual intercourse. During intercourse, special mechanisms in the nervous system prevent the passage of urine into the urethra. Only seminal fluid, prostatic fluid, and sperm pass from the penis into the vagina during ejaculation.

The penis contains a special type of tissue called erectile tissue. This specialized tissue is largely vascular and, when filled with blood, causes the penis to distend into a state of erection. As the vessels fill under pressure from the circulatory system, the penis becomes a large, rigid organ that can enter the vagina. Certain spinal injuries and some diseases can cause a painful continuous erection called **priapism**.

FRONT VIEW   SIDE VIEW

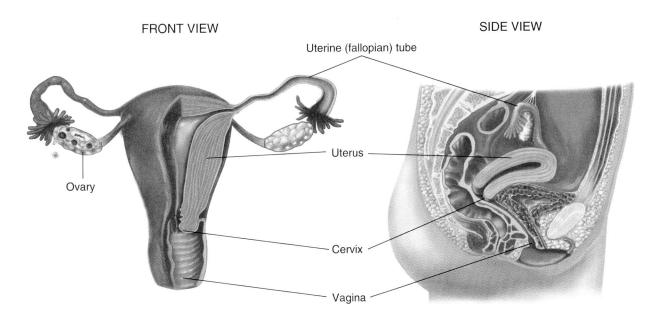

Uterine (fallopian) tube

Ovary

Uterus

Cervix

Vagina

Figure 4-51   The female reproductive system consists of the ovaries, fallopian tubes, uterus, cervix, and vagina.

The Female Reproductive System and Organs

The female reproductive organs include the ovaries, fallopian tubes, uterus, cervix, and vagina (▲ **Figure 4-51**). The **ovaries**, like the testicles, produce sex hormones and specialized cells for reproduction. The female sex hormones are absorbed directly into the bloodstream. A specialized ovum, or egg cell, is produced regularly during the adult female's reproductive years. The ovaries release a mature egg approximately every 28 days. This egg travels through the fallopian tubes to the uterus.

The **fallopian tubes** connect with the uterus and carry the ovum into the cavity of this organ. The uterus is pear-shaped and hollow, with muscular walls. The narrow opening from the uterus to the vagina is the cervix. The **vagina** (birth canal) is a muscular distensible tube that connects the uterus with the vulva (the external female genitalia). The vagina receives the penis during sexual intercourse, when semen is deposited in it. The sperm in the semen may pass into the uterus and fertilize an egg, causing pregnancy. Should the pregnancy come to completion at the end of nine months, the baby will pass through the vagina and be born. The vagina also channels the menstrual flow from the uterus out of the body.

Prep Kit

Ready for Review

To do your work as an EMT-B, you must have a working knowledge of human anatomy so that you can communicate with hospital personnel and other health care providers. You must be able to identify superficial landmarks of the body and know what lies underneath the skin so that you can perform an accurate assessment. Hospital personnel will use these terms to ask you questions about a patient; therefore, it is critical for the well-being of your patient that you learn them and can use them correctly.

Vital Vocabulary

abdomen The body cavity that contains the major organs of digestion and excretion.

abduction Motion of a limb away from the midline.

acetabulum The depression on the lateral pelvis where its three component bones join, in which the femoral head fits snugly.

Adam's apple The firm prominence in the upper part of the larynx formed by the thyroid cartilage. It is more prominent in men than in women.

adduction Motion of a limb toward the midline.

agonal respirations Slow, gasping respiration, sometimes seen in dying patients.

alveoli The air sacs of the lungs in which the exchange of oxygen and carbon dioxide takes place.

anatomic position The position of reference in which the patient stands facing you, arms at the side, with the palms of the hands forward.

angle of Louis A ridge on the sternum that lies at the level where the second rib is attached to the sternum; provides a constant and reliable bony landmark on the anterior chest wall.

anterior The front surface of the body; the side facing you in the standard anatomic position.

anterior superior iliac spines The bony prominences of the pelvis (ilium) at the front on each side of the lower abdomen just below the plane of the umbilicus.

aorta The principal artery leaving the left side of the heart and carrying freshly oxygenated blood to the body.

apex (plural: apices) The tip or the topmost portion of a structure.

appendix A small tubular structure that is attached to the lower border of the cecum in the lower right quadrant of the abdomen.

arteriole The smallest branch of an artery leading to the vast network of capillaries.

atrium Upper chamber of the heart.

autonomic nervous system The part of the nervous system that regulates functions, such as digestion and sweating, that are not controlled voluntarily.

ball-and-socket joint A joint that allows internal and external rotation as well as bending.

biceps The large muscle that covers the front of the humerus.

bilateral A body part that appears on both sides of the midline.

bile ducts Ducts that convey bile between the liver and the intestine.

blood pressure (BP) The pressure that the blood exerts against the walls of the arteries as it passes through them.

brachial artery The major vessel in the upper extremity that supplies blood to the arm.

brain The controlling organ of the body and center of consciousness; functions include perception, control of reactions to the environment, emotional responses, and judgment.

brain stem The area of the brain between the spinal cord and cerebrum, surrounded by the cerebellum; controls functions that are necessary for life, such as respirations.

capillary vessels The fine end-divisions of the arterial system that allow contact between cells of the body tissues and the plasma and red blood cells.

carotid artery The major artery that supplies blood to the head and brain.

carpometacarpal joint The joint between the wrist and the metacarpal bones; the thumb joint.

cecum The first part of the large intestine, into which the ileum opens.

central nervous system (CNS) The brain and spinal cord.

cerebellum One of the three major subdivisions of the brain, sometimes called the "little brain"; coordinates the various activities of the brain, particularly body movements.

cerebrum The largest part of the three subdivisions of the brain, sometimes called the "gray matter"; made up of several lobes that control movement, hearing, balance, speech, visual perception, emotions, and personality.

cervical spine The portion of the spinal column consisting of the first seven vertebrae that lie in the neck.

circulatory system The complex arrangement of connected tubes, including the arteries, arterioles, capillaries, venules, and veins, that moves blood, oxygen, nutrients, carbon dioxide, and cellular waste throughout the body.

clavicle The collarbone; it is lateral to the sternum and medial to the scapula.

coccyx The last three or four vertebrae of the spine; the tailbone.

connecting nerves Nerves that connect the sensory and motor nerves.

costal arch A bridge of cartilage that connects the ends of the sixth through tenth ribs with the lower portion of the sternum.

costovertebral angle An angle that is formed by the junction of the spine and the tenth rib.

cranium The area of the head above the ears and eyes; the skull. The cranium contains the brain.

cricoid cartilage A firm ridge of cartilage that forms the lower part of the larynx.

cricothyroid membrane A thin sheet of fascia that connects the thyroid and cricoid cartilages that make up the larynx.

deep Further inside the body and away from the skin.

dermis The inner layer of the skin, containing hair follicles, sweat glands, nerve endings, and blood vessels.

diaphragm A muscular dome that forms the undersurface of the thorax, separating the chest from the abdominal cavity. Contraction of the diaphragm (and the chest wall muscles) brings air into the lungs. Relaxation allows air to be expelled from the lungs.

diastole The relaxation, or period of relaxation, of the heart, especially of the ventricles.

digestion The processing of food that nourishes the individual cells of the body.

distal Structures that are farther from the trunk or nearer to the free end of the extremity.

dorsal The posterior surface of the body, including the back of the hand.

dorsalis pedis artery The artery on the anterior surface of the foot between the first and second metatarsals.

endocrine system The complex message and control system that integrates many body functions, including the release of hormones.

epidermis The outer layer of skin, which is made up of cells that are sealed together to form a watertight protective covering for the body.

epiglottis A thin, leaf-shaped valve that allows air to pass into the trachea but prevents food or liquid from entering.

esophagus A collapsible tube that extends from the pharynx to the stomach; contractions of the muscle in the wall of the esophagus propel food and liquids through it to the stomach.

extend To straighten.

fallopian tube Long, slender tube that extends from the uterus to the region of the ovary on the same side, and through which the ovum passes from ovary to uterus.

fascia A sheet or band of tough fibrous connective tissue; lies deep under the skin and forms an outer layer for the muscles.

femoral artery The principal artery of the thigh, a continuation of the external iliac artery. It supplies blood to the lower abdominal wall, external genitalia, and legs. It can be palpated in the groin area.

femoral head The proximal end of the femur, articulating with the acetabulum to form the hip joint.

femur The thighbone; longest and one of the strongest bones in the body.

flex To bend.

floating ribs The eleventh and twelfth ribs, which do not attach to the sternum through the costal arch.

foramen magnum A large opening at the base of the skull through which the brain connects to the spinal cord.

Fowler's position The position in which the patient is sitting up with the knees bent.

gallbladder A sac on the undersurface of the liver that collects bile from the liver and discharges it into the duodenum through the common bile duct.

genital system The male and female reproductive systems.

greater trochanter A bony prominence on the proximal lateral side of the thigh, just below the hip joint.

hair follicles The small organs in the skin that produce hair.

heart A hollow muscular organ that receives blood from the veins and propels it into the arteries.

heart rate (pulse) The wave of pressure that is created by the heart's contracting and forcing blood out the left ventricle and into the major arteries.

hinge joints Joints that can bend and straighten but cannot rotate; they restrict motion to one plane.

humerus The supporting bone of the arm.

hypoxic drive A "backup system" to control respiration; senses drops in the oxygen level in the blood.

iliac crest The rim, or wing, of the pelvic bone.

ilium One of three bones that fuse to form the pelvic ring.

inferior The part of the body, or any body part, nearer to the feet.

inferior vena cava One of the two largest veins in the body; carries blood from the lower extremities and the pelvic and the abdominal organs into the heart.

inguinal ligament The tough, fibrous ligament that stretches between the lateral edge of the pubic symphysis and the anterior superior iliac spine.

involuntary muscle Muscle that continues to contract, rhythmically, regardless of the conscious will of the individual.

ischium One of three bones that fuse to form the pelvic ring.

joint (articulation) The place where two bones come into contact.

joint capsule The fibrous sac with synovial lining that encloses a joint.

kidneys Two retroperitoneal organs that excrete the end products of metabolism as urine and regulate the body's salt and water content.

large intestine The portion of the digestive tube that encircles the abdomen around the small bowel, consisting of the cecum, the colon, and the rectum.

lateral Parts of the body that lie farther from the midline. Also called outer structures.

ligament A band of the fibrous tissue that connects bones to bones. It supports and strengthens a joint.

liver A large solid organ that lies in the right upper quadrant immediately below the diaphragm; it produces bile, stores sugar for immediate use by the body, and produces many substances that help regulate immune responses.

lumbar spine The lower part of the back, formed by the lowest five non-fused vertebrae; also called the dorsal spine.

lumbar vertebrae Vertebrae of the lumbar spine.

mandible The bone of the lower jaw.

manubrium The upper quarter of the sternum.

mastoid process A prominent bony mass at the base of the skull behind the ear.

maxillae The upper jawbones that assist in the formation of the orbit, the nasal cavity, and the palate, and lodge the upper teeth.

medial Parts of the body that lie closer to the midline; also called inner structures.

metabolism The sum of all the physical and chemical processes of living organisms; the process by which energy is made available for the uses of the organism.

midaxillary line An imaginary vertical line drawn through the middle of the axilla (armpit), parallel to the midline.

midclavicular line An imaginary vertical line drawn through the middle portion of the clavicle and parallel to the midline.

midline An imaginary vertical line drawn from the middle of the forehead through the nose and the umbilicus (navel) to the floor.

motor nerves Nerves that carry information from the central nervous system to the muscles of the body.

mucous membranes The lining of body cavities and passages that communicate directly or indirectly with the environment outside the body.

mucus The opaque, sticky secretion of the mucous membranes that lubricates the body openings.

musculoskeletal system The bones and voluntary muscles of the body.

myocardium The heart muscle.

nasopharynx The part of the pharynx that lies above the level of the roof of the mouth, or soft palate.

nervous system The system that controls virtually all activities of the body, both voluntary and involuntary.

occiput The most posterior portion of the cranium.

orbit The eye socket, made up of the maxilla and zygoma.

oropharynx A tubular structure that extends vertically from the back of the mouth to the esophagus and trachea.

ovary A female gland that produces sex hormones and ova (eggs).

palmar The front region of the hand.

pancreas A flat, solid organ that lies below the liver and the stomach; it is a major source of digestive enzymes and produces the hormone insulin.

parietal regions The areas between the temporal and occiput regions of the cranium.

patella The kneecap; a specialized bone that lies within the tendon of the quadriceps muscle.

perfusion The circulation of blood within an organ or tissue in adequate amounts to meet the cells' current needs.

peripheral nervous system The part of the nervous system that consists of 31 pairs of spinal nerves and 12 pairs of cranial nerves. These peripheral nerves may be sensory nerves, motor nerves, or connecting nerves.

peristalsis The wave-like contraction of smooth muscle by which the ureters or other tubular organs propel their contents.

pinna The external, visible part of the ear.

plantar The bottom of the foot.

plasma A sticky, yellow fluid that carries the blood cells and nutrients and transports cellular waste material to the organs of excretion.

platelets Tiny, disk-shaped elements that are much smaller than the cells; they are essential in the initial formation of a blood clot, the mechanism that stops bleeding.

pleura The serous membrane covering the lungs and lining the thoracic cavity, completely enclosing a potential space known as the pleural space.

pleural space The potential space between the parietal pleura and the visceral pleura. It is described as "potential" because under normal conditions, the lungs fill this space.

posterior The back surface of the body; the side away from you in the standard anatomical position.

posterior tibial artery The artery just posterior to the medial malleolus; supplies blood to the foot.

priapism A continuous and painful erection of the penis caused by certain spinal injuries and some diseases.

Prep Kit Continued.

prone position The position in which the body is lying face down.

prostate gland A small gland that surrounds the male urethra where it emerges from the urinary bladder; it secretes a fluid that is part of the ejaculatory fluid.

proximal Structures that are closer to the trunk.

pubic symphysis A hard bony prominence that is found in the midline in the lowermost portion of the abdomen.

pubis One of three bones that fuse to form the pelvic ring.

pulmonary artery The major artery leading from the right ventricle of the heart to the lungs; it carries oxygen-poor blood.

pulmonary veins The four veins that return oxygenated blood from the lungs to the left atrium of the heart.

pulse The wave of pressure created as the heart contracts and forces blood out the left ventricle and into the major arteries.

quadrants The way to describe the sections of the abdominal cavity. Imagine two lines intersecting at the umbilicus dividing the abdomen into four equal areas.

radial artery The major artery in the forearm; it is palpable at the wrist on the thumb side.

radius The bone on the thumb side of the forearm.

rectum The lowermost end of the colon.

red blood cells Cells that carry oxygen to the body's tissues; also called erythrocytes.

renal pelvis A cone-shaped collecting area that connects the ureter and the kidney.

respiratory system All the structures of the body that contribute to the process of breathing, consisting of the upper and lower airways and their component parts.

retroperitoneal Behind the abdominal cavity.

sacrum One of three bones (sacrum and two pelvic bones) that make up the pelvic ring; consists of five fused sacral vertebrae.

salivary glands The glands that produce saliva to keep the mouth and pharynx moist.

scalp The thick skin covering the cranium, which usually bears hair.

scapula The shoulder blade.

sebaceous glands Glands that produce an oily substance called sebum, which discharges along the shafts of the hairs.

semen Seminal fluid ejaculated from the penis and containing sperm.

seminal vesicles Storage sacs for sperm and seminal fluid, which empty into the urethra at the prostate.

sensory nerves The nerves that carry sensations of touch, taste, heat, cold, pain, or other modalities from the body to the central nervous system.

shock position The position that has the head and torso (trunk) supine and the lower extremities elevated 8" to 12". This helps to increase blood flow to the brain; also referred to as *modified Trendelenburg's* position.

shoulder girdle The proximal portion of the upper extremity, made up of the clavicle, the scapula, and the humerus.

skeletal muscle Muscle that is attached to bones and usually crosses at least one joint; striated, or voluntary, muscle.

skeleton The framework that gives us our recognizable form; also designed to allow motion of the body and protection of vital organs.

small intestine The portion of the digestive tube between the stomach and the cecum, consisting of the duodenum, jejunum, and ileum.

smooth muscle Nonstriated, involuntary muscle; it constitutes the bulk of the gastrointestinal tract and is present in nearly every organ to regulate automatic activity.

somatic nervous system The part of the nervous system that regulates activities over which there is voluntary control.

spinal cord An extension of the brain, composed of virtually all the nerves carrying messages between the brain and the rest of the body. It lies inside of, and is protected by, the spinal canal.

sternocleidomastoid muscles The muscles on either side of the neck that allow movement of the head.

sternum The breastbone.

striated muscle Muscle that has characteristic stripes, or striations, under the microscope; voluntary, or skeletal, muscle.

subcutaneous tissue Tissue, largely fat, that lies directly under the dermis and serves as an insulator of the body.

superficial Closer to or on the skin.

superior The part of the body, or any body part, nearer to the head.

superior vena cava One of the two largest veins in the body; carries blood from the upper extremities, head, neck, and chest into the heart.

supine position The position in which the body is lying face up.

sweat glands The glands that secrete sweat.

systole The contraction, or period of contraction, of the heart, especially that of the ventricles.

temporal regions The lateral portions on each side of the cranium.

temporomandibular joint The joint where the mandible meets with the temporal bone of the cranium just in front of each ear.

testicle A male genital gland that contains specialized cells that produce hormones and sperm.

thoracic cage The chest or rib cage.

thoracic spine The 12 vertebrae that lie between the cervical vertebrae and the lumbar vertebrae. One pair of ribs is attached to each of the thoracic vertebrae.

thorax The chest cavity that contains the heart, lungs, esophagus, and great vessels (the aorta and the two venae cavae).

thyroid cartilage A firm prominence of cartilage that forms the upper part of the larynx; the Adam's apple.

tibia The shinbone, the larger of the two bones of the lower leg.

topographic anatomy The superficial landmarks of the body that serve as guides to the structures that lie beneath them.

torso The trunk without the head and limbs.

trachea The windpipe; the main trunk for air passing to and from the lungs.

Trendelenburg's position The position in which the body is supine with the head lower than the feet.

triceps The muscle in the back of the upper arm.

ulna The inner bone of the forearm, on the side opposite the thumb.

ulnar artery One of the major arteries of the forearm; it can be palpated at the wrist on the ulnar side (at the base of the fifth finger).

ureter A small, hollow tube that carries urine from the kidneys to the bladder.

urethra The canal that conveys urine from the bladder to outside the body.

urinary bladder A sac behind the pubic symphysis made of smooth muscle that collects and stores urine.

urinary system The organs that control the discharge of certain waste materials filtered from the blood and excreted as urine.

vagina A muscular distensible tube that connects the uterus with the vulva (the external female genitalia); also called the birth canal.

vasa deferentia (vas deferens) The spermatic duct of the testicles; also called vas deferens.

ventral The anterior surface of the body.

ventricle Lower chamber of the heart.

vertebrae The 33 bones that make up the spinal column.

voluntary muscle Muscle that is under direct voluntary control of the brain and can be contracted or relaxed at will; skeletal, or striated, muscle.

white blood cells Blood cells that play a role in the body's immune defense mechanisms against infection; also called leukocytes.

xiphoid process The narrow, cartilaginous lower tip of the sternum.

zygomas The quadrangular bones of the cheek, articulating with the frontal bone, the maxillae, the zygomatic processes of the temporal bone, and the great wings of the sphenoid bone.

www.emtb.com

Assessment in Action

You and your partner are dispatched to a shooting. En route to the scene you hear officers respond. On arrival you find the perpetrator in custody and the scene safe. You find a 21-year-old man lying on his back.

He has one gunshot wound in the right arm, just above the elbow, and one to the chest about 1 inch below the right nipple. He tells you that he "hurts" and is having difficulty breathing.

1. Which organs lie directly under the gunshot wound in his chest?
   A. Liver and lung
   B. Spinal cord and lung
   C. Stomach and liver
   D. Spleen and lung

2. On the basis of this injury and the possible damage to organs directly underneath, you would most likely suspect that the patient is at risk for developing difficulty breathing and:
   A. a bowel obstruction.
   B. vomiting and diarrhea.
   C. paralysis.
   D. severe internal bleeding.

3. Using anatomical terms, the gunshot wound to the elbow was located:
   A. proximal to the shoulder.
   B. in the distal humerus.
   C. in the proximal humerus.
   D. in the distal femur.

4. Using anatomical terms, the entrance wound to the chest was on the:
   A. anterior chest wall, superior to the right nipple.
   B. posterior chest wall, inferior to the right nipple.
   C. anterior chest wall, inferior to the right nipple.
   D. posterior chest wall, superior to the right nipple.

5. Your patient fell, suffering pain in his left forearm just past the antecubital space. Because of the tendons and ligaments located in the area and the location of his pain, which of the following actions is likely related to his injury?
   A. Cannot raise his shoulder
   B. May have pain in his collarbone
   C. Cannot bend his elbow
   D. May have associated pain in his hand

6. A 30-year-old man was playing soccer when the ball forcibly struck him in the lower left part of the chest, hard enough to break two of his anterior ribs. Besides his lungs, what other organ has a high likelihood of injury in this area?
   A. Liver
   B. Heart
   C. Pancreas
   D. Spleen

7. A fall resulting in blunt trauma to the tip of the shoulder has a frequent incidence of injury to what other bone?
   A. Sternum
   B. Clavicle
   C. Ulna
   D. Tibia

8. Blunt trauma to the abdomen resulting in solid organ injury has a high likelihood of causing:
   A. infection later on.
   B. associated chest injury.
   C. bleeding internally.
   D. injury to the vertebra.

Challenging Questions

9. The alveoli are surrounded by a network of tiny blood vessels. These vessels are called pulmonary capillaries. If a clot blocked circulation to a portion of the pulmonary capillaries, what would you hear if you listened to lung sounds?

10. Injury to the kidney may not be recognized outside the hospital. However, if the injury is enough to cause blood to collect in the renal pelvis, how might the injury be recognized?

Points to Ponder

You are arriving on the scene of a motor vehicle crash and as you start to survey the scene you recognize one of the vehicles is a good friend's. It has been hit "broadside" and it appears that someone ran a red light. The damage to both cars is significant. As you approach, you can see that your friend has a serious head injury and open fractures of the humerus and femur. Your friend appears to be alone in the car although the infant seat is in the rear seat. All you can think of is "Who will raise the baby if your friend dies?" You look into the other car and see two patients. One appears unconscious and the other is moaning and moving around. How would you handle this situation? Would you treat your friend or the other patients? Would you tell your partner what is happening? Who could you turn to for support if your friend died?

Issues Treating People You Know, Support Systems and CISD, Communicating With Your Partner, Stress in EMS.

Online Outlook

As an EMT-B, you must have a good understanding of basic human anatomy and physiology. Improve your knowledge by completing Exercise 4 at **www.emtb.com**.

www.emtb.com

Baseline Vital Signs and SAMPLE History

Cognitive

1. Identify the components of vital signs (p 130).
2. Describe the methods to obtain a breathing rate (p 130).
3. Identify the attributes that should be obtained when assessing breathing (p 130).
4. Differentiate between shallow, labored, and noisy breathing (p 131).
5. Describe the methods to obtain a pulse rate (p 134).
6. Identify the information obtained when assessing a patient's pulse (p 134).
7. Differentiate between a strong, weak, regular, and irregular pulse (p 134).
8. Describe the methods to assess skin color, temperature, and condition (capillary refill in infants and children) (p 134).
9. Identify normal and abnormal skin colors (p 134).
10. Differentiate between pale, blue, red, and yellow skin color (p 135).
11. Identify the normal and abnormal skin temperature (p 135).
12. Differentiate between hot, cool, and cold skin temperature (p 135).
13. Identify normal and abnormal skin conditions (p 135).
14. Identify normal and abnormal capillary refill in infants and children (p 135).
15. Describe the methods to assess the pupils (p 142).
16. Identify normal and abnormal pupil size (p 142).
17. Differentiate between dilated (big) and constricted (small) pupil size (p 141).
18. Differentiate between reactive and nonreactive pupils and equal and unequal pupils (p 141).
19. Describe the methods to assess blood pressure (p 136).
20. Define systolic pressure (p 137).
21. Define diastolic pressure (p 137).
22. Explain the difference between auscultation and palpation for obtaining a blood pressure (p 138).
23. Identify the components of the SAMPLE history (p 143).
24. Differentiate between a sign and a symptom (p 129).
25. State the importance of accurately reporting and recording the baseline vital signs (p 130).
26. Discuss the need to search for additional medical identification (p 143).

Affective

27. Explain the value of performing the baseline vital signs (p 130).
28. Recognize and respond to the feelings patients experience during assessment (p 128).
29. Defend the need for obtaining and recording an accurate set of vital signs (p 130).
30. Explain the rationale of recording additional sets of vital signs (p 142).
31. Explain the importance of obtaining a SAMPLE history (p 143).

Psychomotor

32. Demonstrate the skills involved in assessment of breathing (p 130).
33. Demonstrate the skills associated with obtaining a pulse (p 133).
34. Demonstrate the skills associated with assessing the skin color, temperature, condition, and capillary refill in infants and children (p 134).
35. Demonstrate the skills associated with assessing the pupils (p 142).
36. Demonstrate the skills associated with obtaining blood pressure (p 137).
37. Demonstrate the skills that should be used to obtain information from the patient, family, or bystanders at the scene (p 128).

You are the EMT

En route to the hospital, the senior EMT-B on the squad asks for another check on the patient's vital signs. Another EMT-B on the call questions the order as he asks, "Do you really want me to recheck them again so soon? I just checked them 5 minutes ago." A terse, "Yes, please" reply gets him started on his task.

This chapter introduces the essential care concept relative to obtaining and evaluating a patient's baseline vital signs and the SAMPLE history. It will also help you answer the following questions:

1. Why are serial vital signs necessary when caring for seriously ill or injured patients?

2. How can the SAMPLE history that is obtained in the field setting be of value to the emergency department staff at the receiving hospital?

Baseline Vital Signs and SAMPLE History

As an EMT-B, you must perform a quick but thorough assessment to identify a patient's needs and to provide proper emergency medical care. Patient assessment includes many steps and is the most complex skill that you will learn in the EMT-B course. To make the task easier, it is helpful to identify and discuss the key components and skills of patient assessment before you learn the entire process.

As you begin your assessment, you must gather and record some key information about the patient. You will also need to obtain and evaluate the patient's vital signs. The injuries, illnesses, or symptoms that lead to the call to 9-1-1 and the history of what occurred before and since the call was made are key pieces of information that you will have to obtain by asking a series of questions. You must also learn about the patient's past medical history and overall health.

This chapter begins by defining the chief complaint and signs and symptoms. It then explains what key information about the patient you need to obtain at the start of the assessment and why you need it. It also describes each of the vital signs and provides a step-by-step explanation of how to obtain each. Both normal and abnormal vital signs are discussed. The chapter ends with a description of the SAMPLE history.

Gathering Key Patient Information

During the assessment, you will be using your eyes, ears, nose, hands, and a few basic medical instruments to obtain information about your patient. You will need to know which questions to ask and how to ask them

▼ Figure 5-1. By using your deductive powers, you will be able to interpret the meaning and implications of your findings and the information that you have gathered. When assessing the patient, you will have to look, listen, feel, and think. Your scene size-up or the information that is given to you by a first responder or relative when you arrive at the scene should make it immediately apparent whether you were called to the scene because of an accident with injuries or an acute medical problem.

First, find out the patient's name. You will need to know the patient's name so that you can properly address the patient. Unless an adult patient is a close

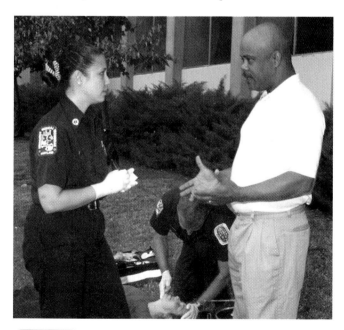

Figure 5-1 You must know how to gather information about the scene and the patient by using your senses and by asking relevant questions.

friend or relative of yours, you should address him or her as "Mr.," "Ms.," "Miss," or "Mrs.," followed by the patient's last name. You may ask the patient how he or she wishes to be called. Often, relatives or staff members of a nursing home or other extended care facility address elderly patients by their first names. You should not use such a familiar mode of address. If the patient's name is difficult to pronounce, you can simply say "Sir" or "Ma'am" instead, to convey a similar respectful and professional manner.

You should try to address children by their first name, especially the name they are customarily called, such as "Johnny," "Betty," or "Joey." Even infants and toddlers who do not yet respond verbally can recognize their name and may be less anxious when it is used.

If an unaccompanied patient is disoriented or unconscious, you should look in his or her wallet or purse for a driver's license or other piece of identification that will tell you the patient's name. At the same time, you should check for any hospital identification or medical alert card. *Always* look for patient identification in the presence of another EMT or law enforcement officer at the scene.

Age and gender are also important considerations in assessing a patient. Some conditions and illnesses are found predominantly in younger patients; others are commonly found only in older patients. Some conditions are prevalent in a certain age group in adult men but in a different age group in women. Some are more prevalent in one gender, and some are limited exclusively to either male or female patients. In addition, the normal range of some of the vital signs will be different for different age groups of children, adults, and elderly patients.

Chief Complaint

The reason that a patient or others call 9-1-1 is vital information. This reason is called the patient's **chief complaint**. In the most literal definition, chief complaints are the major signs and symptoms that the patient reports when asked, "What seems to be the matter?" or "What's wrong?" A patient who responds "My chest hurts" is stating the chief complaint. What you see must also be considered in determining the chief complaint. If the patient's response demonstrates that he or she is having significant difficulty breathing, "difficulty breathing" should be included in the chief complaint as if the patient had reported it verbally. In some protocols, a chief complaint also includes any significant gross, apparent injuries.

The problems or feelings the patients report to you, such as, "I feel dizzy," "My leg hurts," or "Ow, that hurts a lot!" are called **symptoms** (▼ **Figure 5-2A**). These cannot be felt or observed by others. The severity of a symptom is subjective because it is based on the patient's interpretation and tolerance. **Signs** are objective conditions that can be seen, heard, felt, smelled, or measured by you or others (▼ **Figure 5-2B**). Wounds, external bleeding, marked deformities, respirations, and pulse are all signs.

Figure 5-2 **A.** A symptom is a condition that the patient feels and tells you about.

B. A sign is a condition that you can observe about the patient.

Signs and symptoms that occurred before you arrived, such as dizziness that resulted in a loss of consciousness, may be reported by the patient or others at the scene. Because signs and symptoms are essential to understanding the sequence of events and may include signs that are no longer present, they are important parts of the patient history. You should always report how and/or when the signs and symptoms began. This information is important because the reason that signs and symptoms develop often differs, depending on the situation.

Baseline Vital Signs

The initial assessment is a rapid evaluation of the patient's general condition to identify any potentially life-threatening conditions. The brain and other vital organs require constant oxygen. Significant problems with breathing or circulation must be considered potentially life-threatening conditions. A critical problem or deficit in any of the body's other vital systems or functions will progressively affect and be reflected by changes in the respiratory, circulatory, and central nervous systems. Therefore, the status of these systems serves as your guideline for evaluating and measuring the patient's general condition.

Vital signs are the key signs that are used to evaluate the patient's initial general condition. The first set of vital signs that you obtain is called the *baseline vital*

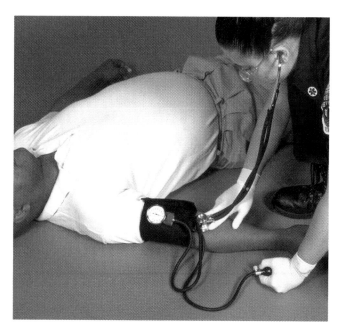

Figure 5-3 Baseline vital signs are key signs that are used to establish the patient's initial condition.

EMT-B Tips

Obtaining the respirations or pulse rate

When obtaining a patient's respirations or pulse rate, count the number of breaths or beats in a 30-second period and then multiply by 2. This method produces a significantly more reliable figure than you would get if you counted for only 15 seconds and multiplied by 4. With either method, the result will always be an even number.

signs. By periodically reassessing the vital signs and comparing the findings with the baseline set, you will be able to identify any significant trends in the patient's condition, particularly whether the patient's condition is becoming worse (▼ Figure 5-3).

Because key indicators include a quantitative (numeric) objective measurement, you will always include the patient's respirations, pulse, and blood pressure when taking and evaluating the vital signs. Other key indications of the patient's respiratory, cardiovascular, and central nervous system status include evaluation of the following:

- Skin temperature and condition in adults
- Capillary refill in children
- Pupillary reaction
- Level of consciousness

Respirations

A patient who is breathing without assistance is said to have **spontaneous respirations** or spontaneous ventilations. Each complete breath includes two distinct phases: inspiration and expiration. During inspiration (inhalation), the chest rises up and out, drawing oxygenated air into the lungs. During expiration (exhalation), the chest returns to its original position, releasing air with an increased carbon dioxide level out of the lungs. Inhalation and exhalation times occur in a 1:3 ratio; the active inhalation phase lasts one third the amount of time of the passive exhalation phase.

Breathing is a continuous process in which each breath regularly follows the last with no notable interruption. Breathing is normally a spontaneous automatic process that occurs without conscious thought, visible effort, marked sounds, or pain. You will assess breathing by watching the patient's chest rise and fall, feeling for air through the mouth and nose during exhalation, and listening to breath sounds with a stethoscope over each lung. Chest rise and breath sounds should be equal on both sides of the chest. A conscious patient who is speaking has spontaneous respirations.

When assessing respirations, you must determine the rate, quality (character), and depth of the patient's breathing.

RATE. Respirations are determined by counting the number of breaths in a 30-second period and multiplying by 2. The result equals the number of breaths per minute. For accuracy, you should count each breath at the same point in its cycle. This is most easily done by counting each peak chest rise. Although you can see peak chest rise, it is easier to place your hand on the patient's chest and feel it. However, be aware that a conscious patient who knows that you are evaluating his or her breathing will often override the automatic rate and depth by breathing more slowly and deeply. To prevent this from happening, you should check respirations in a conscious, alert patient without making the patient aware of what you are evaluating. This can be easily done by first taking a radial pulse and then, without releasing the wrist or otherwise suggesting a change, counting the chest rise that you see or feel as the patient's forearm rises and falls with the movement of the chest (▼ **Figure 5-4**). If the patient coughs, yawns, sighs, or talks during the 30-second period, you should wait a few seconds and start again. (▶ **Table 5-1**) shows the normal range of respiratory rates of patients who are at rest.

> When assessing respirations, you must determine the rate, depth, and quality (character) of the patient's breathing.

QUALITY. You can determine the quality or character of respirations as you are counting. (▼ **Table 5-2**) shows four ways in which the quality or character can be described.

TABLE 5-1 Normal Ranges for Respirations

Age	Range
Adults	12 to 20 breaths/min
Children	15 to 30 breaths/min
Infants	25 to 50 breaths/min

TABLE 5-2 Characteristics of Respirations

Normal	Breathing is neither shallow nor deep
	Equal chest rise and fall
	No use of accessory muscles
Shallow	Slight chest or abdominal wall motion
Labored	Increased breathing effort
	Use of accessory muscles
	Possible gasping
	Nasal flaring, supraclavicular and intercostal retractions in infants and children
Noisy	Increase in sound of breathing, including snoring, wheezing, gurgling, crowing, grunting and stridor

Figure 5-4   Assess respirations in a conscious patient by first taking a radial pulse and then, without releasing the patient's wrist, counting the chest rise and fall for 30 seconds.

Rhythm. While counting the patient's respirations, you should also note the rhythm. If the time from one peak chest rise to the next is fairly consistent, respirations are considered regular. If respirations vary or change frequently, they are considered irregular. When you document the vital signs, be sure to note whether the patient's respirations were regular or irregular.

Effort. Normally, breathing is an effortless process that does not affect a patient's speech, posture, or positioning. Speech is a good indicator of whether a conscious patient is having difficulty breathing. A patient who can speak smoothly without unusual extra pauses is breathing normally. However, a patient who can speak only one word at a time or must stop every two to three words to catch his or her breath is having significant difficulty breathing. Patients who are having marked difficulty breathing will instinctively assume a posture in which it is easier for them to breathe. There are two common postures that indicate that the patient is trying to increase airflow. The first is called the **tripod position**. In this position, a patient sits leaning forward on outstretched arms with the head and chin thrust slightly forward and is having sufficient difficulty breathing that a significant conscious effort is required (▼ **Figure 5-5**). The second is most commonly seen in children—the **sniffing position**. The patient sits upright with the head and chin thrust slightly forward and the patient appears to be sniffing.

Breathing that becomes progressively more difficult requires progressively more effort. When you can see

Figure 5-5   A patient in the tripod position will sit leaning forward on outstretched arms with the head and chin thrust forward slightly.

Pediatric Needs

Chest rise in a small child is less marked than that in an adult. However, a small child's abdomen moves more with each breath than an adult's does. Place your hands on the outer margin of the lower anterior chest to feel the chest wall and abdominal movement, and determine whether the depth is normal, shallow, or deep. In a patient of any age, if it is difficult to gauge the depth of breathing from the chest movement, note instead the amount of air that you feel is exhaled with each breath.

that effort, the patient's breathing is described as **labored breathing**.

Initially, labored breathing is characterized by the patient's position, concentration on breathing, and the increased effort and depth of each breath. As breathing becomes more labored, accessory muscles in the chest and neck are used, and the patient may make grunting sounds with each breath. In infants and small children, nasal flaring and supraclavicular and intercostal retractions (indentation above the clavicles and in the spaces between the ribs) are commonly associated with labored breathing. Sometimes, the patient may be gasping.

Infants and small children will continue to have labored breathing for a sustained period, will then often become exhausted, and finally will no longer have the strength to maintain the necessary energy to breathe. In infants and small children, cardiac arrest is generally caused by respiratory arrest.

Noisy breathing. Normal breathing is silent or, in a very quiet environment, accompanied only by the sounds of air movement at the mouth and nose. Through a stethoscope, normal breath sounds include only the sound of air movement through the bronchi accompanied by a soft, low-pitched murmur. Breathing accompanied by other sounds indicates a significant respiratory problem. When the airway is partially obstructed by a foreign body or swelling, you may hear **stridor**, a harsh, high-pitched, crowing sound. If you can hear bubbling or gurgling, the patient probably has fluid in the airway. You may hear other sounds, including wheezes, snoring, gurgling, or bubbling. The presence of any of these indicates that a serious respiratory problem exists. With a complete airway obstruction, the patient will not be able to move any air and will no longer be able to cough or talk.

A patient who coughs up thick, yellowish or greenish sputum (matter from the lungs) most likely has an advanced respiratory infection. A patient with a chest injury may cough up blood or a frothy whitish or pinkish foam-like sputum. A patient with congestive heart failure may also cough up a frothy sputum. The presence of either substance, regardless of its cause, indicates that an urgent, potentially critical cardiovascular and respiratory problem exists. The patient's condition may deteriorate rapidly to a point at which the patient can no longer breathe.

DEPTH. The amount of air that the patient is exchanging depends on both the rate and the **tidal volume**, the amount of air that is exchanged with each breath. The depth of the breath determines whether the tidal volume is normal, less than normal, or more than normal. Respirations are described as shallow when the movement of the chest wall and air that you feel exhaled with each breath is less than normal. Deep respirations occur when chest movement and exhaled air are significantly greater than normal. You should document when the patient's respirations are shallow or deep; however, you do not have to record a normal depth of breathing.

Pulse

With each heartbeat, the ventricles contract, forcefully ejecting blood from the heart and propelling it into the arteries. The **pulse** is the pressure wave that occurs as each heartbeat causes a surge in the blood circulating through the arteries. The pulse is most easily felt at a pulse point where a major artery lies near the surface and can be pressed gently against a bone or solid organ. To *palpate* (feel) the pulse, hold together your index and long fingers and place their tips over a pulse point, pressing gently against the artery until you feel intermittent pulsations. Sometimes, you may have to slide your fingertips a little to each side and press again until you feel a pulse. When palpating a pulse, do not allow your thumb to touch the patient. If you do so, you may mistake the strong pulsing circulation in your thumb for the patient's pulse.

In responsive patients who are older than 1 year, you should palpate the radial pulse at the wrist ▶ **Figure 5-6A** . In unresponsive patients older than 1 year, you should palpate the carotid pulse in the neck ▶ **Figure 5-6B** . When palpating the carotid pulse, you should place the fingertips of your index and long fingers along the carotid artery in the groove between the trachea and the neck muscle. Use caution when palpating the carotid pulse in a responsive patient, especially an elderly patient. Only gentle pressure on one side of the neck

should be used. Never press on the carotid arteries on both sides of the neck at the same time. Doing so can cut off circulation to the brain.

In infants, both the radial and carotid pulses are difficult to locate. Because of the infant's soft, immature trachea, palpating the carotid pulse is not recommended. Palpate the brachial pulse, located at the underside of the upper arm, in children younger than 1 year ▼ **Figure 5-7** . With the infant lying supine,

Figure 5-6 **A.** To palpate the radial pulse, place the tips of your first two fingers over the radial artery, pressing gently until you feel intermittent pulsations. **B.** To palpate the carotid pulse, place the tips of your first two fingers over the carotid artery, pressing gently until you feel intermittent pulsations.

Figure 5-7 To palpate the brachial pulse in an infant, press firmly along the brachial artery at the underside of the upper arm.

you can access the brachial pulse by elevating the arm over the infant's head. Because most infants have chubby arms, you need to press your adjacent fingertips firmly along the brachial artery, which lies parallel to the long axis of the upper arm, to be able to palpate the pulse.

Your first consideration when taking a pulse is to determine whether the patient has a palpable pulse or is pulseless. When taking the pulse, you should assess and report its rate, strength, and regularity.

RATE. To obtain the pulse rate in most patients, you should count the number of pulses felt in a 30-second period and then multiply by 2. A pulse that is weak and difficult to palpate, irregular, or extremely slow should be palpated and counted for a full minute. A pulse rate is counted as beats per minute; however, in reporting the pulse rate, it is not necessary to state or write "beats per minute" after the number.

The pulse rate in most adults (at rest) averages around 72 beats/min. However, pulse rate can vary significantly from person to person. In the well-conditioned athlete or in individuals taking heart medications such as beta-blockers, the pulse rate may be considerably lower. A pulse rate between 60 and 100 beats/min is considered normal in adults. The average pulse rate in children is generally higher. (▼ **Table 5-3**) shows the normal ranges of pulse rates.

In assessing the pulse rate in an adult patient, a rate that is greater than 100 beats/min is described as **tachycardia**, and a rate of less than 60 beats/min is described as **bradycardia**.

STRENGTH. You should always report the pulse's strength whenever reporting or recording the pulse. The pulse is generally palpated at the radial or carotid arteries in adults and at the brachial artery in infants, because it is normally strong and easily palpable at these locations. Therefore, if the pulse feels of normal strength, you should describe it as being strong. You should describe a stronger than normal pulse

as "bounding" and a pulse that is weak and difficult to feel as "weak" or "thready." With a little experience, you will be able to make the necessary distinctions easily.

REGULARITY. When assessing the quality of the pulse, you must also determine whether it is regular or irregular. When the interval between each ventricular contraction of the heart is short, the pulse is rapid. When the interval is longer, the pulse is slower. No matter what the rate, the interval between each contraction should be the same, and the pulse that results should occur at a constant, regular rhythm. You should note and document this rhythm as regular.

The rhythm is considered irregular if the heart periodically has a premature or late beat or if a pulse beat is missed. Some individuals have a chronically irregular pulse; however, if an irregular pulse is found in a patient with signs and symptoms that suggest a cardiovascular problem, the patient likely needs advanced cardiac assessment and life support. Therefore, depending on your protocols, you should call for ALS backup, arrange for an intercept, or initiate prompt transport to definitive care.

The Skin

The condition of the patient's skin can tell you a lot about the patient's peripheral circulation and perfusion, blood oxygen levels, and body temperature. When assessing the skin, you should evaluate its color, temperature, and moisture.

COLOR. Assessing the skin helps you to determine the adequacy of perfusion. **Perfusion** is the circulation of blood within an organ or tissue. Adequate perfusion meets the cells' current needs; inadequate perfusion will cause cells and tissues to die.

Many blood vessels lie near the surface of the skin. The skin's color is determined by the blood circulating through these vessels and the amount and type of pigment that is present in the skin. Blood is red when it is adequately saturated with oxygen. As a result, skin in lightly pigmented individuals is pinkish. The pigmentation in most individuals will not hide changes in the skin's underlying color, regardless of the individual's race. In patients with deeply pigmented skin, changes in color may be apparent only in certain areas, such as the fingernail beds, the mucous membranes in the mouth, the lips, the underside of the arm and palm (which are usually less pigmented), and the **conjunctiva** of the eyes. The conjunctiva is the delicate membrane lining the eyelids and it covers the exposed surface of the eye. In addition, the palms of the hands and soles of the feet should be assessed in infants and children.

TABLE 5-3 Normal Ranges for Pulse Rate	
Age	**Range, beats/min**
Adults	60 to 100
Children	80 to 120
Toddlers	90 to 150
Newborns	120 to 160

Poor peripheral circulation will cause the skin to appear pale, white, ashen, or gray, possibly with a waxy translucent appearance like a white candle. Abnormally cold or frozen skin may also appear this way. When the blood is not properly saturated with oxygen, it appears bluish. Therefore, in a patient with insufficient air exchange and low levels of oxygen in the blood, the blood and vessels become bluish, and the lips, mucous membranes, nail beds, and skin over the blood vessels appear blue or gray. This condition is called **cyanosis** ▼ **Figure 5-8** .

High blood pressure may cause the skin to be abnormally flushed and red. In some patients with extremely high blood pressure, all the visible blood vessels will be so full that the skin will appear to be a dark reddish-purple. A patient with carbon monoxide poisoning or a significant fever, heatstroke, sunburn, mild thermal burns, or other conditions in which the body is unable to properly dissipate heat will also appear to have red skin.

Changes in skin color may also result from chronic illness. Liver disease or dysfunction may cause **jaundice**, resulting in the patient's skin and **sclera** turning yellow. The sclera is the normally white portion of the eye.

TEMPERATURE. Normally, the skin is warm to the touch. When the patient has a significant fever, sunburn, or hyperthermia, the skin feels hot to the touch. The skin will feel cool when the patient is in early shock, has mild hypothermia, or has inadequate perfusion. The skin will feel cold when the patient is in profound shock, has hypothermia, or has frostbite.

Body temperature is normally measured with a thermometer in the hospital. However, in the field, feeling the patient's forehead with the back of your hand is usually adequate to determine whether the patient's temperature is elevated or depressed ▼ **Figure 5-9** .

MOISTURE. Dry skin is normal. Skin that is wet, moist (often called diaphoretic), or excessively dry and hot suggests a problem. In the early stages of shock, the skin will become slightly moist. Skin that is only slightly moist but not covered excessively with sweat is described as clammy, damp, or moist. When the skin is bathed in sweat, such as after strenuous exercise or when the patient is in shock, the skin is described as wet or **diaphoretic**.

Because the skin's color, temperature, and moisture are often related signs, you should consider them together. When recording or reporting your assessment of the skin, you should first describe the color, then the temperature, and last, whether the skin is dry, moist, or wet. For example, you could say or write, "Skin: pale, cool, and clammy."

Capillary Refill

Capillary refill is a test that evaluates the ability of the circulatory system to restore blood to the capillary system. When evaluated in an uninjured limb, capillary refill reflects the patient's perfusion. Capillary refill time is often affected by the patient's body temperature, position, and medications. To test capillary refill, place your thumb on the patient's fingernail with your fingers on the underside of the patient's finger, and gently compress ▶ **Figure 5-10A** . The blood will be forced from the capillaries in the nail bed. When you remove the pressure applied against the tip of the patient's finger, the nail bed will remain blanched and

Figure 5-8 Cyanosis occurs when the patient has low levels of oxygen in the blood.

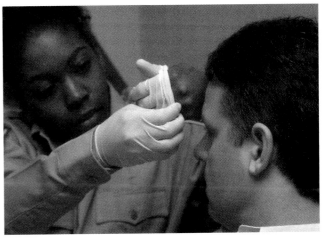

Figure 5-9 Assess skin temperature by feeling the patient's forehead with the back of your hand.

white for a brief period. As the underlying capillaries refill with blood, the nail bed will be restored to its normal pink color.

Capillary refill should be both prompt and pink. With adequate perfusion, the color in the nail bed should be restored to its normal pink within 2 seconds, or about the time it takes to say "capillary refill" at a normal rate of speech (▼ **Figure 5-10B**). You should report and document the capillary refill as normal, "CRT=2" or "CRT>2." You should suspect poor peripheral circulation when capillary refill takes more than 2 seconds or the nail bed remains blanched. In this instance, you should report and document the capillary refill as delayed.

A bluish color may indicate that the capillaries are refilling with blood drawn from the veins rather than with fresh, oxygenated blood from the arteries, making the test invalid. You should also consider the capillary refill test invalid if the patient is in or has been exposed to a cold environment or if the patient is elderly. In both situations, delayed capillary refill is normal.

To assess capillary refill in infants and children younger than 6 years, press on the skin or nail bed, and determine how long it takes for the pink color to return. As with adults, normal capillary refill takes less than 2 seconds.

Blood Pressure

Adequate blood pressure is necessary to maintain proper circulation and perfusion of the vital organ cells. <u>**Blood pressure (BP)**</u> is the pressure of circulating blood against the walls of the arteries. A decrease in the blood pressure may indicate one of the following:

EMT-B Tips

Capillary refill is most reliable as a perfusion indicator.

- Loss of blood or its fluid components
- Loss of vascular tone and sufficient arterial constriction to maintain the necessary pressure even without any actual fluid or blood loss
- A cardiac pumping problem

When any of these conditions occurs and results in a drop in circulation, the body's compensatory mechanisms are activated, the heart and pulse rates increase, and the arteries constrict. Normal blood pressure is maintained, and by decreasing the blood flow to the skin and extremities, available blood volume is temporarily redirected to the vital organs so that they remain adequately perfused. However, as shock progresses, and the body's defense mechanisms can no longer keep up, the blood pressure will fall. *Decreased blood pressure is a late sign of shock and indicates that the critical decompensated phase has begun.* Any patient with a markedly low blood pressure has inadequate pressure to maintain proper perfusion of all the vital organs and needs to have his or her blood pressure and perfusion restored immediately to a normal level.

Figure 5-10 **A.** To test capillary refill, gently compress the fingertip until it blanches.

B. Release the fingertip, and count until it returns to its normal pink color.

When the blood pressure becomes elevated, the body's defenses act to reduce it. Some individuals have chronically high blood pressure from progressive narrowing of the arteries that occurs with age, and during an acute episode, their blood pressure may increase to even higher levels. Head injury or a number of other conditions may also cause blood pressure to rise to very high levels. Abnormally high blood pressure may result in a rupture or other critical damage in the arterial system.

You should measure blood pressure in all patients older than 3 years.

Blood pressure contains two key separate components: systolic pressure and diastolic pressure. **Systolic pressure** is the increased pressure that is caused along the artery with each contraction (systole) of the ventricle and the pulse wave that it produces. **Diastolic pressure** is the residual pressure that remains in the arteries during the relaxing phase of the heart's cycle (diastole), when the left ventricle is at rest. Systolic pressure represents the maximum pressure to which the arteries are subjected, and the diastolic pressure represents the minimum amount of pressure that is always present in the arteries.

Early blood pressure gauges contained a column of mercury and a linear scale that was graduated in millimeters. Even though different gauges are used today, the blood pressure is still measured in millimeters of mercury (mm Hg). Blood pressure is reported as a fraction in the form systolic pressure over diastolic pressure. Therefore, if the patient's systolic pressure is 120 and the diastolic pressure is 78, you would record it as "BP 120/78 mm Hg." You would report the patient's blood pressure verbally as "BP is 120 over 78."

EQUIPMENT FOR MEASURING BLOOD PRESSURE. You will use a sphygmomanometer (blood pressure cuff) to apply pressure against the artery when measuring the blood pressure. The sphygmomanometer contains the following components:

- A wide outer cuff designed to be fastened snugly around the entire arm or leg
- An inflatable wide bladder sewn into a portion of the cuff
- A ball-pump with a one-way valve that allows air to enter and a turn-valve that can be closed or, when opened, will allow air to be released at a controlled speed from the cuff
- A pressure gauge calibrated in millimeters of mercury, which indicates the pressure that exists in the cuff that is being applied against the underlying artery

> Blood pressure contains
> two key separate components:
> systolic pressure and diastolic pressure.

Most agencies carry at least three sizes of blood pressure cuffs: adult, thigh, and pediatric ▼ **Figure 5-11** . The normal size cuff is designed to wrap around the arm 1–1.5 times and take up ²/₃ the length from the armpit to the crease in the elbow of most adults. Use a thigh cuff with patients who are obese or have exceptionally well-developed arm muscles or to take the blood pressure of the thigh in patients who have injuries in both arms. Use a small pediatric cuff with children and exceptionally small adults.

You must be sure to select the appropriately sized cuff. A cuff that is too small may result in falsely high readings; a cuff that is too large may result in falsely low readings.

AUSCULTATION. **Auscultation** is the method of listening to sounds within organs with a stethoscope. You will usually measure blood pressure by auscultation ▶ **Skill Drill 5-1** . Follow these steps:

1. **With the patient's arm extended** with the palm up, place the cuff so that it lies across the upper arm and is located with its distal edge about 1″ above the crease at the inside of the patient's elbow. Make sure the center of the inflatable bladder, which is usually marked by an arrow on the cuff, lies over the brachial artery. Next, wrap

Figure 5-11   Three sizes of blood pressure cuffs: thigh, adult, and pediatric.

SkillDrill 5-1   Obtaining a Blood Pressure by Auscultation or Palpation

Apply the cuff snugly.

Palpate the brachial artery.

Place the stethoscope and grasp the ball-pump and turn-valve.

Close the valve and pump to 20 mm Hg above the point at which you stop hearing pulse sounds. Note the systolic and diastolic pressures as you let air escape slowly.

Open the valve and quickly release remaining air.

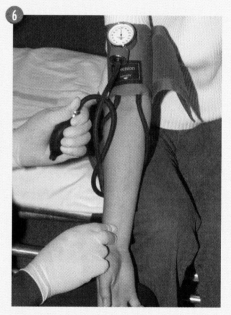

When using the palpation method, you should place your fingertips on the radial artery so that you feel the radial pulse.

the ends so that the cuff surrounds the upper arm snugly but not tightly. Secure the cuff with the Velcro fastener attached to it, making sure to rub your hand over the entire area where the two sides of the Velcro fastener are in contact. Once the cuff has been properly secured around the upper arm, the arm should be held at about the same level as the heart **(Step 1)**.

2. **Palpate the brachial artery** (in the antecubital fossa, the anterior aspect of the elbow) to determine where to place the stethoscope **(Step 2)**.

3. **Place the diaphragm of the stethoscope over the artery,** and hold it firmly pressed against the artery with the fingers of your nondominant hand. Hold the rubber ball-pump in the palm of your other hand and the turn-valve between your thumb and first finger **(Step 3)**.

4. **Close the valve tightly, and pump the ball-pump** until you no longer hear pulse sounds. Continue pumping to increase the cuff's pressure by an additional 20 mm Hg. Next, slowly turn the valve, opening it until air is steadily escaping from the

cuff and you see the needle of the gauge slowly drop. Watch the gauge, and listen carefully. Note the patient's systolic pressure as the reading on the gauge at which the "taps" or "thumps" of the pulse waves can first be heard clearly. As the pressure in the cuff is progressively reduced, pulse sounds will continue for a time, then suddenly disappear. Note the patient's diastolic pressure as the reading on the gauge at which the sounds stopped **(Step 4)**.

5. As soon as the pulse sounds stop, **open the valve, and release the remaining air quickly.** Once you have finished measuring the blood pressure, you should document your findings and the time at which the blood pressure was taken. Blood pressure is most often measured by auscultation with the patient in a sitting or semi-sitting position. Be sure to note whether a different method or position was used. Occasionally, when a patient's blood pressure is very low, you will continue to hear pulse sounds from the reading at which they started all the way until the gauge has reached 0. When this occurs, you should record the diastolic pressure as "0" or "all the way down" to indicate that it was not measurable by stethoscope **(Step 5)**.

PALPATION. The auscultation method will be difficult or impossible to use in a very noisy environment and may produce inaccurate findings. The palpation method, which is examination by touch that does not depend on your ability to hear sounds, should be used in these cases (◄ **Skill Drill 5-1, Step 6**).

To measure blood pressure by palpation, secure the appropriately sized cuff around the patient's upper arm in the manner previously described. With your non-dominant hand, palpate the patient's radial pulse on the same arm as the cuff, without moving your fingertips once you have located it, until you have completed taking the blood pressure. While holding the ball-pump in your other hand, close the turn-valve and rapidly inflate the cuff to 200 mm Hg. As the cuff inflates, you will no longer feel the pulse under your fingertips. Open the turn-valve so that air slowly escapes from the cuff, and carefully observe the gauge. When you can again feel the radial pulse under your fingertips, you should note the reading on the gauge as the patient's systolic blood pressure. You will not be able to determine the diastolic pressure with this method. Next, open the turn-valve further, and completely deflate the cuff. Document your findings including the time, and note that the pressure was taken by palpation. On your patient care report, you can record the blood pressure as "120/P."

EMT-B Tips

Record blood pressure readings with the time. Note the arm on which you took the measurement, and the patient's position if other than sitting or semi-sitting. For a blood pressure by palpation, you can abbreviate: "120/P."

NORMAL BLOOD PRESSURE. Blood pressure levels vary with age and gender. (▼ **Table 5-4**) serves as a guideline for normal blood pressure ranges.

A patient has **hypotension** when the blood pressure is lower than the normal range and **hypertension** when the blood pressure is higher than the normal range.

Typically, you will see children less frequently than adults; therefore, you might not remember the normal ranges for the various age groups. You might wish to carry a chart with you that lists normal blood pressure ranges and other vital signs.

CRITICAL HYPOTENSION. You must assume that a patient who has a critically low blood pressure can no longer compensate sufficiently to maintain adequate perfusion. (▼ **Table 5-5**) shows the point at which blood pressure is considered to be critically low.

TABLE 5-4 Normal Ranges for Blood Pressure

Age	Range
Adults	100 to 140 mm Hg (systolic)
	60 to 90 mm Hg (diastolic)
Children (ages 1 to 8 years)	80 to 110 mm Hg (systolic)
Infants (newborn to to age 1 year)	60 mm Hg (systolic)

TABLE 5-5 Minimum Acceptable Systolic Blood Pressures

Adults/Adolescents	100 mm Hg or less
Children	70 mm Hg or less

EMT-B Tips

AVPU scale

The **AVPU scale** is a rapid method of assessing the patient's level of consciousness using one of the following four terms:

A Awake and **A**lert
V Responsive to **V**erbal Stimulus
P Responsive to **P**ain
U **U**nresponsive

You should determine whether a patient is awake and alert.

A patient who is not awake and alert but who is aroused and responds to your voice by opening his or her eyes, moaning, speaking, or moving is responding to verbal stimulus. A patient who does not respond to your normal speaking voice but who responds to your yelled voice is responding to loud verbal stimulus. Be sure to note how the patient responded. Tap a patient who is hearing impaired with your fingers repeatedly. If the patient responds, note that the patient is hearing impaired but responds to being tapped.

To determine whether a patient who does not respond to verbal stimuli will respond to a painful stimulus, you should gently but firmly pinch the patient's skin (▶ **Figure 5-12**). A patient who moans or withdraws is responding to painful stimulus. Be sure to note the type and location of the stimulus and how the patient responded.

Figure 5-12 To assess whether a patient will respond to a painful stimulus, gently but firmly pinch the patient's skin. This can be done at the neck or on the earlobe.

If the patient does not respond to a painful stimulus on one side, try to elicit a response on the other side. Note that a patient who remains flaccid without moving or making a sound is unresponsive.

In assessing the patient's general circulation, the blood pressure, pulse, skin temperature, and capillary refill should *not* be assessed in an injured limb. However, once you have obtained these vital signs from an uninjured limb, you might wish to compare the distal skin temperature, quality of the distal pulse, and/or capillary refill time in the injured limb with those found on the uninjured side. This information is useful in evaluating whether the injury may have compromised the circulation in the injured limb.

Level of Consciousness

The patient's level of consciousness (LOC) is considered a vital sign because the status of the central nervous system is reflected by it. However, in the early assessment, you need to ascertain only the apparent gross level of consciousness by determining whether the patient is awake and alert with an unaltered LOC, conscious but with an altered LOC, or unconscious.

As you assess a patient, you must determine the appropriateness of a response by how well it demon-strates the patient's understanding and mental activity, not how well it reflects your definition of socially acceptable behavior.

When a patient is conscious with a lower level of consciousness, the body's defense mechanisms may no longer be able to compensate adequately, possibly indicating that inadequate perfusion and oxygenation or a chemical or neurologic problem is adversely affecting the brain and its ability to function. A lowered level of consciousness in a conscious patient can also be caused by medications, drugs, alcohol, or poisoning.

Your assessment of a patient who is unconscious when you arrive should be focused initially on airway, breathing, and circulation, and then on identifying other emergency care that the patient may need. Sustained unconsciousness should warn you that a critical respiratory, circulatory, or central nervous system problem or deficit may exist, and you must assume that the patient has a potentially critical injury or potentially life-threatening condition. Therefore, after rapidly assessing the patient and providing

A - Alert
V - Responsive to Verbal stimulus
P - Responsive to Pain
U - Unresponsive

emergency treatment, you should package the patient and provide rapid transport to the hospital.

The <u>Glasgow Coma Scale</u> is a method of assessing a patient's level of consciousness by scoring the patient's response to eye opening, motor response, and verbal response (▼ **Figure 5-13**).

PUPILS. The diameter and reactivity to light of the patient's pupils reflect the status of the brain's perfusion, oxygenation, and condition. The pupil is a circular opening in the center of the pigmented iris of the eye. The pupils are normally round and of approximately equal size and serve as optical diaphragms, adjusting their size depending on the available light. In normal room light, the pupil appears to be midsize. With less light, the pupils dilate, allowing more light to enter the eye, making it possible to see even in dim

light. With high light levels or when a bright light is suddenly introduced, the pupils instantly constrict, allowing less light to enter, protecting the sensitive receptors in the inner eye from damage (▼ **Figure 5-14A**). When a brighter light is introduced into one eye (or higher levels of light enter one eye only), both pupils should constrict equally to the appropriate size for the pupil receiving the most light.

In the absence of any light, the pupils will become fully relaxed and dilated (▼ **Figure 5-14B**). When light is introduced, each eye sends sensory signals to the brain indicating the level of light it is receiving. Pupil size is regulated by a series of continuous motor commands that the brain automatically sends through the oculomotor nerves to each eye, causing both pupils to constrict to the same appropriate size. Normally, pupil size changes instantly to any change in light level.

GLASGOW COMA SCALE

Eye Opening

Spontaneous	4
To Voice	3
To Pain	2
None	1

Verbal Response

Oriented	5
Confused	4
Inappropriate Words	3
Incomprehensible Words	2
None	1

Motor Response

Obeys Command	6
Localizes Pain	5
Withdraws (pain)	4
Flexion (pain)	3
Extension (pain)	2
None	1

Glasgow Coma Score Total	**15**

(**Figure 5-13**) The Glasgow Coma Scale.

(**Figure 5-14**) **A.** Constricted pupils. **B.** Dilated pupils. **C.** Unequal pupils.

You must assume the patient has depressed brain function as a result of either central nervous system depression or injury if the pupils react in any of the following ways:

- Become fixed with no reaction to light
- Dilate with introduction of a bright light and constrict when the light is removed
- React sluggishly instead of briskly
- Become unequal in size   ◀ **Figure 5-14C**
- Become unequal in size when a bright light is introduced into or removed from one eye

Depressed brain function can be produced by the following situations:

- Injury of the brain or brain stem
- Trauma or stroke
- Brain tumor
- Inadequate oxygenation or perfusion
- Drugs or toxins (central nervous system depressants)

Opiates, which are one category of central nervous system depressants, cause the pupils to constrict so significantly, regardless of light, that they become so small as to be described as pinpoint. Intracranial pressure from intracranial bleeding may cause sufficient pressure against the oculomotor nerve on one side that the motor commands can no longer pass from the brain to that eye. When this occurs, the eye no longer receives commands to constrict, and its pupil becomes fully dilated and fixed. This is described as a blown pupil.

Pupils may be dilated, may be unequal as a result of medication placed into one or both eyes or from an injury or condition of the eye, or may not be reacting appropriately.

The letters PEARRL serve as a useful guide in assessing the pupils. They stand for the following:

P = **P**upils

E = **E**qual

A = **A**nd

R = **R**ound

R = **R**egular in size

L = react to **L**ight

You can report patients with normal pupils as "Pupils are equal, round, and regular in size, and react properly to light" or "pupils = PEARRL." Describe any abnormal findings using the longer form, such as "Pupils are equal and round, the left pupil is fixed and dilated, the right pupil is regular in size and reacts to light."

Reassessment of the Vital Signs

The vital signs that you obtain serve two important functions. The first set establishes an important initial measurement of the patient's respiratory and cardiovascular systems and the quality of perfusion and oxygenation of the brain and other vital organs. The initial vital signs serve as a key baseline.

Throughout your care of the patient, you should monitor the patient's vital signs for any changes from your initial findings. You should reassess and record vital signs at least every 15 minutes in a stable patient and at least every 5 minutes in an unstable patient. You should also reassess and record vital signs following all medical interventions. This ongoing comparative assessment is an important indicator of whether your interventions have restored the patient's vital functions to an acceptable range or are at least preventing further deterioration. Reassessment also indicates whether you should consider more aggressive intervention whenever deterioration continues.

Obtaining a SAMPLE History

Once you have provided emergency care and are ready to further examine the patient, you should try to obtain a key brief history, or **SAMPLE history**. As part of the assessment of every patient, you should ask the following questions, using the word SAMPLE as a guideline:

- **S**igns and **S**ymptoms of the episode: What signs and symptoms occurred at onset of the incident? Does the patient report pain?

- **A**llergies: Is the patient allergic to any medication, food, or other substance? What reactions did the patient have to any of them? If the patient has no known allergies, you should note this on the run report as "no known allergies" or "nka."

- **M**edications: What medications was the patient prescribed? What dosage was prescribed? How often is the patient supposed to take the medication? What prescription and over-the-counter medications has the patient taken in the last 12 hours? How much was taken and when?

- **P**ertinent past history: Does the patient have any history of medical, surgical, or trauma occurrences? Has the patient had a recent accident, fall, or blow to the head?

> You should reassess and record vital signs at least every 15 minutes in a stable patient and at least every 5 minutes in an unstable patient.

- **L**ast oral intake: When did the patient last eat or drink? What did the patient eat or drink and how much was consumed? Did the patient take any drugs or drink alcohol? Has there been any other oral intake in the last 4 hours?

- **E**vents leading to the injury or illness: What are the key events that led up to this incident? What occurred between the onset of the incident and your arrival? What was the patient doing when this illness started? What was the patient doing when this injury happened?

With practice, you will be able to obtain, document, and report a meaningful brief history. Be sure to ask the patient and bystanders for information. If the patient is unconscious, look for a medical identification tag or for a medical information card in the patient's wallet or purse. *Always* look for patient identification in the presence of another EMT or law enforcement officer at the scene.

decorticate - Bring arms into body
decerebrate - Stretch arms, arch back.
More severe.

Prep Kit

Ready for Review

Whenever you are called to the scene of an illness or injury, you should find out the patient's chief complaint. Your assessment of the patient should include rapidly evaluating the patient's general condition and identifying any potentially life-threatening injuries or conditions. Baseline vital signs are the key signs that you will use to evaluate the patient's general condition. You will be assessing the patient's respirations, pulse, skin, blood pressure, level of consciousness, and pupils.

After you have initially assessed the patient and obtained the baseline vital signs, you should reassess the patient for any changes from your initial findings.

In addition to determining the chief complaint and assessing the patient's general condition, you should try to obtain a SAMPLE history from the patient or bystanders. By asking several important questions, you will be able to determine the patient's signs and symptoms, allergies, medications, pertinent past history, last oral intake, and the events leading up to the incident.

Vital Vocabulary

auscultation A method of listening to sounds within an organ with a stethoscope.

AVPU scale A method of assessing level of consciousness by determining whether the patient is awake and alert, responsive to verbal stimulus or pain, or unresponsive; used principally in the initial assessment.

blood pressure (BP) The pressure of circulating blood against the walls of the arteries.

bradycardia Slow heart rate, less than 60 beats/min.

capillary refill A test that evaluates the ability of the circulatory system to restore blood to the capillary system.

chief complaint The reason a patient called for help. Also, the patient's response to questions such as "What's wrong?" or "What happened?"

conjunctiva The delicate membrane lining the eyelids and covering the exposed surface of the eye.

cyanosis A bluish-gray skin color that is caused by reduced levels of oxygen in the blood.

diaphoretic Characterized by profuse sweating.

diastolic pressure The pressure that remains in the arteries during the relaxing phase of the heart's cycle (diastole) when the left ventricle is at rest.

Glasgow Coma Scale A method of assessing a patient's level of consciousness by scoring the patient's response to eye opening, motor response, and verbal response.

hypertension Blood pressure that is higher than the normal range.

hypotension Blood pressure that is lower than the normal range.

jaundice A yellow skin or sclera color that is caused by liver disease or dysfunction.

labored breathing Breathing that requires visibly increased effort; characterized by grunting, stridor, and use of accessory muscles.

perfusion Circulation of blood within an organ or tissue.

pulse The pressure wave that occurs as each heartbeat causes a surge in the blood circulating through the arteries.

SAMPLE history A brief history of a patient's condition to determine signs and symptoms, allergies, medications, pertinent past history, last oral intake, and events leading to the injury or illness.

sclera The white portion of the eye.

sign An objective finding that can be seen, heard, felt, smelled, or measured.

sniffing position An unusually upright position in which the patient's head and chin are thrust slightly forward.

spontaneous respirations Breathing in a patient that occurs with no assistance.

stridor A harsh, high-pitched, crowing inspiratory sound, such as the sound often heard in acute laryngeal (upper airway) obstruction.

symptom A subjective finding that the patient feels but that can be identified only by the patient.

systolic pressure The increased pressure along an artery with each contraction (systole) of the ventricle.

tachycardia Rapid heart rhythm, more than 100 beats/min.

tidal volume The amount of air that is exchanged with each breath.

tripod position An upright position where the patient leans forward onto two arms stretched forward and thrusts the head and chin forward.

vital signs The key signs that are used to evaluate the patient's overall condition, including respirations, pulse, blood pressure, level of consciousness, and skin characteristics.

Assessment in Action

A 36-year-old patient complains that she "does not feel well." She is alert and oriented but you note that she is sitting in a tripod position. She appears pale but her lips are gray and her skin is pale, cool, and clammy.

She has no allergies but has a history of asthma and is on a Proventil inhaler. She has a blood pressure of 162/98 mm Hg, a pulse rate of 102 beats/min, and respirations of 28 breaths/min.

1. The A in SAMPLE History refers to:
   A. age.
   B. affect.
   C. attitude.
   D. allergies.

2. The tripod position usually suggests that the patient may have:
   A. difficulty sitting up.
   B. difficulty lying down.
   C. difficulty breathing.
   D. weakness or dizziness.

3. In this patient, which of the following assessment signs suggests poor perfusion?
   A. BP of 162/98
   B. Gray lips
   C. Pulse 102
   D. Tripod position

4. When getting a history, you note that she can only talk in two- to three-word sentences. Other signs of difficulty breathing you should be looking for include:
   A. accessory muscle use.
   B. difficulty sitting up.
   C. extremity paralysis.
   D. flushed face.

5. Of all the signs of difficulty breathing, which are specific for a child?
   A. Cyanosis
   B. Nasal flaring
   C. Mottled skin
   D. Fever

6. Finding the brachial pulse in an infant may be made easier by:
   A. placing the infant in a sitting position.
   B. lowering the infant's arm.
   C. raising the infant's arm.
   D. tilting the infant's head down.

7. This patient's BP is a little high. One thing that can cause a false high blood pressure is:
   A. a cuff that is too small.
   B. a cuff that is too large.
   C. using the bell of the stethoscope.
   D. using the diaphragm of the stethoscope.

8. This patient is alert, oriented, and squeezes your hands when asked. Her Glasgow Coma Scale score would be:
   A. 0   C. 10
   B. 3   D. 15

Challenging Questions

9. If a patient can talk in a complete sentence, what assumption can be made about tidal volume?

10. When a patient is verbally unresponsive, why should a painful stimulus be tried on both sides of the body?

Points to Ponder

Your regular partner is on vacation and you are teamed with a "part-timer" that fills in for your agency. You are dispatched to a complaint of abdominal pain. When you arrive, the apartment is on the third floor of the building and your partner complains about having to take the stretcher up three flights of stairs. The patient is quite obese and your partner says "just our luck" as you enter the room. The patient describes her pain and you explain that you are going to "feel" her abdomen and you ask her to tell you if anything hurts. Your partner mumbles "good luck" as you approach the patient's abdomen. Hoping to keep him quiet, you suggest that he take a set of vitals. He replies that "there is no way he can get a blood pressure cuff around that arm" and that he is not going all the way back down to the rig for the "huge cuff." How and when would you deal with your partner?

Issues Patient Respect, Personal Biases and Prejudices, Appropriate Discussions in Front of Non-EMS Personnel.

Online Outlook

If time permits, you should attempt to learn the patient's SAMPLE history. Improve your ability to identify SAMPLE information by completing Exercise 5 at **www.emtb.com**.

Lifting and Moving Patients

Objectives

Cognitive

1. Define body mechanics (p 148).
2. Discuss the guidelines and safety precautions that need to be followed when lifting a patient (p 150).
3. Describe the safe lifting of cots and stretchers (p 152).
4. Discuss the guidelines and safety precautions for carrying patients and/or equipment (p 156).
5. Discuss one-handed carrying techniques (p 153).
6. Describe correct and safe carrying procedures on stairs (p 154).
7. State the guidelines for reaching and their application (p 157).
8. Describe correct reaching for log rolls (p 159).
9. State the guidelines for pushing and pulling (p 160).
10. Discuss the general considerations of moving patients (p 161).
11. State three situations that may require the use of an emergency move (p 161).
12. Identify the following patient-carrying devices (p 172):
    - Wheeled ambulance stretcher
    - Portable ambulance stretcher
    - Stair chair
    - Scoop stretcher
    - Long spine board
    - Basket stretcher
    - Flexible stretcher

Affective

13. Explain the rationale for properly lifting and moving patients (p 148).

Psychomotor

14. Working with a partner, prepare each of the following devices for use, transfer a patient to the device, properly position the patient on the device, move the device to the ambulance, and load the patient into the ambulance: wheeled ambulance stretcher, portable ambulance stretcher, stair chair, scoop stretcher, long spine board, basket stretcher, and flexible stretcher (p 148).
15. Working with a partner, demonstrate techniques for the transfer of a patient from an ambulance stretcher to a hospital stretcher (p 168).

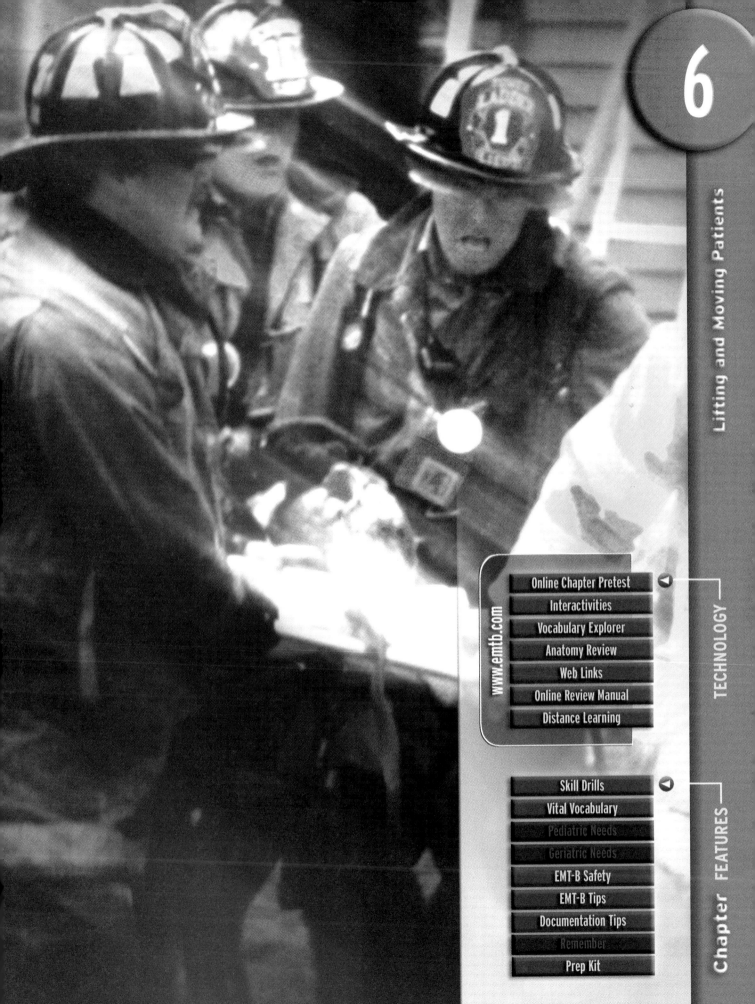

TECHNOLOGY

www.emtb.com

Online Chapter Pretest
Interactivities
Vocabulary Explorer
Anatomy Review
Web Links
Online Review Manual
Distance Learning

Chapter FEATURES

Skill Drills
Vital Vocabulary
Pediatric Needs
Geriatric Needs
EMT-B Safety
EMT-B Tips
Documentation Tips
Remember
Prep Kit

At shift change, you are greeted by someone other than your regular partner, Jason. When you ask for details, you find out that Jason hurt his back while loading a patient during an overtime shift the day before and is expected to be off for the next few days.

The majority of the patients encountered in the field will require some combination of lifting and moving on your part. This chapter will cover the principles and key concepts that you should follow when performing these activities, as well as help you answer the following questions:

1. Why are proper body mechanics and clear communications key elements of safe lifting and moving activities?

2. What's the reason for every ambulance carrying such a wide variety of devices for lifting and moving patients?

Lifting and Moving Patients

You will have to move the patient several times to provide emergency medical care in the field and transport the patient to the emergency department. Often, you will have to move the patient into a different position or location. Once you have assessed the patient and provided emergency care, you and your team will have to move the patient onto a long backboard or cot. Then you must move the patient to the waiting ambulance and load the patient into the patient compartment. After you arrive at the hospital, you must unload the patient, move him or her to the correct examining room, and transfer the patient from the cot to the emergency department bed. To avoid injury to the patient, yourself, or your partners, you will have to learn how to lift and carry the patient properly, using proper body mechanics and a power grip. To be able to move a patient safely and properly in the various situations that you will encounter in the field, you will have to learn how to perform emergency body drags and lifts, rapidly move a patient from a car onto the cot, assist a patient from a chair or bed onto the cot, and lift a patient from the floor onto the cot. In addition, you will need to move a patient from the bed onto the cot or carry a patient up or down stairs. You and your team will have to know how to place a patient with a suspected spinal injury onto a long backboard and package patients with and without suspected spinal injury. At times, you and your team will need to move a patient who weighs more than 300 lb or carry a patient on a trail or across rugged terrain. You will need to know the special techniques for loading and unloading the cot and transferring the patient from the cot to an examining table or bed in the emergency department.

Lifting and carrying are dynamic processes. To ensure that no individual suddenly bears unexpected, dangerous weight and to reduce the risk of injury to an EMT-B or the patient, you must know where rescuers should be positioned and how to give and receive lifting commands so that all parties act simultaneously. You will also need to know how to prepare patient-moving devices, such as a wheeled ambulance stretcher (also called an ambulance cot or simply "the cot"), stair chair, backboard, scoop stretcher, folding ambulance stretcher, basket stretcher, or flexible stretcher, and when and how to use them. This chapter will cover lifting, carrying, and reaching techniques as well as principles of moving patients, including emergency, urgent, and nonurgent moves. In addition, different types of equipment and patient positioning will be discussed in detail.

Body Mechanics

Anatomy Review

The shoulder girdle rests on the rib cage and is supported by the vertebrae that lie inferior to it. The arms are connected to and hang from the shoulder girdle. When the person is standing upright, the individual weight-bearing vertebrae are stacked on top of each other and aligned over the sacrum. The sacrum is both the mechanical weight-bearing base of the spinal column and the fused central posterior section of the pelvic girdle.

When a person is standing upright, the weight of anything being lifted and carried in the hands is

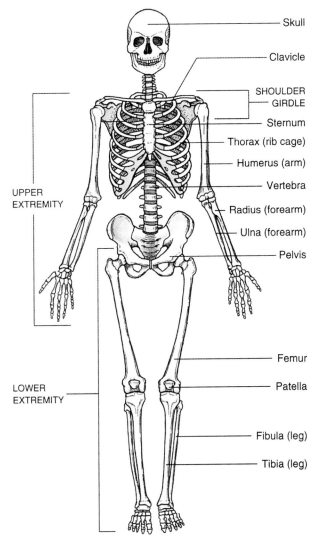

- Skull
- Clavicle
- SHOULDER GIRDLE
- Sternum
- Thorax (rib cage)
- Humerus (arm)
- Vertebra
- Radius (forearm)
- Ulna (forearm)
- Pelvis
- Femur
- Patella
- Fibula (leg)
- Tibia (leg)

UPPER EXTREMITY

LOWER EXTREMITY

Figure 6-1 When you are standing upright, the weight of anything that you lift and carry in your hands is borne by the shoulder girdle, the spinal column, the pelvis, and the legs.

reflected onto the shoulder girdle, the spinal column inferior to it, the pelvis, and then the legs (◄ **Figure 6-1**). In lifting, if the shoulder girdle is aligned over the pelvis and the hands are held close to the legs, the force that is exerted against the spine occurs in an essentially straight line down the strong-stacked vertebrae in the spinal column. Therefore, with the back properly maintained in an upright position, very little strain occurs against the muscles and ligaments that keep the spinal column in alignment, and significant weight can be lifted and carried without injury to the back (▼ **Figure 6-2**). However, you may injure your back if you lift with your back curved or, even if straight, bent significantly forward at the hips (▼ **Figure 6-3**). With the back in either of these positions, the shoulder girdle lies significantly anterior to the pelvis, and the force of lifting is exerted primarily across, rather than down, the spinal column. When this occurs, the weight is supported by the muscles of the back and ligaments that run from the base of the skull to the pelvis, keeping the spinal column in alignment, rather than by each vertebral body and disk resting on those aligned below it. In addition, the upper spine and torso serve as a lever so that the force that is exerted against the muscles and ligaments in the lumbar and sacral regions, as a result of the mechanical advantage produced, is many times that of the combined weight of your upper body and the object you are lifting. Therefore, the first key rule of lifting is to always keep the back in a straight, upright (vertical) position and to lift without twisting.

When lifting, you should spread your legs about 15″ apart (shoulder width) and place your feet so that your

Figure 6-2 If your body is properly aligned when you lift, the line of force exerted against the spine occurs in an essentially straight line down the vertebrae. In this way, the strong-stacked vertebrae support the lift.

Figure 6-3 You may be injured if you lift with your back curved, as the lifting force is exerted primarily across, rather than down, the spinal column. When this occurs, the muscles of the back, not the vertebrae, are supporting the lift.

center of gravity is properly balanced between them. Then, with the back held upright, bring your upper body down by bending the legs. Once you have properly grasped the patient or cot and made any necessary adjustments in the location of your feet, lift the patient by raising your upper body and arms and by straightening your legs until you are again standing. Because the leg muscles are exercised by walking, climbing stairs, or running, they are well developed and extremely strong. Therefore, as well as being the safest way to lift, lifting by extending the properly placed flexed legs is also the most powerful way to lift. This method is appropriately called a **power lift**. The power lift position is also useful for individuals who have weak knees or thighs.

Even if the back is held properly upright, the same adverse force across the spinal column and leverage against the lower back will occur if you lift a heavy object with your arms outstretched so that your hands are significantly anterior to the plane described by the front of the torso. Therefore, you should *never* lift a patient or other heavy object while reaching any significant distance in front of your torso or face. Whenever you are lifting or carrying a patient, be sure to hold your arms so that your hands are almost immediately adjacent to the plane described by your anterior torso (the anterior torso and imaginary lines extended vertically above and below it). Always keep the weight that you are lifting as close to your body as possible.

Lateral force across the spine and sideways leverage against the lower back must also be avoided. If you lift with only one arm or with the arms extended more to one side than the other, more force will be exerted against one side of the shoulder girdle than the other, causing lateral force to be exerted across the spinal column. To prevent this, keep your arms approximately the same distance apart as when hanging at each side of the body, with the weight distributed equally and properly centered between them. If the weight is not balanced between both arms or properly centered between the shoulders when you are preparing to lift, turn your body and/or move to the left or right until the weight is properly balanced and centered. To lift safely and produce the maximal power lift, you should take the following steps (▶ **Skill Drill 6-1**):

1. **Tighten your back in its normal upright position** and use your abdominal muscles to lock it in a slight inward curve.

2. **Spread your legs apart about 15″**, and bend your legs to lower your torso and arms.

3. **With arms extended down each side of the body,** grasp the cot or backboard with your hands held palm up and just in front of the plane described by the anterior torso and imaginary lines extending vertically from it to the ground.

4. **Adjust your orientation and position** until the weight is balanced and centered between both arms **(Step 1)**.

5. **Reposition your feet** as necessary so that they are about 15″ apart with one slightly farther forward and rotated so that you and your center of gravity will be properly balanced between them. Be sure to straddle the object, keep your feet flat, and distribute your weight to the balls of the feet or just behind them **(Step 2)**.

6. **With the arms extended downward,** lift by straightening your legs until you are fully standing. Make sure your back is locked in and that your upper body comes up before your hips **(Step 3)**.

Reverse these steps whenever you are lowering the cot. Always remember to avoid bending at the waist.

Your safety, as well as that of the other EMT-Bs and the patient, depends on the use of proper lifting techniques and having and maintaining a proper hold when lifting or carrying a patient. If you do not have proper hold of the cot, or of the patient in a body lift, you will not be able to bear a proper share of the weight, and there is an increased chance that you can suddenly lose your grasp with one or both hands. If you temporarily lose your grasp with one or both hands, the position and weight distribution of the cot change suddenly, and the other members of the team must quickly reach beyond a safe distance to avoid dropping the patient. As a result, sudden excessive force may be placed across each one's spine, causing lower back injury.

You should use the **power grip** to get the maximum force from your hands whenever you are lifting a patient

Skill Drill 6-1 Performing the Power Lift

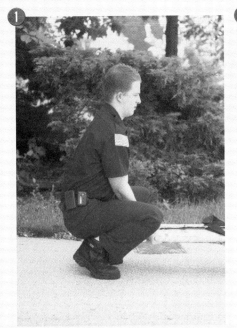

① Lock your back into an upright, inward curve.
Spread and bend your legs.
Grasp the backboard, palms up and just
in front of you.
Balance and center the weight between
your arms.

② Position your feet, straddle the object, and
distribute weight.

③ Straighten your legs and lift, keeping your back
locked in.

▶ **Figure 6-4** . The arm and hand have their greatest
lifting strength when facing palm up. Whenever you
grasp a cot or backboard, your hands should be at least
10" apart. Each hand should be inserted under the
handle with the palm facing up and the thumb extended
upward. You should then advance the hand until the
thumb prevents further insertion and the cylindrical
handle lies firmly in the crease of the curved palm. Curl
your fingers and thumb tightly over the top of the
handle. All your fingers should be at the same angle. To
have the proper power grip, make sure that the underside of the handle is fully supported on your curved
palm with only the fingers and thumb preventing it from
being pulled sideways or upward out of the palm.

If you must lift the object higher once you have lifted
by extending your legs, you will be able to "curl" the
object higher by using your biceps to flex the arms
while maintaining the power grip and weight supported
in the palms.

Figure 6-4 To perform the power grip, grasp the handle of the
litter with your palms up and your thumb extending up. Make sure
your hands are about 10" apart and that your fingers are all at
the same angle. The underside of the handle should be fully
supported by the palm of your hand.

Figure 6-5 When lifting a patient by a bedsheet, you should center the patient on the sheet and tightly roll up the fabric on each side. This produces a cylindrical handle that provides a strong way to grasp the fabric.

Figure 6-6 The diamond carry requires four rescuers, one each at the head of the backboard, the foot end, and each side of the patient's torso.

You should *never* grasp a cot or backboard with the hand placed palm down over the handle. In lifting with the palm down, the weight is supported by the fingers rather than the palm. This hand orientation places the tips of the fingers and thumb under the handle. If the weight forces them apart, your grasp on the handle will be lost.

When lifting a patient by a sheet or blanket, you should center the patient on the sheet and tightly roll up the excess fabric on each side. This produces a cylindrical handle that provides a strong, secure way to grasp the fabric (▲ **Figure 6-5**).

When directly lifting a patient, you should tightly grip the patient in a place and manner that will ensure that you will not lose your grasp on the patient.

Weight and Distribution

Whenever possible, you should use a device that can be rolled to move a patient. However, in case a wheeled device is not available, you must make sure that you understand and follow certain guidelines for

carrying a patient on a cot. (▼ **Table 6-1**) shows the guidelines.

If a patient is supine on a backboard or is lying or in a semi-sitting position on the cot, his or her weight is not equally distributed between the two ends of the device. Between 68% and 78% of the body weight of a patient in a horizontal position is in the torso. Therefore, more of the patient's weight rests on the head half of the device than on the foot half.

A patient on a backboard or cot should be lifted and carried by four rescuers in a **diamond carry**, with one EMT-B at the head end of the device, one at the foot end, and one at each side of the patient's torso (▲ **Figure 6-6**) and (▶ **Skill Drill 6-2**). Follow these steps to perform the diamond carry:

1. To best balance the weight, the EMT-Bs at each side should be located so that they are able to grasp the board or stretcher with one hand adjacent to the distal edge of the patient's pelvis and the other midthorax. **All four lift the device while facing in toward the patient** (Step 1).

TABLE 6-1 Guidelines for Carrying a Patient on a Cot

- Be sure that you know or can find out the weight to be lifted and the limitations of the team's abilities.
- Coordinate your movements with those of the other team members while constantly communicating with them.
- Do not twist your body as you are carrying the patient.

- Keep the weight that you are carrying as close to your body as possible while keeping your back in a locked-in position.
- Be sure to flex at the hips, not at the waist, and bend at the knees, while making sure that you do not hyperextend your back by leaning back from your waist.

Skill Drill 6-2   Performing the Diamond Carry

Position yourselves facing the patient.

After the patient has been lifted, the EMT-B at the foot turns to face forward.

EMT-Bs at the side each turn the head-end hand palm down and release the other hand.

EMT-Bs at the side turn toward the foot end.

2. **Once the device has been lifted,** the EMT-B at the foot end turns around to face forward **(Step 2)**.

3. **The EMT-B at each side** should turn the head-end hand palm down and then release the other hand **(Step 3)**.

4. **The EMT-Bs at the sides turn toward the patient's feet.** All four should be facing the same direction and will be walking forward when carrying the patient **(Step 4)**.

A patient on a backboard or stretcher should be carried feet first to place the lightest load on the EMT-B at the patient's feet, who, to walk forward, must turn and grasp the handles with his or her back to the device.

Carrying the patient feet first will also allow a conscious patient to see in the direction of movement.

It is important that you and your team use the correct lifting techniques to lift the cot. You must also make sure that your team members are of the same approximate height and strength.

One method of lifting and carrying a patient on a backboard is the one-handed carrying technique ▶ **Skill Drill 6-3**. With this method, four or more EMT-Bs each use one hand to support the backboard so that they are able to face forward as they are walking. Here are the steps:

1. **Before lifting the backboard,** be sure that at least two EMT-Bs are on each side of the backboard facing each other and using both hands **(Step 1)**.

Skill Drill 6-3   Performing the One-Handed Carrying Technique

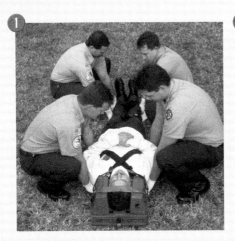

Face each other and use both hands.

Lift the backboard to carrying height.

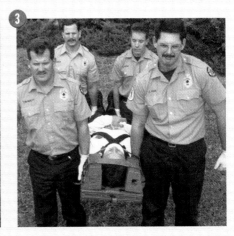

Turn in the direction you will walk and switch to using one hand.

2. **Lift the backboard** to carrying height using correct lifting techniques including a locked-in back **(Step 2)**.

3. Once you have lifted the backboard to carrying height, you and your partners **turn in the direction you will be walking** and switch to using one hand **(Step 3)**.

Be sure to pick up and carry the backboard with your back in the locked-in position. If you need to lean to either side to compensate for a weight imbalance, you have probably exceeded your weight limitation. If this occurs, you may need to add helpers or reevaluate the carry, or you might injure yourselves or drop the patient.

A diamond carry is more stable than a carry in which there are two EMT-Bs at each side of the backboard with no one at the patient's head or feet. With two EMT-Bs at each side, each EMT-B can only hold the backboard or cot with one hand when turned to face in the same direction. However, both carrying methods are recommended and widely used in the field.

The diamond carry is recommended when a patient must be carried in a building ▶ Figure 6-7 . If you must carry a patient through a narrow doorway or hallway, simply stop and have all the EMT-Bs turn until each is again facing in toward the patient. Then, by taking small, slow steps, you can move through the doorway. If the doorway is too narrow for the EMT-Bs at the sides of the backboard to fit through, have one go through the doorway before the backboard or stretcher. As the other three EMT-Bs slowly move through the doorway, the EMT-B who walked through before the backboard should grasp the backboard from the other side of the doorway before the EMT-B who is still at the side of the backboard reaches the doorway and must let go.

Sometimes, if a doorway, hallway, or stairwell is very narrow, it will only be possible to carry the backboard or stretcher from the head and foot ends. When this occurs, the EMT-Bs who were lifting and carrying at each side should relocate to help those at each end. One should move next to the EMT-B at the head end and share the load with him or her. The other should move in front of and grasp the belt of the EMT-B carrying the foot end, and steady and guide him or her.

When you must carry a patient up or down a flight of stairs or other significant incline, use a stair chair if possible. When you must use a backboard or stretcher, be sure that the patient is anatomically secured to the device in such a way that he or she cannot slide significantly when the stretcher is at an angle ▶ Skill Drill 6-4 :

1. **Apply a strap** that passes tightly across the upper torso and through each armpit, but not over the arms, to hold the patient in place while leaving the arms free. The strap is secured to the handles at both sides of the backboard so that it cannot slide toward the foot end of the board. Strap the patient securely to the backboard **(Step 1)**.

SkillDrill 6-4 Carrying a Patient on Stairs

Strap the patient securely.

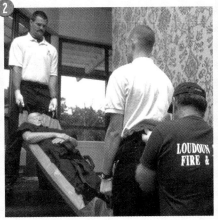

Carry a patient down stairs with the foot end first, head elevated.

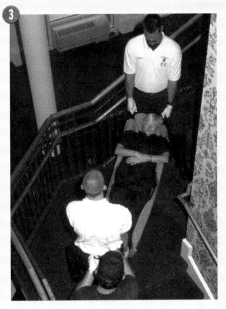

Carry the head end first going up stairs.

2. **When you carry the patient down stairs** or an incline, make sure the backboard or stretcher is carried with the foot end first so that the head end is elevated higher than the foot end. The straps will prevent the patient from sliding down or off the backboard **(Step 2)**.

3. **When you carry a patient up stairs** or an incline, the elevated head end of the backboard or stretcher should go first **(Step 3)**.

Whenever possible, you should use the patient's armpits as similar anatomic anchors and support points when you use a direct body lift or drag to move the patient or when assisting a patient who can stand.

The **wheeled ambulance stretcher** or cot, which is a specially designed cot that can be rolled along the ground, weighs between 40 and 70 lb, depending on its design and features ▶ **Figure 6-8** . Because its

Figure 6-7 Carrying a patient through a narrow doorway or hallway. **A.** Stop and turn in to face the patient until you move through the passage. **B.** If the doorway or hallway is very narrow, the EMT-Bs at the side will need to move. One should move next to the EMT-B at the head end and share the load. The other should move in front of and support the back of the EMT-B carrying the foot end to steady and guide him or her through the passage.

weight must be added to that of the patient, it is generally not taken up or down stairs or to other locations where the patient must be carried rather than rolled for any significant distance. When the patient is upstairs, you should bring the wheeled ambulance stretcher to the ground floor landing and prepare it for the patient. You should then take either a wheeled stair chair or a backboard upstairs. Both of these devices are considerably lighter than a wheeled cot and may be used to carry the patient down to the waiting cot. Use a wheeled **stair chair** to bring a conscious patient down to the waiting cot if the patient's condition allows him or her to be placed in a sitting position (▼ **Figure 6-9**). Once the cot has been reached, transfer the patient from the stair chair onto the cot. When the patient is in cardiac arrest, must be moved in a lying position, or must be immobilized, secure the patient onto a backboard. A **backboard**, which is a device that provides support to patients whom you suspect have hip, pelvic, spinal, or lower extremity injuries, is also called a spine board, trauma board, or longboard (▼ **Figure 6-10**). You can then carry the patient on the backboard down the stairs to the prepared cot. Once you reach the cot, place both the board and patient on the cot and secure them with additional straps.

Directions and Commands

To safely lift and carry a patient, you and your team must anticipate and understand every move, and each move must be executed in a coordinated manner. The team leader should indicate where each team member is to be located and rapidly describe the sequence of steps that will be performed to ensure that the team knows what is expected of it before any lifting is initiated. If you must lift and move the patient through a number of separate stages, the team leader should first give an abbreviated

EMT-B Tips

Since lifting and moving techniques require a team leader to coordinate and direct the process, it will save time and prevent confusion to establish either informal practices or formal procedures that tell all team members—in advance—who will be in charge of these activities.

overview of the stages, followed by a more detailed explanation of each stage just before it will occur.

Orders that will initiate the actual lifting or moving or any significant changes in movement should be given in two parts: a preparatory command and a command of execution. For example, if the team leader says "All ready to stop. STOP!," the "All ready to stop" will get your attention, identify who should act, and prepare them to act; the declarative "STOP!" will indicate the exact moment for execution. Commands of execution should be delivered in a louder voice. Often, a countdown is helpful when you need to lift a patient. To avoid confusion in using a countdown, always clarify whether "three" is to be a part of the preparatory command or whether it is to serve as the order to execute. You can say "We're going to lift on three. One-two-THREE!" or "I'm going to count to three and then we're going to lift. One-two-three-LIFT!"

Additional Lifting and Carrying Guidelines

You should estimate how much the patient weighs before attempting to lift him or her. Commonly, adult patients weigh between 100 and 210 lb. If you use the correct technique, you and one other EMT-B should be able to safely lift this weight. Depending on your

Figure 6-8 The wheeled ambulance stretcher is specially designed to roll along the ground.

Figure 6-9 A wheeled stair chair can be used to transfer a conscious patient up or down a flight of stairs.

Figure 6-10 A backboard is used to transfer patients who must be moved in a supine or immobilized position.

individual strength, you and another EMT-B may be able to safely lift an even heavier patient. However, because it is quite a bit safer to have four rescuers lift, you should try to use four rescuers whenever the available resources allow. *You should know how much you can comfortably and safely lift and should not attempt to lift a proportional weight (the share of the weight that you will bear) that exceeds this amount.* If you find that lifting the patient places strain on you, call for the lifting to be stopped and the patient to be lowered. You should then obtain additional help before again attempting to lift the patient. Be sure to communicate clearly and frequently with your partner and other rescuers whenever you are lifting a patient.

You should *not* attempt to lift a patient who weighs more than 250 lb with fewer than four rescuers, regardless of individual strength. Protocols should include a method to rapidly summon additional help to lift and carry such a patient or, as in the case of a cardiac arrest, provide and maintain the necessary care in the field and when moving and transporting the patient. In addition, you must know, or be able to find out, the weight limitations of the equipment you are using and how to handle patients who exceed the weight limitations. Special techniques, equipment, and resources generally are required to move any patient who weighs more than 300 lb to the ambulance. These resources should be summoned when you arrive.

Because more than half of a patient's weight is distributed to the head end of the backboard or cot, the strongest of the available EMT-Bs should be located at the head end of the device. Even with four or more EMT-Bs carrying the patient, the strain on the EMT-B carrying the head end of the device will be increased when you must negotiate a narrow area or flight of stairs. In carrying a patient up or down a flight of stairs, proportionally greater weight will also be distributed to the EMT-B who is carrying the foot end when the backboard or cot becomes angled because of the incline. You should anticipate this and, in such cases, make sure the two strongest EMT-Bs are positioned at the head and foot ends of the board. Because of the incline of the stairway, if one of the two EMT-Bs is considerably taller than the other, it will be easier if the shorter of the two is at the head end and the taller is at the foot end.

The dynamics that are involved in carrying a patient down a flight of stairs or for any significant distance will not allow you to carry as much proportional weight as you can to safely lift or support the patient during a move onto a nearby backboard or cot. Therefore, if you feel that you are approaching your maximum lifting capacity as you are moving the patient onto a backboard

or cot, you should not attempt to lift and carry the patient for any significant distance or down a flight of stairs. You can again attempt to lift and carry the patient after you have decreased the amount of proportional weight you will be carrying by changing your position on the device or that of the others on the team or have obtained additional help.

You should try to use a stair chair instead of a cot, whenever possible, to carry a patient down stairs.

Follow the steps in ▶ **Skill Drill 6-5** :

1. **Secure the patient to the stair chair with straps.** At a minimum, use a lap belt at the hips and a strap around the chest. You should also use some method to secure the arms and hands so the patient does not reach out to grasp something and throw the carrying team off balance **(Step 1)**.

2. **Rescuers take their places around the patient** seated on the chair: one at the head and one at the foot. The rescuer at the head will give directions to coordinate the lift and carry **(Step 2)**.

3. **A third rescuer precedes the two carrying the chair** to open doors, spot them on stairs, and so on. For lengthy carries, the third responder can also rotate into the carrying team to provide breaks for the other two **(Step 3)**.

4. **When reaching landings and other flat intervals** in the carry, lower the chair to the ground and roll it rather than carrying. When reaching the level where the cot awaits, roll the chair into position next to the cot in preparation for transferring the patient **(Step 4)**.

As with other carries, always remember to keep your back in a locked-in position and to flex at the hips, not the waist. You should also bend at the knees and keep the patient's weight and your arms as close to your body as possible. Try to avoid any unnecessary lifting and carrying of the patient. If an assist, log roll, or body drag will not harm or jeopardize the patient, use one to move the patient onto the backboard or cot.

Principles of Safe Reaching and Pulling

When you use a body drag to move a patient, the same basic body mechanics and principles apply as when lifting and carrying. Your back should always be locked and straight, not curved or bent laterally, and you should avoid any twisting so that the vertebrae remain in normal alignment. When you are reaching overhead, avoid hyperextending your back. When you are pulling a patient who is on the ground, you should always

Skill Drill 6-5   Using a Stair Chair

1

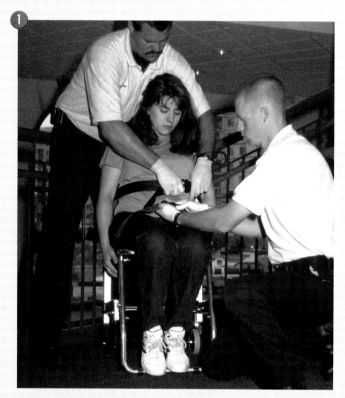

Position and secure the patient on the chair.

2

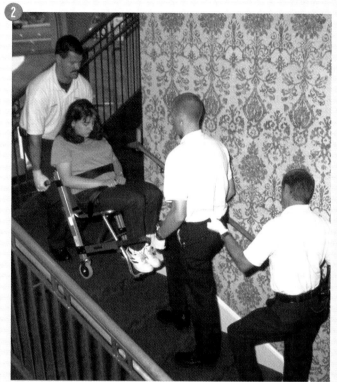

Take your places at the head and foot of the chair.

3

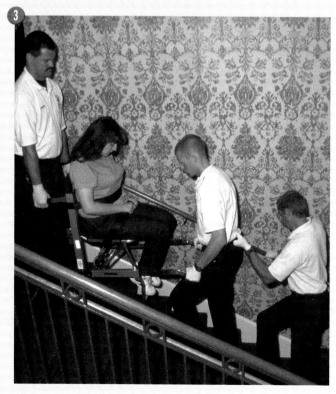

A third rescuer precedes and "backs up" the rescuer carrying the foot.

4

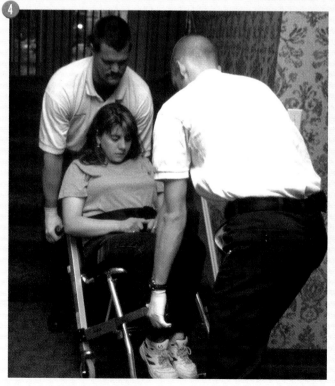

Lower the chair to roll on landings, or for transfer to the cot.

Figure 6-11 Reaching and pulling safely. **A.** Kneel to pull a patient who is on the ground. **B.** When pulling, your elbows should only extend just beyond the anterior torso. **C.** Bend your knees to pull a patient who is at a different height than you are. **D.** Position your feet or knees to balance the force of pull.

kneel to minimize the distance that you will have to lean over (▲ **Figure 6-11A**). To keep your reach within the recommended distance, reach forward and grasp the patient so that your elbows are just beyond the anterior torso (▲ **Figure 6-11B**). When you are pulling a patient who is at a different height from you, bend your knees until your hips are just below the height of the plane across which you will be pulling the patient (▲ **Figure 6-11C**). During pulling, you should extend your arms no more than about 15″ to 20″ in front of your torso. Reposition your feet (or knees, if kneeling) so that the force of pull will be balanced equally between both arms and the line of pull will be centered between them (▲ **Figure 6-11D**). Pull the patient by slowly flexing your arms. When you can pull no farther because your hands have reached the front of your torso, stop and move back another 15″ to 20″. Then, when properly positioned, repeat the steps. You should alternate between pulling the patient by flexing your arms and then repositioning yourself so that your arms are again extended with your hands about 15″ in front of your torso. By not moving yourself and the patient simultaneously, you will prevent undesirable jostling of the patient and the chance that sudden unscheduled force will occur across your spine. You should also try to prevent injury to yourself by avoiding situations that involve strenuous effort lasting more than 1 minute.

If you must drag a patient across a bed, you will have to kneel on the bed to avoid reaching beyond the recommended distance. Then follow the steps described until the patient is within 15″ to 20″ of the bed's edge (Figure 6-11). You can then complete the drag while standing at the side of the bed. Rather than dragging the patient by his or her clothing, use the sheet or blanket under the patient for this purpose.

Unless the patient is on a backboard, transfer a patient from the cot to a bed in the emergency department or the patient's hospital room with a body drag. With the cot at the same height as the bed and held firmly against its side, you and another EMT-B should kneel on the hospital bed and, in the manner previously described, drag the patient in increments until he or she is properly centered on the bed. When transferring the patient onto a narrow examining table, rather than kneeling on the table, you can usually drag the patient while standing against the opposite side.

Sometimes during a body drag, you and another EMT-B may have to pull the patient with one of you on each side of the patient. You will have to alter the usual pulling technique to prevent pulling sideways and producing adverse lateral leverage against your lower back. You should position yourself by kneeling just beyond the patient's shoulder and facing toward his or her groin (▶ **Figure 6-12A**). By extending one arm across and in front of your chest, you can grasp the armpit and, with the other arm extended in front and to the side of the torso, the patient's belt. Then, by raising your elbows and flexing your arms, you can pull the patient with the line of force at the minimum angle possible (▶ **Figure 6-12B**).

Generally, when log rolling a patient onto his or her side, you will initially have to reach farther than 18″ (▶ **Figure 6-13**). To minimize this distance, kneel as close to the patient's side as possible, leaving only enough room so that your knees will not prevent the patient from being rolled. When you lean forward, keep your back straight, and lean solely from the hips. Be sure to use your shoulder muscles to help with the roll. To minimize the amount of time you are extended like this and to support the patient's weight, roll the patient without stopping until the patient is resting on his or her side.

Figure 6-12 A body drag with an EMT-B on each side of the patient. **A.** Kneel just beyond the patient's shoulder facing his or her groin. Extend one arm across and in front of your chest, and grasp the armpit. Extend your other arm in front and to the side of the patient's torso, and grasp the patient's belt. **B.** Raise your elbows, and flex your arms to pull the patient.

Some EMS experts consider that, during a log roll, you should pull rather than push the patient. Local protocols will guide your training in this area.

When you are rolling the wheeled ambulance stretcher, make sure that it is elevated **▼ Figure 6-14** . Pull the stretcher from the foot end. Make sure your arms are held close to your body, and be careful to avoid reaching significantly behind you or hyperextending your back. Your back should be locked, straight, and untwisted. While you are walking and pulling the stretcher, bend slightly forward at the hips. As you walk, your legs are pulled back with the feet on the ground, your pelvis is moved forward, and the movement of the pelvis is transferred to the stretcher through your straight torso and firmly held arms. You should try to keep the line of the pull through the center of your body by bending your knees.

A second EMT-B should guide the head end and assist you by pushing with his or her arms held with the elbows bent so that the hands are about 12" to 15" in front of the torso. To protect your elbows from injury, you should never push an object with your arms fully extended in a straight line and the elbows locked. When you push with the elbow bent but firmly held from bending further, the strong muscles of the arm serve as a shock absorber if the wheels or foot end of the stretcher strikes an obstacle that causes its progress to be suddenly slowed or stopped. You must be sure that you push from the area of your body that is between the waist and shoulder. If the weight you are pushing is lower than your waist, you should push from a kneeling position. Be careful that you do not push or pull from an overhead position.

Figure 6-13 When placing a patient onto a backboard, roll the patient onto his or her side. Kneel as close to the patient's side as possible, leaving only enough room so that your knees will not prevent the patient from being rolled. Lean forward, keeping your back straight and leaning solely from the hips. Use your shoulder muscles to help with the roll.

Figure 6-14 A wheeled ambulance stretcher should be elevated. You should pull the stretcher from the foot end with your arms held close to your body and without hyperextending your back. A second EMT-B should guide the head, assisting you by pushing with the arms held so that the elbows are bent and the hands 12" to 15" in front of the torso.

General Considerations

Moving a patient should normally be done in an orderly, planned, and unhurried fashion. This approach will protect both you and the patient from further injury and reduce the risk of worsening the patient's condition when he or she is moved. At a minimum, on most calls you will have to lift and carry the patient to the wheeled ambulance stretcher, move the stretcher and patient to the ambulance, and load the stretcher into the patient compartment.

You will often have to include several additional steps to place the patient onto a backboard and/or carry him or her down a flight of stairs. You will also have to add a stop at the top of the stairway so that everyone can reposition for carrying the patient down the stairs. Repositioning usually requires lowering the backboard to the ground and lifting it again when all EMT-Bs are in their proper places. If you are carrying the patient in a stair chair, the additional step occurs after you have descended the stairs and reached the stretcher. At that point, you will have to assist or lift the patient from the stair chair onto the stretcher.

You should carefully plan ahead and select the methods that will involve the least lifting and carrying. Remember to always consider whether there is an option that will cause less strain to you and the other EMT-Bs.

Emergency Moves

You should use an **emergency move** to move a patient before initial assessment and care are provided when there is some potential danger, and you and the patient must move to a safe place to avoid possible serious harm or death. The presence of fire, explosives, or hazardous materials and your inability to protect the patient from other hazards or gain access to others in a vehicle who need lifesaving care are all situations in which you should use an emergency move.

The only other time you should use an emergency move is if you cannot properly assess the patient or provide immediate potentially critical emergency care because of the patient's location or position.

If you are alone and danger at the scene makes it necessary for you to use an emergency move, regardless of a patient's injuries, you should use a drag to pull the patient along the long axis of the body. This will help to keep the spinal column in line as much as possible.

When performing an emergency move, one of your primary concerns is the danger of aggravating an existing spinal injury. Remember that it is impossible to remove a patient quickly from a vehicle while providing as much protection to the spine as you would give by using an immobilization device. However, if you follow certain guidelines during the move, you can usually move a patient from a life-threatening situation without causing further injury to the patient.

You can move a patient on his or her back along the floor or ground by using one of the following methods.

- Pull on the patient's clothing in the neck and shoulder area ► **Figure 6-15A**.

- Place the patient onto a blanket, coat, or other item that can be pulled ► **Figure 6-15B**.

- Rotate the patient's arms so that they are extended straight on the ground beyond his or her head, grasp the wrists, and, with the arms elevated above the ground, drag the patient ► **Figure 6-15C**.

- Place your arms under the patient's shoulders and through the armpits, and, while grasping the patient's arms, drag the patient backward ► **Figure 6-15D**.

If you are alone and must remove an unconscious patient from a car, you should first move the patient's legs so they are clear of the pedals and are against the seat. Then rotate the patient so that his or her back is positioned facing the open car door. Next, place your arms through the armpits and support the patient's head against your body ► **Figure 6-16A**. While supporting the patient's weight, drag the patient from the seat. If the legs and feet clear the car easily, you can rapidly drag the patient to a safe location by continuing this method ► **Figure 6-16B**. If the legs and feet do not clear the car easily, you can slowly lower the patient until he or she is lying on his or her back next to the car, clear the legs from the vehicle, and, as previously described, use a long-axis body drag to move the patient a safe distance from the vehicle.

You should use one-person techniques to move a patient only if a potentially life-threatening danger exists and you are alone or, because of the pressing nature of the danger, your partner is moving a second patient simultaneously. Additional one-rescuer drags, carries, and lifts are shown in ► **Figure 6-17**.

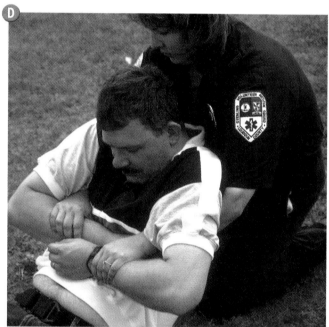

Figure 6-15 Dragging methods. **A.** Emergency clothes drag. **B.** Blanket drag. **C.** Arm drag. **D.** Arm-to-arm drag.

Figure 6-16 One-person technique for moving an unconscious patient from a car. **A.** Grasp the patient under the arms. **B.** Pull the patient down into a supine position.

Figure 6-17 One-rescuer drags, carries, and lifts. **A.** Front cradle. **B.** Firefighter's drag. **C.** One-person walking assist. **D.** Firefighter's carry. **E.** Pack strap.

Urgent Moves

An urgent move may be necessary for moving a patient with an altered level of consciousness, inadequate ventilation, or shock (hypoperfusion). An extreme weather condition may also make an urgent move necessary. In some cases, patients must be urgently moved from the location or position in which they are found. When a patient who is sitting in a car or truck must be urgently moved, you should use the rapid extrication technique.

Rapid Extrication Technique

The long backboard, short backboard, and vest-type devices are known as immobilization devices. Normally, you would use an extrication-type vest or half-backboard device to immobilize a seated patient with a suspected spinal injury before removing the patient from the car. However, using either of these devices usually requires between 6 and 8 minutes, in some cases even longer. By using the **rapid extrication technique** instead, the patient can be moved from sitting in the car to lying supine on a backboard

TABLE 6-2 Situations in Which to Use the Rapid Extrication Technique

- The vehicle or scene is unsafe.
- The patient cannot be properly assessed before being removed from the car.
- The patient needs immediate intervention that requires a supine position.
- The patient's condition requires immediate transport to the hospital.
- The patient blocks the EMT-B's access to another seriously injured patient.

in 1 minute or less. (▲ Table 6-2) describes the situations in which you should use the rapid extrication technique.

In such cases, the delay that occurs in applying an extrication-type vest or half-board is contraindicated. However, the manual support and immobilization that you provide when using the rapid extrication technique produce a greater risk of spine movement. You should not use the rapid extrication technique if no urgency exists.

The rapid extrication technique requires a team of three EMT-Bs who are knowledgeable and practiced in the procedure. You should take the following steps when using the rapid extrication technique

▶ **Skill Drill 6-6** :

1. **First EMT-B applies manual in-line support** of the patient's head and cervical spine from behind. Support may be applied from the side, if necessary, by reaching through the driver's side doorway **(Step 1)**.

2. **Second EMT-B serves as team leader** and, as such, gives the commands until the patient is supine on the backboard. Because Second EMT-B lifts and turns the patient's torso, he or she must be physically capable of moving the patient. Second EMT-B works from the driver's side doorway. If First EMT-B is also working from that doorway, Second EMT-B should stand closer to the door hinges toward the front of the vehicle. Second EMT-B applies a cervical immobilization device and performs the initial assessment **(Step 2)**.

3. **Second EMT-B provides continuous support** of the patient's torso until the patient is supine on

the backboard. Once Second EMT-B takes control of the torso, usually in the form of a body hug, he or she should not let go of the patient for any reason. Some type of cross-chest shoulder hug usually works well, but you will have to decide what method works best for you on any given patient. You must remember that you cannot simply reach into the car and grab the patient; this will only twist the patient's torso. You must rotate the patient as a unit.

4. **Third EMT-B works from the front passenger's seat** and is responsible for rotating the patient's legs and feet as the torso is turned, ensuring that they are free of the pedals and any other obstruction. With care, Third EMT-B should first move the patient's nearer leg laterally without rotating the patient's pelvis and lower spine. The pelvis and lower spine rotate only as Third EMT-B moves the second leg during the next step. Moving the nearer leg early makes it much easier to move the second leg in concert with the rest of the body. After Third EMT-B moves the legs together, they should be moved as a unit **(Step 3)**.

These first four steps of the rapid extrication technique direct the team to their starting positions and responsibilities. First EMT-B applies in-line support and immobilization of the head and neck. Second EMT-B gives orders and supports the torso. Third EMT-B moves and supports the patient's legs. The team is now ready to move the patient.

5. **The patient is rotated 90°** so that the back is facing out the driver's door and the feet are on the front passenger's seat. This coordinated movement is done in three or four short, quick "eighth turns." Second EMT directs each quick turn by saying, "Ready, turn" or "Ready, move." Hand position changes should be made between moves.

6. **In most cases, First EMT-B will be working from the back seat.** At some point, either because the doorpost is in the way or because he or she cannot reach farther from the back seat, First EMT-B will be unable to follow the torso rotation. At that time, Third EMT-B should assume temporary in-line support of the head and neck until First EMT-B can regain control of the head from outside the vehicle. If a fourth EMT-B is present, Fourth EMT-B stands next to Second EMT-B. Fourth EMT-B takes control of the head and neck from outside the vehicle

without involving Third EMT-B. As soon as the change has been made, the rotation can continue **(Step 4)**.

7. **Once the patient has been fully rotated,** the backboard should be placed against the patient's buttocks on the seat. Do not try to wedge the backboard under the patient. If only three EMT-Bs are present, be sure to place the backboard within arm's reach of the driver's door before the move so that the board can be pulled into place when needed. In such cases, the far end of the board can be left on the ground. When a fourth EMT-B is available, First EMT-B exits the rear seat of the car, places the backboard against the patient's buttocks, and maintains pressure in toward the vehicle from the far end of the board. (Note: When the door opening allows, some EMT-Bs prefer to insert the backboard onto the car seat before the patient is rotated.)

8. **As soon as the patient has been rotated** and the backboard is in place, Second EMT-B and Third EMT-B lower the patient onto the board while supporting the head and torso so that neutral alignment is maintained. First EMT-B holds the backboard until the patient is secured **(Step 5)**.

9. **Next, Third EMT-B must move across the front seat** to be in position at the patient's hips. If Third EMT-B stays at the patient's knees or feet, he or she will be ineffective in helping to move the body's weight. The knees and feet follow the hips.

10. **Fourth EMT-B maintains manual in-line support** of the head and now takes over giving the commands. If a fourth EMT-B is not present, you can direct a volunteer to assist you. Second EMT-B maintains direction of the extrication. Second EMT-B stands with his or her back to the door, facing the rear of the vehicle. The backboard should be immediately in front of Third EMT-B. Second EMT-B grasps the patient's shoulders or armpits. Then, on command, Second EMT-B and Third EMT-B slide the patient 8" to 12" along the backboard, repeating this slide until the patient's hips are firmly on the backboard **(Step 6)**.

11. **At that time, Third EMT-B gets out of the vehicle** and moves to the opposite side of the backboard, across from Second EMT-B. Third EMT-B now takes control at the shoulders,

and Second EMT-B moves back to take control of the hips. On command, these two EMT-Bs move the patient along the board in 8" to 12" slides until the patient is placed fully on the board **(Step 7)**.

12. **First (or Fourth) EMT-B continues to maintain manual in-line support** of the head. Second EMT-B and Third EMT-B now grasp their side of the board, and then carry it and the patient away from the vehicle onto the prepared cot nearby **(Step 8)**.

In some cases, you will be able to rest the head end of the backboard on the cot while the patient is moved onto the backboard. In others, you will not. Once the backboard and patient have been placed on the cot, you should begin lifesaving treatment immediately. If you used the rapid extrication technique because the scene was dangerous, you and your team should immediately move the cot a safe distance away from the vehicle before you assess or treat the patient.

The steps of the rapid extrication technique must be considered a general procedure to be adapted as needed. Two-door cars differ from four-door models. Larger cars differ from smaller compact models, pickup trucks, and full-size sedans and four-wheel-drive vehicles. You will handle a large, heavy adult differently from a small adult or child. Every situation will be different—a different car, a different patient, and a different crew. Your resourcefulness and ability to adapt are necessary elements to successfully perform the rapid extrication technique.

Nonurgent Moves

When both the scene and the patient are stable, you should carefully plan how to move the patient. If your patient move is rushed or not well planned, it may result in discomfort or injury to the patient, you, and your team. Before you attempt any move, the team leader must be sure that there are enough personnel, any obstacles have been identified or removed, the proper equipment is available, and the procedure and path to be followed have been clearly identified and discussed.

In nonurgent situations, you and your team may choose one of several methods for lifting and carrying a patient. Three general methods are presented here, which may serve as a basis for your plan. You may adapt these procedures to meet your needs on a case-by-case basis.

Skill Drill 6-6   Performing Rapid Extrication Technique

First EMT-B provides in-line manual support of the head and cervical spine.

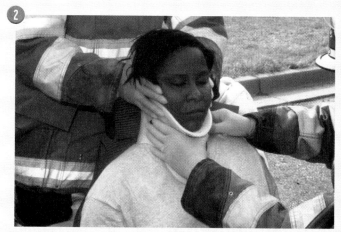

Second EMT-B gives commands, applies a cervical collar, and performs the initial assessment.

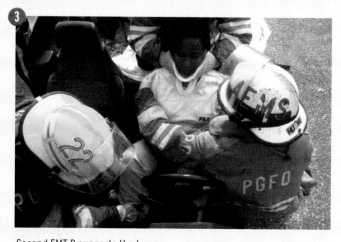

Second EMT-B supports the torso.
Third EMT-B frees the patient's legs from the pedals and moves the legs together, without moving pelvis or spine.

Second and Third EMT-Bs rotate the patient as a unit in several short, coordinated moves.
First EMT-B (relieved by Fourth EMT-B or bystander as needed) supports the head and neck during rotation (and later steps).

Direct Ground Lift

The **direct ground lift** is used for patients with no suspected spinal injury who are found lying supine on the ground. You should use this lift when you have to lift and carry the patient some distance to be placed on the cot. If you find the patient semi-prone or lying on his or her side, you should first roll the patient onto his or her back. Ideally, the direct ground lift should be performed by three EMT-Bs; however, it can be done with only two. The direct ground lift is performed as follows:

1. **Line up on one side of the patient** with First EMT-B at the patient's head, Second EMT-B at the patient's waist, and Third EMT-B at the patient's knees. All EMT-Bs kneel on one knee, preferably the same knee ▶ **Figure 6-18A**.

2. **The patient's arms should be placed on his or her chest if possible.**

3. **First EMT-B places one arm under the patient's neck and shoulders** and cradles the patient's head. First EMT-B then places the other arm under the patient's lower back.

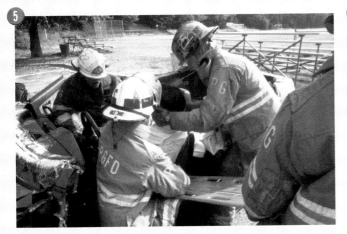

First (or Fourth) EMT-B places the backboard on the seat against patient's buttocks.
Second and Third EMT-Bs lower the patient onto the long spine board.

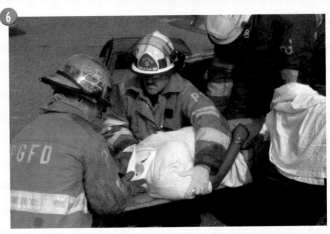

Third EMT-B moves to an effective position for sliding the patient.
Second and Third EMT-Bs slide the patient along the backboard in coordinated, 8" to 12" moves until the hips rest on the backboard.

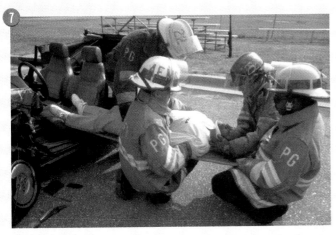

Third EMT-B exits the vehicle, moves to the backboard opposite Second EMT-B, and they continue to slide the patient until patient is fully on the board.

First (or Fourth) EMT-B continues to stabilize the head and neck while Second and Third carry the patient away from the vehicle.

4. **Second EMT-B places both arms under the waist,** and the first and third EMT-Bs slide their arms either up to the midback or down to the buttocks as appropriate.

5. **Third EMT-B places one arm under the patient's knees** and the other above the buttocks.

6. **On command, the team lifts the patient** up to knee level as each EMT-B rests an arm on his or her knee (▶ **Figure 6-18B**).

7. **As a team and on signal,** each EMT-B rolls the patient in toward his or her chest. Again on signal, the team stands and carries the patient to the cot (▶ **Figure 6-18C**).

8. **The steps are reversed** to lower the patient onto the cot.

Figure 6-18   The direct ground lift. **A.** Line up on one side of the patient, with one EMT-B at the head, one at the waist, and one at the patient's knees. Place the patient's arms on his or her chest. **B.** On command, lift the patient to knee level. **C.** On command, roll the patient toward your chest, then stand and carry the patient to the cot.

Extremity Lift

The extremity lift may also be used for patients with no suspected extremity or spinal injuries who are supine or in a sitting position on the ground. The extremity lift may be especially helpful when the patient is in a very narrow space or there is not enough room for the patient and a team of EMTs to stand side by side.

Communication is the key to success with this lift. You and your partner must coordinate your movements through direct verbal commands. You should perform the extremity lift as follows (▶ **Skill Drill 6-7**):

1. **First EMT-B kneels behind the patient's head** as Second EMT-B kneels at the patient's feet. The two EMT-Bs are facing each other.

2. **The patient's hands should be crossed** over his or her chest.

3. **First EMT-B places one hand** under each of the patient's armpits. First EMT-B grasps the patient's wrists and pulls the upper torso until the patient is in a sitting position **(Step 1)**.

4. **First EMT-B reaches his or her arms** through the patient's armpits and grasps the patient's forearms, or his or her own wrists.

5. **Second EMT-B moves to a position** between the patient's legs, facing in the same direction as the patient, and slips his or her hands under the patient's knees **(Step 2)**.

6. **Both EMT-Bs move up to a standing position** and make sure they are balanced with a good grip on the patient.

7. **As the EMT-B at the head gives the command,** both stand fully upright and move the patient to the stretcher **(Step 3)**.

You will be less likely to injure yourself if you bend at the hips and knees and use your legs for lifting. However, this lift and carry method increases pressure on the patient's chest, so the patient may be uncomfortable in this position.

Transfer Moves

There are several ways to transfer the patient from a bed onto the cot.

DIRECT CARRY. Transfer a supine patient from a bed to the cot using the direct carry method. Position the cot parallel to the bed, with the head of the cot at the foot of the bed. Be sure that you prepare the cot by unbuckling the straps and remove any other items from it (▶ **Figure 6-19A**). Both you and your partner should face the patient while standing between the bed and the cot. You should slide one arm under the patient's neck and cup the patient's shoulder. Your partner should slide his or her hand under the patient's hip and lift slightly. You should then slide your other arm under the patient's back, and your partner should place both arms underneath the patient's hips and calves (▶ **Figure 6-19B**). Slide the patient to the edge of the bed, and lift and curl the patient toward your chests. You and your partner should then rotate to the cot and gently place the patient onto it (▶ **Figure 6-19C**).

DRAW SHEET METHOD. To move the patient onto a cot, use the draw sheet method. Place the cot next to the bed, making sure it is at the same height as the bed and rails are lowered and straps are unbuckled. Be sure to hold the cot to keep it from moving. Loosen the bottom

Skill Drill 6-7 Extremity Lift

1
Patient's hands are crossed over the chest.
First EMT-B grasps patient's wrists or forearms and pulls patient to a sitting position.

2
When the patient is sitting, First EMT-B passes his or her arms through patient's armpits and grasps the patient's opposite (or his or her own) forearms or wrists.
Second EMT-B kneels between the legs, facing the feet, and places his or her hands under the knees.

3
Both EMT-Bs rise to crouching.
On command, both lift and begin to move.

Figure 6-19 The direct carry method. **A.** Bring the cot in parallel to the bed with the patient's feet facing the head of the cot. Secure the cot to prevent it from rolling. **B.** Lift the patient in a smooth, coordinated fashion. Slowly walk the patient around, and position him or her over the cot. **C.** Slowly and gently lower the patient onto the cot.

Figure 6-20 The draw sheet method. **A.** Log roll the patient onto a sheet or blanket. **B.** Bring the cot in parallel to the bed. Gently pull the patient to the edge of the bed. **C.** Transfer the patient to the cot.

sheet underneath the patient, or log roll the patient onto a blanket ◄ **Figure 6-20A** . Reach across the cot, and grasp the sheet or blanket firmly at the patient's head, chest, hips, and knees ◄ **Figure 6-20B** . Gently slide the patient onto the cot ◄ **Figure 6-20C** .

OTHER CARRIES. Other carries are performed in the following manner:

- Place a backboard next to the patient and, after using a log roll or slide to move the patient onto the backboard, secure the patient and lift and carry the backboard to the nearby prepared cot.

- Insert the halves of a scoop stretcher under each side of the patient, and fasten the two sides together. Lift and carry the patient to the nearby prepared cot. Follow the steps below ► **Skill Drill 6-8** . (Note that you can also log roll a patient onto a scoop stretcher that is already locked together.)

1. **With the scoop stretcher separated,** measure the length of the scoop and adjust to the proper length **(Step 1)**.

2. **Position the stretcher,** one side at a time. One EMT-B lifts the patient's side slightly by pulling on the far hip and upper arm, while the other EMT-B slides the stretcher into place **(Step 2)**.

3. **Lock the stretcher ends together** by engaging their locking mechanisms one at a time and continuing to lift the patient slightly as needed to avoid pinching **(Step 3)**.

4. **Apply and tighten straps** to secure the patient to the scoop stretcher before transferring to the cot **(Step 4)**.

- Assist an able patient to the edge of the bed, and, placing the patient's legs over the side, help the patient to sit up. Move the cot so that its foot end touches the bed near the patient. Help the patient to stand and rotate so that he or she can sit down on the center of the cot. Lift the patient's legs, and rotate them onto the cot while your partner lowers the torso onto the cot.

To avoid the strain of unnecessary lifting and carrying, you should use the draw sheet method or assist an able patient to the cot whenever possible.

To move a patient from the ground or the floor onto the cot you should use one of the following methods:

- Lift and carry the patient to the nearby prepared cot using a direct body carry.

- Use a log roll or long-axis drag to place the patient onto a backboard, and then lift and carry the backboard to the cot. Place both the backboard and the patient onto the cot.

- Use a scoop stretcher.

- Log roll the patient onto a blanket ▼ **Figure 6-21A** , centering the patient on the blanket and rolling up the excess material on each side. Lift the patient by the blanket, and carry him or her to the nearby cot ▼ **Figure 6-21B** .

Figure 6-21 Log rolling a patient on the ground. **A.** Log roll the patient onto a blanket. **B.** Lift the blanket and transfer the patient to the cot.

SkillDrill 6-8   Using a Scoop Stretcher

Adjust stretcher length.

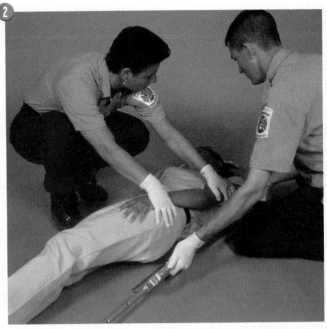

Lift patient slightly and slide stretcher into place, one side at a time.

Lock the stretcher ends together, avoiding pinching.

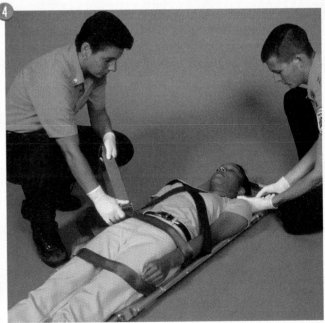

Secure the patient and transfer to the cot.

The wheeled ambulance stretcher, or cot, is the most commonly used device to move and transport patients.

Figure 6-22 Moving a patient from a chair to a wheelchair. **A.** Slide your arms through the patient's armpits, and grasp the patient's crossed forearms. Second EMT-B grasps the patient's legs at the knees. **B.** Gently lift the patient into the locked wheelchair.

If a patient is sitting in a chair and cannot assist you, transfer the patient from the chair to a wheelchair ▲ **Figure 6-22** .

Patient-Moving Equipment

The Wheeled Ambulance Stretcher

The wheeled ambulance stretcher, or cot, is the most commonly used device to move and transport patients. Only when you must transport two patients in the same ambulance should it be necessary to transport one patient on a folding stretcher or backboard placed on the long squad bench.

Most patients are placed directly on the cot. However, you will need to place and secure patients with a possible spinal injury or multiple system trauma onto a backboard. Patients who may need CPR or must be carried down (or up) a flight of stairs while supine should also be placed on a backboard. The backboard and patient are then secured onto the cot.

You can use a stair chair to carry a patient who can tolerate being in a sitting position down a flight of stairs to the prepared cot, which is waiting in the lower hallway. You should then transfer the patient from the chair to the cot.

In most instances, it is best if you pull the foot end of the cot while your partner guides it from the head end. When the cot must be carried, it is best if four rescuers are available to carry it. There is more stability with a four-person carry, and the carry requires less strength. One EMT-B should be positioned at each corner of the cot to provide an even lift. A four-person carry is much safer if the cot must be moved over rough ground. If only two EMT-Bs are available, or if limited space will allow room for only two EMT-Bs to carry the cot, there is risk that the cot will become unbalanced. In a two-person carry, the two EMT-Bs should stand facing each other, with one person at the head end of the cot and the other at the foot end. With this type of carry, one EMT-B will have to walk backward.

FEATURES. The modern cot is available in a number of different models, which may include different features ▼ **Figure 6-23** . Before going on a call, you should be fully familiar with the specific features of the cot that your ambulance carries. You must know where the controls to adjust and lock each feature are located and how each works.

Figure 6-23 An ambulance stretcher (cot).

The cot has a specific head end and foot end. The cot has a strong horizontal rectangular tubular metal main frame to which all of its other parts are attached. The cot should be pulled, pushed, and lifted only by its main frame or handles, which are attached to the main frame specifically for this purpose.

On most models, a second tubular frame made up of three sections is attached within or above the main frame. A metal plate is fastened to each of the three sections between its sides. This plate serves as the platform on which the cot mattress and patient are supported. The head section runs from the head end of the cot to near the center of the cot, where the patient's hips will be. Hinges at the area where the hips will be allow the head end to be elevated and the patient's back to be positioned at any desired angle from flat to fully upright. The head end of the cot is designed to be elevated or moved down only when a tilt control is purposely released. At all other times, the back will remain locked at the position in which it was placed. The frame and plates that lie from the hips to the foot end of the cot are divided into two hinged sections. These sections may be connected so that the foot end can be drawn in toward the knees, causing the frame and plates to hinge upward under the patient's knees to elevate them as desired. This feature is not found in all models.

A retractable guardrail is attached along the central portion of the main frame of the cot at each side and is lowered out of the way when a patient is being loaded onto the cot. Once the patient has been properly placed on the cot, the handle is drawn up and locked in an elevated position perpendicular to the surface of the cot. The patient cannot roll off either side of the cot even if a securing strap becomes released. The guardrail at each side can be lowered only if its locking handle is released.

The underside of the main frame of the cot is supported on a folding undercarriage that has a smaller horizontal rectangular frame and four large rubber casters at its bottom end. The folding undercarriage is designed so that the litter can be adjusted to any height

from about 12" above the ground, which is the desired height when the stretcher is secured in the ambulance, to 32" to 36" above the ground, which is the desired height when the stretcher is being rolled. Because you are able to lock the cot at any height between its lowest height and its fully extended height, it can be locked at the same height as any bed or examining table to allow the patient to be slid from one to the other. This permits you to transfer the patient without the need for any additional lifting. The controls for folding the undercarriage are designed so that the cot remains locked at its present height when the controls are not being activated. As an additional safety feature on most cots, the main frame must be slightly lifted so that the undercarriage becomes unweighted before it will fold, even if the control is pulled. Therefore, if the handle is accidentally pulled, the elevated cot will not suddenly drop. Controls for elevating and lowering most cots are located at the foot end and at one or both sides. You and your partner must use the proper lifting mechanics to lift the wheeled ambulance stretcher.

The mattress on a cot must be fluid resistant so that it does not absorb any type of potentially infectious material, including water, blood, or other body fluid.

MOVING THE COT. Whenever a patient has been placed onto the cot, one EMT-B must hold the main frame to make sure that it cannot roll. When the cot is elevated, the main frame and the patient extend considerably beyond the wheels at both the head end and foot end of the cot. Therefore, whenever a patient is on an elevated cot, you must ensure that it is held firmly between two hands at all times so that even if the patient moves, the cot cannot tip (▼ **Figure 6-24**).

Figure 6-24 Make sure that you hold the main frame of the cot when it is elevated so that even when the patient moves, the cot does not tip.

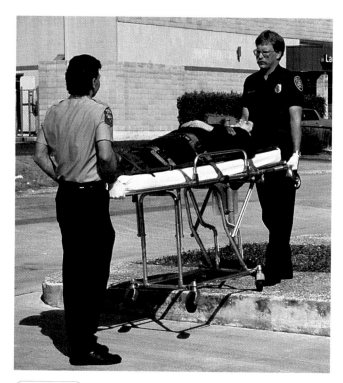

Figure 6-25 You need not retract the undercarriage of the cot when lifting it over a curb, single step, or obstacle of similar height.

If the loaded cot must be carried down a short flight of steps, be sure to first retract the undercarriage; however, this is not necessary when the cot must be lifted over a curb, single step, or obstacle of a similar height (▲ **Figure 6-25**). Remember, if the patient must be carried up or down a full flight or several flights of stairs, you should prepare the cot and leave it on the ground floor at the bottom (or top) of the stairs. Use a backboard or stair chair to carry the patient up or down the stairs to the waiting cot.

These are the steps to load the cot into an ambulance (▶ **Skill Drill 6-9**):

1. **Tilt the head end of the main frame upward** and place it into the patient compartment with the wheels on the floor. The two additional wheels that extend just below the head end are attached to the main frame and will enable this movement **(Step 1)**.

2. **With the patient's weight supported** by these two head-end wheels and the EMT-B at the foot end of the cot, move to the side of the main frame and release the undercarriage lock to lift the undercarriage up to its fully retracted position. The wheels of the undercarriage and the two on the head end of the main frame will now be on the same level **(Step 2)**.

3. **Simply roll the cot** the rest of the way into the back of the ambulance, where it will rest on all six wheels **(Step 3)**.

4. **Secure the cot** in the ambulance with the strong clamps that fasten around the undercarriage when the cot is pushed into them. The clamps are located in a rack on the floor or side of the patient compartment **(Step 4)**.

The clamps will hold the cot in place until they are released at the hospital. You can control and release the clamps with a single handle that is positioned so that you can activate it when standing on the ground at the open back doors of the ambulance when the cot is to be unloaded. The cot is designed to be rolled on regular flat surfaces. If the patient must be moved over a lawn or other irregular surface, you must lift and carry the cot over the terrain.

An IV pole is attached to many cots. The IV pole can be unfolded or extended above the main frame to hold an IV bag above the patient while you move the cot to the ambulance. Some wheeled ambulance stretchers even include a carrier to hold an electrocardiogram (ECG) monitor or automated external defibrillator (AED) and portable oxygen unit. If the model you use does not include these features, you will have to secure the portable oxygen unit and ECG monitor or AED to the top surface of the cot mattress at the patient's legs.

The extra wheels below the head end of the main frame of the cot are not featured on some older or less expensive wheeled ambulance stretchers. These cots are not self-loading. When you reach the back of the ambulance with such a cot, you must lower it until the undercarriage is in its lowest retracted position and then, with you and your partner at each side of the cot, lift it to the height of the floor of the ambulance and roll it into the track that locks it into place. (▼ **Table 6-3**) shows the guidelines that you must follow to load the cot into the ambulance.

TABLE 6-3 Guidelines for Loading the Cot into the Ambulance

- Make sure there is sufficient lifting power.

- Follow the manufacturer's directions for safe and proper use of the cot.

- Make sure that all cots and patients are fully secured before you move the ambulance.

Skill Drill 6-9   Loading a Cot into an Ambulance

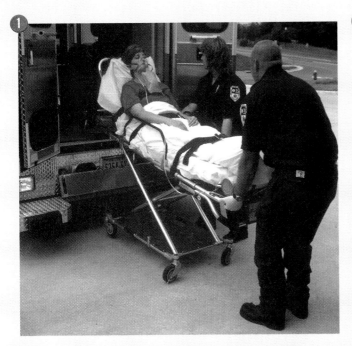

Tilt the head of the cot upward, and place it into the patient compartment with the wheels on the floor.

Second rescuer on the side of the cot releases the undercarriage lock and lifts undercarriage.

Roll the cot into the back of the ambulance.

Secure the cot to the brackets mounted in the ambulance.

Portable/Folding Stretchers

A **portable stretcher** is a stretcher with a strong rectangular tubular metal frame and rigid fabric stretched across it ▶ **Figure 6-26** . Portable stretchers do not have a second multipositioning frame or adjustable undercarriage. Some models have two wheels that fold down about 4″ underneath the foot end of the frame and legs of a similar length that fold down from the head end at each side. The wheels make it easier to move the loaded stretcher. The legs should not be used as handles.

Some portable stretchers can be folded in half across the center of each side so that the stretcher is only half its usual length during storage. Many ambulances carry a portable stretcher to use if a patient is in an area that is difficult to reach with a wheeled ambulance stretcher or a second patient must be transported on the squad bench of the ambulance.

A portable stretcher weighs much less than a wheeled stretcher and does not have a bulky undercarriage. However, because most models do not have wheels, you and your team must support all of the patient's weight and any equipment along with the weight of the stretcher.

Flexible Stretchers

Several types of **flexible stretchers**, such as the SKED, Reeves, or Navy stretcher, are available and can be rolled up across either the stretcher's width or, in the case of the SKED, its length, so that the stretcher becomes a smaller tubular package for storage and carrying ▶ **Figure 6-27** . When you must carry the equipment a considerable distance from the nearest place that the ambulance can be

Figure 6-26 A portable stretcher.

Figure 6-27 A flexible stretcher.

located, this is an important consideration. A flexible stretcher forms a rigid stretcher that conforms around the patient's sides and does not extend beyond them. When these stretchers are extended, they are particularly useful when you must remove a patient from or through a confined space. The SKED stretcher can also be used if the patient must be belayed or rappelled by ropes.

The flexible stretcher is the most uncomfortable of all the various devices; however, it provides excellent support and immobilization. When the stretcher is wrapped around the patient and the straps are secured, the patient is completely immobilized. The stretcher can then be lowered by rope or slid down a flight of stairs by resting it on the front edge of each step.

Backboards

Backboards are long, flat boards made of rigid, rectangular material ▼ **Figure 6-28** . Backboards were originally made of wood but are now made of other materials as well, mostly plastic. They are used to carry patients and to immobilize supine patients with suspected spinal injury or other multiple trauma. Backboards can also be used to move patients out of awkward places. They are 6′ to 7′ long and are commonly used for patients who are found lying down. Parallel to the sides and ends of the backboard are a number of long holes that are about ½″ to 1″ from the outer edge. These holes form handles and handholds so that the board can be easily grasped, lifted, and carried. The handles and adjacent holes also allow straps used to secure and immobilize the patient to the backboard to be secured to each side and end of the backboard at any needed location.

For many years, backboards were made of thick marine plywood whose surface was sealed with polyurethane or another marine varnish. Wooden backboards are still used in some places. If wooden backboards are used, you must follow infectious control procedures before you can reuse the backboards.

Figure 6-28 A long backboard.

Where wooden backboards are no longer used, they have generally been stored so that they will be available in the event of a multiple-casualty situation. Newer backboards are made of plastic materials that will not absorb blood or other infectious substances.

You can use a short backboard, called either a short backboard or a half-board, to immobilize the torso, head, and neck of a seated patient with a suspected spinal injury until you can immobilize the patient on a backboard. Short backboards are 3′ to 4′ long. The original short wooden backboard has generally been replaced with a vest-type device that is specifically designed to immobilize the patient until he or she is moved from a sitting position to supine on a backboard ▼ **Figure 6-29** . The vest-type devices are easier to use than the wooden backboard.

Basket Stretchers

You should use a rigid **basket stretcher**, often called a Stokes litter, to carry a patient across uneven terrain from a remote location that is inaccessible by ambulance or other vehicle ▼ **Figure 6-30** . If you suspect that the patient has a spinal injury, you should first immobilize him or her on a backboard and then place the backboard into the basket stretcher. Once you have reached the ambulance and wheeled ambulance stretcher, you can remove the patient and backboard from the basket stretcher and place them on the cot.

Basket stretchers either are made of plastic with an aluminum frame or have a full steel frame that is connected by a woven wire mesh. The wire basket is very uncomfortable for the patient unless the wire is padded. Either type can be used to carry a patient across fields, rough terrain, or trails or on a toboggan, boat, or all-terrain vehicle. Basket stretchers surround and support the patient, yet their design allows water to drain through holes in the bottom. Basket stretchers are also used for technical rope rescues and some water rescues. Not all basket stretchers are rated or appropriate for each of these specialized rescue uses. The types of basket stretchers that are acceptable for specialized rescue must be determined by individuals with additional special training.

Scoop Stretcher

The **scoop stretcher**, or split litter, is designed to be split into two or four pieces ▼ **Figure 6-31** . These sections are fitted around a patient who is lying on the

Figure 6-29 Vest-type short immobilization devices.
A. KED. **B.** Oregon-type backboard.

Figure 6-30 A basket stretcher.

Figure 6-31 A scoop stretcher.

ground or another relatively flat surface. The parts are reconnected, and the patient is lifted and placed on a long backboard or stretcher. A scoop stretcher may be used for patients who have been struck by a motor vehicle.

A scoop stretcher is efficient; however, both sides of the patient must be accessible. You must also pay special attention to the closure area beneath the patient so that clothing, skin, or other objects are not trapped. As with the long backboard, you must fully stabilize and secure the patient before moving him or her; however, you cannot slip a scoop stretcher under the long axis of the patient's body. Scoop stretchers are narrow, well constructed, and compact and have excellent body support features but are not adequate when used alone for standard immobilization of a spinal injury. You and your team should practice often with a scoop stretcher to be ready for using it with a patient.

Stair Chairs

Stair chairs are folding aluminum frame chairs with fabric stretched across them to form a seat and seat back ▶ Figure 6-32). They have fold-out handles to help you carry their head and foot ends up or down a flight of stairs, and most have rubber wheels at their back with casters in front so that they can be rolled along the floor and make turns. Stair chairs

Figure 6-32) A stair chair.

serve as an adjunct for moving a patient up or down stairs to the ground floor, where the prepared wheeled ambulance stretcher is waiting. You can roll the stair chair on the floor until you reach the stairwell, then carry it (rather than roll and bump it) up or down the stairs. Once you reach the ground floor, you can roll it to the waiting cot and assist or lift the patient onto the cot.

Be sure to follow manufacturer's directions for maintenance, inspection, repair, and upkeep for any device that you use as patient-handling equipment.

Moving and Positioning the Patient

Every time you have to move a patient, you must take special care that neither you, your team, nor the patient is injured. Patient packaging and handling are technical skills that you will learn and perfect through practice and training.

Training and practice are required to use all the equipment that is described in this chapter. You must master the skills necessary for their use and understand the advantages and limitations of each device. Practice each technique with your team often so that when you must move a patient, you can perform the move quickly, safely, and efficiently. After each patient transfer, you and your team should evaluate the appropriateness of the technique that you used, as well as your technical skill in completing the transfer. You must also be sure to maintain your equipment according to the manufacturer's instructions. Using clean, well-maintained equipment is but one part of providing high-quality patient care.

After you deliver the patient to the emergency department, you and your team must begin preparing for your next call. Review the positive points about the transport. Discuss changes that would improve the next run. This process of review and evaluation identifies the following:

- Procedures that need more practice
- Equipment that needs to be cleaned or repaired
- Skills that you need to review or acquire

Most important, a critical review helps you and your team to become more confident and better-skilled EMT-Bs.

Certain patient conditions, such as head injury, shock, spinal injury, and pregnancy, call for special lifting and moving techniques. Patients with chest pain or difficulty breathing should sit in a position of comfort, as long as they are not hypotensive. Patients with suspected spinal injuries must be immobilized on a long backboard. Patients who are in shock should be packaged and moved in a supine position or with their legs elevated 6″ to 12″. Pregnant patients who are hypotensive should be positioned and transported on their left sides. Move an unresponsive patient with no suspected spinal injury into the recovery position by rolling the patient onto his or her side without twisting the body. Transport a patient who is nauseated or vomiting in a position of comfort, but be sure that you are positioned appropriately to manage the airway.

Prep Kit

Ready for Review

The first key rule of lifting is to always keep your back in an upright position and lift without twisting. You can lift and carry significant weight without injury as long as your back is in the proper upright position.

The power lift is the safest and most powerful way to lift. The safety of you, your team, and the patient depends on the use of proper lifting techniques and maintaining a proper hold when lifting or carrying a patient. If you do not have a proper hold, you will not be able to bear your share of the weight, or you may lose your grasp with one or both hands and possibly cause a lower back injury to one or more EMT-Bs.

It is always best to move a patient on a device that can be rolled. However, if a wheeled device is not available, you must understand and follow certain guidelines for carrying a patient on a cot. You must constantly coordinate your movements with those of the other team members and make sure that you communicate with them.

When lifting a cot, you must make sure that you and your team use correct lifting techniques. You and your team should also be of similar height and strength.

If you must carry a loaded backboard or cot up or down stairs or other inclines, be sure that the patient is tightly secured to the device to prevent sliding. Be sure to carry the backboard or cot foot end first so that the patient's head is elevated higher than the feet.

Directions and commands are an important part of safe lifting and carrying. You and your team must anticipate and understand every move and execute it in a coordinated manner. The team leader is responsible for coordinating the moves.

You should try to use four rescuers whenever resources allow. You should also know how much you can comfortably and safely lift and not attempt to lift more than this amount. Rapidly summon additional help to lift and carry a weight that is greater than you are able to lift.

The same basic body mechanics apply for safe reaching and pulling as for lifting and carrying. Keep your back locked and straight, and avoid twisting. Do not hyperextend your back when reaching overhead.

You should normally move a patient with nonurgent moves, in an orderly, planned, and unhurried fashion, selecting methods that involve the least amount of lifting and carrying. At times, you may have to use an emergency move to move a patient before providing initial assessment and care. You should perform an urgent move if a patient has an altered level of consciousness, inadequate ventilation or shock, or in extreme weather conditions.

The wheeled ambulance stretcher, or cot, is the most commonly used device to move and transport patients. Other devices that are used to lift and carry patients include portable stretchers, flexible stretchers, backboards, basket stretchers (Stokes litters), scoop stretchers, and stair chairs.

Whenever you are moving a patient, you must take special care so that neither you, your team, nor the patient is injured. You will learn the technical skills of patient packaging and handling through practice and training. Training and practice are also required to use all the equipment that is available to you. You must practice each technique with your team often so that you are able to perform the move quickly, safely, and efficiently.

Vital Vocabulary

backboard A device that is used to provide support to a patient who is suspected of having a hip, pelvic, spinal, or lower extremity injury. Also called a spine board, trauma board, or longboard.

basket stretcher A rigid stretcher commonly used in technical and water rescues that surrounds and supports the patient yet allows water to drain through holes in the bottom. Also called a Stokes litter.

diamond carry A carrying technique in which one EMT-B is located at the head end, one at the foot end, and one at each side of the patient; each of the two EMT-Bs at the sides uses one hand to support the stretcher so that all are able to face forward as they walk.

direct ground lift A lifting technique that is used for patients who are found lying supine on the ground with no suspected spinal injury.

emergency move A move in which the patient is dragged or pulled from a dangerous scene before initial assessment and care are provided.

extremity lift A lifting technique that is used for patients who are supine or in a sitting position with no suspected extremity or spinal injuries.

flexible stretcher A stretcher that is a rigid carrying device when secured around a patient but can be folded or rolled when not in use.

portable stretcher A stretcher with a strong rectangular tubular metal frame and rigid fabric stretched across it.

power grip A technique in which the litter or backboard is gripped by inserting each hand under the handle with the palm facing up and the thumb extended, fully supporting the underside of the handle on the curved palm with the fingers and thumb.

power lift A lifting technique in which the EMT-B's back is held upright, with legs bent, and the patient is lifted when the EMT-B straightens the legs to raise the upper body and arms.

rapid extrication technique A technique to move a patient from a sitting position inside a vehicle to supine on a backboard in less than 1 minute when conditions do not allow for standard immobilization.

scoop stretcher A stretcher that is designed to be split into two or four sections that can be fitted around a patient who is lying on the ground or other relatively flat surface; also called a split litter.

stair chair A lightweight folding device that is used to carry a conscious, seated patient up or down stairs.

wheeled ambulance stretcher A specially designed stretcher that can be rolled along the ground. A collapsible undercarriage allows it to be loaded into the ambulance. Also called the cot or an ambulance cot.

www.emtb.com

Assessment in Action

During a routine call, you needed to help carry the patient on the cot down some sidewalk steps to the ambulance. It was narrow and awkward. About halfway down you felt the patient start to slip as the weight of the cot shifted.

To prevent the patient from falling, you found yourself bending forward to restrain the patient as you tried to lift the cot. You prevented the patient from falling, but afterward your back felt stiff. The following questions refer to this situation.

1. In this situation, which of the following methods would be best to prevent the patient from slipping while moving?
   A. Keep the cot level at all times.
   B. Have more people help you carry the cot.
   C. Secure the patient with straps at the armpits and groin.
   D. Take the patient down head first.

2 In this situation, the center of gravity was not properly balanced when lifting. How could you ensure a proper position for the center of gravity?
   A. Place your legs about 15" apart with your pelvis centered.
   B. Place your legs about 15" apart with your pelvis slightly to the left.
   C. Place your legs 30" apart with your pelvis and right leg slightly ahead.
   D. Place your legs 30" apart with your pelvis and right leg slightly behind.

3. When the back is maintained in an upright position while lifting, where is the majority of force transmitted?
   A. To the muscles and ligaments of the spine
   B. Along the stacked vertebrae
   C. Against the pelvic ring
   D. To the parallel arms

4. In this situation, what are possible alternatives for moving the patient that would help to avoid this situation? Use a/an:
   A. emergency one-person technique.
   B. wheeled stair-chair.
   C. wooden backboard.
   D. rapid extrication technique.

5. Once you have lifted a cot using good body mechanics, if you need to lean to either side to compensate for a weight imbalance, you have probably:
   A. exceeded your weight limit.
   B. assumed the heavier end of the stretcher.
   C. exceeded your height limit.
   D. exceeded your arm length.

6. The safest and most powerful method of lifting is the:
   A. body twist.
   B. power lift.
   C. power grip.
   D. clean and jerk.

7. To obtain the maximum force from your hands when lifting a patient, you should grasp the litter with your hands at least:
   A. 10" apart, palm down.
   B. 10" apart, palm up.
   C. 15" apart, with one palm up, one down.
   D. 15" apart, with palm up.

8. One of the best ways to move a patient from a bed to the cot is to use:
   A. one of the emergency moves.
   B. the extremity lift.
   C. a draw sheet.
   D. the scoop stretcher.

Challenging Questions

9. In this situation, your back felt stiff after the lifting incident. Why?

10. Why is the sacrum considered the mechanical weight-bearing base of the spinal column?

11. Twisting while pulling or lifting is one of the most frequent causes of back injury for EMTs. Why does this so frequently occur?

Points to Ponder

You are transporting a terminally ill cancer patient home from the hospital for hospice care. She is heavily medicated to control pain and has received "extra" to help her through the transport. She is semiconscious but has stable breathing and pulse. The door to the patient's house is up five steep stairs and then a sharp turn. There is not enough room on the landing for the stretcher so your partner is standing in some bushes and holding the stretcher above his head. Suddenly your partner trips in the shrubs and falls. You catch the stretcher before it falls completely down, but it received a very hard bump as it fell. Your patient moaned but did not regain consciousness. Because of the medications and current medical problems it is hard to tell if the patient was injured by the fall. The patient's husband is in the house and did not see it happen. How would you deal with this? Would you return the patient to the hospital for examination? Who, if anyone, would you report this to?

Issues Best Care for Patients, Making and Admitting Mistakes, Preventing Accidents, Ethics in EMS.

Online Outlook

Seven patient-carrying devices were discussed in this chapter. To improve your knowledge of this equipment, complete Exercise 6 at www.emtb.com.

www.emtb.com

Airway

2

Section

Airway

Objectives

Cognitive

1. Name and label the major structures of the respiratory system on a diagram (p 187).
2. List the signs of adequate breathing (p 192).
3. List the signs of inadequate breathing (p 192).
4. Describe the steps in performing the head tilt-chin lift maneuver (p 195).
5. Relate mechanism of injury to opening the airway (p 193).
6. Describe the steps in performing the jaw-thrust maneuver (p 195).
7. State the importance of having a suction unit ready for immediate use when providing emergency care (p 199).
8. Describe the techniques of suctioning (p 200).
9. Describe how to artificially ventilate a patient with a pocket mask (p 209).
10. Describe the steps in performing the skill of artificially ventilating a patient with a bag-valve-mask device while using the jaw-thrust maneuver (p 211).
11. List the parts of a bag-valve-mask system (p 210).
12. Describe the steps in performing the skill of artificially ventilating a patient with a bag-valve-mask device for one and two rescuers (p 211).
13. Describe the signs of adequate artificial ventilation using the bag-valve-mask device (p 212).
14. Describe the signs of inadequate artificial ventilation using the bag-valve-mask device (p 212).
15. Describe the steps in ventilating a patient with a flow-restricted, oxygen-powered ventilation device (p 213).
16. List the steps in performing the actions taken when providing mouth-to-mouth and mouth-to-stoma artificial ventilation (p 215).
17. Describe how to measure and insert an oropharyngeal (oral) airway (p 197).
18. Describe how to measure and insert a nasopharyngeal (nasal) airway (p 198).
19. Describe how to perform the Sellick maneuver (cricoid pressure) (p 213).
20. Define the components of an oxygen delivery system (p 202).
21. Identify a nonrebreathing face mask and state the oxygen flow requirements needed for its use (p 207).
22. Describe the indications for using a nasal cannula versus a nonrebreathing face mask (p 207).
23. Identify a nasal cannula and state the flow requirements needed for its use (p 208).
24. Identify the patients for whom pulse oximetry will be appropriate to apply (p 208).*
25. List the conditions that will result in an inaccurate reading for the pulse oximeter (p 208).*
26. State measures that the EMT-B can take to ensure an accurate reading for the pulse oximeter (p 208).*

Affective

27. Explain the rationale for basic life support, artificial ventilation, and airway protective skills taking priority over most other basic life support skills (p 186).
28. Explain the rationale for providing adequate oxygenation through high inspired oxygen concentrations to patients who, in the past, may have received low concentrations (p 210).
29. Explain the rationale for applying pulse oximetry (p 208).*
30. Explain the rationale for applying cricoid pressure (p 213).*

Psychomotor

31. Demonstrate the steps in performing the head tilt-chin lift maneuver (p 195).
32. Demonstrate the steps in performing the jaw-thrust maneuver (p 195).
33. Demonstrate the techniques of suctioning (p 200).
34. Demonstrate the steps in providing mouth-to-mouth artificial ventilation with body substance isolation (barrier shields) (p 209).
35. Demonstrate how to use a pocket mask to artificially ventilate a patient (p 209).
36. Demonstrate the assembly of a bag-valve-mask unit (p 210).
37. Demonstrate the steps in performing the skill of artificially ventilating a patient with a bag-valve-mask device for one and two rescuers (p 210).
38. Demonstrate the steps in performing the skill of artificially ventilating a patient with a bag-valve-mask device while using the jaw-thrust maneuver (p 211).
39. Demonstrate artificial ventilation of a patient with a flow-restricted, oxygen-powered ventilation device (p 214).
40. Demonstrate how to artificially ventilate a patient with a stoma (p 214).
41. Demonstrate how to insert an oropharyngeal (oral) airway (p 197).
42. Demonstrate how to insert a nasopharyngeal (nasal) airway (p 198).
43. Demonstrate how to perform the Sellick maneuver (cricoid pressure) (p 213).*
44. Demonstrate the correct operation of oxygen tanks and regulators (p 202).
45. Demonstrate the use of a nonrebreathing face mask and state the oxygen flow requirements needed for its use (p 207).
46. Demonstrate the use of a nasal cannula and state the flow requirements needed for its use (p 207).
47. Demonstrate how to artificially ventilate the infant and child patient (p 209).
48. Demonstrate oxygen administration for the infant and child patient (p. 210)
49. Demonstrate application of the pulse oximetry probe (p 208).*

   * These are noncurriculum objectives

Airway

TECHNOLOGY

www.emtb.com

Online Chapter Pretest
Web Links
Vocabulary Explorer
Interactivities
Anatomy Review
Online Review Manual
Distance Learning

Chapter FEATURES

Skill Drills
Vital Vocabulary
Pediatric Needs
Geriatric Needs
EMT-B Safety
EMT-B Tips
Documentation Tips
Remember
Prep Kit

"Medic 3, respond to the north field at the Metro Softball complex for a girl having difficulty breathing." You arrive to find a very pale, frightened-looking girl sitting upright in the dugout, struggling to breathe.

Approximately one out of every four calls to EMS are either airway or respiratory related. This chapter will help prepare you for these frequently encountered calls in addition to helping you answer the following questions:

1. Why does airway and breathing assessment and care have such a prominent position in the realm of an EMT-B's scope of practice?

2. Is it necessary that you be familiar with all the airway equipment on your ambulance, or just that which you personally like to use?

Airway

The single most important step in caring for any patient is to make sure that he or she can breathe. The patient who cannot breathe properly is not delivering oxygen to body tissues and cells, which need a constant supply of oxygen to survive. Within seconds of being deprived of oxygen, the heart may not beat normally.

Oxygen reaches body tissues and cells through two separate but related processes: breathing and circulation. As we inhale, oxygen moves from the atmosphere into our lungs, then passes from the air sacs in the lungs into the capillaries to oxygenate the blood. The blood, enriched with oxygen, travels through the body by the pumping action of the heart. At the same time, carbon dioxide, produced by cells in the tissues of the body, moves from the blood into the air sacs. The carbon dioxide then leaves our bodies as we exhale.

As an EMT-B, you must be able to locate the parts of the respiratory system, understand how the system works, and be able to recognize which patients are breathing adequately and which ones are breathing inadequately. This will enable you to determine how best to treat your patient.

This chapter will review the anatomy and physiology of the respiratory system, that is, the parts of the system and how they work. It will then describe how to assess patients quickly and carefully to determine their airway and ventilation status. The equipment, procedures, and guidelines that you will need to manage a patient's airway and breathing are described in detail. You will learn several ways to open a patient's airway and specific techniques for removing foreign objects or fluids that may be blocking the airway. Because artificial airway equipment can have serious results if used improperly, the chapter will thoroughly discuss airway adjuncts, oxygen therapy devices, and artificial ventilation methods.

Anatomy of the Respiratory System

The respiratory system consists of all the structures in the body that make up the airway and help us breathe, or ventilate (▶ **Figure 7-1**). Structures that help us breathe include the diaphragm, the muscles of the chest wall, accessory muscles of breathing, and the nerves from the brain and spinal cord to those muscles. **Ventilation** is the exchange of air between the lungs and environment. The diaphragm and muscles of the chest wall are responsible for the regular rise and fall of the chest that accompany normal breathing.

Structures of the Airway

The **airway** is divided into both upper and lower airways. The upper airway consists of the nose, mouth, throat (pharynx), and a structure called the epiglottis. The epiglottis is a leaf-shaped structure above the larynx that prevents food and liquid from entering the larynx during swallowing. The portion of the throat behind the nose is the nasopharynx; the portion behind the mouth is the oropharynx.

The lower airway consists of the larynx, trachea, main bronchi, smaller bronchi, and the alveoli, small sacs where the actual exchange of oxygen and carbon dioxide occur.

The lower airway begins with the larynx (voice box/vocal cords). The cricoid cartilage is a firm cartilage ring that forms the lower part of the larynx. The trachea is directly connected to the larynx. The main bronchi and smaller bronchioles branch off from the trachea, extending into each lung. Eventually the smaller bronchioles end in the alveoli.

The chest (thoracic cage) contains the lungs, one in each half (▶ **Figure 7-2**). The lungs hang freely within the chest cavity. Between the lungs is a space called the

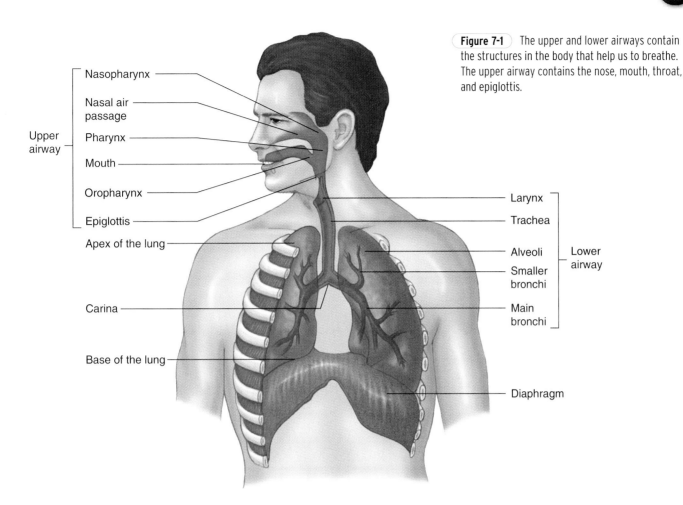

Figure 7-1 The upper and lower airways contain the structures in the body that help us to breathe. The upper airway contains the nose, mouth, throat, and epiglottis.

Upper airway

Nasopharynx

Nasal air passage

Pharynx

Mouth

Oropharynx

Epiglottis

Apex of the lung

Carina

Base of the lung

Larynx

Trachea

Alveoli

Smaller bronchi

Main bronchi

Lower airway

Diaphragm

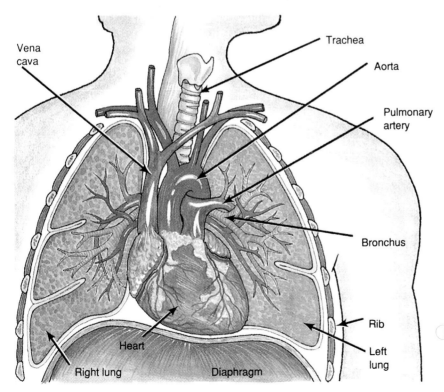

Vena cava

Trachea

Aorta

Pulmonary artery

Bronchus

Rib

Left lung

Heart

Right lung

Diaphragm

pneumo = air/lungs
pector = chest
Brady = Slow
tachy = fast
Pnea = breathing
eu = good
dys = difficult/painful
a = without
apneumo = not breathing

Figure 7-2 The thoracic cage contains important anatomic structures for respiration, including the lungs, the heart, the great vessels (the vena cava and aorta), the trachea, and the major bronchi.

mediastinum, which is surrounded by tough connective tissue. This space contains the heart, the great vessels, the esophagus, the trachea, the major bronchi, and many nerves. The mediastinum effectively separates the right lung space from the left lung space. The boundaries of the thorax are the rib cage anteriorly, superiorly, and posteriorly and the diaphragm inferiorly.

Structures of Breathing

The diaphragm is a skeletal muscle because it is attached to the costal arch and the vertebrae. It is considered a specialized muscle because it functions as both a voluntary and an involuntary muscle. It acts as a voluntary muscle whenever we take a deep breath, cough, or hold our breath—actions that we control. However, unlike other skeletal or voluntary muscles, the diaphragm also performs an automatic function. Breathing continues while we sleep and at all other times. Even though we can hold our breath or temporarily breathe more quickly or slowly, we cannot continue these variations in breathing indefinitely. When the concentration of carbon dioxide rises within the blood, the automatic regulation of breathing resumes under the control of the brain stem.

The lungs, because they have no muscle tissue, cannot move on their own. They need the help of other structures to be able to expand and contract as we inhale and exhale. Therefore, the ability of the lungs to function properly is partially dependent on the movement of the chest and supporting structures. These structures include the thorax, the thoracic cage (chest), the diaphragm, the intercostal muscles, and the accessory muscles of breathing.

Inhalation

The active, muscular part of breathing is called **inhalation**. As we inhale, air enters the body through the trachea. This air travels to and from the lungs, filling and emptying the alveoli. During inhalation, the diaphragm and intercostal muscles contract. When the diaphragm contracts, it moves down slightly and enlarges the thoracic cage from top to bottom. When the intercostal muscles contract, they raise the ribs up and out. As we inhale, the combined actions of these structures enlarge the thorax in all directions. Take a deep breath to see how your chest expands.

The air pressure outside the body, called the atmospheric pressure, is normally higher than the air pressure within the thorax. As we inhale and the thoracic cage expands, the air pressure within the thorax decreases a bit more, creating a slight vacuum. This drives air in through the trachea and fills the lungs. When the air

pressure outside equals the air pressure inside, air stops moving. Gases, such as oxygen, will move from an area of high pressure to an area of lower pressure until the pressures are equal. At this point, the air stops moving, and we stop inhaling. **Tidal volume**, a measure of the depth of breathing, is the amount of air that is moved during one breath. Minute volume is tidal volume times respiratory rate, or the amount of air moved through the lungs in 1 minute.

It may help you to understand this if you think of the thoracic cage as a bell jar in which balloons are suspended. In this example, the balloons are the lungs. The base of the jar is the diaphragm, which moves up and down slightly with each breath. The ribs, which are the sides of the jar, maintain the shape of the chest. The only opening into the jar is a small tube at the top, similar to the trachea. During inhalation, the bottom of the jar moves down slightly and decreases pressure in the jar, creating a slight vacuum. As a result, the balloons fill with air (▼ **Figure 7-3**).

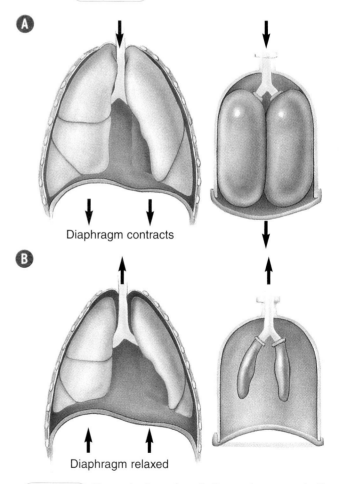

Diaphragm contracts

Diaphragm relaxed

Figure 7-3 The mechanisms of respiration can be compared with that of a bell jar. **A.** Inhalation and chest expansion, anatomic (left) and bell jar (right). **B.** Exhalation and chest contraction, anatomic (left) and bell jar (right).

Exhalation

Unlike inhalation, exhalation does not normally require muscular effort. During <u>exhalation</u>, the diaphragm and the intercostal muscles relax. In response, the thorax decreases in size, and the ribs and muscles assume a normal resting position. When the size of the thoracic cage decreases, air in the lungs is compressed into a smaller space. The air pressure within the thorax then becomes higher than the pressure outside, and air is pushed out through the trachea.

Let's return to the example of the bell jar. During exhalation, the bottom of the jar (the diaphragm) moves up, returning to its normal resting position. This movement increases air pressure within the jar. With this increase in pressure, the sides of the jar contract, and the balloons empty.

Remember that air will reach the lungs only if it travels through the trachea. This is why clearing and maintaining an open airway are so important. Clearing the airway means removing obstructing material, tissue, or fluids from the nose, mouth, or throat. Maintaining the airway means keeping the airway open so that air can enter and leave the lungs freely (▼ **Figure 7-4**).

Air may also pass into the chest cavity through another opening in the throat or chest wall as a result of trauma, keeping air from reaching the alveoli. In Chapter 27, Chest Injuries, you will learn how to recognize and manage these conditions.

Physiology of the Respiratory System

All living cells need energy to survive. Cells take energy from nutrients through a series of chemical processes. The name given to these processes as a whole is <u>metabolism</u>. During metabolism, each cell combines nutrients and oxygen and produces energy and waste products, primarily water and carbon dioxide.

Each living cell in the body requires a supply of oxygen and a regular means of getting rid of waste (carbon dioxide). The body provides these through respiration. Some cells need a constant supply of oxygen to survive. Other cells in the body can tolerate short periods without oxygen and still survive. For example, after 4 to 6 minutes without oxygen, brain cells and cells in the nervous system may be severely and permanently damaged and may even die (▼ **Figure 7-5**). Dead brain cells can never be replaced. However, cells in the kidney may be without oxygen for 45 minutes or more and still survive. This is why certain organ transplants are possible.

Normally, the air that we breathe contains 21% oxygen and 78% nitrogen. Small amounts of other gases make up the remaining 1%.

The Exchange of Oxygen and Carbon Dioxide

As blood travels through the body, it supplies oxygen and nutrients to various tissues and cells. Oxygen

Figure 7-4 Air reaches the lungs only if it travels through the trachea. Maintaining the airway means keeping the airway open so that air can enter and leave the lungs freely.

TIME IS CRITICAL!
- 0 to 1 minute: cardiac irritability
- 0 to 4 minutes: brain damage not likely
- 4 to 6 minutes: brain damage possible
- 6 to 10 minutes: brain damage very likely
- More than 10 minutes: irreversible brain damage

Figure 7-5 Cells need a constant supply of oxygen to survive. Some cells may be severely and permanently damaged after 4 to 6 minutes without oxygen.

passes from the blood through the capillaries to tissue cells, while carbon dioxide and cell waste pass in the opposite direction: from tissue cells through capillaries to the blood (▼ **Figure 7-6**).

Each time we inhale, the alveoli receive a supply of oxygen-rich air. The alveoli are surrounded by a network of tiny pulmonary capillaries. These capillaries are, in fact, located in the walls of the alveoli. This means that the air in the alveoli and the blood in the capillaries are separated only by two very thin layers of wall tissue. Each time we exhale, the carbon dioxide from the bloodstream travels across the same two layers of tissue to the alveoli and is expelled into the atmosphere.

Oxygen and carbon dioxide pass rapidly across the walls of the alveoli and the capillaries through diffusion. **Diffusion** is a passive process in which molecules move from an area with higher concentration of molecules to an area of lower concentration. For example, when we walk into a kitchen and it smells like a rotten egg, that is because the molecules of hydrogen sulfide gas have moved spontaneously from an area of high concentration near the egg to fill the whole space. Molecules of oxygen move from the alveoli into the blood because there are fewer oxygen molecules in the blood. In the same way, molecules of carbon dioxide move from the blood into the alveoli because there are fewer carbon dioxide molecules in the alveoli (▶ **Figure 7-7**).

Normally this is a very slow process. However, the alveoli produce a chemical, called surfactant, that makes the diffusion of carbon dioxide and oxygen much faster and more efficient. Anything that removes surfactant (such as water from a drowning) will cause acute respiratory distress.

Figure 7-7 With diffusion, molecules of oxygen move from the alveoli into the blood, because there are fewer oxygen molecules in the blood. Similarly, molecules of carbon dioxide move from the blood into the alveoli, because there are fewer carbon dioxide molecules in the alveoli.

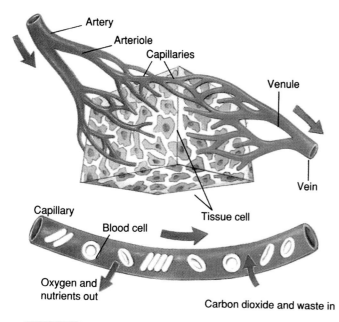

Figure 7-6 Oxygen passes from the blood through capillaries to tissue cells. Carbon dioxide passes from tissue cells through capillaries to the blood.

The blood does not use all the inhaled oxygen as it passes through the body. So the air that we exhale contains 16% oxygen and 3% to 5% carbon dioxide; the rest is nitrogen ▼ Figure 7-8 . Therefore, when you provide artificial ventilations to a patient who is not breathing, that patient is receiving a 16% concentration of oxygen with each of your exhaled breaths.

The Control of Breathing

The area of the brain stem that controls breathing is deep within the skull, in one of the best-protected parts of the nervous system. The nerves in this area act as sensors, reacting primarily to the level of carbon dioxide in the arterial blood. If the levels of carbon dioxide are too high or too low, the brain automatically adjusts breathing. This happens very quickly, in just one breath. Again, this is why you cannot hold your breath indefinitely or breathe rapidly and deeply for very long. In a healthy person, the stimulus to breathe is referred to as the normal respiratory drive.

When the level of carbon dioxide becomes too high, the brain stem sends nerve impulses down the spinal cord that cause the diaphragm and the intercostal muscles to contract. This increases our breathing, or respirations. The higher the level of carbon dioxide in the blood, the stronger the impulses to cause breathing. Once the carbon dioxide returns to an acceptable level, the strength and frequency of respiration decrease.

We also have a "backup system" to control respiration, called the **hypoxic drive**. This system stimulates breathing when oxygen levels fall (hypoxia). However, the nerves in the brain, the walls of the aorta, and the carotid arteries that act as oxygen sensors are easily satisfied with minimal levels of oxygen. Therefore, the hypoxic drive is much less sensitive and less powerful than the carbon dioxide sensors in the brain stem.

HYPOXIA. Hypoxia is an extremely dangerous condition in which the body's tissues and cells do not have enough oxygen; unless it is reversed, patients may die in a matter of moments. **Hypoxia** develops quickly in the vital organs of patients who are not breathing adequately, as well as in those who are not breathing at all. Inadequate breathing means that the person cannot move enough air into the lungs with each breath to meet the body's needs.

Patients who are breathing inadequately will show varying signs and symptoms of inadequate breathing (hypoxia). The onset and the degree of tissue damage will depend on the quality of ventilations. The signs of hypoxia may include mental status changes, the use of accessory muscles for breathing, difficulty breathing, possibly chest pain, and, late in the process, cyanosis. Early signs include nervousness, irritability, apprehension, fast heart rate (tachycardia), and fear. Conscious patients will complain of shortness of breath and may not be able to talk in complete sentences. The best time to give a patient oxygen is before any signs and symptoms appear.

The following conditions are commonly associated with hypoxia:

- **Heart attack (myocardial infarction).** Ischemia within the heart muscle from myocardial infarction occurs when there is inadequate circulation of oxygen-carrying blood to the tissues of the heart.

- **Pulmonary edema.** →swelling Fluid accumulates in the lungs, making the transfer of oxygen to the blood from the alveoli less efficient.

- **Acute narcotic overdose.** Respirations may become decreased and shallow.

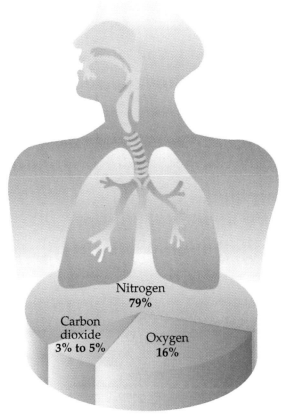

Nitrogen
79%

Carbon
dioxide
3% to 5%

Oxygen
16%

Components of Exhaled Air

Figure 7-8   Exhaled air contains 16% oxygen and 3% to 5% carbon dioxide; 79% is nitrogen.

- **Inhalation of smoke and/or toxic fumes.** These substances cause pulmonary edema and destroy lung tissue, causing problems with gas exchange.

- **Stroke (cerebrovascular accident).** The cause of hypoxia in a stroke patient may be due to facial paralysis and poor control of respirations and heart rhythms by the brain.

- **Chest injury.** Pain interferes with full chest wall expansion, thus limiting the amount of gases that are exchanged. Lung damage can also prevent efficient gas exchange.

- **Shock (hypoperfusion).** Shock often occurs as a result of injuries involving substantial blood loss. With the loss of red blood cells, not enough oxygen is available to the tissues.

- **Chronic obstructive pulmonary disease (chronic bronchitis and emphysema).** Chronic irritation of the lungs and air passages produces alveolar damage and poor gas exchange.

- **Asthma.** Narrowing of respiratory passages and buildup of mucus causes air trapping and poor gas exchange.

All hypoxic patients, whatever the cause of their condition, should be treated with high-flow supplemental oxygen. The method of oxygen delivery will vary, depending on the cause and the severity of the hypoxia.

Patient Assessment

Recognizing Adequate Breathing

Earlier, we compared breathing to an expandable bell jar with a movable bottom. You can also think of a normal breathing pattern as a bellows system. Breathing should appear easy, not labored. As with a bellows used to move air to start a fire, breathing should be a smooth flow of air moving into and out of the lungs. Signs of normal (adequate) breathing for adult patients are listed below:

- A normal rate and depth (between 12 and 20 breaths/min) for adults

- A regular pattern of inhalation and exhalation

- Clear and equal lung sounds on both sides of the chest (<u>bilateral</u>)

- Regular and equal chest rise and fall (chest expansion)

- Adequate depth (tidal volume)

Recognizing Inadequate Breathing

An adult who is awake, alert, and talking to you has no immediate airway or breathing problems. However, you should always have supplemental oxygen close at hand to assist with breathing if this becomes necessary. An adult who is breathing normally will have respirations of 12 to 20 breaths/min (▼ **Table 7-1**). The adult patient who is breathing either much slower (fewer than 8 breaths/min) or much faster (more than 24 breaths/min) should be evaluated for inadequate breathing.

A patient with inadequate breathing may appear to be working hard to breathe. This type of breathing pattern is called <u>labored breathing</u>. It requires effort and, especially among children, may involve the accessory muscles. Accessory muscles are secondary muscles of respiration. They include the neck muscles (sternocleidomastoid), the chest pectoralis major muscles, and the abdominal muscles (▼ **Figure 7-9**).

TABLE 7-1 Normal Respiration Rate Ranges	
Adults	12 to 20 breaths/min
Children	15 to 30 breaths/min
Infants	25 to 50 breaths/min

Figure 7-9 The accessory muscles of breathing are used when a patient is having difficulty breathing, not for normal breathing. These include the sternocleidomastoid, pectoralis major, and abdominal muscles.

Documentation Tips

The respiratory status of the patient is so important that it should be noted at the beginning of your radio report, after mental status. Any changes during treatment or transport should be immediately reported to the receiving hospital. Respiratory status along with any changes should also be documented in your patient care report.

These muscles are not used in normal breathing. More information about recognizing labored breathing and respiratory distress in children may be found in Chapters 31 and 32. Signs of inadequate breathing in adult patients are as follows:

- Respiratory rate of less than 8 breaths/min or greater than 24 breaths/min

- Accessory muscle use

- Skin pulling in around the ribs during inspiration (**retractions**)

- Pale, cyanotic, or cool (clammy) skin

- Irregular (uneven) pattern of inhalation and exhalation

- Lung sounds that are decreased, unequal, or "wet"

- Labored breathing

- Shallow and/or uneven chest rise and fall

- Two- or three-word sentences spoken

Cheyne-Stokes breathing

Figure 7-10 Cheyne-Stokes breathing shows irregular respirations followed by a period of apnea.

You should also be aware that a patient may appear to be breathing after the heart has stopped. These occasional, gasping breaths are called **agonal respirations**. They occur when the respiratory center in the brain continues to send signals to the breathing muscles. These respirations are not adequate, since they are slow and generally shallow. You will need to provide artificial ventilations to patients with agonal respirations.

Some patients may have irregular respiratory breathing patterns that are related to a specific patient condition. An example of this is Cheyne-Stokes respirations, which are often seen in patients with stroke and patients with serious head injuries (▼ Figure 7-10). Cheyne-Stokes respirations are an irregular respiratory pattern in which the patient breathes with an increasing rate and depth of respiration that is followed by a period of **apnea**, or lack of spontaneous breathing, followed again by the pattern of increasing rate and depth. Serious head injuries may also cause changes in the normal respiratory rate and pattern of breathing. The changes may be noted as irregular respirations that may or may not have an identifiable pattern.

Patients with inadequate breathing have inadequate minute volume and need to be treated immediately. This is most easily recognized in patients who are unable to speak in complete sentences when at rest. Emergency medical care includes airway management, supplemental oxygen, and ventilatory support.

Opening the Airway

Emergency medical care begins with ensuring an open airway. The patient's airway and breathing status are the first steps in your initial assessment for a very good reason: Unless you can immediately open and maintain an airway, you will not be able to deliver appropriate patient care.

When you respond to a call and find an unconscious patient, you need to assess and determine immediately whether the patient has an open airway and breathing is adequate. In order to open the airway and to assess breathing, the patient needs to be in the supine position. If your patient is found in the prone (lying face down) position, he or she must be properly positioned to allow for assessment of airway and breathing and to begin CPR should it be necessary. The patient should be log rolled as a unit so the head,

Skill Drill 7-1 Positioning an Unconscious Patient

Support the head while your partner straightens the patient's legs.

Have your partner place his or her hand on the patient's far shoulder and hip.

Roll the patient as a unit with the person at the head calling the count to begin the move.

Open and assess the patient's airway and breathing status.

neck, and spine all move together without any twisting ▲ Skill Drill 7-1.

1. **Kneel beside the patient.** Have your partner kneel far enough away so that the patient, when rolled toward you, does not come to rest in your lap. Rapidly straighten the patient's legs and move the nearer arm across the patient's chest to minimize movement. Place your hands behind the back of the patient's head and neck to provide in-line stabilization of the cervical spine **(Step 1)**.

2. **Have your partner** place his or her hands on the patient's far shoulder and hip **(Step 2)**.

3. **As you call the count** to control movement, have your partner turn the patient toward you by pulling on the far shoulder and hip. Control the head and neck so that they move as a unit with the rest of the torso. In this way, the head and neck stay in the same vertical plane as the back. This single motion will minimize aggravation of any spinal injury. At this point, you should apply a cervical collar. Replace the patient's farther arm back at his or her side **(Step 3)**.

4. **Once the patient is positioned,** maintain an open airway and check for breathing **(Step 4)**.

Figure 7-11 The most common airway obstruction is the patient's own tongue, which falls back into the throat when the muscles of the throat and tongue relax.

Figure 7-12 The head tilt-chin lift maneuver is a simple technique for opening the airway in a patient without a suspected cervical spine injury.

In an unconscious patient, the most common airway obstruction is the patient's own tongue, which falls back into the throat when the muscles of the throat and tongue relax ▲ Figure 7-11 . Dentures (false teeth), blood, vomitus, mucus, food, or other foreign objects may also create a blockage. Therefore, you should always have a suction device available to help clear and maintain a patent airway.

Head Tilt-Chin Lift Maneuver

Opening the airway to relieve an obstruction can often be done quickly and easily by simply tilting the patient's head back and lifting the chin in what is known as the **head tilt–chin lift maneuver**. For patients who have not sustained trauma, this simple maneuver is sometimes all that is needed for the patient to resume breathing.

To perform the head tilt-chin lift maneuver, follow these steps:

1. With the patient in a supine position, position yourself beside the patient's head.

2. Place one hand on the patient's forehead, and apply firm backward pressure with your palm to tilt the patient's head back. This extension of the neck will move the tongue forward, away from the back of the throat, and clear the airway if the tongue is blocking it.

3. Place the tips of the fingers of your other hand under the lower jaw near the bony part of the chin. Do not compress the soft tissue under the chin, as this may block the airway.

4. Lift the chin upward, bringing the entire lower jaw with it, helping to tilt the head back. Do not use your thumb to lift the chin. Lift so that the teeth are nearly brought together, but avoid closing the mouth completely. Continue to hold the forehead to maintain the backward tilt of the head ▲ Figure 7-12 .

Jaw-Thrust Maneuver

The head tilt-chin lift will open the airway in most patients. If you suspect a cervical spine injury, use the jaw-thrust maneuver. The **jaw-thrust maneuver** is a technique to open the airway by placing the fingers behind the angle of the jaw and lifting the jaw upward. You can easily seal a mask around the mouth while doing the jaw-thrust maneuver. This is the method of choice for patients with suspected cervical spine injury. See Chapter 30, Head and Spine Injuries, for a more detailed discussion of these types of injuries.

Perform the jaw-thrust maneuver in an adult in the following manner ▶ Skill Drill 7-2 :

1. **Kneel above the patient's head.** Place your fingers behind the angles of the lower jaw, and forcefully move the jaw upward. Use your thumbs to help position the lower jaw to allow breathing through the mouth as well as the nose **(Step 1)**.

2. The completed maneuver should open the airway with the mouth slightly open and the jaw jutting forward **(Step 2)**.

SkillDrill 7-2 Performing the Jaw-Thrust Maneuver

①

Kneeling above the patient's head, place your fingers behind the angles of the lower jaw, and forcefully move the jaw upward. Use your thumbs to help position the lower jaw.

②

The completed maneuver should look like this.

Once the airway has been opened, the patient may start to breathe on his or her own. Assess whether breathing has returned by using the look, listen, and feel technique (▶ **Figure 7-13**).

With complete airway obstruction, there will be no movement of air. However, you may see the chest and abdomen rise and fall considerably with the patient's frantic attempts to breathe. This is why the presence of chest wall movement alone does not indicate breathing is present. Regular chest wall movement indicates a respiratory effort is present. Observing chest and abdominal movement is often difficult with a fully clothed patient. You may see little, if any, chest movement even with normal breathing. This is particularly true in some patients with chronic lung disease. You must begin artificial ventilation immediately if you use the three-part approach—look, listen, and feel—and discover that there is no movement of air.

Basic Airway Adjuncts

The primary function of an airway adjunct is to prevent obstruction of the upper airway by the tongue and allow the passage of air and oxygen to the lungs.

Oropharyngeal Airways

An **oropharyngeal (oral) airway** has two principal purposes. The first is to keep the tongue from blocking the upper airway. The second is to make it easier to suction the airway if necessary. Both functions are made possible by an opening down the center or along either side of the oropharyngeal airway (▶ **Figure 7-14**). This type of airway is often used in conjunction with bag-valve-mask (BVM) ventilation.

An oropharyngeal airway should be inserted promptly in unconscious patients who have no gag reflex. These patients may or may not be breathing on their own. The **gag reflex** is a protective reflex

(**Figure 7-13**) The look, listen, and feel technique is used to assess whether breathing has spontaneously returned.

Skill Drill 7-3 Inserting an Oral Airway

Size the airway by measuring from the patient's earlobe to the corner of the mouth.

Open the patient's mouth with the cross-finger technique. Hold the airway upside down with your other hand. Insert the airway with the tip facing the roof of the mouth.

Rotate the airway 180°. Insert the airway until the flange (the trumpet-shaped flare) rests on the patient's lips and teeth. In this position, the airway will hold the tongue forward.

mechanism that prevents food and other particles from entering the airway. If you try to insert an oral airway in a patient with a gag reflex, the result may be vomiting or a spasm of the vocal cords. An oral airway is also a safe, effective way to help maintain the airway of the patient with a possible spinal injury. The use of an oral airway may make manual airway maneuvers such as the head tilt-chin lift and the jaw-thrust easier to maintain.

Figure 7-14 An oral airway is used for unconscious patients who have no gag reflex. It works to keep the tongue from blocking the airway and to make suctioning the airway easier.

You must be very clear on when and how this device is used. **▲ Skill Drill 7-3** shows the steps for inserting an oral airway. If the oropharyngeal airway is not the proper size or is inserted incorrectly, it could actually push the tongue back into the pharynx, blocking the airway. The following steps should be used when inserting an oropharyngeal airway:

1. **To select the proper size,** measure from the patient's earlobe to the corner of the mouth on the side of the face **(Step 1)**.

2. **Open the patient's mouth** with the cross-finger technique. Hold the airway upside down with your other hand. Insert the airway with the tip facing the roof of the mouth **(Step 2)**.

3. **Rotate the airway 180°. When inserted properly,** the airway will rest in the mouth with the curvature of the airway following the contour of the tongue. The flange should rest against the lips or teeth, with the other end opening into the pharynx **(Step 3)**.

Take care to avoid injuring the hard palate as you insert the airway. Roughness can cause bleeding, which may aggravate airway problems or even cause vomiting.

Skill Drill 7-4   Inserting an Oral Airway With a 90° Rotation

Depress the tongue so the tongue remains forward.

Insert the oral airway sideways from the corner of the mouth, until the flange reaches the teeth.

Rotate the oral airway at a 90° angle. Remove the tongue blade as you exert gentle backward pressure on the oral airway, until it rests securely in place against the lips and teeth.

If you encounter difficulty while inserting the oral airway, an alternative method may be used by following these steps (▲ Skill Drill 7-4):

1. **Use a tongue blade** to depress the tongue, ensuring that the tongue remains forward **(Step 1)**.

2. **Insert the oral airway sideways** from the corner of the mouth, until the flange reaches the teeth **(Step 2)**.

3. **Rotate the oral airway** at a 90° angle, removing the tongue blade as you exert gentle backward pressure on the oral airway, until it rests securely in place against the lips and teeth **(Step 3)**.

In some instances, a patient may become responsive and regain the gag reflex after you have inserted an oral airway. If this occurs, gently remove the airway by pulling it out, following the normal curvature of the mouth and throat. Be prepared for the patient to vomit.

Pediatric Needs

In children, the alternative method of inserting an oral airway, using a tongue blade to hold the tongue down while inserting the airway, is the only acceptable method. Because the airways of children are undeveloped, rotating an oropharyngeal airway in the posterior pharynx may cause damage. For more discussion on pediatric airways, see Chapter 32.

Have suction available, and log roll the patient onto his or her side to allow any fluids to drain out.

Nasopharyngeal Airways

A **nasopharyngeal (nasal or trumpet) airway** is usually used with a patient who has an intact gag reflex and is not able to maintain an airway (▶ Figure 7-15). Patients with an altered mental status or those who have just had a seizure may also benefit from this type of airway. If a patient has sustained severe trauma to the head or face, you should consult medical control before inserting a nasopharyngeal airway. Extreme care must be used with such trauma patients. If the airway is accidentally pushed through the hole caused by a fracture of the base of the skull, it may penetrate through the cranium and into the brain.

This type of airway is usually better tolerated by patients who have an intact gag reflex. It is not as likely as the oropharyngeal airway to cause vomiting. You should coat the airway well with a water-soluble lubricant before it is inserted. Be aware that slight bleeding may occur even when the airway is inserted properly. However, you should never force the airway into place.

Follow these steps to ensure correct placement of the nasopharyngeal airway (▶ Skill Drill 7-5):

1. **Before inserting the airway,** be sure you have selected the proper size. Measure from the tip of the patient's nose to the earlobe.

Skill Drill 7-5 Inserting a Nasal Airway

Size the airway by measuring from the tip of the nose to the patient's earlobe. Coat the tip with a water-soluble lubricant.

Insert the lubricated airway into the larger nostril with the curvature following the floor of the nose and the bevel towards the septum.

Gently advance the airway.

Continue until the flange rests against the skin. If you feel any resistance or obstruction, remove the airway and insert it into the other nostril.

Figure 7-15 A nasal airway is better tolerated by patients who have an intact gag reflex.

In almost all individuals, one nostril is larger than the other **(Step 1)**.

2. **The airway should be placed** in the larger nostril, with the curvature of the device following the curve of the floor of the nose **(Step 2)**.

3. **Advance the airway gently** **(Step 3)**.

4. **When completely inserted,** the flange rests against the nostril. The other end of the airway opens into the posterior pharynx **(Step 4)**.

If the patient becomes intolerant of the nasal airway, you may have to remove it. Gently withdraw the airway from the nasal passage.

Disadvantages of the nasal airway include the following:

- May be contraindicated in severe head or facial trauma
- May traumatize delicate nasal membranes, causing bleeding
- May not be able to insert if the patient has a history of fractured nasal bones

Suctioning

You must keep the airway clear so that you can ventilate the patient properly. If the airway is not clear, you will force the material into the lungs and possibly cause a complete airway obstruction. Therefore, suctioning is

EMT-B Safety

A mask and protective eyewear should be worn whenever airway management involves suctioning. Body fluids can become aerosolized, and exposure to the mucous membranes of the EMT-B's mouth, nose, and eyes can easily occur.

Skill Drill 7-6 Suctioning a Patient's Airway

Make sure the suctioning unit is properly assembled and turn on the suction unit.

Measure the catheter from the corner of the mouth to the earlobe.

Open the patient's mouth and insert the catheter to the depth measured.

Apply suction in a circular motion as you withdraw the catheter. Do not suction an adult for more than 15 seconds.

your next priority. If you have any doubt about the situation, remember this rule: If you hear gurgling, the patient needs suctioning!

Suctioning Equipment

Portable, hand-operated, and fixed (mounted) suctioning equipment is essential for resuscitation (▶ **Figure 7-16**). A portable suctioning unit must provide enough vacuum pressure and flow to allow you to suction the mouth and oropharynx effectively. Hand-operated suctioning units with disposable chambers are reliable, effective, and relatively inexpensive. A fixed suctioning unit should generate air flow of more than 40 L/min and a vacuum of more than 300 mm Hg when the tubing is clamped.

A suctioning unit should be fitted with the following:

- Wide-bore, thick-walled, nonkinking tubing
- Plastic, semirigid pharyngeal suction tips, called **tonsil tips** or Yankauer tips
- Nonrigid plastic catheters, called French or whistle-tip catheters
- A nonbreakable, disposable collection bottle
- A supply of water for rinsing the tips

You should make sure that the suction yoke, the collection bottle, water for rinsing, and the suction tube are easily accessible at the patient's head.

A **catheter** is a hollow, cylindrical structure that drains or delivers fluids. Tonsil tips are the best kind of catheter for suctioning the pharynx in adults and the

preferred method for infants and children. These plastic tips have a large diameter and are somewhat rigid, so they do not collapse. Tips with a curved contour allow for easy, rapid placement in the pharynx (▶ **Figure 7-17**). Be careful not to touch the back of the airway. This can activate the gag reflex, cause vomiting, and increase the possibility of **aspiration**.

You should use extreme caution when suctioning a conscious or semiconscious patient. Put the tip in only as far as you can visualize. Be aware that suctioning may induce vomiting in these patients.

To properly suction a patient (▲ **Skill Drill 7-6**):

1. **Turn on the assembled suction unit** (Step 1).

2. **Insert the catheter** to the correct depth by measuring the catheter from the corner of the patient's mouth to the edge of the earlobe (Step 2).

3. **Before applying suction,** open the patient's mouth using the cross-finger technique or by pulling the jaw, and insert the tip of the catheter to the depth measured (Step 3).

4. **Apply suction** in a circular motion as you withdraw the catheter. Do not suction an adult for more than 15 seconds (Step 4).

Soft plastic, nonrigid catheters, sometimes called French or whistle-tip catheters, are used to suction the nose and liquid secretions in the back of the mouth and in situations in which you cannot use a rigid catheter, such as for a patient with a **stoma** (▶ **Figure 7-18**).

Remember

Suctioning Time Limits

Adult	15 seconds
Child	10 seconds
Infant	5 seconds

For example, a patient could break off a tooth on a rigid catheter, whereas a flexible catheter may be worked along the cheeks without injury. Before you insert any catheter, make sure to measure for the proper size. Use the same technique as you would use when measuring for an oropharyngeal or nasopharyngeal airway. Never insert a catheter past the base of the tongue, as this may result in gagging and vomiting.

You should clean and decontaminate your suctioning equipment after each use according to the manufacturer's guidelines. You should also inspect this equipment regularly to make sure it is in proper working condition. Switch on the suction, clamp the tubing, and make sure that the unit generates a vacuum of more than 300 mm Hg. Check that a battery-charged unit has charged batteries.

Figure 7-16 Suctioning equipment is essential for resuscitation. **A.** Hand operated. **B.** Fixed unit. **C.** Portable unit.

Techniques of Suctioning

Follow these steps to operate the suction unit:

1. Check the unit for proper assembly of all its parts. Turn on the suctioning unit. Select and attach the appropriate catheter to the tubing. Use a bulb suction or soft catheter set at the low to medium setting when suctioning the nose.

2. Measure the catheter to ensure that you do not allow it to be inserted too deeply.

3. Open the patient's mouth using the cross-finger technique or the jaw-thrust maneuver. Insert the suction tip along the roof of the mouth until you reach the pharynx. Do not use suction unless it is absolutely necessary. Insert the tip only to the base of the tongue.

4. After the tip is in place, apply suction as you withdraw the suction tip from the pharynx and mouth. Move the suction tip from side to side.

Never suction for more than 15 seconds at one time for adult patients, 10 seconds for children, and 5 seconds for infants. Suctioning removes oxygen from the airway

Figure 7-17 Tonsil-tip catheters are the best for suctioning, as they have wide diameter tips and are somewhat rigid.

Figure 7-18 French, or whistle-tip, catheters are used in situations in which rigid catheters cannot be used, such as with a patient who has a stoma or if the patient's teeth are clenched.

along with obstructive material. Rinse the catheter and tubing with water to prevent clogging of the tube with dried vomitus or other secretions. Repeat suctioning only after the patient has been ventilated and re-oxygenated.

At times, a patient may have secretions or vomitus that cannot be suctioned quickly and easily. There are also some suction units that are unable to effectively remove solid objects such as teeth, foreign bodies, and food. In these instances, you should remove the catheter from the patient's mouth, log roll the patient to the side, and then clear the mouth carefully with your gloved finger. A patient may also produce frothy secretions as quickly as you can suction them from the airway. In this situation, you might need to alternate hyperventilation with suctioning. However, note that hyperventilation is not appropriate if vomitus or other particles are present.

Maintaining the Airway

The **recovery position** is used to help maintain a clear airway in a patient who has not had traumatic injuries and is breathing on his or her own with a normal rate and adequate tidal volume (depth of breathing). Take the following steps to put the patient in the recovery position:

1. Roll the patient onto the left side so that head, shoulders, and torso move at the same time without twisting.

2. Place the patient's extended left arm and right hand under his or her cheek (▶ Figure 7-19).

Once patients have resumed spontaneous breathing after being resuscitated, the recovery position will prevent the aspiration of vomitus. However, this position is not appropriate for patients with suspected spinal trauma, nor is it adequate for patients who are unconscious and require airway management. You must reposition such patients to provide access to the airway.

Supplemental Oxygen

You should always give supplemental oxygen to patients who are breathing inadequately because they are not getting enough oxygen to their lungs.

Some tissues and organs, such as the heart, the central nervous system, lungs, kidneys, and liver, need a constant supply of oxygen to function normally. **Never withhold oxygen from any patient who may benefit from it, even if you must assist ventilations.**

Use high-concentration oxygen in any cardiac and/or respiratory arrest situation, whether the patient is an infant or an adult.

Supplemental Oxygen Equipment

In addition to knowing when and how to give supplemental oxygen, you must understand how oxygen is stored and the various hazards associated with its use.

OXYGEN CYLINDERS. The oxygen that you will give to patients is usually supplied as a compressed gas in green, seamless steel or aluminum cylinders. Some bottles may be silver or chrome with a green area around the valve stem on top. Newer bottles are often made of lightweight aluminum or spun steel; older bottles are much heavier.

Check to make sure that the cylinder is labeled for medical oxygen. You should look for letters and numbers stamped into the metal on the collar of the cylinder (▼ Figure 7-20). Of particular importance are the month and year stamps, which indicate when the bottle was last tested.

Figure 7-19   In the recovery position, the patient is rolled onto the left side.

Figure 7-20   Oxygen tanks for medical use will have a series of letters and numbers stamped into the metal on the collar of the cylinder.

Oxygen cylinders are available in several sizes. The two sizes that you will most often use are the D (or super D) and M cylinders (▶ **Figure 7-21**). The D (or super D) cylinder can be carried from your unit to the patient. The M tank remains on board your unit as a main supply tank. Other sizes that you will see are A, E, G, H, and K (▼ **Table 7-2**).

The length of time you can use an oxygen cylinder depends on the pressure in the cylinder and the flow rate. A method of calculating cylinder duration is shown in (▼ **Table 7-3**).

SAFETY CONSIDERATIONS. Compressed gas cylinders must be handled very carefully because their contents are under pressure. Cylinders are fitted with pressure regulators to make sure that patients receive the right amount and type of gas. Make sure that the correct pressure regulator is firmly attached before you transport the cylinders. A puncture or hole in the tank can cause the cylinder to become a deadly missile. Do not handle a cylinder by the neck assembly alone. Cylinders should be secured with mounting brackets when they are stored on the ambulance. Oxygen cylinders that are in use during transport should be positioned and secured to prevent the tank from falling or from damage occurring to the valve-gauge assembly.

(**Figure 7-21**) The cylinders that are most commonly found on an ambulance are the D (or super D) and M size cylinders.

TABLE 7-2 Oxygen Cylinder Sizes Carried on the Ambulance	
Size	**Volume, L**
D	350
Super D	500
E	625
M	3,000
G	5,300
H, A, K	6,900

TABLE 7-3 Oxygen Cylinders: Duration of Flow

Formula:

$$\frac{(\text{Gauge pressure in psi} - \text{the safe residual pressure}) \times \text{constant}}{\text{Flow rate in L/min}} = \text{duration of flow in minutes}$$

RESIDUAL PRESSURE = 200 psi

CYLINDER CONSTANT

D = 0.16	G = 2.41
E = 0.28	H = 3.14
M = 1.56	K = 3.14

Determine the life of an M cylinder that has a pressure of 2000 psi and a flow rate of 10 L/min.

$$\frac{(2000-200) \times 1.56}{10} = \frac{2808}{10} = 281 \text{ min, or 4 h 41 min}$$

PIN-INDEXING SYSTEM. The compressed gas industry has established a **pin-indexing system** for portable cylinders to prevent an oxygen regulator from being connected to a carbon dioxide cylinder, a carbon dioxide regulator from being connected to an oxygen cylinder, and so on. In preparing to administer oxygen, always check to be sure that the pinholes on the cylinder exactly match the corresponding pins on the regulator.

The pin-indexing system features a series of pins on a yoke that must be matched with the holes on the valve stem of the gas cylinder. The arrangement of the pins and holes varies for different gases according to accepted national standards (▼ **Figure 7-22**). Other gases that are supplied in portable cylinders, such as acetylene, carbon dioxide, and nitrogen, use regulators and flowmeters that are very similar to those used with oxygen. Each cylinder of a specific gas has a given pattern and a given number of pins. These safety measures make it impossible for you to attach a cylinder of nitrous oxide to an oxygen regulator. The oxygen regulator will not fit.

The outlet valves on D size or smaller cylinders are designed to accept yoke-type pressure-reducing gauges, which conform to the pin-indexing system (▼ **Figure 7-23**). The safety system for large cylinders is known as the **American Standard System**. In this system, cylinders larger than D sizes are equipped with threaded gas outlet valves. The inside and outside thread sizes of these outlets vary depending on the gas in the cylinder. The cylinder will not accept a regulator

valve unless it is properly threaded to fit that regulator. The purpose of these safety devices is the same as in the pin-indexing system: to prevent the accidental attachment of a regulator to a wrong cylinder.

PRESSURE REGULATORS. The pressure of gas in a full oxygen cylinder is approximately 2,000 psi. This is far too much pressure to be safe or useful for your purposes. Pressure regulators reduce the pressure to a more useful range, usually 40 to 70 psi. Most pressure regulators that are in use today reduce the pressure in a single stage, although multistage regulators do exist. A two-stage regulator will reduce the pressure first to 700 psi and then to 40 to 70 psi.

After the pressure is reduced to a workable level, the final attachment for delivering the gas to the patient is usually one of the following:

- A quick-connect female fitting that will accept a quick-connect male plug from a pressure hose or ventilator or resuscitator

- A flowmeter that will permit the regulated release of gas measured in liters per minute

HUMIDIFICATION. Some EMS systems provide humidified oxygen to patients during transport (▼ **Figure 7-24**). However, humidified oxygen is usually indicated only for long-term oxygen therapies. Dry oxygen is not considered harmful for short-term use. Therefore, many EMS systems do not use humidified oxygen in the prehospital

Figure 7-22 The locations of the pin-indexing safety system holes in a cylinder valve face. Each cylinder of a specific gas has a given pattern and a given number of pins.

Figure 7-23 A yoke-type pressure-reducing gauge is used with a small oxygen cylinder.

Figure 7-24 Giving humidified oxygen may be preferred with long transport times. However, the use of this type of oxygen delivery system is not universal for all EMT-Bs.

Figure 7-25 Pressure-compensated flowmeters contain a float ball that rises or falls according to the gas flow within the tube. It must be maintained in an upright position for an accurate reading.

setting. Always refer to medical control or local protocols for guidance involving patient treatment issues.

FLOWMETERS. Flowmeters are usually permanently attached to pressure regulators on emergency medical equipment. The two types of flowmeters that are commonly used are pressure-compensated flowmeters and Bourdon-gauge flowmeters.

A pressure-compensated flowmeter incorporates a float ball within a tapered calibrated tube. The float rises or falls according to the gas flow within the tube. The flow of gas is controlled by a needle valve located downstream from the float ball. This type of flowmeter is affected by gravity and must always be maintained in an upright position for an accurate flow reading ◀ **Figure 7-25** .

The Bourdon-gauge flowmeter is commonly used because it is not affected by gravity and can be used in any position. It is actually a pressure gauge that is calibrated to record flow rate ▼ **Figure 7-26** . The major disadvantage of this flowmeter is that it does not compensate for backpressure. Therefore, it will usually record a higher flow rate when there is any obstruction to gas flow downstream.

Operating Procedures

Before placing an oxygen cylinder into service ▶ **Skill Drill 7-7** :

1. **Inspect the cylinder** and its markings. If the cylinder was commercially filled, it will have a plastic seal around the valve stem covering the opening in the stem. Remove the seal, and inspect the opening to make sure that it is free of dirt and other debris. The valve stem should not be sealed or covered with adhesive tape or any petroleum-based substances. These can

Figure 7-26 The Bourdon-gauge flowmeter is not affected by gravity and can be used in any position.

contaminate the oxygen and can contribute to spontaneous combustion when mixed with the pressurized oxygen.

"Crack" the cylinder by quickly opening and then reclosing the valve to help make sure that dirt particles and other possible contaminants do not enter the oxygen flow. *Never face the tank toward yourself or others when cracking the cylinder.* Open the tank by attaching a tank key to the valve and rotating the valve counterclockwise. You should be able to hear clearly the rush of oxygen coming from the tank. Close the tank by rotating the valve clockwise **(Step 1)**.

2. **Attach the regulator/flowmeter** to the valve stem after clearing the opening. On one side of the valve stem, you will find three holes. The larger one, on top, is a true opening through which the oxygen flows. The two smaller holes below it do not extend to the inside of the tank. They provide stability to the regulator. Following the design of a pin-indexing system, these two holes are very precisely located in positions that are unique to oxygen cylinders.

   Above the pins on the inside of the collar is the actual port through which oxygen flows from the cylinder to the regulator. A metal or plastic O-ring is placed around the oxygen port to optimize the airtight seal between the collar of the regulator and the valve stem **(Step 2)**.

3. **Place the regulator collar** over the cylinder valve, with the oxygen port and pin-indexing pins on the side of the valve stem that has the three holes. Open the screw bolt just enough to allow the collar to fit freely over the valve stem. Move the regulator so that the oxygen port and the pins fit into the correct holes on the valve stem. The screw bolt on the opposite side should be aligned with the dimpled depression. As you hold the regulator securely against the valve stem, tighten the screw bolt until the regulator is firmly attached to the cylinder. At this point, you should not see any open spaces between the sides of the valve stem and the interior walls of the collar **(Step 3)**.

4. **With the regulator firmly attached,** open the cylinder and read the pressure level on the regulator gauge. Most portable cylinders have a maximum pressure of approximately 2,000 psi. Most EMS services consider a cylinder with less than 500 to 1000 psi to be too low to keep in service.

Skill Drill 7-7 Placing an Oxygen Cylinder Into Service

Using an oxygen wrench, turn the valve counterclockwise to "crack" the cylinder.

Attach the regulator/flowmeter to the valve stem using the two pin-indexing holes and make sure that the washer is in place over the larger hole.

Align the regulator so that the pins fit snugly into the correct holes on the valve stem and hand tighten the regulator.

Attach the oxygen connective tubing to the flowmeter.

Learn your department's policies in this regard and follow them.

The flowmeter will have either a second gauge or a selector dial that indicates the oxygen flow rate. Several popular types of devices are widely used. Attach the selected oxygen device to the flowmeter by connecting the universal oxygen connective tubing to the "Christmas tree" nipple on the flowmeter. Most oxygen delivery devices come with this tubing permanently attached. Some oxygen masks do not. You must add this tubing to the oxygen delivery device if it is not attached **(Step 4)**.

Open the flowmeter to the desired flow rate. Flow rates will vary based on the oxygen delivery device being used. Remember that you must be completely familiar with the equipment before attempting to use it on a patient. Once the oxygen is flowing at the desired rate, apply the oxygen device to the patient and make any necessary adjustments. Monitor the patient's reaction to the oxygen and to the oxygen device, and periodically recheck the regulator gauge to make sure there is sufficient oxygen in the cylinder. Disconnect the tubing from the flowmeter nipple and turn off the cylinder valve when oxygen therapy is complete, or when the patient has been transferred to the hospital and has been switched to the hospital's

oxygen system. In a few seconds, the sound of oxygen flowing from the nipple will cease. This indicates that all the pressurized oxygen has been removed from the flowmeter. Turn off the flowmeter. The gauge on the regulator should read zero with the tank valve closed. This confirms that there is no pressure left above the valve stem. As long as there is a pressure reading on the regulator gauge, it is not safe to remove the regulator from the valve stem.

Hazards of Supplemental Oxygen

Oxygen does not burn or explode. However, it does support combustion. The more oxygen is around, the faster the combustion process. A small spark, even a glowing cigarette, can become a flame in an oxygen-rich atmosphere. Therefore, you must keep any possible source of fire away from the area while oxygen is in use. Make sure the area is adequately ventilated, especially in industrial settings where hazardous materials may be present and where sparks are easily generated. Be extremely cautious in any enclosed environment in which oxygen is being administered, as an oxygen-rich environment increases the chance of fire if a spark or flame is introduced. A bystander who is smoking or sparks from a vehicle extrication are possible ignition sources. Never leave an oxygen cylinder standing unattended. The oxygen can be knocked over, injuring the patient or damaging the equipment.

Oxygen Delivery Equipment

In general, the oxygen delivery equipment that is used in the field should be limited to nonrebreathing masks, BVM devices, and nasal cannulas, depending on local protocol. However, you may encounter other devices during transports between medical facilities.

Nonrebreathing Mask

The <u>nonrebreathing mask</u> is the preferred way of giving oxygen in the prehospital setting. With a good mask-to-face seal, it is capable of providing up to 90% inspired oxygen.

The nonrebreathing mask is a combination mask and reservoir bag system. The mask is similar to a simple face mask. Oxygen fills a reservoir bag that is attached to the mask by a one-way valve. The system is called a nonrebreathing mask because the exhaled gas escapes through flapper valve ports at the cheek areas of the mask (▼ **Figure 7-27**). The valve also prevents the patient from rebreathing exhaled gases as the gas in the reservoir bag flows into the mask during inhalation.

In this system, you must be sure that the reservoir bag is full before the mask is placed on the patient. Adjust the flow rate so that the bag does not fully collapse when the patient inhales. This is about two-thirds of the bag volume, or 10 to 15 L/min. Use a smaller reservoir bag with infants and children, as they will inhale a smaller volume.

Nasal Cannula

A <u>nasal cannula</u> delivers oxygen through two small, tubelike prongs that fit into the patient's nostrils

EMT-B Tips

Oxygen Delivery Devices

Device	Flow Rate	% of Oxygen Delivered
Nasal cannula	1-6 L/min	24%-44%
Nonrebreathing mask	10-15 L/min	up to 90%
BVM device with reservoir	15 L/min-flush	nearly 100%

(▼ **Figure 7-28**). This device can provide 24% to 44% inspired oxygen when the flowmeter is set at 1 to 6 L/min. For the comfort of your patient, flow rates above 6 L/min are not recommended with the nasal cannula.

The nasal cannula delivers dry oxygen directly into the nostrils. Therefore, when you anticipate a long transport time, you should consult medical control about humidification.

A nasal cannula has limited use in the prehospital care setting. For example, a patient who breathes through the mouth or who has a nasal obstruction will get little or no benefit from a nasal cannula. You may consider using this device with patients whom you believe to be stable and not hypoxic, but *always* use a nonrebreathing mask with patients in unstable condition who are breathing on their own. Always try to give high-flow oxygen through a nonrebreathing

Figure 7-27) The nonrebreathing mask contains flapper valve ports at the cheek areas of the mask to prevent the patient from rebreathing exhaled air.

Figure 7-28) The nasal cannula delivers oxygen directly through the nostrils.

mask if you suspect that a patient may have hypoxia, coaching him or her as necessary. If the patient will not tolerate a nonrebreathing mask, you will have to use a nasal cannula, which some patients find more comfortable. As always, a good assessment of your patient will guide your decision.

Pulse Oximetry

Pulse oximetry is a recent assessment tool used to evaluate the effectiveness of oxygenation. The pulse oximeter is a photoelectric device that monitors the oxygen saturation of hemoglobin (the iron-containing portion of the red blood cell to which oxygen attaches) in the capillary beds. Parts that make up the pulse oximeter include a monitor and sensing probe (▼ Figure 7-29). The sensing probe clips onto a finger or ear lobe. The light source must have unobstructed access to a capillary bed, so fingernail polish should be removed. Results appear as a percentage on the display screen. Normally, pulse oximetry values will be greater than 95% on room air, with the majority being between 98% and 100%.

The goal of any oxygen therapy is to increase oxygen saturation to normal levels. This device is a useful assessment tool to determine the effectiveness of oxygen therapy, bronchodilator therapy, and use of the BVM device in certain conditions. However, the pulse oximeter does *not* take the place of good assessment skills and should *not* prevent the application of oxygen to any patient who complains of difficulty breathing regardless of the pulse oximetry value.

Because the device presumes adequate perfusion and numbers of red blood cells, anything that causes vasoconstriction (such as hypoperfusion or cold

Figure 7-29 The pulse oximeter is a device that measures the saturation of oxygen in the blood.

EMT-B Tips

Methods of Ventilation
(listed in order of preference)

- Mouth-to-mask
- Two-person BVM device
- One-person BVM device

extremities) or loss of red blood cells (such as bleeding or anemia) will result in inaccurate or misleading values. The device also presumes that oxygen is saturating hemoglobin. Therefore, any chemical that displaces oxygen (such as carbon monoxide) will cause misleading values.

The pulse oximeter is a useful tool as long as the EMT-B remembers that the device is only a tool, not a substitute for a good assessment. The device should not be used when hypoperfusion or known anemia is present, carbon monoxide or exposure to other toxic inhalants has occurred, or the patient's extremities are cold.

Assisted and Artificial Ventilation

Obviously, a patient who is not breathing needs artificial ventilation and supplemental oxygen. But the same is true of patients who are breathing inadequately, that is, fewer than 8 breaths/min or more than 24 breaths/min. The literature varies regarding the number of breaths/min that is considered inadequate; however, most sources state that fewer than 8 breaths/min or more than 24 to 30 breaths/min is considered inadequate. Keep in mind that fast, shallow breathing can be as dangerous as very slow breathing. Fast, shallow breathing moves air primarily in the larger airway passages (dead air space) and does not allow for adequate exchange of air and carbon dioxide in the alveoli. Patients with inadequate breathing require assisted ventilations.

Although you do not need any special equipment to provide simple artificial or assisted ventilation, remember to follow BSI precautions as needed.

Once you determine that a patient is not breathing or needs assisted ventilations, you should begin artificial ventilation immediately. With a patient who is not breathing, there are several ways to do this, some of which require equipment. The methods that an EMT-B may use to provide artificial ventilation include the one- or two-person BVM device, mouth-to-mask ventilation, and the flow-restricted, oxygen-powered ventilation device. Note, however, that ventilation with a flow-restricted, oxygen-powered ventilation device and mouth-to-mask ventilation are now being used less often than in the past.

Mouth-to-Mouth and Mouth-to-Mask Ventilation

As you learned in your CPR course, mouth-to-mouth ventilations are now routinely done with a barrier device, such as a mask. A **barrier device** is a protective item that features a plastic barrier placed on a patient's face with a one-way valve to prevent the back flow of secretions, vomitus, and gases. Barrier devices provide adequate BSI. Mouth-to-mouth ventilations without a barrier device should be provided only in extreme conditions. Performing mouth-to-mask ventilations with a pocket mask with a one-way valve is a safer method of ventilation to prevent possible disease transmission ▼ **Figure 7-30** .

A mask with an oxygen inlet provides oxygen during mouth-to-mask ventilation to supplement the air from your own lungs. Remember that the gas you exhale contains 16% oxygen, more than enough to maintain the patient's life. With the mouth-to-mask system, however, the patient gets the additional benefit of significant oxygen enrichment with inspired air. This system also frees both your hands to help keep the airway open and helps you to provide a better seal between the mask and the face.

The mask may be shaped like a triangle or a doughnut, with the apex (top) placed across the

Figure 7-30 Barrier devices such as a plastic shield or a pocket mask with a one-way valve provide adequate BSI.

bridge of the nose. The base (bottom) of the mask is placed in the groove between the lower lip and the chin. In the center of the mask is a chimney with a 15-mL connector.

Follow these steps to use mouth-to-mask ventilation ▶ **Skill Drill 7-8** :

1. **Kneel at the patient's head.** Open the airway using the head tilt-chin lift maneuver or the jaw-thrust maneuver if indicated. Connect the one-way valve to the face mask. Place the mask on the patient's face. Make sure the top is over the bridge of the nose and the bottom is in the groove between the lower lip and the chin. Grasp the patient's lower jaw with your first three fingers on each hand. Place your thumbs on the dome of the mask. Make an airtight seal by applying firm pressure between the thumbs and the fingers. Maintain an upward and forward pull on the lower jaw with your fingers to keep the airway open **(Step 1)**.

2. **Take a deep breath and exhale** through the open port of the one-way valve. Breathe slowly into the patient's mask for 2 seconds **(Step 2)**.

3. **Remove your mouth,** and watch for the patient's chest to fall during passive exhalation **(Step 3)**.

You know that you are providing adequate ventilations if you see the patient's chest rise and fall. Feel for resistance of the patient's lungs as they expand. You should also hear and feel air escape as the patient exhales. Make sure that you are providing the correct number of breaths per minute for the patient's age.

To increase the oxygen concentration, administer high-flow oxygen at 15 L/min through the oxygen inlet valve. This, when combined with your exhaled breath, will deliver approximately 55% oxygen to the patient.

The mask also works well for patients breathing on their own who need supplemental oxygen but not

SkilDrill 7-8   Performing Mouth-to-Mask Ventilation

1 Once the patient's head is properly positioned, place the mask on the patient's face. Seal the mask to the face using both hands.

2 Exhale slowly into the open port of the one-way valve for 2 seconds as you watch for chest rise.

3 Watch the patient's chest fall during exhalation.

full ventilatory assistance. The mask may have an elastic strap for use with these patients.

The BVM Device

Both mouth-to-mouth and mouth-to-mask ventilations can provide large volumes of inspired air—up to 4 L per breath, more than a patient needs. But with mouth-to-mouth ventilation, the concentration of oxygen delivered to the patient is only 16%. With mouth-to-mask ventilation connected to high-flow oxygen, the concentration of oxygen, at best, is only 55%.

At the same oxygen flow rate (10 to 15 L/min) as the mask alone, a **BVM device** with an oxygen reservoir can deliver nearly 100% oxygen (▶ **Figure 7-31**). Most BVM devices on the market today include modifications or accessories (reservoirs) that permit the delivery of oxygen concentrations approaching 100%. However, the device can deliver only as much volume as you can squeeze out of the bag by hand. The BVM device provides less tidal volume than mouth-to-mask ventilation; however, it delivers a much higher oxygen concentration. The BVM device is the most common method used to ventilate patients in the field. An experienced EMT-B will be able to supply adequate tidal volumes with a BVM device. Be sure to practice on ventilation manikins several times before using a BVM device on a patient.

A BVM device should be used when you need to deliver high concentrations of oxygen to patients who are not ventilating adequately. The device is also used for patients in respiratory arrest, cardiopulmonary arrest, and respiratory failure. The BVM device may be used with or without oxygen. However, the most efficient use is with supplemental oxygen and a reservoir. You should use an oral or nasal airway adjunct in conjunction with the BVM device.

COMPONENTS. All adult BVM devices should have the following components:

- A disposable self-refilling bag
- No pop-off valve, or if one is present, the capability of disabling the pop-off valve

Figure 7-31 A BVM device with an oxygen reservoir can deliver nearly 100% oxygen if a good seal between the mouth and mask is achieved and if supplemental oxygen is used.

EMT-B Tips

Volume Capabilities of the BVM device

Size	Amount, mL
Adult	1,200-1,600
Pediatric	500-700
Infant	150-240

The volume of air (oxygen) to deliver to the patient is based upon one key observation—chest rise and fall.

- An outlet valve that is a true valve for nonre-breathing

- An oxygen reservoir that allows for high oxygen concentration delivery

- A one-way, no-jam inlet valve system that provides an oxygen inlet flow at a maximum of 30 L/min with standard 15/22mm fittings for face mask and endotracheal (or other advanced airway adjunct) connection

- A transparent face mask

- Ability to perform under extreme environmental conditions, including extreme heat or cold

The total amount of gas in the reservoir bag of an adult BVM device is usually 1,200 to 1,600 mL. The pediatric bag contains 500 to 700 mL, and the infant bag holds 150 to 240 mL.

The volume of air (oxygen) to deliver to the patient is based upon one key observation—chest rise and fall. In most situations, you will be using the BVM device attached to high-flow oxygen (15 L/min or more). When using the BVM device with high-flow oxygen on an adult patient, you should squeeze the bag enough to deliver a volume of 400 to 600 mL (approximately 6 to 7 mL/kg) over 2 seconds. When oxygen is not available, higher tidal volume amounts are required—700 to 1,000 mL (approximately 10 mL/kg) over 2 seconds. By delivering smaller tidal volumes when the BVM device is used with oxygen, the risk of gastric distention (and associated complications of vomiting and aspiration) is reduced.

There are two issues to consider with this approach. It is not practical for the EMT-B to accurately measure tidal volumes in milliliters per kilogram for each patient ventilated in the field. There is also a significant risk of hypoxia when ventilating with smaller volumes. For these reasons, the key is to watch for good chest rise and fall—let this observation be your key for the amount to deliver.

TECHNIQUE. Whenever possible, you and your partner should work together to provide BVM device ventilation. One EMT-B can maintain a good mask seal by securing the mask to the patient's face with two hands while the other EMT-B squeezes the bag. Ventilation using a BVM device is a challenging skill: it may be very difficult for one EMT-B to maintain a proper seal between the mask and the face with one hand while squeezing the bag well enough to deliver adequate air to the patient. This skill can be difficult to maintain if you do not have many opportunities to practice the skill. Effective one-person BVM device ventilation requires considerable experience.

Follow these steps to use the two-person BVM device technique:

1. Kneel above the patient's head. If possible, your partner should be at the side of the head to bag the patient while you hold a seal between the mask and the patient's face with two hands. (This assumes that you have enough personnel to do everything else that needs to be done at the same time, such as chest compressions, putting the stretcher in place, or helping to lift the patient onto the stretcher.)

2. Maintain the patient's neck in an extended position unless you suspect a cervical spine injury. In that case, you should immobilize the patient's head and neck and use the jaw-thrust maneuver. Have your partner hold the head, or, if you are alone, use your knees to immobilize the head.

3. Open the patient's mouth, and suction as needed. Insert an oropharyngeal or nasopharyngeal airway to maintain an open airway.

4. Select the proper mask size.

5. Place the mask on the patient's face. Make sure the top is over the bridge of the nose and the

EMT-B Tips

Indications That Artificial Ventilation Is Adequate

Equal chest rise and fall with ventilation

Ventilations delivered at the appropriate rate

- 12/min for adults
- 20/min for infants and children

Heart rate returns to normal range

Indications That Artificial Ventilation Is Inadequate

Minimal or no chest rise and fall

Ventilations are delivered too fast or too slow for patient's age

Heart rate does not return to normal range

bottom is in the groove between the lower lip and the chin. If the mask has a large, round cuff around the ventilation port, center the port over the patient's mouth. Inflate the collar to obtain a better fit and seal to the face.

6. Bring the lower jaw up to the mask with your ring finger and little finger. This will help to maintain an open airway. If you think the patient may have a spinal injury, make sure your partner immobilizes the cervical spine as you move the lower jaw.

7. Hold the mask in position by placing the thumbs over the top part of the mask and the index and middle fingers over the bottom half. Make sure you do not grab the fleshy part of the neck, as you may compress structures and create an airway obstruction.

8. Connect the bag to the mask if you have not already done so.

9. Hold the mask in place while your partner squeezes the bag with two hands until the patient's chest rises. Continue squeezing the bag once every 5 seconds for adults and once every 3 seconds for infants and children (▼ Figure 7-32).

10. If you are alone, hold your index finger over the lower part of the mask, and secure the upper part of the mask with your thumb. This is known as the C-clamp and will maintain the seal. Use the head tilt-chin lift maneuver to make sure the neck is extended. Squeeze the bag in a rhythmic manner once every 5 seconds with your other hand. Continue squeezing the bag once every 5 seconds for adults and once every 3 seconds for infants and children (▼ Figure 7-33).

When using the device to assist respirations, you should squeeze the bag as the patient tries to breathe in, ideally achieving a more normal rate and depth of respiration.

As you are assisting ventilations with a BVM device, you should evaluate how well the patient is breathing. You will know that artificial ventilation is not adequate

Figure 7-32 With two-person BVM device ventilation, you should hold the mask in place while your partner squeezes the bag with two hands until the patient's chest rises.

Figure 7-33 Maintain the seal of the mask to the face using the C-clamp if you must ventilate alone.

if the patient's chest does not rise and fall with each ventilation, the breathing rate is too slow or too fast, or the heart rate does not return to normal. If the patient's chest does not rise and fall, you may need to reposition the head, use an airway adjunct, or use **cricoid pressure**.

When using a BVM device or any other ventilation device, be alert for **gastric distention**, inflation of the stomach with air. To prevent or alleviate distention, use the **Sellick maneuver**. To perform the Sellick maneuver, have an additional rescuer apply cricoid pressure on the patient by placing the thumb and index finger on either side of the cricoid cartilage (at the inferior border of the larynx) and pressing down. By occluding the esophagus, this will: 1) inhibit the flow of air into the stomach, thus reducing gastric distention, and 2) reduce the chance of aspiration by helping block the flow of gastric contents up the esophagus. Cricoid pressure should only be performed on unconscious patients.

If the patient's stomach seems to be rising and falling, you should reposition the head and use cricoid pressure. In a patient with possible spinal injury, you should reposition the jaw rather than the head. If too much air is escaping from under the mask, reposition the mask for a better seal. If the patient's chest still does not rise and fall after you have made these corrections, check for an airway obstruction. If an obstruction is not present, you should attempt ventilations with another airway device.

Advanced airway techniques are beneficial when a good seal is difficult to maintain, the patient has a cervical spine injury, or the patient's condition warrants. These techniques are described in Chapter 38, Advanced Airway Management.

Figure 7-34   A flow-restricted oxygen-powered ventilation device can provide up to 100% oxygen.

> A BVM device should be used when you need to deliver high oxygen concentrations to patients who are not ventilating adequately.

The BVM device may also be used in conjunction with an endotracheal tube or with other airway adjunct devices such as the Esophageal Tracheal Combitube, the Pharyngeotracheal Lumen Airway, the Laryngeal Mask Airway, and the Trach-light.

Flow-Restricted, Oxygen-Powered Ventilation Devices

Another method of providing artificial ventilation is with flow-restricted, oxygen-powered ventilation devices. These devices are widely available and have been used in EMS for several years. However, recent findings suggest that they should not be used routinely due to the high incidence of gastric distention and possible damage to structures within the chest cavity. Flow-restricted, oxygen-powered devices *should not* be used on infants and children or on patients with suspected cervical spine or chest injury. *Cricoid pressure must be maintained whenever flow-restricted, oxygen-powered ventilation devices are used to ventilate a patient.* This will help to reduce the amount of gastric distention, the most common and significant side effect of the device.

COMPONENTS. Flow-restricted, oxygen-powered ventilation devices should have the following components ◀ Figure 7-34 :

- A peak flow rate of 100% oxygen at up to 40 L/min

- An inspiratory pressure safety release valve that opens at approximately 60 cm of water and vents any remaining volume to the atmosphere or stops the flow of oxygen

- An audible alarm that sounds whenever you exceed the relief valve pressure

- The ability to operate satisfactorily under normal and varying environmental conditions

- A trigger (or lever) positioned so that both your hands can remain on the mask to provide an airtight seal while supporting and tilting the patient's head and keeping the jaw elevated

Learning how to use these devices correctly requires proper training and considerable practice. As with BVM devices, you must make sure there is an airtight fit between the patient's face and mask. The amount of pressure that is necessary to ventilate a patient adequately will vary according to the size of the patient, the patient's lung volume, and the condition of the lungs. A patient with chronic obstructive pulmonary disease (COPD) will need greater pressure to receive a given volume than would be necessary for a patient with normal lungs. Pressures that are too great can cause a **pneumothorax**. Flow-restricted, oxygen-powered ventilation devices are not recommended for use on patients with COPD, chest injury, or on infants and children. Always follow local medical protocols carefully when you use these devices.

Special Considerations

Gastric Distention

Gastric distention occurs when artificial ventilation fills the stomach with air. Although it most commonly affects children, it also affects adults. Gastric distention is most likely to occur when you blow or ventilate too forcefully or too often in artificial ventilation or when the airway is obstructed as a result of a foreign body or improper head position. For this reason, you are instructed to give slow, gentle breaths during artificial ventilation over 2 seconds in the adult patient. Slight gastric distention is not of concern; however, severe inflation of the stomach is dangerous because it may cause vomiting and increase the risk of aspiration

during CPR. Gastric distention can also significantly reduce the lung volume by elevating the diaphragm. Gastric distention is a common side effect of flow-restricted, oxygen-powered ventilation devices—a key reason why this device is not highly recommended.

If the patient's stomach becomes distended as a result of rescue breathing, you should recheck and reposition the airway, apply cricoid pressure, and then watch for rise and fall of the chest wall as you perform rescue breathing. Continue slow rescue breathing without attempting to expel the stomach contents. Applying manual pressure over the patient's upper abdomen will likely result in vomiting. If vomiting does occur, turn the patient's entire body to the side, suction and/or wipe out the mouth with your gloved hand, and return the body back to a supine position so that you can continue CPR.

Stomas and Tracheostomy Tubes

BVM device ventilation must also be used for patients who have had a laryngectomy (surgical removal of the larynx). These patients have a permanent tracheal **stoma** (an opening in the neck that connects the trachea directly to the skin) ▼ **Figure 7-35** . It may be seen as an opening at the center, at the front and base of the neck. Many of these patients will have other openings in the neck, according to the type of operation performed. You should ignore any opening other than the midline tracheal stoma. The midline opening is the only one that can be used to put air into the patient's lungs.

Figure 7-35 A tracheal stoma typically lies in the midline of the neck. The midline opening is the only one that can be used to deliver oxygen to the patient's lungs.

Figure 7-36 Use a BVM device to ventilate a patient with a tracheostomy tube.

Neither the head tilt-chin lift nor the jaw-thrust maneuver is required for ventilating a patient with a stoma. If the patient has a tracheostomy tube, you should ventilate through the tube with a BVM device and 100% oxygen (◄ **Figure 7-36**). If the patient has a stoma and no tube is in place, use an infant or child mask with your BVM device to make a seal over the stoma. Seal the patient's mouth and nose with one hand to prevent a leak of air up the trachea when you ventilate through a stoma. Release the seal of the patient's mouth and nose for exhalation. This allows the air to exhale through the upper airway.

If you are unable to ventilate a patient who has a stoma, try suctioning the stoma and the mouth with a French or soft tip catheter before giving the patient artificial ventilation through the mouth and nose. If you seal the stoma during ventilations, the ability to artificially ventilate the patient in this way may be improved, or it may help to clear any obstructions.

Foreign Body Airway Obstruction

A foreign body that *completely* blocks the airway in a patient is a true emergency that will result in death if not treated immediately. In an adult, sudden foreign body airway obstruction usually occurs during a meal. In a child, it occurs while eating, playing with small toys, or crawling around the house. An otherwise healthy child who has sudden difficulty breathing has probably aspirated a foreign object.

By far, the most common airway obstruction in an unconscious patient is the tongue, which relaxes back into the throat. There are other causes of airway obstruction that do not involve foreign bodies in the airway. These include swelling (from infection or acute allergic reactions) and trauma (tissue damage from injury). With airway obstruction from medical conditions such as infection and acute allergic reactions, repeated attempts to clear the airway as if there were a foreign body will be unsuccessful and potentially dangerous. These patients require specific emergency medical care for their condition and rapid transport to the hospital.

Recognition

Early recognition of airway obstruction is crucial for the EMT-B to be able to provide emergency medical care effectively. Obstruction from a foreign body can

In an adult, sudden airway obstruction by a foreign object usually occurs during a meal. In a child, it occurs while eating, playing with small toys, or crawling around the house.

result in either a **partial airway obstruction** or a **complete airway obstruction**.

Patients with a partial airway obstruction are still able to exchange air, but will have varying degrees of respiratory distress. Great care must be taken to prevent a partial airway obstruction from becoming a complete airway obstruction. The patient will usually have noisy breathing and may be coughing. You should assess the patient and determine whether the patient has **good air exchange** or **poor air exchange**.

With good air exchange, the patient can cough forcefully, although you may hear wheezing between coughs. As long as the patient can breathe, cough forcefully, or talk, you should not interfere with the patient's efforts to expel the foreign object on his or her own. Continue to monitor the patient closely and encourage the patient to continue coughing. Abdominal thrusts are usually not effective for dislodging a partial obstruction. Attempts to remove the object manually could force the object farther down into the airway and cause a complete obstruction. Continually reassess the patient's condition and be prepared to provide treatment if the air exchange becomes poor or a partial obstruction becomes a complete obstruction.

With poor air exchange, the patient has a weak, ineffective (not forceful) cough and may have increased difficulty breathing, stridor (a high-pitched noise heard primarily on inspiration), and cyanosis. You must quickly recognize this situation and provide care. *For patients with partial airway obstruction with poor air exchange, treat immediately as if there is a complete airway obstruction.*

Patients with complete airway obstruction cannot breathe, talk, or cough. One sure sign of a complete obstruction is the sudden inability to speak or cough during or immediately after eating. The person may clutch or grasp his or her throat (universal distress signal), begin to turn cyanotic, and have extreme

EMT-B Tips

Possible Causes of Airway Obstruction

Relaxation of the tongue in an unconscious patient

Aspirated vomitus (stomach contents)

Foreign objects—food, small toys, dentures

Blood clots, bone fragments, or damaged tissue after an injury

Airway tissue swelling—infection, allergic reaction

difficulty breathing (▼ **Figure 7-37**). There is little or no air movement. Ask the conscious patient, "Are you choking?" If the patient nods "yes," provide immediate treatment. If the obstruction is not cleared quickly, the amount of oxygen in the patient's blood will decrease dramatically. If not treated, the patient will become unconscious and then die.

Some patients with a complete airway obstruction will be unconscious during your initial assessment. You may not know that an airway obstruction is the cause of their condition. There are many other causes of unconsciousness and respiratory failure, including stroke, heart attack, seizures, and drug overdoses. A complete and thorough patient assessment by you, therefore, is key in providing appropriate emergency medical care.

Any person found unconscious must be managed as if he or she has a compromised airway. You must first open the airway and provide artificial ventilation if the patient is not breathing (▼ **Figure 7-38**). If, after opening the airway, you are unable to ventilate the patient after several attempts (no chest rise and fall), you feel resistance when ventilating, or pressure is felt (poor lung compliance), consider the possibility of an airway obstruction. **Lung compliance** is the ability of the alveoli to expand when air is drawn in on inhalation; poor lung compliance is the inability of the alveoli to fully expand on inhalation.

Emergency Medical Care for Foreign Body Airway Obstruction

Perform the head tilt-chin lift maneuver to clear an obstruction that is caused by the tongue and throat muscles relaxing back into the airway in any person who is found unconscious, has inadequate breathing or is not breathing, and is not suspected of having spinal trauma. If spinal trauma is suspected, you should open the airway with a jaw-thrust maneuver. Large pieces of vomited food, mucus, loose dentures, or blood clots in the mouth should be swept forward and out of the mouth with your gloved index finger. Once available, suctioning should be used to maintain a clear airway.

The Heimlich maneuver (abdominal thrusts) is the most effective method of dislodging and forcing an object out of the airway. Residual air, which is always present in the lungs, is compressed upward and used to expel the object. You should use the Heimlich maneuver followed by finger sweeps and attempts to ventilate in the adult patient with a complete airway obstruction. Specific techniques for the removal of foreign body

Figure 7-37 The universal sign of choking is a person who grasps his or her throat, turns cyanotic, and has difficulty breathing.

Figure 7-38 Securing and maintaining the airway and ensuring adequate breathing are the first, most important steps in caring for an unconscious patient.

airway obstruction in infants, children, and adults are reviewed in detail in Chapter 39.

If you are unable to clear a complete airway obstruction with your initial attempts, begin rapid transport and continue your efforts at relief of the obstruction with abdominal thrusts, finger sweeps, and attempts at ventilation en route to the hospital.

Remember to treat patients with a partial airway obstruction with *poor air exchange* as if they had a complete obstruction.

Patients with a partial airway obstruction with good air exchange should be monitored closely for change to a complete obstruction. If the patient is unable to clear the obstruction and remains conscious, support (or let the patient control) the airway position that is most efficient and comfortable. Provide supplemental oxygen and transport to the hospital.

Dental Appliances

Many dental appliances can cause an airway obstruction. If a dental appliance, such as a crown or bridge, dentures, or even a piece or section of braces, has become loose, you should manually remove it before providing ventilations. Simple manual removal may relieve the obstruction and allow the patient to breathe on his or her own.

Providing BVM device or mouth-to-mask ventilations is usually much easier when dentures can be left in place. Leaving the dentures in place provides more "structure" to the face and will generally assist you in being able to provide a good face-to-mask seal. However, loose dentures make it much more difficult to perform artificial ventilation by any method and can easily obstruct the airway. Therefore, dentures and dental appliances that do not stay in place should be removed. Dentures and appliances may become loose or be completely out of place following an accident or as you are providing care. Periodically reassess the patient's airway to make sure the devices are firmly in place.

Facial Bleeding

Airway problems can be especially challenging in patients with serious facial injuries ▼ **Figure 7-39** . Because the blood supply in the face is so rich, injuries to the face can result in severe tissue swelling and bleeding into the airway. Control bleeding with direct pressure and suction as necessary. Facial injuries are discussed in detail in Chapter 26.

Figure 7-39 Airway problems can be especially challenging in patients with serious facial injuries.

Prep Kit

Ready for Review

The respiratory system includes the diaphragm, the muscles of the chest wall, and the accessory muscles of breathing. The term "airway" usually means the upper airway, which includes the respiratory structures above the vocal cords. Clearing the airway means removing obstructing material; maintaining the airway means keeping it open. Patients who are breathing inadequately show signs of hypoxia, a dangerous condition in which the body's tissues and cells do not have enough oxygen. Adequate breathing features a normal rate of 12 to 20 breaths/min, a regular pattern of inhalation and exhalation, bilateral clear and equal lung sounds, and regular and equal chest rise and fall. Patients with inadequate breathing need to be treated immediately. Emergency medical care includes airway management, supplemental oxygen, and ventilatory support.

Basic techniques for opening the airway include the head tilt-chin lift maneuver and the jaw-thrust maneuver. One basic airway adjunct is the oropharyngeal or oral airway, which keeps the tongue from blocking the airway in unconscious patients with no gag reflex. If the oral airway is not the proper size or is inserted incorrectly, it can actually push the tongue back into the pharynx, causing an obstruction. Another basic airway adjunct is the nasopharyngeal or nasal airway, which is usually used with patients who have a gag reflex.

Suctioning is the next priority after opening the airway. Semirigid tonsil tips are the best catheters to use when suctioning the pharynx; soft plastic catheters are used to suction the nose and liquid secretions in the back of the mouth. The recovery position is used to help maintain the airway in patients without traumatic injuries who are breathing on their own.

You should always give supplemental oxygen to patients who are not breathing on their own or who have inadequate breathing. Handle compressed gas cylinders very carefully; their contents are under pressure. Always make sure the correct pressure regulator is firmly attached before transporting a cylinder. The pin-indexing safety system features a series of pins on a yoke that must be matched with the holes on the valve stem of the gas cylinder. Pressure regulators reduce the pressure of gas in an oxygen cylinder to between 40 and 70 psi. Pressure-compensated flowmeters and Bourdon-gauge flowmeters permit the regulated release of gas measured in liters per minute. When oxygen therapy is complete, disconnect the tubing from the flowmeter nipple and turn off the cylinder valve, then turn off the flowmeter. As long as there is a pressure reading on the regulator gauge, it is not safe to remove the regulator from the valve stem. Keep any possible source of fire away from the area while oxygen is in use.

Nasal cannulas and the far more effective nonrebreathing masks are used most often to deliver oxygen in the field; always try to use the latter with patients who you suspect may have hypoxia. Nonrebreathing masks can provide over 90% inspired oxygen. Pulse oximetry, an assessment tool to evaluate the effectiveness of oxygenation, does not take the place of a good assessment. This measurement depends on adequate perfusion to the capillary beds and is inaccurate when the patient is cold, in shock, or exposed to carbon monoxide.

The methods of providing artificial ventilation include a one- and two-person BVM device, mouth-to-mask ventilation, and a flow-restricted, oxygen-powered ventilation device. The flow-restricted, oxygen-powered ventilation device, however, is not a recommended ventilation device by most standards. Combined with your own exhaled breath, mouth-to-mask ventilation will give your patient up to 55% oxygen; a BVM device with an oxygen reservoir can deliver nearly 100% oxygen.

When you are providing artificial ventilations, remember that ventilating or blowing too forcefully can cause gastric distention. Slow, gentle breaths during artificial ventilation and use of cricoid pressure can help to prevent gastric distention. Also consider patients who have a tracheal stoma or a tracheostomy tube. You will need to ventilate these patients through the tube or the stoma.

Foreign body airway obstruction usually occurs during a meal in an adult, or while a child is eating, playing with small objects, or crawling about the house. The earlier you recognize any airway obstruction, the better. You must learn to recognize the difference between airway obstruction caused by a foreign object and that caused by a medical condition.

A complete airway obstruction can be removed by the Heimlich maneuver, finger sweeps, manual removal of the object, and attempts to ventilate. Treat patients with a partial airway obstruction with poor air exchange as if they had a complete obstruction. Patients with partial airway obstruction and good air exchange should be closely monitored.

Check for loose dental appliances in a patient before assisting ventilations. Loose appliances should be removed to prevent them from obstructing the airway.

Vital Vocabulary

agonal respirations Occasional, gasping breaths that occur after the heart has stopped.

airway The upper airway tract or the passage above the larynx, which includes the nose, mouth, and throat.

American Standard System A safety system for size D or larger oxygen cylinders, designed to prevent the accidental attachment of a regulator to a cylinder containing the wrong type of gas.

apnea Periods of not breathing.

aspiration The introduction of vomit or other foreign material into the lungs.

bag-valve-mask (BVM) device A device with face mask attached to a ventilation bag containing a reservoir and connected to oxygen; delivers more than 90% supplemental oxygen.

barrier device A protective item, such as a pocket mask with a valve, that limits exposure to a patient's body fluids.

bilateral A body part or condition that appears on both sides of the midline.

catheter A hollow, cylindrical structure that drains or delivers fluids.

complete airway obstruction Occurs when a foreign body completely obstructs the patient's airway. Patients cannot breathe, talk, or cough.

cricoid pressure Pressure on the cricoid cartilage; applied to inhibit gastric distention and aspiration of vomitus in the unconscious patient.

diffusion A process in which molecules move from an area of higher concentration of molecules to an area of lower concentration.

exhalation The part of the breathing process in which the diaphragm and the intercostal muscles relax, forcing air out of the lungs.

gag reflex A normal reflex mechanism that causes retching; activated by touching the soft palate or the back of the throat.

gastric distention A condition in which air fills the stomach as a result of high volume and pressure during artificial ventilation.

good air exchange A term used to distinguish the degree of distress in a patient with a partial airway obstruction. With good air exchange, the patient is still conscious and able to cough forcefully, although wheezing may be heard.

head tilt-chin lift maneuver A combination of two movements to open the airway by tilting the forehead back and lifting the chin; used for non-trauma patients.

hypoxia A dangerous condition in which the body tissues and cells do not have enough oxygen.

hypoxic drive Backup system to control respirations when oxygen levels fall.

inhalation The active, muscular part of breathing that draws air into the airway and lungs.

ischemia A lack of oxygen that deprives tissues of necessary nutrients.

jaw-thrust maneuver Technique to open the airway by placing the fingers behind the angle of the jaw and bringing the jaw forward; used when a patient may have a cervical spine injury.

labored breathing Breathing that requires more than normal effort; may be slower or much faster than normal.

lung compliance The ability of the alveoli to fully expand when air is drawn in on inhalation.

metabolism The chemical processes that provide the cells with energy from nutrients.

nasal cannula An oxygen delivery device in which oxygen flows through two small, tubelike prongs that fit into the patient's nostrils.

nasopharyngeal (nasal or trumpet) airway Airway adjunct inserted into the nostril of a conscious patient who is not able to maintain a natural airway.

nonrebreathing mask A combination mask and reservoir bag system that is the preferred way to give oxygen in the prehospital setting; delivers up to 90% inspired oxygen.

oropharyngeal (oral) airway Airway adjunct inserted into the mouth to keep the tongue from blocking the upper airway and to make suctioning the airway easier.

partial airway obstruction Condition in which an obstruction leaves the patient able to exchange some air, but also causes some degree of respiratory distress.

pin-indexing system A system established for portable cylinders to ensure that a regulator is not connected to a cylinder containing the wrong type of gas.

pneumothorax A partial or complete accumulation of air in the pleural space.

poor air exchange A term used to distinguish the degree of distress in a patient with a partial airway obstruction. With poor air exchange, the patient has a weak, ineffective cough, increased difficulty breathing, possible cyanosis, and may produce a high-pitched noise on inhalation (stridor).

pulse oximetry An assessment method that measures oxygen saturation of hemoglobin in the capillary beds.

recovery position A side-lying position used to maintain a clear airway in patients without injuries.

retractions Movements in which the skin pulls in around the ribs during inspiration.

Sellick maneuver A technique that is used to prevent gastric distention in which pressure is applied on the cricoid cartilage.

stoma Opening in the neck that connects the trachea directly to the skin.

tidal volume The amount of air moved during one breath.

tonsil tip A large, semirigid suction tip recommended for suctioning the pharynx; also called a Yankauer tip.

ventilation Exchange of air between the lungs and the air of the environment, either spontaneously by the patient or with assistance from an EMT-B.

www.emtb.com

Assessment in Action

Your squad receives a call for "a person not breathing" at the Thunder Tube water slide at Splash Magic Water Park. Four minutes later you and your partner find a 35-year-old man in swim trunks lying unresponsive by the side of the pool. A lifeguard is attempting ventilations.

The patient is pale and still wet. You note abdominal distention with each breath but no chest rise and fall. Because of that you suspect there is little air getting into his lungs and gastric distention is present. Your partner immediately gets out the suction, oral airway, and BVM devices. You ask the lifeguard to stop rescue breathing so you can assess the patient. You note that the man's face is pale and his skin is cold. You remember that dusky skin indicates poor oxygenation. Your partner checks the airway and begins to suction while you check for a pulse. There is a weak carotid pulse. The lifeguard tells you that after the man fell into the pool and didn't come up, he went in to get him. You note a small abrasion at the top of the head. Because of the abrasion you suspect spinal trauma. Your partner inserts an oral airway and begins to ventilate the patient at a rate of about 20 breaths/min. Because of suspected spinal trauma, your partner stabilizes the patient's head between his knees while he ventilates. Because of the high risk of aspiration from gastric distention, you apply cricoid pressure while monitoring his pulse. There is good chest rise and fall. After about 30 seconds of ventilation, his carotid puse is stronger. While your partner continues to manage his airway, spinal immobilization equipment is readied, and with help, the patient is loaded into the ambulance for transport.

1. Which of the following techniques for opening the airway would have been appropriate in this situation?
   A. Head tilt-chin lift
   B. Jaw-thrust
   C. Jaw thrust-head tilt

2. Without knowing what type of gastric contents were present, which suction device would you initially have ready for this situation?
   A. French or whistle-tip catheter
   B. Tonsil tip or Yankauer tip catheter

3. How long should suction be applied at any one time?
   A. 15 seconds
   B. 30 seconds
   C. 45 seconds
   D. 60 seconds

4. What is the proper way to measure an oral airway?
   A. From the earlobe to the nose
   B. From the angle of the jaw to the nose
   C. From the earlobe to the corner of the mouth
   D. From the angle of the jaw to the corner of the mouth

5. An oral airway was used in this situation. What is its primary function?
   A. Prevents regurgitation
   B. Determines responsiveness
   C. Keeps the tongue forward
   D. Keeps the jaw forward

6. If the patient had started to gag when the oral airway was inserted, what would have been an appropriate action to take?
   A. Insert a nasopharyngeal airway.
   B. Start to ventilate with the BVM device.
   C. Wait for the spasm to relax and try again.
   D. Remove the oral airway.

7. What were the signs that ventilations were successful in this patient?
   A. There was good chest rise and fall.
   B. His skin was cool.
   C. His pulse became stronger.
   D. His abdominal wall was distended.

8. The lifeguard was attempting rescue breathing but there was no rise and fall of the chest wall. In this situation, what measures should have been done to correct that?
   A. Hyperextend the head.
   B. Perform the head tilt-chin lift maneuver.
   C. Perform the jaw-thrust maneuver.
   D. Place him in the recovery position.

Challenging Questions

9. This patient initially presented with a weak carotid pulse. After about 30 seconds of ventilations, his pulse got stronger. Why?

10. If this patient had inhaled pool water from his near-drowning, what would interfere with oxygen getting to his red blood cells?

11. Why is suspected cervical spine injury such a threat to a patient's ability to breathe?

You receive a call for assistance for the customer of a local retailer who special- izes in antique books. On arrival, you find a 38-year-old man sitting on the floor hunched over; you immediately notice that he seems to be breathing very fast.

As you begin to question him, he can only speak in short three- and four-word bursts. He manages to tell you that he had been looking at old books for the last hour when his chest started to tighten up, probably from the dust, he says. As he continues, you find that he is allergic to penicillin, uses a Ventolin inhaler, and he has a history of hypertension and asthma. Your partner obtains his vital signs, which show a blood pressure of 152/90 mm Hg, a regular pulse of 122 beats/min, and shallow respirations of 34 breaths/min.

1. Of the following interventions, which would be the most appropriate at this time?
   A. Initiate CPR immediately.
   B. Open and assess the patient's airway.
   C. Insert a properly sized oropharyngeal airway.
   D. Apply oxygen using a nonrebreathing mask.

2. What signs/symptoms tell you his respirations are inadequate?
   A. Inability to talk in complete sentences
   B. Rapid respiratory rate
   C. Complaint of chest tightening
   D. All of the above

3. What is important about this patient's history?
   A. Ventolin inhaler and asthma
   B. Looking for books for an hour
   C. Allergy to penicillin
   D. Hypertensive with no medication for the condition

Challenging Question

4. What is important about scene safety for this patient?

Points to Ponder

You are dispatched to a "traffic stop" where you find that the local law enforcement agency has a person subdued. The person is on his side and you immediately notice that he is cyanotic. You ask the law enforcement officers to release him so that you may examine him better and they refuse. They explain that he was quite violent, requiring three people to control him, but that he has been less aggressive since they subdued him. Your partner says that the patient has decreased level of consciousness and labored breathing. The officers still decline to release the patient. What would you do? Would you report this and if so to whom? How might reporting this affect your relationship with law enforce- ment in the future?

Issues Scene Safety, Best Patient Care, Relationships with other Emergency Services, Reporting Channels.

Online Outlook

The respiratory system is a very important part of the body. It delivers oxygen to the lungs and allows carbon dioxide to be removed. To learn more about the anatomy and physi- ology of the respiratory system, complete Exercise 7 at www.emtb.com.

www.emtb.com

Patient Assessment

3

Section

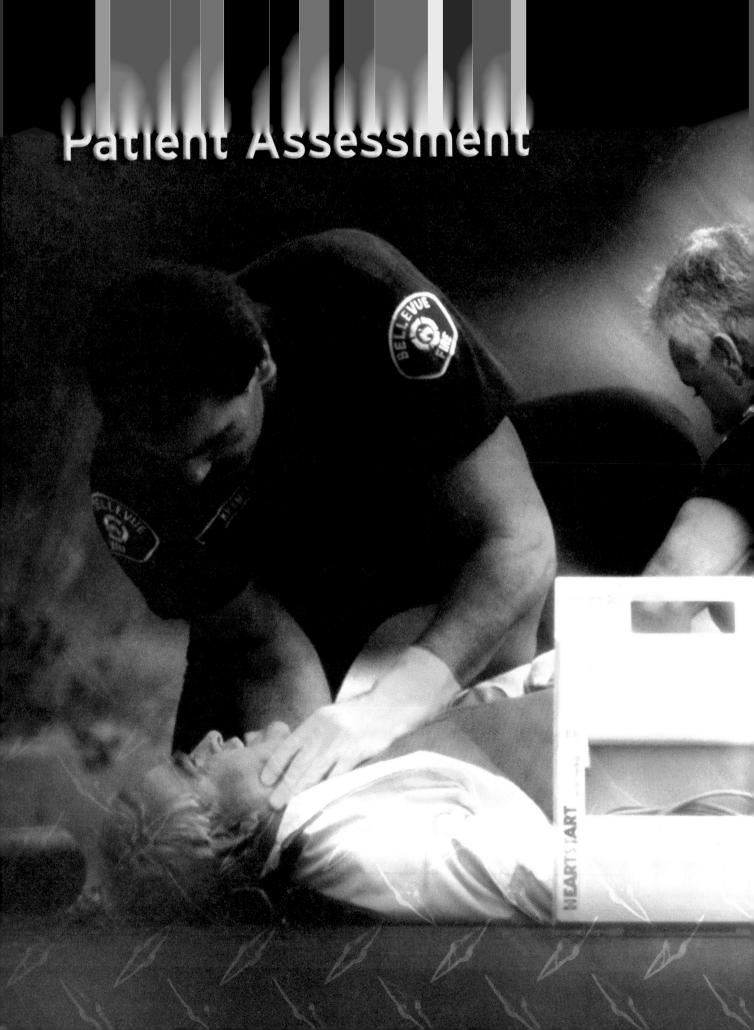

Patient Assessment

TECHNOLOGY

www.emtb.com

- Online Chapter Pretest ◄
- Interactivities
- Vocabulary Explorer
- Anatomy Review
- Web Links
- Online Review Manual
- Distance Learning

Chapter FEATURES

- Skill Drills ◄
- Vital Vocabulary
- Pediatric Needs
- Geriatric Needs
- EMT-B Safety
- EMT-B Tips
- Documentation Tips
- Remember
- Prep Kit

Patient Assessment

4. Describe the areas included in the rapid trauma assessment and discuss what should be evaluated (p 248).

5. Differentiate when the rapid assessment may be altered in order to provide patient care (p 248).

6. Discuss the reason for performing a focused history and physical exam (p 246).

Affective

7. Recognize and respect the feelings that patients might experience during assessment (p 248).

Psychomotor

8. Demonstrate the rapid trauma assessment that should be used to assess a patient based on mechanism of injury (p 248).

Focused History and Physical Exam: Medical Patients

Cognitive

1. Describe the unique needs for assessing an individual with a specific chief complaint with no known prior history (p 258).

2. Differentiate between the history and physical exam that are performed for responsive patients with no known prior history and responsive patients with a known prior history (p 258).

3. Describe the unique needs for assessing an individual who is unresponsive (p 262).

4. Differentiate between the assessment that is performed for a patient who is unresponsive or has an altered mental status and other medical patients requiring assessment (p 262).

Affective

5. Attend to the feelings that these patients might be experiencing (p 258).

Psychomotor

6. Demonstrate the patient care skills that should be used to assist a patient who is responsive with no known history (p 258).

7. Demonstrate the patient care skills that should be used to assist a patient who is unresponsive or has an altered mental status (p 263).

Detailed Physical Exam

Cognitive

1. Discuss the components of the detailed physical exam (p 267).

2. State the areas of the body that are evaluated during the detailed physical exam (p 267).

3. Explain what additional care should be provided while performing the detailed physical exam (p 266).

4. Distinguish between the detailed physical exam that is performed on a trauma patient and that of the medical patient (p 266).

Affective

5. Explain the rationale for the feelings that these patients might be experiencing (p 266).

Psychomotor

6. Demonstrate the skills involved in performing the detailed physical exam (p 267).

Ongoing Assessment

Cognitive

1. Discuss the reason for repeating the initial assessment as part of the ongoing assessment (p 274).

2. Describe the components of the ongoing assessment (p 274).

3. Describe trending of assessment components (p 275).

Affective

4. Explain the value of performing an ongoing assessment (p 274).

5. Recognize and respect the feelings that patients might experience during assessment (p 274).

6. Explain the value of trending assessment components to other health professionals who assume care of the patient (p 275).

Psychomotor

7. Demonstrate the skills involved in performing the ongoing assessment (p 274).

Your unit is dispatched to the driver's license testing center for "a man acting strangely." Upon arrival, you find a 52-year-old man wandering about with an obvious altered mental status. Once you get his attention, you and your partner begin your assessment to see whether you can identify the cause.

Good patient care is directly linked to good patient assessment. This chapter will cover this most essential of all EMT-B skills along with helping you answer the following questions:

1. Why is patient assessment considered one of the cornerstones of prehospital care?

2. Is there a difference between the assessment of a trauma patient and a patient with a medical condition? If so, what is it?

About This Chapter

This chapter will provide a clear and comprehensive approach to patient assessment. A flowchart has been developed to provide a quick, visual reference to guide you through the patient assessment process. The chapter has been divided into six sections. Every section is color coded and numbered for easy reference. The Patient Assessment Flowchart is repeated at every section to show you "at a glance" where you are in the patient assessment process.

Special care has been taken to reflect the EMT-B National Standard Curriculum, but enhancement information will prepare you for your work in the field. You will also find the special patient assessment needs of pediatric patients in Chapter 31 and geriatric patients in Chapter 34.

> Scene Size-Up
>
> Initial Assessment
>
> Focused History and Physical Exam: Trauma Patients
>
> Focused History and Physical Exam: Medical Patients
>
> Detailed Physical Exam
>
> Ongoing Assessment

Patient Assessment

From a practical point of view, prehospital emergency care is simply a series of decisions about treatment and transport. The process that guides decision making in EMS is based on your patient assessment findings. For you to make good decisions about how to best care for your patient, you must start by gathering information as you progress through the Patient Assessment process, as listed below:

- Perform the scene size-up.
- Perform an initial assessment.
- Provide spinal immobilization if necessary.
- Identify and treat life-threatening conditions.
- Perform a focused history and physical exam.
- Provide transport for a patient with an obvious life-threatening condition.
- Perform a detailed physical exam on the scene on a patient with no life-threatening conditions.
- Reassess vital signs.
- Perform ongoing assessments.

Patient Assessment

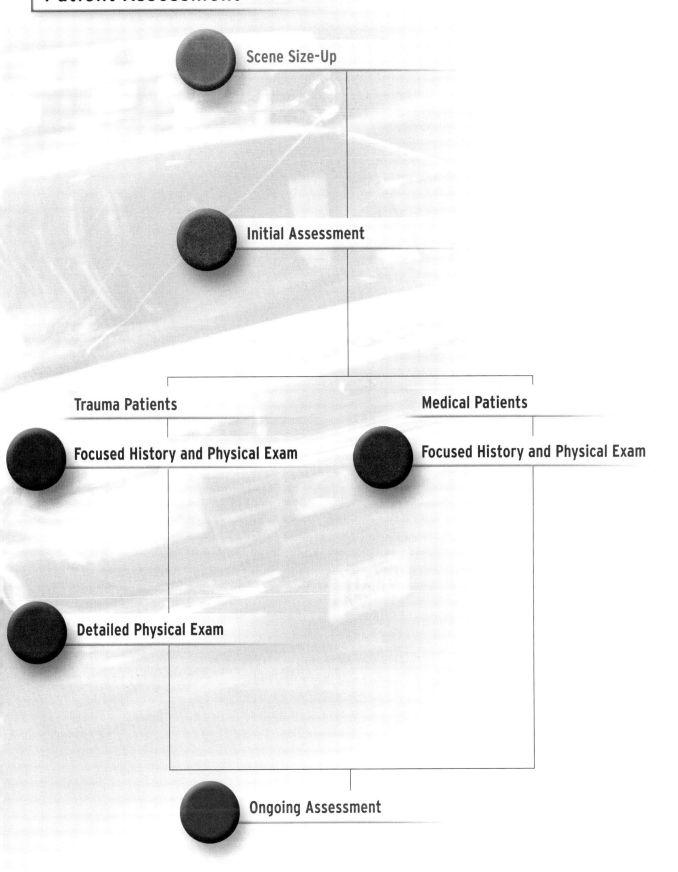

Scene Size-Up

Initial Assessment

Trauma Patients

Focused History and Physical Exam

Medical Patients

Focused History and Physical Exam

Detailed Physical Exam

Ongoing Assessment

Scene Size-Up

Upon arriving at the scene, it is essential to perform a scene size-up. The <u>scene size-up</u> is a quick assessment of the scene and the surroundings that will provide you and your partner with as much information as possible about the safety of the scene, any mechanism of injury, and the nature of the illness before you enter and begin patient care. (▶ **Table 8-1**) lists the components of the scene size-up. Your first step at any scene is to make sure that you and your partner are safe. Never become a victim yourself.

Body Substance Isolation

On every emergency call, you need to be sure to wear the proper protective equipment since this equipment will reduce your risk of exposure to communicable disease. The best way to reduce your risk of exposure is to follow <u>body substance isolation (BSI)</u> precautions. The concept of BSI assumes that all body fluids present a possible risk for infection.

Before you step out of the unit, you and your partner must be wearing the proper protective equipment.

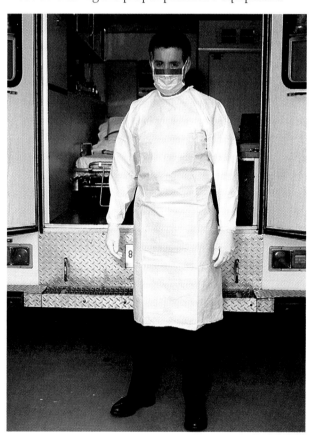

Figure 8-1 Proper protective equipment is vital when you are called to a scene in which there is a lot of blood or other body fluids.

TABLE 8-1 Scene Size-Up
Body Substance Isolation
Scene Safety
Determine Mechanism of Injury/Nature of Illness
Determine Number of Patients
Request Additional Assistance
Consider C-Spine Immobilization

Protective gloves are always indicated. Eye protection, masks, and gowns may also be indicated if there is a lot of blood or other body fluids in the patient area (▼ **Figure 8-1**). Eye protection is needed when there may be a risk that blood or other body fluids will splatter or become airborne. You should put on a mask and gown, if needed and dictated by your protocol, before you enter the area immediately around the patient. If the scene involves hazardous materials or fire, wear the appropriate gear for the situation or do not enter the scene.

Scene Safety

Scene safety is an assessment focused on ensuring the well-being of the EMT-B. You cannot help your patient if you become a victim yourself.

Personal Protection

Look for the following possible dangers before you step out of the unit (▼ **Figure 8-2**):

- Oncoming traffic
- Unstable surfaces (eg, wet or icy patches, loose gravel, slopes)

Figure 8-2 Before you step out of your unit, be sure to evaluate the scene for any hazards.

Patient Assessment

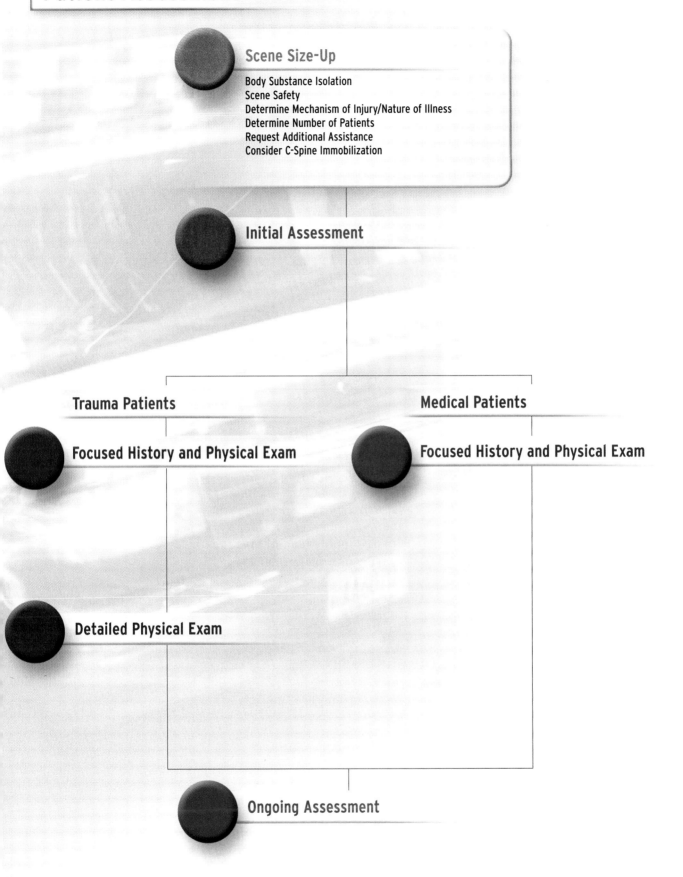

Scene Size-Up

Body Substance Isolation
Scene Safety
Determine Mechanism of Injury/Nature of Illness
Determine Number of Patients
Request Additional Assistance
Consider C-Spine Immobilization

Initial Assessment

Trauma Patients

Focused History and Physical Exam

Medical Patients

Focused History and Physical Exam

Detailed Physical Exam

Ongoing Assessment

- Leaking gasoline or diesel fuel
- Downed electrical lines
- Hostile bystanders/potential for violence
- Fire or smoke
- Possible hazardous or toxic materials
- Other dangers at crash or rescue scenes
- Crime scenes

You should park your unit in a place that will offer you and your partner the greatest safety but also rapid access to the patient and your equipment (▼ Figure 8-3). In many instances, law enforcement will be at the scene before you arrive. If that is the case, you should talk with them before entering the scene. Make sure to follow local protocol if the scene is a crime scene. Also be sure to have law enforcement accompany you if the patient is a suspect in the crime. Consider your unit a safe haven. You are no help to the patient if you enter the scene without first protecting yourself and your partner.

Your next concern is the safety of the patient(s) and bystanders. This is not an easy task. Bystanders can become a problem when they try to help or direct your care. Protect yourself and bystanders alike by moving them to a safe area or assigning them a specific task.

Making an Unsafe Scene Safe

Occasionally, you and your partner will not be able to enter a scene safely. This may be due to the need for extrication, possible hazardous conditions, or the presence of multiple patients that you cannot handle alone. These situations seem very difficult when you want to provide medical care to sick or injured patients. However, your safety and that of your partner are more

Figure 8-3 Park your unit in a place that is safe, yet allows for rapid access to the patient and your equipment. If law enforcement is already on the scene, make sure to check in with them first.

EMT-B Safety

Assessing the safety of a scene before entering may be the single most important way in which emergency responders can attend to their own well-being. Subtle signs of danger not recognized and neutralized—or avoided—at this point can grow much more threatening without being noticed once you shift your attention to patient assessment and care. Initial scene assessment usually makes the difference between a manageably safe scene and one that could spin dangerously out of control without further warning.

important. If you need more help in staging the scene, do not hesitate to ask for it. Be as specific as possible about the type of help you need. Remember that it takes time for additional resources, such as an extrication team, law enforcement, or another EMS unit, to arrive at the scene.

Determine Mechanism of Injury/Nature of Illness

One of the great dangers in performing the prehospital assessment is giving in to the temptation to categorize your patient immediately as either a trauma patient or a medical patient. Remember, the fundamentals of good patient assessment do not change, despite the unique aspects of trauma and medical care. Careful evaluation of the scene, including the possible mechanism of injury and/or the nature of illness, along with the other information that you gather will help you to lean in one direction or the other. Family members, bystanders, and law enforcement can often tell you what prompted the call to 9-1-1. After you have completed your assessment, you will come to a conclusion as to whether your patient's main problem is medical or traumatic in origin.

Determine from the patient why EMS was activated. You might also need to rely on information provided by family or bystanders.

Determine how many patients are involved. If there are more patients than your unit can effectively handle, request additional assistance. Call for additional help before making contact with patients or beginning triage. You are less likely to call for help once you are involved in patient care.

Mechanism of Injury

As an EMT-B, you will be called to motor vehicle crashes or other situations in which patients may have sustained life-threatening traumatic injuries. To care for these patients properly, you must understand how traumatic injuries occur, or the **mechanism of injury**. With a traumatic injury, the body has been exposed to some force or energy that has resulted in a temporary injury, permanent damage, or even death (▼ **Figure 8-4**).

As you might expect, certain parts of the body are more easily injured than others. The brain and the spinal cord are very fragile and easy to injure. Fortunately, they are protected by the skull, the vertebrae, and several layers of soft tissues. The eyes are also easily injured. Even small forces on the eye may result in serious injury. The bones and certain organs are stronger and can absorb small forces without resulting injury. The net result of this information is that you can use the mechanism of injury as a kind of guide to predict the potential for a serious injury by evaluating three factors: the amount of force applied to the body, the length of time the force was applied, and the areas of the body that are involved.

You will commonly hear the terms "blunt trauma" and "penetrating trauma." With **blunt trauma**, the force of the injury occurs over a broad area, and the skin is usually not broken (▶ **Figure 8-5A**). However, the tissues and organs below the area of impact may be damaged. With **penetrating trauma**, the force of the injury occurs at a small point of contact between the skin and the object (▶ **Figure 8-5B**). The object pierces the skin and creates an open wound that carries a high potential for infection. The severity of injury depends on the characteristics of the penetrating object, the amount of force or energy, and the part of the body affected.

MOTOR VEHICLE CRASHES. In motor vehicle crashes, the amount of force that is applied to the body is directly

related to the speed of the crash. As the speed of a crash increases, the forces that are exerted on the patient increase as well. Therefore, patients should be assessed according to the area of the body that was most likely injured. Your evaluation should also be based, to some extent, on the patient's position in the car, the use of seat belts, and how the patient's body shifts during the crash (▶ **Figure 8-6**). Drivers are typically at higher risk for serious injury than passengers because of the potential for striking the steering wheel with the chest, abdomen, or head. Front seat passengers may also be injured by striking the dashboard.

Risk for serious injury also varies depending on whether seat belts are used and whether they are worn properly. Unbelted victims are at much higher risk for a number of other injuries because they may be catapulted throughout the car. As they go "up and over" or "down and under," they may strike the sides, roof, floor, dashboard, steering wheel, or windshield. Even worse, the unrestrained victim may be ejected from the vehicle,

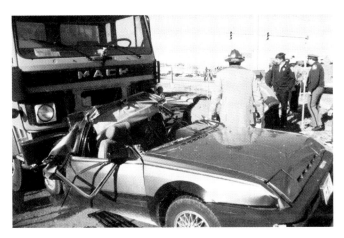

Figure 8-4 With traumatic injuries, the patient has been exposed to some force or energy that results in injury or even possibly death. You can learn a great deal about that force by simply looking at the mechanism of injury.

Figure 8-5 **A.** With blunt trauma, the force of the injury occurs over a broad area, and the skin is not broken. **B.** With penetrating trauma, an object pierces the skin and creates an open wound.

dramatically increasing the risk of head injury, spinal cord injury, and possibly death.

FALLS. In falls, the amount of force that is applied to the body is directly related to the distance fallen. However, the area of the body injured is very hard to predict. Falls from significant heights are high-energy force falls, and patients should be evaluated accord-

Figure 8-6 **A.** Injury to the lower extremities and pelvis can occur when the knee strikes the dashboard. **B.** Injury to the chest and abdomen occurs when the patient's chest and/or abdomen strikes the steering wheel.

ingly. Any patient who has fallen more than three times his or her own height, or greater than 15′ to 20′, should be considered at risk for serious injury. With children, a fall of two to three times their height, or approximately 10′ or more, is potentially lethal.

If the patient's condition is stable, you should attempt to determine exactly what happened during the fall. When possible, you should also identify what the patient landed on and how he or she landed. This information, which may be gleaned from the patient and/or bystanders, may help you to predict what areas of the body might be the most seriously injured.

GUNSHOT AND STAB WOUNDS. Penetrating trauma, often the result of a gunshot or stab injury, is also very difficult to assess because there is little external evidence of the actual damage. The amount of force that is applied to the body in a gunshot wound is most directly related to the caliber of the weapon and the distance the weapon was from the patient when it was fired. Point-blank or high-caliber gunshot wounds are high-force injuries. By comparison, the force that is exerted on the patient in stab injuries is minimal, even though these injuries can still be lethal.

The area of the body that is involved in penetrating trauma may be very difficult to predict. In gunshot wounds, the area that is involved may be predicted by creating an imaginary line between the **entrance wound** (▼ **Figure 8-7A**) and the **exit wound** (▼ **Figure 8-7B**), if one exists, although this is only an approximation at best. However, it is important to remember that bullets may bounce off dense bones or organs in the body, making the exact path almost impossible to determine. Some bullets are even designed to tumble or break apart after they enter the body.

Figure 8-7 **A.** Entrance wound from a gunshot. **B.** Exit wound from a gunshot.

In stab wounds, the body area that is involved can be estimated by looking at the location of entrance and the length of the instrument that was used in the stabbing, if known. Remember that you can only estimate the extent of the injury. An assailant may have moved the weapon in a back-and-forth motion after it entered the patient.

Nature of Illness

As an EMT-B, you will care for as many medical patients as trauma patients. For trauma patients you examine the mechanism of injury as part of your scene size-up. For medical patients, you must examine the nature of the illness. There are similarities between the mechanism of injury and the nature of illness. Both require you to search for clues regarding how the incident occurred. You must make an effort to determine the general type of illness, or **nature of illness**. This is often best described by the patient's **chief complaint**: the reason EMS was called. In order to quickly determine the nature of the illness, talk with the patient, family, or bystanders about the problem. But at the same time, use your senses to check the scene for clues as to the possible problem. You may see open or spilled medicine containers, poisonous substances, or unsanitary living conditions. You may smell an unusual, or strong, odor, such as the odor of fresh paint in a closed room. You may hear a hissing sound, such as a leak from a home oxygen system. Keep these observations of the scene in mind as you begin to assess the patient.

Determine Number of Patients

As part of your scene size-up, it is essential that you accurately determine the total number of patients. This determination is critical for your estimate of the need for additional resources, such as the HazMat team or a specialized rescue group. You should ask yourself the following questions when considering the need for additional resources:

- How many patients are there?
- What is the nature of their condition?
- Who contacted EMS?
- Is this a possible crime scene in which evidence may need to be preserved?
- Are hazardous materials, such as chemicals or leaking fuel, involved?
- Does the scene pose a threat to your or your patient's safety?

Figure 8-8 With multiple patients, you should call for additional resources and then begin triage.

When there are multiple patients, you should call for additional units immediately and then begin triage (▲ **Figure 8-8**). **Triage** is a process of identifying the severity of each patient's condition. Once that is accomplished, you can begin to establish treatment and transport priorities. One EMT-B, usually the most experienced, should be assigned to perform triage. This process will help you to provide care and allocate your personnel and equipment resources most effectively and efficiently in a multiple-patient situation. If there is a large number of patients or if patient needs are greater than the available resources, put your local mass-casualty plan into action.

In these situations, you should always call for additional resources, such as law enforcement, the fire department, rescue units, ALS, and even utilities as soon as possible. It is never wrong to call for backup, even if the extra units are sent back. Remember, you are less likely to ask for help after you begin patient care because at that point, you are part of the scene, particularly at a motor vehicle crash in which patients require spinal immobilization.

Initial Assessment

uring the scene size-up, you speculated about the patient's condition, based on dispatch information, and asked and answered questions about scene safety. These steps are critically important, particularly in light of their role in ensuring your safety. However, patient assessment actually begins when you come into contact with the patient.

The **initial assessment** has a single, critical, all-important goal: to identify and initiate treatment of immediate or potential life threats. Information concerning life-threatening conditions comes from a variety of places, such as the visual appearance of the patient, the patient's chief complaint, or the mechanism of injury when trauma is involved. As you approach the scene and, ultimately, the patient, you will form a general impression of the patient. The **general impression** is based on your immediate assessment of the environment, the presenting signs and symptoms, mechanism of injury in a trauma patient, and the patient's chief complaint. (▲ **Table 8-2**) lists the components of the Initial Assessment.

Form a General Impression of the Patient

The general impression is important, because it helps you to determine the priorities of care, identify the mechanism of injury (if trauma was involved), assess the potential for life-threatening conditions, and judge the reliability of the information the patient is providing (▼ **Figure 8-9**).

(**Figure 8-9**) As you approach the patient, form a general impression of his or her overall condition.

TABLE 8-2 Initial Assessment
Form General Impression of the Patient
Assess Mental Status
Assess the Airway
Assess Breathing
Assess Circulation
Identify Priority Patients

As you approach the scene, note the patient's position, check to see whether the patient is moving or still, awake or unconscious, bleeding or not. Look for the mechanism of injury or the nature of the illness. Listen to what the patient and bystanders have to say. Make note of odors that suggest chemical hazards, smoke, or alcohol on the patient's breath. You can feel for pulses, pain, and deformities when you reach the patient. If the patient is responsive, try to learn as much as possible about what is wrong before you begin your examination. At this time, you should tell the patient your name, identify yourself as an EMT, and explain that you are there to help. You should learn the patient's age, race, gender, and chief complaint and continue to ask questions and talk to a responsive patient throughout the entire assessment.

You must answer the following questions to begin to form your general impression:

- Does the patient appear to have a life-threatening condition? Clues could include unconsciousness, obvious difficulty breathing, severe external bleeding, and either cyanotic (blue) or very pale skin color. If you suspect a life-threatening condition, provide immediate care and transport.

- Was the patient injured by trauma? If so, what was the mechanism of injury? On the basis of the mechanism of injury, would you expect the patient to be severely injured? If so, assume the worst and begin treatment, including spinal immobilization.

- Does the patient appear coherent and able to answer questions? If not, you need to rely more heavily on your physical assessment skills and/or the information that you can learn from others.

Patient Assessment

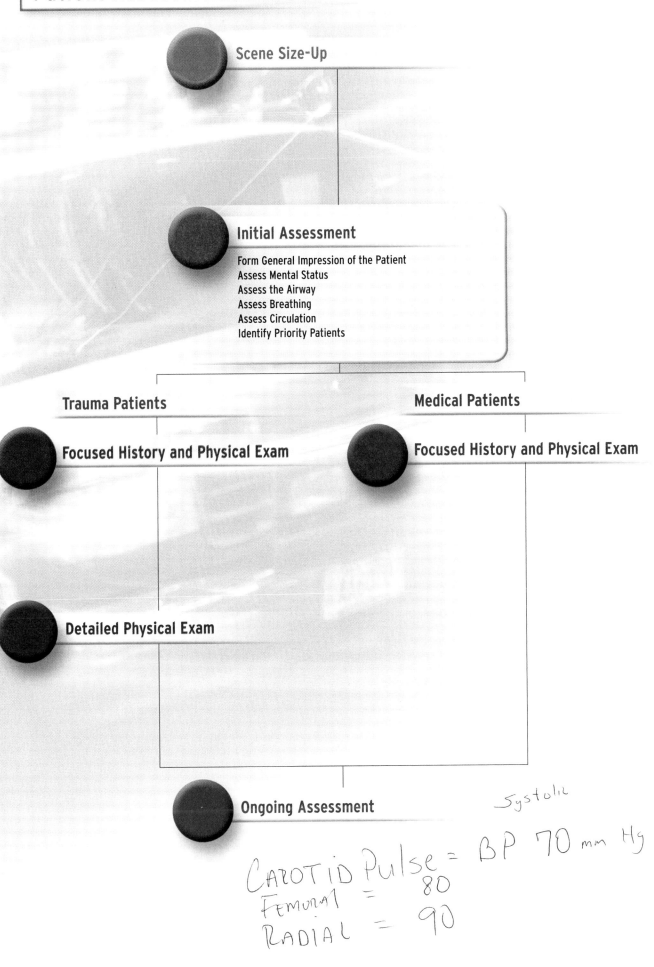

Scene Size-Up

Initial Assessment

Form General Impression of the Patient
Assess Mental Status
Assess the Airway
Assess Breathing
Assess Circulation
Identify Priority Patients

Trauma Patients

Focused History and Physical Exam

Medical Patients

Focused History and Physical Exam

Detailed Physical Exam

Ongoing Assessment

Systolic

CAROTID Pulse = BP 70 mm Hg
FEMURAL = 80
RADIAL = 90

Distinguishing Between Medical and Trauma Patients

Remember that as an EMT-B, you will be called to treat an almost infinite number of different patient problems. Some patients will have a problem that is not related to a crash or trauma; these patients are typically referred to as medical patients (for example, those with chest pain or having difficulty breathing). Others will have been injured in an incident such as a fall, a motor vehicle crash, or a shooting. These patients are usually considered trauma patients. In some situations, this distinction will be obvious. If the primary problem appears to be traumatic in origin, you will want to assume the worst and begin treatment, including spinal immobilization. However, quite frequently, it will not. For instance, a patient who falls at a long-term care facility could simply be treated as a trauma patient; however, it is also possible that the fall was caused by a medical condition such as an episode of fainting, a stroke, or even a heart attack. You will learn that it is not usually easy or prudent to label patients as medical or trauma until you have finished your assessment. In many cases, medical emergencies and trauma go hand in hand.

For this reason, the assessment process does not encourage you to differentiate immediately between medical and trauma patients. Rather, the assessment process begins by assuming that all patients may have both medical and trauma aspects to their condition. Through the assessment process, you will develop an understanding of the patient's problems, both medical and traumatic, and will begin treatment on the basis of that understanding. This approach is both simpler and safer than an approach that starts with an unsupported assumption that the patient is either medical or trauma. As each call unfolds, your patient's primary problem will become apparent.

This rather general assessment is your opportunity to evaluate "the big picture" before you focus on the patient's specific needs, so use all of your senses in observing the scene and patient.

The first steps in caring for any patient focus on finding and treating the most life-threatening illnesses and injuries (▶ Figure 8-10). Through all of these avenues, you need to ask and get answers to the following questions:

- Does the patient have an altered level of consciousness?
- Does the patient have an obstructed airway?
- Does the patient have inadequate breathing?

- Does the patient have inadequate circulation?
- Does the patient have the potential to develop any of these problems?
- Does the patient have the potential for a spinal cord injury?

Figure 8-10   Performing the initial assessment. **A.** Observe the patient to form a general impression. **B.** Assess the patient's mental status. **C.** Assess the mental status of a child.

EMT-B Tips

People call 9-1-1 during some of the most difficult times of their lives. In some cases, they call because of a serious illness or injury. In others, they call because the patient or family is frightened, overwhelmed, or unable to cope with a more minor problem any longer. The patient is often fatigued, sick, frightened, angry, or sad, and the family often shares some or all of these feelings. Regardless of the exact nature of the call, the patient, family, and bystanders expect you to bring comfort, control, and resolution of these problems—emotional and physical.

In many ways, good communication skills are as important as technical proficiency, if not more so. Each step in the assessment process can be impeded by poor communication, and each can be enhanced by a good connection between you and the patient and family. Here are five tips that can vastly improve your communication skills during the assessment process:

1. **Do whatever you can, quickly, to make yourself and the patient comfortable.** Patients are uncomfortable communicating with someone who is standing over them, pacing, or looking away. When time permits, sit down and/or position yourself near the patient, introduce yourself, and ask the patient's name (▶ **Figure 8-11**). This simple action signals the patient that you have time to talk; it opens the channels of communication as nothing else will. At the same time, be conscious of the patient's personal space. Do not move in too quickly. Ask the patient whether there is something you can do to make him or her more comfortable. Caring gestures and good body language are a visible demonstration of your care and concern.

2. **Actively listen to the patient.** In many cases, patients will be able to tell you what is wrong with them if you are paying attention and are truly listening. You can use several skills to actively listen, including leaning in toward the patient, taking selective notes, and periodically repeating back important points to the patient to ensure that you understood correctly. Active listening is often more difficult than it might seem, because scenes are often noisy and chaotic, and you will be receiving information from the patient, the family, your partner, and other EMS, fire, or law enforcement individuals on the scene. Try to screen them out for a few minutes so that you can truly listen to the patient; it will pay big dividends.

3. **Make eye contact with the person with whom you are speaking.** Eye contact signals that you are listening, so the patient is more likely to open up. An added benefit is that you will see facial expressions that, in some cases, communicate more clearly than the patient's words. For instance, you might see a facial grimace of pain or the averted eyes indicating embarrassment. Note that some cultures are uncomfortable with or offended by direct eye contact. Be sure to be familiar with the cultural background of citizens in your area.

Figure 8-11 Position yourself near the patient, at eye level when possible, to begin to establish a relationship with the patient.

4. **Base your initial questions on the patient's complaints.** No one likes to think that he or she is "just another patient." But that is what you communicate if you always ask the same questions of every patient, regardless of their complaints. If you ask questions about their Medicare number while they are trying to tell you about their pain, you are communicating that you are not really interested in their problem. Talk about their problem first, then ask paperwork questions.

5. **Before you start treatment, stop for a moment and mentally summarize** what you have learned and what you are going to do, then tell the patient. By providing necessary information to the patient and family, you help to relieve their anxiety and fear. This will also give them an opportunity to give you additional information if you have missed something.

You should spend your entire EMS career fine-tuning your patient assessment skills, as they are the cornerstone of high-quality prehospital care. A poor assessment almost always results in substandard patient care. Be sure to focus some of your energy on improving the communication process. You will make it easier for patients to feel comfortable around you, which will help them to give honest, direct answers to your questions. As a result, you will get better assessment information in less time.

If the answer to any of these questions is "yes," you need to take immediate action to resolve or prevent the life-threatening condition by performing one of the following: opening the airway, assisting ventilation, giving supplemental oxygen, controlling severe bleeding, performing spinal immobilization, providing transport, or calling for an ALS unit to assist or assume responsibility for patient care.

Approach to the Assessment Process

Remember, after developing a general impression of the patient, you should begin your assessment and care in this order of importance:

A = Airway
B = Breathing
C = Circulation

In all cases, your assessment of the patient's airway, breathing, and circulation (ABCs) will govern the extent of your treatment at the scene. Always give priority to emergency care of the ABCs to ensure life- and limb-saving treatment. Remember to assess the nature of the illness or the mechanism of injury as part of the assessment process.

Assess Mental Status

Evaluating a patient's mental status is important as this reflects the functioning of the brain. Remember to maintain spinal immobilization if needed. Many conditions may alter brain function and hence the level of consciousness. You will learn about many of these conditions as you progress through the EMT-B course.

Mental status and level of consciousness can be evaluated in just a few seconds by using two separate tests: responsiveness and orientation. The test for **responsiveness** assesses how well a patient responds to external stimuli, including verbal stimuli (sound), and painful stimuli (touch, such as pinching the patient's earlobe). For a patient who is alert and responding to verbal stimuli, you should next evaluate orientation.

Orientation tests assess mental status by checking the patient's memory of person (his or her name), place (the current location), time (the current year, month, and approximate date), and event (what happened). These four questions were not selected at random. They evaluate long-term memory (name and place if the patient is at home), intermediate-term memory (place and time), and short-term memory (event). If the patient knows these facts, the patient is said to be "alert and fully oriented." If a patient is does not know one of these facts, he or she is considered not fully oriented. Loss of intermediate- and long-term memory (person and place) is thought to be related to more severe problems than loss

of short-term memory. Collectively, your evaluation of the patient's responsiveness and orientation will paint a picture of the overall mental status.

Responsiveness can be evaluated by using the **AVPU** scale:

- **Alert.** The patient's eyes open spontaneously as you approach, and the patient appears aware of and responsive to the environment. The patient appears to follow commands, and the eyes visually track people and objects.

- **Responsive to Verbal Stimulus.** The patient's eyes do not open spontaneously. However, the patient's eyes do open to verbal stimuli, and the patient is able to respond in some meaningful way when spoken to.

- **Responsive to Pain.** The patient does not respond to your questions but moves or cries out in response to a painful stimulus. This response is tested by gently but firmly pinching the patient's earlobe (▶ **Figure 8-12A**), by pressing down on the bone above the eye (▶ **Figure 8-12B**), or by pinching the muscles of the neck (▶ **Figure 8-12C**). The sternal rub, although advocated in CPR training, is not recommended because it may be inaccurate in patients with cervical spine injuries. The use of ammonia "smelling salts" is also not recommended. An appropriate response is moaning or pushing away or withdrawing from the pinch. Use of extremely painful stimuli is never appropriate.

- **Unresponsive.** The patient does not respond to any stimuli.

If you are in doubt about whether a patient is truly unconscious, assume the worst and treat appropriately.

An altered mental status (patient is determined to be any level of responsiveness other than "alert") may be caused by a wide variety of conditions, including head

Figure 8-12 **A.** Gently but firmly pinch the patient's earlobe. **B.** Press down on the bone above the eye. **C.** Pinch the muscles of the neck.

trauma, hypoxemia, hypoglycemia, stroke, cardiac problems, or drug use. If the patient has an altered mental status, you should rapidly complete the initial assessment and be prepared to give high-flow supplemental oxygen, consider spinal immobilization if trauma is suspected, and initiate transport. Support the ABCs as required, and continually reassess for changes in the patient's condition.

Assess the Airway

As you move through the steps of assessment, you must always be alert for signs of respiratory compromise or airway obstruction. Regardless of the cause, airway obstruction may result in inadequate or absent air flow into and out of the lungs, which may cause permanent damage to the brain, heart, and lungs or may even result in death.

Responsive Patients

Patients of any age who are responsive and are talking or crying have an open airway. However, watching and listening to how patients speak, particularly those with respiratory problems, may provide important clues about the adequacy of their airway and breathing status.

If you identify an airway problem, stop the assessment process, and open the airway using the head tilt-chin lift or jaw-thrust maneuver. Although airway and breathing problems are not the same, their signs and symptoms often overlap. A patient who can speak only two to three words without pausing to take a breath, a condition known as **two- to three-word dyspnea**, has a severe breathing problem. The presence of retractions or the use of the **accessory muscles** (secondary muscles)

of respiration is also a sign of inadequate breathing. **Nasal flaring** and use of the accessory muscles indicate that a child has inadequate breathing. Finally, obviously labored breathing is also a sign of airway or breathing difficulties.

Any of these signs may signal an immediate or pending airway and/or breathing problem. You should be prepared to open the airway, administer supplemental oxygen, assist ventilation, and initiate transport.

Unresponsive Patients

With an unresponsive patient or one with a decreased level of consciousness, you should immediately assess the patency of the airway. If it is clear, you can continue your assessment. If the airway is not clear, your next priority is to open it using the head tilt-chin lift or jaw-thrust maneuver. Airway obstruction in an unconscious patient is most commonly due to relaxation of the tongue muscles back into throat. Dentures, blood clots, vomitus, mucus, food, or other foreign objects may also create a blockage. Signs of airway obstruction in an unconscious patient include the following:

- Obvious trauma, blood, or other obstruction
- Noisy breathing, such as bubbling, gurgling, crowing, or other abnormal sounds (Normal breathing is quiet.)
- Extremely shallow or absent breathing (Airway obstruction may cause impaired breathing.)

To open the airway, positioning depends on the patient's age and size. For medical patients, perform the head tilt-chin lift maneuver. For trauma patients or

> Airway obstruction in an unconscious patient is most commonly due to relaxation of the tongue muscles back into throat.

those with illness of an unknown nature, the cervical spine should be stabilized and immobilized, and, if necessary, the jaw-thrust maneuver should be performed.

Assess Breathing

As you assess the patient's breathing, look at how much work it takes for the patient to breathe. Normal respirations are not unusually shallow or excessively deep, and their rate varies widely in adults, anywhere from 12 to 20 breaths/min. Shallow respirations can be identified by movement of the chest wall. Conversely, deep respirations cause a great deal of chest wall rise and fall and often can be heard as large volumes of air moving into and out of the patient's lungs. As you assess the patient, ask yourself the following questions:

- Are the patient's respirations shallow or deep?
- Does the patient appear to be choking?
- Is the patient cyanotic (blue)?
- Is the patient moving air into and out of the lungs as the chest rises and falls?

If a patient seems to have difficulty breathing, you should immediately reevaluate the airway. Once the airway is open, you should consider assisting ventilation with a BVM device or applying oxygen with a nonrebreathing mask for all patients with respirations greater than 24/min or less than 8/min.

Any patient with a decreased level of consciousness, respiratory distress, or poor skin color should also receive high-flow oxygen. If there is no risk of spinal cord injury, the patient should remain in a comfortable position that supports breathing; this is typically sitting up with the legs dangling. In any patient who has a possible risk for spinal injury, you should immobilize the cervical spine, ensuring that respirations are not compromised.

You should give supplemental oxygen via a nonrebreathing mask at 15 L/min. Any patient whom you identify as having immediate or potential airway or breathing problems should be given supplemental oxygen. Never withhold oxygen from any patient at the scene!

Use the look, listen, and feel technique to evaluate how well an unconscious patient is breathing. If the patient does not appear to be breathing or has an inadequate airway, start airway management immediately, and assist ventilation. The look, listen, and feel technique may be more difficult in infants and small children because they have so little chest wall movement during respirations.

In most cases, a spinal injury should be considered a possibility for any unresponsive trauma patient. These patients must be rolled or moved as a single unit onto a flat surface or backboard. The timing for this maneuver depends on the patient's position when you find him or her. If the patient must be moved to access the face or manage the airway, it should be done immediately. Otherwise, you should log roll the patient after you attend to the ABCs. Remember, you must move the head, neck, torso, and legs as a unit without any unnecessary bending or twisting.

Once the patient is properly positioned and the airway is open and clear, you should begin to treat and support the patient's breathing. For patients with inadequate breathing, provide high-flow oxygen by a nonrebreathing mask or assist ventilations with a BVM device if necessary. If the patient is in respiratory arrest, ventilate with a BVM device and high-flow oxygen.

Assess Circulation

Assessing circulation helps you to evaluate how well blood is circulating to the major organs, including the brain, lungs, heart, kidneys, and rest of the body. A variety of problems can impair circulation, including blood loss, shock, and conditions that affect the heart and major blood vessels. Circulation is evaluated by assessing the presence and qualities of the pulse, identifying external bleeding, and evaluating skin condition.

If the patient has a pulse but is not breathing, continue providing ventilations at a rate of 12 breaths/min for an adult, or 20 breaths/min for an infant or child. Continue to monitor the pulse to evaluate the effectiveness of your ventilations. If at any time the pulse is lost, start CPR immediately and apply the AED if indicated.

Assess the Pulse

The rate, rhythm, and strength of the patient's pulse will give you a rough idea of the overall status of the patient's cardiac function. The pulse is one of the vital signs that you should reassess often in most patients, even en route to the hospital.

Pediatric Needs

You can feel the pulse of a child at the carotid artery, as in an adult. However, palpating this pulse in an infant may present a problem. Because an infant's neck is often very short and fat, and its pulse is often quite fast, you may have a hard time finding the carotid pulse. Therefore, in infants younger than 1 year, you should palpate the brachial artery to assess the pulse. Normal pulse rates for children are shown in (▼ **Table 8-3**).

TABLE 8-3 Normal Pulse Rates in Infants and Children

Age	Range (beats/min)
Newborn: birth to 1 month	120 to 160
Infant: 1 month to 1 year	100 to 160
Toddler: 1 to 3 years	90 to 150
Preschool-age: 3 to 6 years	80 to 140
School-age: 6 to 12 years	70 to 120
Adolescent: 12 to 18 years	60 to 100
Over 18 years	Adult normal ranges (60 to 100)

If you cannot **palpate** a pulse in an unresponsive patient, begin CPR. The AED should be used on medical patients who are at least 8 years old and weigh more than 55 lb and who have been assessed to be unresponsive, not breathing, and pulseless.

Assess and Control External Bleeding

The next step is to identify any major external bleeding. In some instances, blood loss can be very rapid and can quickly result in shock and even death. Therefore, this step demands your immediate attention as soon as the patient's airway is secured and breathing is stabilized. Signs of blood loss include active bleeding from wounds and/or evidence of bleeding such as blood on the clothes or near the patient. Serious bleeding from a large vein may be characterized by steady blood flow. Bleeding from an artery is characterized by a spurting flow of blood. When you evaluate an unconscious patient, do a sweep for blood by quickly and lightly running

your gloved hands from head to toe, pausing periodically to see whether your gloves are bloody.

Controlling external bleeding is often very simple. In almost all instances, direct pressure with your gloved hand and a sterile bandage over the wound will control bleeding. This pressure stops the flow of blood and helps the blood to **coagulate**, or clot naturally. Remember your BSI precautions whenever you may be exposed to blood or other body fluids.

Most often, bleeding can be adequately controlled by using direct pressure, along with elevating the extremity if bleeding is from the arms or legs. When direct pressure and elevation are not successful, you may apply pressure directly over arterial pressure points.

Evaluate Skin Color, Temperature, and Condition

Assessing the skin is one of the most important and most readily accessible ways of evaluating circulation. You should assess the patient's skin color, temperature, and moisture, as well as look for bleeding.

COLOR. Skin color depends on pigmentation and blood oxygen levels, as well as the amount of blood circulating through the vessels of the skin. For this reason, skin color is a valuable assessment tool. The normal skin color of lightly pigmented people is pinkish. Deeply pigmented skin may hide color changes that result from illness or injury. Therefore, you should look for changes in color in areas of the skin that have less pigment: the fingernail beds, the **sclera** (white of the eyes), the **conjunctiva** (lining of the eyelid), and the mucous membranes of the mouth. Normal skin color, particularly of the conjunctivae and mucous membranes, is pinkish. Skin colors that should alert you to possible medical problems include **cyanosis** (blue), flushed (red), pale (white), and **jaundice** (yellow).

TEMPERATURE. The skin is actually an organ, and like all other organs, it has many functions. It helps maintain the water content of the body, acts as insulation and protection from infection, and also plays a role in regulation of body temperature. Normal body temperature is 98.6°F (37°C), but it can change as a result of illness or injury. Assess the skin temperature by touching the patient's skin with your wrist or the back of your hand (▶ **Figure 8-13**).

CONDITION. Finally, determine whether the patient's skin is dry or moist. The skin is normally warm and dry. Cool or cold, moist, clammy skin suggests shock. Hot skin may indicate an abnormally elevated body temperature or fever.

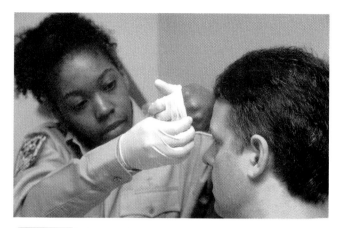

Figure 8-13 Assess skin temperature by touching the patient's skin with the back of your ungloved hand.

CAPILLARY REFILL. Another way to assess circulation is to check capillary refill, especially in infants and children. **Capillary refill** is the ability of the circulatory system to restore blood to the capillaries after circulation has been interrupted. Test capillary refill by squeezing the patient's fingernail bed until the area blanches (turns white). Next release the fingernail bed, and watch for it to return to a normal color. The area should return to its normal color within 2 seconds. If the area remains white or becomes blue, you know that circulation is inadequate, at least in the area being tested.

Capillary refill can be checked in children by squeezing the entire arm or leg at a distal point and observing the return to normal color. Although capillary refill is a quick and very general way to evaluate circulation, it is important to remember that other conditions, not related to the body's circulation, may also slow capillary refill. These conditions include the patient's age and gender, as well as exposure to a cold environment (**hypothermia**), frozen tissue (**frostbite**), or injuries to bones or muscles that cause local circulatory compromise.

RESTORING CIRCULATION. If a patient has inadequate circulation, you must take immediate action to restore or improve circulation, control severe bleeding, and improve oxygen delivery to the tissues. The apparent absence of a palpable pulse in a responsive patient is not caused by cardiac arrest. Therefore, do not begin CPR or use an AED on a responsive patient. However, if you cannot feel a pulse in an unresponsive adult patient, you should immediately begin CPR and, whenever possible and indicated, prepare to defibrillate. Remember to follow BSI precautions, which may include use of a barrier device for ventilation, gloves,

and perhaps protective eyewear. Follow these four steps in a patient who has no pulse and is unresponsive:

1. **Immediately begin CPR** until an AED is available.

2. **Apply and operate the AED** as quickly as possible (defibrillation is your first priority) if the patient is 8 years or older and weighs more than 55 lb. Local protocols may vary on the age and weight requirements for AED use.

3. **If the cardiac arrest is associated** with an obvious, apparently catastrophic traumatic event, perform CPR without preparing for use of the AED. Traumatic arrests do not typically respond to defibrillation. Treatment should include initiation of airway control, ventilation, and chest compressions, followed by transport to the hospital. Immediate transport to a trauma center is the most valuable therapy for the patient in traumatic cardiac arrest.

4. **Initiate use of the AED** in association with CPR, if in doubt about a traumatic origin of the arrest.

Continued impaired circulation is devastating to the body's cells because it denies the cells of vital oxygen, which is necessary for cell function. CPR and bleeding control are intended to maintain or improve circulation. Oxygen delivery is improved through the administration of supplemental oxygen. Any patient with impaired circulation should receive high-flow oxygen via a nonrebreathing mask or assisted ventilations to improve oxygen delivery at the cellular level.

Identify Priority Patients

Once you have completed the initial assessment, you have to make some decisions about patient care. You should have already addressed life-threatening injuries and/or illnesses as they are found. Next, you must identify priority patients, or those who need other interventions and/or immediate transport ▶ **Figure 8-14**.

Patients with one of the following conditions are considered high priority and should be transported immediately or be considered for ALS backup:

- Poor general impression
- Unresponsive with no gag or cough reflexes
- Responsive but unable to follow commands
- Difficulty breathing
- Pale skin or other signs of poor perfusion
- Complicated childbirth

- Uncontrolled bleeding
- Severe pain in any area of the body
- Severe chest pain, especially when the systolic blood pressure is less than 100 mm Hg
- Inability to move any part of the body

Correct identification of high-priority patients is an essential aspect of the initial assessment and helps to improve patient outcome.

While initial treatment is important, it is essential to remember that immediate transport is one of the keys to the survival of any high-priority patient. Transport should be initiated as soon as is practical and possible. Once you have completed the initial assessment and made a transport decision, you can turn to the focused history and physical exam.

From here you proceed to the appropriate focused history and physical exam based on your current assessment of whether the cause of the patient's problem is a trauma or medical emergency, or both.

Figure 8-14 Identifying priority patients.

Focused History and Physical Exam: Trauma Patients

You now have information from both the scene size-up and initial assessment. These have provided you with valuable information about the scene, allowing you to anticipate what you will find and prepare for hazards. You have stabilized any life-threatening conditions, perhaps provided spinal immobilization, and initiated transport.

How do you proceed now? Your patient may have, almost literally, one or more of a million different problems. How do you identify, prioritize, and treat this variety of potential problems?

Goals of the Focused History and Physical Exam

The **focused history and physical exam** help you to focus on specific problems. They have three goals:

1. Identify the patient's chief complaint.
   - What happened to this patient?

2. Understand the specific circumstances surrounding the chief complaint.
   - What circumstances were associated with the event?
   - Is the mechanism of injury a high risk for serious injuries?

3. Direct further physical examination.
   - What problems can be identified through the physical exam?

The focused history and physical exam, like the entire assessment process, guides you to take actions that will stabilize or relieve the patient's problems. Depending on the answers to these questions, you should be prepared to return to the initial assessment if potentially life-threatening conditions are identified, perform spinal immobilization, provide transport or coordinate transfer of the patient to an ALS unit, and/or treat problems that you identify during the exam.

Patients who call 9-1-1 following an acute event may have any number of problems—medical, traumatic, or a combination of both. Assess and manage all patients in the same systematic fashion. However, as each case unfolds, it will often become apparent that the call is predominantly traumatic or medical in nature. When this occurs, you should focus your assessment on the medical or traumatic aspects of the case.

Once you have identified that a patient has sustained a traumatic injury, you need to rapidly make some important treatment and transport decisions. This is because some traumatic injuries are life threatening and cannot be treated in the field. These patients have the best chance for survival if they arrive at an appropriate hospital, usually a trauma center if available, for definitive care within 60 minutes of the time of injury. You will often hear this period of time called the Golden Hour. The **Golden Hour** is the time from injury to definitive care, during which treatment of shock or traumatic injuries should occur because survival potential is the best (▼ **Figure 8-15**). After the first 60 minutes, the body has increasing difficulty in compensating for traumatic injuries. For this reason, you should spend as little time as possible on the scene with patients who have sustained significant or severe trauma. Aim to assess, package, and begin transporting the patient no later than 10 minutes after arrival on the scene, except in cases of difficult extrication. (▶ **Table 8-4**) lists the components of the focused history and physical exam for the trauma patient.

Reconsider the Mechanism of Injury

As part of the scene size-up, you evaluated the mechanism of injury before you began treatment. At this point in the assessment process, you should look at the mechanism again to ensure that you have not missed important information. Understanding the mechanism of injury helps you to understand the severity of the patient's problem and provide invaluable information to hospital staff as well. Some patients have experienced a significant mechanism of injury; others clearly have not.

Initial hospital stabilization 20 minutes

Discovery of incident and activation of EMS 20 minutes

EMS packaging and transport 10 minutes

"The Golden Ten Minutes" Initial assessment and intervention

EMS intervention

Figure 8-15 The Golden Hour is the time during which treatment of shock or traumatic injuries is most critical and the potential for survival is best.

Patient Assessment

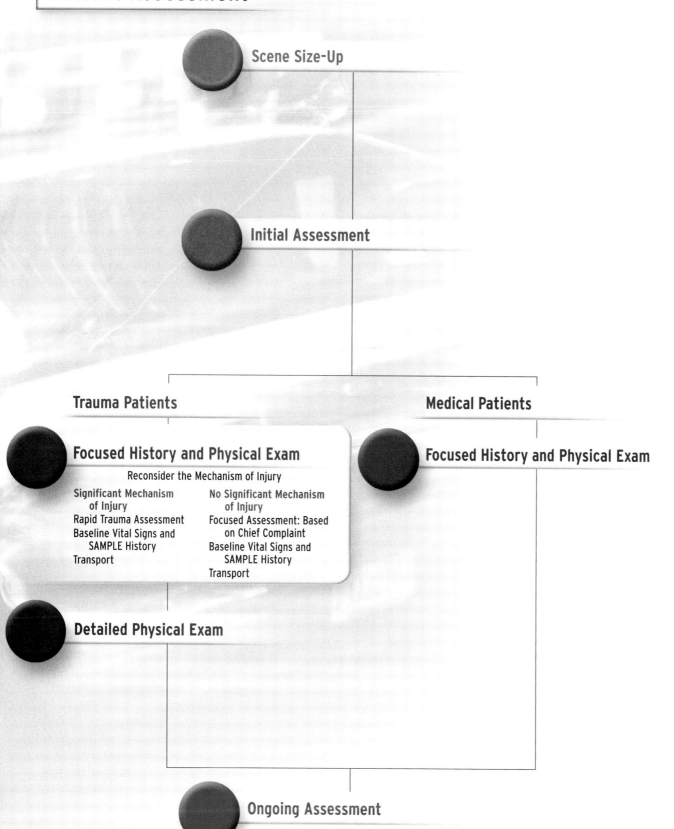

Scene Size-Up

Initial Assessment

Trauma Patients

Medical Patients

Focused History and Physical Exam

Reconsider the Mechanism of Injury

Significant Mechanism of Injury	No Significant Mechanism of Injury
Rapid Trauma Assessment	Focused Assessment: Based on Chief Complaint
Baseline Vital Signs and SAMPLE History	Baseline Vital Signs and SAMPLE History
Transport	Transport

Focused History and Physical Exam

Detailed Physical Exam

Ongoing Assessment

TABLE 8-4 Focused History and Physical Exam: Trauma Patients

Reconsider the Mechanism of Injury	
Trauma Patients With Significant Mechanism of Injury	**Trauma Patients With No Significant Mechanism of Injury**
Rapid Trauma Assessment	Focused Assessment: Based on Chief Complaint
Baseline Vital Signs and SAMPLE History	Baseline Vital Signs and SAMPLE History
Transport	Transport

Significant Mechanism of Injury

Recall that significant mechanisms of injury include the following:

- Ejection from a vehicle
- Death in the passenger compartment
- Fall greater than 15′ to 20′
- Vehicle rollover
- High-speed vehicle collision
- Vehicle-pedestrian collision
- Motorcycle crash
- Unresponsiveness or altered mental status following trauma
- Penetrating trauma to the head, chest, or abdomen

Infant and Child Considerations

Significant mechanisms of injury for children include the above with the following additions or modifications:

- Fall greater than two to three times their height
- Bicycle crash

Hidden Injuries

Seat belts and airbags have significantly reduced the death and disability that are associated with motor vehicle crashes. However, you should be aware that seat belts and airbags can also cause injuries. When evaluating a patient who was involved in a motor vehicle crash, you should look for and ask questions to determine whether seat belts and/or an airbag was involved.

SEAT BELTS. Seat belts have prevented many thousands of injuries and have saved countless numbers of lives. Patients who otherwise would have been thrown out of a smashed car owe their lives to seat belts. However, if the force of a crash is great enough, patients can have bruises under the seat belts and possible internal injuries, although these injuries are less severe than the injuries the patients would have if they had not been wearing seat belts. Seat belts that are worn improperly across the abdomen rather than across the pelvic bones increase the potential for internal injuries (▼ Figure 8-16). Lap seat belts must be worn so that they lie below the iliac crests, snugly up against the hip joints. If the seat belt is worn too high, sudden slowing or an abrupt stop may result in abdominal injuries. Occasionally, injuries

Figure 8-16 **A.** Injury may occur if the seat belt is placed too far above the iliac crest. **B.** A sudden stop could cause compression of the organs between the belt and the spine. **C.** The proper location of the seat belt is at the hip joints.

of the lumbar spine can occur, even if the patient is wearing the seat belt properly.

Lap belts and shoulder belts are now commonly combined into a single unit. Some cars still have separate lap and shoulder belts. Used alone, shoulder belts can cause injuries to the head, chest, ribs, and liver.

AIRBAGS. Airbags represent a great advance in automotive safety. Before airbags were common, individuals in head-on crashes would typically have significant facial injuries and bleeding—clear, visible signs that they had been injured. With airbags, patients occasionally have facial burns or respiratory problems from the chemical process that causes the airbag to expand, or they may have abrasions from the airbag itself. However, with airbags and seat belts, patients may or may not have visible injuries. Remember, patients who have been involved in serious crashes may initially look uninjured but still may have internal injuries.

When an airbag deploys, a patient who is not wearing a seat belt can still go up and over, or down and under, the steering column. You should always look under a deployed airbag to see whether the steering wheel is bent or deformed in any way (▼ **Figure 8-17**). Remove the patient from the car, using spinal precautions. If the steering wheel is bent or deformed, you should suspect possible internal injuries. Injuries may also be possible if the steering wheel is not bent or deformed. The general health of the patient, the patient's age, and other factors can also impact the likelihood for internal injuries.

During your hand-off report at the hospital, make sure that you tell hospital personnel whether seat belts were worn and whether the airbag deployed.

Figure 8-17 If an airbag has deployed, you should lift the airbag and check the steering wheel to see whether it is bent.

Trauma Patients With Significant Mechanism of Injury

The rapid trauma assessment should be performed on any patient with significant mechanism of injury, to identify life-threatening injuries. The purpose of this assessment is to zero in on the patient's problems, and identify potentially life-threatening conditions, which will direct your physical exam. The rapid trauma assessment should be performed on responsive and unresponsive patients alike. Remember, you can use a responsive patient as a resource; you should ask him or her about symptoms throughout your assessment.

An integral part of this assessment is evaluation using the simple mnemonic "DCAP-BTLS." For each area of the body, you should quickly look and feel for Deformities, Contusions, Abrasions, Punctures/Penetrations, Burns, Tenderness, Lacerations, and Swelling (DCAP-BTLS). Remember, you should interrupt your assessment to treat any immediately or potentially life-threatening conditions. Once these conditions have been treated, you may continue with your assessment.

Rapid Trauma Assessment

As you prepare for the rapid trauma assessment, consider your transport decision and request ALS backup if appropriate. Follow the steps in (▶ **Skill Drill 8-1**):

1. **Continue spinal immobilization** while you check the patient's ABCs for any changes in status since the initial assessment and evaluate mental status.

2. **Assess the head,** looking and feeling for DCAP-BTLS and crepitus (Step 1).

3. **Assess the neck,** looking and feeling for DCAP-BTLS, jugular vein distention, and crepitus (Step 2).

4. **Apply a cervical spinal immobilization collar** (Step 3).

5. **Assess the chest,** looking and feeling for DCAP-BTLS, paradoxical motion, and crepitus. You should also assess for breath sounds (Step 4).

6. **Assess the abdomen,** looking and feeling for DCAP-BTLS, rigidity (firm or soft), and distention (Step 5).

7. **Assess the pelvis,** looking and feeling for DCAP-BTLS. If there is no pain, gently compress the pelvis downward or inward to determine tenderness or instability (Step 6).

8. **Assess all four extremities,** looking and feeling for DCAP-BTLS. Also assess and compare bilaterally for distal pulses, sensation, and motor function **(Step 7)**.

9. **Roll the patient with spinal precautions,** and assess the posterior aspect of the body, looking and feeling for DCAP-BTLS **(Step 8)**.

10. **Assess baseline vital signs and SAMPLE history (Step 9)**.

Recognizing a possible spinal injury is one of your principal responsibilities as an EMT-B. You should assume a spinal injury in any patient who has a mechanism that reflects or suggests a significant history of trauma, is intoxicated and may have been traumatized, is unconscious, complains of neck/spine pain following a traumatic event, or cannot move or feel in any or all four extremities following a traumatic event. Immediately begin manual immobilization of the spine. Consider requesting ALS backup or transporting the patient with priority status. Also reevaluate the patient's mental status. Finally, be sure to expose significant trauma patients so you can completely assess and treat the patient. You cannot treat what you cannot see.

Head, Neck, and Cervical Spine

Look for abnormalities of the head, neck, and cervical spine. Gently feel the head and the back of the neck for deformity, tenderness, or crepitus, also checking as you feel for any bleeding. **Crepitus** is the grating or grinding that is often felt or heard when two ends of a broken bone rub together, or the crackling sound produced by air bubbles under the skin. Ask a responsive patient if he or she feels any pain or tenderness. Next, check the neck for signs of trauma, swelling, or bleeding. Feel the skin of the neck for air under the skin, known as **subcutaneous emphysema**, as well as any abnormal lumps or masses. It is particularly important to evaluate the neck before covering it with a cervical collar. Also look for pronounced or distended jugular veins. This is normal in a patient who is lying down; however, their presence in the patient who is sitting up suggests some problem with blood returning to the heart. Report and record your findings carefully. Do not move on to the next step until you are sure that the airway is secure and you have initiated or continued spinal immobilization.

Chest

Next, look at and feel over the chest area for injury or signs of trauma, including bruising, tenderness, or swelling. Watch the chest rise and fall with breathing.

Normal breathing causes both sides of the chest to rise and fall together. Look for abnormal breathing signs, including **retractions** (when the skin pulls in around the ribs during inspiration) or **paradoxical motion** (when only one section rises on inspiration while another area of the chest falls).

Retractions indicate that the patient has some condition, usually medical, that is impairing the flow of air into and out of the lungs. Paradoxical motion is associated with a fracture of several ribs (flail), causing a section of chest to move independently from the rest of the chest. Feel for grating of bones as the patient breathes. Crepitus is associated with rib fractures. Feel over the chest for subcutaneous emphysema, especially in cases of severe blunt chest trauma.

If the patient reports difficulty breathing or has evidence of trauma to the chest, listen to **breath sounds**. This helps you to evaluate air movement in and out of the lungs. To listen, you need a stethoscope. Make sure that you place the earpieces facing forward in your ears. The position of the patient will determine the way you proceed to check for breathing (**▼ Figure 8-18**).

Figure 8-18 **A.** Listen to breath sounds from the patient's back if possible, over the apices, the bases, and the major airways. **B.** If the patient is immobilized or in a supine position, listen from the front.

Skill Drill 8-1   Performing a Rapid Trauma Assessment

Check ABCs, continue spinal immobilization, and assess mental status. Assess the head.

Assess the neck.

Apply a cervical collar.

Assess the chest, including breath sounds.

Assess the abdomen.

Assess the pelvis.

Continued on page 252.

Skill Drill 8-1 Performing a Rapid Trauma Assessment—continued.

Assess the extremities.

Log roll the patient and assess the back.

Assess baseline vitals and SAMPLE history.

Here's how and where to listen:

- First, remember that you can almost always hear breath sounds better from the patient's back. So if the patient's back is accessible, listen there. If you have immobilized the patient or if the patient is in a supine position, listen from the front.

- Listen over the upper lungs (apices), the lower lungs (bases), and over the major airways (mid-clavicular and midaxillary lines).

- Lift the clothing, or slide the stethoscope under the clothing. When you listen over clothing, you are hearing primarily the sound of the stethoscope sliding over the fabric, because the breath sounds are muted by the clothing.

- Place the diaphragm of the stethoscope firmly to best hear the breath sounds.

What are you listening for? Your goal is to hear and document the presence or absence of breath sounds in the three regions described. If you believe that the breathing is abnormal, reassess breathing, and then ensure that the patient is receiving oxygen and, if appropriate, assisted ventilation.

Abdomen

Look at the abdomen for any obvious injuries, bruising, and bleeding. Be sure to feel over both the front and the back of the abdomen, evaluating for tenderness and any bleeding. As you feel all around the abdomen, use the terms "firm," "soft," "tender," or "distended" (swollen) to report your findings. If the patient is awake and alert, ask about pain as you perform the exam. Do not palpate obvious soft-tissue injuries, and be careful not to palpate too hard.

Pelvis

Look for any signs of obvious injury, bleeding, or deformity. If the patient reports no pain, gently press inward and downward on the pelvic bones. Do not rock the pelvis, since this motion may move an unstable spine. If you feel any movement or crepitus, or the patient reports pain or tenderness, it may indicate severe injury. Injuries to the pelvis and surrounding abdomen may bleed profusely, so continue to monitor the patient's skin color and vital signs, and be sure that you are giving supplemental oxygen.

Extremities

Look for cuts, bruises, swelling, obvious injuries, and bleeding. Next, feel along each extremity for deformities. Ask the patient about any tenderness or pain. As you evaluate the extremities, check for pulses and motor and sensory function:

- **Pulse:** Check the distal pulses on the foot (dorsalis pedis or posterior tibial) and wrist (radial). Also check circulation. Evaluate the skin color in the hands or feet. Is it normal? How does it compare with the skin color of the other extremities? Pale or cyanotic skin may indicate poor circulation in the extremity.

- **Motor function:** Ask the patient to wiggle his or her fingers or toes. An inability to move a single extremity can be the result of a bone, muscle, or nerve injury. Inability to move several extremities may be a sign of a brain abnormality or spinal cord injury. Verify that spinal precautions are in place.

- **Sensory function:** Evaluate normal feeling in the extremity by asking the patient to close his or her eyes. Gently squeeze or pinch a finger or toe, and ask the patient to identify what you are doing. The inability to feel sensation in the extremity may indicate a local nerve injury. Inability to feel in several extremities may be a sign of spinal cord injury. Recheck to be sure that you have begun and/or are maintaining spinal immobilization.

Back

Feel the back for tenderness, deformity, and open wounds. If you are placing the patient on a backboard, it is particularly important that you check the back as you log roll the patient onto the backboard. Ensure that you keep the spine in line at all times as you log roll the patient onto his or her side. Carefully palpate the spine from the neck to the pelvis for tenderness or deformity, and look for obvious injuries, including bruising and bleeding.

Baseline Vital Signs and SAMPLE History

After you have completed the rapid trauma assessment, it is time to obtain baseline vital signs and a **SAMPLE history**.

The baseline vital signs provide useful information about the overall functions of the patient's heart and lungs. They may be an important part of the focused examination if your patient appears to have problems related to blood loss, circulation, or breathing. In other cases, you may simply document the vital signs as baseline information. If the patient's condition is stable, you should reassess the vital signs every 15 minutes until you reach the emergency department. If the patient is unstable, you should reassess at a minimum of every 5 minutes, or as often as the situation permits, looking for trends in the patient's condition. ▶ **Table 8-5** through ▶ **Table 8-10** provide more information on baseline vital signs.

Do not be falsely reassured by apparently normal vital signs. The body has amazing abilities to compensate for severe injury or illness, especially in children and young adults. Even patients with severe medical or traumatic conditions may initially present with fairly normal vital signs. However, the body eventually loses its ability to compensate, and the vital signs may deteriorate rapidly, especially in children. In fact, this tendency for the vital signs to fall rapidly as the patient decompensates is the reason that it is important to frequently recheck and record the vital signs.

TABLE 8-5 Determining the Quality of Breathing

Normal	• Breathing is neither shallow nor deep. • Average chest wall motion • No use of accessory muscles
Shallow	• Slight chest or abdominal wall motion
Labored	• Increased breathing effort • Grunting, stridor • Use of accessory muscles • Gasping for air • Nasal flaring, supraclavicular and intercostal retractions (in infants and children)
Noisy	• Increase in sound of breathing, including snoring, wheezing, gurgling, and crowing

TABLE 8-6 Normal Respiratory Rates (breaths/min)

Adults	12 to 20
Children	18 to 34
Infants	30 to 60

TABLE 8-7 Average Pulse Rates (beats/min)

Adults	60 to 100
Children	70 to 140
Toddlers	90 to 150
Infants	100 to 160

TABLE 8-8 Assessing the Skin

Color	Possible Cause	Temperature/Moisture	Possible Cause
Pink	• Normal color	Warm	• Normal condition
Ashen/Pale Face and/or Skin on Extremities	• Hypovolemia • Hypoxia	Hot	• Significant fever • Sunburn • Hyperthermia • Heavy exercise/ sweating
Gray-Blue (cyanotic)	• Insufficient air exchange • Low blood oxygen levels (Hypoxia)	Cool	• Early shock • Heat exhaustion
Flushed	• High blood pressure • Carbon monoxide poisoning • Significant fever • Heatstroke • Sunburn • Allergic reaction	Cold	• Profound shock • Hypothermia • Frostbite
		Dry	• Normal condition
Jaundice	• Liver disease or dysfunction	Clammy, Damp, or Moist	• Shock

TABLE 8-9 Systolic Blood Pressure Readings

Expected	Readings	Critically Low Readings	
Adult Men	Add 100 to the patient's age, up to 150 mm Hg	Male Adults/Adolescents	90 mm Hg or less
Adult Women	Add 90 to the patient's age, up to 150 mm Hg	Female Adults/Adolescents	80 mm Hg or less
Children	Add 70 to 2 times the patient's age in years	Children	70 mm Hg or less

TABLE 8-10 Pupillary Reactions

Appearance	Possible Cause
Round/equal size	Normal condition
Fixed with no reaction to light	Depressed brain function (head injury/stroke)
Fully dilated and fixed (blown pupil)	Intracranial bleeding
Dilate with bright light, constricted with low light	Depressed brain function
Constricted	Drugs (opiates)
Sluggish reaction	Depressed brain function
Unequal in size	Depressed brain function
	Medication placed in eye
	Injury or condition of the eye

For many EMT-Bs, taking the patient history seems to be a bewildering series of questions that seem to bear little or no relationship to the patient's need for help. This becomes worse with patients who have had many medical problems; taking their history is time consuming and often yields little or no information that is useful to you. However, this does not need to be the case. Remember that the mnemonic SAMPLE includes the following elements:

- Signs and Symptoms of the episode
- Allergies, particularly to medications
- Medications, including prescription, over-the-counter, and recreational (illicit) drugs
- Pertinent past history, particularly involving similar episodes in the past
- Last oral intake, including food and/or drinks. This is particularly important if the patient may need surgery or if diabetic.
- Events leading up to the episode, which may include precipitating factors

Transport

Your next steps are to provide the necessary emergency medical care and then to provide transport to the emergency department.

Trauma Patients With No Significant Mechanism of Injury

You will not need to perform such a complete exam on most of your patients. After you have completed the initial assessment and care for any actual or potentially life-threatening conditions, you should focus on anything associated with the patient's chief complaint.

Focused Assessment: Chief Complaint

Once you are sure that the ABCs are stable, move to the patient's specific injury site or **chief complaint**: the patient's description of "what is wrong." In many cases, especially with trauma, this is logical. For example, if the patient reports ankle pain, you should check the ankle. Note, though, that nontraumatic complaints may be a little less obvious. Here are specific items to assess with some common chief complaints:

- **Chest pain:** Evaluate the skin, pulse, and blood pressure. Look for injuries to the chest and listen to the breath sounds.

- **Shortness of breath:** Evaluate the skin, pulse, blood pressure, and rate and depth of respirations. Look for signs of airway obstruction, as well as trauma to the neck and chest. Listen carefully to the breath sounds.

- **Abdominal pain:** Evaluate the skin, pulse, and blood pressure. Look for trauma to the abdomen, and palpate the abdomen to identify any tenderness.

- **Any pain associated with bones or joints:** Evaluate the skin, movement, and sensation adjacent to and below the affected area. Expose the injury site.

- **Dizziness:** Evaluate the skin, pulse, blood pressure, and rate and quality of respirations. Monitor the level of consciousness and orientation carefully. Check the head for signs of trauma.

Next, examine any noticeable abnormalities. This could be something you noticed during the initial assessment and focused history, such as a laceration, a deformed bone, a weakness on one side, or abnormal pupils. Avoid being distracted by these conditions while caring for life threats; it is easy to let a big cut or deformity draw your attention away from more important, potentially life-threatening problems.

However, once you have evaluated and treated life-threatening conditions and have examined the chief complaint, you can come back to any minor problems you found previously. Be sure to ask the patient questions about the abnormality while you are evaluating it. In some cases, deformities or abnormalities may be long term and unrelated to the patient's present condition. For example, a patient who has had a stroke may have a weakness on one side for months following the stroke; it is not a new problem, and is not likely to be related to the patient's current call to EMS.

Once you have assessed for problems that are potentially life threatening, related to the chief complaint or specific injury site, and evaluated abnormalities, you may begin to perform the focused assessment. As we have noted before, plan ahead for BSI precautions; if bleeding is possible (and it is for most patients), be sure your gloves are on before you begin the focused examination. Next, follow the order and components of the rapid trauma assessment, focusing on the specific area of injury or complaint.

Baseline Vital Signs and SAMPLE History

As you know, baseline vital signs provide useful information about the overall functions of the patient's heart and lungs. Remember, if the patient's condition is stable, you should reassess the vital signs every 15 minutes until you reach the emergency department. If the patient is unstable, you should reassess at a minimum of every 5 minutes, or as often as the situation permits. Also obtain a SAMPLE history if possible.

Transport

Your next steps are to provide the necessary emergency medical care addressing the chief complaint and then to provide transport to the emergency department. Remember, the patient's spine should be immobilized if you suspect significant trauma or if there is a mechanism of injury that would make you suspect a spinal injury.

Documentation

Baseline findings during this examination document how the patient looked during your assessment. For all trauma patients, regardless of whether or not the mechanism of injury is significant, your written report should include documentation of the following:

- The skin color, temperature, and moisture
- Initial assessment findings
- Baseline vital signs and subsequent vital signs and SAMPLE history
- The circulation, sensation, and movement in all extremities
- Breath sounds

Other Considerations

Remember, for many patients, you will need to assess the entire body because of the potential severity of their condition. The following patients require a complete rapid trauma assessment, coupled with short scene time and immediate transport to the hospital:

- Any patients who experienced a significant mechanism of injury
- Any patients who are unresponsive or disoriented, since they cannot contribute to the focused history or exam
- Any patients who are extremely intoxicated from drugs or alcohol and cannot reliably contribute to the focused history or exam
- Any patients with a complaint that cannot be identified or clearly understood by using a focused exam should receive a more complete exam

Focused History and Physical Exam: Medical Patients

Evaluate Responsiveness

Early in the assessment process, you need to begin evaluating the patient's problem. In most cases, the patient is alert and able to discuss the problem with you. However, in some cases, the patient may be confused, intoxicated, unable to speak your language, or unconscious. In such a situation, you should immediately proceed to the rapid medical assessment. ▶ **Table 8-11** lists the components of the focused history and physical exam for the medical patient.

History of Illness

The patient's response to general questions such as "What's wrong?" or "What happened?" is the chief complaint (▼ **Figure 8-19**). This response is what drives your assessment of the history of the present illness (focused history) and the physical exam in the medical patient. The chief complaint is the problem that is bothering the patient the most.

If possible, take the time to sit down and help the patient to get comfortable. Now is the time to listen, as you develop an increased understanding of the patient's real condition. Be careful not to jump to conclusions regarding the chief complaint because of what you have

TABLE 8-11 Focused History and Physical Exam: Medical Patients	
Evaluate Responsiveness	
Responsive Patient	**Unresponsive Patient**
History of Illness (OPQRST)	Rapid Medical Assessment
SAMPLE History	Baseline Vital Signs
Focused Physical Exam: Based on Chief Complaint	SAMPLE History
	Reevaluate Transport Decision
Baseline Vital Signs	
Reevaluate Transport	

seen or heard about the patient. In many cases, the chief complaint will not be obvious; it may even be different from what the dispatcher reported. When this occurs, stay flexible. Treat the patient's problem rather than simply reacting to the dispatch report. Nevertheless, the chief complaint represents what is bothering the patient and will help you to focus your history and physical exam. If the patient cannot tell you what is wrong, perhaps because of a language barrier, altered mental status, or severe respiratory difficulty, you may learn the chief complaint from a family member or bystander or from your observations of the scene and patient actions. However, remember that information directly from the patient is far more valuable. You should try, whenever possible, to speak directly to the patient.

As you listen to the patient, you might want to make some brief notes to aid your memory and assist with documentation after the call. You should attempt to record the chief complaint in a few of the patient's own words. Be sure to note if your information comes from someone other than the patient.

OPQRST

As you learn about the chief complaint, you should broaden your knowledge to include the circumstances surrounding the complaint. You can remember the six most important circumstances by using the letters **OPQRST**, which stand for Onset, Provoking Factors, Quality, Radiation, Severity, and Time.

ONSET. The onset refers to when the patient's problem first began. You should ask the patient when the problem first started or when the incident occurred

Figure 8-19 The patient's initial response to the question "What's wrong?" is the chief complaint.

Patient Assessment

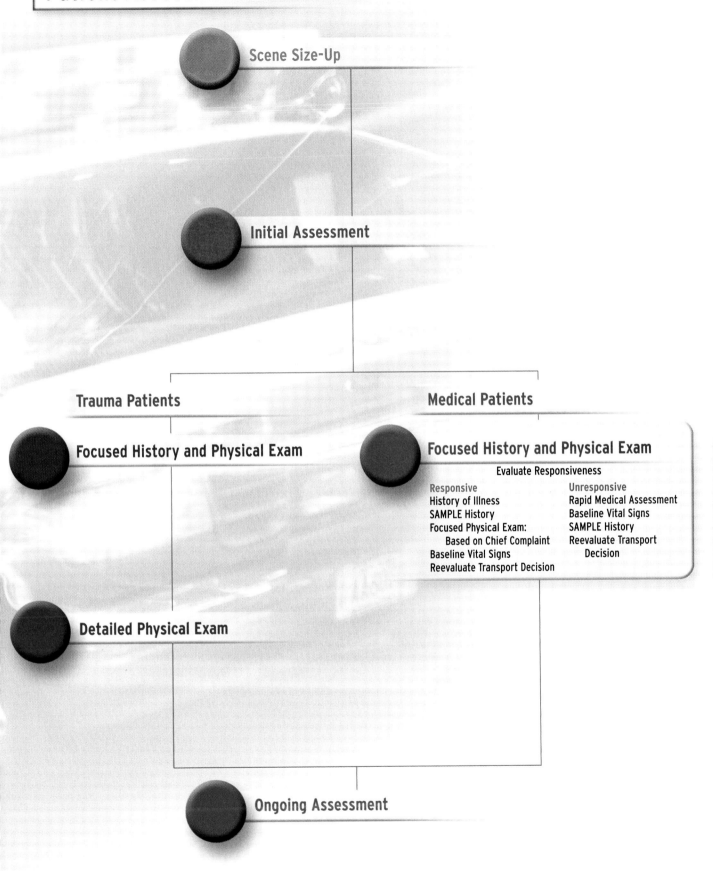

Scene Size-Up

Initial Assessment

Trauma Patients

Focused History and Physical Exam

Medical Patients

Focused History and Physical Exam

Evaluate Responsiveness

Responsive
History of Illness
SAMPLE History
Focused Physical Exam:
    Based on Chief Complaint
Baseline Vital Signs
Reevaluate Transport Decision

Unresponsive
Rapid Medical Assessment
Baseline Vital Signs
SAMPLE History
Reevaluate Transport
    Decision

Detailed Physical Exam

Ongoing Assessment

and how long ago the patient first noticed the problem. If the patient reports that the problem started a long time ago (days or weeks), you should also ask, "What made you finally call now?" In most cases, the patient will note a sudden worsening of the problem or an additional problem that compounded the first one. For example, a patient who has experienced shortness of breath for the past 3 days may have called because of an onset of chest pain an hour ago. You often will not learn about this second problem unless you ask.

For patients with traumatic problems, there may be a delay between when they were hurt and when they called. Again, ask them why they delayed, and what finally caused them to call. The information that they give you may be valuable to you or the hospital staff.

PROVOKING FACTORS. Learning about provoking factors can be extremely helpful in determining the cause and severity of problems. Provoking factors include anything that seems to bring on the problem or that seems to makes the problem better or worse. You should also ask the patient what makes the problem better or worse.

The answer to these questions often helps you to appreciate the potential cause. For instance, shortness of breath that started when the patient climbed a set of stairs may be respiratory or cardiac in origin. However, shortness of breath that started after the patient was struck in the chest by a baseball might be the result of fractured ribs or internal injury. These questions are often the clues to hidden medical problems in traumatic incidents, such as the patient who reports that she fell down the stairs because she felt "really dizzy."

QUALITY OF PAIN. The patient's description of pain may be very useful to hospital staff who are trying to determine the cause. For instance, patients who are having a heart attack classically describe their chest pain as "squeezing" or "pressure," although they may also say things like, "I feel funny," for lack of having a better description. To learn about the quality of pain, ask the patient to describe the pain or explain what the pain feels like to them.

Patients will often initially say, "I don't know," or "It's hard to describe." Once again, the key is for you to be patient. If you wait, most patients will ultimately describe the quality of their pain. Carefully document the patient's own words; these may be very significant to other providers who become involved in the patient's care. Some patients have limited vocabulary when it comes to their bodies; it may be best to let them simply point to their pain, rather than describe it. Ask patients to point to the area of pain, describe the area of pain,

---

Documentation Tips

Your documentation of any pain complaint should include a description in the patient's words, as well as your findings from the other OPQRST questions. Record all pain complaints in detail; not all pain symptoms are "classic"; the exact description may help hospital personnel arrive make the diagnosis in a case that is not typical.

---

or describe pain anywhere else associated with the problem. If the patient still cannot describe the pain, or if the patient cannot speak, you might consider offering several descriptions of pain and letting the patient choose. For instance, you might ask, "Which of these words best describes your pain: Sharp or dull? Burning, stabbing, crushing, or throbbing?"

You can learn a great deal about the patient's problem through these questions. For instance, a patient who points to a single place for his or her pain has what is known as **focal pain** ▶ Figure 8-20A. Many problems, such as fractures or inflammations, are classically focal. However, some patients cannot point to a single location. Instead, they often move their finger around in a circle as they are asked to point to their pain. These patients are experiencing **diffuse pain** ▶ Figure 8-20B. A number of conditions, including heart attack and internal bleeding, are typically diffuse.

RADIATION OF PAIN OR DISCOMFORT. Patients can often provide clues about the cause of their problems by describing the region or location of any pain or discomfort. **Radiation** refers to any additional area where the pain or discomfort may also be present ▶ Figure 8-20C. The presence of radiating pain will not alter your treatment very much; however, physicians and nurses caring for the patient in the hospital may be very interested in hearing about areas of radiation. For example, a patient who is having a heart attack may report chest pain that radiates to the left arm and jaw. Document carefully what you learn.

Be careful how you ask about radiation of pain. Most patients will not understand if you ask, "Does your pain radiate anywhere else?" And asking, "Does your pain go (or travel) anywhere else?" might confuse the patient. After all, who ever heard of pain "traveling"? The best way to ask patients about radiation is to ask, "Do you have pain or discomfort anywhere else?"

SEVERITY. Severity refers to the patient's perception of "how bad" the current incident is in comparison to

Focal pain

Diffuse pain

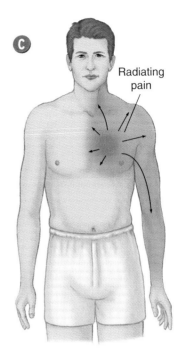

Radiating pain

Figure 8-20   **A.** Focal pain. **B.** Diffuse pain. **C.** Radiating pain.

others. In some cases, particularly when the patient has experienced the problem before, his or her perception provides extremely useful information. For example, a patient with asthma may be very helpful by comparing this episode with other previous asthma attacks. However, if the problem has never occurred, the patient's perception may not be very useful except as a guide to whether it is getting worse or better during transport. To assess severity, you may ask the following questions:

- "How bad is this episode in comparison to previous ones?" (if the problem is chronic or recurring).

- "What happened the last time you had an episode this bad?" (if the problem is chronic or recurring).

- "How would you rate this problem in numbers, if 1 is normal and 10 is the worst pain or discomfort you can imagine?"

For patients with chronic problems, obtaining the answer to the question "What happened the last time you had an episode this bad?" is invaluable. In most cases, patients have been found to be very accurate in their self-assessments of severity. For instance, a patient with asthma might tell you that the last time he had an attack this bad, he was in the hospital for 2 weeks. The patient's comments tell you that this episode is extremely serious and that you should complete your assessment and provide immediate transport. At the other extreme, the patient might tell you that he was kept in the emer-

gency department for about an hour and then discharged. Obviously, these two episodes are very different in urgency, and you can adjust your plans for treatment and transport accordingly.

Another way to evaluate changes in the patient's condition during your treatment and transport is to use a numeric scoring system. For example, a patient with an apparent broken leg might initially tell you that the pain is an 8 on a scale of 1 to 10. After you splint the leg and begin transport, you should recheck the patient's perception. If the pain is now a 9, you might consider changing the position of the leg or using an ice pack. However, if the pain level is now reportedly a 5, you know that the treatment is effective, at least for now. Remember, patients perceive pain in different ways, so it is inappropriate to compare one patient's numeric score with another patient's score.

TIME. The final set of questions provides information about when the problem began and if the patient has experienced the problem on other occasions. You might want to find out whether the problem has been constant or intermittent. If the patient states that the problem is intermittent, ask about what seemed to make it better or worse.

The answers to these questions will further help you and other health professionals involved with the patient's care to understand the nature of the problem. Some conditions, such as those involving abdominal organs, have classically intermittent pain. Other problems, such as fractures, typically have constant pain.

Remember

Common Chief Complaints and Focused Physical Exams

- Chest pain. Evaluate skin, pulse, and blood pressure. Look for trauma to the chest, and listen to breath sounds.

- Abdominal pain. Evaluate skin, pulse, and blood pressure. Look for trauma to the abdomen, and palpate the abdomen to identify any tender spots.

- Shortness of breath. Evaluate skin, pulse, blood pressure, and rate and depth of respirations. Assess for airway obstruction. Listen carefully to breath sounds.

- Dizziness. Evaluate skin, pulse, blood pressure, and adequacy of respirations. Monitor the level of consciousness and orientation carefully. Check the head for signs of trauma.

- Any pain associated with bones or joints. Evaluate skin, pulse, movement, and sensation adjacent and distal to the affected area.

The SAMPLE History

Once you have obtained a clearer picture of the patient's chief complaint and have explored it using the OPQRST questions, you should obtain a SAMPLE history. Recall that the purpose of this history is to gather information about the patient's past medical experiences. The elements of the SAMPLE history are repeated below for your review.

- **S**igns and Symptoms of the episode

- **A**llergies, particularly to medications

- **M**edications, including prescription, over-the-counter, and recreational (illicit) drugs

- **P**ast medical history, particularly involving similar episodes in the past

- **L**ast oral intake, including food and/or drinks. This is particularly important if the patient may need surgery.

- **E**vents leading up to the episode.

Be sure to ask whether the patient has any other problems that you should know about. This question is useful in that it provides the patient with an opportunity to tell you something about apparently unrelated previous medical problems. In most cases, this will serve as useful background information. Occasionally, it will provide you and hospital staff with essential information,

such as when you discovered that the patient who fell for no apparent reason has a history of diabetes. This information suggests the possibility that the fall was caused by a complication of the diabetes.

No matter what you have learned about the patient's past history, you need to be aware of certain medical problems that the patient may have forgotten to mention. These conditions might help to explain the current episode or could affect your treatment decisions or those made by ALS or at the hospital. As you conclude the SAMPLE history, ask the patient the following questions:

1. "Have you ever been told that you have a heart condition?"

2. "Have you ever been told that you have asthma, emphysema, or any other problems with your lungs?"

3. "Have you ever been told that you have seizures?"

These three questions will prevent you from missing important, potentially life-threatening cardiac, respiratory, or neurologic conditions. If the patient answers "yes" to any of these three questions, reevaluate the chief complaint in light of this new information. If you have time, return to the history questions to learn more about the nature of the problem.

The Focused Physical Exam

Now that you have learned about the chief complaint, using OPQRST, and have obtained a thorough history, you should perform a focused exam.

The key to this examination is to emphasize the priorities that you learned during the history. Be logical, and investigate problems that you identified during the initial assessment and focused history.

CHIEF COMPLAINT. Once you know that the ABCs are stable, move to the patient's chief complaint. Remember to assess the following chief complaints carefully, as described previously:

- **Chest pain.** Evaluate the skin color, pulse, and blood pressure. Look for trauma to the chest, and consider listening to the breath sounds.

- **Shortness of breath.** Evaluate the skin color, pulse, blood pressure, and rate and depth of respirations. Look for airway obstruction, as well as trauma to the neck and chest. Listen carefully to the breath sounds.

- **Abdominal pain.** Evaluate the skin color, pulse, and blood pressure. Look for trauma to the abdomen, and palpate the abdomen to identify any particularly tender spots.

- **Any pain associated with bones or joints.** Evaluate the skin color, movement, and sensation adjacent to and below the affected area.
- **Dizziness.** Evaluate the skin color, pulse, blood pressure, and adequacy of respirations. Monitor the level of consciousness and orientation carefully. Check the head for signs of trauma.

ABNORMALITIES. Next, examine anything that has a noticeable abnormality. Sometimes, during the initial assessment and focused history, you will see something that is obviously abnormal. It may be a laceration, a deformed bone, a weakness on one side, abnormal eyes, or some other abnormality. Avoid being distracted by these conditions; it is easy to let a big cut or deformity draw your attention away from more important, potentially life-threatening problems.

However, once you have evaluated and treated life-threatening conditions and have examined chief complaints, you can come back to these. Be sure to ask the patient questions about the abnormality while you are evaluating it. Remember that deformities or abnormalities may be long-term and unrelated to the patient's present condition. For example, a patient who has had a stroke may have a weakness on one side for months after the stroke; it is not a new problem, and it is not likely to be related to the patient's current call for EMS.

Baseline Vital Signs

As you know, baseline vital signs provide useful information about the overall functions of the patient's heart and lungs. Remember that if the patient's condition is stable, you should reassess the vital signs every 15 minutes until you reach the emergency department. If the patient is unstable, you should reassess at a minimum of every 5 minutes, or as often as the situation permits.

Reevaluate Transport Decision

Your next steps are to provide the necessary emergency medical care addressing the chief complaint and then to re-evaluate your transport decision.

Documentation

Documenting your assessment findings helps identify and track trends in the patient's condition and to help hospital staff provide definitive treatment. Your report for the responsive medical patient should include documentation of the following:

- The skin color, temperature, and moisture
- Findings from the initial assessment
- Baseline vital signs (pulse, blood pressure, respirations, temperature) and SAMPLE history
- The sensation and movement in all extremities
- Breath sounds

Evaluate the Unresponsive Patient

Sometimes, new EMT-Bs ask how to assess the chief complaint and history in an unresponsive patient (▼ **Figure 8-21**). The answer is simple: In many cases, you cannot.

With unresponsive patients, you never get to that part of the focused history and physical exam. Instead, you should focus your attention on opening and maintaining the airway, immobilizing the spine, assisting with ventilations, administering supplemental oxygen, controlling bleeding, providing CPR if necessary, and providing immediate transport to an appropriate facility. These priorities reflect the importance of the ABC approach to the initial assessment.

If you have successfully stabilized the ABCs, you ask chief complaint and SAMPLE history questions of a family member or bystander while en route to the hospital. Never delay transport of a critical patient to take a history from family members (or from the patient, for that matter) at the scene.

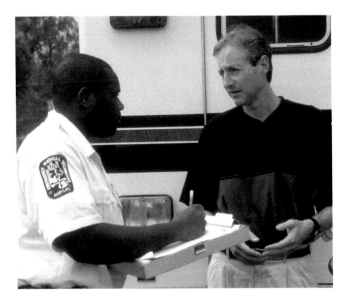

Figure 8-21 If the patient is unresponsive, obtain the chief complaint and any other pertinent history from family members or bystanders.

SkillDrill 8-2 Performing a Rapid Medical Assessment: Unresponsive Patient

Assess the head.

Assess the neck.

Assess the chest.

Assess the abdomen.

Assess the pelvis.

Assess the extremities.

Assess the back.

Rapid Medical Assessment

If you have successfully stabilized the ABCs on any patient who is unconscious, confused, or unable to relate the chief complaint adequately, you should perform a rapid assessment, using the mnemonic "DCAP-BTLS" and following the order of the rapid trauma assessment. The purpose of the rapid medical assessment is to identify existing or potentially life-threatening conditions quickly. Follow the brief sequence of assessment steps shown in ◀ **Skill Drill 8-2** :

1. **Assess the head** for DCAP-BTLS and crepitus **(Step 1)**.

2. **Assess the neck** for DCAP-BTLS, jugular vein distention, and crepitus **(Step 2)**.

3. **Assess the chest** for DCAP-BTLS, paradoxical motion, and crepitus **(Step 3)**.

4. **Assess the abdomen** for DCAP-BTLS, rigidity, and distention **(Step 4)**.

5. **Assess the pelvis** for DCAP-BTLS **(Step 5)**.

6. **Assess all four extremities** for DCAP-BTLS **(Step 6)**.

7. **Assess the back** for DCAP-BTLS **(Step 7)**.

Baseline Vital Signs

Baseline vital signs should be obtained after this exam to provide information for assessing trends in patient conditions. Remember, if the patient's condition is stable, you should reassess the vital signs every 15 minutes until you reach the emergency department. If the patient is unstable, you should reassess at a minimum of every 5 minutes, or as often as the situation permits, looking for trends in the patient's condition.

History of Illness/SAMPLE History

As previously stated, determining the history of the illness and the SAMPLE history is not easy with an unresponsive patient, because your best source of information (the patient) cannot speak to you. But you can still rely somewhat on witnesses, such as family members who were present at the time the victim became unresponsive.

Family members are normally aware of medical conditions such as diabetes, seizure, stroke, heart disease, or respiratory disease. Family members may also be able to provide information relative to the SAMPLE history. For example, they may be able to describe the signs and symptoms the patient had before becoming unresponsive. A family member is also likely to know if the patient has any allergies, is using any medication, or has experienced previous similar incidents. A family member caring for an elder can identify the last time the patient had a meal, as well as events leading up to the loss of consciousness.

Bystanders, especially family members, who are with the patient prior to the time that he or she becomes unresponsive can provide some valuable information. For example, a family member may be able to tell you that the patient has type I diabetes and has taken his insulin, but has also been ill for the past 24 hours, has vomited, and has not eaten normally. The family member may also be able to describe signs of lethargy, confusion, and pale, moist skin that the patient exhibited before losing consciousness.

Re-evaluate Transport Decision

Your next steps are to provide the necessary emergency medical care and then to provide transport to the emergency department. Remember, the patient's spine should be immobilized if you suspect significant trauma or if there is a mechanism of injury that would make you suspect a spinal injury.

Documentation

Documenting your baseline findings during this examination is important to track trends in the patient's condition and to help hospital staff provide definitive treatment. Your report for the unresponsive medical patient should include documentation of the following:

- The skin color, temperature, and moisture

- Findings from the initial assessment

- Baseline vital signs (pulse, blood pressure, respirations, temperature) and SAMPLE history (from bystanders)

- Breath sounds

Detailed Physical Exam

Recall that the assessment process began with anticipation and hazard preparation when you received the dispatch information and performed the scene size-up. Then you performed the initial assessment, in which you identified and treated life-threatening conditions. If trauma was a factor in your patient's situation, you also initiated spinal immobilization. When indicated, you followed up on the initial assessment by performing a focused history and a rapid assessment. You also provided transport if your patient had an obvious life-threatening condition. On the basis of what you learned from the history, you assessed selected areas of the patient's body. You have also taken at least one set of vital signs.

At this point, in most cases you are already en route to the hospital. If you are still on the scene, it is because the patient does not have any life-threatening conditions and you have not found the cause for the patient's complaints. In the case of a trauma patient with a significant mechanism of injury, you are en route but may still have unanswered questions. In either case, this is the time to perform the detailed physical exam. (▲ **Table 8-12**) lists the components of the Detailed Physical Exam. The goals of this exam are to further explore problems that were identified during the focused history and physical exam and to possibly identify the cause of complaints that were not identified during the focused history and physical exam. In most cases, it is the trauma patient with a significant mechanism of injury who receives the detailed exam, because getting the patient to a hospital took priority over performing a detailed exam at the scene.

To achieve the goals of the **detailed physical exam**, you must simply ask and answer one question: "What additional problems can be identified through a detailed physical exam?" The detailed physical exam will provide you with more information about the nature of the patient's problem. Depending on what is learned, you should be prepared to do the following:

- Return to the initial assessment if a potentially life-threatening condition is identified. (This is unlikely this late in the exam, but it is always possible. Remember, stay focused on the ABCs.)

- Perform spinal immobilization if neck or back pain or abnormality in sensation or movement is identified. (Again, this is unlikely this late in the exam.)

Table 8-12 Detailed Physical Exam
Detailed Physical Exam using DCAP-BTLS
Baseline Vital Signs

- Modify any treatment that is under way on the basis of any new information.

- Provide treatment for problems that were identified during the exam.

- Provide transport to an appropriate facility, or call for ALS backup.

The detailed physical exam is a more in-depth examination that builds on the focused physical exam. The patient and the particular injury will determine the need for this exam. Many of your patients will not receive a detailed physical exam, either because it will be irrelevant or unnecessary or because it is not possible given the time constraints.

Most patients have isolated problems that can be adequately evaluated earlier in the assessment process. You will identify the problem and treat it, making a more detailed physical exam of the entire body unnecessary. If you do perform a detailed physical exam in these patients, it will be to further explore what you learned during the rapid assessment.

A few patients will have life-threatening conditions that were identified during the initial assessment. You may spend all of your time with these patients, stabilizing ABCs, which means you will never have a chance to perform a detailed assessment.

You will perform a detailed exam only on stable patients with problems that cannot be identified earlier in the patient assessment process. In most cases, these patients have extremely minor, obscure, or isolated problems, which is why you did not identify them earlier. Regardless of the exact situation, the detailed physical exam is usually performed en route to the hospital, since you could literally spend hours on the scene trying to identify these problems.

Steps of the Detailed Physical Exam

Here, organized by body region, are some additional assessments that you might want to perform during the detailed exam. As you evaluate each region, visualize and palpate to find evidence of signs of injury, again

Patient Assessment

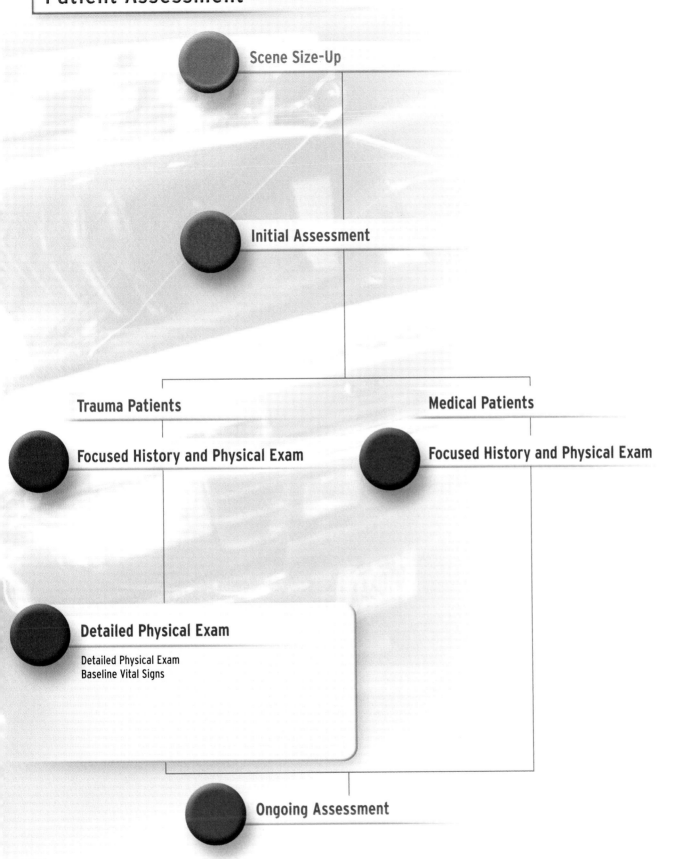

Scene Size-Up

Initial Assessment

Trauma Patients

Focused History and Physical Exam

Medical Patients

Focused History and Physical Exam

Detailed Physical Exam

Detailed Physical Exam
Baseline Vital Signs

Ongoing Assessment

using the mnemonic "DCAP-BTLS." Follow the steps in
▶ **Skill Drill 8-3**):

1. **Look at the face** for obvious lacerations, bruises, or deformities **(Step 1)**.

2. **Inspect the area around the eyes and eyelids** **(Step 2)**.

3. **Examine the eyes** for redness and for contact lenses. Assess the pupils using a penlight **(Step 3)**.

4. **Pull the patient's ear forward** to assess for bruising (Battle's sign) **(Step 4)**.

5. **Use the penlight to look for drainage** or blood in the ears **(Step 5)**.

6. **Look for bruising and lacerations about the head.** Palpate for tenderness, depressions of the skull, and deformities **(Step 6)**.

7. **Palpate the zygomas** for tenderness or instability **(Step 7)**.

8. **Palpate the maxillae (Step 8)**.

9. **Palpate the mandible (Step 9)**.

10. **Assess the mouth for obstructions,** foreign bodies (including loose teeth or dentures), bleeding, lacerations, or deformities and cyanosis **(Step 10)**.

11. **Check for unusual odors** on the patient's breath **(Step 11)**.

12. **Look at the neck** for obvious lacerations, bruises, and deformities **(Step 12)**.

13. **Palpate the front and the back of the neck** for tenderness and deformity **(Step 13)**.

14. **Look for distended jugular veins.** Note that distended neck veins are not necessarily significant in a patient who is lying down **(Step 14)**.

15. **Look at the chest** for obvious signs of injury before you begin palpation. Be sure to watch for movement of the chest with respirations **(Step 15)**.

16. **Gently palpate over the ribs** to elicit tenderness. Avoid pressing over obvious bruises or suspected rib fractures **(Step 16)**.

17. **Listen for breath sounds** over the midaxillary and midclavicular lines **(Step 17)**.

18. **Listen also at the bases and apices of the lungs** **(Step 18)**.

19. **Look at the abdomen and pelvis** for obvious lacerations, bruises, and deformities **(Step 19)**.

20. **Gently palpate the abdomen** for tenderness. If the abdomen is unusually tense, you should describe the abdomen as rigid **(Step 20)**.

21. **Gently compress the pelvis** from the sides to assess for tenderness **(Step 21)**.

22. **Gently press the iliac crests** to elicit instability, tenderness, or crepitus **(Step 22)**.

23. **Inspect all four extremities** for DCAP-BTLS, and medic alert anklets or bracelets. Also assess distal pulses and motor and sensory function in all extremities **(Step 23)**.

24. **Assess the back for tenderness or deformities.** Remember, if you suspect a spinal cord injury, use spinal precautions as you log roll the patient **(Step 24)**.

Head, Neck, and Cervical Spine

A more detailed exam of these areas could include a careful check of the head, face, scalp, ears, eyes, nose, and mouth for abrasions, lacerations, and contusions. Examine the eyes and eyelids, checking for redness and for contact lenses. Use a penlight to check whether the pupils are equal and reactive, and look for any fluid drainage or blood, particularly around the ears and nose. Also check for foreign objects and/or blood in the anterior chamber of the eye. Look for bruising or discoloration around the eyes (raccoon eyes) or behind the ears (Battle's sign); these signs may be associated with head trauma.

Next, palpate gently but firmly around the face, scalp, eyes, ears, and nose for tenderness, deformity, or instability. Tenderness or abnormal movement of bones often signals a serious injury and may cause upper airway obstruction. Monitor the airway carefully in these patients. Look and feel inside the mouth next. Loose or broken teeth or a foreign object may block the airway. Remember, be cautious when inserting your fingers into a patient's mouth. It's much safer if a bite block is used. You should also look for lacerations, swelling, bleeding, and any discoloration in the mouth and the tongue. Smell the patient's breath. Any unusual odors, such as a strong alcohol odor or fruity breath odor, should be reported and recorded.

Palpate the front and back of the neck for tenderness and deformity. The sensation of crackling or popping, not unlike palpating the bubbles in bubble-pack packing material, is called subcutaneous emphysema; it indicates that air is leaking into the space under the skin. Usually, this means that the patient has a pneumothorax or has damaged the larynx. Also look for

SkillDrill 8-3   Performing the Detailed Physical Exam

Observe the face.

Inspect the eyelids and the area around the eyes.

Examine the eyes for redness, contact lenses. Check pupil function.

Look behind the ear for Battle's sign.

Check the ears for drainage or blood.

Observe and palpate the head.

Palpate the zygomas.

Palpate the maxillae.

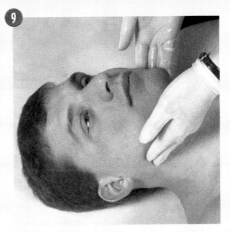

Palpate the mandible.

Continued.

Skill Drill 8-3   Performing the Detailed Physical Exam—continued.

10 Assess the mouth.

11 Check for unusual breath odors.

12 Inspect the neck.

13 Palpate the neck, front and back.

14 Observe for jugular vein distention.

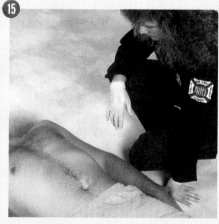

15 Inspect the chest and observe breathing motion.

16 Gently palpate the ribs.

17 Listen to anterior breath sounds (midaxillary, midclavicular).

18 Listen to posterior breath sounds (bases, apices).

Skill Drill 8-3 Performing the Detailed Physical Exam—continued.

Observe the abdomen and pelvis.

Gently palpate the abdomen.

Gently compress the pelvis from the sides.

Gently press the iliac crests.

Inspect the extremities; assess distal circulation and motor sensory function.

Log roll the patient and inspect the back.

distended jugular veins. This is normal in a patient who is lying down; however, their presence in the patient who is sitting up may suggest some type of condition related to the heart.

Chest

Throughout the patient assessment process, you should monitor the patient's breathing. If you have not already done so, you should carefully palpate the patient's chest. Feel for crepitus, as this occurs with a ruptured airway, pneumothorax, or rib fractures. Also evaluate the movement of the chest wall during breathing. Paradoxical motion of the chest wall means that your patient has a flail chest and might need supplemental oxygen and/or assisted ventilation. You might also wish to perform a more detailed evaluation of the patient's breath sounds. Listening at the apices, at the midclavicular lines bilater-

ally, at the bases, and at the midaxillary lines bilaterally, check for the specific sounds of breathing. You may be able to identify one of the following:

- Normal breath sounds. These are clear and quiet on both inspiration and expiration.

- Wheezing breath sounds. These suggest an obstruction of the lower airways. Wheezing is a high-pitched squeal that is most prominent on expiration.

- Wet breath sounds. These may indicate cardiac failure. A moist crackling, usually on both inspiration and expiration, is called <u>rales</u>, or crackles.

- Congested breath sounds. These may suggest the presence of mucus in the lungs. Expect to hear a low-pitched, noisy sound that is most prominent on expiration. This sound may be referred to as <u>rhonchi</u>, or "low wheezing." The patient often reports a productive cough associated with this sound.

- A crowing sound. This is often heard without a stethoscope and may indicate that the patient has an airway obstruction in the neck or upper part of the chest. Expect to hear a brassy, crowing sound that is most prominent on expiration. This sound may be referred to as **stridor**.

Abdomen

During the detailed physical exam, you may perform a more complete examination of the abdomen. As you feel all around the abdomen, use the terms firm, soft, tender, or distended (swollen) to report your findings. Some patients may tense the abdomen as you feel it.

Pelvis

If you have not previously identified any pelvic injury, recheck the pelvis to identify pain, tenderness, instability, and crepitus; all may indicate a fractured pelvis and the potential for shock.

Extremities

If you have not already done so, you should carefully evaluate the extremities for any signs of trauma, again using the DCAP-BTLS method. You should also evaluate the distal circulation, sensation, and movement. If you have already identified an injury, regular evaluation of the circulation, sensation, and movement below the injury will allow you to be sure that the injury has not compromised neurovascular status.

Back

During the rapid assessment, if performed, you should have visualized and palpated the patient's back for signs of trauma, especially near the spine. You must use spinal precautions when logrolling the patient for assessment of back injuries. The presence of spinal deformity or pain suggests that—if you have not already done so—the patient requires spinal immobilization. Look for and document any other conditions that you find on the back.

Baseline Vital Signs

Sometimes, you will be so busy establishing and maintaining the ABCs that you will not have a chance to get the patient's vital signs. That is as it should be. Nothing should take priority over the airway, breathing, and circulation. However, whenever possible, it is important to get a set of baseline vitals at some time during your patient encounter. If you have not assessed the vital signs, now is the time.

Ongoing Assessment

Unlike the detailed physical exam, the **ongoing assessment** is performed on all patients during transport. Its purpose is to ask and answer the following questions:

- Is treatment improving the patient's condition?
- Has an already identified problem gotten better? Worse?
- What is the nature of any newly identified problems?

The ongoing assessment helps you to monitor changes in the patient's condition. If the changes are improvements, simply continue whatever treatment you are providing. However, in some instances, the patient's condition will deteriorate. When this happens, you should be prepared to modify treatment as appropriate and then begin new treatment on the basis of the problem identified. (▼ **Table 8-13**) lists the components of the Ongoing Assessment.

Steps of the Ongoing Assessment

The procedure for the ongoing assessment is simply to repeat the initial assessment and the focused assessment and to check the intervention steps that pertain to the problems you are treating. These steps should be repeated and recorded every 15 minutes for a stable patient and every 5 minutes for an unstable patient (▶ **Figure 8-22**). Remember to use your judgment when timing the ongoing assessments. Some patients may require more frequent assessments.

The steps of the ongoing assessment are as follows:

1. Repeat the initial assessment.

- Reassess mental status.
- Maintain an open airway.
- Monitor the patient's breathing.

TABLE 8-13 Ongoing Assessment
Repeat the Initial Assessment
Reassess Vital Signs
Repeat Focused Assessment
Check Interventions

Patient Assessment

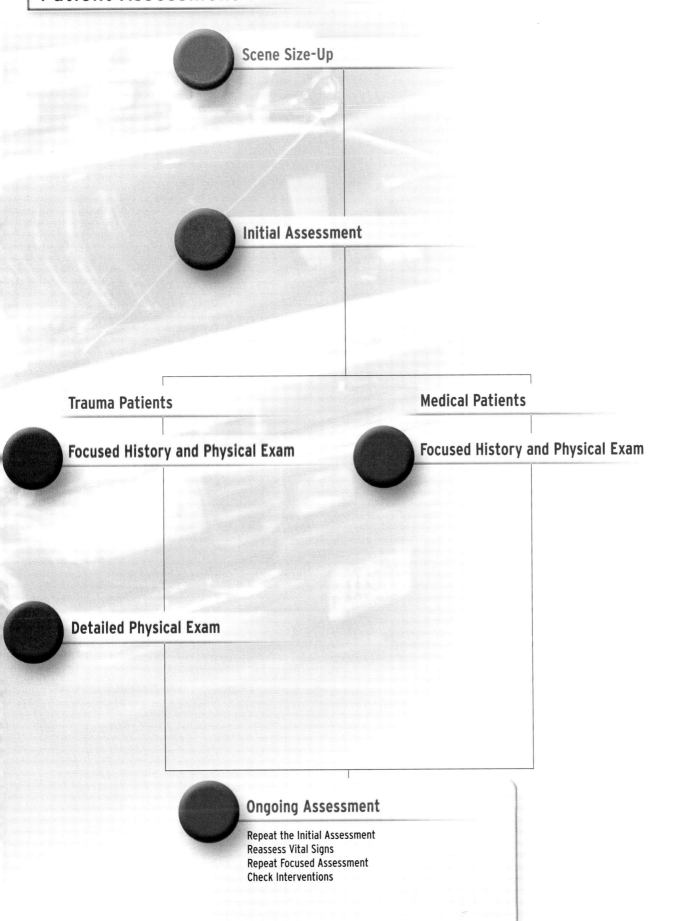

Scene Size-Up

Initial Assessment

Trauma Patients

Focused History and Physical Exam

Medical Patients

Focused History and Physical Exam

Detailed Physical Exam

Ongoing Assessment

Repeat the Initial Assessment
Reassess Vital Signs
Repeat Focused Assessment
Check Interventions

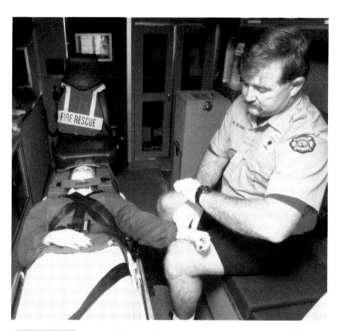

Figure 8-22 During the ongoing assessment, repeat your initial assessment, recheck vital signs, and recheck interventions every 5 minutes if the patient is unstable and every 15 minutes if the patient is stable.

- Reassess pulse rate and quality.

- Monitor skin color and temperature.

- Reestablish patient priorities.

2. Reassess and record vital signs.

3. Repeat your focused assessment regarding patient complaint or injuries, including questions about the patient's history.

4. Check interventions.

- Ensure adequacy of oxygen delivery/artificial ventilation.

- Ensure management of bleeding.

- Ensure adequacy of other interventions.

Repeat the Initial Assessment

The first step is to repeat the initial assessment. If you have been treating the ABCs, you need to continue monitoring these essential functions. It is particularly important to reassess mental status; changes can be initially subtle and then rapidly decline.

Reevaluate any conditions that you have been treating. Reassess the patient's skin color, wound, or anything for which you have begun treatment. If the patient's condition remains stable, great. But, you may discover a need to change a dressing, tighten a strap, or turn up the oxygen. Do it now.

Reassess Vital Signs

Be sure that the patient's vital signs have not changed. Record these so that your documentation is accurate and complete. If the vital signs have changed, evaluate what may have happened and what you should do about it.

Repeat Focused Assessment

As you transport your patient, remember to ask the patient about the chief complaint. Is the chest pain getting better or worse? Is leg pain improving with treatment or staying about the same? If you asked the patient to rate symptoms on a 1 to 10 scale, ask for another rating.

Check Interventions

Reevaluate any interventions you started. Take a moment to make certain that the oxygen is still flowing, that the backboard straps are still tight, that the bleeding has been controlled, and that the airway is still open. Things often change in the uncontrolled prehospital environment, so this is a good time to be sure that your treatments are still "working" the way you expect.

Becoming An Expert

You may notice at times that experienced EMT-Bs and paramedics seem to have a "sixth sense" when it comes to some patients. They seem to be able to recognize severe problems even before they have completed their initial assessment. This clinical intuition is one of the hallmarks of the expert EMT that you can develop as you progress through your career-if you pay attention and work at it.

The aspects of clinical intuition include the following:

- The ability to recognize patterns. Intuitive EMTs immediately recognize clinical patterns that they have seen before. For example, you may immediately recognize that a pale, diaphoretic patient looks like another patient you have seen in severe shock.

- Common sense understanding. Experienced, intuitive EMTs who use their knowledge and experience also use common sense in their assessment and treatment. For instance, they refrain from starting CPR on a responsive patient even though they cannot feel a pulse.

- The ability to sense what is important. Good EMTs know how to track problems that are truly important. They avoid the tendency to get lost in unimportant problems and stay focused on the ones that truly matter. For instance, a forehead laceration will not distract them from the serious cardiac problem that caused a fall.

- Deliberate rationally. Good EMTs use their intuition to help them make decisions, but they always temper it by asking, "What if I'm wrong?" For example, a patient who was in a serious motor vehicle crash but has no complaints and appears normal is probably fine. An experienced EMT-B might believe that the patient has no serious injuries and probably does not require spinal immobilization. However, the answer to the question "What if I'm wrong?" could be "Disastrous: permanent spinal cord injury and paralysis." The experienced EMT-B decides to immobilize.

How can you improve your own intuitive powers? First, you need some experience. The truth is that you will not become intuitive until you have been involved in patient care for some time and have evaluated and treated a number of patients.

By following a systematic approach to patient assessment, using your intuition and common sense, and really listening to the patient, you will learn to make good decisions about the treatment and transport of the many patients you will care for in your career.

Prep Kit

Ready for Review

The assessment process begins with the scene size-up, which identifies real or potential hazards. The patient should not be approached until these hazards have been dealt with in a way that eliminates or minimizes risk to both the EMTs and the patient(s).

The initial assessment is performed on all patients. It identifies any life-threatening conditions to the airway, breathing, and circulation (ABCs). Any life threats identified must be treated before moving to the next step of the assessment.

The rapid assessment is performed quickly on any patient who is unconscious or unable to articulate the nature of the problem to identify injuries or illnesses. When injuries and conditions are found, they should be prioritized and treated as appropriate.

The focused history and physical exam are performed on all patients once their ABCs are stabilized. The focused history and physical exam identify potentially life-threatening conditions and help you to identify and explore the patient's chief complaint. In most cases, the focused history and physical exam will provide adequate information to enable you to initiate treatment.

The detailed physical exam is performed on a select group of patients. It helps you to further understand problems that were identified during the focused exam and may also be used to evaluate problems that cannot be identified using the focused exam. The detailed physical exam should be performed en route to the hospital.

The ongoing assessment is also performed on all patients. It gives you an opportunity to reevaluate problems that are being treated and to recheck treatments to be sure that they are still being delivered correctly. Information from the ongoing assessment may be used to change treatment plans.

As you can see, the assessment process is both systematic and dynamic. All patients will be evaluated by using these same steps. However, because of the ability of the focused history and physical exam to center your actions on the major problems, each of your assessments will be slightly different, depending on the needs of the patient. The result will be a process that will enable you to quickly identify and treat the needs of all patients, both medical and traumatic, in a way that meets their unique needs.

Points to Ponder

You are dispatched to an unconscious woman at a downtown park, known to be a collection site for homeless people. When you arrive there are a few people standing around that point to the woman. When you ask what happened you are told that someone "beat her up." The woman is lying face down, is quite dirty and smells of body odor, vomit, and urine. When you shake her gently she moans but does not awaken. You reach under her head to see if you can feel her breathing and find that she has vomited. How would this situation affect your patient assessment? Would you be as thorough? Would you trust medical history information from these bystanders?

Issues Patient Respect, Personal Biases and Prejudices, Thorough and Consistent Patient Assessment.

Online Outlook

During the initial assessment (ABCs), life-threatening conditions are identified and their management is begun. You can learn more about the initial assessment by following the Trauma Assessment link at **www.emtb.com**.

Vital Vocabulary

accessory muscles The secondary muscles of respiration.

AVPU A method of assessing a patient's level of consciousness by determining whether a patient is Awake and alert, responsive to Verbal stimulus or Pain, or Unresponsive; used principally in the initial assessment.

blunt trauma A mechanism of injury in which force occurs over a broad area and the skin is not usually broken.

body substance isolation (BSI) An infection control concept and practice that assumes that all body fluids are potentially infectious.

breath sounds An indication of air movement in the lungs, usually assessed with a stethoscope.

capillary refill A test that evaluates distal circulatory system function by squeezing (blanching) blood from an area such as a nail bed and watching the speed of its return after releasing the pressure.

chief complaint The reason a patient called for help; also, the patient's response to general questions such as "What's wrong?" or "What happened?"

coagulate To form a clot to plug an opening in an injured blood vessels and stop blood flow.

conjunctiva The delicate membrane that lines the eyelids and covers the exposed surface of the eye.

crepitus A grating or grinding sensation caused by fractured bone ends or joints rubbing together; also air bubbles under the skin that produce a crackling sound or crinkly feeling.

cyanosis Bluish-gray skin color that is caused by reduced oxygen levels in the blood.

DCAP-BTLS A mnemonic for assessment in which each area of the body is evaluated for Deformities, Contusions, Abrasions, Punctures/Penetrations, Burns, Tenderness, Lacerations, and Swelling.

detailed physical exam The part of the assessment process in which a detailed area-by-area exam is performed on patients whose problems cannot be readily identified or when more specific information is needed about problems identified in the focused history and physical exam.

diffuse pain Pain that is not identified as being specific to a single location.

entrance wound The area of the body where a penetrating trauma occurs. In knife or gunshot wounds, this would be the area where the bullet or blade entered. Also seen in serious electrical injuries.

exit wound The area of the body where a penetrating trauma exited. In gunshot wounds, this would be the area where the bullet exited.

focal pain Pain that is easily identified as being specific to a single location.

focused history and physical exam The part of the assessment process in which the patient's major complaints or any problems that are immediately evident are further and more specifically evaluated.

frostbite Damage to tissues as the result of exposure to cold; frozen or partially frozen body parts.

general impression The overall initial impression that determines the priority for patient care; based on the patient's surroundings, the mechanism of injury, signs and symptoms, and the chief complaint.

Golden Hour The time from injury to definitive care, during which treatment of shock or traumatic injuries should occur because survival potential is the best.

hypothermia A condition in which the internal body temperature falls below 95°F (35°C) after exposure to a cold environment.

initial assessment The part of the assessment process that helps you to identify any immediately or potentially life-threatening conditions so that you can initiate lifesaving care.

jaundice A yellow skin color that is seen in patients with liver disease or dysfunction.

mechanism of injury The way in which traumatic injuries occur; the forces that act on the body to cause damage.

nasal flaring Flaring out of the nostrils, indicating that there is an airway obstruction.

nature of illness Effort to determine the general type of illness.

ongoing assessment The part of the assessment process in which problems are reevaluated and responses to treatment are assessed.

orientation The mental status of a patient as measured by memory of person (name), place (current location), time (current year, month, and approximate date), and event (what happened).

OPQRST The six pain questions: Onset, Provoking factors, Quality, Radiation, Severity, Time.

palpate Examine by touch.

paradoxical motion The motion of the chest wall that is detached in a flail chest; the motion is exactly the opposite of normal motion during breathing: in during inhalation, out during exhalation.

penetrating trauma A mechanism of injury in which force occurs in a small point of contact between the skin and the object. The skin is broken and the potential for infection is high.

radiation A continuation of an area of pain or discomfort distal to the site of the origin of the pain; gives the sensation that the pain is moving (radiating) away from the origin.

rales Cracking, rattling breath sound that signals fluid in the air spaces of the lungs; also called crackles.

responsiveness The way in which a patient responds to external stimuli, including verbal stimuli (sound), tactile stimuli (touch), and painful stimuli.

retractions Movements in which the skin pulls in around the ribs during inspiration.

rhonchi Coarse, low-pitched breath sounds heard in patients with chronic mucus in the airways.

SAMPLE history A key brief history of a patient's condition to determine Signs/Symptoms, Allergies, Medications, Pertinent past history, Last oral intake, and Events leading to the illness/injury.

scene size-up A quick assessment of the scene and the surroundings made to provide information about its safety and the mechanism of injury or nature of illness, before you enter and begin patient care.

sclera The white portion of the eye; the tough outer coat that gives protection to the delicate, light-sensitive, inner layer.

stridor A harsh, high-pitched inspiratory sound that is often heard in acute laryngeal (upper airway) obstruction; may sound like crowing and be audible without a stethoscope.

subcutaneous emphysema The presence of air in soft tissues, causing a characteristic crackling sensation on palpation.

triage The process of establishing treatment and transportation priorities according to severity of injury and medical need.

two- to three-word dyspnea A severe breathing problem in which a patient can speak only two to three words at a time without pausing to take a breath.

www.emtb.com

Assessment in Action

You and your partner are dispatched with an Engine Company to a fire at a residence. Firefighters take only minutes to isolate the fire in the kitchen and put it out. Firefighters tell you a frying pan full of grease caught fire spreading up the wall to the cupboards. Your patient is a female, in her early 20s. She was found on the floor of the kitchen and brought immediately to you. She responds only by moaning when you pinch her fingers. Her pupils are dilated and barely reactive. Her face is pale with soot present. Her skin feels warm and moist but her lips are gray. You note burns on her hands and lower arms but no other wounds. Vital signs include a regular pulse of 130/min, respirations of 26 breaths/min, and a blood pressure of 104/66 mm Hg.

1. Appropriate BSI precautions for this situation would include:
   A. gloves and goggles.
   B. gloves and mask.
   C. gloves.
   D. mask and goggles.

2. Which of the following terms would best describe the patient's current level of consciousness?
   A. Alert and oriented
   B. Responsive to pain
   C. Semiconscious
   D. Unresponsive

3. Which of the following characteristics of the patient's skin would suggest that the patient is not getting adequate oxygen?
   A. Pale
   B. Gray lips
   C. Warm
   D. Moist

4. Your general assessment suggests that your immediate action should be to:
   A. call for additional help.
   B. apply oxygen.
   C. dress her burns.
   D. apply spinal immobilization.

5. Part of your rapid trauma assessment includes listening for breath sounds. If there were nothing preventing you, the best place to listen for accurate breath sounds is:
   A. from the back, over the shirt.
   B. from the front, over the shirt.
   C. from the back, under the shirt.
   D. from the front, under the shirt.

6. A SAMPLE history for this patient would include:
   A. finding her unconscious, in the room where a fire started.
   B. documenting that she has burns.
   C. any medications found in the house.
   D. the suspicion that she was getting ready to eat.

7. In this patient, it is especially important to check which of the following?
   A. Back
   B. Abdomen
   C. Mouth
   D. Burns

Challenging Questions

8. From the little information you have, what is most likely causing her unconsciousness?

9. Immediate treatment is included during the initial and ongoing assessment. What immediate treatment is necessary for this patient?

10. During your assessment you note wheezing in all lobes. What is the most likely cause of her wheezing?

Patient Assessment

Scene Size-Up

Body Substance Isolation
Scene Safety
Determine Mechanism of Injury/Nature of Illness
Determine Number of Patients
Request Additional Assistance
Consider C-Spine Immobilization

Initial Assessment

Form General Impression of the Patient
Assess Mental Status
Assess the Airway
Assess Breathing
Assess Circulation
Identify Priority Patients

Trauma Patients

Medical Patients

Focused History and Physical Exam

Reconsider the Mechanism of Injury

Significant Mechanism of Injury	No Significant Mechanism of Injury
Rapid Trauma Assessment	Focused Assessment: Based on Chief Complaint
Baseline Vital Signs and SAMPLE History	Baseline Vital Signs and SAMPLE History
Transport	Transport

Focused History and Physical Exam

Evaluate Responsiveness

Responsive	Unresponsive
History of Illness	Rapid Medical Assessment
SAMPLE History	Baseline Vital Signs
Focused Physical Exam: Based on Chief Complaint	SAMPLE History
Baseline Vital Signs	Reevaluate Transport Decision
Reevaluate Transport Decision	

Detailed Physical Exam

Detailed Physical Exam
Baseline Vital Signs

Ongoing Assessment

Repeat the Initial Assessment
Reassess Vital Signs
Repeat Focused Assessment
Check Interventions

Communications and Documentation

TECHNOLOGY

www.emtb.com

- Online Chapter Pretest
- Interactivities
- Vocabulary Explorer
- Anatomy Review
- Web Links
- Online Review Manual
- Distance Learning

Chapter FEATURES

- Skill Drills
- Vital Vocabulary
- Pediatric Needs
- Geriatric Needs
- EMT-B Safety
- EMT-B Tips
- Documentation Tips
- Remember
- Prep Kit

As the above example illustrates, good documentation is not just for billing purposes. This chapter focuses on the areas of documentation and medical communications, and will also help you to answer the following questions:

1. What are the primary reasons that a pre-arrival radio report is given to the receiving hospital?

2. Are there advantages/disadvantages to using a narrative-style patient care report rather than a "fill in the bubble"-style format?

Communications and Documentation

Effective communication is an essential component of prehospital care. Radio and telephone communications link you and your team with other members of the EMS, fire, and law enforcement communities. This link helps the entire team to work together more effectively and provides an important layer of safety and protection for each member of the team. You must know what your system can and cannot do, and you must be able to use your system efficiently and effectively. You must be able to send precise, accurate reports about the scene, the patient's condition, and the treatment that you provide.

Verbal communications are also a vital skill for EMT-Bs. Your verbal skills will enable you to gather information from the patient and bystanders. They will also make it possible for you to effectively coordinate the variety of responders who are often present at the scene. Excellent verbal communications are also an integral part of transferring the patient's care to the nurses and physicians at the hospital. You must possess good listening skills to fully understand the nature of the scene and the patient's problem. You must also be able to organize your thoughts to quickly and accurately verbalize instructions to the patient, bystanders, and other responders. Finally, you must be able to organize and summarize the important aspects of the patient's presentation and treatment when reporting to the hospital staff.

Written communications complete the process. Written communications, in the form of a written patient care report, provide you with an opportunity to communicate the patient's story to others who may participate in the patient's care in the future. Adequate reporting and accurate records ensure the continuity of patient care. Complete patient records also guarantee proper transfer of responsibility, comply with the requirements of health departments and law enforcement agencies, and fulfill your organization's administrative needs. Reporting and record keeping duties are an essential aspect of patient care, although they are performed only after the patient's condition has been stabilized.

This chapter describes the skills that you need to be an effective communicator. It begins by identifying the kinds of equipment that are used, along with standard radio operating procedures and protocols. Next, the roles of the Federal Communications Commission (FCC) in EMS are described. The chapter concludes with a discussion of a variety of effective methods of verbal communications and guidelines for appropriate written documentation of patient care.

Communications Systems and Equipment

As an EMT-B, you must be familiar with two-way radio communications and have working knowledge of the mobile and hand-held portable radios that are used in your unit. You must also know when to use them and what to say when you are transmitting.

Base Station Radios

The dispatcher usually communicates with field units by transmitting through a fixed radio base station that is controlled from the dispatch center. A **base station** is any radio hardware containing a transmitter and receiver that is located in a fixed place ▶ Figure 9-1 . The base station may be used in a single place by an operator speaking into a microphone that is connected directly to the equipment. It also works remotely through telephone lines or by radio from a communications center. Base stations may include dispatch centers, fire stations, ambulance bases, or hospitals.

A two-way radio consists of two units: a transmitter and a receiver. Some base stations may have more than one transmitter and/or more than one receiver. They may also be equipped with one multi-channel transmitter and several single channel receivers. A **channel** is an assigned frequency or frequencies that are used to carry voice and/or data communications. Regardless of the number of transmitters and receivers, they are commonly called base radios or stations. Base stations usually have more power (often 100 watts or more) and higher, more efficient antenna systems than mobile or portable radios. This increased broadcasting range allows the base station operator to communicate with field units and other stations at much greater distances.

The base radio must be physically close to its antenna. Therefore, the actual base station cabinet and hardware are commonly found on the roof of a tall building or at the bottom of an antenna tower. The base station operator may be miles away in a dispatch center or hospital, communicating with the base station radio by dedicated lines or special radio links. A **dedicated line**, also known as a hot line, is always open or under the control of the individuals at each end. This type of line is immediately "on" as soon as you lift the receiver and cannot be accessed by outside users.

Mobile and Portable Radios

In the ambulance, you will use both mobile and portable radios to communicate with the dispatcher and/or medical control. An ambulance will often have more than one mobile radio, each on a different frequency ▶ Figure 9-2 . One radio may be used to communicate with the dispatcher or other public safety agencies. A second radio is often used for communicating patient information to medical control.

A mobile radio is installed in a vehicle and usually operates at lower power than a base station.

Figure 9-1 A base station consists of radio hardware containing a transmitter and a receiver that is located in a fixed place. Some have more than one transmitter and/or more than one receiver.

Figure 9-2 Some ambulances have more than one mobile radio, to allow communications with mutual aid agencies and other jurisdictions.

Most **VHF (very high frequency)** mobile radios operate at 100 watts of power. Radios that operate at 800 MHz are very common in EMS systems. **UHF (ultra-high frequency)** mobile radios usually have only 40 watts of power. Cellular telephones operate on 3 watts of power or less. Mobile antennas are much closer to the ground than base station antennas, so communications from the unit are typically limited to 10 to 15 miles over average terrain.

Portable radios are hand-carried or hand-held devices that operate at 1 to 5 watts of power ▶ Figure 9-3 . Since the entire radio can be held in your hand, when in use the antenna is often no higher than the EMT who is using the radio. The transmission range of a portable radio is more limited than that of mobile or base station radios. Portable radios are essential in

Figure 9-3 A portable radio is essential if you need to communicate with the dispatcher or medical control when you are away from the ambulance.

helping to coordinate EMS activities at the scene of a multiple-casualty incident. They are also helpful when you are away from the ambulance and need to communicate with dispatch, another unit, or medical control.

Repeater-Based Systems

A **repeater** is a special base station radio that receives messages and signals on one frequency and then automatically retransmits them on a second frequency. Because a repeater is a base station (with a large antenna), it is able to receive lower-power signals, such as those from a portable radio, from a long distance away. The signal is then rebroadcast with all the power of the base station **▼ Figure 9-4** . EMS systems that use repeaters usually have outstanding system-wide communications and are able to get the best signal from portable radios. There are also mobile repeaters that may be found in ambulances or placed in various areas around an EMS system area.

Digital Equipment

Although most people think of voice communications when they think of two-way radios, digital signals are also a part of EMS communications. Some EMS systems use telemetry to send an ECG from the unit to the hospital. With **telemetry**, electronic signals are converted into coded, audible signals. These signals can then be transmitted by radio or telephone to a receiver at the hospital with a decoder. The decoder converts the signals back into electronic impulses that can be displayed on a screen or printed. Another example of telemetry is a fax message.

Digital signals are also used in some kinds of paging and tone alerting systems because they transmit faster than spoken words and allow more choices and flexibility.

Cellular Telephones

Cellular telephones are becoming more common in EMS communications systems **► Figure 9-5** . These telephones are simply low-power portable radios that communicate through a series of interconnected repeater stations called "cells" (hence the name "cellular"). Cells are linked by a sophisticated computer system and connected to the telephone network. Cellular telephones are also popular with other public safety agencies, particularly as more cell sites are constructed in rural areas.

Unlike typical two-way mobile communications, which have free access, a cellular system charges fees for its use. Your system can buy portable or mobile radios on the local EMS frequency and use them at no cost. However, buying a cellular telephone is only half of the process of being able to use it. A cellular telephone cannot simply access the telephone network. The user must be assigned a specially coded number that the cellular system's computers will recognize. It is that access and the amount of time a user spends on the telephone for which the cellular system charges.

Figure 9-4 A message is sent from the control center by a land line to the transmitter. The radio carrier wave is picked up by the repeater for rebroadcast to outlying units. Return radio traffic is picked up by the repeater and rebroadcast to the control center.

Figure 9-5 Use of cellular phones is becoming more common in EMS communications systems.

However, once you are connected to the network, you can call any other telephone in the world and can send voice, data, and telemetry signals.

Many cellular systems make equipment and air time available to EMS services at little or no cost as a public service. The public is often able to call 9-1-1 or other emergency numbers on a cellular telephone free of charge. However, this easy access may result in overloading and jamming of cellular systems in mass-casualty and disaster situations.

As with all repeater-based systems, a cellular telephone is useless if the equipment fails, loses power, or is damaged by severe weather or other circumstances. Like all voice radio communications systems, cellular telephones can be easily overheard on scanners. A **scanner** is a radio receiver that searches or "scans" across several frequencies until the message is completed. Although cellular telephones are more private than most other forms of radio communications, they can still be overheard. Therefore, you must always speak in a professional manner every time you use any form of an EMS communications system.

Other Communications Equipment

Ambulances and other field units are usually equipped with an external public address system. This system may be a part of the siren or the mobile radio. The intercom between the cab and the patient compartment may also be a part of the mobile radio. These components do not involve radio wave transmission, but you must understand how they work and practice using them before you really need them.

EMS systems may use a variety of two-way radio hardware. Some systems operate VHF equipment in the **simplex** (push to talk, release to listen) mode. In this mode, radio transmissions can occur in either

direction but not simultaneously in both. When one party transmits, the other can only receive and then wait for the other party to finish before he or she can reply. Other systems conduct **duplex** (simultaneous talk-listen) communications on UHF frequencies and also use cellular telephones. In the full duplex mode, radios can transmit and receive communications simultaneously on one channel. This is sometimes called "a pair of frequencies." A number of VHF and UHF channels, commonly called **MED channels**, are reserved exclusively for EMS use. However, hundreds of other commercial, local government, and fire services frequencies are also used for EMS communications.

Some EMS systems rely on dedicated lines (hot lines) as control links for their remotely located base stations and antennas. Other systems are more simply configured and require no off-site control links. No matter what type of equipment is used, all EMS communications systems have some basic limitations. Therefore, you must know what your equipment can and cannot do.

The ability for you to communicate effectively with other units or medical control depends on how well the weaker radio can "talk back." Base and repeater station radios often have much greater power and higher antennas than mobile or portable units do. This increased power affects your communications in two ways. First, their signals are generally heard and understood from a much greater distance than the signal produced from a mobile unit. Second, their signals are received clearly from a much greater distance than is possible with a mobile or portable unit. Remember, when you are at the scene, you may be able to clearly hear the dispatcher or hospital on your radio, but you may not be heard or understood when you transmit.

Even small changes in your location can significantly affect the quality of your transmission. Also remember that the location of the antenna is critically important for clear transmission. Commercial aircraft flying at 37,000′ can transmit and receive signals over hundreds of miles, yet their radios have only a few watts of power. The "power" comes from their 37,000′-high antenna.

At times, you may be able to communicate with a base station radio but you will not be able to hear or transmit to another mobile unit that is also communicating with that base. Repeater base stations eliminate such problems. They allow two mobile or portable units that cannot reach each other directly to communicate through the repeater, using its greater power and antenna.

The success of communications depends on the efficiency of your equipment. A damaged antenna or microphone often prevents high-quality

You must always speak in a professional manner every time you use the EMS communications system.

communications. Check the condition and status of your equipment at the start of each shift, and then correct or report any problems.

Radio Communications

All radio operations in the United States, including those used in EMS systems, are regulated by the **Federal Communications Commission (FCC)**. The FCC has jurisdiction over interstate and international telephone and telegraph services and satellite communications-all of which may involve EMS activity.

The FCC has five principal EMS-related responsibilities:

1. **Allocating specific radio frequencies for use by EMS providers.** Modern EMS communications began in 1974. At that time, the FCC assigned 10 MED channels in the 460- to 470-MHz (UHF) band to be used by EMS providers. These UHF channels were added to the several VHF frequencies that were already available for EMS systems. However, these VHF frequencies had to be shared with other "special emergencies" uses, including school buses and veterinarians. In 1993, the FCC created an EMS-only block of frequencies in the 220-MHz portion of the radio spectrum.

2. **Licensing base stations and assigning appropriate radio call signs for those stations.** An FCC license is usually issued for 5 years, after which time it must be renewed. Each FCC license is granted only for a specific operating group. Often, the longitude and latitude (locations) of the antenna and the address of the base station determine the call signs.

3. **Establishing licensing standards and operating specifications for radio equipment used by EMS providers.** Before it can be licensed, each piece of radio equipment must be submitted by its manufacturer to the FCC for type acceptance, based on established operating specification and regulations.

4. **Establishing limitations for transmitter power output.** The FCC regulates broadcasting power to reduce radio interference between neighboring communications systems.

5. **Monitoring radio operations.** This includes making spot field checks to help ensure compliance with FCC rules and regulations.

The FCC's rules and regulations fill many volumes and are written in technical and legal language. Only a very small section (part 90, subpart C) deals with EMS communication issues. You are not responsible for reading these detailed and often confusing documents. For appropriate guidance on technical issues, contact your EMS system supervisor. In fact, many EMS systems look to radio and telephone communications experts for advice on technical issues.

Responding to the Scene

EMS communication systems may operate on several different frequencies and may use different frequency bands. Some EMS systems may even use different radios for different purposes. However, all EMS systems depend on the skill of the dispatcher. The dispatcher receives the first call to 9-1-1 (▼ **Figure 9-6**). You are part of the team that responds to calls once the dispatcher notifies your unit of an emergency.

The dispatcher has several important responsibilities during the alert and dispatch phase of EMS communications. The dispatcher must do all of the following:

- Properly screen and assign priority to each call (according to predetermined protocols).

- Select and alert the appropriate EMS response unit(s).

- Dispatch and direct EMS response unit(s) to the correct location.

Figure 9-6 The dispatcher receives the first call to 9-1-1.

- Coordinate EMS response unit(s) with other public safety services until the incident is over.

- Provide emergency medical instructions to the telephone caller so that essential care (eg, CPR) may begin before the EMTs arrive (according to predetermined protocols).

When the first call to 9-1-1 comes in, the dispatcher must try to judge its relative importance to begin the appropriate EMS response using emergency medical dispatch protocols. First, the dispatcher must find out the exact location of the patient and the nature and severity of the problem. The dispatcher asks for the caller's telephone number, the patient's age and name, and other information, as directed by local protocol. Next, some description of the scene, such as the number of patients or special environmental hazards, is needed.

From this information, the dispatcher will assign the appropriate EMS response unit(s) on the basis of local protocols to determine the level and type of response and the following:

- The dispatcher's perception of the nature and severity of the problem

- The anticipated response time to the scene

- The level of training (first responder, BLS, ALS) of available EMS response unit(s)

- The need for additional EMS units, fire suppression, rescue, a HazMat team, air medical support, or law enforcement

The dispatcher's next step is to alert the appropriate EMS response unit(s) (▶ **Figure 9-7**). Alerting these units may be done in a variety of ways. The dispatch radio system may be used to contact units that are already in service and monitoring the channel. Dedicated lines (hot lines) between the control center and the EMS station may also be used.

The dispatcher may also page EMS personnel. Pagers are commonly used in EMS operations to alert on- and off-duty personnel. **Paging** involves the use of a coded tone or digital radio signal and a voice or display message that is transmitted to pagers (beepers) or desktop monitor radios. Paging signals may be sent to alert only certain personnel or may be blanket signals that will activate all the pagers in the EMS service. Pagers and monitor radios are convenient because they are usually silent until their specific paging code is received. Alerted personnel contact the dispatcher to confirm the message and receive details of their assignments.

Once EMS personnel have been alerted, they must be properly dispatched and sent to the incident. Every EMS system should use a standard dispatching procedure. The dispatcher should give the responding unit(s) the following information:

- The nature and severity of the injury, illness, or incident

- The exact location of the incident

- The number of patients

- Responses by other public safety agencies

- Special directions or advisories, such as adverse road or traffic conditions or severe weather reports

- The time at which the unit or units are dispatched

Your unit must confirm to the dispatcher that you have received the information and that you are en route to the scene. Local protocol will dictate whether it is the job of the dispatcher or your unit to notify other public safety agencies that you are responding to an emergency. In some areas, the emergency department is also notified whenever an ambulance responds to an emergency.

Figure 9-7 You will be assigned to a scene by the dispatcher.

You should report any problems during your response to the dispatcher. You should also inform the dispatcher that you have arrived at the scene. The arrival report to the dispatcher should include any obvious details that you see during scene size up. For example, you might say, "Dispatcher, Medic One is on scene at Main Street with a two-vehicle collision."

All radio communications during dispatch, as well as other phases of operations, must be brief and easily understood. Although speaking in plain English is best, many areas find that 10 codes are shorter and simpler for routine communications. The development and use of such codes require strict discipline. When used improperly or not understood, codes create confusion rather than clear it up.

Communicating with Medical Control and Hospitals

The principal reason for radio communication is to facilitate communication between you and medical control (and the hospital). Medical control may be located at the receiving hospital, another facility, or sometimes even in another city or state. You must, however, consult with medical control to notify the hospital of an incoming patient, to request advice or orders from medical control, or to advise the hospital of special situations.

It is important to plan and organize your radio communication before you push the transmit button. Remember, a concise, well-organized report demonstrates your competence and professionalism in the eyes of all who hear your report. Well-organized radio communications with the hospital will engender confidence in the receiving facility's physicians and nurses, as well as others who are listening. In addition, the patient and family will be comforted by your organization and ability to communicate clearly. A well-delivered radio report puts you in control of the information, which is where you want to be.

Hospital notification is the most common type of communication between you and the hospital. The purpose of these calls is to notify the receiving facility of the patient's complaint and condition ▶ **Figure 9-8**. On the basis of this information, the hospital is able to prepare staff and equipment appropriately to receive the patient.

GIVING THE PATIENT REPORT. The patient report should follow a standard format established by your EMS system. The patient report commonly includes the following seven elements:

1. **Your unit identification and level of services.** Example: "Brimfield Medical 71-BLS."

2. **The receiving hospital and your estimated time of arrival.** Example: "Robinson Memorial Hospital, ETA 10 minutes," or "patient transport code" according to local protocols.

3. **The patient's age and gender.** Example: "A 33-year-old woman." The patient's name should not be given over the radio because it may be overheard. This is a violation of the patient's confidentiality.

4. **The patient's chief complaint or your perception of the problem and its severity.** Example: "The patient complains of pain in the right lower leg."

5. **A brief history of the patient's current problem.** Example: "The patient fell down the steps." Other important history information that may pertain to the current problem should also be included, such as "The patient has diabetes and takes insulin."

6. **A brief report of physical findings.** This report should include level of consciousness, the patient's general appearance, pertinent

Figure 9-8 Giving the patient report should be done in an objective, accurate, professional manner.

abnormalities noted, and vital signs. Example: "The patient is alert and oriented and has normal color and warm skin. Her right lower leg is swollen and tender. Her blood pressure is 132 over 84, pulse is 72, and respirations 14."

7. **A brief summary of the care given and any patient response.** Example: "We have immobilized the injured leg in a padded cardboard splint. The patient is now on a backboard. She still has motor, sensory, and circulatory function distal to the injured area. She also reports a decrease in pain since the splint was applied."

Be sure that you report all patient information in an objective, accurate, and professional manner. People with scanners are listening. You could be successfully sued for slander if you describe a patient in a way that injures his or her reputation.

THE ROLE OF MEDICAL CONTROL. The delivery of EMS involves an impressive array of assessments, stabilization, and treatments. In some cases, you may assist patients in taking medications. Intermediate and advanced EMTs go beyond this level by initiating medication therapy based on the patient's presenting signs. For logical, ethical, and legal reasons, the delivery of such sophisticated care must be done in association with physicians. For this reason, every EMS system needs input and involvement from physicians. One or more physicians, including your system or department medical director, will provide medical direction (medical control) for your EMS system. Medical control is either off-line (indirect) or online (direct), as authorized by the medical director. Medical control guides the treatment of patients in the system through protocols, direct orders and advice, and post-call review.

Depending upon how the protocols are written, you may need to call medical control for direct orders (permission) to administer certain treatments, to determine the transport destination of patients, or to be allowed to stop treatment and/or not transport a patient. In these cases, the radio or cellular phone provides a vital link between you and the expertise available through the base physician.

To maintain this link 24 hours a day, 7 days a week, medical control must be readily available on the radio at the hospital or on a mobile or portable unit when you call (▶ **Figure 9-9**). In most areas, medical control is provided by the physicians who work at the receiving hospital. However, many variations have developed across the country. For example, some EMS units

receive medical direction from one hospital even though they are taking the patient to another hospital. In other areas, medical direction may come from a free-standing center or even from an individual physician. Regardless of your system's design, your link to medical control is vital to maintain the high quality of care that your patient requires and deserves.

CALLING MEDICAL CONTROL. You can use the radio in your unit or a portable radio to call medical control. A cellular telephone can also be used. Regardless of the type of communication, you should use a channel that is relatively free of other radio traffic and interference. There are a number of ways to control access on ambulance-to-hospital channels. In some EMS systems, the dispatcher monitors and assigns appropriate, clear medical control channels. Other EMS systems rely on special communications operations, such as CMEDs (Centralized Medical Emergency Dispatch) or resource coordination centers, to monitor and allocate the medical control channels.

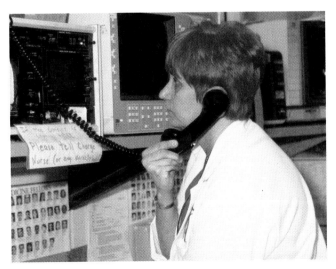

Figure 9-9 Medical control must be readily available on the radio at the hospital.

Because of the large number of EMS calls to medical control, your radio report must be well organized and precise and must contain only important information. In addition, because you need specific directions on patient care, the information that you provide to medical control must be accurate. Remember, the physician on the other end bases his or her instructions on the information that you provide.

You should never use codes when communicating with medical control unless you are directed by local protocol to do so. You should use proper medical terminology when giving your report. Never assume that medical control will know what a "10-50" or "Signal 70" means. Most medical control systems handle many different EMS agencies and will most likely not know your unit's special codes or signals.

To ensure complete understanding, once you receive an order from medical control, you must repeat the order back, word for word, and then receive confirmation. Whether the physician gives an order for medication or a specific treatment or denies a request for a particular treatment, you must repeat the order back word for word. This "echo" exchange helps to eliminate confusion and the possibility of poor patient care. Orders that are unclear or seem inappropriate or incorrect should be questioned. Do not blindly follow an order that does not make sense to you. The physician may have misunderstood or may have missed part of your report. In that case, he or she may not be able to respond appropriately to the patient's needs.

INFORMATION ABOUT SPECIAL SITUATIONS. Depending on your system's procedures, you may initiate communication with one or more hospitals to advise them of an extraordinary call or situation. For instance, a small rural hospital may be better able to respond to multiple victims of a highway crash if it is notified when the ambulance is first responding. At the other extreme, an entire hospital system must be notified of any disaster, such as a plane or train crash, as early as possible to enable activation of its staff call-in system. These special situations might also include HazMat situations, rescues in progress, mass-casualty incidents, or any other situation that might require special preparation on the part of the hospital. In some areas, mutual aid frequencies may be designated in mass-casualty incidents so that responding agencies can communicate with one another on a common frequency.

When notifying the hospital(s) of any special situations, keep the following in mind: The earlier the notification, the better. You should ask to speak to the charge nurse or physician in charge, as he or she is best able to

mobilize the resources necessary to respond. Also, whenever possible, provide an estimate of the number of individuals who may be transported to the facility. Be sure to identify any conditions the patient(s) might have that require special needs, such as burns or hazardous materials exposure, to assist the hospital in preparation. In many cases, hospital notification is part of a larger disaster or HazMat plan. Follow the plan for your system.

Standard Procedures and Protocols

You must use your radio communications system effectively from the time you acknowledge a call until you complete your run. Standard radio operating procedures are designed to reduce the number of misunderstood messages, to keep transmissions brief, and to develop effective radio discipline. Standard radio communications protocols help both you and the dispatcher to communicate properly ▶ Table 9-1 . Protocols should include guidelines specifying a preferred format for transmitting messages, definitions of key words and phrases, and procedures for troubleshooting common radio communications problems.

The "call up" from one unit to another begins by identifying the called unit first, followed by the unit calling, such as "Dispatch, this is Medic One." This exchange alerts the dispatcher to listen for both the identity of the unit calling and the message.

Reporting Requirements

Proper use of the EMS communications system will help you to do your job more effectively. From acknowledgment of the call until you are cleared from the medical emergency, you will use radio communications. You must report in to dispatch at least six times during your run:

1. **To acknowledge the dispatch information** and to confirm that you are responding to the scene

2. **To announce your arrival at the scene**

3. **To announce that you are leaving** the scene and are en route to the receiving hospital. (At this point, you typically should also state the number of patients being transported, your estimated arrival time at the hospital, and the run status.)

4. **To announce your arrival at the hospital** or facility

5. **To announce that you are clear of the incident** or hospital and available for another assignment

6. **To announce your arrival back at quarters** or other off-the-air location

TABLE 9-1 Guidelines for Effective Radio Communication

1. **Monitor the channel before transmitting** to avoid interfering with other radio traffic.

2. **Plan your message before pushing the transmit switch.** This will keep your transmissions brief and precise. You should use a standard format for your transmissions.

3. **Press the push-to-talk (PTT) button on the radio,** then wait for 1 second before starting your message. Otherwise, you might cut off the first part of your message before the transmitter is working at full power.

4. **Hold the microphone 2″ to 3″ from your mouth.** Speak clearly, but never shout into the microphone. Speak at a moderate, understandable rate, preferably in a clear, even voice.

5. **Identify the person or unit you are calling** first, then identify your unit as the sender. You will rarely work alone, so say "we" instead of "I" when describing yourself.

6. **Acknowledge a transmission as soon as you can** by saying, "Go ahead" or whatever is commonly used in your area. You should say, "Over and out," or whatever is commonly used in your area when you are finished. If you cannot take a long message, simply say, "Stand by" until you are ready.

7. **Use plain English.** Avoid meaningless phrases ("Be advised"), slang, or complex codes. Avoid words that are difficult to hear, such as "yes" and "no." Use "affirmative" and "negative."

8. **Keep your message brief.** If your message takes more than 30 seconds to send, pause after 30 seconds and say, "Do you copy?" The other party can then ask for clarification if needed. Also, someone else with emergency traffic can break through if necessary.

9. **Avoid voicing negative emotions,** such as anger or irritation, when transmitting. Courtesy is assumed, making it unnecessary to say "please" or "thank you," which wastes air time. Listen to other communications in your system to get a good idea of the common phrases and their uses.

10. **When transmitting a number with two or more digits, say the entire number first** and then each digit separately. For example, say, "sixty-seven," followed by "six-seven."

11. **Do not use profanity on the radio.** It is a violation of FCC rules and can result in substantial fines and even loss of your organization's radio license.

12. **Use EMS frequencies for EMS communications.** Do not use these frequencies for any other type of communications.

13. **Reduce background noise as much as possible.** Move away from wind, noisy motors, or tools. Close the window if you are in a moving ambulance. When possible, shut off the siren during radio transmissions.

14. **Be sure other radios on the same frequency are turned down** to avoid feedback.

While en route to and from the scene, you should report to the dispatcher any special hazards or road conditions that might affect other responding units. Report any unusual delay, such as road blocks, traffic, or construction. Once you are at the scene, you may request additional EMS or other public safety assistance and then help to coordinate their response.

During transport, you must periodically reassess the patient's overall condition, vital signs, and response to care provided. You should immediately report any significant changes in the patient's condition, especially if the patient seems worse. Medical control can then give new orders and prepare to receive the patient.

Maintenance of Radio Equipment

Like all other EMS equipment, radio equipment must be serviced by properly trained and equipped personnel. Remember that the radio is your lifeline to other public safety agencies (who function to protect you), as well as medical control, and it must perform under emergency conditions. Radio equipment that is operating properly should be serviced at least once a year. Any equipment that is not working properly should be immediately removed from service and sent for repair.

Sometimes, radio equipment will stop working during a run. Your EMS system must have several

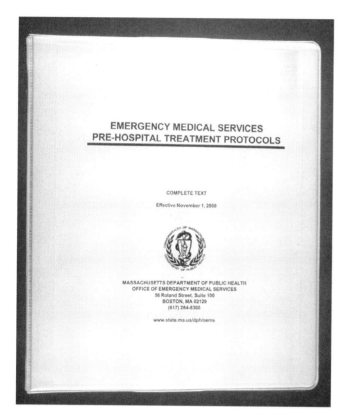

Figure 9-10 Standing orders are protocols developed by the medical director that outline specific directions, permissions, and prohibitions regarding patient care.

backup plans and options. The goal of a backup plan is to make sure that you can maintain contact when the usual procedures do not work. There are quite a few options.

The simplest backup plan relies on written standing orders. **Standing orders** are written documents that have been signed by the EMS system's medical director ▲ **Figure 9-10** . These orders outline specific directions, permissions, and sometimes prohibitions regarding patient care. By their very nature, standing orders do not require direct communication with medical control. When properly followed, standing orders or formal protocols have the same authority and legal status as orders given over the radio. They exist to one extent or another in every EMS system and can be applied to all levels of EMS providers.

Verbal Communications

As an EMT-B, you must master many communication skills, including radio operations and written communications. Verbal communications with the patient, the family, and the rest of the health care team are an essential part of high-quality patient care. And as an EMT-B, you must be able to find out what the patient needs and then tell others. Never forget that you are the vital link between the patient and the remainder of the health care team.

Communicating with Other Health Care Professionals

EMS is the first step in what is often a long and involved series of treatment phases. Effective communication between the EMT-B and health care professionals in the receiving facility is an essential cornerstone of efficient, effective, and appropriate patient care.

Your reporting responsibilities do not end when you arrive at the hospital. In fact, they have just begun. The transfer of care officially occurs during your oral report at the hospital, not as a result of your radio report en route. Once you arrive at the hospital, a hospital staff member will take responsibility of the patient from you ▶ **Figure 9-11** . Depending on the hospital and the condition of the patient, the training of the person who takes over the care of the patient varies. However, you may transfer the care of your patient only to someone with at least your level of training. Once a hospital staff member is ready to take responsibility for the patient, you must provide that person with a formal oral report of the patient's condition.

Giving a report is a longstanding and well-documented part of transferring the patient's care from one provider to another. Your oral report is usually given at the same time that the staff member is doing something for the patient. For example, a nurse or physician may be looking at the patient, beginning assessment, or helping you to move the patient from the stretcher to an examination table. Therefore, you must report important information in a complete, precise way. The following six components must be included in the oral report:

1. **The patient's name** (if you know it) and the chief complaint, nature of illness, or mechanism of injury. Example: "This is Mr. Campbell. His wife told us that he has been acting confused all day."

2. **A summary of the information** that you gave in your radio report. Example: "He has a history of high blood pressure and had a stroke 4 years ago. He has little permanent damage from the stroke. His wife states that he is usually alert and oriented."

3. **Any important history** that was not given already. Example: "His wife told us that he takes his medicine regularly. On the way in, she told us that Mr. Campbell's medicine was just changed 2 days ago."

Figure 9-11 Once you arrive at the hospital, a staff member will take responsibility for the patient from you.

Figure 9-12 Maintaining eye contact with your patient builds trust and lets the patient know that he or she is your first priority.

4. **The patient's response to treatment** given en route. It is especially important to report any changes in the patient or the treatment provided since your radio report. Example: "We started oxygen by nonrebreathing face mask at 10 L/min. His LOC improved, and he started to fight the mask. We were able to get him to hold the mask next to his mouth and nose for the rest of the trip."

5. **The vital signs assessed** during transport and after the radio report. Example: "His vitals during transport were blood pressure 184 over 110, pulse 96, respirations 22. They are generally unchanged since we reported earlier."

6. **Any other information** that you may have gathered that was not important enough to report sooner. Information that was gathered during transport, any patient medications you have brought with you, and any other details about the patient that was provided by family members or friends may be included. Example: "Mrs. Jones's husband rode in with us. Her daughter is coming from home and should be here soon."

Communicating with Patients

Your communication skills will be put to the test when you communicate with patients and/or families in emergency situations. Remember that someone who is sick or injured is scared and might not understand

what you are doing and saying. Therefore, your gestures, body movements, and attitude toward the patient are critically important in gaining the trust of both patient and family. These Ten Golden Rules will help you to calm and reassure your patients:

1. **Make and keep eye contact** with your patient at all times (▲ **Figure 9-12**). Give the patient your undivided attention. This will let the patient know that he or she is your top priority. Look the patient straight in the eye to establish **rapport**. Establishing rapport is building a trusting relationship with your patient. This will make the job of caring for the patient much easier for both you and the patient.

2. **Use the patient's proper name** when you know it. Ask the patient what he or she wishes to be called. Never use terms such as "Honey," or "Dear." Avoid using a patient's first name unless the patient is a child or the patient asks you to use his or her first name. Rather, use a courtesy title, such as "Mr. Peters," "Mrs. Smith," or "Ms. Butler." If you do not know the patient's name, refer to him or her as "sir" or "ma'am."

3. **Tell the patient the truth.** Even if you have to say something very unpleasant, telling the truth is better than lying. Lying will destroy the patient's trust in you and decrease your own confidence. You might not always tell the patient

everything, but if the patient or a family member asks a specific question, you should answer truthfully. A direct question deserves a direct answer. If you do not know the answer to the patient's question, say so. For example, a patient may ask, "Am I having a heart attack?" "I don't know" is an adequate answer.

4. **Use language that the patient can understand.** Do not talk up or down to the patient in any way. Avoid technical medical terms that the patient might not understand. For example, ask the patient whether he or she has a history of "heart problems." This will usually result in more accurate information than if you ask about "previous episodes of myocardial infarction" or a "history of cardiomyopathy."

5. **Be careful of what you say about the patient to others.** A patient might hear only part of what is said. As a result, the patient might seriously misinterpret (and remember for a long time) what was said. Therefore, assume that the patient can hear every word you say, even if you are speaking to others and even if the patient appears to be unconscious or unresponsive.

6. **Be aware of your body language** ▶ **Figure 9-13** . Nonverbal communication is extremely important in dealing with patients. In stressful situations, patients may misinterpret your gestures and movements. Be particularly careful not to appear threatening. Instead, position yourself at a lower level than the patient when practical. Remember that you should always, always conduct yourself in a calm, professional manner.

7. **Always speak slowly, clearly, and distinctly.** Pay close attention to your tone of voice.

8. **If the patient is hearing impaired, speak clearly,** and face the person so that he or she can read your lips. Do not shout at a person who is hearing impaired. Shouting will not make it any easier for the patient to understand you. Instead, it may frighten the patient and make it even more difficult for the patient to understand you. Never assume that an elderly patient is hearing impaired or otherwise unable to understand you. Also, never use baby talk with elderly patients or with anyone but babies.

9. **Allow time for the patient to answer** or respond to your questions. Do not rush a patient unless there is immediate danger. Sick and injured people may not be thinking clearly and

may need time to answer even simple questions. This is especially true in treating elderly patients.

10. **Act and speak in a calm, confident manner** while caring for the patient. Make sure that you attend to the patient's pains and needs. Try to make the patient physically comfortable and relaxed. Find out whether the patient is more comfortable sitting or lying down. Is the patient cold or hot? Does the patient want a friend or relative nearby?

Patients literally place their lives in your hands. They deserve to know that you can provide medical care and that you are concerned about their well-being.

Communicating with Elderly Patients

According to US Census Data, almost 35 million individuals are older than 65 years. It is projected that by the year 2030, the elderly population will be greater than 70 million. A person's actual age might not be the most important factor in making him or her "elderly." It is more important to determine a person's functional age. The functional age relates to the person's ability to function in daily activities, the person's mental state, and activity pattern.

Most elderly people think clearly, can give you a clear medical history, and can answer your questions

Figure 9-13 Watch your body language, as patients may misinterpret your gestures, movements, and stance.

▼**Figure 9-14**). Do not assume that an elderly patient is senile or confused. Remember, though, that communicating with some elderly patients is extremely difficult. Some may be hostile, irritable, and/or confused. Others may have difficulty hearing or seeing you. You need great patience and compassion when you are called upon to care for such a patient. Think of the patient as someone's grandmother or grandfather—or even as yourself when you reach that age.

Approach an elderly patient slowly and calmly. Allow plenty of time for the patient to respond to your questions. Watch for signs of confusion, anxiety, or impaired hearing or vision. The patient should feel confident that you are in charge and that everything possible is being done for him or her.

Elderly patients often do not feel much pain. An elderly person who has fallen or been injured may report no pain. In addition, elderly patients might not be fully aware of important changes in other body systems. As a result, be especially vigilant for objective changes—no matter how subtle—in their condition. Even minor changes in breathing or mental state may signal major problems.

Remember to attend to an elderly patient's family members and friends. Seeing a loved one taken away in an ambulance can be a particularly frightening experience. Take a few minutes to explain to an elderly patient's spouse or family what is being done and why such action is being taken. When possible (which is more often than you'd think), give the patient some time to pack a few personal items before leaving for the hospital. Be sure to get any hearing aids, glasses, or dentures packed before departure; it will make the patient's hospital stay much more pleasant. You should

> Patients deserve to know that you can provide medical care and that you are concerned about their well-being.

document on the prehospital care report that these items accompanied the patient to the hospital and were given to a specific staff person in the emergency department.

Communicating with Children

Everyone who is thrust into an emergency situation becomes frightened to some degree. However, fear is probably most severe and most obvious in children. Children may be frightened by your uniform, the ambulance, and the number of people who have suddenly gathered around. Even a child who says little may be very much aware of all that is going on.

Familiar objects and faces will help to reduce this fright. Let a child keep a favorite toy, doll, or security blanket to give the child some sense of control and comfort. Having a family member or friend nearby is also helpful. When not impractical due to the child's condition, it is often helpful to let the parent or an adult friend hold the child during your evaluation and treatment. However, you will have to make sure that this person will not upset the child. Sometimes, adult family members are not helpful because they become too upset by what has happened. An overly anxious parent or relative can make things worse. Be careful about selecting the proper adult for this role.

Children can easily see through lies or deceptions, so you must always be honest with them. Make sure that you explain to the child over and over again what and why certain things are happening. If treatment is going to hurt, such as applying a splint, tell the child ahead of time. Also tell the child that it will not hurt for long and that it will help "make it better."

Respect a child's modesty. Both little girls and little boys are often embarrassed if they have to undress or be undressed in front of strangers. This anxiety often intensifies during adolescence. When a wound or site of injury has to be exposed, try to do so out of sight of strangers. Again, it is extremely important to tell the child what you are doing and why you are doing it.

You should speak to a child in a professional yet friendly way. A child should feel reassured that you are there to help in every way possible. Maintain eye contact

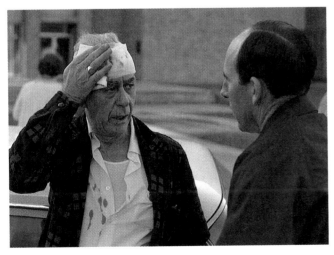

Figure 9-14)   You need a great deal of compassion and patience when caring for the elderly, but do not assume that the patient is senile or confused.

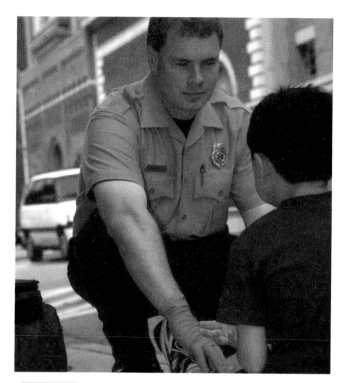

Figure 9-15   Maintain eye contact with a child to let the child know that you are there to help and that you can be trusted.

with a child, as you would with an adult, to let the child know that you are helping and that you can be trusted ◄ **Figure 9-15**). It is helpful to position yourself at their level so that you do not appear to tower above them.

Communicating with Hearing-Impaired Patients

Patients who are hearing impaired or deaf are usually not ashamed or embarrassed by their disability. Often, it is the people around a deaf or hearing-impaired person who have the problem coping. Remember that you must be able to communicate with hearing-impaired patients so that you can provide necessary or even lifesaving care.

The vast majority of hearing-impaired patients have normal intelligence. Hearing-impaired patients can usually understand what is going on around them, provided that you can successfully communicate with them. Most patients who are hearing impaired can read lips to some extent. Therefore, you should place yourself in a position so that the patient can see your lips. Many hearing-impaired patients have hearing aids to help them communicate. Be careful that hearing aids are not lost during an accident or fall. Not only are they extremely expensive, hearing aids will often make it easier to communicate. Hearing aids may also be forgotten if the patient is confused or ill. Look around, or ask the patient or the family about a hearing aid.

Remember the following five steps to help you efficiently communicate with patients who are hearing impaired:

1. **Have paper and a pen available.** This way, you can write down questions and the patient can write down answers, if necessary. Be sure to print so that your handwriting is not a communications barrier.

2. **If the patient can read lips,** you should face the patient and speak slowly and distinctly. Do not cover your mouth or mumble. If it is night or dark, consider shining a light on your face.

3. **Never shout.**

4. **Be sure to listen carefully,** ask short questions, and give short answers. Remember that although many hearing-impaired patients can speak distinctly, some cannot.

5. **Learn some simple phrases in sign language.** For example, knowing the signs for "sick," "hurt," and "help" may be useful if you cannot communicate in any other way ► **Figure 9-16** .

Communicating with Visually Impaired Patients

Like hearing-impaired patients, visually impaired and blind patients have usually accepted and learned to deal with their disability. Of course, not all visually impaired patients are completely blind. Many can perceive light and dark or can see shadows or movement. Ask the patient whether he or she can see at all. Also remember that, as with other patients who have disabilities, you should expect that visually impaired patients have normal intelligence.

As you begin caring for a visually impaired patient, explain everything that you are doing in detail as you are doing it. Be sure to stay in physical contact with the patient as you begin your care. Hold your hand lightly on the patient's shoulder or arm. Try to avoid sudden movements. If the patient can walk to the ambulance, place his or her hand on your arm, taking care not to rush. Transport any mobility aids, such as a cane, with the patient to the hospital. A visually impaired person may have a guide dog. Guide dogs are easily identified by their special harnesses. They are trained not to leave their masters and not to respond to strangers ► **Figure 9-17**). A visually impaired patient who is conscious can tell you about the dog and give instructions for its care. If circumstances permit, bring the guide dog to the hospital with the patient. If the dog has to be left behind, you should arrange for its care.

Figure 9-16 Learn simple phrases in sign language.
A. Sick. **B.** Hurt. **C.** Help.

Figure 9-17 A guide dog is easily identified by its special harness.

Communicating with Non-English-Speaking Patients

As part of the focused history and physical exam, you must obtain a medical history from the patient. You cannot skip this step simply because the patient does not speak English. Most patients who do not speak English fluently will still know certain important words or phrases.

Your first step is to find out how much English the patient can speak. Use short, simple questions and simple words whenever possible. Avoid difficult medical terms. You can help patients to better understand if you point to specific parts of the body as you ask questions.

In many areas, particularly large urban centers, major segments of the population do not speak English. Your job will be much easier if you learn some common words and phrases in their language, especially common medical terms. Pocket cards are available that show the pronunciation of these terms. If the patient does not speak any English, find a family member or friend to act as an interpreter.

Written Communications and Documentation

Along with your radio report and verbal report, you must also complete a formal written report about the patient before you leave the hospital. You might be able to do the written report en route, if the trip is long enough and the patient needs minimal care. Usually, you will finish the written report after you have transferred the care of the patient to a hospital staff member. Be sure to leave the report at the hospital before you leave.

Minimum Data Set

The information that you collect during a call becomes part of the patient's record. The national EMS community has identified a minimum data set that should enable communication and comparison of EMS runs between agencies, regions, and states. The minimum data set includes both patient information and administrative information (▶ **Figure 9-18**). The patient information that is included in the minimum data set is:

- Chief complaint
- Level of consciousness (AVPU) or mental status
- Systolic blood pressure for patients older than 3 years
- Capillary refill for patients younger than 6 years
- Skin color and temperature
- Pulse
- Respirations and effort

The administrative information that is included in the minimum data set should be as follows:

- The time that the incident was reported
- The time that the EMS unit was notified
- The time that the EMS unit arrived at the scene
- The time that the EMS unit left the scene
- The time that the EMS unit arrived at the receiving facility
- The time that patient care was transferred

You will begin gathering the patient information as soon as you reach the patient. Continue collecting information as you provide care until you arrive at the hospital.

Prehospital Care Report

Prehospital care reports help to ensure efficient continuity of patient care. This report describes the nature of the patient's injuries or illness at the scene and the initial

Figure 9-18 The minimum data set includes both patient information and administrative information.

treatment you provide. Although this report might not be read immediately at the hospital, it may very well be referred to later for important information. The prehospital care report serves the following six functions:

1. Continuity of care
2. Legal documentation
3. Education
4. Administrative
5. Research
6. Evaluation and continuous quality improvement

A good prehospital care report documents the care that was provided and the patient's condition on arrival at the scene. It also documents any changes in the patient's condition upon arrival at the hospital. The information in the report also proves that you have provided proper documentation. In some instances, it also shows that you have properly handled unusual or uncommon situations. Both objective and subjective information is included in this report. It is critical that you document everything in the clearest manner possible. If a patient brings legal action against you, you and your prehospital care report will have to go to court. Consider using the old adage of "if you didn't write it, it didn't happen."

These reports also provide valuable administrative information. For example, the report provides information for patient billing. It can also be used to evaluate response times, equipment usage, and other areas of administrative responsibility.

Data may be obtained from the prehospital care forms to analyze causes, severity, and types of illness or injury requiring emergency medical care. These reports may also be used in an ongoing program for evaluation of the quality of patient care. All records are reviewed periodically by your system. The purpose of this review is to make sure that trauma triage and/or other prehospital care criteria have been met.

There are many requirements on a prehospital care report ▶ **Table 9-2** . Often, these requirements vary from jurisdiction to jurisdiction, mainly because so many agencies obtain information from them. There is no universally accepted form.

Types of Forms

You will most likely use one of two types of forms. The first type is the traditional written form with check boxes and a narrative section. The second type is a computerized version in which you fill in information using an electronic clipboard or similar device. If your service uses written forms, be sure to fill in the boxes completely, and avoid making stray marks on the sheet. Make sure that you are familiar with the specific procedures for collecting, recording, and reporting the information in your area.

If you must complete a narrative section, be sure to describe what you see and what you do. Be sure to include significant negative findings and important observations about the scene. Do not record your conclusions about the incident. For example, you may write, "The patient admits to drinking today." This is a clear description that does not make any judgments

TABLE 9-2 Components of Prehospital Care Report
• Patient's name, gender, date of birth, and address
• Dispatched as
• Chief complaint
• Location of the patient when first seen (including specific details, especially if the incident is a car crash or criminal activity is suspected)
• Rescue and treatment given before your arrival
• Signs and symptoms found during your patient assessment
• Care and treatment given at the site and during transport
• Baseline vital signs
• SAMPLE history changes in vital signs and condition
• Date of the call
• Time of the call
• Location of the call
• Time of dispatch
• Time of arrival at the scene
• Time of leaving the scene
• Time of arrival at the hospital
• Patient's insurance information
• Names and/or certification numbers of the EMT-Bs who responded to the call
• Name of the base hospital involved in the run
• Type of run to the scene: emergency or routine

about the patient's condition. However, a report that says, "The patient was drunk," makes a conclusion about the patient's condition. Also avoid radio codes, and use only standard abbreviations. When information is of a sensitive nature, note the source of the information. Be sure to spell words correctly, especially medical terms. If you do not know how to spell a particular word, find out how to spell it, or use another word. Also be sure to record the time with all assessment findings.

Remember that the report form itself and all the information on it are considered confidential documents. Be sure that you are familiar with state and local laws concerning confidentiality. All prehospital forms must be handled with care and stored in an appropriate manner once you have completed them. After you have completed a report, distribute the copies to the appropriate locations, according to state and local protocol. In most instances, a copy of the report will remain at the hospital and will become a part of the patient's record.

Reporting Errors

Everyone makes mistakes. If you leave something out of a report or record information incorrectly, do not try to cover it up. Rather, write down what did or did not happen and the steps that were taken to correct the situation. Falsifying information on the prehospital report may result in suspension and/or revocation of your certification/license. More important, falsifying information results in poor patient care, because other health care providers have a false impression of assessment findings or the treatment given. Document only the vital signs that were actually taken. If you did not give the patient oxygen, do not chart that the patient was given oxygen.

If you discover an error as you are writing your report, draw a single horizontal line through the error, initial it, and write the correct information next to it (▶ **Figure 9-19**). Do not try to erase or cover the error with correction fluid. This may be interpreted as an attempt to cover up a mistake.

If an error is discovered after you submit your report, draw a single line through the error, preferably in a different color ink, initial it, and date it. Make sure to add a note with the correct information. If you left out information accidentally, add a note with the correct information, the date, and your initials.

When you do not have enough time to complete your report before the next call, you will need to fill it out later.

Documenting Refusal of Care

Competent adult patients have the right to refuse treatment (▶ **Figure 9-20**). If you are faced with this situation, you must inform medical control immediately. Before you leave the scene, try to persuade the patient to go to the hospital, and consult medical direction as directed by local protocol. Also make sure that the patient is able to make a rational, informed decision and is not under the influence of alcohol or other drugs or the effects of an illness or injury. Explain to the patient why it is important to be examined by a physician at the hospital. Also explain what may happen if the patient is not examined by a physician. If the

patient still refuses, suggest other means for the patient to obtain proper care. Explain that you are willing to return. If the patient still refuses, document any assessment findings and emergency medical care given, then have the patient sign a refusal form. You should also have a family member, police officer, or bystander sign the form as a witness. If the patient refuses to sign the refusal form, have a family member, police officer, or bystander sign the form verifying that the patient refused to sign.

Be sure to complete the prehospital report, including the patient assessment findings. Also include a description of the care that you wished to provide for the patient. You must also include a statement explaining that you informed the patient of the possible consequences of failure to accept care, including potential death, and alternative methods of obtaining the care that you suggested.

Special Reporting Situations

In some instances, you may be required to file special reports with appropriate authorities. These may include incidents involving gunshot wounds, dog bites, certain infectious diseases, or suspected physical, sexual, or substance abuse. Learn your local requirements for reporting these incidents. Failure to report them may have legal consequences. It is important that the report be accurate, objective, and submitted in a timely manner. Also remember to keep a copy for your own records.

Another special reporting situation is a mass-casualty incident (MCI). The local MCI plan should have some means of recording important medical information temporarily (such as a triage tag that can be used later to complete the form). The standard for completing the form in an MCI is not the same as for a typical call. Your local plan should have specific guidelines.

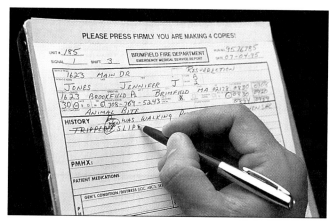

Figure 9-19 If you make a mistake in writing your report, the proper way to correct it is to draw a single horizontal line through the error, initial it, and write the correct information next to it.

RELEASE FROM RESPONSIBILITY WHEN PATIENT REFUSES IV THERAPY

This is to certify that I, _____, am refusing IV treatment. I acknowledge
patient's name
that I have been informed of the risk involved and hereby release the emergency medical services
provider(s), the physician consultant, and the consulting hospital from all responsibility for any
ill effects which may result from this action.

Witness _____ Signed _____
                                                        patient name or nearest relative

Witness _____ _____
                                                        relationship

---

RELEASE FROM RESPONSIBILITY WHEN PATIENT REFUSES SERVICE

This is to certify that I, _____, am refusing the services offered by the
patient's name
emergency medical services provider(s). I acknowledge that I have been informed of the risk
involved and hereby release the emergency medical services provider(s), the physician consultant,
and the consulting hospital from all responsibility for any ill effects which may result from this action.

Witness _____ Signed _____
                                                        patient name or nearest relative

Witness _____ _____
                                                        relationship

---

RELEASE FROM RESPONSIBILITY WHEN PATIENT REFUSES SERVICES
BUT ACCEPTS TRANSPORT

This is to certify that I, _____, am refusing _____
patient's name
_____. I acknowledge that I have been informed of the risk involved
and hereby release the emergency medical services provider(s), the physician consultant, and the
consulting hospital from all responsibility for any ill effects which may result from this action.
However, I do accept transportation to a medical facility.

Witness _____ Signed _____
                                                        patient name or nearest relative

Witness _____ _____
                                                        relationship

---

Figure 9-20 A competent adult patient has the right to refuse medical treatment and must sign a refusal form.

Prep Kit

Ready for Review

Excellent communication skills are crucial in relaying pertinent information to the hospital before arrival. Radio and telephone communication links you and your team to other members of the EMS, fire, and law enforcement communities. This enables your entire team to work together more effectively. It is your job to know what your communication system can and cannot handle. You must be able to communicate effectively by sending precise, accurate reports about the scene, the patient's condition, and the treatment that you provide.

There are many different forms of communication that an EMT-B must understand and be able to use. First, you must be familiar with two-way radio communications and have a working knowledge of mobile and hand-held portable radios. You must know when to use them and what type of information you can transmit. Remember, the lines of communication are not always exclusive; therefore, you should speak in a professional manner at all times.

In addition to radio and oral communications with hospital personnel, EMT-B's must have excellent person-to-person communication skills. You should be able to interact with the patient and any family members, friends, or bystanders. It is important for you to remember that people who are sick or injured may not understand what you are doing or saying. Therefore, your body language and attitude are very important in gaining the trust of both the patient and family. You must also take special care of individuals such as children, the elderly, and hearing-impaired, visually impaired, and non-English-speaking patients.

Along with your radio report and oral report, you must also complete a formal written report about the patient before you leave the hospital. This is a vital part of providing emergency medical care and ensuring the continuity of patient care. This information guarantees the proper transfer of responsibility, complies with the requirements of health departments and law enforcement agencies, and fulfills your administrative needs. Reporting and record-keeping duties are essential, but they should never come before the care of a patient.

Vital Vocabulary

base station Any radio hardware containing a transmitter and receiver that is located in a fixed place.

cellular telephone A low-power portable radio that communicates through an interconnected series of repeater stations called "cells."

channel An assigned frequency or frequencies that are used to carry voice and/or data communications.

dedicated line A special telephone line that is used for specific point-to-point communications; also known as a "hot line."

duplex The ability to transmit and receive simultaneously.

Federal Communications Commission (FCC) The federal agency that has jurisdiction over interstate and international telephone and telegraph services and satellite communications, all of which may involve EMS activity.

MED channels VHF and UHF channels that the FCC has designated exclusively for EMS use.

paging The use of a radio signal and a voice or digital message that is transmitted to pagers ("beepers") or desktop monitor radios.

rapport A trusting relationship that you build with your patient.

repeater A special base station radio that receives messages and signals on one frequency and then automatically retransmits them on a second frequency.

scanner A radio receiver that searches or "scans" across several frequencies until the message is completed; the process is then repeated.

simplex Single-frequency radio; transmissions can occur in either direction but not simultaneously in both; when one party transmits, the other can only receive, and the party that is transmitting is unable to receive.

standing orders Written documents, signed by the EMS system's medical director, that outline specific directions, permissions, and sometimes prohibitions regarding patient care; also called protocols.

telemetry A process in which electronic signals are converted into coded, audible signals; these signals can then be transmitted by radio or telephone to a receiver at the hospital with a decoder.

UHF (ultra-high frequency) Radio frequencies between 300 and 3,000 MHz.

VHF (very high frequency) Radio frequencies between 30 and 300 MHz; the VHF spectrum is further divided into "high" and "low" bands.

Points to Ponder

You are new with an agency and on your third shift you respond to a nearby "rest home" for a patient transfer. The patient walks over to the stretcher and lies down. You notice that your partner marks nonambulatory on the run sheet. When you ask her about it she says, "They told us to mark nonambulatory so Medicare will pay." In this agency, both EMTs sign the run sheet. What would you do? Would you sign the run sheet?

Issues Ethics in EMS, Risk of Losing Your Job for What Is Right, Management Relationships, Rules/Regulations and Laws Outside of EMS.

Online Outlook

The Federal Communications Commission (FCC) has five main EMS-related responsibilities. To learn more about the FCC's role in EMS, complete Exercise 9 at www.emtb.com.

www.emtb.com

Assessment in Action

You have been dispatched to a cardiac arrest. At the scene a family member tells you that your patient, a 44-year-old man, collapsed suddenly at home. He has a history of lung cancer but is not taking medication, and he has no allergies. The family members talk about looking for a "Do Not Resuscitate" order but cannot find it. They begin to fight among themselves about whether to have treatment given. Because of the family's indecision and the absence of a DNR, you apply the AED and it tells you "no shock indicated." You begin CPR and transport. En route to the hospital you give a radio report.

1. The receiving hospital asks you to repeat your report because they are having a hard time understanding you. Measures to take to ensure that you are understood while speaking include which of the following?
   A. Hold the microphone 2" to 3" from your mouth and then wait for about 1 second after pressing the push-to-talk button before you start talking.
   B. Hold the microphone 3" to 5" from your mouth, raise your voice, and talk immediately after pressing the push-to-talk button.
   C. Hold the microphone very close to your mouth, raise your voice, and talk immediately after pressing the push-to-talk button.
   D. Hold the microphone 5" to 7" from your mouth and wait for 10 to 15 seconds after pressing the push-to-talk button before talking.

2. In this situation you initiated and continued treatment without calling the hospital or contacting medical control. This method of authorized patient care is termed:
   A. a direct physician order.
   B. standing orders.
   C. radio protocols.
   D. communicating orders.

3. You want to alert the hospital regarding the family issues with this patient so you choose to use a dedicated line. Using a dedicated line means:
   A. the line is immediately "on" as soon as you lift the receiver and cannot be accessed by outside users.
   B. the line is immediately "on" and can be accessed by a scanner.
   C. the line must be accessed by a specified number or "code" but cannot be accessed by outside users.
   D. the line must be accessed by a specified number or "code" and can be accessed by a scanner.

4. When you arrive at the receiving hospital you must give a verbal report of the incident in a complete, precise manner. Which of the following contains all the components necessary for an oral report regarding this incident?
   A. This is Mr. Jones, he collapsed at home. He has a history of cancer of the brain. His family states there is a DNR but were unable to find it. We started CPR and brought him directly here.
   B. This is Mr. Jones. He is a cancer patient and was found unresponsive by his family. They have a DNR but were unable to find it. We did CPR with no response. A defibrillator was applied.
   C. This is Mr. Jones. He has a history of lung cancer and was found unresponsive with no vital signs. He has been unresponsive to CPR. The defibrillator stated "no shock indicated."
   D. Mr. Jones was found unresponsive, pulseless, and apneic. He has a history of cancer, his family argued over whether or not to resuscitate, there was some question of a DNR but we didn't see it. We applied the AED and got "no shock indicated." We continued CPR, and there has been no response.

You are called to the scene of a elderly adult male who was wandering around the neighborhood. Your patient is alert but only communicates by gesturing with his hands. His skin is normal, pulse of 82 beats/min, respirations of 16 breaths/min, and blood pressure of 150/84 mm Hg. You notice bilateral hearing aids. There is no sign of trauma.

5. Which of the following would be appropriate actions that could help you communicate with this patient?
   A. Raise your voice in case he is deaf.
   B. Allow more time for him to respond.
   C. Speak quickly and briskly so he will not misunderstand.
   D. Position yourself directly in front of him when you talk.

6. After a short time you realize that this patient is trying to gesture in sign language. One of the best ways to maintain ongoing communication with this patient is to:
   A. know the name and number of someone who knows sign language.
   B. continue speaking in a loud tone of voice and face the patient.
   C. stand directly in front of the patient and introduce yourself.
   D. have paper and pen available so both of you can write.

7. You are dispatched to a person who has fallen. On arrival you immediately notice a large dog sitting beside your patient. The dog has a heavy harness with a handle. Your patient tells you that she has trouble seeing and that her dog must go with her to the hospital because she is not close to home. Which of the following is the most appropriate action to take?
   A. Have a law enforcement officer take the dog.
   B. Have the humane society take the dog.
   C. Take the dog to the hospital with your patient.
   D. Find a bystander to take the dog.

8. You have made an error on your patient care report form. The best method to correct that error would be to:
   A. cross it out and mark over it.
   B. draw a line through it and initial it.
   C. erase it and start over.
   D. use correction fluid and mark over it.

Challenging Questions

9. A tornado hit your community. You have cell phones for your main communication device. What are the potential problems that might occur when cellular telephones are used in this situation?

10. Your adult patient refuses to go to the hospital with you despite your efforts to convince him otherwise. After ensuring that he is alert and oriented, you explain what consequences might occur due to his refusal, encourage him to call you back if he runs into any trouble, and have him sign the refusal form. Why is it so necessary that you explain the consequences of his actions?

www.emtb.com

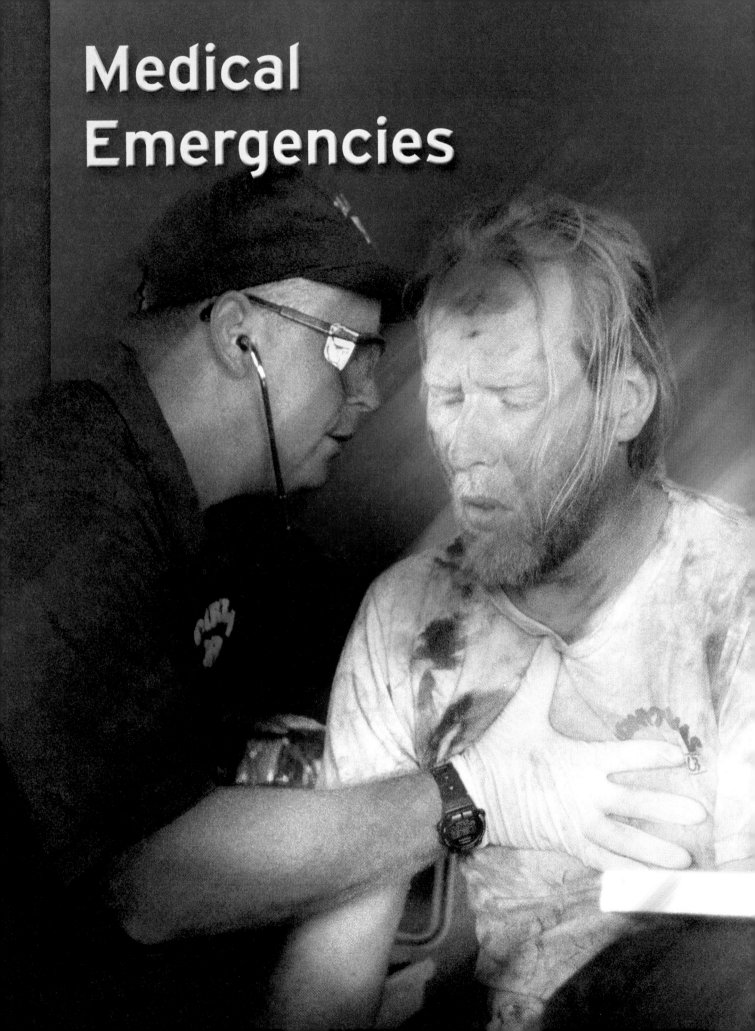

Medical Emergencies

Section

4

General Pharmacology

Objectives

Cognitive

1. Identify which medications will be carried on the unit (p 312).
2. State the medications carried on the unit by the generic name (p 312).
3. Identify the medications with which the EMT-B may assist the patient with administering (p 314).
4. State the medications the EMT-B can assist the patient with by the generic name (p 314).
5. Discuss the forms in which medications may be found (p 310).

Affective

6. Explain the rationale for the administration of medications (p 308).

Psychomotor

7. Demonstrate general steps for assisting the patient with self-administration of medications (p 315).
8. Read the labels and inspect each type of medication (p 318).

TECHNOLOGY

www.emtb.com

- Online Chapter Pretest
- Interactivities
- Vocabulary Explorer
- Anatomy Review
- Web Links
- Online Review Manual
- Distance Learning

Chapter FEATURES

- Skill Drills
- Vital Vocabulary
- Pediatric Needs
- Geriatric Needs
- EMT-B Safety
- EMT-B Tips
- Documentation Tips
- Remember
- Prep Kit

You are the EMT

"Medic 5, please respond to Reynolds High School in the art room for a girl with an unknown medical problem." As you are heading to the art room, a friend of the patient meets you and tells you that her friend broke up with her boyfriend last night and that she thinks she may have taken some pills in a suicide attempt. Later in the call, you contact medical control, which gives an order for activated charcoal to be given.

Medication administration by EMT-Bs is a relatively recent expansion of the scope of their duties, and one that has come with increased responsibilities. This chapter presents the key concepts of basic pharmacology and will also help you answer the following questions:

1. Why must EMT-Bs have a working knowledge of any medication they may administer or help a patient in taking?

2. What are the nine routes by which medications are commonly given? List why each choice might be made.

General Pharmacology

Administering medications is a serious business. Used appropriately, a medication may alleviate pain, ease suffering, and improve a patient's well-being. However, used inappropriately, medication may cause harm and even death. As an EMT-B, you will be responsible for administering certain medications to patients and helping them to self-administer others. You will ask patients about their medications allergies, and you will report this information to hospital personnel. To act without understanding how medications work is to place patients and yourself in danger.

This chapter describes the various forms of medications, the different ways in which they can be administered, and how they work. It then takes a close look at each of the six medications you may be called upon to administer or help patients to self-administer.

How Medications Work

Pharmacology is the study of the properties (characteristics) and effects of drugs and medications. Although these two terms are often used interchangeably, "drugs" may make some people think of narcotics or illegal substances. For this reason, you should try to use the word "medications," especially when interviewing patients and families. In general terms, a medication is a chemical substance that is used to treat or prevent disease or relieve pain.

The **dose** is the amount of the medication that is given. The dose depends on the patient's size or age; adults and children will get different amounts of the same medication. It also depends on the desired action of the medication. The **action** is the therapeutic effect that a medication is expected to have on the body. For example, nitroglycerin relaxes the walls of the blood vessels and may dilate the arteries. This increases the blood flow, and thus the supply of oxygen, to the heart muscle. In this way, nitroglycerin relieves the squeezing or crushing pain that occurs with the cardiac condition called angina. Nitroglycerin is therefore indicated for chest pain associated with angina. **Indications** are the therapeutic uses for a particular medication.

There are times when you should not a give a patient medication, even if it is indicated for that person's condition. Such situations are called **contraindications**. A medication is contraindicated when it would either harm the patient or have no positive effect on the patient's condition. For example, giving activated charcoal is indicated when a patient has swallowed a poison. Generally, activated charcoal, premixed with water, is used to prevent the body from absorbing a poison. However, activated charcoal would be contraindicated if the patient were unconscious and could not swallow.

Side effects are any actions of a medication other than the desired ones. Side effects may occur even when a medication is administered properly. For example, giving epinephrine to a patient who is having an allergic reaction should dilate the bronchioles and decrease wheezing. However, two side effects of epinephrine are cardiac stimulation and constriction of the arteries, which may elevate the patient's heart rate and blood pressure. These side effects are predictable; others are not.

Medication Names

A medication may have many different names. A **trade name** is the brand name that a manufacturer gives to a medication, such as Tylenol or Lasix. As a proper noun, a trade name begins with a capital letter. Trade names are used in every aspect of our daily lives, not just in medications. Well-known examples include Jell-O gelatin, Band-Aid adhesive bandages, and Hershey chocolate candy. A medication may have many different trade names, depending on how many companies manufacture it. Advil, Nuprin, and Motrin all are trade names for the same generic medication: ibuprofen.

The **generic name** of a medication (such as ibuprofen) is usually its original chemical name, which is not capitalized. Sometimes a medication is called by its generic name more often than by any of its trade names. For example, you may hear the term "nitroglycerin" used more often than the trade names Isordil and Nitrostat. All medications that are licensed for use in the United States are listed by their generic names in the *United States Pharmacopoeia*.

Medications may be **prescription medications** or **over-the-counter (OTC) medications**. Prescription medications are distributed to patients only by pharmacists according to a physician's order. OTC medications may be purchased directly from a wholesale or retail source, such as a discount store or supermarket, without a prescription. In recent years, the number of prescription medications that have become available OTC has increased dramatically. Therefore, many of the problems that are attributable to prescription medications may become more common. You may also come into contact with patients who have taken "street" drugs such as heroin or cocaine. Although street drugs lack the pharmaceutical purity of OTC or prescribed medications, they still are pharmacologically active and will cause an effect.

Routes of Administration

Absorption is the process by which medications travel through body tissues until they reach the bloodstream. There are nine routes of medication delivery into the body.

- **Intravenous (IV) injection**. "Intravenous" means "into the vein." Medications that need to enter the bloodstream immediately may be injected directly into a vein. This is the fastest way to deliver a chemical substance, but the IV route cannot be used for all chemicals. For example, aspirin, oxygen, or charcoal cannot be given by the IV route.

- **Oral**. Many medications are taken by mouth, **per os (PO)**, and enter the bloodstream through

---

EMT-B Safety

A needle withdrawn from a patient's skin after giving an injection is assumed to be contaminated with potentially infectious fluids. Handle contaminated "sharps" accordingly and dispose of them immediately according to your service's procedures for preventing infectious exposures.

---

the digestive system. This process often takes as much as 1 hour.

- **Sublingual (SL)**. "Sublingual" means "under the tongue." Medications that take the SL route, such as nitroglycerin tablets, are absorbed by the venous plexus under the tongue and enter the bloodstream through the oral mucous membranes within minutes. This route is not only faster, it protects medications from chemicals in the digestive system, such as acids that can weaken or inactivate them.

- **Intramuscular (IM) injection**. "Intramuscular" means "into the muscle." Usually, medications that are administered via IM injection are absorbed quickly, because muscles have a lot of blood vessels. Some types of medications, though, are designed for a slower, sustained release from the muscle. Many such medications have the prefix "depo" in their names, meaning that they form a depository in the muscle after being injected. However, not all medications can be administered intramuscularly. Intramuscular injections can cause damage to muscle tissue and result in uneven, unreliable absorption. This is especially true in people who are experiencing decreased tissue perfusion or shock.

- **Intraosseous (IO)**. "Intraosseous" means "into the bone." Medications that are delivered via this route reach the blood through the bone marrow. To get medication into the marrow requires drilling a needle through the bone cortex. Because this is painful, the IO route of delivery is used most often in patients who are unconscious as a result of cardiac arrest or extreme shock. Most commonly, the IO route is reserved for children who have less available (or difficult to access) IV sites.

- **Subcutaneous (SC) injection**. "Subcutaneous" means "beneath the skin." An SC injection is given into the tissue between the skin and the muscle. Because there is less blood here than in the muscles, medications that are delivered via this route are generally absorbed more slowly, and their effects last longer. An SC injection is a useful way to deliver medications that cannot be taken by mouth, as long as they do not irritate or damage the tissue. Commonly, a daily insulin shot is given this way to a patient with diabetes. Also, epinephrine can be given by this route.

- **Transcutaneous**. Transcutaneous means "through the skin." Some medications can be absorbed transcutaneously, such as "nicotine patches" in individuals who are trying to quit smoking. On occasion, a medication that comes in another form is administered transcutaneously to achieve a slower, longer-lasting effect. An example is an adhesive patch containing nitroglycerin.

- **Inhalation**. Some medications are inhaled into the lungs so that they can be absorbed into the blood more quickly. Others are inhaled because they actually work in the lungs. Generally, inhalation helps to minimize the effects of the medication in other body tissues. Such medications come in the form of aerosols, fine powders, or sprays.

- **Per rectum (PR)**. "Per rectum" means "by rectum." This route of delivery is frequently used with children because of easier administration and more reliable absorption. (Children often

regurgitate some or all of a medication.) For similar reasons, many medications that are used for nausea and vomiting come in a rectal suppository form. Some medications to control seizures are administered PR when it is impossible to administer them intravenously.

▼ Table 10-1 lists the words that are used for routes of medication delivery, along with their meanings.

Medication Forms

The form that a medication comes in usually dictates its route of delivery. For instance, a tablet or a spray cannot be delivered through a needle. The manufacturer chooses the form to ensure the proper route of the medication, the timing of its release into the bloodstream, and its effects on the target organs or body systems. As an EMT-B, you should be familiar with the following seven medication forms.

Tablets and Capsules

Most medications that are given by mouth to adult patients are in tablet or capsule form ▶ Figure 10-1 . Capsules are gelatin shells filled with powdered or liquid medication. If the capsule contains liquid, the shell is sealed and usually soft. If the capsule contains powder, the shell can usually be pulled apart. Tablets often contain other materials that are mixed with the medication and compressed under high pressure.

Some tablets are designed to dissolve very quickly in small amounts of liquid so that they can be given sublingually and absorbed rapidly. An example is the

TABLE 10-1 Routes of Administration: Words and Their Meanings

This Word . . .	From These Latin Words . . .	Means
Inhalation	inhalatio (drawing air into the lungs)	inhaling or breathing in
Intramuscular (IM)	intra (into) and muscularis (of the muscles)	into muscle
Intraosseous (IO)	intra (into) and ossa (bone)	into bone
Intravenous (IV)	intra (into) and venosus (of the veins)	into vein
Per os (PO)	per (by) and os (mouth)	by mouth
Per rectum (PR)	per (by) and rectum (rectum)	by rectum
Subcutaneous (SC)	sub (under) and cutis (skin)	under the skin
Sublingual (SL)	sub (under) and lingua (relating to the tongue)	under the tongue
Transcutaneous	trans (through) and cutis (skin)	through the skin

sublingual nitroglycerin tablet used for chest pain by patients with cardiac conditions. These medications are especially useful in emergency situations. Generally, a medication that must be swallowed is less useful in an emergency, since the digestive tract provides a slower route of delivery. For example, an oral pain medication is less useful than an IV pain medication when pain relief is needed within minutes.

Solutions and Suspensions

A **solution** is a liquid mixture of one or more substances that cannot be separated by filtering or allowing the mixture to stand. Solutions can be given by almost any route. When given by mouth, solutions may be absorbed from the stomach fairly quickly because the medication is already dissolved. Solutions that irritate the stomach may be given rectally, applied topically to the skin, sprayed sublingually, or inhaled. For example, you may need to help in the sublingual delivery of a nitroglycerin spray (▼ **Figure 10-2**). Many solutions can be given as an IV, IM, or SC injection. If a patient has a severe allergic reaction, you may help to administer a solution of epinephrine subcutaneously, using an auto-injector.

Figure 10-1 Tablets and capsules are typically taken by mouth and enter the bloodstream through the digestive system.

Many substances do not dissolve well in liquids. Some of these can be ground into fine particles and evenly distributed throughout a liquid by shaking or stirring. This type of mixture is called a **suspension**. An example is activated charcoal, which you may give to patients who have taken overdoses of certain medications or ingested certain poisons.

Suspensions separate if they stand or are filtered. It is very important that you shake or swirl a suspension before administering it to ensure that the patient receives the right amount of medication. For example, if you are a parent, you may have had to shake a suspension of oral antibiotic before giving it to your child.

Suspensions usually are administered by mouth but sometimes are given rectally. Occasionally, suspensions are applied directly to the skin to treat skin problems. You may have used calamine lotion in this way. Injectable suspensions are given via IM or SC injection only. Certain hormone shots or vaccinations are given this way because of the suspended particles. They cannot be given via IV injection because the suspended particles do not remain dissolved.

Metered-Dose Inhalers

If liquids or solids are broken into small enough droplets or particles, they can be inhaled. A **metered-dose inhaler (MDI)** is a miniature spray canister, used to direct such substances through the mouth and into the lungs (▼ **Figure 10-3**). An MDI delivers the same amount of medication each time it is used. Since an inhaled medication usually is a suspension, the MDI must be shaken vigorously before the medication is administered. MDIs are often used by patients with respiratory illnesses such as asthma or emphysema.

Topical Medications

Lotions, creams, and ointments all are **topical medications**, that is, they are applied to the surface of the skin

Figure 10-2 Nitroglycerin, which is prescribed for chest pain, is often given sublingually (SL) as a spray or a tablet.

Figure 10-3 Some medications are inhaled into the lungs with a metered-dose inhaler so that they can be absorbed into the bloodstream more quickly.

and affect only that area. Lotions contain the most amount of water, while ointments contain the least. You have probably noticed that OTC lotions are oilier than prescribed lotions. This is a result of a smaller amount of water used in the preparation, resulting in a slower rate of absorption of the medication. For example, hand lotions usually are absorbed faster than facial creams. Calamine lotion, on the other hand, is an example of a medical lotion. Creams, in turn, are absorbed faster than ointments such as Neosporin first-aid ointment. Hydrocortisone cream, to diminish skin itching, is an example of a medical cream that can also be given in ointment form.

Transcutaneous Medications

Transdermal medications are designed to be absorbed through the skin, or transcutaneously. Medications such as nitroglycerin paste usually have properties or delivery systems that help to dilate the blood vessels in the skin and thus speed absorption into the bloodstream. In contrast to most topical medicines, which work directly on the application site, transdermal medications are usually intended for systemic (whole-body) effects. A note of caution: If you touch such a medication with your bare skin while administering it, you will absorb it just as readily as the patient will.

Newer delivery systems for transcutaneous medications include the adhesive patch. Patches attach to the skin and allow even absorption of a medication for many hours (▼ **Figure 10-4**). Both prescription and OTC medications come in this form. Two common examples are nitroglycerin and nicotine.

Gels

A gel is a semi-liquid substance that is administered orally through capsules or plastic tubes. Gels usually have the consistency of paste or creams but are transparent (clear). "Gelatinous" means thick and sticky, like

As an EMT-B, you should be familiar with the dosage forms.

gelatin. Depending on your local medical directives, as an EMT-B, you may give oral glucose in gel form to a patient with diabetes (▼ **Figure 10-5**).

Gases for Inhalation

Gaseous medications are neither solid nor liquid and most often are delivered in an operating room (OR). The medication that is most commonly used in gas form outside the OR is oxygen. You might not think of oxygen as a medication because it is all around us and we all use it. However, in its concentrated form, it is a potent medication that has systemic effects, that is, effects throughout the body (▶ **Figure 10-6**). You will usually administer oxygen through a non-rebreather mask, or occasionally through a nasal cannula.

Medications Carried on the EMS Unit

The three medications that may be carried on the EMS unit are oxygen, oral glucose, and activated charcoal. Used wisely, each can be a powerful tool. Keep in mind, however, that you may deliver these medications only according to standing orders in a protocol (off-line medical control) or a direct order (online medical control).

Oxygen

All cells need oxygen to function properly. The heart and brain, especially, cannot function for long if oxygen levels go down, which is why oxygen was chosen as an

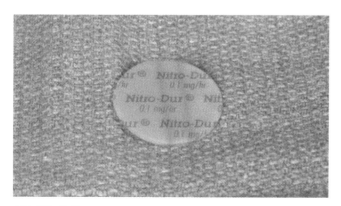

Figure 10-4 Some medications are transcutaneous, or administered through the skin, such as the nitroglycerin patch shown.

Figure 10-5 Oral glucose, used in diabetic emergencies, is available in both gel and tablet form.

Documentation Tips

When documenting the use of oxygen, include the liter flow rate and the type of device used. For instance: "Nonrebreathing mask at 12 L/min." Also document the patient's response to oxygen administration.

on-board medication for EMS units. If a patient is not breathing or is having trouble getting air into the lungs, you should administer supplemental oxygen. In general, you will be giving oxygen via a nonrebreathing mask at 10 to 15 L/min (or via nasal cannula at 2 to 6 L/min if the patient does not tolerate a nonrebreather mask). However, if the patient is not breathing, you must also provide artificial ventilations, so you will need to use the BVM device. Oxygen is usually delivered at 15 L/min with this technique.

Outside a hospital, the nonrebreathing mask is the preferred method of giving oxygen to patients who are experiencing significant respiratory difficulties or shock. With a good mask-to-mouth seal, this mask can provide up to 90% inspired oxygen ▼ Figure 10-7 . With a nasal cannula, oxygen flows through two small, tubelike prongs that fit into the patient's nostrils. This device can provide up to 44% inspired oxygen if the flowmeter is set at 6 L/min.

Remember that, although oxygen itself does not burn, it allows other things to burn. If there is extra oxygen in the air, objects will burn more easily. So make sure there are no open flames, lit cigarettes, or sparks in the area in which you are administering oxygen.

Remember

Know These Medications

Under the US Department of Transportation's 1994 EMT-Basic National Standard Curriculum, an EMT-B is allowed to administer or help patients self-administer the following six medications.

You may be called upon to administer these medications:
- Oxygen
- Activated charcoal
- Oral glucose

You may help patients self-administer these medications:
- Epinephrine
- Metered Dose Inhaler Medications
- Nitroglycerin

However, you may administer or help to administer these medications only under the following conditions:
- A licensed physician gives you a direct order to administer a medication, and/or the local medical protocols under which you are working permit you to administer that medication. Some local protocols exclude one or more of the six medications listed above.
- The local medical protocols under which you are working include standing orders for the use of a medication in defined situations. It is imperative that you do not give or help patients take any other medications under any circumstances.

Figure 10-6 Oxygen is a potent medication that you will typically give through a nonrebreathing mask.

Figure 10-7 A nonrebreathing mask is the preferred method of giving oxygen, as it provides up to 90% inspired oxygen.

Activated Charcoal

Many poisoning emergencies involve overdoses of medications taken by mouth. Fortunately, many medications adsorb activated charcoal, which keeps the medications from being absorbed by the body. <u>Adsorption</u> means to bind to or stick to a surface. <u>Activated charcoal</u> is ground into a very fine powder to provide the greatest possible surface area for binding. You will probably carry a container with a premixed suspension of activated charcoal powder and water in the EMS unit, if allowed by local protocol ▼ Figure 10-8 .

The bond between medication and charcoal is not permanent. Because the medication may break free and be absorbed into the bloodstream if activated charcoal remains in the digestive system throughout a normal day, charcoal is frequently suspended with another medication called sorbitol (a complex sugar). This suspension has a laxative effect that causes the entire mixture, including the medication, to move quickly through the digestive system.

Activated charcoal is given by mouth. Although sorbitol sweetens the suspension, the black charcoal makes it look unappealing. For this reason, you should use

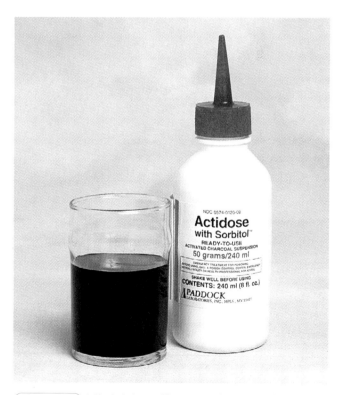

Figure 10-8 Activated charcoal is a suspension that is often used for patients who have taken a medication overdose or swallowed a poison.

a covered container and ask the patient to drink the fluid through a straw.

Oral Glucose

Glucose is a sugar that our cells use as fuel. Although some cells can use other sugars, brain cells must have glucose. If the level of glucose in the blood gets too low, a person can lose consciousness, have seizures, and ultimately die.

The medical term for an extremely low blood glucose level is <u>hypoglycemia</u>. Hypoglycemia can be caused by an excess of insulin, which is taken to control blood glucose levels. Patients with diabetes who use insulin regularly understand the effects of this medication on the body. If they ever inject more insulin than the body can use, hours later they may need to eat a candy bar or drink a sugared cola to try to counteract the insulin's action. The <u>oral glucose</u> that is carried in the EMS unit can counteract the effects of hypoglycemia (abnormally low blood glucose) in the same way as a candy bar or sweet drink, but faster. This is because common table sugar (sucrose) and fruit sugars (fructose) are complex sugars and must be broken down before they can be absorbed. Glucose is a simple sugar that is readily absorbed by the bloodstream.

Hospital personnel and paramedics can give glucose through an IV line. As an EMT-B, you can give glucose only by mouth. Glucose is available as a gel designed to be spread on the mucous membranes between the cheek and gum; however, absorption through this route is not as reliable as with injection. Because the patient may be conscious one moment and unconscious the next, you must be very careful when administering oral glucose. If the patient is unable to swallow well, you should not give glucose, as it might be accidentally inhaled into the lungs.

Patient-Assisted Medications

The three prescribed medications that you may help patients self-administer are epinephrine, metered-dose inhaler medications, and nitroglycerin. These medications, prescribed by doctors for self-administration by patients, have risks as well as benefits, and you must understand them.

Epinephrine

Epinephrine is the main hormone that controls the body's fight-or-flight response. It is released inside the body when there is sudden stress, such as during

Geriatric Needs

Geriatric patients often take many medications. They might also save medications left over from prior medical conditions. Make every effort to identify which medications are current and what conditions they are being used to treat. Ask family members to help distinguish current from outdated medications, or look at the expiration dates on the medication labels. Take either a list of the current medications or the drugs themselves with you to the emergency department.

Elderly patients can become confused about their medication regimen. Uncertainty as to whether or not they missed a dose may cause the patients to repeat the medication, possibly leading to an overdose. If you think an overdose has occurred, contact medical control.

Remember, medications can interact with each other, creating potentially harmful conditions for the patient. Even though a medication may be indicated for a special condition, it might be contraindicated in the presence of another medication. For example, if the patient is taking the heart medication propranolol (Inderal) and has an acute episode of shortness of breath, any asthma remedy might be rendered ineffective by the heart medication.

The new medication sildenafil (Viagra) can have potentially fatal interactions with common heart medications. Ask a patient who has been prescribed nitroglycerin if he has used Viagra within the previous 24 hours. Report this to medical control.

While medications do help people to recover from acute conditions and adjust to chronic diseases, they can pose serious problems for the geriatric patient. You should distinguish current from prior medications, suspect accidental or intentional overdoses, and be prepared for potentially lethal medication interactions. Document all findings and inform medical control.

Documentation Tips

When documenting a medication, the proper form includes the name of the medication, dose and route, and vital signs before and after administration. For instance:

10:30 am—VS: P 88, R 18, BP 128/68—nitro, 0.4 mg SL
10:35 am—VS: P 80, R 18, BP 124/60

Epinephrine has the following characteristics:
- Secreted naturally by adrenal glands
- Decreases muscle tone of bronchiole tree
- Dilates passages in lungs
- Constricts blood vessels
- Increases heart rate and blood pressure

ADMINISTERING EPINEPHRINE BY METERED-DOSE INHALER. Asthma, also known as "reactive airway disease," can be a life-threatening condition. Therefore, some patients use epinephrine inhalers to relieve bronchial spasms quickly. The trade names of some of these inhalers include Primatene Mist, Bronitin Mist, Bronkaid Mist, and Medihaler-Epi. Since epinephrine tends to increase heart rate and blood pressure, most patients with asthma also use certain chemical cousins of epinephrine that produce fewer side effects. Metaproterenol (Alupent or Metaprel) and albuterol (Proventil or Ventolin) both work more on the bronchial spasms and less on the cardiovascular system.

ADMINISTERING EPINEPHRINE BY INJECTION. Patients who know that they are allergic to insect stings often carry epinephrine for SC or IM injections, just in case they are stung. In these individuals, insect venom causes the body to release histamine, which lowers blood pressure by relaxing the small blood vessels and allowing them to leak. The release of histamine may also cause wheezing from bronchial spasms and swelling of the airway tissues (edema), which make it difficult for the patient to breathe. Epinephrine acts as a specific antidote to histamine, countering both of these harmful effects. It constricts the blood vessels, allowing blood pressure to rise and reducing the swelling. In the lungs, it has the opposite effect; it dilates these passages, so the flow of air is less restricted. You can also expect the patient's heart rate to increase after administration of epinephrine.

You may be trained to administer SC and IM injections of epinephrine, depending on local protocol.

exercise or when the patient becomes suddenly scared. Because epinephrine is secreted by the adrenal glands, it is also known as adrenaline. Epinephrine has different effects on different body tissues and is used as a medication in several forms. Generally, **epinephrine** will increase heart rate and blood pressure and decrease the muscle tone of the bronchiole tree. Therefore, it can ease breathing problems caused by the bronchiole spasms that are common in asthma and allergic reactions. In a person who is close to anaphylactic shock as a result of an allergic reaction, epinephrine may also help to maintain the patient's blood pressure.

Remember that an SC injection puts the epinephrine into the tissue between the skin and the muscle. Therefore, it is usually helpful to pinch the skin lightly to lift it away from the muscle. A syringe used for SC injections has a short, thin needle, typically between 1/2" and 5/8" long. The syringe for IM use has a longer, thicker needle that is between 1 and 1 1/2" long so that it can reach into the muscle.

Follow these steps for either an SC or an IM injection:

1. Before giving an injection, prepare the skin with an appropriate antiseptic (▼ Figure 10-9A).

2. Insert the needle into the skin (or muscle). For an SC injection, pinch the skin while inserting the needle at a 45-degree angle (▼ Figure 10-9B). Then draw the syringe's plunger back slightly before injecting the medication.

3. Check to see whether any blood seeps into the syringe. If it does, you have accidentally placed the needle in a small blood vessel and will need to withdraw the needle and start again using the same syringe (assuming that the skin remains sterilized).

4. If no blood returns when you pull back on the needle, push the plunger on the syringe to inject the medication.

5. Once the needle has been injected into the patient's skin, it becomes contaminated with potential viruses and other infectious agents from the patient. Appropriate disposal precautions must be taken.

Epinephrine may also be dispensed from an auto-injector, which automatically delivers a preset amount of the medication (▼ Figure 10-10). This is the method that you will most likely use. Pressing the device into the skin activates the mechanism. Regardless of the method used, epinephrine causes a burning sensation where it is injected, and the patient's heart rate will increase after the injection.

Metered-Dose Inhaler Medications

Sometimes, a respiratory condition such as asthma is not severe enough to require the use of epinephrine. In such cases, patients may use one of the epinephrine cousins that is more narrowly focused on the lungs. These medications are delivered with a metered-dose inhaler. An MDI requires a great deal of coordination, something that may be in short supply when an individual is having trouble breathing. Patients must aim properly and spray just as they start to inhale. An adapter, which fits over the inhaler like a sleeve, can be used; however, most of the medication tends to end up on the roof of the patient's mouth. To avoid misdirecting the spray, many physicians prescribe "spacer"

Figure 10-9 Administering an SC or IM injection. **A.** Cleanse the skin. **B.** Insert the needle then draw the plunger back slightly.

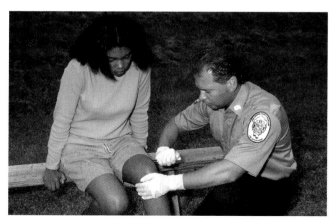

Figure 10-10 An Epi-Pen auto-injector may be used to administer a preset dose of epinephrine.

devices for use with the inhaler ▼**Figure 10-11**. The inhaler fits into an opening on one end of the spacer's chamber, and the mouthpiece fits on the other end. The patient sprays the prescribed dose into the chamber and then breathes in and out of the mouthpiece until the mist is completely inhaled.

Activate the spray by pressing the canister into the adapter just as the patient starts to inhale. If relief is not achieved, wait about 3 minutes and repeat this sequence. Above all, it is important to ensure that the patient inhales all the medication in a single-sprayed dose.

Nitroglycerin

Many patients with cardiac conditions carry some form of fast-acting nitroglycerin to relieve the pain of angina. Nitroglycerin is the same substance as TNT (trinitrotoluene), which is why the term "nitro" is used both in medicine and the explosives industry. Fortunately, the forms of nitroglycerin that you will use have been stabilized so that they are not explosive.

If you have ever run for a prolonged period of time, you probably remember that your muscles developed a painful, heavy, burning sensation. This is because the demand for oxygen to those muscles exceeded the supply. When heart muscle develops a similar pain, it is called angina pectoris. The cause is the same: not enough oxygen, in this case because of a blockage or narrowing in the blood vessels that supply the heart. Occasionally, the cause is a spasm in these blood vessels. Unlike the runner with sore legs, of course, the heart muscle cannot stop and rest until the pain goes away.

The purpose of **nitroglycerin** is to increase blood flow by relieving the spasms or causing the arteries to dilate. It does this by relaxing the muscular walls of the coronary arteries and veins. Nitroglycerin also relaxes

Figure 10-11 Some inhalers have spacer devices to better direct the medication spray.

veins throughout the body, so less blood is returned to the heart and the heart does not have to work as hard each time it contracts. In short, blood pressure is decreased. Because of this, however, it is important that you always take the patient's blood pressure before administering nitroglycerin. If the systolic blood pressure is less than 100 mm Hg, the nitroglycerin may have the harmful effect of lowering the blood flow to the heart's own blood vessels. Even a patient who has adequate blood pressure should sit or lie down with head elevated before taking this medication. If the patient is standing, he or she may faint when blood flow to the brain is reduced as the nitroglycerin starts to work. If a significant drop in the patient's blood pressure (15 to 20 mm Hg) occurs and the patient suddenly feels dizzy or sick, lay the patient down and raise the legs.

During a heart attack (myocardial infarction, or MI), a blood clot forms in a narrowed coronary artery, blocking the blood flow to a section of the heart muscle. If the blockage is not cleared in time, that section of the heart muscle will die. If nitroglycerin no longer brings relief to a person in whom it has previously worked, the person may be experiencing an MI instead of an angina attack. Therefore, it is important to know how much nitroglycerin a patient has needed in the past to relieve chest pain and how much has been taken during the current emergency. Always report this information to medical control. Remember, you cannot administer this medication without clearance from medical control or standing orders.

Nitroglycerin has the following effects:

- Relaxes the muscular walls of coronary arteries and veins

- Less blood is returned to the heart

- Decreases blood pressure

- Relaxes veins throughout the body

- Often causes a mild headache after administration

ADMINISTERING NITROGLYCERIN BY TABLET. Nitroglycerin is usually taken sublingually: The patient places a tiny tablet under the tongue, where it dissolves. The tablet should create a slight tingling or burning sensation. If the nitroglycerin has lost its usual "bite," it may have lost potency because of aging or improper storage. Be sure to check the expiration date on the bottle.

Sublingual nitroglycerin tablets should be stored in their original glass container with the cap screwed on tightly. Note that what looks like cotton in the container is actually rayon. If real cotton is placed in the container, it can absorb nitroglycerin, thus reducing the tablets' potency. Other medications placed in the container can likewise rob nitroglycerin of its power. If you notice any signs of improper storage, be sure to include that information in the patient's medical history.

ADMINISTERING NITROGLYCERIN BY METERED-DOSE SPRAY. Some patients who take nitroglycerin use a metered-dose spray, which deposits medication on or under the tongue. Each spray is equivalent to one tablet. To ensure direct, proper dosing on the bottom of the tongue, do not use a spacer with the metered-dose canister when delivering nitroglycerin by this method.

Whether using the tablets or the metered-dose spray, you should wait 5 minutes for a response before repeating. Closely monitor the patient's vital signs, particularly the blood pressure.

General Steps in Administering Medication

As an EMT-B, you must be familiar with the five general steps of administering any medication to a patient:

1. **Obtain an order from medical control.** This order may be given to you directly, through online medical control via telephone or radio. Or it may be indirect, through protocols that contain standing orders for the administration of certain medications. For example, your system may use a protocol that describes how the medical director wants you to deal with a patient who is having respiratory difficulties. Part of this protocol may direct you to use a nonrebreathing mask to deliver oxygen to such a patient at 15 L/min. You may do this without calling online medical control if the patient meets the criteria of the protocol.

2. **Verify the proper medication and prescription.** You have received and confirmed the medication order and determined that the patient is still a candidate for the medication. You must now make sure that the medication you are about to deliver is the correct medication. Carefully read the label. If it is the patient's own prescription, the bottle may show the trade name or the generic name. If you have any questions at all, contact on-line medical control. Make sure that the medication is, indeed, the patient's own and does not belong to a friend or relative. You should never give a medication to a patient that

has been prescribed for someone else. The only exception to this rule is if you are ordered to do so by medical control and you are sure that they understand that the medication does not belong to the patient.

3. **Verify the form, dose, and route of the medication.** You have confirmed your order and verified that the medication is the one you want to give. Now you must make sure that the form of the medication, the dose, and the route are all compatible with the order you received. For example, suppose that you are told to give the patient a sublingual nitroglycerin tablet. The patient's nitroglycerin tablet bottle is empty, but he has another bottle of nitroglycerin capsules. These are to be swallowed four times a day. The medication is the same, but the form, dose, and route of delivery are different from the order given. You may not substitute the capsules for the tablets without specific orders from medical control.

4. **Check the expiration date and condition of the medication.** The last step before administering a medication is to make sure it has not expired. Prescription and OTC medications alike should have an expiration date on their labels. Check the date. If no date can be found, you should examine the medication with suspicion. In addition, if you find discoloration, cloudiness, or particles in a liquid medication, you should not use it. If a patient with asthma gives you an MDI and the expiration date on it is smudged, you should not use it.

5. **Reassess the vital signs, especially heart rate and blood pressure, at least every 5 minutes or as the patient's condition changes.**

6. **Document.** Remember the EMS rule: The work is not done until the paperwork is done. Once the medication has been delivered, you must document your actions and the patient's response. This includes the time you gave the medication as well as the name, dose, and route of administration. Did the patient improve, get worse, or not change at all? Were there any side effects? A second EMS rule says, "if you did not write it down, it did not happen." If your performance should ever be questioned, documentation is your best defense.

Remember

General Steps in Administering Medication

1. Obtain an order from medical control.
2. Verify the proper medication and prescription.
3. Verify the form, dose, and route of the medication.
4. Check the expiration date and condition of the medication.
5. Reassess the vital signs, especially heart rate and blood pressure, at least every 5 minutes or as the patient's condition changes.
6. Document.

Pediatric Needs

Children are not small adults, especially when it comes to the administration of medications. The approach to this population differs from that of the adult. First the dosages will be different. Sometimes they are smaller; sometimes, however, they can be larger. This has to do with the way that children metabolize medications. Most of the assisted medications will be smaller doses. Let's look at epinephrine, for example: The dose for the adult is 0.3 to 0.5 mg and the child will be given 0.2 to 0.3 mg. The approach to the injection is also different, the injection for an adult will be in the lateral thigh and the child will be in the medial thigh. Location of the injection has to do with the development of blood vessels and muscle mass in the thigh. So to avoid hitting a blood vessel, to ensure the larger spectrum of the muscle, and to ensure proper distribution of the medication, it is important to use the medial thigh in the infant and small child. When administering an MDI to children, they may not have the coordination needed to use an inhaler. It will be easier if a spacer device is added to the inhaler to ensure the child receives the full benefit of the medicine. The last and most important issue around medication administration in children is the affective side. Children are not cognitively or emotionally the same as adults. Therefore it may require you a little more time and effort to explain each procedure. It is also in your best interest to tell the child the truth. It is very important to gain the trust of the child in the short time you have to bond with him or her.

But what if the same patient is also having chest pain "just like my other heart attack"? In that case, you may be able to apply the oxygen, but you may have to call medical control or follow standing orders before helping to administer the patient's nitroglycerin spray. Knowing and understanding the local protocols under which you will be working are absolutely essential.

In addition to getting approval to administer a medication, you must verify the online order, which means that you should restate the name of the medication, the dose to be given, and the route of administration to medical control. Verifying the order will help to reduce the chance of a miscommunication leading to the administration of an inappropriate medication.

Next, you must reconfirm that the patient can tolerate the medication. For example, suppose that you have received and verified the order to give one sublingual nitroglycerin tablet to a patient with a cardiac condition. While you were getting the order, however, the patient began to sweat more and became less responsive. A repeat blood pressure reading is 80/60 mm Hg. Using your knowledge about nitroglycerin, you would decide not to give the medication. Instead, you would notify medical control of the changes in the patient's condition and seek further orders.

Prep Kit

Ready for Review

Medications come in seven different forms: tablets and capsules, solutions and suspensions, metered-dose inhalers, topical medications, transdermal medications, gels, and gases. They may be administered through nine different routes: intravenous, intramuscular, or subcutaneous injection; orally; sublingually; intraosseously; transcutaneously; by inhalation; and by rectum. In all but the intravenous injection route, the medication is absorbed into the bloodstream through various body tissues. These routes of administration often determine the speed with which the medication takes effect.

Three medications are typically carried on the EMS unit: oxygen, oral glucose, and activated charcoal. There are three additional medications that the EMT-B may help the patient self-administer: metered-dose inhaler medications, nitroglycerin, and epinephrine. Remember, though, that these may differ depending on local protocol. The administration of any medication requires approval by medical control, either through direct orders given on-line or standing orders that are part of the local protocols.

There are five steps to follow in administering medications, four of which occur before you give the medication: Obtain an order from medical control, verify the proper medication, verify the dose and route, and check the expiration date of the medication. The fifth step is to accurately document the patient's history, assessment, treatment, and response.

Vital Vocabulary

absorption The process by which medications travel through body tissues until they reach the bloodstream.

action The therapeutic effect of a medication on the body.

activated charcoal An oral medication that binds and adsorbs ingested toxins in the gastrointestinal tract, for treatment of some poisonings and medication overdoses. Charcoal ground into a very fine powder that provides the greatest possible surface area for binding medications that have been taken by mouth; it is carried on the EMS unit.

adsorption To bind or stick to a surface.

contraindication Situations in which a medication should not be given because it would not help or may actually harm a patient.

dose The amount of medication given on the basis of the patient's size and age.

epinephrine Medication that increases heart rate and blood pressure but also eases breathing problems by decreasing muscle tone of the bronchiole tree; the EMT-B may be allowed to help the patient self-administer the medication.

gel A semi-liquid substance that is administered orally through capsules or plastic tubes.

generic name The original chemical name of a medication (in contrast to one of its "trade names"); not capitalized.

hypoglycemia An abnormally low blood glucose level.

indication A therapeutic use for a specific medication.

inhalation Breathing into the lungs; a medication delivery route.

intramuscular (IM) injection Injection into a muscle; a medication delivery route.

intraosseous (IO) Into the bone; a medication delivery route.

intravenous (IV) injection Injection directly into a vein; a medication delivery route.

metered-dose inhaler (MDI) A miniature spray canister through which droplets or particles of medication may be inhaled.

nitroglycerin Medication that increases cardiac perfusion by blood flow by causing arteries to dilate; the EMT-B may be allowed to help the patient self-administer the medication.

oral By mouth; a medication delivery route.

oral glucose A simple sugar that is readily absorbed by the bloodstream; it is carried on the EMS unit.

over-the-counter (OTC) medications Medications that may be purchased directly by a patient without a prescription.

oxygen A gas that all cells need in order to metabolize; the heart and brain, especially, cannot function without oxygen.

per os (PO) Through the mouth; a medication delivery route; same as oral.

per rectum (PR) Through the rectum; a medication delivery route.

pharmacology The study of the properties and effects of medications.

prescription medications Medications that are distributed to patients only by pharmacists according to a physician's order.

side effects Any effects of a medication other than the desired ones.

solution A liquid mixture that cannot be separated by filtering or allowing the mixture to stand.

sublingual (SL) Under the tongue; a medication delivery route.

suspension A mixture of ground particles that are distributed evenly throughout a liquid but do not dissolve.

subcutaneous (SC) injection Injection into the tissue between the skin and muscle; a medication delivery route.

topical medications Lotions, creams, and ointments that are applied to the surface of the skin and affect only that area; a medication delivery route.

trade name The brand name that a manufacturer gives a medication; capitalized.

transcutaneous Through the skin; a medication delivery route.

transdermal medications Medications that are designed to be absorbed through the skin (transcutaneously).

Assessment in Action

You have been waiting for the new jump-kits when they finally arrived. Your service has decided to carry activated charcoal and glucose gel in the new kit. In addition to the protocols, your crew has also decided to carry cards on the patient-assisted medications inside the kits.

It is your job to put those cards together. The cards will include information on activated charcoal and glucose gel as well as epinephrine, nitroglycerin, and metered-dose inhalers.

1. The cards will include all information necessary for any EMT to appropriately administer these medications. Which of the following lists give complete information for any medication?
   A. Actions, dose, route of administration, indications, contraindications, and side effects
   B. Dose, indications, contraindications, generic name and prescription name
   C. Indications, contraindications, generic name, side effects, and the local pharmacy
   D. Generic name, trade names, side effects, route of administration, and your medical director's name

2. Appropriate information to include on an information card about activated charcoal includes administration. A good way to administer activated charcoal is to:
   A. pour it in a glass to drink.
   B. sip it through a straw.
   C. chew it as a tablet.
   D. administer it under the tongue.

3. The appropriate method to administer the patient-assisted medication called epinephrine is to:
   A. administer it under the tongue.
   B. chew it as a tablet.
   C. inject it between the skin and muscle.
   D. swallow it as a liquid.

4. Another patient-assisted medication is a metered dose inhaler. Information on the card will include instructions to:
   A. shake well before administering.
   B. refrigerate prior to using.
   C. administer under the tongue.
   D. turn the device upside down.

5. The medication that is used most commonly in the form of a gas outside the hospital environment is:
   A. nitroglycerin.   B. metered-dose inhaler.
   C. oxygen.   D. carbon dioxide.

6. One of the contraindications for oral glucose is the patient who:
   A. is a diabetic.   B. cannot swallow.
   C. has a digestive problem. D. is having chest pain.

7. The other name for epinephrine is:
   A. metaproterenol.   B. albuterol.
   C. nitroglycerin.   D. adrenaline.

Challenging Questions

8. Why are "spacers" used?

9. Why does nitroglycerin have a tendency to lower blood pressure?

Points to Ponder

You are dispatched to an "unconscious patient" to find a middle-aged man, wide-awake, sitting in a living room chair. He is complaining that someone called you and that he does not need any help. He explains that he "just got dizzy and passed out for a second." As you continue your assessment, the only notable finding is that the patient's blood pressure is quite elevated. The patient states that he only takes his blood pressure medicine when his headaches get too bad. In further questioning, he explains that he is supposed to take one tablet twice a day, but it affects his "manhood." You remember from your pharmacology lecture that some blood pressure medication make the patient unable to achieve an erection. He also states that his headaches have been occurring for about three days. Your patient tells you that he "don't need to see no damned doctor" and refuses transport. What are the potential risks for this patient if he does not

take his blood pressure medication as prescribed? How would you counsel him and what would you say? How will you deal with him if he becomes more talkative about his sex life?

Issues Education and Counseling, Refusal of Treatment.

Online Outlook

A medication may have many different names, which may be a bit confusing for you at first. To learn more about trade names and generic names of medications, complete Exercise 10 at the www.emtb.com.

www.emtb.com

Respiratory Emergencies

Objectives

Cognitive

1. List the structure and function of the respiratory system (p 324).
2. State the signs and symptoms of a patient with breathing difficulty (p 327).
3. Describe the emergency medical care of the patient with breathing difficulty (p 335).
4. Recognize the need for medical direction to assist in the emergency medical care of the patient with breathing difficulty (p 335).
5. Describe the emergency medical care of the patient with breathing distress (p 335).
6. Establish the relationship between airway management and the patient with breathing difficulty (p 336).
7. List signs of adequate air exchange (p 337).
8. State the generic name, medication forms, dose, administration, action, indications, and contraindications for the prescribed inhaler (p 336).
9. Distinguish between the emergency medical care of the infant, child, and adult patient with breathing difficulty (p 338).
10. Differentiate between upper airway obstruction and lower airway disease in the infant and child patient (p 339).

Affective

11. Defend EMT-B treatment regimens for various respiratory emergencies (p 335).
12. Explain the rationale for administering an inhaler (p 338).

Psychomotor

13. Demonstrate the emergency medical care for breathing difficulty (p 335).
14. Perform the steps in facilitating the use of an inhaler (p 339).

TECHNOLOGY

www.emtb.com

Online Chapter Pretest
Interactivities
Vocabulary Explorer
Anatomy Review
Web Links
Online Review Manual
Distance Learning

Chapter FEATURES

Skill Drills
Vital Vocabulary
Pediatric Needs
Geriatric Needs
EMT-B Safety
EMT-B Tips
Documentation Tips
Remember
Prep Kit

Your squad is dispatched to a local restaurant for a "sick patron." You arrive to find a 31-year-old woman complaining that she "just can't breathe" and "has a sharp pain in the chest."

Given the frequency with which calls to EMS are related to breathing, it is paramount that an EMT-B be prepared to handle them. This chapter will prepare you to do just that as well as to answer the following questions:

1. What are the most common signs and symptoms of patients with breathing difficulties?

2. What is the relationship between airway management and breathing difficulty?

Respiratory Emergencies

Dyspnea, the feeling of being short of breath, is a complaint that you will encounter often. It is a symptom of many different conditions, from the common cold and asthma to heart failure and pulmonary embolism. You may or may not be able to determine what is causing dyspnea in a particular patient; this can be difficult even for physicians in a hospital setting. Also, several different problems may contribute to a patient's dyspnea at the same time, including some that are serious or life threatening. Even without a definitive diagnosis, however, you may still be able to save a life.

This chapter begins with a basic explanation of how the lungs function. It then looks at common medical problems that can impede normal functioning and cause dyspnea, including acute pulmonary edema, chronic obstructive pulmonary disease, and asthma. You will learn the signs and symptoms of each condition. You should keep all these possible medical problems in mind as you take the patient's history and perform a physical assessment, a process that the chapter describes in detail. The information that you collect will help you to decide on the proper treatment, which differs according to the probable cause of the dyspnea.

Remember, the sensation of not getting enough air can be terrifying, regardless of its cause. As an EMT-B, you should be prepared to treat not just the symptom and the underlying problem, but also the anxiety that it produces.

Anatomy and Function of the Lungs

The respiratory system consists of all the structures of the body that contribute to the breathing process. Important anatomic features include the upper and lower airways, the lungs, and the diaphragm ▶ **Figure 11-1** . Air enters the trachea and moves along the bronchial tubes to the air spaces, called alveoli, where oxygen and carbon dioxide are exchanged.

The principal function of the lungs is respiration, which is the exchange of oxygen and carbon dioxide. The two processes that occur during respiration are inspiration, the act of breathing in or inhaling, and expiration, the act of breathing out or exhaling. During respiration, oxygen is provided to the blood, and carbon dioxide is removed from it. This exchange of gases takes place rapidly in normal lungs at the level of the alveoli. Alveoli are microscopic, thin-walled air sacs that lie against the pulmonary capillary vessels. Oxygen and carbon dioxide must be able to pass freely between the alveoli and the capillaries ▶ **Figure 11-2** . Oxygen entering the alveoli from inhalation passes through tiny passages in the alveolar wall into the capillaries, which carry the oxygen to the heart. The heart pumps the oxygen around the body. Carbon dioxide produced by the body's cells ▶ **Figure 11-3A** returns to the lungs in the blood that circulates through and around the alveolar air spaces. The carbon dioxide diffuses back into the alveoli and travels back up the bronchial tree and out the upper airways during exhalation ▶ **Figure 11-3B** . Again, carbon dioxide is "exchanged" for oxygen, which travels in exactly the opposite direction (during inhalation).

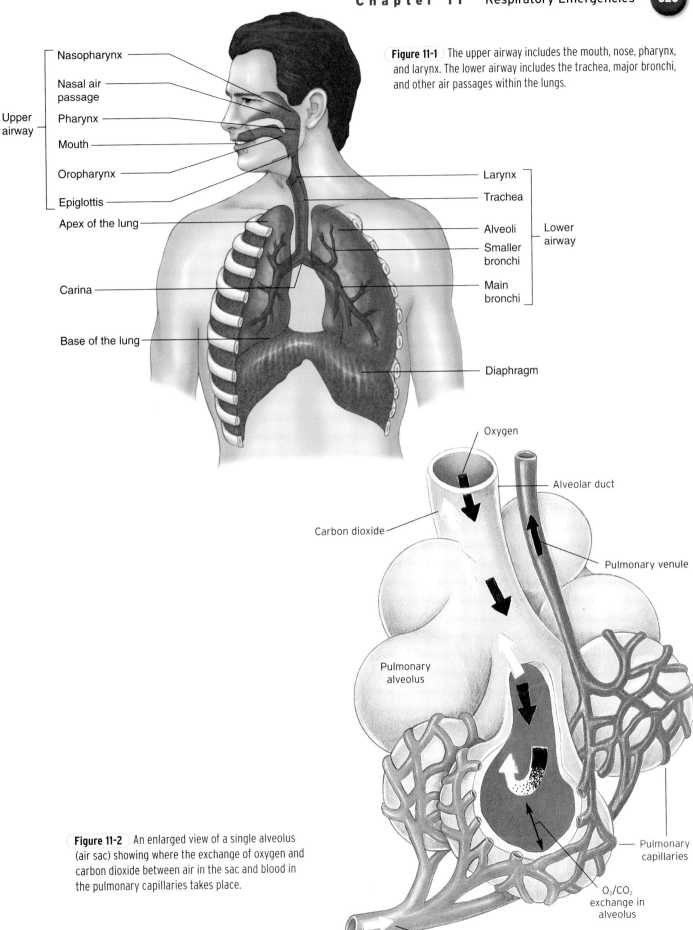

Figure 11-1 The upper airway includes the mouth, nose, pharynx, and larynx. The lower airway includes the trachea, major bronchi, and other air passages within the lungs.

Upper airway
- Nasopharynx
- Nasal air passage
- Pharynx
- Mouth
- Oropharynx
- Epiglottis

Apex of the lung

Carina

Base of the lung

Larynx
Trachea
Alveoli
Smaller bronchi
Main bronchi

Lower airway

Diaphragm

Oxygen

Carbon dioxide

Alveolar duct

Pulmonary venule

Pulmonary alveolus

Pulmonary capillaries

O_2/CO_2 exchange in alveolus

Pulmonary arteriole

Figure 11-2 An enlarged view of a single alveolus (air sac) showing where the exchange of oxygen and carbon dioxide between air in the sac and blood in the pulmonary capillaries takes place.

Pulmonary edema is one of the most common causes of hospital admission in the United States. It is not uncommon for a patient to have repeated bouts.

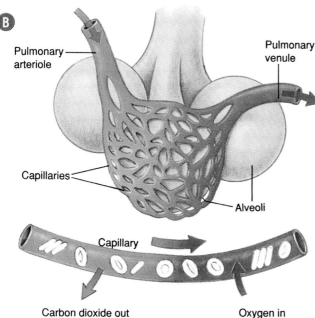

Figure 11-3 The exchange of oxygen and carbon dioxide in respiration. **A.** Oxygen passes from the blood through capillaries to tissue cells. Carbon dioxide passes from tissue cells through capillaries to the blood. **B.** In the lungs, oxygen is picked up by the blood and carbon dioxide is given off.

In most disorders of the lung, one or more of the following situations exists:

- The pulmonary vessels are actually obstructed from absorbing oxygen or releasing carbon dioxide by fluid, infection, or collapsed air spaces.

- The alveoli are damaged and cannot transport gases properly across their own walls.

- The air passages are obstructed by muscle spasm, mucus, or weakened floppy airway walls.

- Blood flow to the lungs is obstructed by blood clots.

- The pleural space is filled with air or excess fluid, so the lungs cannot properly expand.

All these conditions prevent the proper exchange of oxygen and carbon dioxide. In addition, the pulmonary blood vessels themselves may have abnormalities that interfere with blood flow and thus with the transfer of gases.

The brain stem senses the level of carbon dioxide in the arterial blood. The level of carbon dioxide bathing the brain stem is what stimulates a healthy person to breathe. If the level drops too low, the person automatically breathes at a slower rate and less deeply. As a result, less carbon dioxide is expired, allowing carbon dioxide levels in the blood to return to normal. If the level of carbon dioxide in the arterial blood rises above normal, the patient breathes more rapidly and more deeply. When more fresh air (containing no carbon dioxide) is brought into the alveoli, more carbon dioxide diffuses out of the bloodstream, thereby lowering the level.

The following are the characteristics of adequate breathing:

- A normal rate and depth

- A regular pattern of inhalation and exhalation

- Good audible breath sounds on both sides of the chest

- A regular rise and fall movement on both sides of the chest

- Pink, warm, dry skin

The following are signs of inadequate breathing:

- A rate of breathing that is slower than 8 breaths/min or faster than 24 breaths/min

- Muscle retractions above the clavicles, between the ribs, and below the rib cage, especially in children

- Pale or cyanotic skin

- Cool, damp (clammy) skin
- Shallow or irregular respirations
- Pursed lips
- Nasal flaring

The level of carbon dioxide in the arterial blood can rise for a number of reasons. The exhalation process may be impaired by various types of lung disease. The body may also produce too much carbon dioxide, either temporarily or chronically, depending on the disease or abnormality.

If, over a period of years, arterial carbon dioxide levels rise slowly to an abnormally high level and remain there, the respiratory center in the brain, which senses carbon dioxide levels and controls breathing, may work less efficiently. The failure of this center to respond normally to a rise in arterial levels of carbon dioxide is called chronic **carbon dioxide retention**. If the condition is severe, respiration will stop unless there is a secondary drive, called **hypoxic drive**, to stimulate the respiratory center. Fortunately, a second stimulus does develop in patients with chronically high blood carbon dioxide levels, namely, a low level of oxygen in the blood. Low blood oxygen causes the respiratory center to respond and stimulate respiration. If the arterial level of oxygen is then raised, as happens when the patient is given additional oxygen, there is no longer any stimulus to breathe; both the high carbon dioxide and low oxygen drives are lost. Patients with chronic lung diseases frequently have a chronically high level of blood carbon dioxide. Therefore, giving too much oxygen to these patients may actually depress, or completely stop, the respirations. Individuals older than 65 years are especially prone to problems with respiration, either from occult (not obvious) stroke, lung disease, cardiovascular disease, liver disease, or certain medications.

Causes of Dyspnea

Dyspnea is shortness of breath or difficulty breathing. Many different medical problems may cause dyspnea. Be aware that if the problem is severe and the brain is deprived of oxygen, the patient may not be alert enough to complain of shortness of breath. More commonly, altered mental status is a sign of hypoxia of the brain.

Patients often develop breathing difficulty or hypoxia with the following medical conditions:

- Upper or lower airway infection
- Acute pulmonary edema
- Chronic obstructive pulmonary disease (COPD)

EMT-B Safety

If you suspect that a patient has an airborne disease, place a surgical mask (or a NRM if needed) on the patient. When you have specific reason to suspect tuberculosis, do this and also wear a HEPA respirator yourself. See Chapter 2 for detailed discussion on disease transmission precautions.

- Spontaneous pneumothorax
- Asthma or allergic reactions
- Pleural effusion
- Prolonged seizures
- Obstruction of the airway
- Pulmonary embolism
- Hyperventilation
- Severe pain, particularly chest pain

Upper or Lower Airway Infection

Infectious diseases causing dyspnea may affect all parts of the airway. Some cause mild discomfort. Others obstruct the airway to the point that patients require a full range of respiratory support. In general, the problem is always some form of obstruction, either to the flow of air in the major passages (colds, diphtheria, epiglottitis, and croup) or to the exchange of gases between the alveoli and the capillaries (pneumonia). ▶ **Table 11-1** shows infectious diseases that are associated with some degree of dyspnea.

Acute Pulmonary Edema

Sometimes, the heart muscle is so injured after an acute myocardial infarction or other illness that it cannot circulate blood properly. In these cases, the left side of the heart cannot remove blood from the lung as fast as the right side delivers it. As a result, fluid builds up within the alveoli as well as in the lung tissue between the alveoli and the pulmonary capillaries. This accumulation of fluid, called **pulmonary edema**, can develop quickly after a major heart attack. By physically separating alveoli from pulmonary capillary vessels, the edema interferes with the exchange of carbon dioxide and oxygen. There is not enough room left in the lung for slow, deep breaths. The patient usually experiences dyspnea with rapid, shallow respirations. In the most severe instances, you will see a frothy pink sputum at the nose and mouth.

TABLE 11-1 Infectious Diseases Associated with Dyspnea

Disease	Characteristics	Disease	Characteristics
<u>Common Cold</u>	• A viral infection usually associated with swollen nasal mucous membranes and the production of fluid from the sinuses and nose. • Dyspnea is not severe; patients complain of "stuffiness" or difficulty breathing through the nose.	<u>Epiglottitis</u>	• A bacterial infection of the epiglottis that can produce severe swelling of the flap over the larynx. • In preschool and school-aged children especially, the epiglottis can swell to two to three times its normal size (▼ Figure 11-4A). • The airway may become almost completely obstructed, sometimes quite suddenly (▼ Figure 11-4B).
<u>Diphtheria</u>	• Although well controlled in the past decade, it is still highly contagious and serious when it occurs. • The disease causes the formation of a diphtheritic membrane lining the pharynx that is composed of debris, inflammatory cells, and mucus. This membrane can rapidly and severely obstruct the passage of air into the larynx.		
<u>Pneumonia</u>	• An acute bacterial or viral infection of the lung that damages lung tissue, usually associated with fever, cough, and production of sputum. • Fluid also accumulates in the surrounding normal lung tissue, separating the alveoli from their capillaries. (Sometimes, fluid can also accumulate in the pleural space.) • The lung's ability to exchange oxygen and carbon dioxide is impaired. • The breathing pattern in pneumonia does not indicate major airway obstruction, but the patient may experience tachypnea, an increase in the breathing rate, which is an attempt to compensate for the reduced amount of normal lung tissue and for the buildup of fluid.		

Swollen epiglottis

Figure 11-4) Acute epiglottitis. **A.** Epiglottitis is caused by a bacterial infection resulting in severe swelling of the epiglottis. **B.** The epiglottis is massively swollen and almost fully obstructs the airway.

Disease	Characteristics
Epiglottitis **continued**	• **Stridor** (harsh, high-pitched, rough barking inspiratory sounds) may be heard late in the development of airway obstruction.
	• Acute epiglottitis in the adult is characterized by a severe sore throat.
	• The disease is now much less common than it was 20 years ago because of a vaccine that can help to prevent most cases.
Croup	• An inflammation and swelling of the lining of the larynx, the narrowest point of the airway, typically seen in children between ages 6 months and 3 years ▼ **Figure 11-5**.
	• The common signs of croup are stridor and a seal-bark cough, which signal a significant narrowing of the air passage of the larynx that may progress to significant obstruction.
	• Croup often responds well to the administration of humidified oxygen.

Pharynx

Swollen larynx

Esophagus

Figure 11-5 Croup swells the lining of the larynx, which is the narrowest point in a child's airway.

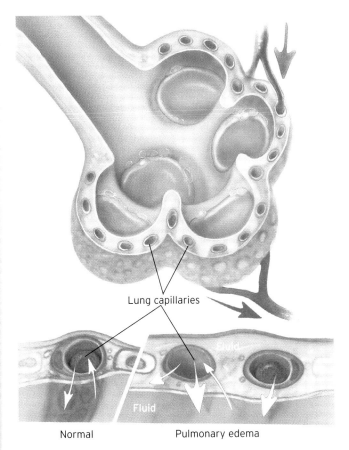

Lung capillaries

Fluid

Fluid

Normal   Pulmonary edema

Figure 11-6 In pulmonary edema, fluid fills the alveoli and separates the capillaries from the alveolar wall, interfering with the exchange of oxygen and carbon dioxide.

In most cases, patients have a longstanding history of chronic congestive heart failure that can be kept under control with medication. However, an acute onset may occur if the patient stops taking the medication, eats food that is too salty, or has a stressful illness, a new heart attack, or an abnormal heart rhythm. Pulmonary edema is one of the most common causes of hospital admission in the United States ▲ **Figure 11-6**. It is not uncommon for a patient to have repeated bouts.

Some patients who have pulmonary edema do not have heart disease. Inhaling large amounts of smoke or toxic chemical fumes can produce pulmonary edema, as can traumatic injuries of the chest. In these cases, fluid collects in alveoli and lung tissue in response to damage to the tissues of the lung or the bronchi.

Chronic Obstructive Pulmonary Disease

Chronic obstructive pulmonary disease (COPD) is a common lung condition, affecting some 10% to 20% of the entire adult population in the United States. It is the end of a slow process, which over several years results in disruption of the airways, the alveoli, and the pulmonary blood vessels. The process itself may be a result of direct lung and airway damage from repeated infections or inhalation of toxic agents such as industrial gases, but most often, it results from cigarette smoking. Although it is well known that cigarettes are a direct cause of lung cancer, their role in the development of COPD is far more significant and less well publicized.

Tobacco smoke is itself a bronchial irritant and can create a **chronic bronchitis**, an ongoing irritation of the trachea and bronchi.

With bronchitis, excess mucus is constantly produced, obstructing small airways and alveoli. Protective cells and lung mechanisms that remove foreign particles are destroyed, further weakening the airways. Chronic oxygenation problems can also lead to right heart failure and fluid retention, such as edema in the leg.

Pneumonia develops easily when the passages are persistently obstructed. Ultimately, repeated episodes of irritation and pneumonia cause scarring in the lung and some dilation of the obstructed alveoli, leading to COPD (▼ **Figure 11-7**).

Another type of COPD is called **emphysema**. Emphysema is a loss of the elastic material around the air spaces as a result of chronic stretching of the alveoli when bronchitic airways obstruct easy expulsion of gases. Smoking can also directly destroy the elasticity of the lung tissue. Normally, lungs act like a spongy balloon that is inflated; once they are inflated, they will naturally recoil because of their elastic nature, expelling gas rapidly. However, when they are constantly obstructed or when the "balloon's" elasticity is diminished, air is no longer expelled rapidly, and the walls of the alveoli eventually fall apart, leaving large "holes" in the lung that resemble a large air pocket or cavity. This condition is called emphysema.

Most patients with COPD have elements of both chronic bronchitis and emphysema. Some patients will have more elements of one condition than the other; few patients will have only emphysema or bronchitis. Therefore, most patients with COPD will chronically produce sputum, have a chronic cough, and have difficulty expelling air from their lungs, with long expiration phases and wheezing.

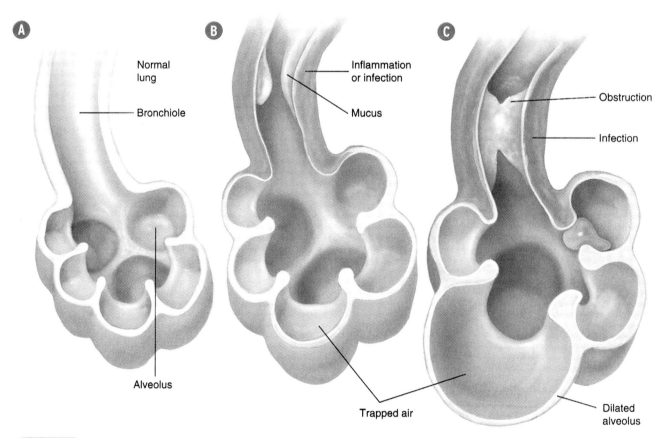

A. Normal lung · Bronchiole · Alveolus

B. Inflammation or infection · Mucus

C. Obstruction · Infection · Trapped air · Dilated alveolus

Figure 11-7 Repeated episodes of irritation and inflammation in the alveoli result in the obstruction, scarring, and some dilation of the alveolar sac characteristic of COPD. **A.** Normal alveolus. **B.** Infection produces mucus and swelling. **C.** A mucous plug creates an obstruction and further dilation of the alveolus.

Patients with COPD cannot handle pulmonary infections well, because the existing airway damage makes them unable to cough up the mucus or sputum produced by the infection. The chronic airway obstruction makes it difficult to breathe deeply enough to clear the lungs. Gradually, the arterial oxygen level falls, and the carbon dioxide level rises. If a new infection of the lung occurs in a patient with COPD, the arterial oxygen level may fall rapidly. In a few patients, the carbon dioxide level may rise high enough to cause sleepiness. These patients require respiratory support and careful administration of oxygen.

Patients with COPD usually are older than 50 years. They will always have a history of recurring lung problems and are almost always long-term cigarette smokers. Patients with COPD may complain of tightness in the chest and constant fatigue. Because air has been gradually and continuously trapped in their lungs in increasing amounts, their chests often have a barrel-like appearance (▼ Figure 11-8). If you listen to the chest with a stethoscope, you will hear abnormal breath sounds. These may include <u>rales</u>, which are crackling, rattling sounds that are usually associated with fluid in the lungs but here are related to chronic scarring of small airways. <u>Rhonchi</u>, which are coarse, gravelly sounds caused by mucus in the airways, and high-pitched, whistling <u>wheezes</u>, which are expiratory sounds common to patients with asthma, may be heard as well. Because of large emphysematous air pockets and diminished airflow, sounds of breathing are frequently hard to hear and may be detected only high up on the posterior chest.

The patient with COPD usually presents with a long history of dyspnea with a sudden increase in shortness of breath. There is rarely a history of chest pain. More often, the patient will remember having had a recent "chest cold" with fever and either inability to cough up mucus or a sudden increase in sputum. If the patient is able to cough up sputum, it will be thick and is often green or yellow. The blood pressure of patients with COPD is normal; however, the pulse is rapid and occasionally irregular. Pay particular attention to the respirations. They may be rapid, or they may be very slow.

Spontaneous Pneumothorax

Normally, the "vacuum" pressure in the pleural space keeps the lung inflated. When the surface of the lung is disrupted, however, air escapes into the pleural cavity, and the negative vacuum pressure is lost; the natural elasticity of the lung tissue causes the lung to collapse. The accumulation of air in the pleural space, which may be partial or complete, is called a **pneumothorax** (▼ Figure 11-9). Pneumothorax is most often caused by trauma, but it can also be caused by some medical conditions without any injury. In these patients, the condition is called a "spontaneous" pneumothorax.

Figure 11-8 Typically, a patient with COPD has a barrel-shaped chest and uses accessory muscles and pursed lips for breathing. Notice, also, that the patient is sitting in the tripod position.

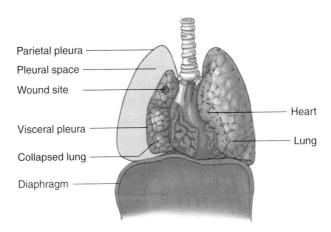

Parietal pleura
Pleural space
Wound site
Visceral pleura
Collapsed lung
Diaphragm
Heart
Lung

Figure 11-9 A pneumothorax occurs when air leaks into the pleural space from an opening in the chest wall or the surface of the lung. The lung collapses as air fills the pleural space and the two pleural surfaces are no longer in contact.

Spontaneous pneumothorax may occur in patients with certain chronic lung infections or in young people born with weak areas of the lung. Patients with emphysema and asthma are at high risk for spontaneous pneumothorax when a weakened portion of lung ruptures, often during coughing. A patient with a spontaneous pneumothorax becomes dyspneic (short of breath) and can complain of **pleuritic chest pain**, a sharp, stabbing pain on one side that is worse during breathing or with certain movement of the chest wall. By listening to the chest with the stethoscope, you can sometimes tell that breath sounds are absent or decreased on the affected side. However, altered breath sounds are very difficult to detect in a patient with severe emphysema. Spontaneous pneumothorax may be the cause of sudden dyspnea in a patient with underlying emphysema.

Asthma and Allergic Reactions

Asthma is an acute spasm of the smaller air passages called bronchioles, associated with excessive mucus production and sometimes with spasm of the bronchiolar muscles (▼ **Figure 11-10**). It is a common but serious disease, affecting about 6 million Americans and killing some 4,000 to 5,000 Americans each year. Asthma produces a characteristic wheezing as patients attempt to exhale through partially obstructed air passages. These same air passages open easily during inspiration. In other words, when patients inhale, breathing appears relatively normal; the wheezing is heard only when they exhale. This wheezing may be so loud that you can hear it without a stethoscope. In other cases, the airways are so blocked that no air movement is heard. In severe cases, the actual work of exhaling is very tiring, and cyanosis and/or respiratory arrest may quickly develop, even within minutes.

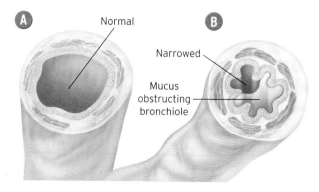

Figure 11-10 Asthma is an acute spasm of the bronchioles.
A. Cross-section of a normal bronchiole. **B.** The bronchiole in spasm; a mucous plug has formed and partially obstructed the bronchiole.

Asthma affects patients of all ages and is usually the result of an allergic reaction to an inhaled, ingested, or injected substance. Note that the substance itself is not the cause of the allergic reaction; rather, it is an exaggerated response of the body's immune system to that substance that causes the reaction. In some cases, however, there is no identifiable substance, or **allergen**, that triggers the body's immune system. Almost anything can be considered an allergen. An allergic response to certain foods or some other allergen may produce an acute asthma attack. Between attacks, patients may breathe normally. In its most severe form, an allergic reaction can produce anaphylaxis and even anaphylactic shock. This, in turn, may cause respiratory distress that is severe enough to result in coma and death. Asthma attacks may also be caused by severe emotional stress, exercise, or respiratory infections.

Most patients with asthma are familiar with their symptoms and know when an attack is imminent. Typically, they will have appropriate medication either with them or at home. You should listen carefully to what these patients tell you; they often know exactly what they need.

ASTHMA AND ANAPHYLACTIC REACTIONS. Patients who do not have asthma may still have severe allergic reactions. The same allergens that may cause asthma attacks may cause anaphylaxis, a reaction characterized by airway swelling and dilation of blood vessels all over the body, which may lower blood pressure significantly. Anaphylaxis may be associated with widespread itching and an asthmalike condition. The airway may swell so much that breathing problems can progress from extreme difficulty in breathing to total airway obstruction in a matter of a few minutes. Most anaphylactic reactions occur within 30 minutes of exposure to the allergen, which can be anything from eating certain nuts to receiving a penicillin injection. For some patients, this may be the first time they had such a reaction to the substance. Therefore, they may not know what caused the swelling and allergic reaction. In other cases, the patient may know of the allergen but not be aware of exposure. In severe cases, epinephrine is the treatment of choice. Oxygen and antihistamines are also useful. As always, medical direction should guide appropriate therapy.

HAY FEVER. A much milder and more common allergy problem is hay fever. This is caused by an allergic reaction to pollen. In some areas of the country where pollen is present in the air throughout the year, hay fever is almost a universal illness. Generally, it does not produce major emergency problems. It does produce a number of difficulties in the upper respiratory tract, such as a stuffy or runny nose and sneezing.

Pleural Effusions

A **pleural effusion** is a collection of fluid outside the lung on one or both sides of the chest; in compressing the lung or lungs, it causes dyspnea (▼ **Figure 11-11**). This fluid may collect in large volumes in response to any irritation, infection, or cancer. Though it can build up gradually, over days or even weeks, patients often report that their dyspnea came on suddenly. Pleural effusions should be considered as a contributing diagnosis in any patient with lung cancer and shortness of breath.

When you listen with a stethoscope to the chest of a patient with dyspnea resulting from pleural effusions, you will hear decreased breath sounds over the region of the chest where fluid has moved the lung away from the chest wall. These patients frequently feel better if they are sitting upright. Nothing will really relieve their symptoms, however, except removal of the fluid, which must be done by a physician in the hospital.

Mechanical Obstruction of the Airway

As an EMT-B, you should always be aware of the possibility that a patient with dyspnea may have a mechanical obstruction of the airway and be prepared to treat it quickly. In semiconscious and unconscious individuals, the obstruction may be the result of aspiration of vomitus or a foreign object (▼ **Figure 11-12A**), or of a position of the head that causes obstruction by the tongue (▼ **Figure 11-12B**). Opening the airway with the head tilt-chin lift maneuver may solve the problem. You should perform this maneuver only after you have ruled out a head or neck injury. If simply opening the airway does not correct the breathing problem, you will have to assess the upper airway for the obstruction.

Always consider upper airway obstruction from a foreign body first in patients who were eating just before becoming short of breath. The same is true of young children, especially crawling babies, who might have swallowed and choked on a small object.

Pulmonary Embolism

An **embolus** is anything in the circulatory system that moves from its point of origin to a distant site and

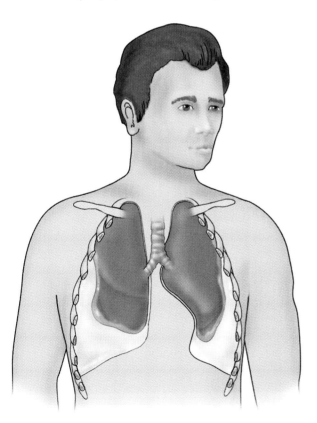

Figure 11-11 With a pleural effusion, fluid may accumulate in large volumes on one or both sides, compressing the lungs and causing dyspnea.

Figure 11-12 **A.** Foreign body obstruction occurs when an object, such as food, is lodged in the airway. **B.** Mechanical obstruction also occurs when the head is not properly positioned, causing the tongue to fall back into the throat.

lodges there, obstructing subsequent blood flow in that area. Beyond the point of obstruction, circulation can be completely cut off or at least markedly decreased, which can result in a serious, life-threatening condition. Emboli can be fragments of blood clots in an artery or vein that break off and travel through the bloodstream. They also can be foreign bodies that enter the circulation, such as a bullet or a bubble of air.

A **pulmonary embolism** is the passage of a blood clot formed in a vein, usually in the legs or pelvis, that breaks off and circulates through the venous system. The large clot moves through the right side of the heart and into the pulmonary artery, where it becomes lodged, significantly decreasing or blocking blood flow (▼ **Figure 11-13**). Even though the lung is actively involved in inhalation and exhalation of air, no exchange of oxygen or carbon dioxide takes place in the areas of blocked blood flow because there is no effective circulation. In this circumstance, the level of arterial carbon dioxide usually rises, and the oxygen level may drop enough to cause cyanosis. More important, blood clots can inhibit circulation and cause significant dyspnea.

Pulmonary emboli may occur as a result of damage to the lining of vessels, a tendency for blood to clot unusually fast, or, most often, slow blood flow in a lower extremity. Slow blood flow in the legs is usually caused by bed rest, which can lead to the collapse of veins. Patients whose legs are immobilized following a fracture or recent surgery are at risk for pulmonary emboli for days or weeks after the incident. Only rarely do pulmonary emboli occur in active, healthy individuals.

Although they are fairly common, pulmonary emboli are difficult to diagnose. They occur about 650,000 times a year in the United States. Ten percent are immediately fatal, but most often, the patient never notices them. Symptoms and signs, when they do occur, include the following:

- Dyspnea
- Acute pleuritic chest pain
- Hemoptysis (coughing up blood)
- Cyanosis
- Tachypnea
- Varying degrees of hypoxia

With a large enough embolus, complete, sudden obstruction of the right heart's output of blood flow can result in sudden death.

Hyperventilation Syndrome

When dyspnea occurs in a patient with no lung abnormalities, it is called hyperventilation syndrome. **Hyperventilation** is defined as overbreathing to the point that the level of arterial carbon dioxide falls below normal. This may be an indicator of major, life-threatening illness. For example, a patient with diabetes who has very high blood glucose levels, a patient who has overdosed with aspirin, or a patient with a severe infection is likely to hyperventilate. In these patients, rapid, deep breathing is the body's attempt to stay alive. The body is trying to compensate for *acidosis*, the buildup of excess acid in the blood or body tissues, resulting from the primary illness. Because carbon dioxide, mixed with water in the bloodstream, can add to the blood's acidity, lowering the level of carbon dioxide helps to compensate for the other acids.

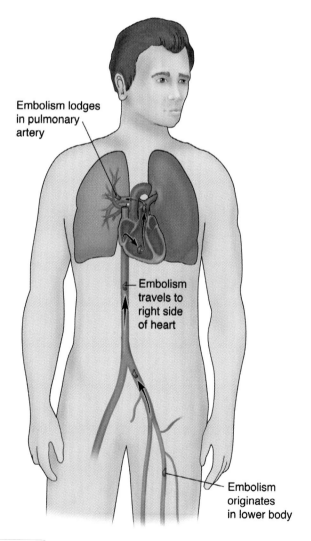

Embolism lodges in pulmonary artery

Embolism travels to right side of heart

Embolism originates in lower body

Figure 11-13 A pulmonary embolus is a blood clot from the vein that breaks off, circulates through the venous system, and moves through the right side of the heart into the pulmonary artery. Here, it can become lodged and significantly obstruct blood flow.

Similarly, in an otherwise healthy person, blood acidity can be diminished by excessive breathing, because it "blows off" too much carbon dioxide. The result is a relative lack of acids. The resulting condition, *alkalosis*, is the buildup of excess base (lack of acids), in the body fluids.

Alkalosis is the cause of many of the symptoms associated with *hyperventilation syndrome*, including anxiety, dizziness, numbness, tingling of the hands and feet, and even a sense of dyspnea despite the rapid breathing. Although hyperventilation can be the response to illness and a buildup of acids, hyperventilation syndrome is not the same thing. Instead, this syndrome occurs in the absence of other physical problems. However, it is very common during psychological stress, affecting some 10% of the population at one time or another. The respirations of an individual who is experiencing hyperventilation syndrome may be as high as more than 40 shallow breaths/min or as low as only 20 very deep breaths/min.

The decision whether hyperventilation is being caused by a life-threatening illness or a panic attack should not be made outside the hospital. All patients who are hyperventilating should be given supplemental oxygen and transported to the hospital, where physicians will make that medical decision.

Emergency Care of Respiratory Emergencies

When taking the initial vital signs of a person with dyspnea, you should pay particular attention to respirations. Always speak with assurance and assume a concerned, professional approach to reassure the patient, who is probably very frightened. You will usually administer oxygen. Take great care in monitoring the respirations as you do so. Reevaluate the respirations and the patient's response to oxygen repeatedly, at least every 5 minutes, until you reach the emergency department. In a person with a chronically high carbon dioxide level (eg, certain patients with COPD), this is critical, because the supplemental oxygen may cause a rapid rise in the arterial oxygen level. This, in turn, may abolish the secondary respiratory oxygen drive and cause respiratory arrest.

Do *not* withhold oxygen for fear of depressing or stopping breathing in a patient with COPD who needs oxygen. Slowing of respirations after administration of oxygen does not necessarily mean that the patient no longer needs the oxygen; he or she may need it even more. If respirations slow and the patient becomes unconscious, you should assist breathing with a BVM.

Geriatric Needs

As we get older, normal aging processes alter the respiratory system and our ability to exchange oxygen and carbon dioxide. If the patient is a smoker, the disease processes of emphysema or chronic bronchitis can hasten or worsen these changes.

Several changes occur as we age. The chest wall, including the muscles and ribs, become less resilient. Additionally, the bronchi and bronchioles lose their muscle mass or tone, and the air sacs (alveoli) become stiffer and less able to recoil (relax and empty) in exhaling. If the chest wall, including muscles and ribs, is weaker or less flexible, the chest cavity cannot expand as easily, and the total amount of air that is allowed into the lungs will be reduced. With decreased recoil of the lungs, alveoli can become distended with air trapped inside. If you are required to ventilate the apneic (nonbreathing) geriatric patient, you will notice that it is more difficult because of increased resistance of the chest and airways as well as reduced compliance of the lungs.

The geriatric patient is at an increased risk of pneumonia or a worsening of asthma or COPD if the airways have lost muscle mass or tone. Secretions might not be expelled from the airways, allowing pneumonia to develop.

The result of normal changes with aging is a reduction of the total amount of air the lungs can hold, air becoming trapped in overstretched alveoli, and increased resistance to air flow into and out of the lungs. Ultimately, all these changes cause a decreased oxygen/carbon dioxide exchange in the respiratory system with reduced oxygen delivery to the cells. Be sure to consider changes in aging that affect the respiratory system, and provide adequate ventilation and oxygenation according to the patient's needs. The geriatric patient may need ventilatory support for conditions that, in the younger adult, are easily accommodated by the respiratory system.

Approach to the Patient in Respiratory Distress

Your first questions are always the same: Is the patient conscious? Is he or she breathing? If not, you must take action. Assess the airway and give two ventilations. As you ventilate, you need to ask another series of questions, as follows:

1. **Is air going into the lungs?** Look for clues in the rise and fall of the chest, the respirations, and the heart rate.

2. **When you squeeze the BVM device, does the chest wall expand?**

3. **When you release the bag, does the chest fall?** If not, something is wrong. Try to reposition the patient and insert an oral airway to keep the tongue from blocking the airway. Reposition the head. Reassess your hand position and face mask seal.

Next, assess the rate at which you are assisting the patient's ventilations. You need to give breaths at roughly the same rate as the patient would if he or she were breathing spontaneously (eg, 12 to 20/min). Rescuers often get excited and ventilate the patient too quickly. Breathing for the patient too rapidly can cause harm. With rapid squeezing of the bag, higher pressures force the air rapidly into the lungs. Higher pressures can fill the stomach, as well as the lungs, with air. If the air and fluid in the stomach come back up the esophagus, vomit may enter the lungs, which can cause a serious form of pneumonia. Adults should be given one breath every 5 seconds. School-aged children need a smaller breath every 3 seconds. Infants need a small breath every 3 seconds. Use appropriately sized BVM device for each.

Finally, assess the pulse. If the patient has a pulse, continue to support respirations. Measure the pulse rate; if it is normal, chances are that the patient is receiving enough oxygen to support life. If the pulse rate is too fast (more than 100/min) or too slow (less than 60/min), the patient may not be getting enough oxygen. Recheck everything. Is the oxygen bottle hooked up to the mask? Is the oxygen turned on? Is the flow rate adequate (10 to 15 L/min)? Is there a good face mask seal? Is the chest rising and falling with each breath? Is the airway blocked with vomit or the tongue?

SIGNS AND SYMPTOMS. If the patient is breathing, you need to decide whether the breathing is adequate. ▶ **Table 11-2** lists the clues that will help you to decide if there is a breathing difficulty.

FOCUSED HISTORY AND PHYSICAL EXAMINATION. After you form your general impression and have completed the initial assessment, ask the patient to describe the problem. Begin by asking an open-ended question: "What can you tell me about your breathing?" Pay close attention to OPQRST: when the problem began (onset), what makes the breathing difficulty worse (provocation), how the breathing feels (quality), and whether the discomfort moves (radiation). How much of a problem is the patient having (severity)? Is the problem continuous or intermittent (time)? If it is intermittent, how long does it last?

Find out what the patient has already done for the breathing problem. Does the patient use a prescribed inhaler? If so, when was it used last? How many doses have been taken? Does the patient use more than one

inhaler? Find out whether the patient has any allergies or history of medication reactions.

INTERVENTIONS. If the patient complains of breathing difficulty, you should administer supplemental oxygen. In general, you do not need to worry about giving too much oxygen. Put a nonrebreathing face mask on the patient and supply oxygen at a rate of 10 to 15 L/min (enough to maintain the reservoir bag) in a patient with severe difficulty breathing. Then continue your assessment. Obtain a set of vital signs and document them.

As was stated previously, there is some concern about suppression of the "hypoxic" drive to breathe in some patients with COPD. Unless these patients are unresponsive, a more conservative approach is suggested. In patients who have longstanding COPD and probable carbon dioxide retention, administration of low-flow oxygen (2 L/min) is a good place to start, with adjustments to 3 L/min, then 4 L/min, and so on until symptoms have improved (for example, the patient has less dyspnea or a better mental status). When in doubt, err on the side of more oxygen, and monitor the patient closely.

Patients who call for help because of breathing difficulty are likely to have had the same trouble before. They probably have prescribed medications to use that are delivered by inhaler. If so, you may be able to help them use it. Consult medical control. Remember to report what the medication is, when the patient last took a puff, how many puffs were used at that time, and what the label states regarding dosage. If medical control permits, you may assist the patient to self-administer the medication. Be certain that the inhaler belongs to the patient, it contains the correct medication, the expiration date has not passed, and the correct dose is being administered. Administer repeat doses of the medication if the maximum dose has not been exceeded and the patient is still experiencing shortness of breath.

If the patient does not have a prescribed inhaler, continue with the focused history and physical exam. Even patients who use their inhaler may continue to get worse. You need to reassess breathing frequently and be prepared to assist ventilations in severe cases. You must assist ventilation in a patient who is having an asthma attack, using slow, gentle breaths. Remember, the problem in asthma is getting the air out of the lungs, not into them. Resist the temptation to squeeze the bag hard and fast. Always assist with ventilations as a last resort, and then provide only about 10 to 12 shallow breaths/min.

Prescribed Inhalers

Some of the most common medications used for shortness of breath are called inhaled beta-agonists, which dilate breathing passages. Typical trade names are

TABLE 11-2 Signs and Symptoms of Inadequate Breathing

- **The patient complains of difficulty breathing.**
- **The patient appears anxious or restless.** This can happen if the brain is not getting enough oxygen for its needs. Check the vital signs.
- **The patient's respiratory rate is too slow** (respirations are less than 8 breaths/min), you may need to assist ventilations with a BVM device.
- **The patient's skin is blue (cyanotic).** The tongue, nailbeds, and inside the lips are good places to look for cyanosis. These all have a large collection of blood vessels and thin skin, making bluish blood easy to see.
- **The patient is wheezing, gurgling, snoring, stridor, or crowing.** Common causes of stridor include a foreign body obstruction and infection.
- **The patient cannot speak more than few words between breaths.** Ask the patient something such as "How are you doing?" If the patient cannot speak at all, he or she probably has a respiratory emergency that will need immediate attention.
- **The patient is using the accessory muscles in the neck to assist breathing.** If the patient is using only the diaphragm to breathe, suspect damage to the nerves that carry breathing commands to the chest muscles; the diaphragm may be getting the command to breathe, but because of spinal cord injury, the chest muscles may not.
- **The patient has an altered mental status associated with shallow or slow breathing.**
- **The patient is coughing excessively,** which might mean that the patient has anything from mild upper respiratory infection or hay fever to pneumonia, asthma, or heart failure.
- **The patient's breathing rhythm is irregular.** Because the brain controls breathing, an irregular breathing rhythm may indicate a head injury. In this case, the patient will probably be unresponsive.
- **The patient is sitting up, leaning forward** with palms flat on the bed or the arms of the chair. This is called the tripod position, because the back and two arms are working together to support the upper body. This position allows the diaphragm the most room to function and helps the patient to use accessory muscles to assist breathing. It is usually a good idea to let the patient stay in the most comfortable position.
- **The chest has a barrel shape.** In certain chronic lung diseases, because air has been gradually and continuously trapped within the lung in increasing amounts, the distance from front to back gets longer, nearly equaling the side-to-side distance. A barrel chest may indicate a long history of breathing problems.
- **The conjunctivae are pale.** Perhaps the patient is short of breath because there are not enough red blood cells to carry oxygen to the tissues.
- **The patient has an increased pulse and respirations** (heart rate more than 100 beats/min or respirations more than 24 breaths/min).

Proventil, Ventolin, Alupent, Metaprel, and Brethine. The generic name for Proventil and Ventolin is albuterol; for Alupent and Metaprel, it is metaproterenol; and for Brethine, it is terbutaline. The action of most of these medications is to relax the muscles that surround the bronchioles in the lungs, leading to enlargement (dilation) of the airways and easier passage of air. Common side effects of inhalers used for acute shortness of breath include increased pulse rate, nervousness, and muscle tremors.

If the patient has a prescribed metered-dose inhaler, read the label carefully to make sure that the medication is to be used for shortness of breath and that it has, in fact, been prescribed by a physician ▶ **Figure 11-14** . When in doubt, consult medical control.

Figure 11-14 Some inhalers have spacer devices to better direct the medication spray.

Documentation Tips

After assisting with the administration of an inhaler treatment, document another set of vital signs as well as the patient's response to the treatment. Be sure to include lung sounds.

Pediatric Needs

Asthma is a common childhood illness. When assessing a pediatric patient, look for retraction of the skin above the sternum and between the ribs. Retractions are typically easier to see in children than in adults. Cyanosis is a late finding in children. Keep in mind that a cough may not be a symptom of a cold; it could signal pneumonia or asthma. Even if you do not hear much wheezing, the presence of a cough can indicate that some degree of reactive airway disease, or an acute asthma attack may be taking place.

The emergency care of a child with shortness of breath is the same as it is for an adult, including the use of supplemental oxygen. However, many small children will not tolerate (or may refuse to wear) a face mask. Rather than fighting with the child, hold the oxygen mask in front of the child's face or ask the parent to hold the mask (▼ **Figure 11-15**). Many children with asthma also will have prescribed hand-held metered-dose inhalers. Use these inhalers just as you would with an adult.

Figure 11-15 Because children may refuse to wear an oxygen mask, you may have to hold the mask in front of the child's face. If the child still refuses, enlist the parents' help.

Before helping a patient to self-administer any metered-dose inhaler medication, make sure that the medication is indicated, that is, the patient has signs and symptoms of shortness of breath. Finally, check that there are no contraindications for its use, such as the following:

- The patient is unable to help coordinate inhalation with depression of the trigger, perhaps because the patient is too confused.
- The inhaler is not prescribed for this patient.
- You did not obtain permission from medical control or local protocol.
- The patient had already met the maximum prescribed dose before your arrival.

ADMINISTRATION OF METERED-DOSE INHALER MEDICATION. To help a patient self-administer medication from an inhaler, follow these steps (▶ **Skill Drill 11-1**) :

1. **Obtain an order** from medical control or local protocol.
2. **Check that you have** the right medication, the right patient, and the right route.
3. **Make sure that the patient is alert** enough to use the inhaler.
4. **Check the expiration date** of the inhaler.
5. **Check to see whether the patient** has already taken any doses.
6. **Make sure the inhaler** is at room temperature or warmer **(Step 1)**.
7. **Shake the inhaler** vigorously several times.
8. **Stop administering** supplemental oxygen and remove any mask from the patient's face.
9. **Ask the patient** to exhale deeply and, before inhaling, to put his or her lips around the opening of the inhaler.
10. **If the patient has a spacer,** use it to allow more effective use of the medication **(Step 2)**.
11. **Have the patient** depress the hand-held inhaler as he or she begins to inhale deeply.
12. **Instruct the patient** to hold his or her breath for as long as is comfortable to help the body absorb the medication **(Step 3)**.
13. **Continue to administer** supplemental oxygen.
14. **Allow the patient** to breathe a few times, then repeat second dose per direction from medical control or local protocol **(Step 4)**.

REASSESSMENT. You need to carefully watch patients with shortness of breath. About 5 minutes after the patient uses an inhaler, obtain the vital signs again and perform a focused reassessment. Ask the patient whether the treatment made any difference. Look at the patient's chest to see whether the patient is still using accessory muscles to breathe. Listen to the patient's speech pattern. Keep in mind that the patient may get

Skill Drill 11-1   Assisting a Patient with a Metered-Dose Inhaler

1 Ensure inhaler is at room temperature or warmer.

2 Remove oxygen mask. Hand inhaler to patient. Instruct about breathing and lip seal. Use a spacer if patient has one.

3 Instruct patient to press inhaler and inhale. Instruct about breath holding.

4 Reapply oxygen. After a few breaths, have patient repeat dose if order/protocol allows.

worse instead of better, and be prepared to assist ventilations with a BVM device.

After helping the patient with the inhaler treatment, transport the patient to the emergency department. While en route, continue to assess the patient's breathing. Try talking to calm and reassure the patient and continue to give supplemental oxygen.

Treatment of Specific Conditions

INFECTION OF THE UPPER OR LOWER AIRWAY. Dyspnea associated with acute infections is quite common. Except for the patient with pneumonia, acute bronchitis, or epiglottitis, it is rarely serious. The acute congestion and stuffiness of a common cold hardly ever require emergency care. Indeed, most people with colds treat themselves with OTC medications. However, individuals with a common cold who have underlying problems such as asthma or heart failure may experience a worsening of their condition as a result of the additional stress of the infection. In addition, cold medications may also have stressful side effects, such as agitation, increased heart rate, and increased blood pressure.

For patients with upper airway infections and dyspnea, administer humidified oxygen (if available). Do not attempt to suction the airway or place an oropharyngeal airway in a patient with suspected epiglottitis. These maneuvers may cause a spasm and complete airway obstruction. Transport the patient promptly to the hospital. Allow the patient to sit in the position that is most comfortable. For someone with epiglottitis, this is usually sitting upright and leaning forward, the "sniffing

position" (▼ Figure 11-16). To force a patient with epiglottitis to lie supine may cause upper airway obstruction that could result in death.

The dyspnea of pneumonia is caused not by upper airway obstruction but by the loss of effective lung volume and a need for more rapid air exchange. Here again, the problem will not be helped by the use of artificial airways but may improve with the administration of oxygen.

ACUTE PULMONARY EDEMA. Dyspnea caused by acute pulmonary edema may be associated with cardiac disease or direct lung damage. In either case, administer 100% oxygen, and, if necessary, carefully suction any secretions from the airway. Provide prompt transport to the emergency department. The best position for a conscious patient who has a myocardial infarction or direct lung injury is the one in which it is easiest to breathe.

Figure 11-16 A child with epiglottis may be more comfortable sitting up and leaning forward.

Usually, this is sitting up. Rarely will you need to use an artificial airway, because no upper airway obstruction problem exists. However, an unconscious patient with acute pulmonary edema may require full ventilatory support, including airway, positive pressure ventilation with oxygen, and suctioning.

CHRONIC OBSTRUCTIVE PULMONARY DISEASE. Patients with COPD may be semiconscious or unconscious from **hypoxia**, a condition in which the body's cells and tissues do not get enough oxygen, or from carbon dioxide retention. They may appear to be in respiratory distress and/or be cyanotic. They may have pursed lips and may be using accessory muscles to breathe, including those in the neck and shoulders.

Assist with the patient's prescribed inhaler if they have one. Transport patients with COPD as promptly as possible to the emergency department, allowing them to sit upright if this is most comfortable (▼ Figure 11-17). Patients with COPD often find breathing difficult when lying down.

SPONTANEOUS PNEUMOTHORAX. Patients with spontaneous pneumothorax may have severe respiratory distress, or they may have no distress at all and complain only of pleuritic chest pain. Provide supplemental oxygen, and provide prompt transport to the hospital. Like most dyspneic patients, those with spontaneous pneumothorax are usually more comfortable sitting up. Monitor the patient carefully, watching for any sudden deterioration in the respiratory status. Be ready to support the airway, assist respirations, and give full cardiopulmonary support if it becomes necessary.

ASTHMA OR ALLERGIC REACTIONS. Many lung problems are incorrectly labeled "asthma"; therefore, your assessment of the patient is critical. A patient who truly has asthma will have a history of repeated episodes of sudden shortness of breath, in which he or she had difficulty exhaling. Confirm whether the patient is able to breathe normally at other times. If possible, ask family members to describe the patient's asthma. Even if they only identify wheezing as a problem, be aware that some forms of heart failure, foreign body aspiration, or toxic fumes inhalation may cause wheezing.

As you assess the patient's vital signs, note that the pulse rate will be normal or elevated, the blood pressure may be slightly elevated, and respirations will be increased. Assist with patient's prescribed inhaler if they have one. Administer oxygen, and allow the patient to sit in an upright position, which makes breathing easier. Be reassuring; tension and anxiety make asthma attacks worse.

Ask questions about how and when the symptoms began, as reactions that follow a bee or wasp sting may progress rapidly to anaphylactic shock. A patient in anaphylactic shock may quickly become unconscious and require assisted ventilations and supplemental oxygen. If the patient is already unconscious upon your arrival, look for a medical identification tag that may provide a clue (▼ Figure 11-18). Unconscious patients require prompt transport to the emergency department.

As you care for the patient, be prepared to suction large amounts of mucus from the mouth and to administer oxygen. If you do suction, do not withhold oxygen for more than 15 seconds for adult patients, 5 seconds for an infant, and 10 seconds for a child. Allow some time for oxygenation between suction attempts. If the patient is unconscious, you may have to provide airway management.

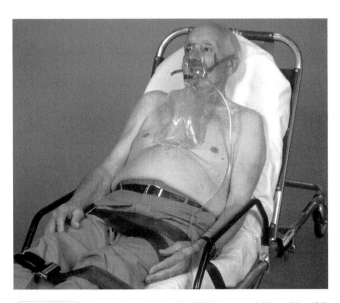

Figure 11-17 Transport a patient with COPD in an upright position if it is most comfortable. Ensure that you continue to monitor the patient.

Figure 11-18 Some patients who are known to be severely allergic to bee stings, certain medications, or other substances often wear a medical identification tag.

If the patient carries medication, such as an epinephrine auto-injector, for an asthma attack or allergic reaction, you may help with its administration, as directed by local protocol (See Figure 10-10). Keep in mind that epinephrine is a very potent agent with a number of significant side effects. Do not give it unless you are certain that the patient is having a severe asthma attack or severe allergic reaction and you know the history of the episode.

A prolonged asthma attack that is unrelieved by epinephrine may progress into a condition known as *status asthmaticus*. The patient is likely to be frightened, frantically trying to breathe, while using all the accessory muscles. Status asthmaticus is a true emergency, and the patient must be given oxygen and transported immediately to the emergency department.

The effort to breathe during an asthma attack is very tiring, and the patient may be exhausted by the time you arrive. An exhausted patient may have stopped feeling anxious or even struggling to breathe. This patient is not recovering; he or she is at a very critical stage and is likely to stop breathing. Aggressive airway management, oxygen administration, and prompt transport are essential in this situation. Tiering with ALS should be considered. Follow local protocol.

PLEURAL EFFUSIONS. Treatment of pleural effusions consists of removal of fluid collected outside the lung, which must be done by a physician in a hospital setting. However, you should provide oxygen and other routine support measures to these patients.

OBSTRUCTION OF THE UPPER AIRWAY. If the patient is a small child or someone who was eating just before dyspnea developed, you may assume that the problem is an inhaled or aspirated foreign body. If the patient is old enough to talk but cannot make any noise, upper airway obstruction is the likely cause.

The first thing to do is clear the upper airway. Then, whether or not you are successful, administer supplemental oxygen and transport the patient promptly to the emergency department.

PULMONARY EMBOLISM. Because a considerable amount of lung tissue may not be functioning, supplemental oxygen is mandatory in a patient with a pulmonary embolism. Place the patient in a comfortable position, usually sitting, and assist breathing as necessary. Hemoptysis, if present, is usually not severe, but any blood that has been coughed up should be cleared from the airway. The patient may have an unusually rapid and possibly irregular heartbeat. Transport the patient to the emergency department promptly. Be aware that pulmonary emboli may cause cardiac arrest.

EMT-B Tips

While one EMT-B is getting oxygen ready, the second EMT-B should try to coach the patient with asthma or COPD to use "pursed-lip" breathing. The increase in back pressure will help air flow through narrowed bronchioles.

HYPERVENTILATION. When you respond to a patient who is hyperventilating, complete an initial assessment and history of the event. Is the patient having chest pain? Is there a history of cardiac problems or diabetes? You must always assume a serious underlying problem even if you suspect that the underlying problem is stress. Do not have the patient breathe into a paper bag, even though it is thought to be the traditional technique for managing hyperventilation syndrome. In theory, breathing into a paper bag causes the patient to rebreathe exhaled carbon dioxide, allowing the level of carbon dioxide in the blood to return to normal. In fact, if the patient is hyperventilating because of a serious medical problem, this maneuver could make things worse. A patient with underlying pulmonary disease who breathes into a bag may become severely hypoxic. Treatment should instead consist of reassuring the patient in a calm, professional manner; supplying supplemental oxygen; and providing prompt transport to the emergency department. Patients who hyperventilate need to be evaluated in the hospital setting.

Prep Kit

Ready for Review

Dyspnea is a common complaint that may be caused by numerous medical problems, including infections of the upper or lower airways, acute pulmonary edema, chronic obstructive pulmonary disease, spontaneous pneumothorax, asthma or allergic reactions, pleural effusions, mechanical obstruction of the airway, pulmonary embolism, and hyperventilation. Each of these lung disorders interferes in one way or another with the exchange of oxygen and carbon dioxide that takes place during respiration. This interference may be in the form of damage to the alveoli, separation of the alveoli from the pulmonary vessels by fluid or infection, obstruction of the air passages, or air or excess fluid in the pleural space. Patients with longstanding lung diseases often have chronically high levels of blood carbon dioxide; in some cases, giving too much oxygen to these patients may depress or stop respirations. However, judicious use of oxygen is always an important priority in patients with dyspnea.

Signs and symptoms of breathing difficulty include unusual breath sounds, including wheezing, stridor, rales, and rhonchi; nasal flaring; pursed lip breathing; cyanosis; inability to talk; use of accessory muscles to breathe; and sitting in the tripod position, which allows the diaphragm the most room to function.

In treating dyspnea, it is important to reassure the patient and provide supplemental oxygen. Remember to maintain the patient in a position that is comfortable for breathing, usually sitting upright. If the patient is not breathing, use a BVM device to assist breathing. If the patient is breathing inadequately, apply oxygen through a nonrebreathing face mask with the oxygen flow set at 10 to 15 L/min. Next, perform a focused history and physical exam, including vital signs. If the patient has a prescribed inhaler or epinephrine auto injector, consult medical control to assist with its use. Then transport the patient to the hospital, monitoring his or her condition on the way. Talking with the patient is a good way to monitor a breathing problem.

Remember, a patient who is breathing rapidly may be getting insufficient oxygen as a result of respiratory distress from a variety of problems, including pneumonia or a pulmonary embolism; trying to "blow off" more carbon dioxide to compensate for acidosis caused by a poison, a severe infection, or a high level of blood glucose; or having a stress reaction. In every case, prompt recognition of the problem, giving oxygen, and prompt transport are essential.

Vital Vocabulary

allergen A substance that causes an allergic reaction.

asthma A disease of the lungs in which muscle spasm in the small air passageways and the production of large amounts of mucus result in airway obstruction.

carbon dioxide retention A condition characterized by a chronically high blood level of carbon dioxide in which the respiratory center no longer responds to high blood levels of carbon dioxide.

chronic bronchitis Irritation of the major lung passageways, from either infectious disease or irritants such as smoke.

chronic obstructive pulmonary disease (COPD) A slow process of dilation and disruption of the airways and alveoli, caused by chronic bronchial obstruction.

common cold A viral infection usually associated with swollen nasal mucous membranes and the production of fluid from the sinuses and nose.

croup An infectious disease of the upper respiratory system that may cause partial airway obstruction and is characterized by a barking cough; usually seen in children.

diphtheria An infectious disease in which a membrane lining the pharynx is formed that can severely obstruct passage of air into the larynx.

dyspnea Shortness of breath or difficulty breathing.

embolus A blood clot or other substance in the circulatory system that travels to a blood vessel where it causes blockage.

emphysema A disease of the lungs in which there is extreme dilation and eventual destruction of pulmonary alveoli with poor exchange of oxygen and carbon dioxide; it is one form of chronic obstructive pulmonary disease (COPD).

epiglottitis An infectious disease in which the epiglottis becomes inflamed and enlarged and may cause upper airway obstruction.

hyperventilation Rapid or deep breathing that lowers blood carbon dioxide levels below normal.

hypoxia A condition in which the body's cells and tissues do not have enough oxygen.

hypoxic drive Backup system to control respirations when oxygen levels fall.

pleural effusion A collection of fluid between the lung and chest wall that may compress the lung.

pleuritic chest pain Sharp, stabbing pain in the chest that is worsened by a deep breath or other chest wall movement; often caused by inflammation or irritation of the pleura.

pneumonia An infectious disease of the lung that damages lung tissue.

pneumothorax A partial or complete accumulation of air in the pleural space.

pulmonary edema A buildup of fluid in the lungs, usually as a result of congestive heart failure.

pulmonary embolism A blood clot that breaks off from a large vein and travels to the blood vessels of the lung, causing obstruction of blood flow.

rales Crackling, rattling breath sounds signaling fluid in the air spaces of the lungs.

rhonchi Coarse breath sounds heard in patients with chronic mucus in the airways.

stridor A harsh, high-pitched, barking inspiratory sound often heard in acute laryngeal (upper airway) obstruction.

wheeze A high-pitched, whistling breath sound, characteristically heard on expiration in patients with asthma or COPD.

Assessment in Action

You receive a call for an adult with difficulty breathing at a local bookstore. On arrival you find one of the customers, a 38-year-old man, sitting up, leaning forward, with his hands braced on his knees. You notice that his neck muscles are straining when he inhales and he appears pale. As you begin to ask him questions he answers in short, three- to four-word phrases. He manages to tell you that he had been looking at old books for the last hour when his chest started to tighten up.

The patient also tells you that he has a history of asthma and uses a Ventolin inhaler, but he left it in his car. The patient also tells you that he is allergic to dust, cats, pollen, and penicillin. Your partner obtains baseline vital signs, which include a pulse of 122 beats/min and regular shallow respirations of 34 breaths/min; and a blood pressure of 152/90 mm Hg. His skin is cool and dry. Lung sounds disclose wheezes in both sides of his chest.

1. Which of the following assessment signs tell you that the patient has difficulty breathing?
   - A. Vital signs and history
   - B. Position and speech
   - C. Vital signs and skin color
   - D. History of allergies

2. The medical term for this patient's chief complaint is:
   - A. apnea.
   - B. dyspnea.
   - C. anoxia.
   - D. hyperventilation.

3. How do you know that this patient has accessory muscle use?
   - A. His neck muscle are straining when he inhales.
   - B. He is sitting in a hunched-over position.
   - C. He is talking in three- to four-word phrases.
   - D. His respiratory rate is 34/minute.

4. This patient is sitting up, leaning forward with his hands braced on his knees. What is this position called?
   - A. Hunched position
   - B. COPD position
   - C. Fowler's position
   - D. Tripod position

5. Another customer offers to let the patient use her inhaler when the patient states that he left his inhaler in the car. The most appropriate course of action would be to:
   - A. thank the other customer and state that the patient needs his own inhaler.
   - B. check the inhaler, then assist the patient with using the customer's inhaler.
   - C. observe the patient as the other customer helps administer the inhaler.
   - D. obtain another set of vital signs, then assist the patient in using the inhaler.

6. The patient finds an almost-empty inhaler in his briefcase and uses it. Which of the following would be considered a side effect of his Ventolin inhaler?
   - A. Symptom relief and bradycardia
   - B. Bradycardia and nervousness
   - C. Nervousness and tachycardia
   - D. Tachycardia and low blood pressure

7. This patient has asthma with wheezes in both sides of his chest. The sound of wheezes in an asthmatic patient is caused by which of the following?
   - A. Enlargement of the pulmonary blood vessels
   - B. Excessive pleural effusions outside the lungs
   - C. Excess fluid and scarring in the lungs
   - D. Excess mucus and spasm of the bronchioles

Challenging Questions

8. En route to the hospital, this patient has a bout of coughing that resulted in a sudden onset of sharp, stabbing pain on one side of his chest wall that is worse during breathing and with certain movement of the chest wall. You listen with a stethoscope and can tell that breath sounds are decreased on that side. What has most likely happened to your patient and why is your patient prone to this problem?

9. Patients with chronic lung diseases frequently have a chronically high level of blood carbon dioxide, which is the normal stimulus to breathe. When that happens, what takes over their stimulus to breathe?

10. If this patient exhibited a barrel chest, what would that tell you in terms of his respiratory problem?

Points to Ponder

You have been with your response agency for about three months and you already recognize the address when you are dispatched to a "female in respiratory distress." You respond at least once a week to Alice, who is a COPD patient. When you arrive, she is wheezing and using auxiliary muscles to breathe. Her home oxygen is on and in use and once again, she is smoking while using her oxygen. She says that this is the first time today, but by the number of butts in the ashtray next to her chair, you know that is not correct. She typically goes to the emergency room and receives a nebulizer treatment and is released for you to pick up another day. Each time, Medicaid pays for the "ride" and you are out of service for over an hour. This trip she even asks if she can smoke in the ambulance. How will you feel about this woman? Will your feelings affect how you interact with her? What often happens to assessment and care of patients who seem to be abusing the health care system?

Issues "Frequent Flyers," Patients who Make Choices We Do Not Agree With, Abuse of the System, Patient Respect.

Online Outlook

The term COPD comprises emphysema and chronic bronchitis. The number of lives that are claimed by chronic lung disease has increased sharply over the past 20 years. To learn more about COPD, complete Exercise 11 at the www.emtb.com.

www.emtb.com

Cardiovascular Emergencies

Objectives

Cognitive

1. Describe the structure and function of the cardiovascular system (p 346).
2. Describe the emergency medical care of the patient experiencing chest pain/discomfort (p 352).
3. List the indications for automated external defibrillation (AED) (p 362).
4. List the contraindications for automated external defibrillation (p 362).
5. Define the role of EMT-B in the emergency cardiac care system (p 346).
6. Explain the impact of age and weight on defibrillation (p 355).
7. Discuss the position of comfort for patients with various cardiac emergencies (p 354).
8. Establish the relationship between airway management and the patient with cardiovascular compromise (p 355).
9. Predict the relationship between the patient experiencing cardiovascular compromise and basic life support (p 356).
10. Discuss the fundamentals of early defibrillation (p 362).
11. Explain the rationale for early defibrillation (p 362).
12. Explain that not all chest pain patients result in cardiac arrest and do not need to be attached to an automated external defibrillator (p 362).
13. Explain the importance of prehospital ACLS intervention if it is available (p 366).
14. Explain the importance of urgent transport to a facility with Advanced Cardiac Life Support if it is not available in the prehospital setting (p 366).
15. Discuss the various types of automated external defibrillators (p 361).
16. Differentiate between the fully automated and the semiautomated defibrillator (p 361).
17. Discuss the procedures that must be taken into consideration for standard operations of the various types of automated external defibrillators (p 363).
18. State the reasons for assuring that the patient is pulseless and apneic when using the automated external defibrillator (p 361).
19. Discuss the circumstances which may result in inappropriate shocks (p 361).
20. Explain the considerations for interruption of CPR when using the automated external defibrillator (p 363).
21. Discuss the advantages and disadvantages of automated external defibrillators (p 360).
22. Summarize the speed of operation of automated external defibrillation (p 362).
23. Discuss the use of remote defibrillation through adhesive pads (p 362).
24. Discuss the special considerations for rhythm monitoring (p 362).
25. List the steps in the operation of the automated external defibrillator (p 363).
26. Discuss the standard of care that should be used to provide care to a patient with persistent ventricular fibrillation and no available ACLS (p 364).
27. Discuss the standard of care that should be used to provide care to a patient with recurrent ventricular fibrillation and no available ACLS (p 364).
28. Differentiate between the single rescuer and multi-rescuer care with an automated external defibrillator (p 364).
29. Explain the reason for pulses not being checked between shocks with an automated external defibrillator (p 363).
30. Discuss the importance of coordinating ACLS trained providers with personnel using automated external defibrillators (p 366).
31. Discuss the importance of postresuscitation care (p 364).
32. List the components of postresuscitation care (p 364).
33. Explain the importance of frequent practice with the automated external defibrillator (p 369).
34. Discuss the need to complete the Automated Defibrillator: Operator's Shift Checklist (p 368).
35. Discuss the role of the American Heart Association (AHA) in the use of automated external defibrillation (p 362).
36. Explain the role medical direction plays in the use of automated external defibrillation (p 369).
37. State the reasons why a case review should be completed following the use of the automated external defibrillator (p 369).
38. Discuss the components that should be included in a case review (p 369).
39. Discuss the goal of quality improvement in automated external defibrillation (p 369).
40. Recognize the need for medical direction of protocols to assist in the emergency medical care of the patient with chest pain (p 369).
41. List the indications for the use of nitroglycerin (p 354).
42. State the contraindications and side effects for the use of nitroglycerin (p 358).
43. Define the function of all controls on an automated external defibrillator, and describe event documentation and battery defibrillator maintenance (p 367).

Affective

44. Defend the reasons for obtaining initial training in automated external defibrillation and the importance of continuing education (p 360).
45. Defend the reason for maintenance of automated external defibrillators (p 367).
46. Explain the rationale for administering nitroglycerin to a patient with chest pain or discomfort (p 354).

Psychomotor

47. Demonstrate the assessment and emergency medical care of a patient experiencing chest pain/discomfort (p 355).
48. Demonstrate the application and operation of the automated external defibrillator (p 363).
49. Demonstrate the maintenance of an automated external defibrillator (p 367).
50. Demonstrate the assessment and documentation of patient response to the automated external defibrillator (p 363).
51. Demonstrate the skills necessary to complete the Automated Defibrillator: Operator's Shift Checklist (p 368).
52. Perform the steps in facilitating the use of nitroglycerin for chest pain or discomfort (p 356).
53. Demonstrate the assessment and documentation of patient response to nitroglycerin (p 356).
54. Practice completing a prehospital care report for patients with cardiac emergencies (p 352).

You are the EMT

"Medic 7, respond to 48 Henderson Drive for a man with 'indigestion.'" En route, dispatch informs you that a first responder squad is on scene performing CPR on the patient who arrested moments after their arrival.

Cardiac-related calls also fall in the category of *daily* emergencies that are handled by EMS systems across the country. This chapter will prepare you to respond to these often catastrophic events and will also help you answer the following questions.

1. What is "cardiac denial," and why is it a factor in the mortality/morbidity of patients with cardiac emergencies?

2. Can you identify the most common presenting cardiac rhythm for patients who experience sudden cardiac death as well as the appropriate EMT-B intervention for it?

Cardiovascular Emergencies

The American Heart Association reports that cardiovascular disease (CVD) claimed 953,110 lives in the United States in 1997. This is 41.2% of all deaths, or 1 of every 2.4 deaths. CVD was about 60% of total mortality, which means that of the more than 2,000,000 deaths from all causes, CVD was listed as a primary or contributing cause on more than 1,406,000 death certificates. Heart disease has been the leading killer of Americans since 1900. This statistic is still true today. As a result, heart disease remains the leading cause of death. Thus, many of your calls will involve some type of cardiac emergency.

It is important for EMS providers to understand that many deaths caused by CVD occur from problems that may have been avoided by people living more prudent lifestyles and by access to improved medical technology. We can help to reduce these numbers of deaths with better public awarness, early access, increased numbers of laypeople trained in CPR, and with public access defibrillation.

This chapter begins with a brief description of the heart and how it works. It then discusses the relationship between chest pain and ischemic heart disease. It explains how to recognize and treat acute myocardial infarction (classic heart attack) and the complications of sudden death, cardiogenic shock, and congestive heart failure. The use of nitroglycerin is described. The last part of the chapter is devoted to the use and maintenance of the automated external defibrillator (AED).

Cardiac Structure and Function

The heart is a relatively simple organ with a simple job. It has to pump blood to supply oxygen-enriched red blood cells to the tissues of the body. The heart is divided down the middle into two sides (left and right) by a wall called the septum. Each side of the heart has an **atrium**, or upper chamber, and a **ventricle**, or lower chamber ▶ **Figure 12-1** . Blood leaves each of the four chambers of the heart through a one-way valve. These valves keep the blood moving through the circulatory system in the proper direction. The largest valve is the **aortic valve**, lying between the left ventricle and the aorta. The **aorta**, the body's main artery, receives the blood ejected from the left ventricle and delivers it to all the other arteries so that they can carry blood to the tissues of the body.

The right side of the heart receives oxygen-poor (deoxygenated) blood from the veins of the body ▶ **Figure 12-2A** . Blood enters into the right atrium from the vena cava, which then fills the right ventricle. After contraction of the right ventricle, blood flows into the pulmonary artery and the pulmonary circulation, where the blood is oxygenated. The left side of the heart receives oxygen-rich (oxygenated) blood from the lungs through the pulmonary veins ▶ **Figure 12-2B** . Blood enters into the atrium, then passes into the left ventricle. This side of the heart is more muscular than the other because it must pump blood into the aorta and all the other arteries of the body.

The heart contains more than muscle tissue. The heart's electrical system, which is distributed throughout the entire heart, controls heart rate and enables the atria

Close to one half of Americans will eventually die as a result of heart disease.

and ventricles to work together (► **Figure 12-3**). Normal electrical impulses begin in the sinus node, just above the atria. The impulses travel across both atria, causing them to contract. Between the atria and the ventricles, the impulses cross over a bridge of special electrical tissue called the atrioventricular (AV) node. Here the signal is slowed down for about one tenth to two tenths of a second to allow blood time to pass from the atria to the ventricles. Then the impulses exit the AV node and spread throughout both ventricles, causing the ventricular muscle cells to contract.

Circulation

To carry out its function of pumping blood, the **myocardium**, or heart muscle, must have a continuous supply of oxygen and nutrients. During periods of physical exertion or stress, the myocardium requires more oxygen, so the heart must increase its output of bloodflow. In the normal heart, the increased need for blood is easily supplied by **dilation**, or widening, of the coronary arteries, which increases blood flow. The **coronary arteries** are the blood vessels that supply blood to the heart muscle. They start at the first part of the aorta, just above the aortic valve. The right coronary artery supplies blood to the right ventricle and, in most people, the bottom part, or inferior wall, of the left ventricle. The left coronary artery divides into two major branches, both of which supply the left ventricle (► **Figure 12-4**).

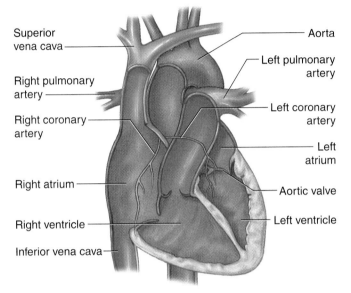

Figure 12-1 The heart is a four-chambered muscle that pumps blood to all parts of the body.

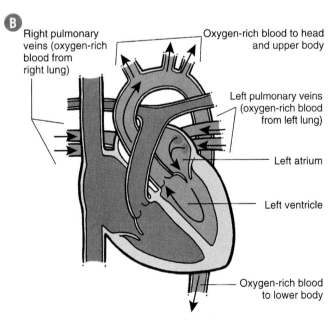

Figure 12-2 **A.** The right side of the heart receives oxygen-poor blood from the veins. **B.** The left side of the heart receives oxygen-rich blood from the lungs through the pulmonary veins.

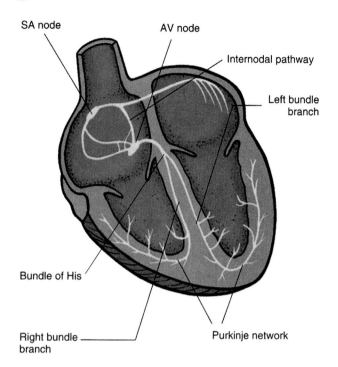

SA node
AV node
Internodal pathway
Left bundle branch
Bundle of His
Right bundle branch
Purkinje network

Figure 12-3 The electrical conduction system of the heart controls most aspects of heart rate and enables the four chambers to work together.

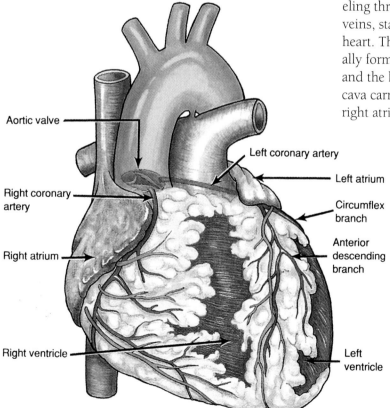

Aortic valve
Right coronary artery
Right atrium
Right ventricle
Left coronary artery
Left atrium
Circumflex branch
Anterior descending branch
Left ventricle

Figure 12-4 The coronary arteries carry the blood supply to the heart.

Two major arteries branching from the upper aorta supply blood to the head and arms. The right and left carotid arteries supply the head and brain with blood. The subclavian arteries (under the clavicles) supply blood to the upper extremities. As the subclavian artery enters each arm, it becomes the brachial artery, the major vessel that supplies blood to each arm. Just below the elbow, the brachial artery divides into two major branches: the radial and ulnar arteries (▸ **Figure 12-5**).

At the level of the navel, the aorta divides into two main branches called the right and left iliac arteries, which supply blood to the groin, pelvis, and legs. As the iliac arteries enter the legs through the groin, they become the right and left femoral arteries. At the level of the knee, the femoral artery divides into the **anterior** (front) and **posterior** (back) tibial artery and the peroneal artery.

After blood travels through the arteries, it enters smaller and smaller vessels, called arterioles and capillaries. The capillaries are tiny blood vessels about one cell thick that connect arterioles to venules. Capillaries, which are found in all parts of the body, allow the exchange of nutrients and waste at the cellular level.

Venules are the smallest branches of veins. After traveling through the capillaries, blood enters the system of veins, starting with the venules, on its way back to the heart. The veins become larger and larger and eventually form the two large venae cavae: the upper vena cava and the lower vena cava. The **superior** (upper) vena cava carries blood from the head and arms back to the right atrium. The **inferior** (lower) vena cava carries blood from the abdomen, kidneys, and legs back to the right atrium. The superior and inferior venae cavae join at the right atrium of the heart, where blood is eventually returned into the pulmonary circulation for oxygenation (▸ **Figure 12-6**).

Blood consists of several types of cells and fluid (▸ **Figure 12-7**). *Red blood cells* are the most numerous and give the blood its color. Red blood cells carry oxygen to the body's tissues and then remove carbon dioxide. Larger *white blood cells* help to fight infection. *Platelets*, which help the blood to clot, are much smaller than either red or white blood cells. *Plasma* is the fluid that the cells float in. It is a mixture of water, salts, nutrients, and proteins.

Blood pressure is the pressure of circulating blood against the walls of the arteries. Systolic blood pressure is the max-

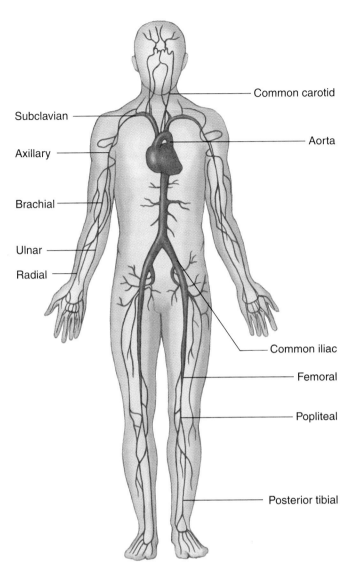

Figure 12-5 The major arteries of the body carry oxygen-rich blood to all parts of the body.

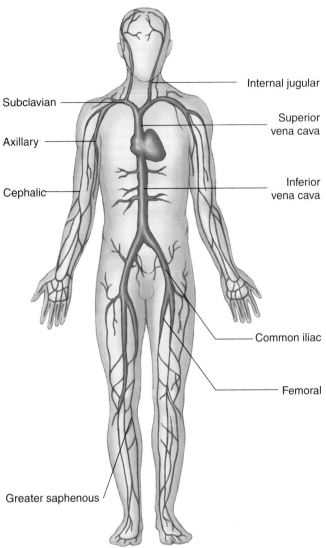

Figure 12-6 The veins carry blood from the body back to the heart, which pumps it through the lungs for oxygenation.

imum pressure exerted by the left ventricle as it contracts. As the left ventricle relaxes, the arterial pressure falls. When the aortic valve closes, blood flow stops. The diastolic blood pressure is the pressure exerted against the walls of the arteries while the left ventricle is at rest. Remember that the top number in a blood pressure reading is the systolic pressure, and the bottom number is the diastolic or resting pressure.

Cardiac Compromise

Chest pain or discomfort that is related to the heart usually stems from a condition called **ischemia**, or insufficient oxygen. Because of a partial or complete blockage of flow through the coronary arteries, heart tissue fails to get enough oxygen and nutrients.

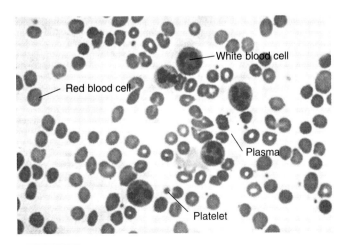

Figure 12-7 Blood consists of several types of cells and fluids, including red blood cells, white blood cells, and platelets.

EMT-B Tips

Pulsation

As the left ventricle contracts, it ejects a forceful wave of blood through the arteries. You can feel that wave in areas where the artery lies over a bone and is near the surface of the skin. This wave is called the pulse. Common places to feel for a pulse include the following (▶ **Figure 12-8**):

- The *carotid pulse* can be felt in the neck, two fingerbreadths on either side of the Adam's apple (thyroid cartilage), and should be taken on side closest to the EMT-B.

- The *femoral pulse* can be felt in the groin, right at the crease dividing the lower abdomen from the leg.

- The *brachial pulse* can be felt on the medial aspect of the elbow, right at the level of the crease. Pulsations also can be palpated on the inside of the arm between the elbow and armpit. This is the pulse that you listen to when you take blood pressure.

- The *radial pulse* can be felt on the thumb side of the wrist, about one finger width above the wrist crease.

- The *posterior tibial pulse* can be felt on the inside of the ankle, just posterior to the medial malleolus. The medial malleolus is the bony bump at the end of the tibia.

- The *dorsalis pedis pulse* can be felt at the top of the foot. This artery is not in the exact same place in all people. To find its pulse, place your hand across the top of the foot just below the ankle crease. Once you feel something that might be a pulse, use your fingertips to confirm that finding.

Practice feeling for these pulses on yourself and on friends and family members.

Figure 12-8 Common pulse points.
  A. The carotid pulse is taken at the neck.
  B. The femoral pulse is felt in the groin area.
  C. The brachial pulse can be felt on the inside of the upper arm.
  D. The radial pulse can be felt on the thumb side of the wrist.
  E. The posterior tibial pulse can be felt on the inside of the ankle.
  F. The dorsalis pedis pulse can be felt at the top of the foot.

The tissue soon begins to starve and, if blood flow is not restored, eventually dies. Ischemic heart disease, then, is disease involving a decrease in blood flow to one or more portions of the heart muscle.

Atherosclerosis

Most often, the low blood flow to heart tissue is caused by coronary artery atherosclerosis. **Atherosclerosis** is a disorder in which calcium and a fatty material called cholesterol build up and form a plaque inside the walls of blood vessels, obstructing flow and interfering with their ability to dilate or contract (▶ **Figure 12-9**). Eventually, atherosclerosis can even cause complete **occlusion**, or blockage, of a coronary artery. Atherosclerosis usually involves other arteries of the body, as well.

The problem begins when the first deposit of cholesterol is laid down on the inside of an artery. This may happen during the teenage years. As a person ages, more of this fatty material is deposited; the **lumen**, or the inside diameter of the artery, narrows. As the cholesterol deposits grow, calcium deposits can form as well. The inner wall of the artery, which is normally smooth and elastic, becomes rough and brittle with these atherosclerotic plaques. Damage to the coronary arteries may become so extensive that they cannot accommodate increased blood flow at times of maximum need.

For reasons that are still not completely understood, a brittle plaque will sometimes develop a crack, exposing the inside of the atherosclerotic wall. Acting like a torn blood vessel, the ragged edge of the crack activates the blood-clotting system, just as it does when an injury has caused bleeding. In this situation, however, the resulting blood clot will partially or completely

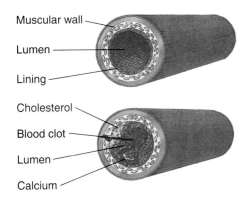

Figure 12-9 In atherosclerosis, calcium and cholesterol build up inside the walls of the blood vessels, causing an obstruction in blood flow to the heart.

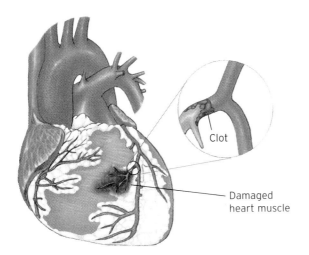

Figure 12-10 An acute myocardial infarction occurs when a blood clot prevents blood flow to an area of the heart muscle. If left untreated, this can result in death of heart tissue.

block the lumen of the artery. Tissues downstream from the blood clot will suffer from lack of oxygen (ischemia). If blood flow is resumed in a short time, the ischemic tissues will recover. However, if too much time goes by before blood flow is resumed, the tissues will die. This sequence of events is known as an **acute myocardial infarction (AMI)**, a classic heart attack ▼ **Figure 12-10** . **Infarction** means the death of tissue. The same sequence may also cause the death of cells in other organs, such as the brain. The death of heart muscle can lead to severe diminishment of the heart's ability to pump or cardiac arrest.

In the United States, coronary artery disease is the number one cause of death for both men and women. The peak incidence of heart disease occurs between ages 40 and 70 years, but it can also strike teens or individuals in their 90s. You must be alert to the possibility that, although less likely, a 26-year-old person with chest pain could actually be having a heart attack, especially if he or she has a higher than usual risk.

Factors that place a person at higher risk for a myocardial infarction are called risk factors. The major controllable factors are cigarette smoking, high blood pressure, elevated cholesterol levels, elevated blood sugar levels (diabetes), lack of exercise, and stress. The major risk factors that cannot be controlled are older age, family history of atherosclerotic coronary artery disease, and male gender.

Angina Pectoris

Chest pain does not always mean that a person is having an AMI. When, for a brief period of time, heart tissues are not getting enough oxygen, the pain is called **angina pectoris**, or angina. Although it can result from a spasm of the artery, angina is most often a symptom of atherosclerotic coronary artery disease. Angina occurs when the heart's need for oxygen exceeds its supply, usually during periods of physical or emotional stress when the heart is working hard. A large meal or sudden fear may also trigger an attack. When the increased oxygen demand goes away (eg, the person stops exercising), the pain typically goes away.

Angina pain is typically described as crushing, squeezing, or "like somebody standing on my chest." It is usually felt in the midchest, under the sternum. However, it can radiate to the jaw, the arms (frequently the left arm), the midback, or the epigastrium (the upper-middle region of the abdomen). The pain usually lasts from 3 to 8 minutes, rarely longer than 15 minutes. It may be associated with shortness of breath, nausea, or sweating. It disappears promptly with rest, supplemental oxygen, or nitroglycerin, all of which increase the supply of oxygen to the heart. Although angina pectoris is frightening, it does not mean that heart cells are dying, nor does it usually lead to death or permanent heart damage. It is, however, a warning that you and the patient should both take seriously. Even with angina, because oxygen supply to the heart is diminished, the electrical system can be compromised and the person is at risk for significant cardiac rhythm problems.

Keep in mind that it can be very difficult even for doctors in hospitals to distinguish between the pain of angina and the pain of a myocardial infarction

Acute Myocardial Infarction

As we have seen, the pain of AMI signals the actual death of cells in the area of the heart where blood flow is obstructed. Once dead, the cells cannot be revived. Instead, they will eventually turn to scar tissue and become a burden to the beating heart. This is why fast action is so critical in treating a heart attack. The sooner the blockage can be cleared, the fewer the cells that may die. About 30 minutes after blood flow is cut off, some heart muscle cells begin to die. After about 2 hours, as many as half of the cells in the area can be dead; in most cases, after 4 to 6 hours, more than 90% of them will be dead. However, studies show that in many cases, opening the coronary artery with either "clot-busting" medications or angioplasty (mechanical clearing of the artery) can prevent damage to the heart muscle if done within the first hour after the onset of symptoms. Therefore, immediate treatment and transport to the emergency department is essential.

AMI is more apt to occur in the larger, thick-walled left ventricle, which needs more blood and oxygen, than in the right ventricle.

The Pain of Acute Myocardial Infarction

The pain of AMI differs from the pain of angina in three ways:

- **It may or may not be caused by exertion** but can occur at any time, sometimes when a person is sitting quietly or even sleeping.

- **It does not resolve in a few minutes;** rather, it can last between 30 minutes and several hours.

- **It may or may not be relieved** by rest or nitroglycerin.

Note that not all patients who are having an AMI experience pain or recognize it when it does occur. In

Documentation Tips

Documenting exactly how a patient describes chest discomfort, in the patient's own words, is a valuable source of information for hospital staff. Remember—OPQRST.

fact, about a third of patients never seek medical attention. This can be attributed, in part, to the fact that people are afraid of dying and do not wish to face the possibility that their symptoms may be serious (cardiac denial). Middle-aged men, in particular, are likely to minimize their symptoms. However, a few patients, particularly elderly individuals or those with diabetes, do not experience any pain during an AMI. Others may feel only mild discomfort and call it "indigestion."

Therefore, when you are called to a scene where the chief complaint is chest pain, complete a thorough assessment, no matter what the patient says. Any complaint of chest discomfort in a person older than age 21 years is a serious matter. In fact, the best thing you can do is to assume the worst.

Consequences of Acute Myocardial Infarction

Acute myocardial infarction can have three serious consequences:

- Sudden death
- Cardiogenic shock
- Congestive heart failure

SUDDEN DEATH. Approximately 40% of all patients with AMI never reach the hospital. Sudden death is usually the result of **cardiac arrest**, in which the heart fails to generate an effective blood flow. Although you cannot feel a pulse in someone experiencing cardiac arrest, the heart may still be twitching, though erratically. The heart is using up energy without pumping. Such an abnormality of heart rhythm is a ventricular **arrhythmia**, known as **ventricular fibrillation**.

A variety of other lethal and nonlethal arrhythmias may follow AMI, usually within the first hour. In most cases, it is premature ventricular contractions (PVCs), or extra beats in the damaged ventricle. PVCs by themselves are a harmless arrhythmia that is common among healthy, as well as sick, individuals. Other arrhythmias are much more dangerous ▶ **Figure 12-11**. These include the following:

- **Tachycardia**: Rapid beating of the heart, 100 beats/min or more.

- <u>Bradycardia</u>: Unusually slow beating of the heart, 60 beats/min or less.

- <u>Ventricular tachycardia (VT)</u>: Rapid heart rhythm, usually at a rate of 150 to 200 beats/min. The electrical activity starts in the ventricle instead of the atrium. This rhythm usually does not allow adequate time between each beat for the left ventricle to fill with blood. Therefore, the patient's blood pressure may fall. He or she may also feel weak or lightheaded or may even become unresponsive. In some cases, the patient may develop worsening chest pain or chest pain that was not there before onset of the arrhythmia. A string of three or more PVCs, back to back, can be called a "run of VT." Most cases of VT will be more sustained and may deteriorate into ventricular fibrillation.

- <u>Ventricular fibrillation</u>: Disorganized, ineffective quivering of the ventricles. No blood gets to the body, and the patient usually becomes unconscious within seconds. The only way to treat this arrhythmia is to electrically defibrillate the heart. To <u>defibrillate</u> means to shock the heart with a specialized electrical current in an attempt to restore a normal rhythmic beat. Defibrillation is highly successful in terms of saving a life if delivered within a minute or two. If a defibrillator is not immediately available, CPR must be initiated to buy a few more minutes for arrival of the AED. Even if CPR is begun right at the time of collapse, chances of survival diminish each minute until defibrillation is accomplished.

If uncorrected, unstable ventricular tachycardia or ventricular fibrillation will eventually lead to <u>asystole</u>, the absence of all heart electrical activity. Without CPR, this may occur within minutes. Because it reflects a long period of ischemia, nearly all patients you find in asystole will die.

CARDIOGENIC SHOCK. Shock is a simple concept but one that few people without medical training really understand. For that reason, Chapter 23 is devoted to a discussion of shock. The discussion of shock in this chapter is limited to that associated with cardiac problems.

For an EMT-B, shock is also a critical concept. Shock is present when body tissues do not get enough oxygen, causing body organs to malfunction. In <u>cardiogenic shock</u>, often caused by a heart attack, the problem is that the heart lacks enough power to force the proper volume of blood through the circulatory system. Cardiogenic shock can occur immediately or as late as 24 hours after the onset of the AMI. The various signs and symptoms of cardiogenic shock are produced by the improper functioning of the body's organs. The challenge for you is to recognize shock in its early stages, when treatment is much more successful.

CONGESTIVE HEART FAILURE. Failure of the heart occurs when the ventricular heart muscle is so damaged that it can no longer keep up with the return flow of blood from the atria. <u>Congestive heart failure (CHF)</u> can occur any time after a myocardial infarction, heart valve damage, or longstanding high blood pressure, but it usually happens between the first few hours and the first few days after an acute myocardial infarction.

Just as the pumping function of the left ventricle can be damaged by coronary artery disease, it can also be damaged by diseased heart valves or chronic hypertension. In any of these cases, when the muscle can no

Figure 12-11 Common heart arrhythmias **A.** Sinus tachycardia **B.** Bradycardia **C.** Ventricular tachycardia (VT) **D.** Ventricular fibrillation (VF) **E.** Asystole

EMT-B Tips

More about shock

Signs and symptoms

- One of the first signs of shock is *anxiety* or *restlessness* as the brain becomes relatively starved for oxygen. The patient may complain of *"air hunger."* Think of the possibility of shock when the patient is yelling, "I can't breathe." Obviously, the patient can breathe, because he or she can talk. However, the patient's brain is sensing that it is not getting enough oxygen.

- As the shock continues, the body tries to send blood to the most important organs, such as the brain and heart, and away from less important organs, such as the skin. Therefore, you may see *pale, clammy skin* in patients with shock.

- As the shock gets worse, the body will attempt to compensate by increasing the amount of blood pumped through the heart. Therefore, the *pulse rate will be higher than normal.* In severe shock the heart rate will usually, but not always, be greater than 120 beats/min.

- Shock can also be characterized by rapid and shallow breathing, nausea and vomiting, and a decrease in body temperature.

- Finally, as the heart and other organs begin to malfunction, the *blood pressure will fall below normal.* A systolic blood pressure less than 90 mm Hg is easy to recognize, but it is a late finding that indicates decompensated shock. Do not assume that shock is not present just because the blood pressure is normal (compensated shock).

Treatment of patients with cardiogenic shock. Take the following steps when treating patients with signs and symptoms of shock:

1. Position the patient comfortably. Most patients with heart failure will be more comfortable in semi-Fowler's position; however, those with low blood pressure may not tolerate a semi-upright position. These patients may be more comfortable and be more alert in a supine position.

2. Administer high flow oxygen.

3. Assist ventilations as necessary.

4. Provide prompt transport to the emergency department.

More about CHF

Signs and symptoms

Watch for the following signs and symptoms in a patient you suspect has CHF:

- The patient finds it easier to breathe when sitting up. When the patient is lying down, more blood is returned to the right ventricle and lungs, causing further pulmonary congestion.

- Often, the patient is mildly or severely agitated.

- Chest pain may or may not be present.

- The patient often has distended neck veins that do not collapse even when the patient is sitting.

- The patient may have swollen ankles from pedal edema (back-up of fluid).

- The patient generally will have a high blood pressure, rapid heart rate, and rapid respirations.

- The patient will usually be using accessory breathing muscles of the neck and ribs, reflecting the additional hard work of breathing.

- The fluid surrounding small airways may produce rales, best heard by listening to either side of the patient's chest, about midway down the back. In severe congestive heart failure, these soft sounds can be heard even at the top of the lung.

Once congestive heart failure develops, it can be treated but not cured. Regular use of medications may alleviate the symptoms. However, these patients often become ill again and are frequently hospitalized. Approximately half will be dead within 5 years of the onset of symptoms.

Treatment of CHF. Treat the patient with congestive heart failure the same way as the patient with chest pain:

1. Take the vital signs, monitor heart rhythm, and give oxygen by nonrebreathing face mask with an oxygen flow of 10 to 15 L/min.

2. Allow the patient to remain sitting in an upright position with the legs down.

3. Be reassuring; many patients with CHF are quite anxious because they cannot breathe.

4. Patients who have had problems with CHF before will usually have specific medications for its treatment. Gather these medications and take them along to the hospital.

5. Nitroglycerin may be of value if the patient's blood pressure is above 100 systolic. If the patient has prescribed nitroglycerin, and medical control advises you to do so, you can administer it sublingually.

6. Prompt transport to the emergency department is essential.

longer contract effectively, the heart tries other ways to maintain an adequate cardiac output. Two specific changes in heart function occur: The heart rate increases, and the left ventricle enlarges in an effort to increase the amount of blood pumped each minute.

When these adaptations can no longer make up for the decreased heart function, congestive heart failure eventually develops. It is called "congestive" heart failure because the lungs become congested with fluid once the heart fails to pump the blood effectively. Blood tends to back up in the pulmonary veins, increasing the pressure in the capillaries of the lungs. When the pressure in the capillaries exceeds a certain level, fluid (mostly water) passes through the walls of the capillary vessels and into the alveoli. This condition is called pulmonary edema. It may occur suddenly, as in AMI, or slowly over months, as in chronic congestive heart failure. Sometimes, patients with an acute onset of CHF will develop severe pulmonary edema, in which the patient has pink, frothy sputum, and severe dyspnea.

Fluid also collects elsewhere in the body, usually in the feet and legs. This is called **pedal edema**. The swelling causes relatively few symptoms other than discomfort. However, chronic pedal edema may indicate underlying heart disease even in the absence of pain or other symptoms.

Signs and Symptoms of Acute Myocardial Infarction

A patient with an acute myocardial infarction may show any of the following signs and symptoms:

- Sudden onset of weakness, nausea, and sweating without an obvious cause
- Chest pain/discomfort that is often crushing or squeezing and that does not change with each breath
- Pain in the lower jaw, arms, or neck
- Sudden arrhythmia with **syncope** (fainting)
- Pulmonary edema
- Sudden death

Physical Findings of AMI and Cardiac Compromise

The physical findings of AMI vary, depending on the extent and severity of heart muscle damage. The following are common:

- **Pulse.** Generally, the pulse rate increases as a normal response to pain, stress, fear, or actual injury to the myocardium. Because arrhythmias are common in AMI, you may feel an irregularity of the pulse.
- **Blood pressure.** Blood pressure may fall as a result of diminished cardiac output and diminished capability of the left ventricle to pump. However, most patients with AMI will have a normal or, most likely, elevated blood pressure.
- **Respiration.** Respirations are usually normal unless the patient has congestive heart failure. In that case, respirations may become rapid and labored.
- **General appearance.** The patient often appears frightened. There may be nausea, vomiting, and a cold sweat. The skin is often ashen gray because of poor cardiac output and the loss of **perfusion**, or blood flow through the tissue. Occasionally, the skin will have a bluish tint, called cyanosis; this is the result of poor oxygenation of the circulating blood.
- **Mental status.** Patients with AMI sometimes experience an almost overwhelming feeling of impending doom. If a patient tells you, "I think I am going to die," pay attention.

Approach to the Patient with Chest Pain

All patient assessments begin by determining whether or not the patient is responsive. If the patient is not responsive and weighs at least 55 lb (25 kg) and is less than 8 years old, you must decide whether or not, on the basis of your local protocols, to use the automated external defibrillator (AED) and begin CPR. If the patient weighs less than 55 lb (usually patients younger than age 8 years), use of the AED is not advised. Generally, the AED should be applied if the patient is pulseless, not breathing (apneic), and unresponsive. If the patient is responsive take the following steps when you are treating a conscious patient who complains of chest discomfort ▶ **Skill Drill 12-1** :

1. **Reassure the patient** and perform the initial assessment. After confirming consciousness and the chief complaint of chest pain, reassure the patient as you prepare to apply oxygen. Act professionally; be calm. Speak to the patient in a normal voice that is neither too loud nor too soft. Let the patient know that trained individuals, including yourself, are present to provide care and that he or she will soon be taken to the hospital. Remember, some patients may act carefree, while others may be demanding. However, most are still frightened. Your professional attitude

may be the single most important factor in winning the patient's cooperation and helping him or her through this event. Patients often have a good idea about what is happening, so do not lie and offer false reassurance. If asked, "Am I having a heart attack?" you can say, "I do not know for sure, but in case you are, we are taking care of you. We are going to help you now by giving oxygen, and we will be taking you to the hospital. You are in good hands."

2. **Apply oxygen.** If available, use pulse oximetry. Apply a nonrebreathing mask at 10 to 15 L/min.

3. **Position the patient.** If you suspect AMI, place the patient in a comfortable position, usually sitting up and well supported. Make sure the patient has no difficulty breathing and has no airway obstruction. Try not to allow the patient to exert himself or herself, strain, or walk. If necessary, lift the patient, using care **(Step 1)**.

4. **Measure and record the patient's vital signs.** As your partner obtains the SAMPLE history, you should take baseline vital signs, including pulse, blood pressure, and the rate and depth of breathing. You must obtain readings for both systolic and diastolic blood pressures. Note the time that the vital signs are taken. Vital signs should be reassessed at least every 5 minutes or as significant changes in the patient's condition occur. It is essential to monitor the patient with a suspected AMI closely, because sudden cardiac arrest is always a risk. If cardiac arrest occurs, you must be ready to begin automated defibrillation or CPR immediately. If an AED is immediately available, use it; if not, perform CPR until the AED is available **(Step 2)**.

5. **Obtain a focused history and physical exam.** Take a brief history from the patient. Friends or family members who are present often have helpful information. Ask them the following questions:

• Has the patient ever had a heart attack before?

• Has the patient been told about having previous heart problems?

• Are there any risk factors for coronary artery disease?

In terms of the physical exam, check the skin color, temperature, and condition. Is it cool, moist? How do the mucous membranes look? Are they pink, ashen, or bluish? Are the lung sounds clear? Are the neck veins distended?

6. **Ask specific questions** about the patient's chest discomfort. Use the OPQRST mnemonic to determine the type of pain ▶ **Table 12-1** .

In addition, ask whether the patient has had the same pain before. If so, ask "Do you take any medications for the pain?" and "Do you have any of the medication with you?" If the patient has had a heart attack or angina before, ask whether this is the same type of pain.

7. **Prepare to assist with prescribed nitroglycerin: Check the medication and its expiration date (Step 3).**

8. **Help the patient administer prescribed nitroglycerin.** Nitroglycerin works in most patients within 5 minutes to relieve the pain of angina. Most patients who have been prescribed nitroglycerin carry a supply with them. Trade names of nitroglycerin include Nitrostat and others. Patients take one dose of nitroglycerin under the tongue whenever they have an episode of angina that does not immediately go away with rest. If the pain is still present after 5 minutes, patients are typically instructed by their doctors to take a second dose. If the second dose does not work, most patients are told to take a third dose and then call for EMS. If the patient has not taken all three doses, you can help to administer the medication, if you are allowed to do so by local protocol **(Step 4)**.

Nitroglycerin comes in several forms: as a small white pill, placed sublingually (under the tongue); as a spray, also taken sublingually; or as a skin patch applied to the chest ▼ **Figure 12-12** . In any form, the effect is the same.

Figure 12-12 Nitroglycerin used to treat AMI comes in many forms, including paste, spray, tablets, and skin patches.

Skill Drill 12-1   Caring for a Conscious Patient with Chest Pain

1

Reassure the patient as you perform the initial assessment.
Apply oxygen.
Place the patient in a comfortable position.

2

Measure and record the baseline vital signs, obtain a SAMPLE History,
and monitor the patient closely.
Obtain a focused history and physical exam.
Ask about the patient's discomfort using OPQRST.

3

Check medication and expiration date.

4

Help the patient administer nitroglycerin.

5

Prepare to transport the patient.
Report to medical control.

Table 12-1 OPQRST Mnemonic for Assessing Pain

- **Onset.** Determine what time the discomfort that motivated the call for help began.

- **Provocation.** Ask what makes the pain or discomfort worse. Is it positional? Does a deep breath or palpation of the chest make it worse? Is the pain steady?

- **Quality.** Ask what type of pain it is. Let the patient use his or her own words to describe what is happening. Try to avoid supplying the patient with only one option. Do not ask "Does it feel like an elephant is sitting on your chest?" Instead, say "Tell me what the pain feels like." If the patient cannot answer an open-ended question, then provide a list of alternatives. "There are lots of different kinds of pain. Is your pain more like a heaviness, pressure, burning, tearing, dull ache, stabbing, or needlelike?"

- **Radiation.** Ask whether the pain travels to another part of the body.

- **Severity.** Ask the patient to rate the pain on a simple scale. Often, a scale ranging from 0 to 10 is used, in which 0 represents no pain at all and 10 represents the worst pain imaginable. Do not use the patient's answer to determine whether the pain has a serious cause. Instead, use it to check whether the pain is getting better or worse. After a few minutes of oxygen or administration of nitroglycerin pill, ask the patient to rate the pain again.

- **Time.** Find out how long the pain lasts when it is present and whether it has been intermittent or continuous.

Nitroglycerin relaxes the muscle of blood vessel walls, dilates coronary arteries, increases blood flow and the supply of oxygen to the heart muscle, and decreases the workload of the heart. Nitroglycerin also dilates blood vessels in other parts of the body and can sometimes cause low blood pressure and/or a severe headache. Other side effects include changes in the patient's pulse rate, including tachycardia and bradycardia. For this reason, you should take the patient's blood pressure within 5 minutes after each dose. If the systolic blood pressure is less than 100 mm Hg, do not give any more medication. Other contraindications include the presence of a head injury, and the maximum prescribed dose has already been given (usually three doses).

If the patient does not have prescribed nitroglycerin, continue with your focused assessment and prepare to transport. Be sure that this process does not consume too much time. Do not delay transport to assist with administration of nitroglycerin. The drug can be given en route. To safely assist the patient with nitroglycerin, follow the steps listed below.

- Obtain an order from medical direction either online or offline protocol.

- Take the patient's blood pressure. Continue with administration of nitroglycerin only if the systolic blood pressure is greater than 100 mm Hg.

- Check that you have the right medication, the right patient, and the right delivery route.

- Check the expiration date of the nitroglycerin.

- Question the patient about the last dose he or she took and its effects. Make sure that the patient understands the route of administration.

- When you give a patient nitroglycerin, you should be prepared to have the patient lie down to prevent fainting if the nitroglycerin substantially lowers the patient's blood pressure (the patient gets dizzy or feels faint).

- Ask the patient to lift his or her tongue. Place the tablet or spray the dose underneath the tongue (while wearing gloves), or have the patient do so.

- Have the patient keep his or her mouth closed with the tablet under the tongue until it is dissolved and absorbed. Caution the patient against chewing or swallowing the tablet.

- Recheck blood pressure within 5 minutes.

- Record each medication and the time of administration.

- Perform continued reassessment.

EMT-B Tips

While your partner is getting the nitroglycerin ready, check to see if the patient's mucous membranes are moist. If not, a mouth rinse before using the pill form of the medication helps ensure that the pill dissolves and the patient gets its full benefit. This is not necessary if you are using the spray form.

After giving nitroglycerin, reassess the patient and note the response to the medication. If the chest pain persists and the patient still has a systolic blood pressure greater than 100 mm Hg, repeat the dose in minutes as authorized by your medical control. In general, a maximum of three doses of nitroglycerin are given for any one episode of chest pain.

9. **Transport the patient.** Early, prompt transport to the emergency department is critical so that newer treatments, such as clot-busting medications or angioplasty, can be initiated. To be most effective, these treatments must be started as soon as possible after the onset of the attack. Therefore, alert the emergency department about the status of your patient and your estimated time of arrival. Report to medical control. Report to the hospital by radio or cellular telephone while en route. Give the patient's history, vital signs, repeat vital signs, medications being taken, and the treatment you are giving. Follow the instructions of your medical control physician. Describe the patient's condition to the emergency department staff on arrival **(Step 5)**.

Heart Operations and Pacemakers

Over the last 20 years, hundreds of thousands of open heart operations were performed to bypass damaged segments of coronary arteries in the heart. In the coronary artery bypass graft (CABG) operation, a blood vessel from the chest or leg is sewn directly from the aorta to a coronary artery beyond the point of the obstruction. Other patients may have had a procedure called percutaneous transluminal coronary angioplasty (PTCA), which aims to dilate, rather than bypass, the coronary artery. In this procedure, usually called an angioplasty or balloon angioplasty, a tiny balloon is attached to the end of a long, thin tube. The tube is introduced through the skin into a large vein, usually in the groin, and then threaded into the narrowed

coronary artery, with radiographs serving as a guide. Once the balloon is in position inside the coronary artery, it is inflated. The balloon is then deflated, and the tube is removed from the body. Sometimes, a metal mesh called a stent is placed inside the artery either instead of or after the balloon. The stent is left in place permanently to help keep the artery from narrowing again.

You will almost certainly have a patient with previous AMI or angina who has had one of these procedures. Patients who have had a bypass graft will have a long surgical scar on their chest from the operation ▼ **Figure 12-13** . Patients who have had an angioplasty or coronary artery stent usually will not. However, newer "keyhole" surgical techniques may not produce a large scar. You should not assume that a patient who has a small scar has not had bypass surgery. Chest pain in a patient who has had any of these procedures should be treated the same as chest pain in patients who have not had any heart surgery. In any event, chest pain in a patient who has undergone either procedure is treated exactly the same as chest pain in a patient who has not. Carry out all the described tasks, and transport the patient promptly to the emergency department of the hospital. If CPR is required, perform it in the usual way, regardless of the scar on the patient's chest. Likewise, if indicated, an AED should be used as well.

Many people with heart disease in the United States have cardiac pacemakers to maintain a regular cardiac rhythm and rate. Pacemakers are inserted when the electrical control system of the heart is so damaged that it cannot function properly. These battery-powered

Figure 12-13 The surgical scar on the patient's chest implies a previous coronary artery bypass graft (CABG) surgery.

Figure 12-14 A pacemaker, which is typically inserted under the skin in the left upper chest, delivers an electrical impulse to regulate heartbeat.

Figure 12-15 An AICD is attached directly to the heart and continuously monitors heart rhythm, delivering shocks as needed. The electricity from the AICD is so low that it has no effect on rescuers.

devices deliver an electrical impulse through wires that are in direct contact with the myocardium. The generating unit is generally placed under a heavy muscle or a fold of skin; it typically resembles a small silver dollar under the skin in the left upper chest ▲ **Figure 12-14** .

Normally, you do not need to be concerned about problems with pacemakers. Thanks to modern technology, an implanted unit will not require replacement or a battery charge for years. Wires are well protected and rarely broken. In the past, pacemakers sometimes malfunctioned when a patient got too close to an electrical radiation source, such as a microwave oven, but this is no longer the case. Every patient with a pacemaker still should be aware of the precautions, if any, that must be taken to maintain its proper functioning.

If a pacemaker does not function properly, as when the battery wears out, the patient may experience syncope, dizziness, or weakness because of an excessively slow heart rate. The pulse ordinarily will be less than 60 beats/min because the heart is beating without the stimulus of the pacemaker and without the regulation of its own electrical system, which may be damaged. In these circumstances, the heart tends to assume a fixed slow rate that is not fast enough to allow the patient to function normally. A patient with a malfunctioning pacemaker should be promptly transported to the emergency department; repair of the problem may require an operation. When an AED is used, the patches should not be placed directly over the

pacemaker. This will ensure a better flow of electricity through the patient's body.

Automatic Implantable Cardiac Defibrillators

More and more patients who survive ventricular fibrillation cardiac arrests have a small automatic implantable cardiac defibrillator (AICD) implanted. Some patients who are at particularly high risk for a cardiac arrest have them as well. These devices are attached directly to the heart and can prolong the lives of certain patients. They continuously monitor the heart rhythm, delivering shocks as needed ▲ **Figure 12-15** . Regardless of whether a patient having an AMI has an AICD, he or she should be treated like all other AMI patients; treatment should include performing CPR and using an AED if the patient goes into cardiac arrest. Generally, the electricity from an AICD is so low that it will have no effect on rescuers and therefore should not be of concern to you.

Automated External Defibrillation

In the late 1970s and early 1980s, scientists developed a small computer that could analyze electrical signals from the heart and determine when ventricular fibrillation was taking place. This development, along with improved battery technology, made possible the automated portable defibrillator, which can automatically administer an electrical shock to the heart when needed.

Pediatric Needs

Heart problems in childhood are uncommon and usually congenital, meaning that the patient was born with the problem. In general, your approach to these patients should be the same as that for an adult. You should attempt to reassure the patient. If possible, administer oxygen. If the patient will not wear a face mask, have the parent hold the oxygen in front of the child's face.

Cardiac arrest in younger children is less common than in older children and is usually caused by a breathing problem. The energy levels of the electrical shock delivered by most AEDs are too high for children who are younger than 8 years or weigh less than 55 lb (25 kg); therefore, do not use an AED on children who fall into either of these categories. Teenagers, who may occasionally have a cardiac arrest related to a heart problem, may benefit from an AED.

AED machines come in models with different features (▼ **Figure 12-16**). All of them require a certain degree of operator interaction, beginning with applying the pads and turning the machine on. The operator also has to push a button to deliver an electrical shock, regardless of the model. Many AEDs use a computer voice synthesizer to advise the EMT which steps to take on the basis of the AED's analysis. Some have a button that tells the computer to analyze the heart's electrical rhythm; other models start doing this as soon as they are turned on. In the United States, the majority of the AEDs are semiautomated. Even though most defibrillators are now semiautomated, we are using the term *automated external defibrillators* (AED) as the general term to describe all of these machines. There are very few actual AED's left; all manufacturers are only producing semiautomated external defibrillators.

AEDs also come equipped to give a monophasic shock or a biphasic shock. Monophasic means to send the energy in one direction, from negative to positive and biphasic means to send the energy in two directions simultaneously. The advantage of biphasic shock is that it produces a more efficient defibrillation and may require a lower energy setting. The energy setting for ventricular fibrillation on a monophasic machine is generally 200 joules to start then moves to 200 or 300 joules, and then to 360 joules. With the biphasic technology the energy can be set at 120 joules for all three shocks and all subsequest shocks after that, or can

start at 120 joules and then escalate to 200 joules. The actual setting of the biphasic machines is still being studied and no recommendations for either is currently supported in the literature.

The computer inside the AED is specially programmed to recognize rhythms that require defibrillation to correct, most commonly ventricular fibrillation. The current programs are extremely accurate. It would be extremely rare for them to recommend a shock when a shock would not be called for, and they rarely fail to recommend one when it would be helpful. Therefore, if the AED recommends a shock, you can believe that it is indicated.

When an error does occur, it is usually the operator's fault. The most common error is not having a charged battery. To avoid this problem, many defibrillator companies have built smarter machines that will warn the operator that the battery is unlikely to work. However, some of the older models do not have this feature. You should check the AED daily and exercise the battery as often as the manufacturer recommends.

Another error occurs when the AED is applied to a patient who is moving. The computer may be unable to tell the difference between electrical signals from the heart and electrical signals from the arms and chest muscles that are moving. The way to avoid this error is to apply the AED only to pulseless, unresponsive patients and to stay clear of the patient (do not touch the patient) during analysis and shocking.

A third error can occur when the AED is applied to a responsive patient with a rapid heart rate. Most computers identify a regular rhythm faster than 150 or 180

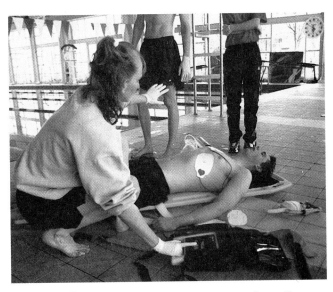

Figure 12-16   AEDs vary in their design, features, and operation.

You should check the AED daily and exercise the battery as often as the manufacturer recommends.

beats/min as ventricular tachycardia, which should be shocked. Sometimes, though, a patient has another heart rhythm that should not be shocked but that is fast enough to confuse the computer. Again, to avoid this problem, you should apply the AED only to unresponsive patients with no pulse.

Automated external defibrillation offers the EMT-B a number of advantages. First, of course, the machine is fast, and it delivers the most important treatment for the patient in ventricular fibrillation: an electrical shock. It can be delivered within 1 minute of the EMT's arrival at the patient's side. Second, you will find that using an AED is easier than performing CPR. ALS providers do not have to be on the scene to provide this definitive care.

Current AEDs offer two other advantages. The shock can be given through remote, adhesive defibrillator pads, which are safer for you than paddles. Also, the pad area is larger than paddles, which means that the transmission of electricity is more efficient. Usually, there are pictures on the pads to remind you where they go on the patient's chest.

Not all patients in cardiac arrest require an electrical shock. Although all patients in cardiac arrest should be analyzed with an AED, some do not have shockable

rhythms (eg, pulseless electrical activity and asystole). Asystole (flatline) indicates that no electrical activity remains. Pulseless electrical activity usually refers to a state of cardiac arrest despite an organized electrical complex. In both cases, CPR should be initiated as soon as possible.

Rationale for Early Defibrillation

Few patients who experience sudden cardiac arrest outside of a hospital survive unless a rapid sequence of events takes place. The chain of survival is a way of describing the ideal sequence of events that can take place when such an arrest occurs.

The four links in the chain of survival are as follows ▼ Figure 12-17 :

- Recognition of early warning signs and immediate activation of EMS

- Immediate bystander CPR

- Early defibrillation

- Early advanced cardiac life support.

If any one of the links in the chain is absent, the patient is more likely to die. For example, few patients benefit from defibrillation when more than 10 minutes elapse before administration of the first shock or if CPR is not performed in the first 2 to 3 minutes. If all links in the chain are strong, the patient has the best possible chance of survival. The link with the most determinant for survival is the third link—early defibrillation.

CPR helps patients in cardiac arrest because it prolongs the period of time during which defibrillation can be effective. Rapid defibrillation has successfully resuscitated many patients with cardiac arrest from ventricular fibrillation. However, defibrillation works

Early access   Early CPR   Early defibrillation   Early advanced care

Figure 12-17 The four links of the chain of survival.
Source: American Heart Association

best if it takes place within 2 minutes of the onset of the cardiac arrest. To try to achieve better survival rates among cardiac arrest victims, many communities are exploring the idea that nontraditional first responders should be trained to administer early defibrillation. These responders would include police officers, security personnel, lifeguards, maintenance workers, and flight attendants. As an EMT-B, you should support these efforts to shorten the time interval until defibrillation. Remember, seconds really do matter when the patient is in cardiac arrest.

Integrating the AED and CPR

Since most cardiac arrests occur in the home, a bystander at the scene may already have started CPR before you arrive. For this reason, you must know how to work the AED into the CPR sequence. Remember that the AED is not very complex; it may not be able to distinguish other movements from ventricular fibrillation. Therefore, do not touch the patient while the AED is analyzing the heart rhythm and delivering shocks. Stop CPR, and let the AED do its job. CPR may be stopped for up to 90 seconds if three shocks are necessary. This is entirely proper; defibrillation is more important than CPR when ventricular fibrillation is present.

Prepare with BSI precautions while you are en route to the scene. Upon arrival at the scene, make sure that the scene is safe for you and your partner to enter. Ask any bystanders or first responders who are performing CPR to stop so that you can apply the AED and defibrillate the patient. Take the following steps if allowed by your local protocols ▶ **Skill Drill 12-2** :

1. **Arrive on scene and perform your initial assessment.** Assess responsiveness. If the patient is responsive, do not apply the AED.

2. **Stop CPR** if it is in progress.

3. **Verify pulselessness and apnea.** Check for breathing and a pulse even if the patient appears to be breathing.

4. If the patient is unresponsive and not breathing or is breathing agonally (slow, gasping breaths), **give two ventilations** using a BVM device or a pocket mask **(Step 1)**.

5. **Have your partner start or resume CPR.**

6. If an AED is close at hand, **prepare the AED pads.**

7. **Turn on the machine (Step 2)**.

8. **Remove clothing from the patient's chest area.** Apply the pads to the chest: one just to the right of the breastbone (sternum) just below the collarbone (clavicle), the other on the left chest with the top of the pad 2″ to 3″ below the armpit. Ensure that the pads are attached to the patient cables (and that they are attached to the AED in some models).

9. **Stop CPR (Step 3)**.

10. **State aloud, "Clear the patient,"** and ensure that no one is touching the patient.

11. **Push the analyze button,** if there is one.

12. **Wait for the computer** in the AED to determine whether a shockable rhythm is present.

13. If a shock is not needed, go to step 18 (CPR only). If a shock is advised, make sure that no one is touching the patient. When the area is clear, **push the shock button.**

14. **After the shock is delivered,** most AEDs will automatically reanalyze the rhythm; if not, push the analyze button again.

15. **If the machine advises a shock, deliver a second shock.**

16. **Reanalyze the rhythm.**

17. **If the machine advises a shock, deliver a third shock (Step 4)**.

18. **Check for a pulse.**

19. **If the patient has a pulse,** check the patient's breathing **(Step 5)**.

20. **If the patient is breathing adequately,** give the patient oxygen via nonrebreathing mask and transport. If the patient is not breathing adequately, use necessary airway adjuncts and proper positioning of the head and jaw to ensure an open airway. Provide artificial ventilations with high-concentration oxygen and transport.

21. **If the patient has no pulse,** perform 1 minute of CPR.

22. **After 1 minute of CPR,** make sure no one is touching the patient. Push the analyze button again (as applicable).

23. **If necessary, repeat one cycle of up to three stacked shocks.**

24. **Transport and check with medical control.**

25. **Continue to support the patient** as needed: ventilate until the patient begins to breathe normally, and continue CPR if needed **(Step 6)**.

If, after any rhythm analysis, the AED advises no shock, check the patient's pulse. If the patient has a pulse, check the patient's breathing. If the patient is breathing adequately, give high-concentration oxygen via nonrebreathing mask and transport. If the patient is not breathing adequately, provide artificial ventilations with high-concentration oxygen via a BVM device and transport. Ensure that appropriate airway techniques are used at all times.

If the patient has no pulse, resume CPR for 1 minute, then have the AED reanalyze the heart rhythm. If the AED advises shock, deliver up to two sets of three stacked shocks. Separate each set of three shocks with 1 minute of CPR.

If the AED advises no shock and the patient has no pulse, resume CPR for 1 minute, then stop and reanalyze the heart rhythm for a third time. If the AED advises shock, deliver up to two sets of three stacked shocks with 1 minute of CPR between the two sets. If the AED still advises no shock, check with medical control, resume CPR, and transport.

If you are the only rescuer at the scene and you have an AED, take the following steps:

1. Perform an initial assessment. Assess responsiveness. If the patient is responsive, do not apply the AED.

2. Verify that the patient has no pulse and is not breathing (or is breathing with inadequate gasping breaths).

3. If the patient is not breathing or is gasping, give two slow breaths using a BVM device or pocket mask.

4. Expose the patient's chest. Apply one pad just to the right of the breastbone (sternum), just below the collarbone (clavicle), and the other on the left side of the chest with the top of the pad 2″ to 3″ below the armpit.

5. Turn on the AED.

6. Push the analyze button, if there is one.

7. Deliver up to three shocks, if indicated.

8. Follow your local protocol. If the AED indicates no need for shocks, provide CPR.

If another person is available who knows CPR, ask for help. You will perform the steps in the same order. The only difference is that the other person can continue CPR while you are getting the AED out and applied to the patient.

After AED Shocks

The care of the patient after the AED delivers its shock depends on your location and EMS system; therefore, you should follow your local protocols. After the AED protocol is completed, the patient is likely to have had one of the following occur:

• Regained a pulse

• No pulse, and the AED indicates that no shock is advised

• No pulse, and the AED indicates that a shock is advised

If you got to the patient quickly and the patient started breathing on his or her own, administer oxygen by nonrebreathing face mask with the oxygen flow set to 10 to 15 L/min. Check the patient's pulse. If the patient has a pulse but is not breathing adequately, assist ventilations, using a BVM device with high-flow oxygen. Prepare for transport, keeping the AED attached to the patient. Recheck the pulse frequently, at least every 30 seconds. In applicable devices, push the analyze button on the AED if the pulse is lost. Commonly, patients who are successfully defibrillated by AED will develop a normal heart rhythm for a while. However, since the heart still is not receiving optimal amounts of oxygen, ventricular fibrillation will often recur.

Patients who fail to regain a pulse on the scene of the cardiac arrest usually do not survive. What you do with these patients will, again, depend on your EMS system. Whether you should transport the patient or wait for ALS to arrive should be in the local protocols established by medical direction. If paramedics or another advanced life support service is responding to the scene, the best option usually is to stay where you are and continue the sequence of shocks and CPR. Administering CPR while patients are being moved or transported is usually not effective. Patients' best chance of survival is if they are

Skill Drill 12-2 AED and CPR

1

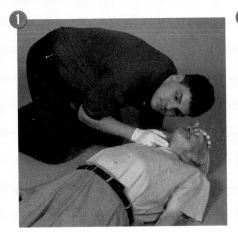

Stop CPR if in progress.
Assess responsiveness.
Check breathing and pulse.
If unresponsive and not breathing adequately,
give two slow ventilations.

2

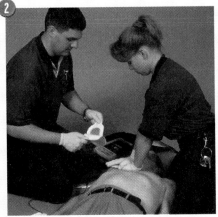

If pulseless, begin CPR.
Prepare the AED pads.
Turn on the AED; begin narrative if needed.

3

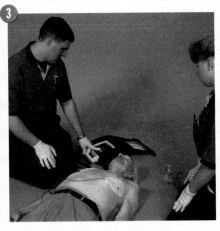

Apply AED pads.
Stop CPR.

4

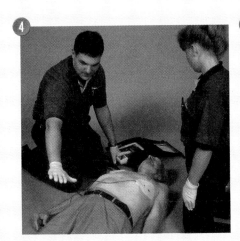

Verbally and visually clear the patient.
Push the Analyze button if there is one.
Wait for the AED to analyze rhythm.
If no shock advised, perform CPR for 1 min.
If shock advised, recheck that all are clear and
push the Shock button.
Push the Analyze button, if needed, to analyze
rhythm again.
Press Shock if advised (second shock).
Push the Analyze button, if needed, to analyze
rhythm again.
Press Shock if advised (third shock).

5

Check pulse.
If pulse is present, check breathing.

6

If breathing adequately, give oxygen and trans-
port. If not, open airway, ventilate, and trans-
port.
If no pulse, perform CPR for 1 minute.
Clear the patient and analyze again.
If necessary, repeat one cycle of up to three
shocks.
Transport and call medical control.
Continue to support breathing or perform CPR,
as needed.

EMT-B Tips

AED operational tips

- One EMT-B operates the defibrillator while another does CPR.
- Defibrillation comes first. Do not apply oxygen or do anything else that delays analysis of rhythm or defibrillation.
- Be familiar with the AED device used by your EMS system.
- Avoid all contact with the patient during analysis of the rhythm.
- State, "Clear the patient" before shocking. Another popular phrase is "I'm clear, you're clear, we're all clear" before delivering shocks.
- In applicable models of AEDs, check the batteries at the beginning of your shift; carry an extra charged battery with your AED.
- Do not use an AED for cardiac arrest in children younger than age 8 years or who weigh less than 55 lb (25 kg).
- Unless indicated otherwise by local protocol, you do not need to perform pulse checks during rhythm analysis; typically, there will be no pulse check between stacked shocks 1 and 2 and stacked shocks 2 and 3.
- Continued airway maintenance and artificial ventilation are of prime importance.

resuscitated where they are found, unless the location is unsafe.

If an advanced life support service is not responding to the scene and your local protocols agree, you should begin transport when one of the following occurs:

- The patient regains a pulse.
- Six to nine shocks are delivered.
- The machine gives three consecutive messages (separated by 1 minute of CPR) that no shock is advised.

If you transport a patient while performing CPR, you need a plan for managing the patient in the ambulance. Ideally, you will have two EMT-Bs in the patient compartment while a third drives. You may deliver additional shocks at the scene or en route with the approval of medical control. Keep in mind that AEDs cannot analyze rhythm while the vehicle is in motion. Nor is it as safe to defibrillate in a moving ambulance. Therefore, you should come to a complete stop if more shocks are needed. Be sure to memorize the protocol of your EMS service so that you will know how to manage patients in this situation (▶ Figure 12-18).

Cardiac Arrest During Transport

If you are traveling to the hospital with an unconscious patient, check the pulse at least every 30 seconds. If a pulse is not present, take the following steps:

1. Stop the vehicle.
2. If the AED is not immediately ready, perform CPR until it is available.
3. Analyze the rhythm.
4. Deliver shocks, if indicated.
5. Continue resuscitation according to your local protocol.

If you are en route with a conscious adult patient who is having chest pain and becomes unconscious, take the following steps:

1. Check for a pulse.
2. Stop the vehicle.
3. If the AED is not immediately ready, perform CPR until it is ready.
4. Analyze the rhythm.
5. Deliver up to three shocks, if indicated.
6. Continue resuscitation according to your local protocol. If a "no shock" message is given and no pulse is present, you should start CPR, then transport.

Coordination with ALS

The time to defibrillation is critical to survival after cardiac arrest. As an EMT-B equipped with an AED, you have the one tool that the dying patient in ventricular fibrillation needs most. Furthermore, it is very hard to hurt someone with an AED. Therefore, if you have an AED available, do not wait for the paramedics to arrive to administer a shock. Waiting might seem like a good idea. It is not. It is throwing away the patient's best chance for survival.

If the patient is unresponsive and does not have a pulse, apply the AED and push the analyze button (if there is one) as quickly as you can. Notify the ALS personnel as soon as possible after you recognize a cardiac arrest, but do not delay defibrillation. After the paramedics arrive at the scene, you should interact with them according to your local protocols.

Safety Considerations

As the operator of the AED, you are responsible for making sure that the electricity injures no one, including yourself. As long as you place the pads in the correct position and make sure no one is touching

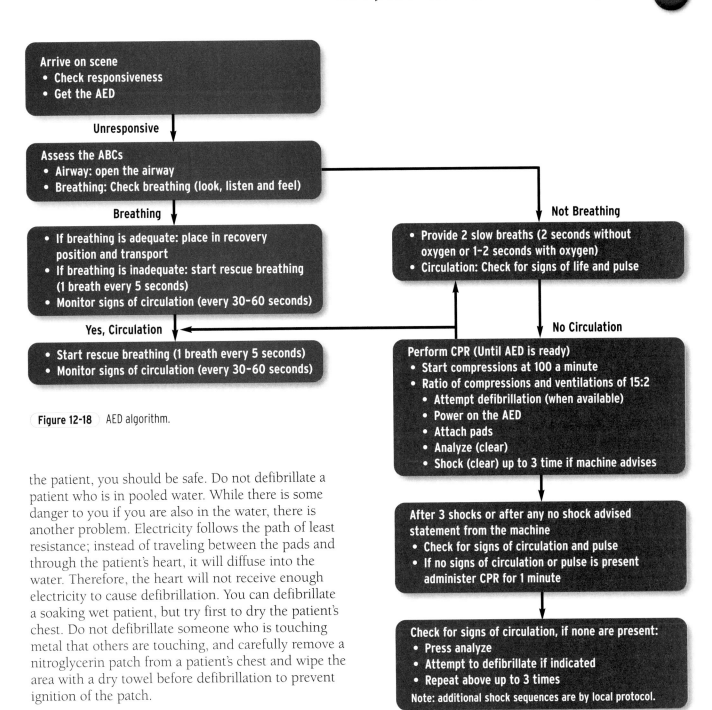

Figure 12-18 AED algorithm.

the patient, you should be safe. Do not defibrillate a patient who is in pooled water. While there is some danger to you if you are also in the water, there is another problem. Electricity follows the path of least resistance; instead of traveling between the pads and through the patient's heart, it will diffuse into the water. Therefore, the heart will not receive enough electricity to cause defibrillation. You can defibrillate a soaking wet patient, but try first to dry the patient's chest. Do not defibrillate someone who is touching metal that others are touching, and carefully remove a nitroglycerin patch from a patient's chest and wipe the area with a dry towel before defibrillation to prevent ignition of the patch.

AED Maintenance

One of your primary missions as an EMT-B is to deliver an electrical shock to a patient in ventricular fibrillation. To accomplish this mission, you need to have a functioning AED. You must become familiar with the maintenance procedures required for the brand of AED your service uses. Read the operator's manual. If your defibrillator does not work on the scene, someone will want to know what went wrong. That person may be your system's administrator, your medical director, the local newspaper reporter, or the

family's attorney. You will be asked to show proof that you maintained the defibrillator properly, and attended any mandatory in-services.

The main legal risk in using the AED is failing to deliver a shock when one was needed. The most common reason for this failure is that the battery did not work, usually because it was not properly maintained. Another problem is operator error. This means not pushing the analyze or shock buttons when the

AUTOMATED EXTERNAL DEFIBRILLATOR
Daily/Shift Inspection Checklist

Serial # _____ Date _____ Time _____

Model # _____ Inspected by _____

Item	Pass	Fail
Exterior/Cables:		
Nothing stored on top of unit		
Carry case intact and clean		
Exterior/LCD screen clean and undamaged		
Cables/connectors clean and undamaged		
Cables securely attached to unit		
Batteries:		
Unit charger is plugged in and operational (if applicable)		
Fully charged battery in unit		
Fully charged spare battery		
Spare battery charger plugged in and operational (if applicable)		
Valid expiration date on both batteries		
Supplies:		
Two sets of electrodes		
Electrodes in sealed packages with valid expiration dates		
Razor		
Hand towel		
Alcohol wipes		
Memory/voice recording device—module, card, microcassette		
Manual override—module, key (if applicable)		
Printer paper (if applicable)		
Operation:		
Unit self-test per manufacturer's recommendation/instructions		
Display (if applicable)		
Visual indicators		
Verbal prompts		
Printer (if applicable)		
Attach AED to simulator/tester:		
Recognizes shockable rhythm		
Charges to correct energy level within manufacturer's specifications		
Delivers charge		
Recognizes nonshockable rhythm		
Manual override system in working order (if applicable)		

Signature:

Figure 12-19 A sample daily checklist for the AED.

machine advises you to do so or failing to apply the AED to a patient in cardiac arrest. Of course, the AED is like any other manufactured item. It can fail, although this is rare. Ideally, you will encounter any such failure while doing routine maintenance, not while caring for a patient in cardiac arrest. Check your equipment, including your AED, at the beginning of each shift. Ask the manufacturer for a checklist (◀ **Figure 12-19**) of items that should be checked daily, weekly, or less often.

If you do have an AED failure while caring for a patient, you must report that problem to the manufacturer and the US Food and Drug Administration. Be sure to follow the appropriate EMS procedures for notifying these organizations.

Medical Direction

Defibrillation of the heart is a medical procedure. While AEDs have made the process of delivering electricity much simpler, there is still a benefit in having a physician's involvement. The medical director of your service should help to teach you how to use the AED. At the very least, he or she should approve the written protocol that you will follow in caring for patients in cardiac arrest. In most states, successful completion of AED training in an EMT-B course is not permitted without approval by state laws, rules, and local medical direction authority.

There should be a review of each incident in which the AED is used. After returning from the hospital or the scene, sit down with the rest of the team and go over what happened. This discussion will help all members of the team to learn from the incident. Review such events by using the written report, any voice-ECG tape recorder, and the device's solid-state memory modules and magnetic tape recordings, if applicable.

There should also be a review of the incident by your service's medical director or quality improvement officer. Quality improvement involves individuals using AEDs and the responsible EMS system managers. This review should focus on speed of defibrillation, that is, the time from call to shock. Few systems will achieve the ultimate goal: shocking 100% of patients within 1 minute of the call. However, all systems continuously work on improving patient care. Mandatory continuing education with skill competency review is generally required for EMS providers, with a continuing competency skill review every 3 to 6 months for the EMT-B.

Geriatric Needs

Like the other body systems, the cardiovascular system undergoes changes as we get older. The heart, like other major organs, will show the effects of aging. As the heart's muscle mass and tone decrease, the amount of blood pumped out of the heart per beat is decreased. The residual (reserve) capacity of the heart is also reduced; therefore, when the vital organs of the body need additional blood flow, the heart cannot meet the need. When blood flow to the tissues is decreased, the organs suffer. If blood flow to the brain is inadequate, the patient may complain of weakness, fatigue, or dizziness and may develop syncope (fainting).

The power to the heart muscle can fail. The heart runs on electricity and has its own electrical system. Under normal conditions, electrical impulses travel throughout the heart resulting in the contraction of the heart muscle and the pumping of blood from the heart's chambers. With aging, the electrical system can deteriorate, causing the heart's contraction to weaken or, if blood flow to the heart muscle is affected, extra beats to form. With a decreased strength of contraction, the heartbeat is weaker and blood flow to the tissues is reduced. If extra beats are produced, the patient's heart rhythm will be irregular. While some irregular heart rhythms are acceptable, others can be potentially lethal.

The arteries are also affected by aging. Arteriosclerosis (hardening of the arteries) can develop, affecting perfusion of the tissues. There is an increased chance of heart attack or stroke from decreased blood flow or plaque formation (atherosclerosis) in the narrowed arteries.

Patients with diabetes can experience reduced circulation to the hands and feet; this makes peripheral pulses harder to detect. It also puts the hands and feet at particular risk for developing infection or ulcerations.

In some older patients, particularly diabetics, chest pain is absent, and the clinical picture can be confused with other, noncardiac conditions.

The cardiovascular system is affected by aging. You should be aware of the changes, seeking to determine what is normal versus what is chronic for the patient as opposed to what is an acute condition. Sometimes, the weakening of the heart muscle, the deterioration of its electrical system, and the hardening of the arteries make the task of assessing and caring for the elderly patient more difficult.

Prep Kit

Ready for Review

The heart is divided down the middle into two sides, right and left, each with an upper chamber called the atrium and a lower chamber called the ventricle. The largest of the four heart valves that keep blood moving through the circulatory system in the proper direction is the aortic valve, which lies between the left ventricle and the aorta, the body's main artery. The heart's electrical system controls heart rate and helps to keep or maintain that the atria and ventricles work together.

During periods of exertion or stress, the myocardium requires more oxygen. This is supplied by dilation of the coronary arteries, which increases blood flow.

Common places to feel for a pulse include the carotid, femoral, brachial, radial, ulnar, posterior tibial, and dorsalis pedis arteries.

Low blood flow to the heart is usually caused by coronary artery atherosclerosis, a disease in which cholesterol plaques build up inside blood vessels, eventually occluding them. Occasionally, a brittle plaque will crack, causing a blood clot to form. Heart tissue downstream suffers from a lack of oxygen and, within 30 minutes, will begin to die. This is called an acute myocardial infarction (AMI), or heart attack. Heart tissues that are not getting enough oxygen but are not yet dying can cause pain called angina. The pain of AMI is different from the pain of angina in that it can come at any time, not just with exertion; it lasts up to several hours, rather than just a few moments; and it is not relieved by rest or nitroglycerin. In addition to crushing chest pain, signs of AMI include sudden onset of weakness, nausea, and sweating; sudden arrhythmia; pulmonary edema; and even sudden death.

Heart attacks can have three serious consequences. One is sudden death, usually the result of cardiac arrest caused by abnormal heart rhythms called arrhythmias. These include tachycardia, bradycardia, ventricular tachycardia, and, most commonly, ventricular fibrillation. The second consequence is cardiogenic shock. Symptoms include restlessness; anxiety; pale, clammy skin; pulse rate higher than normal; and blood pressure lower than normal. Patients with these symptoms should receive oxygen, assisted ventilations as needed, and immediate transport.

The third consequence of AMI is congestive heart failure, in which damaged heart muscle can no longer contract effectively enough to pump blood through the system. The lungs become congested with fluid, breathing becomes difficult, the heart rate increases, and the left ventricle enlarges. Signs include swollen ankles from pedal edema, high blood pressure, rapid heart rate and respirations, rales, and sometimes the pink sputum and dyspnea of pulmonary edema. Treat a patient with CHF as you would a patient with chest pain. Monitor the patient's heart rhythm, give the patient oxygen via nonrebreathing face mask, allow the patient to remain sitting up.

In treating patients with chest pain, obtain a SAMPLE history, following the OPQRST mnemonic to assess the pain; measure and record vital signs; put the patient in a comfortable position, usually sitting up; administer prescribed nitroglycerin and oxygen; and transport the patient, reporting to medical control as you do. If a patient is not responsive and is 8 years or older and weighs at least 55 lb, you must decide whether to use the automated external defibrillator (AED). If the patient weighs less than 55 lb, begin CPR.

The AED requires the operator to apply the pads, power on the unit, analyze the rhythm, and to press the shock button. The computer inside the AED recognizes rhythms that require shocking and will not mislead you. The three most common errors in using certain AEDs are failure to keep a charged battery in the machine, applying the AED to a patient who is moving, and applying the AED to a responsive patient with a rapid heart rate. Do not touch the patient while the AED is analyzing the heart rhythm or delivering shocks. In integrating use of the AED and CPR, you should perform CPR only after giving up to three shocks, if these are all needed. If you still cannot get a pulse, perform CPR for 1 minute. If advanced life support service is responding to the scene, stay where you are and continue the sequence of shocks and CPR. Do not wait for ALS to arrive to begin defibrillation. If ALS is not responding, begin transport after six shocks or after the machine gives three consecutive messages that no shock is advised. If an unconscious patient has a pulse but loses it during transport, you must stop the vehicle, start CPR if the defibrillator is not ready, then apply the AED.

The chain of survival, which is the sequence of events that must happen for a patient with cardiac arrest to have the best chance of survival, includes recognition of early warning signs and immediate activation of EMS, immediate CPR by bystanders, early defibrillation, and early advanced care. Seconds count at every stage.

www.emtb.com

Vital Vocabulary

acute myocardial infarction (AMI) Heart attack; death of heart muscle following obstruction of blood flow to it. Acute in this context means "new" or "happening right now."

angina pectoris Transient (short-lived) chest discomfort caused by partial or temporary blockage of blood flow to the heart muscle.

anterior The front surface of the body; the side facing you in the standard anatomic position.

aorta The main artery, which receives blood from the left ventricle and delivers it to all the other arteries that carry blood to the tissues of the body.

aortic valve The one-way valve that lies between the left ventricle and the aorta. It keeps blood from flowing back into the left ventricle after the left ventricle ejects its blood into the aorta. One of four heart valves.

arrhythmia An irregular or abnormal heart rhythm.

atherosclerosis A disorder in which cholesterol and calcium build up inside the walls of blood vessels, eventually leading to partial or complete blockage of blood flow.

asystole Complete absence of heart electrical activity.

atrium One of two (right and left) upper chambers of the heart. The right atrium receives blood from the vena cava and delivers it to the right ventricle. The left atrium receives blood from pulmonary veins and delivers it to the left ventricle.

bradycardia Slow heart rate, less than 60 beats/min.

cardiac arrest A state in which the heart fails to generate an effective and detectable blood flow; pulses are not palpable in cardiac arrest, even if muscular and electrical activity continues in the heart.

cardiogenic shock A state in which not enough oxygen is delivered to the tissues of the body, caused by low output of blood from the heart. It can be a severe complication of a large acute myocardial infarction, as well as other conditions.

congestive heart failure (CHF) A disorder in which the heart loses part of its ability to effectively pump blood, usually as a result of damage to the heart muscle and usually resulting in a backup of fluid into the lungs.

coronary artery A blood vessel that carries blood and nutrients to the heart muscle.

defibrillate To shock a fibrillating (chaotically beating) heart with specialized electrical current in an attempt to restore a normal rhythmic beat.

dilation Widening of a tubular structure such as a coronary artery.

fibrillation Completely disorganized, ineffective twitching of the heart muscle.

infarction Death of a body tissue, usually caused by interruption of its blood supply.

inferior The part of the body, or any body part, nearer to the feet.

ischemia A lack of oxygen that deprives tissues of necessary nutrients, resulting from partial or complete blockage of blood flow; potentially reversible since permanent injury has not yet occurred.

lumen The inside diameter of an artery or other hollow structure.

myocardium Heart muscle.

occlusion Blockage, usually of a tubular structure such as a blood vessel.

pedal edema Swelling of the feet and ankles caused by collection of fluid in the tissues; a possible sign of congestive heart failure (CHF).

perfusion The flow of blood through body tissues and vessels.

posterior The back surface of the body; the side away from you in the standard anatomical position.

superior The part of the body, or any body part, nearer to the head.

syncope Fainting spell or transient loss of consciousness.

tachycardia Rapid heart rhythm, more than 100 beats/min.

ventricle One of two (right and left) lower chambers of the heart. The left ventricle receives blood from the left atrium (upper chamber) and delivers blood to the aorta. The right ventricle receives blood from the right atrium and pumps it into the pulmonary artery.

ventricular fibrillation Disorganized, ineffective twitching of the ventricles, resulting in no blood flow and a state of cardiac arrest.

ventricular tachycardia Rapid heart rhythm in which the electrical impulse begins in the ventricle (instead of the atrium), which may result in inadequate blood flow and eventually deteriorate into cardiac arrest.

[Handwritten notes:]

SHOCKS

Cardiogenic — pump failure (mi)
Hypovolemic — volume (bleeding)
Anaphylactic — volume (hypotn)
Metabolic — respiratory
Psydogenic — Syncope (respiratory)
Septic
Respiratory
Neurogenic — spinal shock

Assessment in Action

You are dispatched to a private residence for a "man with chest pain." The patient's wife meets you at the door. As she leads you to the bedroom where her husband is lying in bed, she tells you that he has had indigestion for the last hour but about 15 minutes ago he started complaining of chest pain; that's when she called EMS.

As the wife begins introducing her husband, you note that he is very pale, his lips are gray, and sweat is beading up on his forehead. He is clutching his chest and looks at you with frightened eyes. His vital signs include a pulse of 110 beats/min and regular, shallow respirations of 20 breaths/min, and a blood pressure of 98/56 mm Hg. His skin is cold and clammy. He is alert and oriented with a history of gastric reflux disease, hypertension, and angina. He is on nitroglycerin for angina pectoris, Tinormen for hypertension, and Prilosec for gastric reflux. He has no allergies.

1. Chest pain that is cardiac in origin is usually caused by:
   A. too much oxygen to the lungs.
   B. insufficient oxygen to the heart.
   C. excess oxygen to the heart.
   D. trauma to the chest wall.

2. Which of the following signs or symptoms that this patient is exhibiting indicate a high suspicion for cardiac involvement? Chest pain, clutching his chest, and:
   A. pale, cold, clammy skin and blood pressure.
   B. pulse, blood pressure, and respiratory rate.
   C. history of indigestion and now chest pain.
   D. frightened look in his eyes and mental status.

3. The most likely reason this patient has ashen gray skin is because:
   A. his skin is normally that color.
   B. he has poor cardiac output.
   C. his blood pressure is abnormally high.
   D. he is getting ready to vomit.

4. Treatment should include high-flow oxygen and:
   A. lying him flat with his feet elevated.
   B. keeping him in an upright position.
   C. placing him in the recovery position.
   D. applying the AED.

5. This patient has his own nitroglycerin that is current. Your protocols will allow you to use nitro so your partner gets ready to administer it. Appropriate actions include:
   A. rechecking his blood pressure and assisting with administration.
   B. ensuring that his mouth is moist prior to administration.
   C. reminding your partner that his blood pressure is too low.
   D. listening to breath sounds and assisting with administration.

6. When you listen to breath sounds you hear crackles. This suggests that which of the following is present?
   A. Sudden death
   B. Spontaneous pneumothorax
   C. Pulmonary edema
   D. Pulmonary emboli

7. You notice that this patient's neck veins are becoming distended, his color is getting worse, and he is becoming confused. Vital signs are now: pulse 120 and irregular, respirations 28 and labored, blood pressure 90/64. What is happening?
   A. Congestive heart failure
   B. A cerebrovascular accident
   C. An unrelated pulmonary problem
   D. Cardiogenic shock

Challenging Questions

8. This patient cannot lie down. Why?

9. This patient is going into cardiac arrest. Why shouldn't the AED be applied?

10. Why should you encourage patients to lie down after they are given nitroglycerin?

Points to Ponder

You respond to a report of chest pain. The patient is on the third floor of an office building. You are the designated care provider on this call. When you walk into the office you immediately recognize the patient as a man who is inappropriately suing your father and asking for a large financial settlement. It has been an ugly case with very hard feelings on both sides of the lawsuit. The patient is in obvious respiratory distress and has significant chest pain. He immediately recognizes you but does not say anything. How would you deal with this situation? Do you need to document this interaction any differently? Should it be reported and, if so, to whom?

Issues Conflict of Interest, Best Patient Care, Reporting Non-medical Issues.

Online Outlook

In an average lifetime, the heart beats more than two and a half billion times, without ever pausing to rest. Like a pumping machine, the heart provides the power that is needed for life. To learn more about the heart and cardiovascular system, complete Exercise 12 at <u>www.emtb.com</u>.

Neurologic Emergencies

You are the EMT

"Rescue 1, respond to the driver's license station on 17th and Alder for a man who is acting strange." Altered mental status can be caused by a variety of medical and traumatic conditions. It may well be one of the most challenging conditions encountered by an EMT-B.

This chapter will lay the foundation of knowledge necessary for you to provide quality care for patients with neurologic dysfunction and will also help you answer the following questions:

1. Why is the brain so dependent on a continuous supply of oxygen?

2. What is the clinical significance of a patient having a TIA?

Neurologic Emergencies

S troke is the third most common cause of death in the United States, after heart disease and cancer. In the past few years, there has been a revolution in the treatment of stroke. For the most part, emergency treatment had not previously been available for patients with stroke, who typically faced years of painful rehabilitation or lifelong paralysis. Now, emergency physicians, neurologists, and neurosurgeons can help some patients with acute stroke to avoid the most devastating consequences of this disease, assuming that they get to the hospital in time.

Seizures and altered mental status also occur when there is a disorder in the brain. Seizures may occur as a result of a recent or old head injury, a brain tumor, a metabolic problem, or simply a genetic disposition. Your ability to recognize when a seizure has occurred or is occurring is critical for the patient, as it helps to direct appropriate treatment.

Altered mental status is a common presentation in patients with a wide variety of medical problems. Though it is tempting, you should not make assumptions about the cause of altered mental status. Causes range from alcohol intoxication to stroke. Obviously, treatment varies widely as well. Patients with altered mental status present a particular challenge in that they may be difficult to handle and frustrating to treat at times. Your professionalism is paramount in these situations.

The chapter opens with a description of the structure and function of the brain and what goes wrong in the most common causes of brain disorder, including stroke, seizure, and altered mental status. It then discusses the signs and symptoms of each condition. You will learn how to approach and assess a patient

with a brain disorder and why prompt transport to an appropriate medical facility is so important. The chapter then describes key assessment strategies for stroke, seizure, and altered mental status. Appropriate management of each is then discussed.

Brain Structure and Function

The brain is the body's computer. It controls breathing, speech, and all other body functions. All your thoughts, memories, wants, needs, and desires reside in the brain. Different parts of the brain perform different functions. For example, some receive input from the senses, including sight, hearing, taste, smell, and touch; others control the muscles and movement, while others control the formation of speech.

The brain is divided into three major parts: the brain stem, the cerebellum, and the largest part, the cerebrum ▶ Figure 13-1 . The brain stem controls the most basic functions of the body, such as breathing, blood pressure, swallowing, and pupil constriction. Just behind the brain stem, the cerebellum controls muscle and body coordination. It is responsible for coordinating complex tasks that involve many muscles, such as standing on one foot without falling, walking, writing, picking up a coin, or playing the piano.

The cerebrum, located above the cerebellum, is divided down the middle into the right and left cerebral hemispheres. Each hemisphere controls activities on the opposite side of the body and the same side of the face. The front part of the cerebrum controls emotion and thought, and the middle part controls touch and movement. The back part of the cerebrum processes sight. In most people, speech is controlled on the left side of the brain near the middle of the cerebrum.

Figure 13-1 The brain lies well protected within the skull. Its major parts are the cerebrum, the cerebellum, and the brain stem.

Parietal lobe
Temporal lobe
Occipital lobe
Cerebellum
Foramen magnum
Spinal cord
CEREBRUM
Frontal lobe
Brain stem

All the messages traveling to and from the brain travel along nerves. Twelve cranial nerves run directly from the brain to various parts of the head, such as the eyes, ears, nose, and face. All the rest of the nerves join in the spinal cord and exit the brain through a large hole in the base of the skull called the foramen magnum ▶ **Figure 13-2** . At each vertebra in the neck and back, two nerves, called spinal nerves, branch out from the spinal cord and carry signals to and from the body.

Common Causes of Brain Disorder

Stroke is a common cause of brain disorder that is potentially treatable. Other brain disorders include coma, infection, and tumor. Although these specific problems are not covered here, the seizures or altered mental status that often accompany them are discussed. The information in this section will help you better understand, communicate with, and care for patients who have experienced some type of brain disorder.

Stroke

A <u>cerebrovascular accident (CVA)</u> is an interruption of blood flow to the brain that results in the loss of brain function. <u>Stroke</u> is the loss of brain function that results from a CVA and occurs when part of the blood flow to the brain is suddenly cut off. Lacking oxygen, brain cells stop working and begin to die; these dead cells are called <u>infarcted cells</u>. Medical science currently has little to offer these cells once they are dead. However, it may take several hours or more for cell death to occur, even when it appears that severe disability will occur. Also, in some cases, a trickle of blood may still be getting through to the affected area of the brain. This blood may supply enough oxygen to keep alive a larger group of brain cells, called <u>ischemic cells</u>, but not enough to let the cells work properly and perform their given jobs. For example, if ischemic

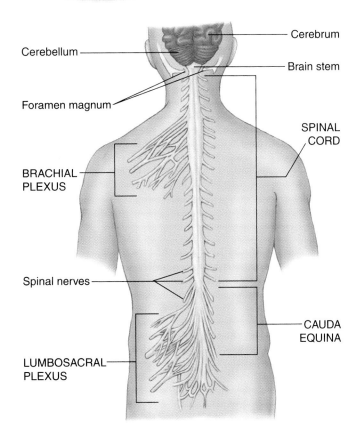

Cerebellum
Foramen magnum
BRACHIAL PLEXUS
Spinal nerves
LUMBOSACRAL PLEXUS
Cerebrum
Brain stem
SPINAL CORD
CAUDA EQUINA

Figure 13-2 The spinal cord is the continuation of the brain stem. It exits the skull at the foramen magnum and extends down to the level of the second lumbar vertebra.

cells are responsible for controlling the left arm, the patient will not be able to move that arm. If normal blood flow is restored to that area of the brain in time, the patient may regain use of the arm.

New therapies, such as "clot busters," have been shown to reverse symptoms and thus abort the stroke, if given within 2 to 3 hours. These therapies may not work for all patients, and they cannot be given to patients with bleeding-type (hemorrhagic) strokes. Nevertheless, until the potential for definitive treatment is ruled out at the hospital, you should proceed under the assumption that the area of the brain can still be saved. The sooner the treatment is begun, the better for the patient.

Interruption of cerebral blood flow may result from <u>thrombosis</u>, clotting of the cerebral arteries; <u>arterial rupture</u>, rupture of a cerebral artery; or <u>cerebral embolism</u>, obstruction of a cerebral artery caused by a clot that was formed elsewhere and traveled to the brain.

There are two main types of stroke: hemorrhagic (usually from arterial rupture) and ischemic (from embolism or thrombosis). Their symptoms are the same, although the events taking place inside the brain are different.

HEMORRHAGIC STROKE. A <u>hemorrhagic stroke</u> occurs as a result of bleeding inside the brain. The free blood then forms a clot, which squeezes the brain tissue next to it. When that tissue is compressed, oxygenated blood cannot get into the area, and the surrounding cells begin to die.

Certain types of patients are at higher risk of hemorrhagic stroke. The patients who are at highest risk are those who have very high or long-term elevated blood pressure that is not treated. After many years of high pressure, the blood vessels in the brain weaken. Eventually, one of the vessels may rupture, and blood will spurt out of the hole and into the brain, increasing the pressure inside the cranium. Proper treatment of high blood pressure can help to prevent this long-term damage to the blood vessels.

Some individuals may have been born with weaknesses, called *aneurysms*, in the walls of the arteries. An aneurysm is a swelling or enlargement of part of an artery, resulting from weakening of the arterial wall. Many of these individuals have a sudden onset of a "bad headache." When a hemorrhagic stroke occurs in an otherwise healthy young person, the likely cause is often a weakness in a blood vessel called a *berry aneurysm*. This type of aneurysm resembles a tiny balloon (or berry) that juts out from the artery. When the aneurysm is overstretched and ruptures, blood spurts into an area around the coverings of the brain called the subarachnoid space. Therefore, these types of strokes are called subarachnoid hemorrhages. Again, patients with this type of stroke experience a sudden severe headache, typically described as the worst headache they have ever had. If the patient seeks medical attention immediately, surgeons may be able to repair the aneurysm.

ISCHEMIC STROKE. When blood flow to a particular part of the brain is cut off by a blockage inside a blood vessel,

the result is an <u>ischemic stroke</u>. This can be from a thrombosis or an embolism that blocks blood flow. As with coronary artery disease, atherosclerosis in the blood vessels is usually the cause. <u>Atherosclerosis</u> is a disorder in which calcium and cholesterol build up, forming a plaque inside the walls of blood vessels. This plaque obstructs blood flow, interfering with the vessel's ability to dilate. Eventually, atherosclerosis can cause complete occlusion (blockage) of an artery (▼ **Figure 13-3**). In other cases, an atherosclerotic plaque in the carotid artery in the neck will rupture. A blood clot will form over the crack in the plaque, sometimes growing big enough to completely block all blood flow through that artery. Deprived of oxygen, parts of the brain supplied by the artery will stop working. Patients with such ischemic strokes will have dramatic symptoms, including loss of movement on the opposite side of the body.

Even if the blockage in the carotid artery is not complete, smaller pieces of the clot may embolize (break off and be carried by the blood flow) deep into the brain. There, a piece of clot will lodge in a branch blood vessel. This cerebral embolism then blocks blood flow (▶ **Figure 13-4**). Depending on the location of the lodged clot, the patient may experience anything from no

Clot

Figure 13-3) Atherosclerosis can damage the wall of a cerebral artery, producing narrowing and a clot. When the vessel is narrowed or completely blocked, blood flow to that part of the brain may be blocked, and the cells begin to die.

symptoms at all to being completely paralyzed and unable to move one side of the body.

TRANSIENT ISCHEMIC ATTACK. In some patients, normal processes in the body will break up a blood clot in the brain. When that happens quickly, blood flow is restored to the affected area, and the patient will regain use of the affected body part. When stroke symptoms go away on their own in less than 24 hours, the event is called a **transient ischemic attack (TIA)**. Some patients call these mini-strokes.

Although most patients with TIAs do well, every TIA is an emergency. It may be a warning sign that a larger, permanent stroke is about to occur. For this reason, all patients with a new TIA should be evaluated by a physician to determine whether preventive action can be taken.

Seizures

A **seizure**, or convulsion, is typically characterized by unconsciousness and a generalized severe twitching of all of the body's muscles that lasts several minutes or longer. This type of seizure is often called a **generalized seizure** or *grand mal seizure*. In other cases, the seizure may simply be characterized by a brief lapse

of attention in which the patient seems to just stare and does not seem to respond to anyone. This type of seizure, called an **absence** (ob-sáhnz) **seizure** or *petit mal seizure*, typically occurs in young children.

CHARACTERISTICS OF SEIZURES. Some seizures occur on only one side of the body. Others begin on one side and gradually progress to a generalized seizure that affects the entire body. Most individuals with lifelong or chronic seizures tolerate these events reasonably well without complications, but in some situations, seizures may signal life-threatening conditions.

Most seizures last 3 to 5 minutes and are followed by a lengthy period (5 to 30 minutes or more) of what is called a **postictal state**, in which the patient remains unconscious and unresponsive. Gradually, in most cases, the patient will begin to recover and awaken. In contrast, a petit mal seizure can last for just a fraction of minute, after which the patient fully recovers immediately with only a brief lapse of memory of the event.

Seizures that recur every few minutes are referred to as **status epilepticus**, also known as status seizures. For obvious reasons, recurring seizures should be considered potentially life-threatening situations in which patients need immediate emergency medical care.

CAUSES OF SEIZURES. Some seizure disorders, such as epilepsy, are congenital, which means that the patient was born with the condition. Other types of seizures may be due to high fevers, structural problems in the brain, or metabolic or chemical problems in the body (▶ **Table 13-1**). Epileptic seizures can usually be controlled with medications such as phenytoin (Dilantin), phenobarbital, or carbamazepine (Tegretol). Patients with epilepsy will often have seizures if they stop taking their medications or if they do not take an adequate dose.

Seizures may also be caused by an area of abnormality in the brain, such as a benign or cancerous tumor, an infection (brain abscess), or a scar from some type of injury. These seizures are said to have a *structural* cause; in other cases, the seizures are *metabolic*. Seizures from a metabolic cause can be caused by abnormal levels of certain blood chemicals (eg, extremely low sodium levels), hypoglycemia (low blood glucose levels), poisons, drug overdoses, or sudden withdrawal from routine and heavy alcohol or sedative drug usage or even from prescribed medications. Dilantin, a drug that is used to control seizures, can cause seizures itself if the person takes too much.

Seizures can also result from sudden high fevers, particularly in children. Such convulsions, known as **febrile seizures**, are usually very unnerving for parents

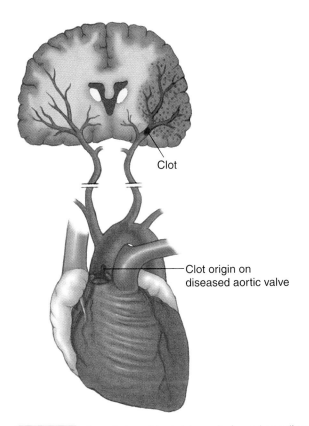

Figure 13-4 An embolus, a blood clot usually formed on a diseased heart valve, can travel through the body's vascular system, lodge in a cerebral artery, and cause a stroke.

TABLE 13-1 Common Causes of Seizures

Type	Cause
Epileptic	Congenital in origin
Structural	Tumor (benign or cancerous)
	Infection (brain abscess)
	Scar from injury
Metabolic	Abnormal blood chemistry
	Hypoglycemia
	Poisoning
	Drug overdose
	Sudden withdrawal from alcohol, medications
Febrile	Sudden high fever

EMT-B Safety

Be on the lookout for patients who may behave violently during the postictal phase. Though most seizure patients pose no threat to EMS responders, signs of alcohol or drug abuse should heighten your awareness of the potential for dangerous behavior.

Documentation Tips

Physician evaluation of a patient who has had a seizure depends heavily on reports of the seizure pattern and changes in that pattern. Record all pertinent information about the seizure in terms of duration, areas of body movement, and possible triggering factors. This requires effective interviewing of available witnesses, family members, or caregivers.

to observe but are generally well tolerated by the child. Nevertheless, you must transport a child who has had a febrile seizure, as this condition needs to be evaluated in the hospital. The fact that a second seizure may occur is very worrisome, and if it occurs, the patient requires rapid hospital evaluation to identify possible causes, such as serious infection within the brain or tissues covering the brain.

THE IMPORTANCE OF RECOGNIZING SEIZURES. Regardless of the type of seizure, it is extremely important for you to recognize when a seizure is occurring or whether one has already occurred. You must also determine whether this episode differs from any previous ones. For example, if the previous seizure occurred on only one side of the body and this seizure occurs over the entire body, some additional or new problem may be involved. In addition to recognizing that seizure activity has occurred and/or that something different may now be occurring, you must also recognize the postictal state as well as the complications of seizures.

Because most seizures involve a vigorous twitching of the muscles, they use a lot of oxygen. This excessive demand consumes oxygen that was being delivered by the circulation to the vital functions of the body. It is similar to a situation in which you exercise vigorously without giving your body a chance to rest. As a result, there is a buildup of acids in the bloodstream, and the patient may turn cyanotic (bluish lips, tongue, and skin) from the lack of oxygen. Often, the seizures themselves

prevent the patient from breathing normally, making the problem worse.

Recognizing seizure activity also means looking at other problems associated with the seizure. For example, the patient may have fallen during the seizure episode and injured some part of the body; head injury is the most serious possibility. Patients having a generalized seizure may become **incontinent**, meaning that they may lose bowel and bladder control. Therefore, one clue that unresponsive or confused patients may have had a seizure is to find that they urinated into their clothing. Although incontinence is possible with other medical conditions, sudden incontinence is very likely a sign that a seizure has occurred.

THE POSTICTAL STATE. Once a seizure has stopped, the patient's muscles relax, becoming almost flaccid, or floppy, and the breathing becomes labored (fast and deep) in an attempt to compensate for the buildup of acids in the bloodstream. By breathing faster and more deeply, the body can balance the acidity in the bloodstream. With a normal circulation and liver function, the acids clear away within minutes, and the patient will begin to breathe more normally. Intuitively, the longer and harder the convulsions are, the longer it will take for this imbalance to correct itself. Likewise, longer and more severe seizures will result in longer postictal unresponsiveness and confusion.

In some situations, the postictal state may be characterized by **hemiparesis**, or weakness on one side of the

> Besides recognizing that a seizure has occurred, it is important to learn whether the pattern has changed. Was this seizure different from previous ones?

body, resembling a stroke. Unlike the typical stroke, hypoxic hemiparesis soon resolves itself. Most commonly, the postictal state is characterized by lethargy and confusion to the point that the patient may be combative and appear angry. You must be prepared for these circumstances, both in your approach to scene control and in your treatment of the patient's symptoms. If the patient's condition does not improve, you should consider other possible underlying problems, including hypoglycemia or infection.

Altered Mental Status

Aside from stroke and seizures, the most common type of neurologic emergency that you will encounter is altered mental status. Simply put, altered mental status means that the patient is not thinking clearly or is incapable of being aroused. In some instances, patients will be unconscious (▼ **Figure 13-5**); in others, they may be alert but confused. The range of problems is wide, and the causes are many, including common problems such as **hypoglycemia** (low blood glucose levels), hypoxemia, intoxication, drug overdose, unrecognized head injury, brain infection, body temperature abnormalities, and uncommon conditions such as brain tumors, glandular abnormalities, and overdoses/poisonings.

HYPOGLYCEMIA. The clinical picture of patients with altered mental status due to hypoglycemia is very complex. Patients can have signs and symptoms that mimic stroke and seizures. Because both oxygen and glucose are needed for brain function, hypoglycemia can mimic conditions in the brain such as those associated with stroke. In these instances, the patient may have hemiparesis, similar to what occurs as a result of a stroke. The principal difference, however, is that a patient who has had a stroke may be alert and attempting to communicate normally, whereas a patient with hypoglycemia almost always has an altered or decreased level of consciousness (▼ **Figure 13-6**).

Patients with hypoglycemia commonly, but not always, take medications that lower blood glucose levels. Thus, if the patient appears to have signs and symptoms of stroke and an altered mental status, you should report your findings to medical control and treat the patient accordingly. Check for and report medications, but remember that not all patients who have diabetes take insulin or other medications to lower their blood glucose levels. Remember, also, that patients with a decreased level of consciousness should not be given anything by mouth. Again, local protocols should guide your actions.

Patients with hypoglycemia can also experience seizures, and you may arrive at the scene to find a patient in a postictal state: confused and disoriented or unresponsive. The mental status of a patient who has had a typical seizure is likely to improve; however, in a patient with hypoglycemia, the mental status is not likely to improve, even after several minutes. Therefore, you should consider the possibility of hypoglycemia in a patient who has had a seizure, especially if the blood glucose tested below normal.

Figure 13-5 A patient with altered mental status can be unconscious in some instances; in others, the patient may be alert but confused.

Figure 13-6 During your assessment of a patient with an altered or decreased level of consciousness, consider the possibility of hypoglycemia.

Likewise, you should consider hypoglycemia in a patient who has altered mental status after an injury such as a motor vehicle crash, even when there is the possibility of an accompanying head injury. As with any other patient, you should look for medical identification bracelets or medications that might confirm your suspicions.

OTHER CAUSES OF ALTERED MENTAL STATUS. Altered mental status can occur as a result of hypoglycemia, but there are many other possibilities as well, including unrecognized head injury or severe alcohol intoxication. Your consideration of other possibilities becomes important because a patient with altered mental status may be combative and refuse treatment and transport. You should be prepared for difficult patient encounters and follow local protocols for dealing with these situations, recognizing the potential for serious underlying problems.

In most cases, a patient who appears intoxicated most likely is just that; however, you must consider other problems as well. Individuals with chronic alcoholism can have abnormalities in liver function and in their blood-clotting and immune systems, which can predispose them to intracranial bleeding, brain and bloodstream infections, and hypoglycemia.

Psychological problems and complications from medications are also possible causes of altered mental status. A person who appears to have a psychological problem may also have an underlying medical condition.

Infections are another possible cause, particularly those involving the brain or bloodstream. Infections in these areas are obviously life threatening and need immediate attention. Patients may not demonstrate typical signs of infection, such as fever, particularly if they are very young or very old or have impaired immune systems.

Altered mental status can also be caused by drug overdose or poisonings; therefore, you should monitor patients closely for accompanying cardiac and breathing problems.

Thus, the presentation of altered mental status varies widely from simple confusion to coma. No matter what the cause, you should consider altered mental status to be an emergency that requires immediate attention even when it appears that the culprit may simply be alcohol intoxication or a minor car crash or fall.

Signs and Symptoms of Brain Disorder

Many different disorders can cause brain or other neurologic symptoms, which can affect level of consciousness, speech, and voluntary muscle control. As a general rule, if the brain problem is caused primarily by disorders in the heart and lungs, the entire brain will be affected. For example, without any blood flow (cardiac arrest), the patient will go into a coma and can have permanent brain damage within minutes, even if CPR is performed immediately. However, if the primary problem is in the brain, such as a poor blood supply to the middle part of the left cerebral hemisphere, the patient may not be able to move some parts of the right side of the body. This might be the right arm, the right leg, or the facial muscles. Low oxygen levels in the bloodstream, due to lung disease, for example, will affect the entire brain, causing anxiety, restlessness, and confusion.

Stroke

LEFT HEMISPHERE PROBLEMS. If the left cerebral hemisphere has been affected, the patient may have a speech disorder called **aphasia**, an inability to produce or understand speech. Speech problems can vary widely. Patients may have trouble understanding speech but can speak clearly. This condition is called receptive aphasia. You can detect this problem by asking the patient a question such as "What day is today?" In response, the patient with aphasia may say, "Green." The speech is clear, but it does not make sense. Other patients will be able to understand the question but cannot produce the right sounds in order to answer. Only grunts or other incomprehensible sounds emerge. These patients have expressive aphasia.

RIGHT HEMISPHERE PROBLEMS. If the right cerebral hemisphere of the brain is not getting enough blood, patients will have trouble moving the muscles on the left side of the body. Usually, they will understand language and be able to speak, but their words may be slurred and hard to understand. This problem is called **dysarthria**.

Interestingly, patients with right hemisphere strokes may be completely oblivious to their problem. If you ask these patients to lift their left arm and they cannot, they will lift their right arm instead. They seem to have forgotten that the left arm even exists. This symptom is called neglect. Patients with a problem affecting the back part of the cerebrum may neglect certain parts of their vision. Generally, this is hard to detect in the field, but you should be aware of the possibility. Try to sit or stand on the patient's good side, since he or she may be unable to see things on the "bad" side.

The problem of neglect causes many patients who have had large strokes to delay seeking help. Strokes are not painful. Therefore, a patient may be unaware that there is a problem until a family member or friend points out that some part of the patient's body is not working correctly.

BLEEDING IN THE BRAIN. Patients who have bleeding in their brain may have very high blood pressure. Sometimes, this is the cause of the bleeding, but many times it is a response to the bleeding: The brain is raising the blood pressure in an attempt to force more oxygen into its injured parts. High blood pressure in stroke patients should not be treated in the field. Quite often, blood pressure will return to normal or may drop significantly on its own.

Other Conditions

The following three conditions may simulate stroke:

- Hypoglycemia
- A postictal state
- Subdural or epidural bleeding (a blood clot near the skull that presses on the brain)

Because both oxygen and glucose are needed for brain metabolism, a patient with hypoglycemia may look like a patient who is having a stroke. You should find out whether the patient has diabetes and takes insulin or a glucose-lowering medication.

A patient in the postictal state may look like a patient who is having a stroke. However, in most cases, a patient having a seizure will recover rapidly, within the next few minutes.

Subdural and epidural bleeding usually occur as a result of trauma. The dura is a leathery covering over the brain, next to the skull. A fracture near the temples may cause an artery to bleed on top of the dura and the resulting clot presses on the brain (▼ **Figure 13-7A**). Onset of this *epidural* bleeding is usually very rapid after injury. In other cases, the veins just below the dura may be torn and bleed, a *subdural* bleed (▼ **Figure 13-7B**).

Onset occurs more slowly, sometimes over a period of several days.

The onset of stroke-like signs and symptoms may be subtle; the original injury may not even be remembered.

Assessing the Patient

Stroke

When you are called to assist a patient with a possible stroke, you should first determine whether the patient is responsive and breathing. Friends and family members may think that the patient has had a stroke when he or she has really had a cardiac arrest.

INITIAL ASSESSMENT. Upon arrival, you should check and care for immediate problems with the patient's ABC. If the patient is responsive and breathing, obtain a history. Also try to speak with relatives or friends who may have seen what happened (▼ **Figure 13-8**). Make a special effort to determine when the patient last appeared to be normal. This will tell physicians in the emergency department whether it is safe to begin certain treatments that must be given in the first hours after onset. Since you may be the only person on the emergency medical team with the opportunity to speak with bystanders, you may be the only one who can make this critical determination. Many times, you will be able to find out only that the patient was normal when he or she went to sleep the night before. Note that in such cases, the time the patient was last seen to be normal was at bedtime, not when the patient awoke with symptoms. Collect or list all medications the patient has taken.

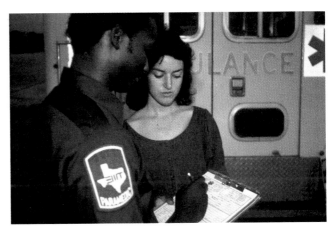

Figure 13-8 Try to speak with family members or bystanders who may have seen what happened. They may also be able to tell you when the patient last appeared "normal."

Figure 13-7 Trauma to the head can result in intracranial bleeding.
A. Bleeding outside the dura and under the skull is epidural.
B. Bleeding beneath the dura but outside the brain is subdural.

Figure 13-9 Make a special effort to establish communication with a patient who may have had a stroke. Look for indications that the patient understands you, such as a glance, gaze, squeeze of the hand, efforts to speak, or nodding of the head.

Although a stroke patient may appear to be unconscious and unable to speak, the patient may still be able to hear and understand what is taking place. Be careful what you say, avoiding all unnecessary or inappropriate remarks. Try to communicate with the patient by looking for indications that the patient can understand you, such as a glance, gaze, motion or pressure of the hand, efforts to speak, or nodding the head. Establishing effective communication can help you to calm the patient and lessen the fear that accompanies an inability to communicate ▲ Figure 13-9.

As you perform the initial assessment, administer supplemental oxygen. Then begin your focused assessment, including vital signs. If necessary, provide assisted ventilation, protect the airway, and suction to prevent aspiration. Remember to check for any history of diabetes, seizure, or recent head injury.

FOCUSED HISTORY AND PHYSICAL EXAM. As soon as possible, perform a neurologic exam as part of your focused physical exam. You should perform at least three key physical tests on patients you suspect of having had a stroke: tests of speech, facial movement, and arm movement. If any one of the three is positive (abnormal), the patient may be having a stroke.

The EMT should utilize the Cincinnati Stroke Scale, which tests speech, facial droop, and arm drift. The entire examination is identified in ▼ Table 13-2.

To test speech, simply ask the patient to repeat a simple phrase such as "The sky is blue in Cincinnati." If the patient does this correctly, you know that he or she both understands and can produce speech. If the patient

TABLE 13-2 Cincinnati Stroke Scale

Test	Normal	Abnormal
Facial Droop (Ask patient to show teeth or smile.)	Both sides of face move equally well.	One side of face does not move as well as the other.
Arm Drift (Ask patient to close eyes and hold both arms out with palms up.)	Both arms move the same, or both arms do not move.	One arm does not move, or one arm drifts down compared with the other side.
Speech (Ask patient to say, "The sky is blue in Cincinnati.")	Patient uses correct words with no slurring.	Patient slurs words, uses inappropriate words, or is unable to speak.

cannot repeat the phrase, the problem may be with either function: understanding speech or producing it.

To test facial movement, ask the patient to show his or her teeth (or gums, if there are no teeth). Watch to see that both sides of the face around the mouth move equally. If only one side is moving well, then you know that something is wrong with the control of the muscles on the other side.

To test arm movement, ask the patient to hold both arms in front of his or her body, palms up toward the sky, with eyes closed and without moving. Over the next 10 seconds, watch the patient's hands. If you see one side drift down toward the ground, then you know that side is weak. If both arms stay up and do not move, then you know that both sides of the brain are working.

If both arms fall to the ground, you have not really learned anything. Perhaps the patient did not understand your instructions. Try the arm test again, but this time move the patient's arms into position yourself. Another possibility to consider is that the patient is having a problem other than stroke. This is likely to be the answer if both sides of the brain are working improperly.

All patients who are victims of a possible stroke should also have a Glasgow Coma Scale performed, which can be seen in ▼ Table 13-3 .

TRANSPORT CONSIDERATIONS. After you have performed the neurologic exam, prepare the patient for transport. You want to spend as little time on the scene as possible. Remember, stroke is an emergency. There may be

Figure 13-10 A patient who has had a stroke should be positioned with the paralyzed side down and well protected with padding. Elevate the head about 6".

treatment available for the patient at the hospital. Place the patient in a comfortable position, usually on one side, with the paralyzed side down and well protected with padding (▲ **Figure 13-10**). The patient's head should be elevated about 6". Continue giving oxygen while en route.

After you begin transport, you should relay the information you have learned to the receiving hospital. Be sure to include the time that the patient was last seen to be normal, the findings of your neurologic examination, and the time you anticipate arriving at the hospital. This information will help the emergency department.

TABLE 13-3 Glasgow Coma Scale

Eye Opening		Best Verbal Response		Best Motor Response	
Spontaneous	4	Oriented conversation	5	Obeys commands	6
In response to speech	3	Confused conversation	4	Localizes pain	5
In response to pain	2	Inappropriate words	3	Withdraws to pain	4
None	1	Incomprehensible sounds	2	Abnormal flexion	3
		None	1	Abnormal extension	2
				None	1

Score: 14-15 Mild dysfunction
Score: 11-13 Moderate to severe dysfunction
Score: 10 or less is severe dysfunction

Figure 13-11   A patient who has had a seizure may be found in the postictal state when you arrive. If this is the case, be sure to ask family members or bystanders to verify that a seizure has occurred and how the seizure developed.

Seizures

You are typically called to care for a patient who has had a seizure because someone actually witnessed the seizure. However, you may also be called to see an unresponsive patient when the patient is found in a postictal state (▲ **Figure 13-11**). In other situations, you may be called to care for a patient who is having seizures and find that the patient actually has some other medical problem, such as cardiac arrest or some psychological problem. Therefore, thorough assessment is key because the information gathered at the scene may be extremely important to the hospital staff who must soon care for the patient.

In most instances, you will arrive sometime after the seizure has occurred, as it only lasts a few minutes. By the time someone recognizes the problem, calls for help, and receives a response, the patient is usually in a postictal state. Thus, you must gather as much information from family or bystanders as possible to verify that a seizure has occurred and to obtain a description of the way the seizure developed.

INITIAL ASSESSMENT. As with any other situation, you should focus on the ABCs upon arrival. The patient may have been eating or chewing gum at the time of the seizure, and so there may be a foreign body obstruction. Bystanders may have tried to put objects in a patient's mouth "to help them breathe better," even though this practice is ill advised. Breathing and circulation should be confirmed as normal or treated as necessary. Again, in the immediate postictal state following

Geriatric Needs

Over time, the brain will gradually deteriorate and shrink as a part of the normal aging process. This can increase the risk of head injury from minor forces, since the brain can bounce off the inside of the skull. A reduced brain mass can also reduce the patient's mental status and capacity. A smaller brain can impair memory function, and with lapses in short-term memory, the geriatric patient can ask the same or similar questions repeatedly.

When you are called to care for an elderly patient with an altered mental status, consider the possibility of a stroke or transient ischemic attack (TIA). At the scene of a motor vehicle crash involving an elderly driver, consider a stroke or TIA as the precipitating factor in the crash. Be alert for an altered mental state or unusual pupil responses in low light (ie, constricted or unequal pupils in dim light).

Beware of headache. Although elderly patients do get tension headaches, they are far less common in the elderly population. You should consider any headache as potentially serious.

As with the general population, the elderly can also sustain seizures. Remember that seizures are not necessarily due to epilepsy. You should consider and assess for the possibility of a drug overdose, stroke, head injury, or central nervous system infection. Status epilepticus in an elderly patient can have harmful effects such as hypoxia, irregular heart rhythm, hypotension, elevated body temperatures, low blood glucose levels, and, if the patient vomits, aspiration.

Remember that the elderly patient is at higher risk for central nervous system illnesses and injuries, including brain injury, TIA, stroke, and seizures. Do not be surprised to find a serious head injury from what you might consider a simple bump on the head.

a major seizure, you should anticipate rapid, deep respirations and an accompanying fast heart rate due to the stress of the severe convulsions. However, both respirations and heart rate should begin to slow to normal rates after several minutes. If not, you might suspect problems beyond the seizure alone.

FOCUSED HISTORY AND PHYSICAL EXAM. You should obtain a SAMPLE history, including whether the patient has a history of seizures. If so, it is important to find out how the patient's seizures typically occur and whether this episode differs in some way from previous episodes. You should also ask what medications the patient has been taking. If the patient takes Dilantin and phenobarbital, he or she most likely has chronic problems. You might find that the patient ran out of medication or stopped taking medication for a while.

If the patient has no history of convulsions and now has a sudden focal (not generalized) seizure, a serious condition, such as brain tumor, intracranial bleeding, or serious infection should be suspected. Assessment is also the time to determine whether the patient takes medications that lower blood glucose, such as insulin or oral hypoglycemic agents. In other situations, you may want to inquire about drug use or exposure to poisons.

As you document the physical signs of seizure, observe for recurrent seizures. If they occur, note whether the seizure starts at a focal part of the body (eg, one arm or one leg) and then progresses to the rest of the body. Most important, evaluate the patient's mental status and monitor it every several minutes to verify progressive improvement. The patient should be checked for injuries, including head lacerations, shoulder dislocations, bitten tongue, and occasional extremity fractures. Also assess for weakness or loss of sensation on one side of the body, and reassess for improvement in such findings.

Altered Mental Status

Although the presentation of altered mental status is relatively straightforward, you should attempt to categorize the severity of the problem and look for accompanying or underlying conditions as you assess the patient. Use the AVPU scale to assess responsiveness.

During your assessment, you should also consider other underlying medical conditions; the most impor-

tant are those that are easily reversible. Therefore, you should consider hypoxemia and hypoglycemia as possible causes. Continually reassess these patients closely for depressed respirations; assist ventilations if needed. Likewise, a patient with a decreased level of consciousness may not be able to protect the airway. Therefore, you should make sure that basic airway maneuvers are followed and suctioning is available (▼ Figure 13-12). Prompt transport is necessary, with close monitoring of vital signs en route.

Coordination with ALS

If paramedics are available, you should request their assistance if the patient is unresponsive or has any signs of airway compromise, particularly if the patient has a history of diabetes.

Emergency Medical Care

Stroke

In most patients with suspected stroke, physicians in the emergency department need to determine whether there is bleeding in the brain. If there is no bleeding, the patient may be a candidate for medication to help break up the blood clot or to help brain cells survive the reduced amount of oxygen. The only reliable way to tell whether there is bleeding is with a special type of X-ray test called computed tomography (CT). Blood is usually easy to see on the CT scan (▼ Figure 13-13).

Figure 13-12 Securing and maintaining the airway in a patient who is unconscious is critical; also be sure to have suction readily available in the event that the patient vomits.

Figure 13-13 A CT scan of a ruptured cerebral aneurysm. The light area represents hemorrhage into the brain tissue (arrows).

Most hospitals have only one CT scanner. The technician who knows how to run the machine may not be in the hospital in the middle of the night. That is why it is important that you recognize the signs and symptoms of stroke. If the emergency department staff knows that you are transporting a patient with a possible stroke, they may be able to call in the technician before you even arrive, or they may decide to delay a CT scan on another patient who has a less critical problem. Keep in mind that most treatments for stroke must be started as soon as possible after the onset of the event (▶ **Table 13-4**). Few, if any, current treatments do any good if they are started more than 3 to 6 hours after the stroke begins. Even if 3 hours have passed, prompt action on your part is essential.

Seizures

In most situations, patients who have had a seizure require definitive evaluation and treatment in the hospital. Even a patient who has a history of chronic epilepsy that is controlled with medications may have an occasional seizure, commonly referred to as a breakthrough seizure. These patients should also be taken to the hospital for observation. At the hospital, blood levels of seizure medications are checked to ensure that patients are receiving the correct dose. Clearly, patients who have just had their first seizure or those with chronic seizures who have had an episode that is "different" require immediate examination to rule out life-threatening conditions. Unless the patient has a well-established history of seizures and is completely alert and oriented, supplemental oxygen is strongly advised, not only to provide extra oxygen but also to prevent the possibility of a recurrent seizure if there is a hypoxic component to the source of the convulsion.

Depending on local protocols, you should assess and treat the patient for possible hypoglycemia (diabetic with altered mental status who takes insulin or oral agents that lower blood glucose levels). If trauma is suspected, provide spinal immobilization. With recurrent seizures, protect the patient from further injury and manage the airway once the seizure ceases.

If you are treating a child who you suspect is having a febrile seizure, you should attempt to lower the child's

---

TABLE 13-4 Tips on Patient Care

- Patients who experience a TIA may have most of the same signs and symptoms as patients with a stroke. These signs and symptoms can last from minutes up to 24 hours. Therefore, the signs of stroke that you note on arrival may gradually disappear. Patients who appear to have had a TIA should be transported for further evaluation.

- Place the patient's affected or paralyzed extremity in a secure and safe position during patient movement and transport.

- Some patients who have had a stroke may be unable to communicate, but they can often understand what is being said around them. Be aware of this possibility.

- New therapies for stroke must be used shortly after the start of symptoms. Minimize time on the scene and notify the receiving hospital as soon as possible.

---

temperature by removing his or her clothing and cooling the child with tepid water, particularly about the head and neck, and then fanning the moistened areas. Be careful not to make the patient shiver, which will increase temperature.

If the patient has been exposed to a toxin or poison, you should safely remove the source if possible. Suction should be readily available in case a patient with a decreased level of consciousness begins to vomit.

In all instances, you should be patient and tolerant with these patients, as many of them are likely to be confused and occasionally frightened. Many patients who experience seizures are frustrated with their condition and may refuse transport. Kindness and professional behavior are required to help convince the patient that transport is necessary for definitive care.

Pediatric Needs

Children can have altered mental status caused by strokes, seizures, and other brain emergencies. However, children who have subarachnoid hemorrhages may not have a berry aneurysm; instead, they may have a congenital problem with the blood vessels in the brain. Children who have sickle cell anemia are at particularly high risk for ischemic stroke. Treat stroke in children the same way that you do in adults.

As was mentioned earlier in this chapter, seizures can result from sudden high fevers, particularly in children. Remember that although febrile seizures are generally well tolerated by children, you must transport these patients to the hospital. The possibility of a second seizure makes transport mandatory so that if other problems develop, the child is in the hospital and can receive immediate definitive care.

If you suspect that a patient with altered mental status has hypoglycemia and you have the ability to test for it, you should do so and treat the patient according to local protocols. Also, these patients require close monitoring, particularly of the airway, en route to the hospital.

Prep Kit

Ready for Review

The cerebrum, the largest part of the brain, is divided into right and left hemispheres, each controlling the opposite side of the body. Different parts of the brain control different functions: The front part of the cerebrum controls emotion and thought; the middle controls touch and movement; the back part of the cerebrum is involved with vision. In most people, speech is controlled on the left side of the brain, near the middle of the cerebrum.

Many different disorders can cause brain or other neurologic symptoms. As a general rule, if the problem is primarily in the brain, only part of the brain will be affected. If the problem is in the heart or lungs, the whole brain will be affected. Stroke is a significant brain disorder because it is common and potentially treatable. Seizures and altered mental status are also common, and you must learn to recognize the signs and symptoms of each. Other causes of neurologic dysfunction include coma, infections, and tumors.

Strokes occur when part of the blood flow to the brain is suddenly cut off; within minutes, brain cells begin to die. Signs and symptoms of stroke include receptive or expressive aphasia, dysarthria, muscle weakness or numbness on one side, facial droop, and sometimes high blood pressure. You should always do at least three neurologic tests on patients you suspect of having a stroke: testing speech, facial movement, and arm movement. In a transient ischemic attack (TIA), normal body processes break up the blood clot, restoring blood flow and ending symptoms in less than 24 hours. However, patients with TIA are at high risk for a permanent stroke. Because current treatments must be administered within 3 to 6 hours (and preferably within 2 hours) of the onset of symptoms to be most effective, you should provide prompt transport. Also, always notify the hospital as soon as possible that you are bringing in a possible stroke patient, so that staff there can prepare to test and treat the patient without delay.

Seizures are characterized by unconsciousness and generalized twitching of all or part of the body. There are types of seizures that you should learn to recognize: generalized, absence, and febrile convulsions. Most seizures last between 3 and 5 minutes and are followed by a postictal state in which the patient may be unresponsive, have labored breathing, and have hemiparesis and may have urinated on himself or herself. It is important for you to recognize the signs and symptoms of seizures so that you can provide emergency department staff with information as you transport the patient.

Altered mental status is also a common neurologic problem that you will encounter as an EMT-B. Signs and symptoms vary widely, as do the causes for this condition. Among the most common causes are hypoglycemia, intoxication, drug overdose, and poisoning. As you assess the patient with altered mental status, do not always assume intoxication; hypoglycemia is just as likely a cause. Prompt transport with close monitoring of vital signs en route is indicated.

Vital Vocabulary

absence seizure Seizure that may be characterized by a brief lapse of attention in which the patient may stare and does not respond. Also known as petit mal seizure.

aphasia The inability to understand or produce speech.

arterial rupture Rupture of a cerebral artery that may contribute to interruption of cerebral blood flow.

atherosclerosis A disorder in which cholesterol and calcium build up inside the walls of blood vessels, forming plaque, which eventually leads to partial or complete blockage of blood flow. An atherosclerotic plaque can also become a site where blood clots can form, break off, and embolize elsewhere in the circulation.

cerebral embolism Obstruction of a cerebral artery caused by a clot that was formed elsewhere in the body and traveled to the brain.

cerebrovascular accident (CVA) An interruption of blood flow to the brain that results in the loss of brain function.

dysarthria The inability to pronounce speech clearly, often due to loss of the nerves or brain cells that control the small muscles in the larynx.

febrile seizures Convulsions that result from sudden high fevers, particularly in children.

generalized seizure Seizure characterized by severe twitching of all the body's muscles that may last several minutes or more; also known as a grand mal seizure.

hemiparesis Weakness on one side of the body.

hemorrhagic stroke One of the two main types of stroke; occurs as a result of bleeding inside the brain.

hypoglycemia A condition characterized by low blood glucose levels.

incontinent Loss of bowel and bladder control due to a generalized seizure.

infarcted cells Cells in the brain that die as a result of loss of blood flow to the brain.

ischemic cells Cells in the brain that receive enough blood after a cerebrovascular accident to stay alive but not to function properly.

ischemic stroke One of the two main types of stroke; occurs when blood flow to a particular part of the brain is cut off by a blockage (eg, a clot) inside a blood vessel.

postictal state Period following a seizure that lasts between 5 and 30 minutes, characterized by labored respirations and some degree of altered mental status.

seizure Generalized, uncoordinated muscular activity associated with loss of consciousness; a convulsion.

status epilepticus A condition in which seizures recur every few minutes, or last more than 5 minutes.

stroke A loss of brain function in certain brain cells that do not get enough oxygen during a CVA. Usually caused by obstruction of the blood vessels in the brain that feed oxygen to those brain cells.

thrombosis Clotting of the cerebral arteries that may result in the interruption of cerebral blood flow and subsequent stroke.

transient ischemic attack (TIA) A disorder of the brain in which brain cells temporarily stop working because of insufficient oxygen, causing stroke-like symptoms that resolve completely within 24 hours of onset.

Assessment in Action

You are dispatched to an elderly woman who has fallen. On arrival, you find a 77-year-old female sitting propped against a street vendor's espresso stand. She appears awake and focuses on you as you approach. Her friend tells you that they were walking by the vendor when your patient seemed to stumble. She was caught by a passerby and eased to the ground. There is no trauma involved.

The patient attempts to answer your questions but her speech is garbled. As you observe her, you note that the left side of her face appears to droop. Her skin is pale, cool, and dry. As you continue with your assessment your partner determines that her vital signs include a pulse of 88 beats/min and irregular, respirations of 16 breaths/min, and a blood pressure of 156/96 mm Hg.

1. The first step in caring for this patient should be to:
   A. ask the patient to try and stand on her own.
   B. obtain a history of her medications.
   C. contact a family member to obtain permission to treat.
   D. ensure that her airway is open and clear.

2. What potentially life-threatening problem is associated with the patient's facial droop?
   A. Serious depression
   B. Impending heart attack
   C. Possible airway compromise
   D. Increasing hyperventilation

3. For any patient with a neurologic problem, specific neurologic assessment should include assessing:
   A. breath sounds, chest rise, and skin color.
   B. speech, facial movement, and arm movement.
   C. skin color, blood pressure, and capillary return.
   D. skin moisture and degree of dehydration.

4. Which of the following is vitally important to determine with this patient?
   A. A history of physical activity prior to the incident
   B. A history of diabetes, seizures, or a head injury
   C. A family history of cardiovascular disease
   D. When she last saw her physician

5. Transport considerations for this patient include which of the following?
   A. Protecting the paralyzed extremities
   B. Elevating her feet and keeping her warm
   C. Placing her in the recovery position
   D. Placing her in a head down position

6. On the way to the hospital her speech becomes clear and distinct and she moves all her extremities to command. At the emergency department she has no complaints and wants to go home. A return of function in this patient suggests that:
   A. she has suffered a very short stroke.
   B. what happened was not a neurologic event.
   C. the patient was faking her signs and symptoms.
   D. she most likely had a transient ischemic attack.

7. This patient has signs and symptoms that suggest a stroke. Stroke patients are also at risk for developing which of the following?
   A. Vomiting
   B. Allergic reactions
   C. Seizures
   D. Diabetic reactions

Challenging Questions

8. Because this patient is having trouble speaking, which part of her body may also be affected?

9. If this patient were taking medication such as Tegretol or Dilantin, what other condition might you suspect?

10. There is a difference between a patient who has suffered an ischemic stroke and a patient who has developed stroke-like symptoms due to a hypoglycemic reaction. What is the difference?

Points to Ponder

You are dispatched to an "unconscious person." When you get to the house a man in his mid-20s answers the door. It quickly becomes noticeable that the man is mentally impaired and is functional at about an 8-year-old level. He leads you to his elderly mother whom you determine may have experienced a stroke. The man is very scared and agitated. He wants to know if his mother is all right. He has no other family. The mother seems stable but unresponsive. How would you calm the son? How much time would you spend on scene with the son? Would you transport the son with the mother?

Issues Special Populations, Personal Biases, Care for Non-Patients at the Scene.

Online Outlook

Different parts of the brain do different things. For example, some parts receive input from the senses, including sight, hearing, taste, smell, and touch; others control the muscles and movement; and still others control the formation of speech. To see many pictures of the brain and learn more about its function centers, complete Exercise 13 at www.emtb.com.

www.emtb.com

The Acute Abdomen

Objectives*

Cognitive

1. Define the term "acute abdomen" (p 394).
2. Identify the signs and symptoms of the acute abdomen and the necessity for immediate transport of patients with these symptoms (p 394).
3. Define the concept of "referred pain" (p 394).
4. Describe the areas of pain or referred pain seen with the common causes of the acute abdomen (p 397).
5. Explain that pain in the abdomen can arise from other body systems (p 398).

Affective

None

Psychomotor

6. Perform a rapid gentle assessment of the abdomen (p 396).

   * All of these objectives are noncurriculum objectives.

TECHNOLOGY

www.emtb.com

| Online Chapter Pretest | ◄ |
| Interactivities |
| Vocabulary Explorer |
| Anatomy Review |
| Web Links |
| Online Review Manual |
| Distance Learning |

Chapter FEATURES

| Skill Drills | ◄ |
| Vital Vocabulary |
| Pediatric Needs |
| Geriatric Needs |
| EMT-B Safety |
| EMT-B Tips |
| Documentation Tips |
| Remember |
| Prep Kit |

You are the EMT

A brief stop for coffee turns into work when a 25-year-old woman just in front of you in the line collapses. Your partner contacts dispatch to advise them as to what's going on while you check out the patient, who is complaining of "terrible stomach pain."

An acute abdomen can be the result of something as minor as indigestion or as life threatening as a ruptured appendix. This chapter will prepare you to properly care for the patient with an acute abdomen as well as help you answer the following questions:

1. What does "referred pain" mean, and is it indicative of a serious problem or not?

2. Is it a requirement that all patients complaining of abdominal pain be transported to the hospital?

The Acute Abdomen

Abdominal pain is a common complaint, but the cause is often difficult to identify, even for a physician. As an EMT-B, you do not need to determine the exact cause of acute abdominal pain. You simply need to be able to recognize a life-threatening problem and act swiftly in response. Remember, the patient is in pain and is probably anxious, requiring all your skills of rapid assessment and emotional support.

This chapter begins by explaining the physiology of the abdomen. It then describes the signs and symptoms of the acute abdomen and explains how to examine the abdomen. Next, it discusses the different causes of the acute abdomen and appropriate emergency medical care.

The Physiology of the Abdomen

Acute abdomen is a medical term referring to the sudden onset of abdominal pain that indicates an irritation of the **peritoneum**, the thin membrane that lines the entire abdominal cavity. This condition, called **peritonitis**, can be caused by an infection, a penetrating abdominal wound, a blunt injury severe enough to damage abdominal organs, and many diseases. In all cases, the major symptom is the same: severe pain. The major clinical signs are abdominal tenderness and distention.

Anatomically, the peritoneum is not one membrane, but two. The *parietal peritoneum* lines the walls of the abdominal cavity; the *visceral peritoneum* covers the surface of each of the organs in the abdominal cavity.

Two different types of nerves supply these two areas of the peritoneum. The parietal peritoneum is supplied by the same nerves from the spinal cord that supply the

skin of the abdomen; it can therefore perceive much the same sensations: pain, touch, pressure, heat, and cold. These sensory nerves can easily identify and localize a point of irritation. In contrast, the visceral peritoneum is supplied by the autonomic nervous system. These nerves are far less able to localize sensation. The visceral peritoneum is stimulated when distention or contraction of the hollow abdominal organs activates the stretch receptors. This sensation is usually interpreted as **colic**, a severe, intermittent cramping pain. Other painful sensations that occur because of an irritated visceral peritoneum may be perceived at a distant point on the surface of the body, such as the back or shoulder. This phenomenon is called **referred pain**.

Referred pain is the result of connections between the body's two separate nervous systems. The spinal cord supplies sensory nerves to the skin and muscles; these nerves are called the somatic nervous system. The autonomic nervous system controls the abdominal organs and the blood vessels. The nerves connecting these two systems cause the stimulation of the autonomic nerves to be perceived as stimulation of the spinal sensory nerves. For example, *acute cholecystitis* (inflammation of the gallbladder) may cause pain in the right shoulder, because the autonomic nerves serving the gallbladder lie near the spinal cord at the same anatomic level as the spinal sensory nerves that supply the skin of the shoulder ▶ **Figure 14-1** .

Signs and Symptoms of Acute Abdomen

Peritonitis typically causes **ileus**, or paralysis of the muscular contractions that normally propel material

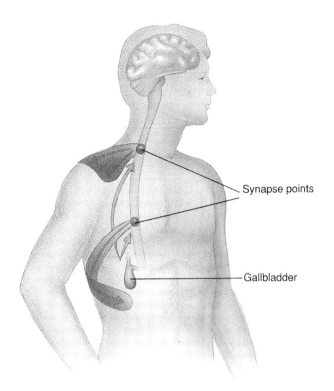

Synapse points

Gallbladder

Figure 14-1   Acute cholecystitis causes referred pain in the shoulder as well as abdominal pain.

through the intestine. The retained gas and feces, in turn, cause abdominal distention. In the presence of such paralysis, nothing that is eaten can pass normally out of the stomach or through the bowel. The only way the stomach can empty itself, then, is by **emesis**, or vomiting. For this reason, peritonitis is almost always associated with nausea and vomiting, usually in that order. These complaints do not point to a particular cause, since they can accompany almost every type of gastrointestinal disease or injury.

Similarly, **anorexia**, loss of hunger or appetite, is a nonspecific symptom. It, too, is an almost universal complaint in gastrointestinal and abdominal disease or injury. In fact, if a patient does not have anorexia, the situation may not be as serious as it otherwise appears.

Peritonitis is associated with a loss of body fluid into the abdominal cavity. The loss of fluid usually results from abnormal shifts of fluid from the bloodstream into body tissues. This decreases the volume of circulating blood and may eventually cause *hypovolemic shock*. This problem can be compounded by massive internal or external bleeding, resulting in severely inadequate perfusion. The patient may have normal vital signs or, if the peritonitis has progressed farther, may have tachycardia and hypotension. When peritonitis is accompanied by hemorrhage, the signs of shock are much more apparent.

> An acute abdomen is characterized by abdominal pain and tenderness.

Fever may or may not be present, depending on the cause of the peritonitis. Patients with **diverticulitis** (an inflammation of small pockets in the colon) or **cholecystitis** may have a substantial elevation in temperature. However, patients with acute **appendicitis** may have a normal temperature until the appendix ruptures and an abscess starts to form.

As we have seen, an acute abdomen is characterized by abdominal pain and tenderness. The pain may be sharply localized or diffuse and will vary in its severity. Localized pain gives a clue to the problem organ or area causing it. Tenderness may be minimal or so great that the patient will not allow you to touch the abdomen.

Another sign of the acute abdomen is tenseness of the abdominal muscles over the irritated area. In some instances, the muscles of the abdominal wall become rigid in an involuntary effort to protect the abdomen from further irritation. This board-like muscle spasm, called **guarding**, can be seen with major problems such as a perforated peptic ulcer or **pancreatitis**. In some situations, patients are comfortable only when lying in one particular position, which tends to relax muscles adjacent to the inflamed organ and thus lessen the pain. Therefore, the position of the patient may provide an important clue. For example, a patient with appendicitis may draw up the right knee. A patient with pancreatitis may lie curled up on one side.

To gauge the degree of distention, simply look at the patient's abdomen. Distention begins shortly after muscular contractions of the bowel have ceased. Pulse and blood pressure may undergo significant change or none at all. These findings usually reflect the severity of the process, its duration, and the amount of fluid lost into the abdomen.

Remember, the patient with peritonitis usually has abdominal pain, even when lying quietly. The patient can be quiet but have difficulty breathing and may take rapid, shallow breaths because of the pain. Usually, you will find tenderness on palpation of the abdomen or when the patient moves. The degree of pain and tenderness is usually related directly to the severity of peritoneal inflammation.

Documentation Tips

An acute abdomen usually indicates peritonitis, in which generalized signs can make it challenging to determine exactly where the problem lies, even for physicians. Knowing abdominal assessment steps well, and recording your findings in detail, are important early factors in the process that leads to diagnosis.

Figure 14-2 Check tenderness or rigidity by gently palpating the abdomen.

The following is a checklist of common signs and symptoms of irritation or inflammation of the peritoneum that you can use to determine whether a patient has an acute abdomen:

- Local or diffuse abdominal pain and/or tenderness
- A quiet patient who is guarding the abdomen (in shock)
- Rapid and shallow breathing
- Referred (distant) pain
- Anorexia, nausea, vomiting
- Tense, often distended, abdomen
- Sudden constipation or bloody diarrhea
- Tachycardia
- Hypotension
- Fever
- Rebound tenderness (hurts less when direct pressure is applied, but very painful when pressure is released)

Use the following steps to assess the abdomen:

1. Explain to the patient what you are about to do.

2. Place the patient in a supine position with the legs drawn up and flexed at the knees to relax the abdominal muscles, unless there is any trauma, in which case the patient will remain supine and immobilized.

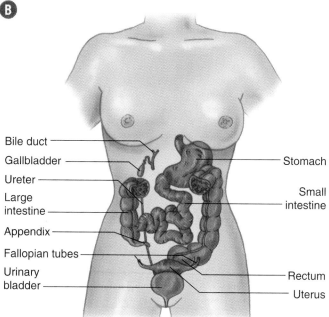

Figure 14-3 The solid and hollow organs of the abdomen. **A.** Solid organs include the liver, spleen, pancreas, kidneys, and ovaries (in women). **B.** Hollow organs include the gallbladder, stomach, small and large intestine, and bladder.

3. Determine whether the patient is restless or quiet; whether motion causes pain; or whether any characteristic position, distention, or obvious abnormality is present.

4. Palpate the four quadrants of the abdomen gently to determine whether it is tense (guarded) or soft ◄ **Figure 14-2** . Leave the suspect quadrant for last.

5. Determine whether the patient can relax the abdominal wall on command.

6. Determine whether the abdomen is tender when palpated.

Although such an examination will yield much information, it should not be prolonged. The physician will do a much more detailed examination in the hospital. Remember to be very gentle when palpating the abdomen. Occasionally, an organ within the abdomen will be enlarged and very fragile, and rough palpation could cause further damage.

Causes of Abdominal Pain

Gastrointestinal and Urinary Tract

The abdominal cavity contains the solid and hollow organs that make up the gastrointestinal, genital, and urinary systems ◄ **Figure 14-3** . Many of these organs, such as the bowel, are covered by visceral peritoneum; parietal peritoneum covers the inside aspect of the

abdominal wall that forms the abdominal cavity. The entire abdominal cavity normally contains a very small amount of peritoneal fluid to bathe the organs. Any condition that allows pus, blood, feces, urine, gastric juice, intestinal contents, bile, pancreatic juice, amniotic fluid, or other foreign material to lie within or adjacent to this cavity can cause an acute abdomen. Technically, organs such as kidneys, ovaries, and other genitourinary structures are *retroperitoneal* (behind the peritoneum) ▼ **Figure 14-4** . However, because they lie next to the peritoneum, problems in these organs can lead to an acute abdomen. Therefore, nearly every kind of abdominal problem can cause an acute abdomen.

Among the common diseases that produce signs of an acute abdomen are acute appendicitis, perforated gastric <u>ulcer</u>, cholecystitis, and diverticulitis. The more common emergency problems, with most common locations of direct and referred pain, are listed in ▼ **Table 14-1** .

Because the parietal peritoneum is richly supplied with very sensitive nerves, disease or inflammation of

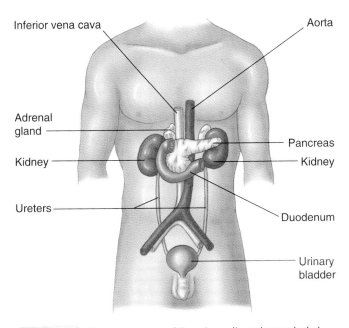

Figure 14-4   The major organs of the retroperitoneal space include the kidneys, ovaries, and other genitourinary structures.

Inferior vena cava

Aorta

Adrenal gland

Kidney

Ureters

Pancreas

Kidney

Duodenum

Urinary bladder

TABLE 14-1 Common Abdominal Conditions

Condition	Localization of Pain
Appendicitis	Around navel (referred); right lower quadrant (direct)
Cholecystitis	Right shoulder (referred); right upper quadrant (direct)
Duodenal Ulcer	Upper midabdomen or upper back
Diverticulitis	Left lower quadrant
Aortic Aneurysm (ruptured or dissecting)	Low back and right lower quadrant
<u>**Cystitis**</u> (inflammation of the bladder)	Lower midabdomen (retropubic)
Kidney Infection	Costovertebral angle
Kidney Stone	Right or left flanks, radiating to genitalia (referred)
Pelvic Inflammation (in women)	Both lower quadrants
Pancreatitis	Upper abdomen (both quadrants); back

Geriatric Needs

The elderly patient is just as susceptible to the acute abdomen as the younger adult is. However, their signs and symptoms might be different. Because of altered pain sensation, the geriatric patient with an acute abdomen may not feel any discomfort or may describe the discomfort as mild, even in severe conditions.

Because the elderly patient has decreased body temperature regulation and response, the patient with an acute abdomen, including peritonitis, may not have a fever. However, if a fever is present, it can be minimal.

Because of the elderly patient's response to the acute abdomen, a delay in identifying the condition and seeking medical attention is possible, putting the patient at risk for complications. You should ask about the patient's medical history, especially the history of recent illness, to identify a potential illness. Ask about abdominal discomfort, when the patient last had a bowel movement, whether she or he was constipated or had diarrhea, when the patient last ate, and whether she or he vomited. Ruling out appendicitis, bowel obstruction, or ruptured bowel can hasten proper treatment and recovery.

organs that lie behind or beneath the abdominal cavity can cause the signs of peritonitis. These signs and symptoms are similar to those produced by actual inflammation within the abdominal cavity. Pancreatitis for example, can produce a severe reaction that is hard to distinguish from a perforated ulcer. Kidney stones that cause colic of the ureter are frequently associated with ileus. Infections of the urinary tract may also cause peritoneal irritation.

Uterus and Ovaries

Gynecologic problems are a common cause of acute abdominal pain. Always consider that a woman with lower abdominal pain and tenderness may have a problem related to her ovaries, fallopian tubes, or uterus.

Abdominal pains may also be related to the normal menstrual cycle. A common lower abdominal pain, often confused with appendicitis but fairly short lived, is called *mittelschmerz*. It is associated with the release of an egg from the ovary, characteristically occurring in the middle of the menstrual cycle, between menstrual periods. Mittelschmerz may also be associated with lower abdominal tenderness. Some women experience painful cramps at the time of their menstrual periods.

In some, the discomfort may be crippling and the menstrual flow severe.

A common cause of an acute abdomen in women is *pelvic inflammatory disease (PID)*, an infection of the fallopian tubes and the surrounding tissues of the pelvis. With PID, acute pain and tenderness in the lower abdomen may be intense and accompanied by a high fever. If you suspect PID, promptly transport the patient to the emergency department for treatment.

Between 1% and 2% of all pregnancies are ectopic. The term *ectopic pregnancy* means that a fertilized egg has come to lie in an area outside the uterus, usually in a fallopian tube. A fallopian tube is simply not large enough to support the growth of a fetus and placenta for more than about 6 to 8 weeks. When the tube ruptures, it produces massive internal hemorrhage and abrupt abdominal pain. In this situation, the acute abdomen may be associated with the onset of hypovolemic shock. This combination mandates immediate transport to the hospital.

Other Organ Systems

The aorta lies immediately behind the peritoneum on the spinal column. In older individuals, the wall of the aorta sometimes develops weak areas that swell to form an **aneurysm**. The development of an aneurysm is rarely associated with symptoms because it occurs slowly, but if the aneurysm ruptures, massive hemorrhage may occur and, with it, the signs of acute peritoneal irritation. The patient may also experience severe back pain, because the peritoneum can, at times, be rapidly stripped away from the wall of the main abdominal cavity by the hemorrhage. Pain can also be associated with the pressure of blood on the back itself. In such instances, bleeding usually leads to profound shock. Again, the association of acute abdominal signs and symptoms with shock requires prompt transportation. Because this is a fragile situation with a large, leaking artery, avoid unnecessary or vigorous palpation of the abdomen. Remember to handle the patient gently during transport.

Pneumonia, especially in the lower parts of the lung, may cause both ileus pain and abdominal pain. In this instance, the problem lies in an adjacent body cavity, but the intense inflammatory response can affect the abdomen. Treat and transport this patient as you would any patient with abdominal pain.

A **hernia** is a protrusion of an organ or tissue through a hole in the body wall covering its normal site. Virtually every organ or tissue in the body will herniate through its covering membranes in certain circumstances. Hernias can occur as a result of the following:

- A congenital defect, as around the umbilicus
- A surgical wound that has failed to heal properly
- Some natural weakness in an area such as in the groin

Hernias always produce a mass or lump that the patient will be aware of. At times, the mass will disappear back into the body cavity in which it belongs. In this case, the hernia is said to be *reducible*. If the mass cannot be pushed back within the body, it is said to be *incarcerated*.

Reducible hernias pose little risk to the patient; some individuals live with them for years. When a hernia is incarcerated, however, its contents may become seriously compressed by the surrounding tissue, eventually compromising the blood supply. This situation, called **strangulation**, is a serious medical emergency. Immediate surgery is required to remove any dead tissue and repair the hernia.

The following signs and symptoms indicate a serious hernia problem:

- The existence of the hernia itself
- A clear statement that a mass that was reducible can no longer be pushed back inside the body
- Pain at the hernia site
- Tenderness when the hernia is palpated
- Red or blue skin discoloration over the hernia

Any of these signs and symptoms, other than the hernia itself, is cause for prompt transport to the emergency department.

Emergency Medical Care

The signs and symptoms of an acute abdomen signal a serious medical or surgical emergency. Ensure that you provide prompt, gentle transport for the patient; do not delay transport. Carry out the following steps as quickly as possible before transport.

1. **Do not attempt to diagnose** the cause of the acute abdomen.

2. **Clear and maintain the airway.**

3. **Anticipate vomiting.**

4. **Administer oxygen.**

5. **Do not give the patient anything by mouth.** Food or fluid will only aggravate many of the symptoms, since intestinal paralysis will prevent it from passing out of the stomach. The presence of food in the stomach will make any emergency surgery more dangerous.

6. **Document all pertinent information:** Onset, Provocation, Quality, Radiation, Severity, Time and treatment (OPQRST). Note the presence of abdominal tenderness, distention, or guarding.

7. **Anticipate the development of hypovolemic shock.** Treat the patient for shock when it is evident.

8. **Make the patient as comfortable** as possible for transport. Conserve body heat with blankets, as needed.

9. **Monitor vital signs;** these may change quickly.

Prep Kit

Ready for Review

The acute abdomen is a medical emergency, requiring prompt but gentle transport. The pain, tenderness, and abdominal distention associated with acute abdomen are signs of peritonitis, which may be caused by any condition that allows pus, blood, feces, urine, gastric juice, intestinal contents, bile, pancreatic juice, amniotic fluid, or other foreign material to lie within or adjacent to the peritoneum. In addition to abdominal disease or injury, problems in the gastrointestinal, genital, and urinary systems may also cause peritonitis. Appendicitis, perforated gastric ulcer, cholecystitis, and diverticulitis are common causes of an acute abdomen. A strangulated hernia is another.

Signs and symptoms of acute abdomen include pain, nausea, vomiting, and a tense, distended abdomen. Pain is common directly over the inflamed area of the peritoneum, or it may be referred to another part of the body. Referred pain occurs because of the connections between the two different nervous systems supplying the parietal peritoneum and the visceral peritoneum.

Your first priorities are to assess airway, breathing, and circulation and then apply oxygen. Next, obtain a pertinent medical history: When did the symptoms begin? How have they changed over time? Where exactly is the pain? What does it feel like? How long does it last and how intense is it? Has there been a loss of fluid volume as a result of vomiting or diarrhea? Take vital signs and gently palpate the abdomen. The presence of abdominal tenderness will confirm the need to transport the patient to the emergency department in an urgent manner.

Do not give the patient with an acute abdomen anything by mouth. In all likelihood, the bowel is paralyzed, making it impossible for food to pass out of the stomach.

Vital Vocabulary

acute abdomen A condition of sudden onset of pain within the abdomen, usually indicating peritonitis; demands immediate medical or surgical treatment.

aneurysm A swelling or enlargement of a part of an artery, resulting from weakening of the arterial wall.

anorexia Lack of appetite for food.

appendicitis Inflammation of the appendix.

cholecystitis Inflammation of the gallbladder.

colic Acute, intermittent cramping abdominal pain.

cystitis Inflammation of the bladder.

diverticulitis Bulging out of intestinal rings in small pockets at weak areas in the muscle walls, creating abdominal discomfort.

emesis Vomiting.

guarding Involuntary muscle contractions (spasm) of the abdominal wall, an effort to protect the inflamed abdomen.

hernia The protrusion of a loop of an organ or tissue through an abnormal body opening.

ileus Paralysis of the bowel, arising from any one of several causes; stops contractions that move material through the intestine.

pancreatitis Inflammation of the pancreas.

peritoneum The membrane lining the abdominal cavity (parietal peritoneum) and covering the abdominal organs (visceral peritoneum).

peritonitis Inflammation of the peritoneum.

referred pain Pain felt in an area of the body other than the area where the cause of pain is located.

strangulation Complete obstruction of blood circulation in a given organ as a result of compression or entrapment, an emergency situation causing death of tissue.

ulcer Abrasion of the stomach or small intestine.

Assessment in Action

You are dispatched in response to a 39-year-old man with abdominal pain. On arrival you find your patient in a small apartment furnished only with a couch, a TV, and a mattress. Beer cans, empty pizza boxes, and alcohol bottles litter the floor. The patient is very pale and is lying on the couch.

He tells you that his stomach has been bothering him for about a week but this morning when he got up to vomit, he got "really dizzy" and noticed pain in his upper left shoulder and neck. In response to your questions, he tells you that the vomit appeared "brownish, like coffee grounds." He has cool, moist skin with a rapid, weak radial pulse. His abdomen is firm and tender to the touch. His vital signs include a pulse of 136 beats/min, respirations of 28 breaths/min, and a blood pressure of 102/78 mm Hg.

1. Which of the following should be done for this patient at this point?
   A. Prepare him for transport.
   B. Apply oxygen by nonrebreathing mask.
   C. Have him lie flat and elevate his legs.
   D. Cover him to keep him warm.

2. What is a normal pulse rate for an adult?
   A. 120-140   B. 100-120
   C. 80-100   D. 60-100

3. Even though this patient's blood pressure is within normal limits, his pulse is too fast. What additional assessment step will help you determine if his perfusion is being maintained adequately?
   A. Listen to his breath sounds. B. Look for edema in his feet.
   C. Test for capillary refill.   D. Check his pupils.

4. When assessing this patient's abdominal pain it is important to ask specific questions about the pain. Which of the following characteristics of his pain will be most helpful to know?
   A. Onset, provocation, quality, radiation, severity, and time
   B. Character, cluster, radiation, positioning, and frequency
   C. Onset, positioning, location, density, and frequency
   D. Severity, timing, constancy, quality, and irritation

5. This patient noticed that when he got up to vomit he got very dizzy and suddenly noticed pain in his neck and shoulder. The term used to describe this pain is:
   A. diffuse pain.   B. referred pain.
   C. focal pain.   D. severe pain.

6. During your assessment of this patient he complains of thirst and asks for a drink of water. Your most appropriate response is to:
   A. allow him to drink small sips of room temperature water.
   B. allow him to drink as much water as he wishes.
   C. ask him if he can wait until he arrives at the hospital.
   D. ask him not to eat or drink anything because he may vomit.

7. The patient's description of the emesis suggests that the patient:
   A. has abused alcohol.   B. has bleeding hemorrhoids.
   C. is vomiting well-digested   D. is vomiting partially digested
      food.   blood.

8. On the basis of the available information, which of the following statements best describes the patient's condition?
   A. The patient is in shock associated with gastrointestinal bleeding.
   B. The patient has a ruptured liver as a result of chronic alcohol abuse.
   C. The patient probably has flu-like symptoms from something he ate.
   D. The patient's condition is a result of alcohol withdrawal syndrome.

Challenging Questions

9. This patient got dizzy when he got up to vomit. Why is this significant information?

10. Because this patient has upper gastrointestinal bleeding, what additional questions would be most appropriate to ask this patient?

Points to Ponder

You respond to a 13-year-old girl with severe abdominal pain. You find the pain to be generalized throughout the abdomen and the abdomen is rigid. Both of her parents are present and confirm that she has no history of abdominal problems. You ask the girl if there is any chance she could be pregnant. Her father becomes quite upset and yells that she is only 13. You notice a change in both the girl's and the father's behavior and willingness to answer questions. You are ready to transport and when the parents go to get their coats, the girl tells you that her father has been raping her and that she thinks she may be pregnant. She is afraid that if her father finds out she is pregnant or if she tells anyone what is happening that he will beat her, like he did before. She asks you not to tell anyone. How do you deal with this information? Do you

report this and if so, to whom? Would you allow the father to go with her in the ambulance? Do you tell the staff in the hospital even though she asked you not to?

Issues Reporting Requirements, Reporting Procedures, Patient Confidentiality, Sexual Abuse, Well-Being of the EMT-B.

Online Outlook

A hernia is a protrusion of an organ or tissue through a hole in the body wall covering its normal site. Virtually every organ or tissue in the body will herniate through its covering membranes in certain circumstances. Learn about the surgical repair of a hernia by completing Exercise 14 at www.emtb.com.

www.emtb.com

Diabetic Emergencies

Objectives

Cognitive

1. Identify the patient taking diabetic medications with altered mental status and the implications of a history of diabetes (p 405).
2. State the steps in the emergency medical care of the patient taking diabetic medicine with an altered mental status and a history of diabetes (p 409).
3. Establish the relationship between airway management and the patient with altered mental status (p 409).
4. State the generic and trade names, medication forms, dose, administration, action, and contraindications for oral glucose (p 409).
5. Evaluate the need for medical direction in the emergency medical care of the diabetic patient (p 409).

Affective

6. Explain the rationale for administering oral glucose (p 405).

Psychomotor

7. Demonstrate the steps in the emergency medical care for the patient taking diabetic medicine with an altered mental status and a history of diabetes (p 410).
8. Demonstrate the assessment and documentation of patient response to oral glucose (p 410).
9. Demonstrate the steps in the use of a glucometer (p 406).*
10. Demonstrate the steps in the administration of oral glucose (p 410).
11. Demonstrate how to complete a prehospital care report for patients with diabetic emergencies (p 299).

   * These are noncurriculum objectives.

You are the EMT

"Squad 18, respond to 10416 South Market Street for an 'unresponsive man.' "

Diabetes is a complicated disease that has an impact on every body system and every organ over the course of a lifetime. This chapter will provide you with the knowledge you'll need to care for the various diabetes-related emergencies you will respond to as an EMT-B. It will also help you answer the following questions:

1. Which diabetic emergency has a sudden onset and which one comes on over a day or more?

2. What is the difference in the presentation (signs and symptoms) of a patient with high blood glucose levels vs. one with low blood glucose levels?

Diabetic Emergencies

Diabetes is a very common disease, affecting about 6% of the population. It is a metabolic disorder in which the hormone that is needed to regulate blood glucose levels is missing or ineffective. Without treatment, blood glucose levels become too high and can cause coma and death. If properly treated, most people with diabetes can live a relatively normal life. However, diabetes can have many severe complications that affect the length and quality of life, including blindness, cardiovascular disease, and kidney failure. Also, treatment to lower high blood glucose levels can overshoot and cause a life-threatening state of hypoglycemia (low blood glucose). Therefore, as an EMT-B, you need to know the signs and symptoms of a blood glucose level that is either too high or too low so that you can administer the proper lifesaving treatment.

This chapter explains two types of diabetes and how they are controlled, including the role of glucose and insulin. You will learn how to distinguish between diabetic coma and insulin shock, which often resemble each other. The chapter discusses how to identify and treat diabetic emergencies in the prehospital setting. Complications, such as seizures, altered mental status, and heart attack are also briefly discussed, as are the emergency medical care for each.

Diabetes
Defining Diabetes

Literally, the word "diabetes" means "a passer through; a siphon." Medically, the term refers to a metabolic disorder in which the body's ability to metabolize simple carbohydrates (blood glucose) is impaired. It is characterized by the passage of large quantities of urine containing glucose, significant thirst, and deterioration of body functions. <u>Glucose</u>, or dextrose, is one of the basic sugars in the body and, along with oxygen, is the primary fuel for cellular metabolism.

The central problem in diabetes is the lack or ineffective action of <u>insulin</u>, a hormone that is normally produced by the pancreas that enables glucose to enter the cells. A <u>hormone</u> is a chemical substance produced by a gland that has special regulatory effects on other body organs and tissues. Without insulin, cells begin to "starve" because insulin is needed, like a key, to let glucose into the cells.

The full name of diabetes is <u>diabetes mellitus</u>, which means "sweet diabetes." This refers to the presence of glucose (sugar) in the urine. Diabetes mellitus is considered a metabolic disorder in which the body cannot metabolize glucose, usually because of the lack of insulin; the result is a wasting of glucose in the urine. *Diabetes insipidus*, a rare condition, also involves excessive urination, but here the missing hormone is one that regulates urinary fluid reabsorption. In this book, the term "diabetes" always refers to diabetes mellitus.

Left untreated, diabetes leads to a wasting of body tissues and death. Even with medical care, some patients with particularly aggressive forms of diabetes will die relatively young from one or more complications of the disease. Most patients with diabetes, however, can live out a normal life span. But they must be willing to adjust their lives to the demands of the disease, especially their eating habits and activities.

Types of Diabetes

Diabetes is a disease with two distinct onset patterns. It may become evident when the patient is a child, or it may develop in later life, usually when the patient is middle-aged.

In **type I diabetes**, most patients do not produce insulin at all; they are insulin dependent (IDDM). They need daily injections of supplemental, synthetic insulin throughout their lives to control blood glucose. Since this is the type of diabetes that strikes children, it used to be called "juvenile diabetes." However, it can, in some cases, develop in later life as well. Patients with type I diabetes are more likely to have metabolic problems and organ damage, such as blindness, heart disease, kidney failure, and nerve disorders.

In **type II diabetes**, which usually appears later in life, patients produce inadequate amounts of insulin. In other cases, they may produce a fairly normal amount but the insulin does not function effectively. Although some patients with non-insulin-dependent diabetes (NIDD) may require some supplemental insulin, most can be treated with diet and non-insulin-type oral medications (hypoglycemic agents), such as chlorpropamide (Diabinase), tolbutamide (Orinase), glyburide (Micronase), and glipizide (Glucotrol). These medications stimulate the pancreas to produce more insulin and thus lower blood glucose. In some cases, these medications can lead to hypoglycemia, particularly when patient activity and exercise levels are too vigorous or excessive. Patients with **hypoglycemia** have an abnormally low level of blood glucose. Non-insulin-dependent diabetes used to be called adult (maturity)-onset diabetes. Again, some patients with non-insulin-dependent diabetes may, in fact, be dependent on insulin.

The two types of diabetes are equally serious, although non-insulin-dependent diabetes is easier to regulate. Both can affect many tissues and functions other than the glucose-regulating mechanism. Both require lifelong medical management. Diabetes is considered to be an autoimmune problem, in which the body becomes allergic to its own tissues and literally destroys them. The severity of diabetes relates to the amount of insulin-producing tissue that is damaged or destroyed, as well as the time of life when the process started.

The Role of Glucose and Insulin

Glucose is the major source of energy for the body, and all cells need it to function properly. Some cells will not function at all without glucose. A constant supply of glucose is as important as oxygen to the brain. Without glucose, or with very low levels, brain cells rapidly suffer permanent damage. With the exception of the brain, insulin is needed to allow glucose to enter individual body cells to fuel their functioning. For this reason, insulin is said to be a "cellular key" ▼ **Figure 15-1** .

Without insulin, glucose from food remains in the blood and gradually rises to extremely high levels. This condition is called **hyperglycemia**. Once the blood glucose levels reach 200 mg/dL or more, or twice the usual amount (normally 80 to 120 mg/dL), excess glucose is excreted by the kidney. This process requires a large amount of water. The loss of water in such large

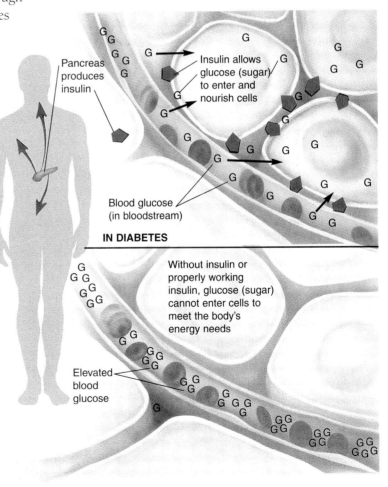

Figure 15-1 Diabetes is defined as a lack of or ineffective action of insulin. Without insulin, cells begin to "starve" because insulin is needed to allow glucose to enter and nourish the cells.

amounts causes the classic symptoms of uncontrolled diabetes, the "3 Ps":

- <u>Polyuria</u>: frequent and plentiful urination
- <u>Polydipsia</u>: frequent drinking of liquid to satisfy continuous thirst (secondary to the loss of so much body water)
- <u>Polyphagia</u>: excessive eating as a result of cellular "hunger"; seen only occasionally

Without glucose to supply energy for cells, the body must turn to other fuel sources. The most abundant is fat. Unfortunately, when fat is used as an immediate energy source, chemicals called *ketones* and *fatty acids* are formed as waste products and are hard for the body to excrete. As they accumulate in blood and tissue, certain ketones can produce a dangerous condition called <u>acidosis</u>. The form of acidosis seen in uncontrolled diabetes is called <u>diabetic ketoacidosis (DKA)</u>, in which an accumulation of certain acids occurs when insulin is not available in the body. Signs and symptoms of diabetic ketoacidosis include vomiting, abdominal pain, and a type of deep, rapid breathing called *Kussmaul respirations*. When the acid levels in the body become too high, individual cells will cease to function. If the patient is not given proper fluid and insulin to reverse fat metabolism and restore use of glucose as a source of energy, ketoacidosis will progress to unconsciousness, diabetic coma, and eventually death.

As we have seen, diabetes mellitus is treatable; however, treatment must be tailored for the individual patient. The trick is to balance constantly the patient's need for glucose with the available supply of insulin by testing either the blood or the urine. In the past, most patients tested their urine daily for the presence of glucose and acetone. *Acetone* is one type of ketone, indicating the presence of ketones in the blood, but its absence does not mean that there are no ketones in the blood. Many patients now measure the level of glucose in the blood instead, using a *blood glucose self-monitoring unit*. This is a much simpler and more accurate procedure: A drop of blood from the fingertip is placed on a thin strip of chemically treated paper. The paper turns color and is compared with a color chart, which matches colors with approximate blood glucose readings (▼ **Figure 15-2A**). The readings are in milligrams per deciliter of blood; remember that the normal blood glucose level is between 80 and 120 mg/dL. Patients can also buy devices for pricking the fingertip with a fine needle, standard tables for reading the strips, or a more elaborate unit that automatically analyzes the test strip and provides a digital readout of the blood glucose level, otherwise known as a glucometer. EMT-Bs are allowed to use test strips or glucometers in some systems across North America (▼ **Figure 15-2B**).

Figure 15-2 **A.** Glucose test strips for blood analysis. **B.** Blood glucose self-monitoring kit with digital meter is a device used by patients at home or by EMT-Bs in some areas.

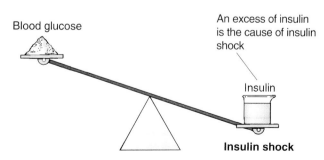

Figure 15-3 The two most common diabetic emergencies, diabetic coma and insulin shock, develop when the patient has either too much or too little glucose in the blood, respectively.

TABLE 15-1 Characteristics of Diabetic Emergencies

	Diabetic Coma	Insulin Shock
History		
Food intake	Excessive	Insufficient
Insulin dosage	Insufficient	Excessive
Onset	Gradual	Rapid, within minutes
Skin	Warm and dry	Pale and moist
Infection	Common	Uncommon
Gastrointestinal Tract		
Thirst	Intense	Absent
Hunger	Absent	Intense
Vomiting	Common	Uncommon
Respiratory System		
Breathing	Rapid, deep (Kussmaul respirations)	Normal or rapid
Odor of breath	Sweet, fruity	Normal
Cardiovascular System		
Blood pressure	Normal to low	Low
Pulse	Normal or rapid and full	Rapid, weak
Nervous System		
Consciousness	Restless merging to coma	Irritability, confusion, seizure, or coma
Urine		
Sugar	Present	Absent
Acetone	Present	Absent
Treatment		
Response	Gradual, within 6 to 12 hours following medication and fluid	Immediately after administration of glucose

Diabetic Coma and Insulin Shock

Two different conditions can lead to a diabetic emergency: diabetic coma (high blood glucose, or extreme hyperglycemia) or insulin shock (low blood glucose, or hypoglycemia) ◄ Figure 15-3 . The signs and symptoms of the two conditions can be quite similar ▲ Table 15-1 . For example, staggering and an intoxicated appearance or complete unresponsiveness are signs and symptoms of both. Note that your assessment of these potential emergencies should not prevent you from providing prompt care and transport as detailed in this chapter. However, in such urgent emergencies, the earlier clues

are gathered, the better for the patient. With specific information about the type of emergency, you can help the hospital to prepare prompt, definitive care for the patient.

DIABETIC COMA. Diabetic coma is a state of unconsciousness resulting from several problems, including ketoacidosis, dehydration because of excessive urination, and hyperglycemia. Too much blood glucose by itself does not always cause diabetic coma, but on some occasions, it can lead to it.

Diabetic coma may occur in the patient who is not under medical treatment, who takes insufficient insulin, who markedly overeats, or who is undergoing some sort of stress, such as an infection, illness, over-exertion, fatigue, or drinking alcohol. Usually, ketoacidosis develops over a period of time lasting from hours to days. The patient may ultimately be found comatose with the following physical signs:

- <u>**Kussmaul respirations**</u>

- Dehydration, as indicated by dry, warm skin and sunken eyes

- A sweet or fruity (acetone) odor on the breath, caused by the unusual waste products in the blood (ketones)

- A rapid, weak ("thready") pulse

- A normal or slightly low blood pressure

- Varying degrees of unresponsiveness

INSULIN SHOCK. In **insulin shock**, the problem is hypoglycemia, insufficient glucose in the blood. When insulin levels remain high, glucose is rapidly taken out of the blood to fuel the cells. If glucose levels get too low, there may be an insufficient amount to supply the brain. If blood glucose remains low, unconsciousness and permanent brain damage can quickly follow.

Insulin shock occurs when the patient has done one of the following:

- Taken too much insulin

- Taken a regular dose of insulin but has not eaten enough food

- Had an unusual amount of activity or vigorous exercise and used up all available glucose

- Has been ill, vomiting, and cannot eat

Insulin shock may also occur after the patient vomits a meal on a day he or she took a regular dose of insulin. At times, insulin shock may occur with no identifiable predisposing factor.

Children who have diabetes may pose a particular management problem. First, their high levels of activity mean that they can use up circulating glucose more quickly than adults do, even after a normal insulin injection. Second, they do not always eat correctly and on schedule. As a result, insulin shock can develop more often and more severely in children than in adult patients.

Insulin shock develops much more quickly than diabetic coma. In some instances, it can occur in a matter of minutes. Hypoglycemia can be associated with the following signs and symptoms:

- Normal or rapid respirations

- Pale, moist (clammy) skin

- Diaphoresis (sweating)

- Dizziness, headache

- Rapid pulse

- Normal to low blood pressure

- Altered mental status, aggressive, confused, lethargic, or unusual behavior

- Anxious or combative behavior

- Hunger

- Seizure, fainting, or coma

- Weakness on one side of the body (may mimic stroke)

Both diabetic coma and insulin shock produce unconsciousness and, in some instances, death. But they call for very different treatment. Diabetic coma is a complex metabolic condition that usually develops over time and involves all the tissues of the body. Correcting this condition may take many hours in a well-controlled hospital setting. Insulin shock, however, is an acute condition that can develop rapidly. A patient with diabetes who has taken his or her standard insulin dose and missed lunch may be in insulin shock before dinner. The condition is just as quickly reversed by giving the patient glucose. Without that glucose, however, the patient will suffer permanent brain damage. Minutes count.

Most individuals with diabetes understand and manage their disease well. Still, emergencies occur. In addition to diabetic coma and insulin shock, patients with diabetes may have "silent," or painless, heart attacks, a possibility that you should always consider. Their only symptom may be "not feeling so well."

DIABETES AND THE ALCOHOLIC. Occasionally, patients in insulin shock or a diabetic coma are thought to be intoxicated, especially if their condition has caused a motor vehicle crash or other incident. Confined by police in a "drunk tank," a patient with diabetes is at risk. In such situations, an emergency medical identification bracelet, necklace, or card may help to save the patient's life. Often, only a blood glucose test performed at the scene or in the emergency department will identify the real problem. In some EMS systems, you will be trained and allowed to perform the blood glucose test at the scene. Otherwise, you must always suspect hypoglycemia in any patient with altered mental status.

Certainly, diabetes and alcoholism can coexist in a patient. But you must be alert to the similarity in symptoms of acute alcohol intoxication and diabetic emergencies. Likewise, hypoglycemia and a head injury can coexist, and you must appreciate the potential even when the head injury is obvious.

Emergency Medical Care

You should ask the following questions of any ill patient who you know has diabetes:

- Do you take insulin or any pills that lower your blood sugar?

- Have you taken your usual dose of insulin (or pills) today?

- Have you eaten normally today?

- Have you had any illness, unusual amount of activity, or stress today?

If the patient has eaten but has not taken insulin, it is more likely that diabetic ketoacidosis is developing. If the patient has taken insulin but has not eaten, the problem is more likely to be insulin shock. A patient with diabetes will often know what is wrong. If the patient is not thinking or speaking clearly (or is unconscious), ask a family member or bystander the same questions.

The first step is to perform an initial assessment to verify that the airway is open. If the patient is not breathing or is having difficulty breathing, open the airway, give oxygen, and assist ventilations. Continue to monitor the airway as you provide care. Perform the focused history and physical exam while your partner obtains the baseline vital signs and SAMPLE history.

When you are assessing a patient whom you suspect might have diabetes, check to see whether he or she has an emergency medical identification symbol: a wallet card, necklace, or bracelet. Or ask the patient or family if the patient has diabetes. Remember, however, that just because a person has diabetes does not mean that the diabetes is causing the current problem. He or she might be having a heart attack, stroke, or other medical emergency. For this reason, you must always do a full, careful assessment, paying attention to the ABCs. Inform medical control that you are at the scene of a diabetic emergency. Ask the patient or family about the patient's last meal and insulin dose.

In the past, EMTs were often advised to place oral glucose gel or glucose tablets under the tongue or in the mouth of the unconscious patient. Very little sugar is actually absorbed in this manner. The risk of choking or aspirating liquid into the lungs probably outweighs the benefits of providing such small amounts of glucose. Therefore, although glucose is very important to give to patients with diabetes with altered mental status, *you*

should not attempt to give anything by mouth to an unconscious patient, even if you suspect insulin shock. These patients need IV glucose, which you are not authorized to give. Your responsibility is to provide prompt transport to the hospital, where the proper care can be given.

What if no one else is present, but you know that the unconscious patient has diabetes? Then you must use your knowledge of the signs and symptoms to decide whether the problem is diabetic coma or insulin shock. Remember, however, this assessment should not prevent you from providing prompt treatment and transport. The primary visible difference will be the patient's breathing: deep, sighing respirations in diabetic coma and normal or rapid respirations in insulin shock. However, the patient with diabetes who is unconscious and having convulsions is more likely to be in insulin shock.

Keep in mind that any unconscious patient may have undiagnosed diabetes. In patients with an altered mental status, you may be able to determine this in the field, if you have the proper equipment to test for blood glucose. Without this critical knowledge, treat this patient as you would any other unconscious individual. Provide emergency medical care, particularly airway management, and prompt transport. At the emergency department, the diabetes and its complication can quickly be diagnosed.

Giving Oral Glucose

Oral glucose is a commercially available gel that dissolves when placed in the mouth ▼ **Figure 15-4** . One toothpaste-type tube of gel equals one dose. Trade names for the gel include Glutose and Insta-Glucose. Glucose gel, which acts to increase blood glucose levels, should be given to any patient with a decreased level of consciousness who has a history of diabetes. The only contraindications to glucose are an inability to swallow

Figure 15-4 Oral glucose is commercially available in gel and tablet form. One tube of gel equals one dose.

or unconsciousness, since aspiration (inhalation of the substance) can occur. Oral glucose itself has no side effects if it is administered properly; however, the risk of aspiration in a patient who does not have a gag reflex can be dangerous. A conscious patient (even if confused) who does not really need glucose will not be harmed by it. Therefore, do not hesitate to give it under these circumstances.

As always, be sure to wear gloves before placing anything into a patient's mouth. After you have confirmed that the patient is conscious and able to swallow, and have obtained an online or off-line order, follow these steps to administer oral glucose (▶ **Skill Drill 15-1**):

1. **Examine the tube** to ensure that it is not open or broken. Check the expiration date **(Step 1)**.

2. **Squeeze the entire tube** onto the bottom third of a bite stick or tongue depressor **(Step 2)**.

3. **Open the patient's mouth.**

4. **Place the tongue depressor** on the mucous membranes between the cheek and gum, with the gel side next to the cheek. Once the gel is dissolved, or if the patient loses consciousness or has a seizure, remove the tongue depressor **(Step 3)**.

Reassess the patient regularly after giving glucose, even if you see rapid improvement in the patient's condition. Watch for airway problems, sudden loss of consciousness, or seizures. Provide prompt transport to the hospital; do not delay transport just to give additional oral glucose.

A patient in insulin shock (rapid onset of altered mental status—hypoglycemia) needs sugar immediately, and a patient in diabetic coma (acidosis, dehydration, hyperglycemia) needs insulin and IV fluid therapy. These patients need prompt transport to the hospital for appropriate medical care.

For the conscious patient in insulin shock, protocols usually recommend oral glucose. These will usually reverse the reaction within several minutes. Do not be afraid to give too much sugar. The problem often will not be solved with just a sip of juice. An entire candy bar or a full glass of sweetened juice is often needed. Do not give sugar-free drinks that are sweetened with saccharin or other synthetic sweetening compounds, as they will have little or no effect. Remember that even if the patient responds after receiving glucose, he or she may still need additional treatment. Therefore, you must transport the patient to the hospital as soon as possible.

When there is any doubt about whether a conscious patient with diabetes is going into insulin shock or

EMT-B Safety

Managing problems related to diabetes and altered mental status poses very little risk to you, because exposure to body fluids is generally very limited. However, some patients can become confused and even aggressive at times. Follow BSI precautions, as you would with any other patient. Always use gloves, and wash your hands carefully after obtaining and checking a blood sample or if you perform airway techniques.

Geriatric Needs

You might encounter an elderly patient who has undiagnosed diabetes. These patients report that they have not been feeling well for a while but have not seen a physician. A patient with undiagnosed diabetes or one who is in denial or ignores the advice of his or her physician may call 9-1-1 when the signs and symptoms become annoying. Nonhealing wounds, blindness, renal failure, and other complications are associated with poorly controlled or uncontrolled diabetes. As an EMT-B, you might be the first to recognize and suggest medical treatment to an elderly patient who might otherwise ignore his or her condition. It is important that you recognize the signs and symptoms of diabetes. As you obtain a SAMPLE history, also ask the patient whether he or she has noticed an increase in the number of ants in the bathroom, especially around the toilet. Ants like sugar, and excess sugar is excreted in the urine. An infestation of ants around the toilet could indicate sugar excreted in the urine and hence elevated blood glucose and the possibility of diabetes.

diabetic coma, most protocols will err on the side of giving glucose, even though the patient may have diabetic ketoacidosis. Untreated insulin shock will result in unconsciousness and can quickly cause significant brain damage or death. Compared with the patient in diabetic ketoacidosis, the patient in insulin shock is in a far more critical condition and far more likely to experience permanent problems. Furthermore, the amount of sugar that is typically given to such a patient is very unlikely to make a patient in diabetic ketoacidosis significantly worse. When in doubt, consult medical control.

Complications of Diabetes

Diabetes is a systemic disease affecting all tissues of the body, especially the kidneys, eyes, small arteries, and peripheral nerves. Therefore, you are likely to be called to treat patients with a variety of complications of

Skill Drill 15-1   Administering Glucose

Make sure that the tube of glucose is intact and has not expired.

Squeeze the entire tube of oral glucose onto the bottom third of a bite stick or tongue depressor.

Open the patient's mouth.
Place the tongue depressor on the mucous membranes between the cheek and the gum with the gel side next to the cheek.

diabetes, such as heart disease, visual disturbances, renal failure, stroke, and ulcers or infections of the feet or toes. With the exception of heart attack and stroke, most of these will not be acute emergencies. Considering that diabetes is a major risk factor for cardiovascular disease, individuals with diabetes should always be suspected of having a potential for heart attack, particularly older patients, even when they do not present with classic symptoms such as chest pain.

Seizures

Although seizures are rarely life threatening, you should consider them very serious, even in patients with a history of chronic seizures, Seizures, which may be brief or prolonged, are caused by fever, infections, poisoning, hypoglycemia, trauma, or decreased levels of oxygen. They can also be idiopathic (of unknown cause) in children. Although brief seizures are not harmful, they may indicate a more dangerous and potentially life-threatening underlying condition. Because seizures can be caused by head injury, consider trauma as a cause. In the patient with diabetes, you should also consider hypoglycemia.

Emergency medical care of seizures includes ensuring that the airway is clear and placing the patient on his or her side if there is no possibility of cervical spine trauma. Do not attempt to place anything in the patient's mouth (eg, a bite stick or oral airway). Be sure to have suctioning equipment ready in case the patient vomits. Provide artificial ventilation if the patient is cyanotic or appears to be breathing inadequately, and provide prompt transport.

Altered Mental Status

Although altered mental status is often caused by complications of diabetes, it may also be caused by a variety of conditions, including poisoning, part of the postseizure state, infection, head injury, and decreased levels of oxygen.

Begin emergency medical care of altered mental status by ensuring that the airway is clear. Be prepared to provide artificial ventilation and suctioning in case the patient vomits, and provide prompt transport.

Relationship to Airway Management

Patients with altered mental status, particularly those who are difficult to awaken, are at risk for losing their gag reflex. When the gag reflex is not working, patients cannot reject foreign materials in their mouth (including vomit), and their tongues will often relax and obstruct the airway. Therefore, you must carefully monitor the airway in patients with hypoglycemia, diabetic coma, or a diabetic complication such as stroke or seizure. Place the patient in a lateral recumbent position, and make sure suction is readily available.

Prep Kit

Ready for Review

Diabetes is a metabolic disorder caused by the lack of insulin, a hormone that enables glucose to enter the cells, where it can be used for energy. Diabetes is typically characterized by excessive urination and resulting thirst, along with deterioration of body tissues. There are two types of diabetes. Type I diabetes, or insulin-dependent diabetes, usually starts in childhood and requires daily insulin to control blood glucose. Type II diabetes, or noninsulin-dependent diabetes, usually develops in middle age and often can be controlled with diet and oral medications. Both are serious systemic diseases, especially affecting the kidneys, eyes, small arteries, and peripheral nerves.

Patients with diabetes have chronic complications that place them at risk for other diseases such as heart attack, stroke, and infections. Most often, however, you will be called upon to treat the acute complications of blood glucose imbalance. These include hyperglycemia (excess blood glucose) and hypoglycemia (not enough blood glucose). Symptoms of hypoglycemia classically include confusion, rapid respirations, pale, moist skin, diaphoresis, dizziness, fainting, and even coma and seizures. This condition, called insulin shock, is rapidly reversible with the administration of glucose or sugar. Without treatment, however, permanent brain damage and death can occur. Hyperglycemia is usually associated with dehydration and ketoacidosis. It can result in diabetic coma, marked by rapid (often deep) respirations; warm, dry skin; a weak pulse; and a fruity breath odor. Hyperglycemia must be treated in the hospital with insulin and IV fluids.

Since either too much or too little blood glucose can result in altered mental status, you must perform a thorough history and patient assessment. When you cannot determine the nature of the problem, it is best to treat the patient for hypoglycemia. Be prepared to give oral glucose to a conscious patient who is confused or has a slightly decreased level of consciousness; however, do not give oral glucose to a patient who is unconscious or otherwise unable to swallow properly or protect his or her own airway. Remember, in all cases, providing emergency medical care and prompt transport is your primary responsibility.

Vital Vocabulary

acidosis A pathologic condition resulting from the accumulation of acids in the body.

diabetes mellitus A metabolic disorder in which the ability to metabolize carbohydrates (sugars) is impaired, usually because of a lack of insulin.

diabetic coma Unconsciousness caused by dehydration, very high blood glucose, and acidosis in diabetes.

diabetic ketoacidosis (DKA) A form of acidosis in uncontrolled diabetes in which certain acids accumulate when insulin is not available.

glucose One of the basic sugars; it is the primary fuel, along with oxygen, for cellular metabolism.

hormone A chemical substance that regulates the activity of body organs and tissues; produced by a gland.

hyperglycemia Abnormally high glucose level in the blood.

hypoglycemia Abnormally low glucose level in the blood.

insulin A hormone produced by the pancreas that enables sugar in the blood to enter the cells of the body; used in synthetic form to treat and control diabetes mellitus.

insulin shock Unconsciousness or altered mental status in a patient with diabetes caused by significant hypoglycemia; usually the result of excessive exercise and activity or failure to eat after a routine dose of insulin.

Kussmaul respirations Deep, rapid breathing; usually the result of an accumulation of certain acids when insulin is not available in the body.

polydipsia Excessive thirst persisting for long periods of time despite reasonable fluid intake; often the result of excessive urination.

polyphagia Excessive eating; in diabetes, the inability to use glucose properly can cause a sense of hunger.

polyuria The passage of an unusually large volume of urine in a given period; in diabetes, this can result from wasting of glucose in the urine.

type I diabetes The type of diabetic disease that usually starts in childhood and requires insulin for proper treatment and control.

type II diabetes The type of diabetic disease that usually starts in later life and often can be controlled through diet and oral medications.

Assessment in Action

A college student returns to his apartment and finds his roommate lying on the bed, unconscious and unresponsive. He immediately calls EMS. When you arrive, you find a 20-year-old man dressed in jogging gear. The patient appears very pale, is unresponsive to any stimuli, and is breathing quickly with no apparent airway problems.

As you check for a pulse, you notice that his skin is cool and clammy. The roommate states that your patient said he was not feeling well at breakfast and promised to eat something later. He also tells you that the patient has no known allergies and does not take any medicine except insulin. Finally, he tells you that the patient began jogging a few weeks ago to try to get back into shape. Baseline vital signs obtained by your partner include a pulse of 128 beats/min, respirations of 28 breaths/min, and a blood pressure of 88/54 mm Hg.

1. The most important part of this patient's history that helps determine your treatment is a history of:
A. unresponsiveness.
B. not feeling well.
C. recent jogging.
D. diabetes.

2. Your protocol allows you to test his blood sugar with a glucometer. On the basis of the rapid onset of symptoms and the history provided by the patient's roommate, you expect the patient's blood glucose level to be:
A. very low.
B. within normal limits.
C. very high.
D. too high to measure.

3. Based on this patient's assessment findings and history, the best position for transport would be:
A. supine.
B. Fowler's.
C. lateral recumbent.
D. prone.

4. Which of the following indicates treatment with oral glucose?
A. A history of diabetes with unconsciousness
B. Altered mental status with a history of diabetes
C. Altered mental status in any adult
D. A history of diabetes in any patient with a complaint

5. Proper administration of oral glucose in a diabetic patient with an altered mental status includes confirming that the patient is conscious and able to swallow and:
A. applying it as a topical ointment.
B. placing it between the cheek and gum.
C. placing it in an inhaler.
D. injecting it in the outer thigh.

6. In situations where oral glucose has been given, what complications should you watch for and be prepared to manage?
A. Airway problems, sudden loss of consciousness, and seizures
B. Sudden loss of consciousness, vomiting, and severe headache
C. A drop in blood pressure, chest pain, and difficulty breathing
D. A rise in blood pressure, severe headache, and chest pain

7. Several months have passed when you are again dispatched to this same patient. On arrival you find that he is awake, alert, and oriented but is very anxious and complaining of chest pain. His color is very pale and he is cool and clammy. Knowing his history of diabetes, insulin injections, and desire to exercise, you should suspect that:
A. he has probably exercised too much and pulled a muscle.
B. this is not related to his diabetes because his mental status is intact.
C. he may very well be having a heart attack and should be treated.
D. this is highly suggestive of a hyperglycemic diabetic reaction.

Challenging Questions

8. Altered mental status in the older diabetic patient may mimic the signs and symptoms of what conditions?

9. What is the biggest difference between insulin shock in an adult and insulin shock in a child?

10. Why is hypoglycemia (insulin shock) considered more of an immediate emergency than hyperglycemia (diabetic coma)?

Points to Ponder

You respond to an elderly woman with a seriously infected foot. Her neighbor called 9-1-1 because she did not know the severity of the problem. The elderly woman is diabetic and the diabetes has led to blindness and amputation of her other foot. For some reason you and the elderly woman "connect" and she trusts you. The woman is very scared that she will have to have this foot amputated also. While transporting her you realize that she is very much like your grandmother. By the time you get to the hospital the woman is very relaxed and you are talking about many different things. Once you are in the emergency department the woman becomes very scared again and asks if you can stay with her until her daughter arrives. What would you tell this woman?

Would you stay with her? Would it be appropriate to come back after your shift and check on her?

Issues Communication, Patient Relationships, Total Patient Care, Understanding Patient's Feelings and Experiences.

Online Outlook

There is a wealth of information about diabetes on the World Wide Web. Explore some of these Internet resources by completing Exercise 15 at www.emtb.com.

www.emtb.com

Allergic Reactions and Envenomations

Objectives

Cognitive

1. Recognize the patient experiencing an allergic reaction (p 416).
2. Describe the emergency medical care of the patient with an allergic reaction (p 419).
3. Establish the relationship between the patient with an allergic reaction and airway management (p 419).
4. Describe the mechanisms of allergic response and the implications for airway management (p 420).
5. State the generic and trade names, medication forms, dose, administration, action, and contraindications for the epinephrine auto-injector (p 420).
6. Evaluate the need for medical direction in the emergency medical care of the patient with an allergic reaction (p 420).
7. Differentiate between the general category of those patients having an allergic reaction, and those patients having an allergic reaction and requiring immediate medical care, including immediate use of an epinephrine auto-injector (p 419).

Affective

8. Explain the rationale for administering epinephrine using an auto-injector (p 420).

Psychomotor

9. Demonstrate the emergency medical care of the patient experiencing an allergic reaction (p 419).
10. Demonstrate the use of an epinephrine auto-injector (p 420).
11. Demonstrate the assessment and documentation of patient response to an epinephrine injection (p 421).
12. Demonstrate proper disposal of equipment (p 420).
13. Demonstrate completing a prehospital care report for patients with allergic emergencies (p 299).

Dispatch receives a call from a frantic mom who keeps screaming, "My son can't breathe and his face is swelling." While most allergic reactions aren't life threatening, they can still be very frightening for the patient and family members.

This chapter will give you the background to help you calmly manage these frantic calls and also help you answer the following questions:

1. Why does the time between exposure and reaction often indicate the severity of an allergic reaction?

2. What is the primary mechanism of an allergic reaction, and how can it have an impact on airway patency?

Allergic Reactions and Envenomations

Every year, at least 1,000 Americans die of acute allergic reactions. In dealing with allergy-related emergencies, you must be aware of the possibility of acute airway obstruction and cardiovascular collapse and be prepared to treat these life-threatening complications. You must also be able to distinguish between the body's usual response to a sting or bite and an allergic reaction, which may require epinephrine. Your ability to recognize and manage the many signs and symptoms of allergic reactions may be the only thing standing between a patient and imminent death.

This chapter begins by describing the five categories of stimuli that may provoke allergic reactions. It then goes into considerable detail about insect stings and the typical reactions to them that occur among people who are, and those who are not, allergic to bees, wasps, yellow jackets, and hornets. You will learn what to look for in assessing patients who may be having an allergic reaction and how to care for them, including administration of epinephrine. The chapter then describes specific bites from poisonous spiders and snakes, ticks, dogs, humans, and marine animals.

Allergic Reactions

Contrary to what many people think, an **allergic reaction**, an exaggerated immune response to any substance, is not caused directly by an outside stimulus, such as a bite or sting. Rather, it is a reaction by the body's immune system, which releases chemicals to combat the stimulus. Among these chemicals are **histamines** and **leukotrienes**. An allergic reaction may be mild and local, involving hives, itching, or tenderness, or it may be severe and systemic, resulting in shock and respiratory failure.

Anaphylaxis is an extreme allergic reaction that is not always life threatening, but it typically involves multiple organ systems. In severe cases, anaphylaxis can rapidly result in death. Two of the most common signs of anaphylaxis are **wheezing**, a high-pitched, whistling breath sound usually resulting from bronchospasm and typically heard on expiration, and widespread **urticaria**, or hives. Urticaria consists of small areas of generalized itching or burning that appear as multiple, small, raised areas on the skin (▼ Figure 16-1).

Given the right person and the right circumstances, almost any substance can trigger the body's immune system and cause an allergic reaction: animal bites, food, latex gloves, or even semen can be an **allergen**. The most common allergens, however, fall into the following five general categories:

Figure 16-1 Urticaria, or hives, may appear following a sting and is characterized by multiple, small, raised areas on the skin. Urticaria may be one of the warning signs of impending anaphylactic reaction.

> Anaphylaxis is a severe allergic reaction that may be life threatening and typically involves multiple organ systems.

- **Insect bites and stings.** When an insect bites you and injects the bite with its venom, the act is called **envenomation** or, more commonly, a sting. The sting of a honeybee, wasp, ant, yellow jacket, or hornet may cause a severe reaction with the swiftness of an injected medication. The reaction may be local, causing swelling and itchiness in the surrounding tissue, or it may be systemic, involving the entire body. Such a total body reaction would be considered an anaphylactic reaction.

- **Medications.** Injection of medications such as penicillin may cause an immediate (within 30 minutes) and severe allergic reaction. However, reactions to oral medications, such as oral penicillin, may be slower in onset (more than 30 minutes) but equally severe. The fact that a person has taken a medication once without experiencing an allergic reaction is no guarantee that he or she will not have an allergic reaction to it the next time around.

- **Plants.** Individuals who inhale dusts, pollens, or other plant materials to which they are sensitive may experience a rapid and severe allergic reaction.

- **Food.** Eating certain foods, such as shellfish or nuts, may result in a relatively slow (more than 30 minutes) reaction that still can be quite severe. The person may be unaware of the exposure or inciting agent.

- **Chemicals.** Certain chemicals, makeup, soap, latex, and various other substances can cause severe allergic reactions.

Insect Stings

There are more than 100,000 species of bees, wasps, and hornets. Deaths from anaphylactic reactions to stinging insects far outnumber deaths from snake bites. The stinging organ of most bees, wasps, yellow jackets, and hornets is a small hollow spine projecting from the abdomen. Venom can be injected through this spine directly into the skin. The stinger of the honeybee is barbed, so the bee cannot withdraw it (▼ **Figure 16-2A**). Therefore, the bee leaves a part of its abdomen embedded with the stinger and dies shortly after flying away. Wasps and hornets have no such handicap; they can sting repeatedly (▼ **Figure 16-2B**). Since these insects usually fly away after stinging, it is often impossible to identify which species was responsible for the injury.

Figure 16-2   Most stinging insects inject venom through a small, hollow spine that projects from the abdomen. **A.** The stinger of the honeybee is barbed and cannot be withdrawn once the bee has stung someone. **B.** The wasp's stinger is unbarbed, meaning that it can inflict multiple stings.

Some ants, especially the fire ant (Formicoidea, ▸ **Figure 16-3A**), also strike repeatedly, often injecting a particularly irritating <u>toxin</u>, or poison, at the bite sites. It is not uncommon for a patient to sustain multiple ant bites, usually on the feet and legs, within a very short period of time ▸ **Figure 16-3B** .

Signs and symptoms of insect stings or bites include sudden pain, swelling, localized heat, and redness in light-skinned individuals, usually at the site of injury. There may be itching and sometimes a <u>**wheal**</u>, which is a raised, swollen, well-defined area on the skin ▸ **Figure 16-4** . There is no specific treatment for these injuries, although applying ice sometimes makes them less irritating. The swelling associated with an insect bite may be dramatic and sometimes frightening to patients. However, these local manifestations are usually not serious.

Because the stinger of the honeybee remains in the wound, it can continue to inject venom for up to 20 minutes after the bee has flown away. In caring for a patient who has been stung by a honeybee, you should gently attempt to remove the stinger and attached muscle by scraping the skin with the edge of a sharp, stiff object such as a credit card ▸ **Figure 16-5** . Generally, you should not use tweezers or forceps, as squeezing may cause the stinger to inject still more venom into the wound. Gently wash the area with soap and water or a mild antiseptic. Try to remove any jewelry from the area before swelling begins. Position the injection site slightly below the level of the heart and apply ice or cold packs to the area, but not directly on the skin, to help relieve pain and slow the absorption of the toxin. Be alert for vomiting or any signs of shock or allergic reaction, and do not give the patient anything by mouth. Place the patient in the shock position and give oxygen if needed. Monitor the patient's vital signs and be prepared to provide further support as needed.

Anaphylactic Reaction to Stings

Approximately 5% of all people are allergic to the venom of the bee, hornet, yellow jacket, or wasp. This type of allergy, which accounts for about 200 deaths per year, can cause very severe reactions, including anaphylaxis. Patients may experience generalized itching and burning, widespread urticaria, wheals, swelling about the lips and tongue, bronchospasm and wheezing, chest tightness and coughing, dyspnea, anxiety, abdominal cramps, and hypotension. Occasionally, respiratory failure occurs.

If untreated, such an anaphylactic reaction can proceed rapidly to death. In fact, more than two thirds of

Figure 16-3 **A.** The fire ant. **B.** Fire ants inject an irritating toxin at multiple sites. Bites are generally found on the feet and the legs and appear as multiple small raised pustules.

Figure 16-4 A wheal is a whitish, firm elevation of the skin that occurs after an insect sting or bite.

Figure 16-5 To remove the stinger of a honeybee, gently scrape the skin with the edge of a sharp, stiff object such as a credit card.

patients who die of anaphylaxis do so within the first half hour, so speed on your part is essential.

Patient Assessment

Begin by performing a scene size-up, which in some cases of can lead you to possible answers. Second, perform your initial assessment. A patient may have bite or sting marks that may identify with other signs and symptoms an allergic reation. Assess baseline vital signs and get a SAMPLE history. Then collect a focused history and perform a physical examination. Allergic symptoms are almost as varied as allergens themselves. Your assessment of the patient experiencing an allergic reaction should include evaluations of the respiratory system, circulatory system, mental status, and the skin ▼ Table 16-1 .

Wheezing occurs because excessive fluid and mucus are secreted into the bronchial passages, and muscles around these passages tighten in reaction to the allergen. Exhalation, normally the passive, relaxed part of breathing, becomes harder as the patient tries to cough up the secretions or move air past the constricted airways. The fluid in the air passages and the constricted bronchi together produce the wheezing sound. Breathing rapidly becomes more difficult, and the patient may even stop breathing. Prolonged respiratory difficulty can cause a rapid heartbeat (tachycardia),

EMT-B Tips

While one EMT-B is getting oxygen ready, the other should be assisting the patient into a supine position with the head and shoulders elevated. This will help perfusion to the brain while easing respiratory effort.

shock, and even death. <u>Stridor</u>, a harsh, high-pitched inspiratory sound, occurs when swelling in the upper airway (near the vocal cords and throat) closes off the airway and can eventually lead to total obstruction.

Remember, the presence of hypoperfusion (shock) or respiratory distress indicates that the patient is having a severe enough allergic reaction to lead to death.

Emergency Medical Care

If the patient seems to be having an allergic reaction, you should give 100% oxygen by nonrebreathing mask as you complete the initial assessment. Perform a focused history and physical examination. Find out whether the patient has a history of allergies, what the patient was exposed to, and how the patient was exposed. Determine what the effects of the exposure have been and how they have progressed. Find out what interventions have been completed. Inform medical control about the patient's

---

TABLE 16-1 Common Signs and Symptoms of Allergic Reaction

Respiratory System

- Sneezing or an itchy, runny nose (initially)
- Tightness in the chest or throat
- Irritating, persistent dry cough
- Hoarseness
- Respirations that become rapid, labored, or noisy
- Wheezing and/or stridor

Circulatory System

- Decrease in blood pressure as the blood vessels dilate
- Increase in pulse rate (initially)
- Pale skin and dizziness, as the vascular system fails
- Loss of consciousness and coma

Skin

- Flushing, itching, or burning skin; especially common over the face and upper chest
- Urticaria over large areas of the body, both internally and externally
- Swelling, especially of the face, neck, hands, feet, and/or tongue
- Swelling and cyanosis or pallor around the lips
- Warm, tingling feeling in the face, mouth, chest, feet, and hands

Other Findings

- Anxiety, a sense of impending doom
- Abdominal cramps
- Headache
- Itchy, watery eyes
- Decreasing mental status

condition, then find out whether the patient has any prescribed, preloaded medications for allergic reactions. If necessary, be prepared to use standard airway procedures and positive pressure ventilation according to the principles identified in Chapter 7.

If the patient appears to be having a severe allergic (or anaphylactic) reaction, you should administer BLS at once and provide prompt transport to the hospital. You may wish to request ALS backup if you work in a tiered response system. In addition to providing oxygen, you should be prepared to maintain an airway or give CPR. Placing ice over the injury site has been thought to slow absorption of the toxin and diminish swelling, but ice packs placed directly on the skin may freeze it and cause more damage. Like any other attempt to reduce swelling with ice, you should be careful not to overdo the icing. In some areas, you may be allowed to assist the patient with epinephrine.

Whether made by the body (adrenaline) or by a drug manufacturer, **epinephrine** works rapidly to raise the pulse rate and blood pressure by constricting the blood vessels. Epinephrine also inhibits the allergic reaction and dilates the bronchioles. All bee sting kits should contain a prepared syringe of epinephrine, ready for intramuscular injection, along with instructions for its use. Your EMS service may or may not allow you to help patients self-administer epinephrine to combat allergic reactions or anaphylaxis. In some places, the medical director may authorize you to carry an epinephrine auto-injector (EpiPen) or to assist patients that have their own EpiPen. The adult system delivers 0.3 mg of epinephrine via an automatic needle and syringe system; the infant/child system delivers 0.15 mg (▶ **Figure 16-6A**).

If the patient is able to use the auto-injector on his or her own, your role is limited to helping. To use, or help the patient use, the auto-injector, you should first **receive a direct order from medical control** or follow local protocols or standing orders. **Follow BSI precautions, and make sure the medication has been prescribed** specifically for that patient. If it has not, do not give the medication: inform medical control, and provide immediate transport. **Finally, make sure the medication is not discolored** or expired.

Once you have done these things, follow the steps in (▶ **Skill Drill 16-1**) to use an auto-injector.

1. **Remove the safety cap** from the auto-injector and, if possible, wipe the patient's thigh with alcohol or some other antiseptic. However, do not delay administration of the drug **(Step 1)**.

2. **Place the tip of the auto-injector** against the lateral part of the patient's thigh, midway between the waist and the knee **(Step 2)**.

Figure 16-6 Patients who experience severe allergic reactions often carry their own epinephrine, which comes predosed in an auto-injector or a standard syringe. **A.** EpiPen auto-injectors (1–unfired adult model, 2–fired junior model). **B.** AnaKit with epinephrine syringe.

3. **Push the injector firmly** against the thigh until the injector activates, about 5 to 10 seconds. This action will help prevent the kick that the spring-loaded syringe can cause when the needle is pulled from the injection site too soon. Hold the injector in place until the medication is injected (10 seconds). **(Step 3)**.

4. **Remove the injector** from the patient's thigh and dispose of it in the proper biohazard container.

5. **Record the time and dose** of injection on your run sheet.

6. **Reassess and record** the patient's vital signs after using the auto-injector.

If the patient is known to be allergic, he or she might carry a commercial bee sting kit (AnaKit) that contains a standard syringe of epinephrine for intramuscular injection (▲ **Figure 16-6B**). If you will administer this

Skill Drill 16-1   Using an Auto-Injector

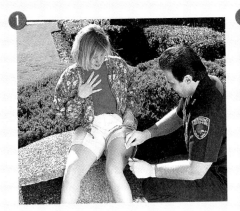

Remove the auto-injector's safety cap and quickly wipe the thigh with antiseptic.

Place the tip of the auto-injector against the lateral thigh.

Push the auto-injector firmly against the thigh and hold it in place until all the medication is injected.

---

epinephrine, make the same general preparations you make for an auto-injector: Get an order, take BSI precautions, and ensure that the medicine is the patient's and is not discolored or expired. Follow the steps in

▶ **Skill Drill 16-2** to administer epinephrine from an AnaKit:

1. **Prepare the injection site** with an alcohol wipe or other antiseptic, if there is time. Remove the needle cover **(Step 1)**.

2. **Hold the syringe upright** so any air inside rises to the base of the needle. Remove the air by slowly depressing the syringe plunger until fluid just slightly squirts from the needle tip **(Step 2)**.

3. **Turn the plunger** one-quarter turn **(Step 3)**.

4. **Insert the needle quickly,** straight into the injection site, deep enough to place the tip into the muscle beneath the skin and subcutaneous fat **(Step 4)**.

5. **Holding the syringe steady,** push the plunger until it stops, to ensure that all medication is injected **(Step 5)**.

6. **Have the patient take the Chlo-Amine tablets** in the kit **(Step 6)**.

7. If you have or can **make a cold pack,** apply it to the site of the sting to reduce swelling and minimize the amount of venom that enters the circulation **(Step 7)**.

Other bee sting kits contain some oral or IV *antihistamines,* agents that block the effect of histamine. These work relatively slowly, within several minutes to 1 hour. Because epinephrine can have an effect within 1 minute, it is the primary way to save the life of someone having a severe anaphylactic reaction.

In some areas of the country, EMT-B squads can administer epinephrine for anaphylaxis. Follow your local protocols or medical direction, but generally you will inject 0.3 to 0.5 mL of 1/1,000 epinephrine solution to an adult weighing more than 50 kg intramuscularly or subcutaneously at intervals of 5 to 15 minutes, as needed. Doses for children vary, ranging from 0.1 to 0.3 mL, depending on the patient's weight. Be aware that the medication may cause significant tachycardia as well as increased anxiety or nervousness. Complete the emergency care outlined above for this patient, and provide prompt transport, closely monitoring vital signs frequently. Remember that all patients with suspected anaphylaxis should be given high-flow, high-concentration oxygen.

Because epinephrine constricts blood vessels, it may cause the patient's blood pressure to rise significantly. Other side effects include tachycardia, pallor, dizziness, chest pain, headache, nausea, and vomiting. All these effects may cause the patient to feel anxious or excited. These side effects are worth the trade-off when epinephrine is used in a life-threatening situation. However, if the patient has no signs of respiratory distress or shock

Skill Drill 16-2 Using an AnaKit

1 Prepare the injection site with antiseptic and remove the needle cover.

2 Hold the syringe upright and carefully use the plunger to remove air.

3 Turn the plunger one-quarter turn.

4 Quickly insert the needle into the muscle.

5 Hold the syringe steady and push the plunger until it stops.

6 Have the patient take the Chlo-Amine tablets provided in the kit.

7 If available, apply a cold pack to the sting site.

after contact with a substance that causes an allergic reaction, continue with the focused history and physical exam. Note that patients who are not wheezing, or who have no signs of respiratory compromise or hypotension, should not be given epinephrine.

Whether or not your emergency treatment includes epinephrine, you should always provide prompt transport for any patient who may be having an allergic reaction or has experienced a poisonous envenomation or bite. Continue to reassess the patient's vital signs en route; remember that signs and symptoms may change rapidly. You may need to give more than one injection of epinephrine if you note that the patient has decreasing mental status, increased breathing difficulty, or a decreasing blood pressure. Be sure to consult medical control first. Current auto-injectors give only one dose,

EMT-B Tips

If your medical director and protocols allow it, and your patient has an inhaler as well as an epinephrine auto-injector, one EMT-B can help administer the inhaler while the other administers the epinephrine.

and a patient who needs more than one dose will need to have more than one injector. As with any patient you are transporting, be prepared to treat for shock, begin BLS measures, or use the AED if necessary.

If the patient's condition improves, provide supportive care, including giving the patient oxygen during transport.

Specific Bites and Envenomations

Spider Bites

Spiders are both numerous and widespread in the United States. Many species of spiders bite. However, only two, the female black widow spider and the brown recluse spider, are able to deliver serious, even life-threatening bites. When you care for a patient who has had some type of bite, be alert to the possibility that the spider may still be in the area, although it is not likely. Remember that your safety is of paramount importance.

BLACK WIDOW SPIDER. The female black widow spider (*Latrodectus*) is fairly large as far as spiders go, measuring approximately 2″ long with its legs extended. It is usually black and has a distinctive, bright red-orange marking in the shape of an hourglass on its abdomen (▼ **Figure 16-7**). The female is larger and more toxic than the male. Black widow spiders are found in every state except Alaska. They prefer dry, dim places around buildings, in woodpiles, and among debris.

The bite of the black widow spider is sometimes overlooked. If the site becomes numb right away, the patient may not even recall being bit. However, most black widow spider bites cause localized pain and symptoms, including agonizing muscle spasms. In some cases, a bite on the abdomen causes muscle spasms so severe that the patient may be thought to have an acute abdomen, possibly peritonitis. The main danger with this type of bite, however, comes from the fact that the black widow's venom is poisonous to nerve tissues (neurotoxic). Other systemic symptoms include dizziness, sweating, nausea, vomiting, and rashes. Tightness in the chest and difficulty breathing develop within 24 hours, as well as severe cramps, with board-like rigidity of the abdominal muscles. Generally, these signs and symptoms subside over 48 hours.

If necessary, a physician can administer a specific **antivenin**, a serum containing antibodies that counteract the venom, but because of a high incidence of side effects, its use is reserved for very severe bites, for the aged or very feeble, and for children younger than

Allergic reactions and responses to bites and stings can progress quickly to the level of life threats. With good care, severe signs and symptoms may subside just as quickly. Doing a multisystem exam and documenting your findings is thus important both before and after treatment. Pay particular attention to skin signs and respiratory, circulatory, and mental function.

5 years. The severe muscle spasms are usually treated in the hospital with IV benzodiazepines such as diazepam (Valium) or lorazepam (Ativan). In general, emergency treatment for a black widow spider bite consists of BLS for the patient in respiratory distress. Much more often, the patient will merely require relief from pain. Transport the patient to the emergency department as soon as possible for treatment of both pain and muscle rigidity. If possible, bring the spider along.

BROWN RECLUSE SPIDER. The brown recluse spider (*Loxosceles*) is dull brown and, at 1″, somewhat smaller than the black widow (▼ **Figure 16-8**). The short-haired body has a violin-shaped mark, brown to yellow in color, on its back. Although it lives mostly in the southern and central parts of the country, the brown recluse may be found throughout the continental United States. The spider takes its name from the fact that it tends to live in dark areas: in corners of old, unused buildings, under rocks, and in woodpiles. In cooler areas, it moves indoors to closets, drawers, cellars, and old piles of clothing.

In contrast to the venom of the black widow spider, the venom of the brown recluse spider is not neurotoxic but cytotoxic; that is, it causes severe local tissue damage. Typically, the bite is not painful at first but becomes so within hours. The area becomes swollen and tender, developing a pale, mottled, cyanotic center and possibly a small blister (▶ **Figure 16-9**). Over the next several days, a scab of dead skin, fat, and debris

Figure 16-7 Black widow spiders are distinguished by their glossy black color and bright orange hourglass marking on the abdomen.

Figure 16-8 Brown recluse spiders are dull brown and have a dark, violin-shaped mark on the back.

Figure 16-9 The bite of a brown recluse spider is characterized by swelling, tenderness, and a pale, mottled cyanotic center. There may also be a small blister on the bite.

will form and dig down into the skin, producing a large ulcer that may not heal unless treated promptly. Transport patients with such symptoms as soon as possible.

Brown recluse spider bites rarely cause systemic symptoms and signs. When they do, the initial treatment is BLS and transportation to the emergency department. Again, it is helpful if you can identify the spider and bring it to the hospital along with the patient.

Snake Bites

Snake bites are a worldwide problem of some significance. More than 300,000 injuries from snake bites occur annually, including 30,000 to 40,000 deaths. The greatest number of the fatalities occur in Southeast Asia and India (25,000 to 30,000) and in South America (3,000 to 4,000). In the United States, 40,000 to 50,000 snake bites are reported annually, about 7,000 of them caused by poisonous snakes. However, snake bite fatalities in the United States are extremely rare, about 15 a year for the entire country.

Of the approximately 115 different species of snakes in the United States, only 19 are venomous. These include the rattlesnake (*Crotalus*), the copperhead (*Agkistrodon contortrix*), the cottonmouth, or water moccasin (*Agkistrodon piscivorus*), and the coral snakes (*Micrurus* and *Micruroides*) ▶ **Figure 16-10** . At least one of these poisonous species is found in every state except Alaska, Hawaii, and Maine. As a general rule, these creatures are timid. They usually do not bite unless provoked, angered, or accidentally injured, as when they are stepped on. There are a few exceptions to these rules. Cottonmouths are often rather aggressive, and very little provocation is needed to annoy a rattlesnake. Coral snakes, by contrast, are very shy and usually bite only when they are being handled.

Most snake bites occur between April and October, when the animals are active, and tend to involve young men who have been drinking alcohol. Texas reports the largest number of bites. Other states with a major concentration of snake bites are Louisiana, Georgia, Oklahoma, North Carolina, Arkansas, West Virginia, and Mississippi. If you work in one of these areas,

Figure 16-10
A. Rattlesnake.
B. Copperhead.
C. Coral snake.
D. Cottonmouth.

you should be thoroughly familiar with the emergency handling of snake bites. Remember, almost any time you are caring for a patient with a snake bite, another snake could come along and create a second victim: you. Therefore, use extreme caution on these calls, and be sure to wear the proper protective equipment for the area.

In general, only a third of snake bites result in significant local or systemic injuries. Often, envenomation does not occur because the snake has recently struck another animal and exhausted its supply of venom.

With the exception of the coral snake, poisonous snakes native to the United States all have hollow fangs in the roof of the mouth that inject the poison from two sacs at the back of the head. The classic appearance of the poisonous snake bite, therefore, is two small puncture wounds, usually about ½" apart, with discoloration, swelling, and pain surrounding them (▼ **Figure 16-11**). Nonpoisonous snakes can also bite, usually leaving a horseshoe of tooth marks. However, some poisonous snakes have teeth as well as fangs, making it impossible to say which kind is responsible for a given set of tooth marks. On the other hand, fang marks are a clear indication of a poisonous snake bite.

PIT VIPERS. Rattlesnakes, copperheads, and cottonmouths are all pit vipers, with triangular-shaped, flat heads (▼ **Figure 16-12**). They take their name from the small pits located just behind each nostril and in front of each eye. The pit is a heat-sensing organ that allows the snake to strike accurately at any warm target, especially in the dark when it cannot see through its vertical, slit-like pupils.

The fangs of the pit viper normally lie flat against the roof of the mouth and are hinged to swing back and forth as the mouth opens. When the snake is striking, the mouth opens wide and the fangs extend; in this way, the fangs penetrate whatever the mouth strikes. The fangs are actually special hollow teeth that act much like hypodermic needles. They are connected to a sac containing a reservoir of venom, which in turn is attached to a poison gland. The gland itself is a specially adapted salivary gland, which produces powerful enzymes that digest and destroy tissue. The primary purpose of the venom is to kill small animals and to start the digestive process prior to their being eaten.

The most common form of pit viper is the rattlesnake. Several different species of rattlesnake can be identified by the rattle on the tail. The rattle is actually numerous layers of dried skin that were shed but failed to fall off, coming to rest against a small knob on the end of the tail. Rattlesnakes have many patterns of color, often with a diamond pattern. They can grow to 6' or more in length.

Copperheads are smaller than rattlesnakes, usually 2' to 3' long, with a reddish coppery color crossed with brown or red bands. These snakes typically inhabit woodpiles and abandoned dwellings, often close to areas of habitation. Although they account for most of the venomous snake bites in the eastern United States, copperhead bites are almost never fatal; however, note that the venom can destroy extremities.

Cottonmouths grow to about 4' in length. Also called water moccasins, these snakes are olive or brown, with black cross-bands and a yellow undersurface. They are water snakes, with a particularly aggressive pattern of behavior. Although fatalities from these snake bites are rare, tissue destruction from the venom may be severe.

The signs of envenomation by a pit viper are severe burning pain at the site of the injury, followed by

Figure 16-11 A snake bite wound from a poisonous snake has characteristic markings: two small puncture wounds about ½" apart, discoloration, and swelling.

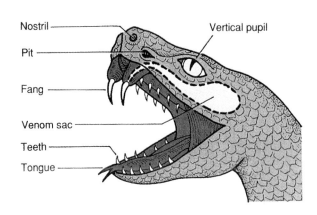

Figure 16-12 Pit vipers have small, heat-sensing organs (pits) located in front of their eyes that allow them to strike at warm targets, even in the dark.

swelling and a bluish discoloration (ecchymosis) in light-skinned individuals that signals bleeding under the skin. These signs are evident within 5 to 10 minutes after the bite has occurred and spread over the next 36 hours. In addition to destroying tissues locally, the venom of the pit viper can also interfere with the body's clotting mechanism and cause bleeding at various distant sites. Other systemic signs, which may or may not occur, include weakness, sweating, fainting, and shock. If the patient has no local signs an hour after being bitten, it is safe to assume that envenomation did not take place. If swelling has occurred, you should mark its edges on the skin. This will allow physicians to assess what has happened, and when it happened, with greater accuracy.

Occasionally, a patient bitten by a snake will faint from fright. The patient will usually regain consciousness promptly when placed in a supine position. Do not confuse a fainting spell with shock. If shock occurs, it will happen much later.

In treating a snake bite from a pit viper, follow these steps to get the patient to the hospital in a timely fashion:

1. Calm the patient; assure him or her that poisonous snake bites are rarely fatal. Have the patient supine, and explain that staying quiet will slow the spread of any venom through the system.

2. Locate the bite area; clean it gently with soap and water or a mild antiseptic. **Do not apply ice to the area.**

3. If the bite occurred on an arm or leg, splint the extremity to decrease movement.

4. Be alert for vomiting, which may be a sign of anxiety rather than the toxin itself.

5. Do not give anything by mouth.

6. If, as rarely happens, the patient was bitten on the trunk, keep him or her supine and quiet and transport as quickly as possible.

7. Monitor the patient's vital signs and mark the skin with a pen over the area that is swollen, proximal to the swelling, to note whether swelling is spreading.

8. If there are any signs of shock, place the patient in the shock position and give oxygen.

9. If the snake has been killed, as is often the case, be sure to bring it with you so that physicians can identify it and administer the proper antivenin.

EMT-B Safety

Evidence of the exact source of an allergic reaction or envenomation may be scarce when you arrive, or bystanders may give you incorrect information. The cause is more likely to pose a risk to responders, and added risk to the patient, if you draw incorrect conclusions about its nature. Keep your eyes and ears open, avoid making unsupported assumptions, and be curious about things that don't quite make sense.

10. Notify the hospital that you are bringing in a snake bite patient; if possible, describe the snake.

11. Transport the patient promptly to the hospital.

If the patient shows no sign of envenomation, provide BLS as needed, place a sterile dressing over the suspected bite area, and immobilize the injury site. All patients with suspected snake bite should be taken to the emergency department, whether they show signs of envenomation or not. Treat the wound as you would any deep puncture wound to prevent infection.

If you work in an area where poisonous snakes are known to live, you should know the local protocol for handling snake bites. You should also know the address of the nearest facility where anti-venin is available. This may be a nearby zoo, the local or public state health department, or a local community hospital.

Coral snakes. The coral snake is a small reptile with a series of bright red, yellow, and black bands completely encircling the body. Many harmless snakes have similar coloring, but only the coral snake has red and yellow bands next to one another, as this helpful rhyme suggests: "Red on yellow will kill a fellow; red on black, venom will lack."

A rare creature that lives primarily in Florida and in the desert Southwest, the coral snake is a relative of the cobra. It has tiny fangs and injects the venom with its teeth by a chewing motion, leaving behind one or more puncture or scratch-like wounds. Because of its small mouth and teeth and limited jaw expansion, the coral snake usually bites its victims on a small part of the body, such as a finger or toe.

Coral snake venom is a powerful toxin that causes paralysis of the nervous system. Within a few hours of being bitten, a patient will exhibit bizarre behavior, followed by progressive paralysis of eye movements and respiration. Often, there are limited or no local symptoms.

Successful treatment, either emergency or long term, depends on positive identification of the snake and support of respiration. Antivenin is available, but most hospitals do not stock it. Therefore, you should notify the hospital of the need for it as soon as possible. The steps for emergency care of a coral snake bite are as follows:

1. Immediately quiet and reassure the patient.

2. Flush the area of the bite with 1 to 2 quarts of warm, soapy water to wash away any poison left on the surface of the skin. **Do not apply ice to the region.**

3. Splint the extremity to minimize movement and the spread of venom at the site.

4. Check the patient's vital signs and continue to monitor them.

5. Keep the patient warm and elevate the lower extremities to help prevent shock.

6. Give supplemental oxygen if needed.

7. Transport the patient promptly to the emergency department, giving advance notice that the patient has been bitten by a coral snake.

8. Give the patient nothing by mouth.

Scorpion Stings

Scorpions are eight-legged arachnids from the biological group Arachnida with a venom gland and a stinger at the end of their tail (▼ Figure 16-13). Scorpions are rare; they live primarily in the southwestern United States and in deserts. With one exception, a scorpion's sting is usually very painful but not dangerous, causing localized swelling and discoloration. The exception is the *Centruroides sculpturatus*. Although it is found naturally in Arizona and New Mexico, as well as parts of Texas, California, and Nevada, it may be kept as a pet by anyone. The venom of this particular species may produce a severe systemic reaction that brings about circulatory collapse, severe muscle contractions, excessive salivation, hypertension, convulsions, and cardiac failure. Antivenin is available but must be administered by a physician. If you are called to care for a patient with a suspected sting from *sculpturatus*, you should

notify medical control as soon as possible. Administer all the elements of BLS and transport the patient to the emergency department as rapidly as possible.

Tick Bites

Found most often on brush, shrubs, trees, sand dunes, or other animals, ticks usually attach themselves directly to the skin (▼ Figure 16-14). Only a fraction of an inch long, they can easily be mistaken for a freckle, especially since their bite is not painful. Indeed, the danger with a tick bite is not from the bite itself, but from the infecting organisms that the tick carries. Ticks commonly carry two infectious diseases: Rocky Mountain spotted fever and Lyme disease. Both are spread through the tick's saliva, which is injected into the skin when the tick attaches itself.

Rocky Mountain spotted fever, which is not limited to the Rocky Mountains, occurs within 7 to 10 days after a bite by an infected tick. Its symptoms include nausea, vomiting, headache, weakness, paralysis, and possibly cardiorespiratory collapse.

Lyme disease has received extensive publicity. It is, after AIDS, the second most rapidly growing infectious disease in the United States. Originally seen only in Connecticut, Lyme disease has now been reported in 35 states. It occurs most commonly in the Northeast, the Great Lake States, and the Pacific Northwest; New York State reports the largest number of cases. The first symptom, a rash that may spread to several parts of the body, begins about 3 days after the bite of an infected tick. The rash may eventually resemble a target bull's-eye pattern in one third of patients (▼ Figure 16-15). After a few more days or weeks, painful swelling of the joints, particularly the knees, occurs. Lyme disease may be confused with rheumatoid arthritis and, like that disease, may result in permanent disability. However, if it is recognized and treated promptly with antibiotics, the patient may recover completely.

Figure 16-14   Ticks typically attach themselves directly to the skin.

Figure 16-15   The rash associated with Lyme disease has a characteristic "bull's eye" pattern.

Figure 16-13   The sting of a scorpion is usually more painful than it is dangerous, causing localized swelling and discoloration.

Tick bites occur most commonly during the summer months, when people are out in the woods wearing little protective clothing. Transmission of the infection from tick to person takes at least 12 hours, so if you are called on to remove a tick, you should proceed carefully and slowly. Do not attempt to suffocate the tick with gasoline or Vaseline or burn it with a lighted match; you will only burn the patient. Instead, using fine tweezers, grasp the tick by the body and pull it straight out of the skin. This method will usually remove the whole tick. Even if part of the tick is left embedded in the skin, the part containing the infecting organisms has been removed. Cleanse the area with disinfectant and save the tick in a glass jar or other container so that it can be identified. Do not handle the tick with your fingers. Provide any necessary supportive emergency care, and transport the patient to the hospital.

Dog Bites and Rabies

Most people who are bitten by dogs do not report the incident to a physician, believing that dog bites are not serious. They can be very serious, however. A dog's mouth is heavily contaminated with virulent bacteria. You should consider all dog bites as contaminated and potentially infected wounds that may require antibiotics, tetanus prophylaxis, and suturing (▼ Figure 16-16). Occasionally, dog bites result in mangled, complex wounds that require surgical repair. For these reasons, all dog bites should be treated by a physician. Place a dry, sterile dressing over the wound, and promptly

Figure 16-16 Dog bite wounds should be examined at the hospital, as these wounds are heavily contaminated with virulent bacteria.

transport the patient to the emergency department. If an arm or leg was injured, splint that extremity. Often, the patient will be extremely upset and frightened, a situation that calls for calm reassurance on your part.

A major concern with dog bites is the spread of *rabies*, an acute, fatal viral infection of the central nervous system that can affect all warm-blooded animals. Although rabies is extremely rare today, particularly with widespread inoculation of pets, it still exists. Stray dogs that have not been inoculated can be carriers of the disease, as can squirrels, bats, foxes, skunks, and raccoons. The virus is in the saliva of a **rabid**, or infected, animal and is transmitted through biting or licking an open wound. Infection can be prevented in a person who has been bitten by such an animal only by a series of special vaccine injections, a painful procedure that must be begun soon after the bite. Since animals that have rabies do not always show it immediately in their behavior, a person's only chance to avoid the vaccine is to find the animal and turn it over to the health department for observation and/or testing. Refer to your local animal control procedures.

Children, particularly young ones, may be seriously injured or even killed by dogs. These dogs are not always vicious or rabid; sometimes, the child had unknowingly provoked the animal. However, you must assume that it may turn and attack you as well. Therefore, you generally should not enter the scene until the animal has been secured by either the police or an animal control officer. Then you may carry out the necessary emergency care and transport the child to the emergency department.

Human Bites

The human mouth, more so than even the dog's, contains an exceptionally wide range of virulent bacteria and viruses. For this reason, you should regard any human bite that has penetrated the skin as a very serious injury. Similarly, any laceration caused by a human tooth can result in a serious, spreading infection (▶ Figure 16-17). Remember this if you have occasion to treat someone who has been punched in the mouth: The person who delivered the punch may also need treatment.

The emergency treatment for human bites consists of the following steps:

1. Promptly immobilize the area with a splint or bandage.

2. Apply a dry, sterile dressing.

3. Provide transport to the emergency department for surgical cleansing of the wound and antibiotic therapy.

Injuries from Marine Animals

Coelenterates, including the fire coral, Portuguese man-of-war, sea wasp, sea nettles, true jellyfish, sea anemones, true coral, and soft coral, are responsible for more envenomations than any other marine animals ▶ Figure 16-18 . The stinging cells of the coelenterate are called nematocysts, and large animals may discharge hundreds of thousands of them. Envenomation causes very painful, reddish lesions in light-skinned individuals extending in a line from the site of the sting. Systemic symptoms include headache, dizziness, muscle cramps, and fainting.

To treat a sting from the tentacles of a jellyfish, a Portuguese man-of-war, various anemones, corals, or hydras, remove the patient from the water and pour any type of alcohol on the affected area. Unlike fresh water, alcohol will inactivate the nematocysts. Do not try to manipulate the remaining tentacles; this will only cause further discharge of the nematocysts. Remove the tentacles by scraping them off with the edge of a sharp, stiff object such as a credit card. Persistent pain may respond to immersion of the area in hot water (110° to 115°F, 43° to 46°C) for 30 minutes. On very rare occasions, a patient may have a systemic allergic reaction to the sting of one of these animals. Treat such a patient for anaphylactic shock. Give BLS, and provide immediate transport to the hospital.

Toxins from the spines of urchins, stingrays, and certain spiny fish such as the lionfish, scorpion fish, or stonefish are heat sensitive ▶ Table 16-2 . Therefore, the best treatment for such injuries is to immobilize the affected area and soak it in hot water for 30 minutes. This will often provide dramatic relief from local pain. However, the patient still needs to be transported to the emergency department, since he or she could develop an allergic reaction or infection, including tetanus.

Figure 16-17 Human bites can result in serious, spreading infection. Thus, patients must be evaluated at the hospital.

TABLE 16-2 Common Marine Envenomations

Dogfish
Dragon fish
Fire coral
Hydroids
Jellyfish
Lionfish
Marine snail
Portuguese man-of-war
Ratfish
Scorpion fish
Sea anemone
Sea urchins
Starfish
Stingray
Stonefish
Tiger fish
Toadfish
Weever fish

Figure 16-18 Coelenterates are responsible for many marine envenomations. **A.** Jellyfish. **B.** Portuguese man-of-war. **C.** Sea anemone.

If you work near the ocean, you should be familiar with the marine life in your area. The emergency treatment of common coelenterate envenomations consists of the following steps:

1. **Limit further discharge** of nematocysts by avoiding fresh water, wet sand, showers, or careless manipulation of the tentacles. Keep the patient calm, and reduce motion of the affected extremity.

2. **Inactivate the nematocysts** by applying alcohol. (Although isopropyl or rubbing alcohol is recommended, virtually any type of alcohol, including high proof liquor or cologne, is effective.)

3. **Remove the remaining tentacles** by scraping them off with the edge of a sharp, stiff object such as a credit card. Do not use your ungloved hand to remove the tentacles, because self-envenomation will occur. Persistent pain may respond to immersion in hot water (110° to 115°F, 43° to 46°C) for 30 minutes.

4. **Provide transport** to the emergency department.

Prep Kit

Ready for Review

An allergic reaction is a response to chemicals the body releases in order to combat certain stimuli, called allergens. Allergic reactions occur most often in response to five categories of stimuli: insect bites and stings, medications, food, plants, and chemicals. The reaction may be mild and local, involving itching, redness, and tenderness; or severe and systemic, including shock and respiratory failure. Anaphylaxis is a life-threatening allergic reaction mounted by multiple organ systems, which must be treated with epinephrine. Wheezing and skin wheals can be signs of anaphylaxis. People who know that they are allergic to bee, hornet, yellow jacket, or wasp venom often carry a bee sting kit that contains epinephrine in an auto-injector. You may help to administer this medication in this form with authorization from medical control. All patients with suspected anaphylaxis require oxygen.

In assessing a person who may be having an allergic reaction, you should check for flushing, itching, and swelling skin, hives, wheezing and stridor, a persistent cough, a decrease in blood pressure, a weak pulse, dizziness, abdominal cramps, and headache.

Poisonous spiders include the black widow spider and the brown recluse spider. Poisonous snakes include pit vipers and coral snakes. A person who has been bitten by a pit viper needs prompt transport; clean the bite area and keep the patient quiet to slow the spread of venom. Notify the hospital as soon as possible if a patient has been bitten by a coral snake, as its venom can cause paralysis of the nervous system, and most hospitals do not have appropriate antivenin on hand.

Patients who have been bitten by ticks may be infected with Rocky Mountain spotted fever or Lyme disease and should see a doctor within a day or two. Remove the tick using a tweezers, and save it for identification.

Dog and human bites can both lead to serious infection and must be treated by a physician. Dogs can carry rabies, a fatal viral infection present in their saliva. Painful vaccine treatment is necessary to prevent rabies in a person who has been bitten by a dog that cannot be captured or identified. Do not try to rescue a child who is being attacked by a dog without the help of police or animal control officers.

Remember that a hundred times more people die every year from allergic reactions to food, bee stings, or medications than from the bites of venomous snakes or marine animals. Many venomous snake bites may be treated with antivenin. Many marine envenomations may benefit from submersion in hot water to deactivate the heat-sensitive toxins. Such treatment may be started in the field at the request of medical control.

Always provide prompt transport to the hospital for any patient who is having an allergic reaction or has been bitten by a poisonous insect or animal. Remember that signs and symptoms can deteriorate rapidly. Carefully monitor the patient's vital signs en route, especially for airway compromise.

Vital Vocabulary

allergen A substance that causes an allergic reaction.

allergic reaction The body's exaggerated immune response to an internal or surface agent.

anaphylaxis An extreme, possibly life-threatening systemic allergic reaction that may include shock and respiratory failure.

antivenin A serum that counteracts the effect of venom from an animal or insect.

envenomation The act of injecting venom.

epinephrine A substance produced by the body (commonly called adrenaline), and a drug produced by pharmaceutical companies that increases pulse rate and blood pressure; the drug of choice for an anaphylactic reaction.

histamine A substance released by the immune system in allergic reactions that is responsible for many of the symptoms of anaphylaxis.

leukotrienes Chemical substances that contribute to anaphylaxis; released by the immune system in allergic reactions.

rabid Describes an animal that is infected with rabies.

stridor A harsh, high-pitched respiratory sound, generally heard during inspiration, that is caused by partial blockage or narrowing of the upper airway.

toxin A poison or harmful substance.

urticaria Small spots of generalized itching and/or burning that appear as multiple raised areas on the skin; hives.

wheal A raised, swollen, well-defined area on the skin resulting from an insect bite or allergic reaction.

wheezing A high-pitched, whistling breath sound, usually caused by a partial airway blockage and typically heard on expiration.

Assessment in Action

You are dispatched to a 14-year-old girl with a possible bee sting. On arrival you find your patient seated against a rock in a park. She was on a nature hike with her middle school class. The teacher tells you the girl is allergic to bee stings and carries medicine for it. Your patient has six obvious stings, two of them on her face. The sting areas are red and swollen, and the girl says that they itch "a lot."

Initial assessment reveals that the patient is awake, anxious, and obeys command. She appears flushed, is breathing loudly and her skin is warm and moist. The patient has a blood pressure of 104/66 mm Hg, respirations of 40 breaths/min and shallow, and a pulse of 142 beats/min.

1. Because this patient has known allergies to bee stings, you should expect that she would carry:
   A. oral antibiotics.
   B. oral glucose gel.
   C. a Proventil inhaler.
   D. an epinephrine auto-injector.

2. An immediate treatment priority for this patient is to ensure adequate:
   A. circulation.
   B. oxygenation.
   C. perfusion.
   D. warmth.

3. The medical term for the patient's red, swollen areas that itch is:
   A. an allergen.
   B. urticaria.
   C. a toxin.
   D. a histamine.

4. When you listen to this patient's breath sounds you hear wheezing. Wheezing is caused by:
   A. swelling of the upper airway passages.
   B. a collection of fluid in the alveoli.
   C. constricted lower airway passages.
   D. fluid in the upper airway passages.

5. During your assessment a bystander brings an ice pack to apply to the area of the bee sting. You know that the biggest problem with applying ice to the area of the sting is:
   A. ice packs directly on the skin may freeze it and cause more damage.
   B. cooling the skin may concentrate the venom causing more tissue damage.
   C. for ice packs to really work they need to be applied for at least a hour.
   D. venom may be activated by the cooling effect causing more of a reaction.

6. Before you finish your assessment, your patient hands you a bee sting kit with an epinephrine auto-injector. The kit has her name on it and has a current date. You know that epinephrine will:
   A. lower the heart rate, lower the BP, and constrict the bronchioles.
   B. raise the heart rate, raise the BP, and dilate the bronchioles.
   C. lower the heart rate, maintain the BP, and have no effect on the bronchioles.
   D. maintain the heart rate, raise the BP, and have no effect on the bronchioles.

7. Your medical control allows you to administer an epinephrine auto-injector. The best place to give the epinephrine auto-injector is the:
   A. medial thigh.
   B. medial humerus.
   C. lateral thigh.
   D. lateral forearm.

8. After having administered epinephrine to this patient, which side effects might you expect?
   A. Apathy, drowsiness, and lack of energy
   B. Confusion, anxiety, and combativeness
   C. Nausea/vomiting, diarrhea, and abdominal pain
   D. Chest pain, headache, and nausea/vomiting

9. Use of this patient-assisted medication requires that certain criteria be met. Which of the following best describes the criteria for use of an epinephrine auto-injector? History of exposure to an allergen and:
   A. a history of severe allergic reactions.
   B. severe respiratory distress or low blood pressure.
   C. wheezing patients speaking in complete sentences.
   D. severe abdominal pain with diarrhea.

Challenging Questions

10. When conducting an assessment on a patient who is experiencing an allergic reaction, what indicators will suggest a high probability of anaphylaxis occurring?

11. When a patient has suffered a bite from a snake or any other animal, the first treatment of the wound is to gently wash or flush it with soap and water. Why?

Points to Ponder

You are enjoying a day off by going for a hike. You are about two hours from where you started when you come across a woman who asks if you can help her. You find out that her friend is a short distance off of the trail and is having trouble breathing. She tells you that he is "allergic to bee stings" and has been stung. When you find the friend, he is unresponsive, barely breathing and showing many signs of anaphylactic shock. You quickly check his pockets and find his "Epi kit." Would you administer the EpiPen? If you are off-duty, are you functioning as an EMT-B? Could the woman give you permission to give the injection? Is administration of epinephrine covered under Good Samaritan laws?

Issues On-Duty Versus Off-Duty Provision of Care, Consent, Local/State Regulations, Good Samaritan Laws, Invasive Procedures.

Online Outlook

Given the right person, almost any substance can trigger the body's immune system and cause an allergic reaction. To learn more about common allergens, complete Exercise 16 at www.emtb.com.

Substance Abuse and Poisoning

Objectives

Cognitive

1. List various ways that poisons enter the body (p 435).
2. List signs and symptoms associated with poisoning (p 435).
3. Discuss the emergency medical care for the patient with possible overdose (p 439).
4. Describe the steps in the emergency medical care for the patient with suspected poisoning (p 439).
5. Establish the relationship between the patient suffering from poisoning or overdose and airway management (p 437).
6. State the generic and trade names, indications, contraindications, medication form, dose, administration, actions, side effects, and reassessment strategies for activated charcoal (p 439).
7. Recognize the need for medical direction in caring for the patient with poisoning or overdose (p 435).

Affective

8. Explain the rationale for administering activated charcoal (p 439).
9. Explain the rationale for contacting medical direction early in the prehospital management of the poisoning or overdose patient (p 434).

Psychomotor

10. Demonstrate the steps in the emergency medical care for the patient with possible overdose (p 439).
11. Demonstrate the steps in the emergency medical care for the patient with suspected poisoning (p 439).
12. Perform the necessary steps required to provide a patient with activated charcoal (p 439).
13. Demonstrate the assessment and documentation of patient response (p 439).
14. Demonstrate proper disposal of the equipment for the administration of activated charcoal (p 439).
15. Demonstrate completing a prehospital care report for patients with a poisoning/overdose emergency (p 299).

www.emtb.com

TECHNOLOGY

Online Chapter Pretest
Interactivities
Vocabulary Explorer
Anatomy Review
Web Links
Online Review Manual
Distance Learning

Chapter FEATURES

Skill Drills
Vital Vocabulary
Pediatric Needs
Geriatric Needs
EMT-B Safety
EMT-B Tips
Documentation Tips
Remember
Prep Kit

"Rescue 6, please respond to the 8th Street bridge and see Officer Gonzalez. You have a possible 'jumper on PCP.'"

Substance abuse has been documented in society for hundreds of years. From small town to large urban center, substance abusers frequently find themselves in need of EMS interventions. This chapter will provide valuable information to help you care for these patients in addition to helping you answer the following questions:

1. Why is any information obtained from substance abusers in regard to the drugs they ingested highly suspicious?

2. Is there a difference in the signs and symptoms of an amphetamine abuser compared with a narcotics abuser? Describe them.

Substance Abuse and Poisoning

Every day, each of us comes into contact with things that are potentially poisonous. This is not surprising when you consider that almost any substance may be a poison in certain circumstances. Different doses can turn even a remedy into a poison. Consider aspirin. When taken in recommended doses, it is a safe and effective analgesic. Too much aspirin, however, can result in death.

Acute poisoning affects some 5 million children and adults each year. Chronic poisoning, often caused by abuse of medications and other substances, including tobacco, is much more common. Fortunately, deaths from poisoning are fairly rare. Rates of death from poisoning for children have decreased steadily since the 1960s, when safety caps were introduced for drug bottles and containers. Deaths from poisoning in adults, though, have been rising, the majority the result of drug abuse.

In this chapter, the term "poisoned" includes both acute and chronic poisonings. As an EMT-B, you must recognize that patients with either type of problem may have a variety of injuries. Although you cannot stop a chronic substance abuse problem, you may be able to prevent death from the acute effects of the poison.

This chapter discusses how to identify the patient who has been poisoned and how to gather clues about the poison. It describes the different ways in which poison is introduced into the body. It then discusses the signs, symptoms, and treatment of specific poisons, including sedatives and **opioids** (medicines with actions similar to morphine). Food poisoning and plant poisoning are also discussed.

Identifying the Patient and the Poison

A **poison** is any substance whose chemical action can damage body structures or impair body function. A poison can be introduced into the body through a variety of means. Poisons act by changing the normal metabolism of cells or by actually destroying them. Poisons may act acutely, as in an overdose of heroin, or chronically, as in years of alcohol or other substance abuse. **Substance abuse** is the knowing misuse of any substance to produce a desired effect (eg, cocaine intoxication).

Your primary responsibility to the patient who has been poisoned is to recognize that a poisoning has occurred. Keep in mind that very small amounts of some poisons can cause considerable damage or death. If you have even the slightest suspicion that a patient has taken a poisonous substance, you should notify medical control and begin emergency treatment at once.

Symptoms and signs of poisoning vary according to the specific agent, as shown in ▶ **Table 17-1**. Some poisons cause the pulse to speed up, while others cause it to slow down; some cause the pupils to dilate, while others cause the pupils to constrict. If respiration is depressed or difficult, cyanosis may occur. Some chemical compounds will irritate or burn the skin or mucous membranes, resulting in burning or blistering. The presence of such injuries at the mouth strongly suggests the **ingestion** (swallowing) of a poison, such as lye. If possible, consider asking the patient the following questions:

- What substance did you take?
- When did you take it (or become exposed to it)?
- How much did you ingest?
- What actions have been taken?
- How much do you weigh?

TABLE 17-1 Toxidromes: Typical Signs and Symptoms of Specific Drug Overdose

Opioid	Hypoventilation/ respiratory arrest Pinpoint pupils (miosis) Sedation/coma Hypotension	**Anticholinergics**	Tachycardia Hyperthermia Hypertension Dilated pupils (mydriasis) Dry skin and mucous membranes Sedation/agitation/seizures/ coma/delirium Decreased bowel sounds
Sympathomimetics	Hypertension Tachycardia Dilated pupils (mydriasis) Agitation/seizures Hyperthermia	**Cholinergics**	Excess defecation/urination Muscle fasciculations Pinpoint pupils (miosis) Excess lacrimation/ salivation Airway compromise Nausea/vomiting
Sedative-Hypnotics	Slurred speech Sedation/coma Hypoventilation Hypotension		

Try to determine the nature of the poison. Objects at the scene may provide clues: an overturned bottle, a needle or syringe, scattered pills, chemicals, even an overturned or damaged plant. The remains of any nearby food or drink may also be important. Place any suspicious material in a plastic bag, and take it to the hospital, along with any containers you find.

Containers can provide critical information. In addition to the name and concentration of the drug, a pill bottle label may list specific ingredients, the number of pills that were originally in the bottle, the name of the manufacturer, and the dose that was prescribed. This information can help emergency department physicians to determine how much has been ingested and what specific treatment may be required. For certain food poisonings, a food container that lists the name and location of the maker or the vendor may be of equal importance in saving the life of the patient and possibly other people.

If the patient vomits, collect the material, called **vomitus**, in a separate plastic bag so that it can be analyzed at the hospital. After providing emergency care, collecting and bagging suspicious materials and vomitus may be the most important thing you can do for the patient.

How Poisons Get Into the Body

Emergency care for the patient who has been poisoned may include a range of actions from reassuring an

EMT-B Tips

Poison Control Centers

There are several hundred poison centers in the United States. The phone number of your local poison control center is typically found on the inside cover of your local phone book. Staff persons at every center have access to information about virtually all of the commonly used medications, chemicals, and substances that could possibly be poisonous. They know the appropriate emergency treatment for each, including the antidote, if there is one. An **antidote** is a substance that will counteract the effects of a particular poison.

If you believe that a patient has been poisoned, you should immediately provide medical control with all relevant information: when the poisoning occurred; a description of the suspected poison, including the amount involved; and the patient's size, weight, and age. If necessary, medical control can contact the regional poison center and relay specific instructions back to you.

A medical toxicologist is a physician who specializes in caring for patients who have been poisoned. About 100 of these specialists work in special hospitals called Medical Toxicology Treatment Centers, located throughout the United States. At times, your medical control may divert a patient who meets certain poisoning criteria to one of these centers instead of to the closest hospital.

You and your medical control center should know the telephone number of your regional poison control center and have it available in case you come upon an unexpected case of poisoning.

anxious parent to instituting CPR. Most often, it will not include administering a specific antidote, because most poisons do not have one. Therefore, in general, the most important treatment for poisoning is diluting and/or physically removing the poisonous agent. How you do this depends on how the poison gets into the patient's body in the first place. Essentially, the four avenues to consider are as follows:

- Ingestion ▼ Figure 17-1A
- Inhalation ▼ Figure 17-1B
- Injection ▼ Figure 17-1C
- Absorption (surface contact) ▼ Figure 17-1D

Injection often can be the most worrisome avenue of poisoning. You can administer oxygen to a patient who has inhaled a poison, and you can give activated charcoal to one who has ingested a poison. You can flood the skin with water and wash out the eyes of one who has contacted a poison. However, it is difficult to remove or dilute injected poisons, a fact that makes these cases especially urgent. On the other hand, all routes of poisoning can be deadly, and each should be thought of as being equally serious.

Always consult medical control before you proceed with the treatment of any poisoning victim.

Ingested Poisons

Approximately 80% of all poisoning is by mouth (ingestion). Ingested poisons include liquids, household cleaners, contaminated food, plants, and, in the majority of cases, drugs. Ingested poisoning is usually accidental in children and, except for contaminated food, deliberate in adults. Plant poisonings are common among children, who like to explore and often bite the leaves of various bushes or shrubs.

Your goal as an EMT-B is to rapidly remove as much of the poison as possible from the gastrointestinal tract. For most poisoning victims, this emergency treatment is sufficient.

In the past, syrup of ipecac was used to cause vomiting, but today it is recommended in only a few situations in which the risk of losing consciousness is clearly ruled out. Because syrup of ipecac induces vomiting, individuals who have ingested substances that may cause diminished alertness over time might vomit and inhale the vomit into the lungs as they lose conscious-

Figure 17-1 There are four routes by which a poison can enter the body. **A.** Ingestion. **B.** Inhalation. **C.** Injection. **D.** Absorption (surface contact).

ness. As a result, syrup of ipecac is usually not carried on ambulances. Today, many EMS systems allow you to carry activated charcoal on your unit. Activated charcoal comes as a suspension that binds to the poison in the stomach and carries it out of the system. Therefore, it is both more effective and safer than syrup of ipecac. Because activated charcoal is an inky, messy fluid, you may have to do some coaxing to get the patient to drink it; try to give it in a covered cup with a straw ▼ **Figure 17-2** . Remember, you should never force this (or any other) liquid into a patient's mouth.

Although every poison will result in a specific set of symptoms and signs, you should always assess the airway, breathing, and circulation of every patient who has been poisoned. Many patients have died as a result of problems with ABC that might have been managed easily. Be prepared to provide aggressive ventilatory support and CPR to a patient who has ingested an opiate, sedative, or barbiturate, each of which can cause depression of the central nervous system (CNS) and slow breathing. Whenever poisoning is involved, you should provide prompt transport to the emergency department. The patient may need IV support and other treatments that can be given only in the hospital. If you work in a tiered system, ALS backup also may be a good idea, as these providers often carry and can administer additional medications and therapies.

Inhaled Poisons

Patients who have inhaled poison, including natural gas, certain pesticides, carbon monoxide, chlorine,

or other gases, should be moved into fresh air immediately ▼ **Figure 17-3** . Depending on how long they were exposed, they may require supplemental oxygen. Always use a self-contained breathing apparatus (SCBA) to protect yourself from poisonous fumes. Remember that once patients are removed from the toxic environment, they are not toxic to you. However, make certain that only trained rescuers remove the patient from the poisonous environment.

Some inhaled poisons, such as carbon monoxide, are odorless and produce severe hypoxia without damaging or even irritating the lungs. Others, such as chlorine, are very irritating and cause airway obstruction and pulmonary edema. The patient may report the following signs and symptoms: burning eyes, sore throat, cough, chest pain, hoarseness, wheezing, respiratory distress, dizziness, confusion, headache, or stridor in severe cases. The patient may also have seizures or an altered mental status. Some inhaled agents cause progressive lung damage, even after the patient is removed from direct exposure; the damage may not be evident for a few hours. Meanwhile, it may take 2 or 3 days or more of intensive care to reestablish normal lung function. For this reason, all patients who have inhaled poison require immediate transport to an emergency department. Be prepared to use supplemental oxygen via nonrebreathing mask and/or ventilatory support with a BVM device, if necessary. Make sure a suctioning unit is available in case the patient vomits. As with other poisonings, it is helpful to bring containers, bottles, and labels when you transport the patient to the hospital.

Figure 17-2   Activated charcoal comes as a premixed suspension that you should give, if local protocol allows, in a covered cup with a straw.

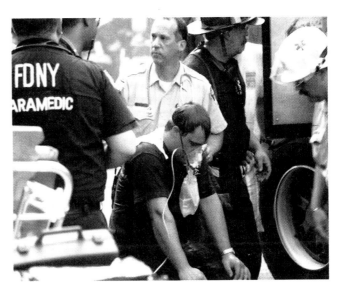

Figure 17-3   Patients who have inhaled poisons need supplemental oxygen and prompt transport to the emergency department.

Injected Poisons

Poisoning by injection is almost always the result of a deliberate drug overdose, such as heroin or cocaine ▼ Figure 17-4 . Contrary to the thinking of television detectives, the only other parties who are likely to have injected a patient with poison are insects and animals.

Signs and symptoms of poisoning by injection can have a multitude of presentations, including weakness, dizziness, fever, chills, easy excitability, or unresponsiveness.

In general, injected poisons are impossible to dilute or remove, as they are usually absorbed quickly into the body or cause intense local tissue destruction. If you suspect that rapid absorption has occurred, monitor the patient's airway, provide high-flow oxygen, and be alert for nausea and vomiting. Remove rings, watches, and bracelets from areas around the injection site if swelling occurs. Prompt transport to the emergency department is essential. Bring all containers, bottles, and labels with the patient to the hospital.

Absorbed (Surface Contact) Poisons

Many corrosive substances will damage the skin, mucous membranes, or eyes, causing chemical burns, tell-tale rashes, or lesions. Acids, alkalis, and some petroleum (hydrocarbon) products are very destructive. Signs and symptoms of absorbed poisoning include a history of exposure, liquid or powder on a patient's skin, burns, itching, irritation, redness of the skin in light-skinned individuals, or typical odors of the substance.

Emergency treatment for a typical contact poisoning includes the following two steps:

EMT-B Safety

To minimize contamination from a patient who has contacted a hazardous substance, one EMT-B should stay fully protected and assist the patient. This EMT-B is considered "contaminated." The other EMT-B should stay clear and have as little contact as possible, to be able to provide what is needed and drive without contaminating equipment and the front of the vehicle.

1. Avoid contaminating yourself or others.

2. Remove the irritating or corrosive substance from the patient as rapidly as possible.

Remove all clothing that has been contaminated with poisons or irritating substances, thoroughly brush off any dry chemicals, flush the skin with running water, then wash the skin with soap and water. When a large amount of material has been spilled on a patient, flooding the affected part for at least 20 minutes may be the fastest and most effective treatment. If the patient has a chemical agent in the eyes, you should irrigate them quickly and thoroughly, at least 5 to 10 minutes for acid substances and 15 to 20 minutes for alkalis. As you irrigate the eyes, make sure that the fluid runs from the bridge of the nose outward ▼ Figure 17-5 .

Many chemical burns occur in industrial settings, where showers and specific protocols for handling surface burns are available. If you are called to such a scene, trained people usually will be there to assist you.

Figure 17-4 Injected poisons are impossible to dilute or remove from the body; therefore, prompt transport to the emergency department is critical.

Figure 17-5 If chemical agents are in the patient's eyes, irrigate the eyes quickly and thoroughly, ensuring that the irrigation fluid runs from the bridge of the nose outward. (Use of a nasal cannula is pictured.)

Do not spend time trying to neutralize substances on the skin with additional chemicals. This may actually be more harmful. Instead, wash the substance off immediately with lots of water.

The only time you should not irrigate the contact area with water is when a poison reacts violently with water, such as contamination with phosphorus or elemental sodium. These substances ignite when they come into contact with water. Instead, brush the chemical off the patient, remove contaminated clothing, and apply a dry dressing to the burn area. Be sure to wear gloves and the proper protective clothing.

Provide prompt transport to the emergency department for definitive care. En route, continue irrigation and provide oxygen if possible.

Emergency Medical Care

External decontamination is important. Remove tablets or fragments from the patient's mouth, wash or brush poison from the patient's skin, and monitor the patient's breathing. Treatment focuses on support: assessing and maintaining the patient's ABCs.

In some cases, you will give activated charcoal to patients who have ingested poison, if approved by medical control or local protocol. Charcoal is not indicated for patients who have ingested an acid, alkali, or petroleum product; who have a decreased level of consciousness; or who are unable to swallow.

Remember that activated charcoal adsorbs, or sticks to, many commonly ingested poisons, preventing the **toxin** (poison) from being absorbed into the body by the stomach or intestines. If local protocol permits, you will likely carry plastic bottles of premixed suspension, each containing up to 50 g of activated charcoal. Some common trade names for the suspension form are InstaChar, Actidose, and LiquiChar. The usual dosage for an adult or child is 1 g of activated charcoal per kilogram of body weight. The usual adult dose is 25 to 50 g, and the usual pediatric dose is 12.5 to 25 g.

Before you give a patient charcoal, obtain approval from medical control. Next, shake the bottle vigorously to mix the suspension. The medication looks like mud, so it is best to cover the outside of the container so that the fluid is not visible, and ask the patient to drink with a straw. You might need to persuade the patient to drink it, particularly if the patient is a child, but never force it. If the patient takes a long time to drink the mixture, you will have to shake the container frequently to keep the medication mixed. Be sure to record the time when you administered the activated charcoal.

The major side effect of ingesting activated charcoal is black stools. If the patient has ingested a poison that causes nausea, he or she may vomit after taking activated charcoal, and the dosage will have to be repeated. As you reassess the patient, be prepared for vomiting, nausea, and possible airway problems.

Specific Poisons

Over time, a person who routinely misuses a substance needs increasing amounts of it to achieve the same result. This is called developing a **tolerance** to the substance. Increasing tolerance can lead to addiction. A person with an **addiction** has an overwhelming desire or need to continue using the agent, at whatever cost, with a tendency to increase the dosage. This does not happen only with the classic drugs of abuse, such as cocaine. Almost any substance can be abused, including laxatives, nasal decongestants, vitamins, and food.

The importance of BSI precautions in caring for victims of drug abuse cannot be stressed enough. Known drug abusers have a fairly high incidence of serious and undiagnosed infections, including HIV and hepatitis. These patients may bite, spit, hit, or otherwise injure you, causing you to come into contact with their blood and other body fluids. Always be sure to wear appropriate protective equipment. A calm, professional approach can defuse frightening situations, but keep your safety and that of your team uppermost in mind. Expect the unexpected and remember: The drug user, not the drug, can pose the greatest threat.

Alcohol

The most commonly abused drug in the United States is alcohol ▶ **Figure 17-6** . It affects people from all walks of life and kills more than 200,000 of them each year. More than 50% of all traffic fatalities or injuries, 67% of murders, and 33% of suicides are related to alcohol, which impairs the capacity to think and function rationally. Alcoholism is one of the greatest national health problems, along with heart disease, cancer, and stroke.

Figure 17-6 Alcohol intoxication causes altered mental status, slowed reflexes, and impaired reaction time.

Alcohol is a powerful CNS depressant. It is both a **sedative**, a substance that decreases activity and excitement, and a **hypnotic**, meaning that it induces sleep. In general, alcohol dulls the sense of awareness, slows reflexes, and reduces reaction time. It may also cause aggressive and inappropriate behavior and lack of coordination. However, a person who appears intoxicated may have other medical problems as well. Look for signs of head trauma, toxic reactions, or uncontrolled diabetes. Severe acute alcohol ingestion may cause hypoglycemia, which may contribute to the symptoms. At the very least, you should assume that all intoxicated patients are experiencing a drug overdose and require thorough examination by a physician. In most states, such patients cannot legally refuse transport.

If a patient exhibits signs of serious CNS depression, you must provide respiratory support. This may be difficult, however, because depression of the respiratory system can also cause **emesis**, or vomiting. The vomiting may be very forceful or even bloody (**hematemesis**), since large amounts of alcohol irritate the stomach. Internal bleeding should also be considered if the patient appears to be in shock (hypoperfusion), as blood might not clot effectively in a patient who has a prolonged history of alcohol abuse.

A patient in alcohol withdrawal may experience frightening hallucinations or **delirium tremens (DTs)**, a syndrome characterized by restlessness, fever, sweating, disorientation, agitation, and even convulsions. These conditions may develop if patients no longer have their daily source of alcohol. Alcoholic hallucinations come and go. A patient with an otherwise fairly clear mental state may see fantastic shapes or figures or hear odd voices. Such auditory and visual hallucinations often precede DTs, which are a much more severe complication.

DTs may develop 1 to 7 days after a person stops drinking or when consumption levels are decreased suddenly. Again, patients may experience one or more of the following signs and symptoms:

- Agitation and restlessness
- Fever
- Sweating
- Confusion and/or disorientation
- Delusions and/or hallucinations
- Seizures

Provide prompt transport for these patients after you have completed your assessment and given necessary care. A person who is experiencing hallucinations or DTs is extremely ill. Should seizures develop, treat them as you would any other seizure. The patient should not be restrained, although you must protect him or her from self-injury. Give the patient oxygen and watch carefully for vomiting. Hypovolemia may develop from sweating, fluid loss, insufficient fluid intake, or vomiting associated with DTs. If you see signs of hypovolemic shock, elevate the patient's feet slightly, clear the airway, and turn the head to one side to minimize the chance of aspiration during transport. These patients may not respond appropriately to suggestions or conversation; they are often confused and frightened. Therefore, your approach should be calm and relaxed. Reassure the patient and provide emotional support.

Opioids

The pain relievers called opioid analgesics are named for the opium in poppy seeds, the origin of heroin, codeine, and morphine. On the list of frequently abused drugs, they have been joined by a number of synthetic opioids, with origins in the laboratory. These include meperidine (Demerol), hydromorphone (Dilaudid), propoxyphene (Darvon), oxycodone (Percocet), hydrocodone (Vicodin), and methadone ▶ **Table 17-2** . Most of these drugs have legitimate medical uses. With the exception of heroin, which is illegal in the United States, many addicts may have started using any of the opioids with an appropriate medical prescription.

These agents are CNS depressants and can cause severe respiratory depression. When administered intravenously, however, they produce a characteristic "high" or "kick." Tolerance develops rapidly, so some users may require massive doses to experience the same high.

In general, emergency medical problems related to opioids are caused by respiratory depression, including a decreased volume of inspired air and decreased respirations. Patients typically appear sedated and cyanotic and have pinpoint pupils.

Treatment includes supporting the airway and breathing. You may try to arouse patients by talking loudly to them or shaking them gently. Always give supplemental oxygen and be prepared for vomiting. Many home remedies are believed to reverse the respiratory depression associated with heroin overdose, including applying ice to the groin or forcing milk into the mouth. *None of these work, and they frequently complicate the clinical picture.* Nevertheless, you should be aware that a patient's friends may have attempted inappropriate methods of resuscitation. The only effective antidote to reverse the symptoms and signs of opioid overdose are certain narcotic antagonists such as naloxone (Narcan). Patients will respond within 2 minutes to naloxone when it is given intravenously. Naloxone is usually administered by paramedics or by physicians at the emergency department.

Sedative-Hypnotic Drugs

Barbiturates and benzodiazepines have been a part of legitimate medications for a long time. They are easy to obtain and relatively cheap. People sometimes solicit prescriptions from several physicians for the same hypnotics or a variety of sedative-hypnotics. These drugs are CNS depressants and alter level of consciousness, with effects similar to those of alcohol so that the patient may appear drowsy, peaceful, or intoxicated ▼ Table 17-3). By themselves, these drugs do not relieve pain, nor do they produce a specific high, although users often take alcohol or an opioid at the same time to boost their effects.

In general, these agents are taken by mouth. Occasionally, however, contents of capsules are suspended or dissolved in water and injected to produce a rather sudden state of ease and contentment. Unfortunately, use of IV sedative-hypnotic drugs quickly induces tolerance, so an individual requires increasingly larger doses. As a result, you are less likely to be called upon to treat

TABLE 17-2 Common Opioid Drugs

Butorphanol (Stadol)

Codeine

Fentanyl derivatives ("China White")

Heroin

Hydrocodone (Hycodan)

Hydromorphone (Dilaudid)

Meperidine (Demerol)

Methadone (Dolophine)

Morphine

Oxycodone (Percodan)

Pentazocine (Talwin)

Propoxyphene (Darvon)

TABLE 17-3 Examples of Sedative-Hypnotic Drugs

Barbiturates	Benzodiazepines	Others
Amobarbital	Alprazolam (Xanax)	Carisoprodol (Soma)
Butabarbital	Chlordiazepoxide (Librium)	Chloral hydrate ("Mickey Finn")
Pentobarbital	Diazepam (Valium)	Cyclobenzaprine (Flexeril)
Phenobarbital	Flunitrazepam (Rohypnol)	Ethchlorvynol (Placidyl)
Secobarbital	Lorazepam (Ativan)	Ethyl alcohol (drinking alcohol)
	Oxazepam (Serax)	Glutethimide (Doriden)
	Temazepam (Restoril)	Hydrocarbon inhalants
		Isopropyl alcohol (rubbing alcohol)
		Meprobamate (Equagesic)

an acute overdose in someone who chronically abuses these drugs. However, you may be called to a scene of an attempted suicide in which the patient has taken large quantities of these drugs. In these situations, patients will have marked respiratory depression and may even be in a coma.

Sedative-hypnotic drugs may also be given to unsuspecting people as a "knock-out" drink, or "Mickey Finn." More recently, drugs such as flunitrazepam (Rohypnol) have been abused as a "date rape drug," causing the unwary individual to become sedated and even unconscious. The individual later begins to awaken, confused and unable to remember what happened.

In general, your treatment of patients who have overdosed with sedative-hypnotics and have respiratory depression is to provide airway clearance, ventilatory assistance, and prompt transport. Give supplemental oxygen and be ready to assist ventilation. You may attempt to stimulate the person by speaking loudly or gently shaking him or her; remember to watch for vomiting.

A specific antidote is available for acute benzodiazepine overdose. It is called flumazenil and is given intravenously. Although it will reverse the sedation and respiratory depression of the benzodiazepine sedative-hypnotics, it will have no effect on the signs and symptoms of overdose from ethyl alcohol or barbiturates. Almost always, flumazenil is administered in the hospital after a physician's assessment. As multi-drug use becomes more common, you may find it increasingly difficult to determine what agents the patients have taken. Your best approach is to treat any obvious injuries or illnesses, keeping in mind that drug use may complicate the picture and make full life support necessary. Focus on ABC, especially the possibility of airway problems (relaxation of the tongue, causing obstruction), vomiting, respiratory depression, and, in severe cases, cardiac arrest.

Abused Inhalants

Many abused inhalants produce several of the same CNS effects as other sedative-hypnotics, but these agents are inhaled instead of ingested or injected. Some of the more common agents include acetone, toluene, xylene, and hexane, which are found in glues, cleaning compounds, paint thinners, and lacquers. Similarly, gasoline and various halogenated hydrocarbons, such as Freon, used as propellants in aerosol sprays, are also abused as inhalants. None of these inhalants is a medication. Since these are products that can be bought in hardware stores, they are commonly abused by teenagers seeking an alcohol-like high.

Always use special care in dealing with a patient who may have used inhalants. Their effects range from mild drowsiness to coma, but unlike most other sedative-hypnotics, these agents may often cause seizures. Also, halogenated hydrocarbon solvents can make the heart supersensitive to the patient's own adrenaline, putting the patient at high risk for sudden cardiac death from ventricular fibrillation; even the action of walking may release enough adrenaline to cause a fatal ventricular arrhythmia. You must try to keep such patients from struggling with you or exerting themselves. Give supplemental oxygen and use a stretcher to move the patient. Prompt transport to the hospital is essential; monitor vital signs en route.

Sympathomimetics

Sympathomimetics are CNS stimulants that frequently cause hypertension, tachycardia, and dilated pupils. A **stimulant** is an agent that produces an excited state. Amphetamine and methamphetamine ("ice") are commonly taken by mouth. They are also injected by abusers in many cases. They typically are taken to make the user "feel good," improve task performance, suppress appetite, or prevent sleepiness. They may just as easily produce irritability, anxiety, lack of concentration, or seizures. Other common examples include phentermine and Benzedrine. Caffeine, theophylline, and phenylpropanolamine (a nasal decongestant) are all mild sympathomimetics. So-called "designer drugs," such as Ecstasy and Eve, are also frequently abused in certain areas of the country.

Sympathomimetic drugs are frequently called "uppers" (▼ Table 17-4). Someone using one of these agents may display disorganized behavior, restlessness, and sometimes anxiety or great fear. Paranoia and delusions are common with sympathomimetic abuse.

Cocaine, also called coke, crack, crystal, snow, freebase, rock, gold dust, blow, and lady, may be taken in a number of different ways. Classically, it is inhaled into

TABLE 17-4 Street Names for Amphetamines		
Adam	Fen-phen	Psychodrine
Bennies	Golden eagle	Speed
Crank	Ice	STP
DOM	MDA	Uppers
Ecstasy	Meth	
Eve		

the nose and absorbed through the nasal mucosa, damaging tissue, causing nosebleeds, and ultimately destroying the nasal septum. It can also be injected intravenously or subcutaneously (skin-popping). Cocaine can be absorbed through all mucous membranes and even across the skin. In any form, the immediate effects of a given dose last less than an hour.

Another method of abusing cocaine is by smoking it. Crack is pure cocaine. It melts at 93°F (34°C) and vaporizes at a slightly higher temperature. Therefore, crack is easily smoked. In this form, it reaches the capillary network of the lungs and can be absorbed into the body in seconds. The immediate outflow of blood from the heart speeds the drug to the brain, so its effect is felt at once. Smoked crack produces the most rapid means of absorption and therefore the most potent effect.

Cocaine is one of the most addicting substances known, more so than heroin or nicotine. Its immediate effects include excitement and euphoria. Acute cocaine overdose is a genuine emergency, as patients are at high risk for seizures and cardiac arrhythmias. Chronic cocaine abuse may cause hallucinations; patients with "cocaine bugs" think that bugs are crawling out of their skin.

In caring for patients who have been poisoned with any of the sympathomimetics, be aware that their severe agitation can lead to tachycardia and hypertension. Patients may also be paranoid, putting you and other health care providers in danger. Law enforcement officers should be at the scene to restrain the patient, if necessary. Do not leave the patient unattended and unmonitored during transport.

All of these patients need to get to the emergency department promptly because of their risk of seizures, cardiac arrhythmias, and stroke. You may see blood pressures as high as 250/150 mm Hg. Give supplemental oxygen and be ready to provide suctioning. If the patient is already having a seizure, you must protect him or her against self-injury.

Marijuana

The flowering hemp plant *Cannabis sativa*, called marijuana, is abused throughout the world. It has been estimated that as many as 20 million people use marijuana daily in the United States. Inhaling marijuana smoke from a cigarette or pipe produces euphoria, relaxation, and drowsiness. It also impairs short-term memory and the capacity to do complex thinking and work. In some people, the euphoria progresses to depression and confusion. An altered perception of time is common, and anxiety and panic can occur. With very high doses, patients experience hallucinations.

A person who has been using marijuana rarely needs transport to the hospital. Exceptions may include someone who is hallucinating, very anxious, or paranoid. However, you should be aware that marijuana is often used as a vehicle to get other drugs into the body. For example, it may be covered with crack or PCP, also known as "angel dust."

Hallucinogens

Hallucinogens alter an individual's sensory perceptions (▼ **Table 17-5**). The classic hallucinogen is lysergic acid diethylamide (LSD). Abuse of another hallucinogen, phencyclidine (PCP, "angel dust") is relatively uncommon among young adults. PCP is a dissociative anesthetic that is easily synthesized and highly potent. Its effectiveness by oral, nasal, pulmonary, and IV routes makes it easy to add to other street drugs. PCP is dangerous, as it causes severe behavioral changes in which individuals often inflict injury to themselves.

All these agents cause visual hallucinations, intensify both vision and hearing, and generally separate the user from reality. The user, of course, expects that the altered sensory state will be pleasurable. Often, however, it can be terrifying. At some point, you are bound to encounter patients who are having a "bad trip." They will usually be hypertensive, tachycardic, anxious, and probably paranoid.

Many of the hallucinogens have sympathomimetic properties. Indeed, your care for a patient who is having a bad reaction to a hallucinogenic agent is the same as that for a patient on a sympathomimetic. Use a calm, professional manner, and provide emotional support.

TABLE 17-5 Commonly Abused Hallucinogens

Bufotenine (toad skin)

Dimethyltryptamine (DMT)

Jimson weed

Lysergic acid diethylamide (LSD)

Marijuana

Mescaline

Morning glory

Nutmeg

Phencyclidine (PCP)

Psilocybin (mushroom)

Do not use restraints unless you or the patient is in danger of injury and then always within the guidelines specified by local authorities. These patients may suddenly experience hallucinations or odd perceptions, so you must watch them carefully throughout transport. Never leave a patient who has taken a hallucinogen unattended and unmonitored.

Anticholinergic Agents

The classic picture of a person who has taken too much of an anticholinergic medication is "hot as a hare, blind as a bat, dry as a bone, red as a beet, and mad as a hatter." These are medications that have properties that, among other effects, block the parasympathetic nerves. Common drugs with a significant anticholinergic effect include atropine, diphenhydramine (Benadryl), jimsonweed, and certain tricyclic antidepressants. With the exception of jimsonweed, these medications usually are not abused drugs but may be taken as an intentional overdose. You will find that it is often difficult to distinguish between an anticholinergic overdose and a sympathomimetic overdose. In both groups of patients, patients may be agitated and tachycardic and have dilated pupils. Once a pure anticholinergic poisoning has been diagnosed, the patient may be treated with physostigmine intravenously by staff in the emergency department, depending on the severity of the situation.

As newer, safer antidepressants such as fluoxetine (Prozac) and sertraline (Zoloft) crowd the market, you can expect to see fewer overdoses of tricyclic antidepressants such as amitriptyline (Elavil) and imipramine (Tofranil). In addition to its anticholinergic effects, a cyclic antidepressant overdose may cause more serious, indeed life-threatening, effects. This is because the medication may block the electrical conduction system in the heart, leading to lethal cardiac arrhythmias. Patients with acute cyclic antidepressant overdose must be transported immediately to the emergency department; they may go from appearing "normal" to seizure and death within 30 minutes. The seizures and cardiac arrhythmias caused by a severe cyclic antidepressant overdose are best treated in the hospital with IV sodium bicarbonate. If you work in a tiered system, you should consider calling for ALS backup when you are en route to the scene.

Cholinergic Agents

The "nerve gases" designed for chemical warfare are cholinergic agents. These agents overstimulate normal body functions that are controlled by parasympathetic nerves, resulting in salivation, mucous secretion, urination, crying, and heart rate. Obviously, you are unlikely to run across these. However, you may well be called to care for patients who have been exposed to one of the

Weapons of Mass Destruction

Although the use of weapons of mass destruction (WMD) still remains more prevalent in wartime and more closely associated with the military, it has become a threat during peacetime and could involve EMT-Bs practicing in civilian life. We have seen WMD used to produce tragedies such as the Oklahoma bombing of a federal building. We now protect ourselves against terrorist attacks at events such as the Olympic games. Protection involves military presence and in the event of an attack, we are equipped with military medical teams and civilian teams, which include the disaster medical assistance teams (DMATs). These DMATs are made up of experts that include physicians, nurses, respiratory therapists, EMT-Bs, paramedics, and clergy. During these events, DMATs are federalized and operate under the Department of Health and Human Services.

Biological, chemical, and nuclear warfare are used for mass destruction. Many different agents are used. Treatment after an attack is typically divided into three zones. The first zone is the red or hot zone, which is usually managed by the military or other highly trained individuals. In the hot zone, patients are triaged and go through early decontamination (called decon). In the next zone, the yellow or warm zone, extensive decontamination takes place by trained individuals. The last zone, the green zone or cold zone, is where EMS will transport the patient. Although EMT-Bs do not manage patients who are in a hot zone, they will have to manage patients after the decontamination team has completed and cleared the patients for transport. EMS providers do not enter the red or yellow area unless they are trained and are wearing the proper clothing. It is important to understand that you should never enter a situation that is potentially dangerous without proper training.

organophosphate insecticides or certain wild mushrooms, which are also cholinergic agents. The signs and symptoms of cholinergic drug poisoning are easy to remember because of the mnemonic DUMBELS:

- **D**efecation
- **U**rination
- **M**iosis (constriction of the pupils)
- **B**ronchorrhea (discharge of mucus from the lungs)
- **E**mesis
- **L**acrimation (tearing)
- **S**alivation

Alternatively, you can use the mnemonic SLUDGE:

- **S**alivation
- **L**acrimation
- **U**rination
- **D**efecation
- **G**I irritation
- **E**ye constriction/Emesis

In poisonings, patients will have excessive amounts of these normal functions and body secretions. In addition, patients may have either bradycardia or tachycardia.

The most important consideration in caring for a patient who has been exposed to an organophosphate insecticide or some other cholinergic agent is to avoid exposure yourself. Because such agents may cling to a patient's clothing and skin, decontamination may take priority over immediate transport to the emergency department. At the hospital, the anticholinergic drug atropine can be used to dry up the patient's secretions. In the meantime, your priority after decontamination is to decrease the secretions in the mouth and trachea that threaten to suffocate the patient, and provide airway support. Depending on your local EMS protocol, this can be treated as a HazMat situation.

Miscellaneous Drugs

While not as common as it was 30 years ago, aspirin poisoning remains a potentially lethal condition. Ingesting too many aspirin tablets, either acutely or chronically, may result in nausea, vomiting, hyperventilation, and ringing in the ears. Patients with this problem are frequently anxious, confused, tachypneic, and in danger of having seizures. They should be transported quickly to the hospital.

Overdosing with *acetaminophen* is also very common, probably because acetaminophen is available in so many different preparations, such as Tylenol. The good news is that acetaminophen is generally not very toxic. A healthy patient could ingest 140 mg of acetaminophen for every kilogram of body weight without serious adverse effects. The bad news is that the symptoms of an overdose generally do not appear until it is too late. For example, massive liver failure may not be apparent for a full week. And patients may not provide the information necessary for a correct diagnosis. For this reason, gathering information at the scene is very important. By finding an empty acetaminophen bottle, you may save a patient's life. If given early enough (before liver failure occurs), a specific antidote may prevent liver damage.

Be extremely careful in dealing with a child who has unintentionally ingested a poisonous substance. Although such incidents usually do not lead to death, family members may be distraught, and your professional attitude will help to ease the tension. Remember, however, that a single swallow of some substances can kill a child ◄ **Table 17-6** .

Some alcohols, including methyl alcohol and ethylene glycol, are even more toxic than ethyl alcohol (drinking alcohol). Although they may be used as a

TABLE 17-6 Fatal Ingested Poisons

Benzocaine

Calcium channel blockers (verapamil, nifedipine, diltiazem)

Camphor

Chloroquine

Hydrocarbon solvents

Lomotil

Methanol/ethylene glycol

Methylsalicylate (oil of wintergreen)

Phenothiazines (Thorazine)

Quinine

Theophylline

Tricyclic antidepressants (amitriptyline [Elavil], imipramine [Tofranil], nortriptyline [Pamelor])

Visine

Geriatric Needs

In an accidental overdose or poisoning, the elderly patient may have become confused about his or her drug regimen. He or she may have forgotten that the medication had been taken, repeating the dose a number of times. Or the patient could have forgotten the doctor's instructions to discard left-over medication and might have taken both the current and the older drug, resulting in an increase in effects or an unwanted drug interaction.

The elderly patient may also intentionally overdose in an attempt to commit suicide. Geriatric patients have been known to ingest common household chemicals such as insecticides, acetaminophen, aspirin, or caustic substances in an attempt to end their lives. Be alert for any indication of an intentional overdose or poisoning, even though the patient might deny an attempted suicide.

In considering any poisoning, remember the basics. Because of the aging process, the routes of administration in the elderly patient pose significant changes in the way the poison is absorbed into the body. In the senior citizen, damage to the stomach could be more severe, since increased gastric acids can alter absorption of the poison.

Additionally, decreased gastric mobility slows absorption by delaying emptying of the stomach and, in the event of caustic substance ingestion, increases injury to the stomach.

If a senior citizen inhales a poison, even in tiny quantities, lung damage can be severe. Consider the decreased lung capacity and ability to exchange oxygen and carbon dioxide in the elderly patient's lungs. Pulmonary function could be worsened to potentially fatal levels with the inhalation of minute amounts of poison.

For poisons that are absorbed by or injected into the skin, reduced circulation to the skin can decrease or delay absorption into the body. Watch for an increased reaction or irritation at the skin site.

In the geriatric patient, the liver may not be able to metabolize the poison as effectively, or the kidneys may not be able to excrete the poison as quickly. In either case, the drug or poison remains in the body for a longer period of time, causing additional tissue damage. When a medication is not metabolized or excreted as quickly as before, the drug could accumulate to toxic levels and, ultimately, become fatal.

---

substitute by the chronic alcoholic who is unable to obtain ethyl alcohol, they are more often taken by someone attempting suicide. In either case, immediate transport to the emergency department is essential. Methyl alcohol is found in dry gas products and Sterno; ethylene glycol is found in some antifreeze products. Both cause a "drunken" feeling. Left untreated, both will also cause severe tachypnea, blindness (methyl alcohol), renal failure (ethylene glycol), and eventually death. Even ethyl alcohol (typical drinking alcohol) can stop a patient's breathing if taken in too high a dose or too fast, particularly in children.

Food Poisoning

The term "ptomaine poisoning" was coined in 1870 to indicate poisoning by a class of chemicals found in rotting food. It is still used today in many news accounts of food poisoning. This is unfortunate, because the term is misleading. Food poisoning is almost always caused by eating food that is contaminated by bacteria.

The food may appear perfectly good, with little or no decay or odor to suggest danger.

There are two main types of food poisoning. In one, the organism itself causes disease; in the other, the organism produces toxins that cause disease ▶ Table 17-7 . A toxin is a poison or harmful substance produced by bacteria, animals, or plants.

One organism that produces direct effects of food poisoning is the *Salmonella* bacterium. The condition called salmonellosis is characterized by severe gastrointestinal symptoms within 72 hours of ingestion, including nausea, vomiting, abdominal pain, and diarrhea. In addition, patients suffering from salmonellosis may be systemically ill with fever and generalized weakness. Some people are carriers of certain bacteria; although they may not become ill themselves, they may transmit diseases, particularly if they work in the food services industry. Usually, proper cooking kills bacteria, and proper cleanliness in the kitchen prevents the contamination of uncooked foods.

The more common cause of food poisoning is the ingestion of powerful toxins produced by bacteria, often in leftovers. The bacterium *Staphylococcus*, a common culprit, is quick to grow and produce toxins in foods that have been prepared in advance and kept too long, even in the refrigerator. Foods prepared with mayonnaise, when left unrefrigerated, are a common vehicle for the development of staphylococcal toxins. Usually, staphylococcal food poisoning results in sudden gastrointestinal symptoms, including nausea, vomiting, and diarrhea. Although time frames may vary from individual to individual, usually these symptoms may start within 2 to 3 hours after ingestion or as long as 8 to 12 hours after ingestion.

The most severe form of toxin ingestion is botulism. This often-fatal disease usually results from eating improperly canned food, in which the spores of *Clostridium* bacteria have grown and produced a toxin. The symptoms of botulism are neurologic: blurring of vision, weakness, and difficulty in speaking and breathing. Symptoms may develop as long as 4 days after ingestion or as early as the first 24 hours.

In general, you should not try to determine the specific cause of acute gastrointestinal problems. After all,

severe vomiting may be a sign of a self-limiting food poisoning, a bowel obstruction requiring surgery, or another poison, such as copper, arsenic, zinc, cadmium, scombrotoxin (fish poison), or Clitocybe or Inocybe mushrooms. Instead, you should gather as much history as possible from the patient, and transport him or her promptly to the hospital. When two or more individuals in one group have the same illness, you should bring along some of the suspected food. In advanced cases of botulism, you may have to assist respirations and give basic life support.

Plant Poisoning

Several thousand cases of poisoning from plants occur each year, some severe. Many household plants are poisonous if ingested, as they may be by children who like to nibble leaves ▼ **Table 17-8**. Some poisonous plants cause local irritation of the skin; others can affect the circulatory system, the gastrointestinal tract, or the

TABLE 17-7 Common Sources of Food Poisoning

Bacillus cereus

Campylobacter

Clostridium botulinum toxin

Clostridium perfringens

Cryptosporidium

Enterococcus

Escherichia coli

Giardia lamblia

Rotavirus

Salmonella

Shigella

Staphylococcus toxin

Vibrio parahaemolyticus

Yersinia enterocolitica

TABLE 17-8 Common Toxic Plants

Scientific Name	Common Name
Abrus precatorius	Jequirity bean/rosary pea
Cicuta species	Water hemlock/wild carrot
Colchicum autumnalel	Autumn crocus
Conium maculatum	Poison hemlock
Convallaria majalis	Lily of the valley
Datura species	Jimsonweed/stinkweed
Dieffenbachia	Dumbcane
Digitalis purpurea	Foxglove
Nerium oleander	Oleander/rose laurel
Nicotiana glauca	Tree tobacco
Phoradendron	Mistletoe
Phytolacca americana	Pokeweed
Rhododendron	Rhododendron/azaleas
Ricinus communis	Castor bean
Solarium nigrum	Nightshade
Zygadenus species	Death camas

Figure 17-7 The toxins in these common poisonous plants are often ingested or absorbed through the skin. **A.** Dieffenbachia. **B.** Mistletoe. **C.** Castor bean. **D.** Nightshade. **E.** Foxglove. **F.** Rhododendron. **G.** Jimson weed. **H.** Death camus. **I.** Pokeweed. **J.** Rosary pea. **K.** Poison ivy. **L.** Poison oak. **M.** Poison sumac.

central nervous system. It is impossible for you to memorize every plant and poison, let alone their effects ▲ Figure 17-7 . You can and should do the following:

1. Assess the patient's airway and vital signs.

2. Notify the regional poison control center for assistance in identifying the plant.

3. Take the plant to the emergency department.

4. Provide prompt transport.

Irritation of the skin and/or mucous membranes is a problem with the common houseplant called dieffenbachia, which resembles "elephant ears." When chewed, a single leaf may irritate the lining of the upper airway enough to cause difficulty in swallowing, breathing, and speaking. In rare circumstances, the airway may be completely obstructed. For this reason, dieffenbachia has been called "dumb cane." Emergency medical treatment of dieffenbachia poisoning includes maintaining an open airway, giving oxygen, and transporting the patient promptly to the hospital for respiratory support. You should continue to assess the patient for airway difficulties throughout transport. If necessary, provide positive pressure ventilation.

Prep Kit

Ready for Review

Poisons act acutely or chronically to destroy or impair body cells. If you believe a patient may have taken a poisonous substance, you should notify medical control and begin emergency treatment at once. This may include administration of an antidote, usually at the hospital, if an antidote exists. It also entails collecting any evidence of the type of poison that was used and bringing it to the hospital; diluting and physically removing the poisonous agent; providing respiratory support; and transporting the patient promptly to the hospital.

A poison can be introduced into the body in one of four ways: ingestion, inhalation, injection, or surface contact (absorption). Approximately 80% of all poisoning is by ingestion, including plants, contaminated food, and most drugs. In general, activated charcoal should be used in these patients. In the case of surface contact poisons, be sure to avoid contaminating yourself. You should then remove all contaminated substances and clothing from the patient, and flood the affected part. Move patients who have inhaled poison into the fresh air; be prepared to use supplemental oxygen via nonrebreathing mask and/or ventilatory support via BVM device. BLS may be needed for some patients, especially those who have injected poison, which is almost always a deliberate act.

People who abuse a substance can develop a tolerance to it, which may lead to addiction. Always use BSI precautions when caring for victims of drug abuse. In addition to alcohol and marijuana, commonly abused drugs fall into seven categories: opioid analgesics, sedative-hypnotics, inhalants, sympathomimetics, hallucinogens, anticholinergics, and cholinergics. Like alcohol, drugs in the first three categories depress the CNS and can cause respiratory depression. You must support the airway in such cases and be prepared for the patient to vomit. Take special care with patients who have used inhalants, since the drugs may cause seizures. Sympathomimetics, including cocaine, stimulate the CNS, causing hypertension, tachycardia, seizures, and dilated pupils. These patients may be paranoid, as may patients who have taken hallucinogens. Anticholinergic medications, often taken in suicide attempts, can cause a person to become hot, dry, blind, red-faced, and mentally unbalanced. An overdose of cyclic antidepressants can lead to cardiac arrhythmias. The symptoms of cholinergic medications, which include organophosphate insecticides, can be remembered by the mnemonic DUMBELS or SLUDGE, for excessive defecation, urination, miosis, bronchorrhea, emesis, lacrimation, and salivation.

Two main types of food poisoning cause gastrointestinal symptoms. In one type, bacteria in the food directly cause disease, such as salmonellosis; in the other, bacteria such as *Staphylococcus* produce powerful toxins, often in leftover food. The most severe form of toxin ingestion is botulism, which can first produce neurologic symptoms as late as 4 days after ingestion. Plant poisoning can affect the circulatory system, the gastrointestinal system, or the central nervous system. Some plants, such as the dieffenbachia, irritate the skin or mucous membranes, and even sometimes cause obstruction of the airway.

Vital Vocabulary

addiction A state of overwhelming obsession or physical need to continue the use of a drug or agent.

antidote A substance that is used to neutralize or counteract a poison.

delirium tremens (DTs) A severe withdrawal syndrome seen in alcoholics who are deprived of ethyl alcohol; characterized by restlessness, fever, sweating, disorientation, agitation, and convulsions; can be fatal if untreated.

emesis Vomiting.

hallucinogen An agent that produces false perceptions in any one of the five senses.

hematemesis Vomiting blood.

hypnotic A sleep-inducing effect or agent.

ingestion Swallowing; taking a substance by mouth.

opioids Any drug or agent with actions similar to morphine.

poison A substance whose chemical action could damage structures or impair function when introduced into the body.

sedative A substance that decreases activity and excitement.

stimulant An agent that produces an excited state.

substance abuse The knowing misuse of any substance to produce some desired effect.

tolerance The need for increasing amounts of a drug to obtain the same effect.

toxin A poison or harmful substance produced by bacteria, animals, or plants.

vomitus Vomited material.

weapons of mass destruction Biological, chemical, and nuclear warfare mediums used for mass destruction, more prevalent in wartime and more closely associated with the military.

Assessment in Action

You are dispatched, along with police, to an unconscious male in a park located about 10 minutes from the hospital. Upon arrival, you find a 20-year-old man on a blanket. His girlfriend is crying and begging him to wake up. You see syringes, a tourniquet, and some spoons on the blanket.

After making sure the scene is safe, you assess your patient. He is unresponsive to painful stimuli. He is very pale, with slow, shallow respirations at 6/min. His pulse is almost too weak to feel, and he has cool, dry skin. You see track marks in both arms. His girlfriend tells you they got some "good stuff" and decided to try it in the park.

1. After scene safety, your first priority for this patient is to:
   A. apply a nonrebreathing mask and take his blood pressure.
   B. insert an oral airway and begin assisting ventilation with a BVM device.
   C. place him in recovery position and keep him warm.
   D. contact medical control for direction.

2. Because of the patient's history of IV drug abuse and presence of track marks on his arms, you would suspect that he is at high risk for which of the following conditions?
   A. HIV, AIDS, and hepatitis
   B. Cancer and pneumonia
   C. COPD, asthma, and allergies
   D. Ulcers, headaches, and GI bleeding

3. A detailed assessment reveals that the patient has pinpoint pupils, a carotid pulse of 136, spontaneous respirations of 6, and a blood pressure of 70/46 mm Hg. His mouth and mucous membranes seem dry. The most likely cause of this patient's overdose is:
   A. opioid or narcotic.
   B. sympathomimetic.
   C. anticholinergic.
   D. hallucinogenic.

4. In this situation it would be appropriate to:
   A. apply a cervical collar and logroll him onto a backboard.
   B. splint the arm he was injecting.
   C. apply the AED.
   D. prepare the suction unit.

5. During transport this patient vomits. Additional actions include:
   A. cleaning the patient prior to arrival.
   B. collecting the vomitus in a plastic bag.
   C. placing absorbent cotton in the patient's mouth.
   D. attempting to ventilate around the vomitus.

6. At the emergency department, the staff person tells you that the patient will be administered an antidote. The best definition for an antidote is a substance that will:
   A. counteract the effects of a particular poison.
   B. potentiate the effects of a particular poison.
   C. have an additive effect to a particular poison.
   D. have an idiosyncratic effect to a particular poison.

7. While you are at the hospital finishing up your paperwork, your partner asks you if activated charcoal should have been given. What should be your response?
   A. We could have given it but transport time was too short.
   B. We didn't give it because we did not have the appropriate equipment.
   C. We could have given it but did not contact the hospital for permission.
   D. We didn't give it because the patient did not meet the criteria.

Challenging Questions

8. Of all the routes for poisoning, which is the most commonly used and why?

9. Patients who have inhaled poisons are moved to fresh air immediately. Why?

Points to Ponder

You are working for a rural agency and have responded to a motorcycle accident where the motorcyclist received a fractured tibia and many abrasions. You have responded to this patient several times in the past for drug-related emergencies and overdoses. He did not appear high at this accident. About 20 minutes into your transport he begins to get agitated and about 30 minutes into transport he starts moving around a lot and wants to get up. He explains that he needs to shoot up or he will go into withdrawal. He explains that his "stuff" is in his backpack that he brought along and asks if you will help him shoot-up. When you tell him that you cannot do that, he asks if you can just stop and get out and he will "take care of it" without you knowing. You still have 90 minutes before arriving at the hospital, and he is becoming more agitated and aggressive. How will you handle this patient? Is there a time that you would let him shoot-up?

Issues Best Patient Care, Safety Issues, Patient Restraints, Personal Biases and Prejudices.

Online Outlook

The National Clearinghouse for Alcohol and Drug Information is a comprehensive source of information on drug abuse and its health consequences. Learn more from this web site by completing Exercise 17 at **www.emtb.com**.

Environmental Emergencies

TECHNOLOGY

www.emtb.com

Online Chapter Pretest
Interactivities
Vocabulary Explorer
Anatomy Review
Web Links
Online Review Manual
Distance Learning

For the first call of your shift, dispatch sends you to the Sudsy Laundromat for a "sick man." You arrive shortly after the call and find a 23-year-old male sitting next to a bench mumbling incoherently.

Irrespective of where you work as an EMT-B, environmental emergencies will be a part of your regular caseload. This chapter will provide information necessary to care for patients with an environmental emergency and help you answer the following questions:

1. How does heat exhaustion differ from heat stroke?
2. Are there differences between the signs and symptoms of a patient with acute hypothermia when compared to a patient with chronic hypothermia?

Environmental Emergencies

Heat and cold can both overwhelm the body's mechanisms for regulating temperature, including sweating and radiation of body heat into the atmosphere. A variety of medical emergencies can result from exposure to heat or cold, particularly in children, the elderly, people with chronic illnesses, and young adults who overexert themselves. There is also a range of medical emergencies that arise from water recreation, and these can sometimes be complicated by the cold. These emergencies include localized injuries and systemic illnesses. As an EMT-B, you can save lives by recognizing and responding properly to these emergencies, most of which require prompt treatment in the hospital.

This chapter describes how the body regulates core temperature, and the ways in which body heat is lost to the environment. It then discusses the various forms of heat-, cold-, and water-related emergencies, including how to diagnose and treat hypothermia, hyperthermia, and diving injuries.

Cold Exposure

Normal body temperature must be maintained within a very narrow range for the body's chemistry to work efficiently. If the body, or any part of it, is exposed to cold environments, these mechanisms may be overwhelmed. Cold exposure may cause injury to individual parts of the body, such as the feet, hands, ears, or nose, or to the body as a whole. When the entire body temperature falls, the condition is called **hypothermia**.

Because heat always travels from a warmer place to a cooler place, the body will tend to lose heat to the environment. The body can lose heat in the following five ways:

- **Conduction** is the direct transfer of heat from a part of the body to a colder object, as when a warm hand touches cold metal or ice, or is immersed in water with a temperature of less than 98°F (37°C). Heat passes directly from the body to the colder object.

- **Convection** occurs when heat is transferred to circulating air, as when cool air moves across the body surface. A person standing outside in windy winter weather, wearing lightweight clothing, is losing heat to the environment mostly by convection.

- **Evaporation** is the conversion of any liquid to a gas, a process that requires energy, or heat. Evaporation is the natural mechanism by which sweating cools the body. This is why swimmers coming out of the water feel a sensation of cold as the water evaporates from their skin. Individuals who exercise vigorously in a cool environment may sweat and feel warm at first, but later, as their sweat evaporates, they can become exceedingly cool.

- **Radiation** is the loss of body heat directly to colder objects in the environment. Because heat always travels from a warm object to a cooler one, a person standing in a cold room will lose heat by radiation.

- **Respiration** causes body heat to be lost, as warm air in the lungs is exhaled into the atmosphere and cooler air is inhaled.

The rate and amount of heat loss by the body can be modified in three ways:

1. **Increase heat production.** One way for the body to increase its heat production is to increase the rate of metabolism of its cells, as occurs in shivering.

2. **Move to an area where heat loss is decreased.** The most obvious way to decrease heat loss from radiation and convection is to move out of a cold environment and seek shelter from wind. Just covering the head will minimize radiation heat loss by up to 70%.

3. **Wear insulated clothing, which helps to decrease heat loss in several ways.** Insulators, such as specific materials or dry, still air, do not conduct heat. Thus, layers of clothing that trap air provide good insulation, as do wool, down, and synthetic fabrics that have small pockets of trapped air. Protective clothing also traps perspiration and prevents evaporation. Sweating without evaporation will not result in cooling.

Hypothermia

Hypothermia literally means "low temperature." It is diagnosed when the **core temperature** of the body—the temperature of the heart, lungs, and vital organs—falls below 95°F (35°C). The body can usually tolerate a drop in core temperature of a few degrees. However, below this critical point, the body loses the ability to regulate its temperature and to generate body heat. Progressive loss of body heat then begins.

To protect itself against heat loss, the body normally constricts blood vessels in the skin; this results in the characteristic appearance of blue lips and/or fingertips. As a secondary precaution against heat loss, the body tends to create additional heat by shivering, which is the active moving of many muscles to generate heat. As cold exposure worsens and these mechanisms are overwhelmed, many body functions begin to slow down. Eventually, the functioning of key organs such as the heart begins to slow. Untreated, this can lead to death.

Hypothermia can develop either quickly, as when someone is immersed in cold water, or more gradually, as when a lost person is exposed to the cold environment for several hours or more. The temperature does not have to be below freezing for hypothermia to occur. In winter, homeless people and those whose homes lack heating may develop hypothermia at higher temperatures. Even in summer, swimmers who remain in the water for a long time are at risk of hypothermia. Like all heat- and cold-related injuries, hypothermia is more common among elderly, pediatric, and ill individuals, who are less able to adjust to temperature extremes. Hypothermia is also common among the very young, who are unable to put on clothes to protect themselves against the cold. Infants and children are small, with a relatively large surface area, and have less body fat than do adults. Also, because of their small muscle mass, children may not be able to shiver as effectively as adults, and infants do not shiver at all.

Patients with injuries or illness, such as burns, shock, head injury, stroke, generalized infection, injuries to the spinal cord, diabetes, and hypoglycemia, are more prone to hypothermia, as are patients who have taken certain drugs or poisons.

SIGNS AND SYMPTOMS. Signs and symptoms of hypothermia generally become progressively more severe as the core temperature falls. Hypothermia generally progresses through four general stages, as shown in ▼ Table 18-1 . Although there is no clear distinction

TABLE 18-1 Characteristics of Systemic Hypothermia				
Core Temperature	90° to 95°F (32° to 35°C)	89° to 92°F (32° to 33°C)	80° to 88°F (27° to 31°C)	<80°F (<27°C)
Signs and Symptoms	Shivering, foot stamping	Loss of coordination, muscle stiffness	Coma	Apparent death
Cardiorespiratory Response	Constricted blood vessels, rapid breathing	Slowing respirations, slow pulse	Weak pulse, arrhythmias, very slow respirations	Cardiac arrest
Level of Consciousness	Withdrawn	Confused, lethargic, sleepy	Unresponsive	Unresponsive

among the stages, the different signs and symptoms of each will help you estimate the severity of the problem. When you assess a patient in the field, you should be able to distinguish between mild and severe hypothermia.

To assess the patient's general temperature, pull back on your glove and place the back of your hand on the patient's skin (▼ **Figure 18-1**). If the skin feels cool, the patient is likely experiencing a generalized cold emergency. If you work in a cold environment, you may carry a hypothermia thermometer, which registers lower core temperatures (▼ **Figure 18-2**). It must be inserted in the rectum for an accurate reading. Note that regular thermometers will not register the temperature of a patient who has significant hypothermia. Mild hypothermia occurs when the core temperature is between 90° and 95°F (32° and 35°C). The patient is usually alert and shivering in an attempt to generate more heat through muscular activity. The patient may jump up and down and stamp his or her feet. Pulse rate

Figure 18-1 To assess a patient's temperature, pull back your glove and place the back of your hand on the patient's skin.

Figure 18-2 A special rectal hypothermia thermometer registers temperatures well below that of a regular thermometer.

Documentation Tips

Recording specific results of your early assessment is particularly valuable in hypothermic patients. If there is a question about beginning CPR, note where you checked the pulse and for how long. Also note the initial body temperature and where it was taken. These points will be important to hospital staff, and will help protect you if medicolegal issues are ever raised.

and respirations are usually rapid. The skin in light-skinned individuals can be red, but may eventually appear pale, then cyanotic. As was noted previously, individuals in a cold environment may have blue lips or fingertips because of the body's constriction of blood vessels at the skin to retain heat.

More severe hypothermia occurs when the core temperature is less than 90°F (32°C). Shivering stops, and muscular activity decreases. At first, small, fine muscle activity such as coordinated finger motion ceases. Eventually, as the temperature falls further, all muscle activity stops.

As the core temperature drops toward 85°F (29°C), the patient becomes lethargic, usually losing interest in continuing to fight the cold. The level of consciousness decreases, and the patient may try to remove his or her own clothes. Poor coordination and memory loss follow, along with reduced or complete loss of sensation to touch, mood changes, and impaired judgment. The patient becomes less communicative, experiences joint or muscle stiffness, and has trouble speaking. The muscles eventually become rigid, and the patient begins to appear stiff or rigid.

If the temperature continues to fall to 80°F (27°C), vital signs slow; the pulse becomes weaker, and respirations slow to shallow or become absent. Cardiac arrhythmias may occur as the blood pressure decreases or disappears.

At a core temperature less than 80°F (27°C), all cardiorespiratory activity may cease, pupillary reaction is slow, and the patient may appear dead. **Never assume that a cold, pulseless patient is dead.** Patients may survive even severe hypothermia, if proper emergency measures are carried out.

EMERGENCY MEDICAL CARE. Even mild degrees of hypothermia can have serious consequences and complications. These include cardiac arrhythmia and blood-clotting abnormalities. Therefore, all patients with hypothermia require immediate transport for evaluation and treatment. Management of hypothermia in the field, regardless of the severity of the exposure, consists of stabilizing the ABCs and preventing further heat loss.

In most cases, you should move the patient from the cold environment to prevent further heat loss. To prevent further damage to the feet, do not allow the patient to walk. Remove any wet clothing, and place dry blankets over and under the patient (▼ Figure 18-3). Always make sure to handle the patient gently so that you will not cause any pain or further injury to the skin. Do not massage the extremities. Do not allow the patient to eat, to use any stimulants, such as coffee, tea, or cola, or to smoke or chew tobacco.

You can give the patient warm, humidified oxygen if you have not already done so as part of the initial assessment. Next, assess the patient's pulse for 30 to 45 seconds, especially before considering CPR. Begin passive rewarming, which includes wrapping the patient in blankets and turning up the heat in the patient compartment of the ambulance.

If the patient is alert and responds appropriately, the hypothermia is mild, and you can begin active rewarming, which includes wrapping the patient in blankets and applying heat packs or hot water bottles to the groin, axillary, and cervical regions. Turn the heat up high in the patient compartment of the ambulance.

You must try to minimize further loss of body heat, especially when you cannot get to a hospital quickly. However, when the patient has moderate or severe hypothermia, you should never try to rewarm the

Figure 18-3 Place dry blankets over and under the hypothermia patient; give warm, humidified oxygen; assess the pulse before considering CPR.

patient actively (placing heat on or into the body). Rewarming too quickly may cause a fatal cardiac arrhythmia that requires defibrillation; for this reason, rewarming should be done in the hospital. Again, your goal is to prevent further heat loss. Remove the patient immediately from the cold environment. Place the patient in the ambulance, and turn up the heat. If you cannot get the patient out of the cold immediately, move him or her out of the wind and away from contact with any object that will conduct heat from the body. Place a protective cover on the patient, and remember that most heat is lost around the head and neck.

If the patient is alert and shivering, you may assume that the hypothermia is relatively mild. If possible, you can give warm fluids by mouth in this case, assuming that the patient can swallow without a problem. Remove all wet clothing, and cover the patient with a blanket. Notify the hospital of the patient's condition so that staff can prepare to start rewarming as soon as you arrive.

When the patient is not shivering and is lethargic, moderate or severe hypothermia is probably present. A special low-temperature thermometer is required to take this patient's temperature, generally done through the rectum. A patient with a moderate form of hypothermia will have a core temperature of less than 90°F (32°C).

If you cannot feel a radial pulse, gently palpate for a carotid pulse and wait for 30 to 45 seconds before you decide that the patient is pulseless.

Physicians disagree about the wisdom of performing BLS (ie, CPR) on a patient with hypothermia who appears to be pulseless. Such a patient actually may be in a kind of "metabolic ice box," having achieved a metabolic balance that BLS may upset. Even a pulse rate of one or two beats per minute indicates cardiac activity, and cardiac activity may spontaneously recover once the core is warmed. However, there is evidence that when correctly done, BLS will increase blood flow to the critical parts of the body. For this reason, some authorities recommend starting BLS on a patient with hypothermia and no pulse. The American Heart Association recommends that CPR be started if the patient has no detectable pulse or breathing. Again, for a patient with hypothermia, this may require a prolonged pulse check. You can perform ventilation with warm, humidified oxygen. Remove wet clothing, and protect the patient from the cold and wind with blankets in a warmer environment.

If you are in an area where hypothermia is a common problem, you should have specific protocols for dealing with this situation. In all cases, consult with medical control.

Management of Cold Exposure in a Sick or Injured Person

All patients who are severely injured are at risk for hypothermia. Keep this in mind when you are evaluating a patient with multiple injuries.

A sick or injured person who has been trapped in a cold environment may develop hypothermia or may already have problems related to cold exposure. Such a person is more susceptible than a healthy person to cold injury. Take the following steps promptly to prevent further cold injury:

1. **Remove wet clothing** and keep the patient dry.

2. **Prevent conduction heat loss.** Move the patient away from any wet or cold surfaces, such as a car frame.

3. **Insulate all exposed body parts,** especially the head, by wrapping them in a blanket or any other available dry, bulky material.

4. **Prevent convection heat loss** by erecting a wind barrier around the patient.

5. **Remove the patient** from the cold environment as promptly as possible.

Regardless of the nature or severity of the cold injury, remember that even an unresponsive patient may be able to hear you. Some patients have told of hearing themselves pronounced dead by someone who had forgotten the old saying: "No one is dead unless he is warm and dead." If you carry an AED, you should consider defibrillation. Although this heart rhythm is unlikely in patients with hypothermia, it can develop in patients who are rewarmed too rapidly.

Local Cold Injuries

Most injuries from cold are confined to exposed parts of the body. The extremities, particularly the feet, and the exposed ears, nose, and face, are especially vulnerable to cold injury (▶ **Figure 18-4**). When exposed parts of the body become very cold but not frozen, the condition is called frostnip, chilblains, or immersion foot (trench foot). When the parts become frozen, the injury is called <u>frostbite</u>.

You should try to find out the duration of the exposure, the temperature to which the body part was exposed, and the wind velocity during exposure. These are important factors in determining the severity of a local cold injury. You should also investigate a number of underlying factors:

- Exposure to wet conditions
- Inadequate insulation from cold or wind
- Restricted circulation from tight clothing or shoes or circulatory disease
- Fatigue
- Poor nutrition
- Alcohol or drug abuse
- Hypothermia
- Diabetes
- Cardiovascular disease
- Older age

In hypothermia, blood is shunted away from the extremities in an attempt to maintain the core temperature. This shunting of blood increases the risk of local cold injury to the extremities, ears, nose, and face. Thus, the patient with hypothermia should also be assessed for frostbite or other local cold injury. The reverse is also true. You must remember that both local and systemic cold exposure problems can occur in the same patient.

FROSTNIP AND IMMERSION FOOT. After prolonged exposure to the cold, the skin may be freezing while the deeper tissues are unaffected. This condition, which often affects the ears, nose, and fingers, is called frostnip. Because frostnip is usually not painful, the patient often is unaware that a cold injury has occurred. Immersion foot, also called trench foot, occurs after prolonged exposure to cold water. It is particularly common in hikers or hunters who stand for a long time in a river or lake. With both frostnip and immersion

Figure 18-4 The extremities and the ears, nose, and face are particularly susceptible to frostbite.

foot, the skin is pale (blanched) and cold to the touch; normal color does not return after palpation of the skin. In some cases, the skin of the foot will be wrinkled, but it can also remain soft. The patient complains of loss of feeling and sensation in the injured area.

As in all other hypothermia cases, the emergency treatment of these less severe local cold injuries consists of removing the patient from the cold, wet environment, but also rewarming the affected part. With frostnip, contact with a warm object may be all that is needed; you can use your hands, your breath, or the patient's own body. During rewarming, the affected part will often tingle and become red in light-skinned individuals. With immersion foot, remove wet shoes, boots, and socks, and rewarm the foot gradually, protecting it from further cold exposure.

FROSTBITE. Frostbite is the most serious local cold injury, because the tissues are actually frozen. Freezing permanently damages cells, although the exact mechanism by which damage occurs is not known. The presence of ice crystals within the cells may cause physical damage. The change in the water content in the cells may also cause changes in the concentration of critical electrolytes, producing permanent changes in the chemistry of the cell. When the ice thaws, further chemical changes occur in the cell, causing permanent damage or cell death, called gangrene (▼ Figure 18-5). If gangrene occurs, the dead tissue must be surgically removed, sometimes by amputation. Following less severe damage, the exposed part will become inflamed, tender to touch, and unable to tolerate exposure to cold.

Frostbite can be identified by the hard, frozen feel of the affected tissues. Most frostbitten parts are hard

and waxy (▼ Figure 18-6). The injured part feels firm to frozen as you gently touch it. Blisters and swelling may be present. In light-skinned individuals with a deep injury that has thawed or partially thawed, the skin may appear red with purple and white, or it may be mottled and cyanotic.

As with a burn, the depth of skin damage will vary. With superficial frostbite, only the skin is frozen; with deep frostbite, the deeper tissues are frozen as well. You may not be able to tell superficial from deep frostbite in the field. Even an experienced surgeon in a hospital setting may not be able to tell until several days have gone by.

EMERGENCY MEDICAL CARE OF LOCAL COLD INJURY. The emergency treatment of local cold injuries in the field should include the following steps:

1. **Remove the patient** from further exposure to the cold.

2. **Handle the injured part gently,** and protect it from further injury.

3. **Administer oxygen,** if this was not already done as part of the initial assessment.

4. **Remove any wet or restricting clothing** over the injured part.

With an early or superficial injury, such as frostnip or immersion foot, splint the extremity and cover it loosely with a dry, sterile dressing. Never rub injured tissues with anything; rubbing just causes further damage. Do not re-expose the injury to cold.

Figure 18-5   Gangrene, or permanent cell death, can occur when tissue is frozen and certain chemical changes occur in the cells.

Figure 18-6   Frostbitten parts are hard and usually waxy to touch.

With a late or deep cold injury, such as frostbite, be sure to remove any jewelry from the injured part and cover the injury loosely with a dry, sterile dressing. Do not break blisters or rub or massage the area. Do not apply heat or rewarm the part. Unlike frostnip and trenchfoot, rewarming of the frostbitten extremity is best accomplished under controlled circumstances in the emergency department. You can cause a great deal of further injury to fragile tissues by attempting to rewarm a frostbitten part. Never apply something warm or hot, such as the exhaust from the ambulance engine or, even worse, an open flame. Do not allow the patient to stand or walk on a frostbitten foot.

Evaluate the patient's general condition for the signs or symptoms of systemic hypothermia. Support the vital functions as necessary, and transport the patient promptly to the hospital.

If prompt hospital care is not available and medical control instructs you to institute rewarming in the field, use a warm-water bath. Immerse the frostbitten part in water with a temperature between 100° and 112°F (38° and 44.5°C). Check the water temperature with a thermometer before immersing the limb, and recheck it frequently during the rewarming process. The water temperature should never exceed 112°F (44.5°C). Stir the water continuously. Keep the frostbitten part in the water until it feels warm and sensation has returned to the skin. Dress the area with dry, sterile dressings, placing them also between injured fingers or toes. Expect the patient to complain of severe pain.

Never attempt rewarming if there is any chance that the part may freeze again before the patient reaches the hospital. Some of the most severe consequences of frostbite, including gangrene and amputation, have occurred when parts were thawed and then refrozen.

Cover the frostbitten part with soft, padded, sterile cotton dressings. If blisters have formed, do not break them. Remember, you cannot accurately predict the outcome of a case of frostbite early in its course. Even body parts that appear gangrenous may recover following proper emergency and hospital treatment.

Cold Exposure and You

As an EMT-B, you are also at risk for hypothermia if you work in a cold environment. If cold weather search-and-rescue operations are a possibility in your assigned areas, you should receive survival training and precautionary tips. You should be thoroughly familiar with local conditions. Be aware of existing and potential weather conditions, and stay on top of changes that are forecast for the area. Make sure proper clothing is avail-

> As with so many hazards, you cannot help others if you do not practice self-protection.

able, and wear it whenever appropriate. Your vehicle, too, must be properly equipped and maintained for a cold environment. As with so many hazards, you cannot help others if you do not practice self-protection. Never allow yourself to become a casualty!

Heat Exposure

Normal body temperature is 98.6°F (37°C). Complicated regulatory mechanisms keep this internal temperature constant, regardless of the **ambient temperature**, the temperature of the surrounding environment. In a hot environment or during vigorous physical activity, when the body itself produces excess heat, the body will try to rid itself of the excess heat. There are several ways of doing this. The two most efficient are sweating (and evaporation of the sweat) and dilation of skin blood vessels, which brings blood to the skin surface to increase the rate of heat radiation. In addition, of course, the person who becomes overheated can remove clothing and try to find a cooler environment.

Ordinarily, the heat-regulating mechanisms of the body work very well, and individuals are able to tolerate significant temperature changes. When the body is exposed to more heat energy than it loses or generates more heat than it can lose, hyperthermia results. **Hyperthermia** is a high core temperature, usually 101°F (38.3°C) or more.

When the body's mechanisms to decrease body heat are overwhelmed and the body is unable to tolerate the excessive heat, illness develops. High air temperature can reduce the body's ability to lose heat by radiation; high humidity reduces the ability to lose heat through evaporation. Another contributing factor is vigorous exercise, during which the body can lose more than 1 L of sweat an hour, causing loss of fluid and electrolytes. Illness from heat exposure can take the following three forms:

- Heat cramps
- Heat exhaustion
- Heatstroke

All three forms of heat illness may be present in the same patient, since untreated heat exhaustion may progress to heatstroke. Heatstroke is a life-threatening emergency.

Persons at greatest risk for heat illnesses are children; the elderly; patients with heart disease, COPD, diabetes, dehydration, and obesity; and those with limited mobility. The elderly, newborns, and infants exhibit poor thermoregulation. Newborns and infants often wear too much clothing. Alcohol and certain drugs, including medications that dehydrate the body or decrease the ability of the body to sweat, also make a person more susceptible to heat illnesses. When you are treating someone for a heat illness, always obtain a medication history.

Heat Cramps

<u>Heat cramps</u> are painful muscle spasms that occur after vigorous exercise. They do not occur only when it is hot outdoors. They may be seen in factory workers and even well-conditioned athletes. The exact cause of heat cramps is not well understood. We know that sweat produced during strenuous exercise, particularly in a warm environment, causes a change in the body's <u>electrolyte</u>, or salt, balance. The result may be a loss of essential electrolytes from the cells. Dehydration may also play a role in the development of muscle cramps. Large amounts of water can be lost from the body as a result of excessive sweating. This loss of water may affect muscles that are being stressed and cause them to go into spasm.

Heat cramps usually occur in the leg or abdominal muscles. When the abdominal muscles are involved, the pain and muscle spasm may be so severe that the patient appears to have an acute abdominal problem. If a patient with a sudden onset of abdominal cramps has been exercising vigorously in a hot environment, you should suspect heat cramps.

Take the following steps to treat heat cramps in the field ▶ **Figure 18-7** :

1. **Remove the patient** from the hot environment, including sunlight, a source of radiant heat gain. Loosen any tight clothing.

2. **Rest the cramping muscles.** Have the patient sit or lie down until the cramps subside.

3. **Replace fluids by mouth.** Use water or a diluted (half-strength) balanced electrolyte solution, such as Gatorade. In most cases, plain water is the most useful. Do not give salt tablets or solutions that have a high salt concentration. The patient already has an adequate amount of electrolytes circulating; they are just not distributed properly. With adequate rest and fluid replacement, the body will adjust the distribution of electrolytes, and the cramps will disappear.

If the cramps do not go away after these measures, transport the patient to the hospital.

Once the cramps are gone, the patient may resume activity. For example, an athlete can return to play once the heat cramps have disappeared. However, heavy sweating may cause the cramps to recur. Hydration by drinking a lot of water is the best preventive and treatment strategy.

Heat Exhaustion

<u>Heat exhaustion</u>, also called *heat prostration* or *heat collapse*, is the most common serious illness caused by heat. It is the result of the body's losing so much water and so many electrolytes through very heavy sweating that hypovolemia (fluid depletion) occurs. For sweating to be an effective cooling mechanism, the sweat must be able to evaporate from the body. Otherwise, the body will continue to produce sweat, with further loss of body water. People standing in the hot sun and particularly those wearing several layers of clothing, such as football fans or parade watchers,

Figure 18-7 A patient with heat cramps should be moved to a cool environment as you begin your assessment and treatment.

may sweat profusely but experience little body cooling. High humidity will also decrease the amount of evaporation that can occur. Individuals working or exerting themselves in poorly ventilated areas are unable to release heat through convection. Thus, people who work or exercise vigorously and those who wear heavy clothing in a warm, humid, or poorly ventilated environment are particularly prone to heat exhaustion.

The signs and symptoms of heat exhaustion and those of associated hypovolemia are as follows:

- Onset while working hard or exercising in a hot, humid, or poorly ventilated environment and sweating heavily

- Onset, even at rest, in the elderly and infant age groups in hot, humid, and poorly ventilated environments or extended time in hot, humid environments

- Cold, clammy skin with ashen pallor

- Dry tongue and thirst

- Dizziness, weakness, or faintness, with accompanying nausea or headache

- Normal vital signs, although the pulse is often rapid and the diastolic blood pressure may be low

- Normal or slightly elevated body temperature; on rare occasions, as high as 104°F (40°C)

To treat the patient follow the steps in
▶ **Skill Drill 18-1** :

1. **Remove any excessive layers of clothing,** particularly around the head and neck **(Step 1)**.

2. **Move the patient promptly** from the hot environment, preferably into the back of the air-conditioned ambulance. If outdoors, move out of the sun.

3. **Give the patient oxygen** if this was not already done as part of the initial assessment.

4. **Encourage the patient to lie down** and elevate the legs (supine position). Loosen any tight clothing and fan the patient for cooling **(Step 2)**.

5. **If the patient is fully alert,** encourage him or her to sit up and slowly drink up to a liter of water, as long as nausea does not develop. Never force fluids by mouth on a patient who is not fully alert, or allow drinking while supine, because the patient could aspirate the fluid into the lungs **(Step 3)**.

If the patient does become nauseated, transport on the side, also to prevent aspiration.

In most cases, these measures will reverse the symptoms, causing the patient to feel better within 30 minutes. But you should prepare to transport the patient to the hospital for more aggressive treatment, such as IV fluid therapy and close monitoring, especially in the following circumstances:

- The symptoms do not clear up promptly.

- The level of consciousness decreases.

- The temperature remains elevated.

- The person is very young, elderly, or has any underlying medical condition, such as diabetes or cardiovascular disease.

6. **Transport the patient on his or her side** if you think the patient may be nauseated and ready to vomit, but make certain that the patient is secured **(Step 4)**.

Heatstroke

Heatstroke, the least common but most serious illness caused by heat exposure, occurs when the body is subjected to more heat than it can handle, and normal mechanisms for getting rid of the excess heat are overwhelmed. The body temperature then rises rapidly to the level at which tissues are destroyed. Untreated heatstroke always results in death.

Heatstroke can develop in patients during vigorous physical activity or when they are outdoors or in a closed, poorly ventilated, humid space. It also occurs during heat waves among individuals (particularly the elderly) who live in buildings with no air conditioning or with poor ventilation. It may also develop in children who are left unattended in a locked car on a hot day.

Many patients with heatstroke have hot, dry, flushed skin because their sweating mechanism has been overwhelmed. However, early in the course of heatstroke, the skin may be moist or wet. Keep in mind that a patient can have heatstroke even if he or she is still sweating. The body temperature rises rapidly in patients with heatstroke. It may rise to 106°F (41°C) or more. As the body core temperature rises, the patient's level of consciousness falls.

Often, the first sign of heatstroke is a change in behavior. However, the patient then becomes unresponsive very quickly. The pulse is usually rapid and strong at first, but as the patient becomes increasingly unresponsive, the pulse becomes weaker and the blood pressure falls.

SkillDrill 18-1   Treating for Heat Exhaustion

Remove extra clothing.

Move the patient to a cooler environment.
Give oxyen.
Place the patient in a supine position, elevate the legs, and fan the patient.

If the patient is fully alert, give water by mouth.

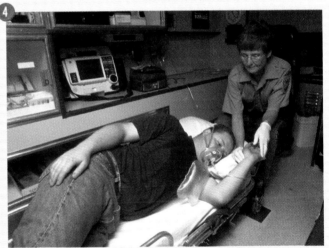

If nausea develops, transport on the side.

Recovery from heatstroke depends on the speed with which treatment is administered, so you must be able to identify this patient quickly. Emergency treatment has one objective: Get the body temperature down by any means available. Take the following steps when treating a patient with heatstroke:

1. **Move the patient** out of the hot environment and into the ambulance.

2. **Set the air conditioning** to maximum cooling.

3. **Remove the patient's clothing.**

4. **Give the patient oxygen** if this was not done as part of the initial assessment.

5. **Apply cool packs** to the patient's neck, groin, and armpits ▶ Figure 18-8 .

6. **Cover the patient** with wet towels or sheets, or spray the patient with cool water and fan him or her to quickly evaporate the dampness on the skin.

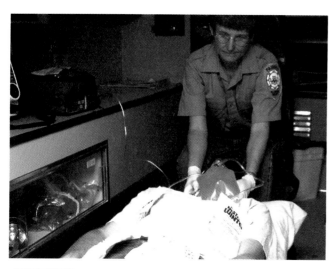

Figure 18-8 As part of treatment of heatstroke, give oxygen and place cool packs about the patient's neck, groin, and armpits.

7. **Aggressively and repeatedly fan** the patient with or without dampening the skin.

8. **Provide immediate transport** to the hospital.

9. **Notify the hospital** as soon as possible so that the staff can prepare to treat the patient immediately on arrival.

Drowning and Near Drowning

<u>Drowning</u> is death from suffocation after submersion in water; <u>**near drowning**</u> is defined as survival, at least temporarily (24 hours), after suffocation in water. Drowning is often the last in a cycle of events caused by panic in the water ▶ **Figure 18-9** . It can happen to anyone who is submerged in water for even a short period of time. Struggling toward the surface or the shore, the person becomes fatigued or exhausted, which leads him or her to sink even deeper. However, drowning also occurs in mop buckets, puddles, bathtubs, and other places where the individual is not completely submerged. Small children can drown in only a few inches of water if unattended.

Inhaling very small amounts of either fresh or salt water can severely irritate the larynx, sending the muscles of the larynx and the vocal cords into spasm, called <u>**laryngospasm**</u>. The average person experiences this to a mild degree when a bit of a drink is inhaled and the patient coughs and seems to be choking for a few seconds. This is the body's attempt at self-preservation, since laryngospasm prevents more water from entering the lungs. But this can be too much of a good thing in

Geriatric Needs

As we age, our bodies can lose their ability to respond to the environment. Older adults undergo changes in their ability to compensate for low or high ambient temperatures. For example, if the ambient temperature rises from 85° to 94°F (29.5° to 34.5°C), the older adult may not recognize the change or be able to compensate for it. Therefore, unless the person is accustomed to the heat, heatstroke can develop relatively quickly.

Shivering, a common effect of hypothermia, is the body's attempt to maintain heat. However, because of a decrease in muscle mass or tone, the hypothermic elderly patient may not shiver. Further, a decrease in muscle mass and body fat means that there is less insulation and protection from the cold. Because of the body's altered response to heat loss and its ability to gain heat, the health care provider might not suspect or report hypothermia. In caring for the geriatric patient in cold climates, be sure to protect the patient against unwanted heat loss. Cover all exposed areas with loose-fitting blankets. Pay particular attention to protecting the patient's head, since heat loss from the head is substantial.

Because of reduced circulation to the skin, heat loss via conduction, convection, and radiation is significantly lower. Additionally, the aging process alters the patient's ability to perspire; therefore, heat loss through evaporation is reduced. Since the elderly patient cannot disperse heat effectively, classic heatstroke can develop rapidly. Typically, the older adult will not go through an initial stage of heat exhaustion. During the summer, you should be acutely aware of the potential for heatstroke and factors that can predispose a patient to heat illness. Factors that increase the possibility of heatstroke include medications, diabetes, alcohol abuse, malnutrition, Parkinsonism, hyperthyroidism, and obesity.

Both hypothermia and hyperthermia can appear in older patients in environmental settings that are subtle unless you are looking for them. These problems appear commonly, for instance, when budget concerns prompt the elderly to keep heat turned down in the winter, or to not use air conditioning in hot weather. Thermal emergencies can develop over a period of time in these indoor, urban environments that may not seem uncomfortable to you.

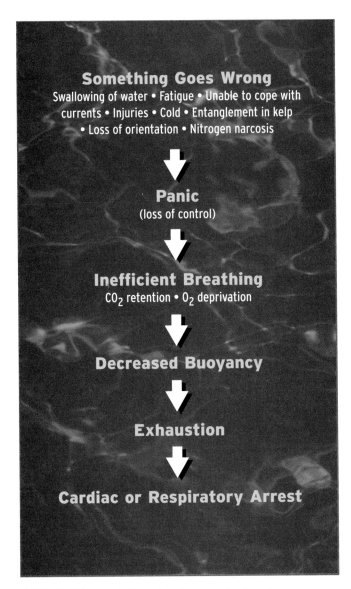

Something Goes Wrong

Swallowing of water • Fatigue • Unable to cope with currents • Injuries • Cold • Entanglement in kelp • Loss of orientation • Nitrogen narcosis

⬇

Panic
(loss of control)

⬇

Inefficient Breathing
CO_2 retention • O_2 deprivation

⬇

Decreased Buoyancy

⬇

Exhaustion

⬇

Cardiac or Respiratory Arrest

Figure 18-9 Panic in the water often precedes drowning.

EMT-B Tips

The cold-water near-drowning patient may require more care than two EMT-Bs can provide by themselves. Airway management and ventilation needs can make it difficult to remove wet clothing, treat hypothermia, or perform further assessment unless additional trained help is available. On this type of response, consider requesting backup before you encounter the patient.

begin as soon as possible, even before the victim is removed from the water. At the same time, you must take care to stabilize and protect the patient's spine when a long fall or dive has occurred (or if this is a possibility when no information is provided). Associated cervical spine injuries are possible, especially in diving mishaps. If the patient does not have a possible spinal injury, you can turn the patient quickly to the left side to allow draining from the upper airway. Note that water will not drain from the lungs. If there is evidence of upper airway obstruction by foreign matter, remove the obstruction manually or, if available, by suction. If necessary, use abdominal thrusts, followed by assisted ventilations. Administer oxygen if this was not done as part of the initial assessment, either by mask for patients who are breathing spontaneously or via BVM device for those requiring assisted ventilation.

Check for a pulse immediately after the patient emerges from the water. It may be difficult to find a pulse because of constriction of the peripheral blood vessels and low cardiac output. Nevertheless, if the pulse is unmeasurable, start CPR if the patient is unresponsive.

Even if resuscitation in the field appears completely successful, you must always transport near-drowning patients to the hospital. Inhalation of any amount of fluid can lead to delayed complications lasting for days or weeks.

Make sure that the patient is kept warm, especially after cold water immersion. Make sure blankets and protection from the environment are provided as needed. If ventilation equipment is not available but oxygen is, you can breathe the oxygen in yourself and give mouth-to-mask ventilation until rescue equipment arrives. In this method, your expired air will have a higher percentage of oxygen.

severe cases such as water submersion, since the patient's lungs cannot be ventilated when significant laryngospasm is present. Instead, progressive hypoxia occurs until the patient becomes unconscious. At this point, the spasm relaxes, making rescue breathing possible. Of course, if the patient has not already been removed from the water, the patient may now inhale deeply, and more water may enter the lungs. In 85% to 90% of cases, significant amounts of water enter the lungs of the drowning victim.

Emergency Medical Care

Treatment begins with rescue and removal from the water. When necessary, artificial ventilation should

EMT-B Safety

You must ensure the safety of rescue personnel before a water rescue can begin. If the patient is conscious and still in the water, you should perform a water rescue. An old saying sums up the basic rule of water rescue: "Reach, throw and row, and *only then go*". First, try to reach for the patient (▶ **Figure 18-10A**). If that does not work, then throw the patient a rope, a life preserver, or any floatable object that is available (▶ **Figure 18-10B**). For example, an inflated spare tire, rim and all, will float well enough to support two people in the water. Next, use a boat if one is available (▶ **Figure 18-10C**). Do not attempt a swimming rescue unless you are trained and experienced in the proper techniques (▶ **Figure 18-10D**). Even then, you should always wear a helmet and a personal flotation device (▶ **Figure 18-11**). Too many well-meaning individuals have themselves become victims while attempting a swimming rescue. In cold climates or cold water locations, rapid hypothermia is a concern as well for rescuers. Be prepared for this potential event.

If you work in a recreation area near lakes, rivers, or the ocean, you must have a prearranged plan for water rescue. This plan should include access to and cooperation with local personnel who are trained and skilled in water rescue; these personnel should help to develop the protocol for water rescue. Because the success of any water rescue depends on how rapidly the patient is removed from the water and ventilated, make sure you always have immediate access to personal flotation devices and other rescue equipment.

Figure 18-10 Basic rules of water rescue. **A.** Reach the person from shore. If you cannot reach the person from shore, wade closer. **B.** If an object that floats is available, throw it to the person. **C.** Use a boat if one is available. **D.** If you must swim to the person, use a towel or board for him or her to hold onto. Do not let the person grab you.

Figure 18-11 When performing a water rescue, you must wear proper personal protective equipment, including a personal flotation device.

Spinal Injuries in Submersion Incidents

Submersion incidents may be complicated by spinal fractures and spinal cord injuries. You must assume that spinal injury exists with the following conditions:

- The submersion has resulted from a diving mishap or long fall.

- The patient is unconscious, and no information is available to rule out the possibility of a mechanism causing neck injury.

- The patient is conscious but complains of weakness, paralysis, or numbness in the arms or legs.

- You suspect the possibility of spinal injury despite what witnesses say.

Most spinal injuries in diving incidents affect the cervical spine. When spinal injury is suspected, the neck must be protected from further injury. This means that you will have to stabilize the suspected injury while the patient is still in the water. Follow the steps in (▶ **Skill Drill 18-2**):

1. **Turn the patient supine.** Two rescuers are usually required to turn the patient safely, although in some cases one rescuer will suffice. Always rotate the entire upper half of the patient's body as a single unit. Twisting only the head, for example, may aggravate any injury to the cervical spine **(Step 1)**.

2. **Restore the airway and begin ventilation.** Immediate ventilation is the primary treatment of all drowning and near-drowning patients. As soon as the patient is face up in the water, use a pocket mask if it is available. Have the other rescuer support the head and trunk as a unit while you open the airway and begin artificial ventilation **(Step 2)**.

3. **Float a buoyant backboard under the patient** as you continue ventilation **(Step 3)**.

4. **Secure the head and trunk to the backboard** to eliminate motion of the cervical spine. Do not remove the patient from the water until this is done **(Step 4)**.

5. **Remove the patient from the water, on the backboard (Step 5)**.

You should never give up on resuscitating a cold-water drowning victim.

6. **Cover the patient with a blanket.** Give oxygen if the patient is breathing spontaneously. Begin CPR if there is no pulse. Effective cardiac compression or CPR is extremely difficult to perform when the patient is still in the water **(Step 6)**.

Recovery Techniques

On occasion, you may be called to the scene of a drowning and find that the patient is not floating or visible in the water. An organized rescue effort in these circumstances calls for personnel who are experienced with recovery techniques and equipment, including snorkel, mask, and scuba gear. <u>Scuba</u> (self-contained underwater breathing apparatus) gear is a system that delivers air to the mouth and lungs at atmospheric pressures that increase with the depth of the dive.

As a last resort, when standard procedures for recovery are unsuccessful, you may have to use a grappling iron or large hook to drag the bottom for the victim. Although the hook could seriously wound the patient, it may be the only effective way to bring him or her to the surface for resuscitation efforts.

Resuscitation Efforts

You should *never* give up on resuscitating a cold-water drowning victim. When a person is submerged in water that is colder than body temperature, heat will be conducted from the body to the water. The resulting hypothermia can protect vital organs from the lack of oxygen. In addition, exposure to cold water will occasionally activate certain primitive reflexes, which may preserve basic body functions for prolonged periods. In one case, a 2¹/₂-year-old girl recovered after being submerged in cold water for at least 66 minutes. Continue full resuscitation efforts until the patient recovers or is pronounced dead by a physician.

Also, whenever a person dives or jumps into very cold water, the **diving reflex**, slowing of the heart rate caused by submersion in cold water, may cause immediate **bradycardia**, a slow heart rhythm. Loss of

Skill Drill 18-2 Stabilizing a Suspected Spinal Injury in the Water

1 Turn the patient to a supine position by rotating the entire upper half of the body as a single unit.

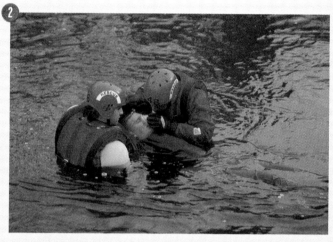

2 As soon as the patient is turned, begin artificial ventilation using the mouth-to-mouth method or a pocket mask.

3 Float a buoyant backboard under the patient.

4 Secure the patient to the backboard.

5 Remove the patient from the water.

6 Cover the patient with a blanket and apply oxygen if breathing. Begin CPR if breathing and pulse are absent.

consciousness and drowning may follow. However, the person may be able to survive for an extended period of time under water, thanks to a lowering of the metabolic rate associated with hypothermia. For this reason, you should continue full resuscitation efforts no matter how long the patient has been submerged.

Diving Emergencies

Most serious water-related injuries are associated with dives, with or without scuba gear. Some of these problems are related to the nature of the dive; others result from panic. Panic is not restricted to the person who is frightened by water. It can happen even to the experienced diver or swimmer.

There are more than 3,000,000 scuba sport divers in the United States, and approximately 200,000 new divers being trained annually. Medical problems relating to scuba diving techniques and equipment are becoming increasingly common. These problems are separated into three phases of the dive: descent, bottom, and ascent.

Descent Emergencies

Descent problems are usually due to the sudden increase in pressure on the body as the person dives deeper into the water. Some body cavities cannot adjust to the increased external pressure of the water; the result is severe pain. The usual areas affected are the lungs, the sinus cavities, the middle ear, the teeth, and the area of the face surrounded by the diving mask. Usually, the pain caused by these "squeeze problems" forces the diver to return to the surface to equalize the pressures, and the problem clears up by itself. A diver who continues to complain of pain, particularly in the ear, after returning to the surface should be transported to the hospital.

A person with a perforated tympanic membrane (ruptured eardrum) may develop a special problem while diving. If cold water enters the middle ear through a ruptured eardrum, the diver may lose his or her balance and orientation. The diver may then shoot to the surface and run into ascent problems.

Emergencies at the Bottom

Problems related to the bottom of the dive are rarely seen. They include inadequate mixing of oxygen and carbon dioxide in the air the diver breathes and accidental feeding of poisonous carbon monoxide into the breathing apparatus. Both are the result of faulty connections in the diving gear. These situations can cause drowning or rapid ascent; they require emergency resuscitation and transport of the patient.

> **Panic is not restricted to the person who is frightened by water. It can happen even to the experienced diver or swimmer.**

Ascent Emergencies

Most of the serious injuries associated with diving are related to ascending from the bottom and are referred to as *ascent problems*. These emergencies usually require aggressive resuscitation. Two particularly dangerous medical emergencies are *air embolism* and *decompression sickness* (also called "the bends").

AIR EMBOLISM. The most dangerous, and most common, emergency in scuba diving is **air embolism**, a condition involving bubbles of air in the blood vessels. Air embolism may occur on a dive as shallow as 6 feet. The problem starts when the diver holds his or her breath during a rapid ascent. The air pressure in the lungs remains at a high level while the external pressure on the chest decreases. As a result, the air inside the lungs expands rapidly, causing the alveoli in the lungs to rupture. The air released from this rupture can cause the following injuries:

- Air may enter the pleural space and compress the lungs (a pneumothorax).

- Air may enter the mediastinum (the space within the thorax that contains the heart and great vessels), causing a condition called *pneumomediastinum*.

- Air may enter the bloodstream and create bubbles of air in the vessels called *air emboli*.

Pneumothorax and pneumomediastinum both result in pain and severe dyspnea. An air embolus will act as a plug and prevent the normal flow of blood and oxygen to a specific part of the body. The brain and spinal cord are the organs most severely affected by air embolism because they require a constant supply of oxygen.

The following are potential signs and symptoms of air embolism:

- Blotching (mottling of the skin)

- Froth (often pink or bloody) at the nose and mouth

- Severe pain in muscles, joints, or abdomen

- Dyspnea and/or chest pain

- Dizziness, nausea, and vomiting

- Dysphasia (difficulty speaking)

- Difficulty with vision

- Paralysis and/or coma

- Irregular pulse and even cardiac arrest

DECOMPRESSION SICKNESS. **Decompression sickness**, commonly called **the bends**, occurs when bubbles of gas, especially nitrogen, obstruct the blood vessels. This condition results from too rapid an ascent from a dive. During the dive, nitrogen that is being breathed dissolves in the blood and tissues because it is under pressure. When the diver ascends, the external pressure is decreased, and the dissolved nitrogen forms small bubbles within those tissues. These bubbles can lead to problems similar to those that occur in air embolism (blockage of tiny blood vessels, depriving parts of the body of their normal blood supply), but severe pain in certain tissues or spaces in the body is the most common problem.

The most striking symptom is abdominal and/or joint pain so severe that the patient literally doubles up or "bends." Dive tables and computers are available to show the proper rate of ascent from a dive, including the number and length of pauses that a diver should make on the way up. However, even divers who stay within these limits can suffer the bends.

Even after a "safe dive," decompression sickness can occur from driving a car up a mountain or flying in an unpressurized airplane that climbs too rapidly to a great height. However, the risk of this diminishes after 24 to 48 hours. The problem is exactly the same as ascent from a deep dive: a sudden decrease of external pressure on the body and release of dissolved nitrogen from the blood that forms bubbles of nitrogen gas within the blood vessels.

You may find it difficult to distinguish between air embolism and decompression sickness. As a general rule, air embolism occurs immediately on return to the surface, whereas the symptoms of decompression sickness may not occur for several hours. The emergency treatment is the same for both. It consists of BLS followed by recompression in a **hyperbaric chamber**, a chamber or a small room that is

Figure 18-12 A hyperbaric chamber, usually a small room, is pressurized to more than atmospheric pressure and used in the treatment of decompression sickness and air embolism.

pressurized to more than atmospheric pressure (▲ **Figure 18-12**). Recompression treatment allows the bubbles of gas to dissolve into the blood and equalizes the pressures inside and outside the lungs. Once these pressures are equalized, gradual decompression can be accomplished under controlled conditions to prevent the bubbles from re-forming.

In treating patients who are suspected of having air embolism or decompression sickness, you should follow these accepted treatment steps:

1. Remove the patient from the water. Try to keep the patient calm.

2. Begin BLS and administer oxygen.

3. Place the patient in a left lateral recumbent position with the head down.

4. Provide prompt transport to the nearest recompression facility for treatment.

Injury from decompression sickness is usually reversible with proper treatment. However, if the bubbles block critical blood vessels that supply the brain or spinal cord, permanent central nervous system injury may result. Therefore, the key in emergency management of these serious ascent problems is to recognize that an emergency exists and treat as soon as possible. Administer oxygen and provide rapid transport.

Other Water Hazards

You must pay close attention to the body temperature of a person who is rescued from cold water. Treat hypothermia caused by immersion in cold water the same way you treat hypothermia caused by cold exposure. Prevent further heat loss from contact with the ground, stretcher, or air, and transport the patient promptly.

A person swimming in shallow water may suffer from **breath-holding syncope**, a loss of consciousness caused by a decreased stimulus for breathing. This happens to swimmers who breathe in and out rapidly and deeply before entering the water in an effort to expand their capacity to stay underwater. While increasing the oxygen level, this hyperventilation lowers the carbon dioxide level. Because an elevated level of carbon dioxide in the blood is the strongest stimulus for breathing, the swimmer may not feel the need to breathe even after using up all the oxygen in his or her lungs. The emergency treatment for a breath-holding syncope is the same as that for a drowning or near drowning.

Injuries caused by boat propellers, sharp rocks, water skis, or dangerous marine life may be complicated by immersion in cold water. In these cases, remove the patient from the water, taking care to protect the spine, and administer oxygen. Apply dressings and splints if indicated, and monitor the patient closely for any signs of immersion or cold injury.

You should be aware that a child who is involved in a drowning or near drowning may be the victim of child abuse. Although it may be difficult to prove, such incidents should be handled according to the rules set up for suspected child abuse.

Prevention

Appropriate precautions can prevent most immersion incidents. Each year, many small children drown in residential pools. All pools should be surrounded by a fence that is at least 6′ high, with slats no farther apart than 3″ and self-closing, self-locking gates. The most common problem is lack of adult supervision, even when attention is not given for a few seconds. Half of all teenage and adult drownings are associated with the use of alcohol. As a health care professional, you should be involved in public education efforts to make people aware of the hazards of swimming pools and water recreation.

Prep Kit

Ready for Review

Cold illness can be either a local or a systemic problem. Local cold injuries include frostbite, frostnip, and immersion foot. Frostbite is the most serious because tissues actually freeze with this injury. All patients with a local cold injury should be removed from the cold and protected from further exposure. You can rewarm frostnipped parts, including immersion foot, with your warm hands or breath. On the other hand, you can cause further damage to a frost-bitten part by attempting to rewarm it in the field. If this is necessary because you cannot transport the patient to the hospital, immerse the part in water at a temperature between 100° and 112°F (38° and 44.5°C).

Patients who are exposed to the cold can also become hypothermic. The key to treating such patients is to stabilize vital functions and prevent further heat loss. Do not attempt to rewarm patients who have moderate to severe hypothermia, because they are prone to developing arrhythmias unless handled very carefully. Even if you cannot find a pulse, do not consider a patient dead until he or she is "warm and dead." Local protocol will dictate whether or not such patients receive CPR or defibrillation in the field.

The body's regulatory mechanisms normally maintain body temperature within a very narrow range around 98.6°F (37°C). The body can increase its core temperature by increasing its metabolism, for example, by shivering. In general, however, body temperature is regulated by losing heat to the atmosphere. This can occur via five mechanisms: conduction, convection, evaporation, radiation, and respiration. Of these, evaporation, convection, and radiation are the most important. The very young and the very old, as well as patients with certain diseases and medication regimens, are at increased risk of heat or cold injuries because their regulatory mechanisms are not as efficient as those of other patients.

Heat illness can take three forms: heat cramps, heat exhaustion, and heatstroke. Heat cramps are painful muscle spasms that occur with vigorous exercise. They usually go away if you remove the patient from the hot environment, rest the affected muscles, and replace lost fluids (by drinking a lot of water).

Heat exhaustion, a more systemic illness, is essentially a form of hypovolemic shock. It occurs when the body loses so much water and so many electrolytes that it becomes dehydrated. Patients with heat exhaustion may be cold and clammy, weak or faint, confused, and have a headache. As with other patients in shock, the pulse is often rapid. Body temperature can be high, and the patient may or may not still be sweating. Treatment includes removing the patient, if feasible, from the heat and treating for mild hypovolemic shock, usually with oral fluids. More often, IV fluids will be necessary.

Heat exhaustion can progress to heatstroke. This is a life-threatening emergency, usually fatal if untreated. Patients with heatstroke may or may not still be sweating, but they will usually be dry and will have high body temperatures. Changes in mental status can include coma. Rapid lowering of the body temperature in the field can save the life of a patient with heatstroke. Fanning dampened skin and placement of cold packs around the neck, armpits, and groin are key.

Drowning and near-drowning incidents can occur even in areas that are not associated with water recreation. The first rule in caring for victims of such incidents is to be sure not to become a victim yourself. Take care to protect the spine when removing patients from the water, since spinal cord injuries, especially cervical spine injuries, are often involved in drownings. Be aware of the possibility of hypothermia, especially in cold water immersions.

While some injuries associated with scuba diving are immediately apparent, others may show up hours later. Most significant injuries occur during ascent. Patients with air embolism or decompression sickness may have pain, paralysis, or altered mental status. Be prepared to transport such patients to a recompression facility with a hyperbaric chamber.

Vital Vocabulary

air embolism Air bubbles in the blood vessels.

ambient temperature The temperature of the surrounding environment.

bends Common name for decompression sickness.

bradycardia Slow heart rate, less than 60 beats/min.

breath-holding syncope Loss of consciousness caused by a decreased breathing stimulus.

conduction The loss of heat by direct contact (eg, when a body part comes into contact with a colder object).

convection The loss of body heat caused by air movement (eg, breeze blowing across the body).

core temperature The temperature of the central part of the body (eg, the heart, lungs, and vital organs).

decompression sickness A painful condition seen in divers who ascend too quickly, in which gas, especially nitrogen, forms bubbles in blood vessels and other tissues; also called "the bends."

diving reflex Slowing of the heart rate caused by submersion in cold water.

drowning Death from suffocation by submersion in water.

electrolytes Certain salts and other chemicals that are dissolved in body fluids and cells.

evaporation Conversion of water or another fluid from a liquid to a gas.

frostbite Damage to tissues as the result of exposure to cold; frozen body parts.

heat cramps Painful muscle spasms usually associated with vigorous activity in a hot environment.

heat exhaustion A form of heat injury in which the body loses significant amounts of fluid and electrolytes because of heavy sweating; also called heat prostration or heat collapse.

heatstroke A life-threatening condition of severe hyperthermia caused by exposure to excessive natural or artificial heat, marked by warm, dry skin; severely altered mental status; and often irreversible coma.

hyperbaric chamber A chamber, usually a small room, pressurized to more than atmospheric pressure.

hyperthermia A condition in which core temperature rises to 101°F (38.3°C) or more.

hypothermia A condition in which core temperature falls below 95°F (35°C) after exposure to a cold environment.

laryngospasm A severe constriction of the larynx and vocal cords.

near drowning Survival, at least temporarily, after suffocation in water.

radiation The direct loss of body heat to colder objects in the environment, or heat gain from warmer objects such as the sun.

respiration The loss of body heat as warm air in the lungs is exhaled into the atmosphere and cooler air is inhaled.

scuba A system that delivers air to the mouth and lungs at various atmospheric pressures, increasing with the depth of the dive; stands for **self-contained underwater breathing apparatus**.

www.emtb.com

Assessment in Action

It is a hot, humid August day and inside the North End Welding Shop, the temperature is more than 120°F. Usually, the employees work for only 50 minutes between breaks. However, one welder was trying to catch up on a difficult job, so he skipped two consecutive breaks and collapsed suddenly. You arrive to find a 23-year-old man sitting on the floor against a wall. The patient reports that he feels weak and dizzy and has abdominal pain, "like someone punched me in the gut."

A coworker who saw the event reports that after he called EMS, he checked on the patient and found that the patient could scarcely respond. The patient states that he has been battling the flu for the last couple of days and has had several episodes of vomiting and diarrhea. Because of that, he has had little to eat or drink. Assessment reveals that the patient has cool, moist skin, a blood pressure of 118/68 mm Hg, a pulse of 126 beats/min, and respirations of 24 breaths/min.

1. The patient's severe muscle cramps have most likely developed because his:
   A. pulse rate is higher than normal.
   B. systolic blood pressure is too low for his body.
   C. respirations are not keeping up with the metabolic need.
   D. electrolytes are depleted, causing muscle cramps.

2. Your first step in caring for this patient should be to:
   A. listen to his breath sounds.
   B. move him to a cooler environment.
   C. administer supplemental oxygen.
   D. obtain more of a medical history.

3. The high temperature in the welding shop has reduced the patient's ability to:
   A. exchange carbon dioxide for oxygen.
   B. exchange oxygen for carbon dioxide.
   C. compensate through breathing.
   D. lose heat from sweating.

4. Once you have moved the patient to the ambulance, you decide to cool him with ice packs. Appropriate application of ice packs includes:
   A. placing them directly in the armpits and groin.
   B. covering them with a washcloth prior to application.
   C. applying to the forehead and face.
   D. covering them with heavy towels prior to application.

5. The patient states that he cannot afford to take the time off and go to the hospital and that he really would like to return to work. At this point you should:
   A. suggest that the patient drive himself home and go to bed.
   B. summon law enforcement and force him to go to the hospital.
   C. encourage the patient to go to the hospital for a complete evaluation.
   D. help the patient out of the ambulance and let him return to work.

You have been called to an apartment where an elderly man was found by a relative unresponsive, lying on his sofa. You notice that it is chilly in the apartment and you must keep your coat on to keep warm. The patient is unresponsive to voice and moans with pain. His skin is pale, cool, and dry. His radial pulse is hard to feel; the carotid is weak and irregular. There are no signs of trauma. Vital signs include an irregular pulse of 62 beats/min, respirations of 8 breaths/min, and a blood pressure of 88/56 mm Hg.

6. A good way to assess this patient's general temperature is to:
   A. pull back your glove and place the back of your hand on the patient's abdomen.
   B. gently pinch the skin on the patient's forehead and observe for delayed movement.
   C. find the thermostat and read the temperature.
   D. pull back your glove and place your hand on his mouth to feel the temperature of exhaled air.

7. This patient's pulse should be assessed for:
   A. 15 seconds and multiply by 4.
   B. 20 seconds and multiply by 3.
   C. 30 seconds and multiply by 2.
   D. 45 to 60 seconds.

8. Management of hypothermia, regardless of the severity, consists of stabilizing the vital functions and:
   A. warming the patient as fast as possible.
   B. preventing further heat loss.
   C. beginning active rewarming.
   D. applying the AED.

9. Appropriate care of this patient includes:
   A. removing all his clothing and wrapping in blankets.
   B. applying heat packs or hot water bottles to the groin.
   C. vigorous massaging of the extremities.
   D. administering warm fluids such as hot chocolate.

Challenging Question

10. This patient is not shivering. What is the significance of that?

Points to Ponder

You are staged at a search for a toddler who walked away from her home. Your partner has agreed to stay with the ambulance while you help search for the child. It is a cold snowy night, and everyone knows that it is unlikely a young child will survive the cold. The child has been missing about 10 hours when you notice her father sitting in an alley holding something. When you approach him you see that he is holding the child and crying. The child is blue, limp and cold and you cannot feel a pulse. You want to take the child and begin resuscitation because you cannot be sure how long she has been unresponsive. The father tells you no, that she is dead and he just wants to hold her and be with her. The father refuses to let go of her and starts to move away from you. How would you handle this situation? Would you force the child from the father? Does the father have the right to refuse treatment? Is the child "saveable?" Who could help you in this case?

Issues   Stages of Grief, Living DNRs, Parental Rights, Consent, Care for Family and Friends, Personal Feelings Regarding Children, EMT's Need to "Do Something."

Online Outlook

Hypothermia can develop either quickly, as when someone is immersed in cold water, or more gradually, as when a lost hunter is exposed to the cold environment for several hours or more. To learn more about preventing and treating hypothermia, complete Exercise 18 at www.emtb.com.

www.emtb.com

Behavioral Emergencies

Objectives

Cognitive

1. Define behavioral emergencies (p 478).
2. Discuss the general factors that may cause an alteration in a patient's behavior (p 479).
3. State the various reasons for psychological crises (p 479).
4. Discuss the characteristics of an individual's behavior which suggest that the patient is at risk for suicide (p 482).
5. Discuss special medicolegal considerations for managing behavioral emergencies (p 483).
6. Discuss the special considerations for assessing a patient with behavioral problems (p 482).
7. Discuss the general principles of an individual's behavior which suggest that the patient is at risk for violence (p 486).
8. Discuss methods to calm behavioral emergency patients (p 480).

Affective

9. Explain the rationale for learning how to modify your behavior toward the patient with a behavioral emergency (p 478).

Psychomotor

10. Demonstrate the assessment and emergency medical care of the patient experiencing a behavioral emergency (p 481).
11. Demonstrate various techniques to safely restrain a patient with a behavioral problem (p 485).

TECHNOLOGY

www.emtb.com

- Online Chapter Pretest
- Interactivities
- Vocabulary Explorer
- Anatomy Review
- Web Links
- Online Review Manual
- Distance Learning

Chapter FEATURES

- Skill Drills
- Vital Vocabulary
- Pediatric Needs
- Geriatric Needs
- EMT-B Safety
- EMT-B Tips
- Documentation Tips
- Remember
- Prep Kit

The police department contacts dispatch to request an ambulance to the 35th street train station for a man who has locked himself in the bathroom and is threatening to kill himself.

Behavioral emergencies can be very challenging calls for a variety of reasons. This chapter will give you insights into how you can safely and effectively manage these calls in addition to helping you answer the following questions:

1. Is law enforcement always necessary at scenes for patients with an altered mental status?

2. What type of information gathered during the patient history might suggest to you that there is a high risk for suicide?

Behavioral Emergencies

As an EMT-B, you can expect to deal often with patients undergoing a psychological or behavioral crisis. The crisis may be due to the emergency situation, mental illness, mind-altering substances, stress, or many other causes. This chapter discusses various kinds of behavioral emergencies, including those involving overdoses, violent behavior, and mental illness. You will learn how to assess a person who exhibits signs and symptoms of a behavioral emergency and what kind of emergency care may be required in these situations. The chapter also covers legal concerns in dealing with disturbed patients. Finally, it describes how to identify and manage the potentially violent patient, including the use of restraints.

Myth and Reality

~~Everyone~~ Jason Foster has mental illness problems at some point in life, some more severe than others. Perfectly healthy people may have some of the symptoms and signs of mental illness from time to time. Therefore, you should not jump to the conclusion that you are mentally disturbed when you behave in certain ways that are discussed in this chapter. For that matter, you also should not jump to this conclusion about a patient in any given situation.

The most common misconception about mental illness is that if you are feeling "bad" or "depressed," you must be "sick." That is simply untrue. There are many perfectly justifiable reasons for feeling depressed, including divorce, loss of a job, and the death of a relative or friend. For the teenager who just broke up with his girlfriend of 12 months, it is altogether normal to withdraw from ordinary activities and to feel "blue." This is a normal reaction to a crisis situation. However, when a person finds that Monday morning blues last until Friday, week after week, he or she may indeed have a behavioral problem.

Many people believe that all individuals with mental health disorders are dangerous, violent, or otherwise unmanageable. This is untrue. Only a small percentage of those with mental health problems fall into these categories. As an EMT-B, however, you may be exposed to a higher proportion of violent patients. After all, you are seeing people who are, by definition, considered to be having an emergency; otherwise, you probably would not be seeing them. You are there because family members or friends felt unable to manage the patient by themselves. This may be a result of the use or abuse of drugs or alcohol. It may be that the patient has a long history of mental illness and is reacting to a particularly stressful event.

While you cannot determine what has caused a person's behavioral problem, you may be able to predict that the person will become violent. The ability to predict violence is an important assessment tool for the EMT-B.

Defining Behavioral Emergencies

Behavior is what you can see of a person's response to the environment: his or her actions. Sometimes, it is obvious what a person is responding to: A person is punched, and he or she runs away or bursts into tears or hits back. Sometimes, it is less clear, as when someone is depressed for very complex reasons.

Most of the time, individuals respond to the environment in reasonable ways. Over the years, they have learned to adapt to a variety of situations in daily life, including stresses and strains. This is called *adjustment*. There are times, however, when the stress is so great that the normal ways of adjusting do not work. When this happens, a person's behavior is likely to change, even if only temporarily. The new behavior may not be appropriate, or normal.

The definition of a **behavioral crisis** or emergency is any reaction to events that interferes with the **activities of daily living (ADL)** or has become unacceptable to the patient, family, or community. For example, when someone experiences an interruption of the daily routine, such as washing, dressing, and eating, chances are his or her behavior has become a problem. For that person, at that time, a behavioral emergency may exist. If the interruption of daily routine tends to recur on a regular basis, the behavior is also considered a *mental health* problem. It is then a pattern, rather than an isolated incident.

For example, a person who experiences a panic attack after having a heart attack is not necessarily mentally ill. Likewise, you would expect a person who is fired from a job to have some sort of reaction, often sadness and depression. These behavioral problems are short-term and isolated events. However, the person who reacts with a fit of rage, attacking people and property or going on a "bender" for a week, has gone beyond what society considers appropriate or normal behavior. That person is clearly undergoing a behavioral emergency. Usually, if an abnormal or disturbing pattern of behavior lasts for at least a month, it is regarded as a matter of concern from a mental health standpoint. For example, chronic **depression**, a persistent feeling of sadness and despair, may be a symptom of a mental or physical disorder. This type of long-term problem would be labeled a mental health disorder.

A person who is no longer able to respond appropriately to the environment may be having what is called a psychological or psychiatric emergency. When a psychiatric emergency arises, the patient may show agitation or violence or become a threat to himself, herself, or others. This is more serious than a more typical behavioral emergency that causes inappropriate behavior such as interference with ADL or intolerable actions. An immediate threat to the person involved or to others in the immediate area, including family, friends, bystanders, and EMT-Bs should be considered a psychiatric emer-

Documentation Tips

The medicolegal issues associated with responses to behavioral emergencies put added emphasis on thorough and specific documentation. Record detailed, objective findings that support the conclusion of abnormal behavior (withdrawn, won't talk, crying uncontrollably) and quote the patient's own words when appropriate. ("Life isn't worth it any more," or "The voices are telling me to kill people"). Avoid judgmental statements; these create the impression that you based your care on personal bias rather than the patient's needs.

gency. For example, a person might respond to the death of a spouse by attempting suicide. On the other hand, although this is a major life disruption, it does not have to involve violence or harm to an individual. Disruption can take many forms; not all involve violence nor are they all psychiatric emergencies.

The Magnitude of Mental Health Problems

According to the National Institutes of Mental Health, at one time or another, one in five Americans has some type of **mental disorder**, an illness with psychological or behavioral symptoms that may result in an impairment in functioning. It can be caused by a social, psychological, genetic, physical, chemical, or biologic disturbance.

Pathology: Causes of Behavioral Emergencies

Although sudden grief, emotional conflicts, and other psychological problems can cause behavioral emergencies, sudden illness, recent trauma, drug or alcohol intoxication, and diseases of the brain, such as Alzheimer's disease, can produce abnormal behavior as well. Likewise, altered mental status can arise from low levels of blood glucose, lack of oxygen, inadequate blood flow to the brain, and excessive heat or cold. As an EMT-B, you are not responsible for diagnosing the underlying cause of a behavioral or psychiatric emergency. However, you should know the two basic categories of diagnosis a physician will use: organic (physical) and functional (psychological).

Organic brain syndrome is a temporary or permanent dysfunction of the brain caused by a disturbance in the physical or physiologic functioning of brain tissue, such as the disturbances listed above.

> You should know the two basic types of underlying causes of behavioral emergencies: organic (physical) and functional (psychological).

That is, something has gone wrong in the way the organ itself is working. For example, low levels of blood glucose could cause organic brain syndrome. A **functional disorder** is one in which the abnormal operation of an organ cannot be traced to an obvious change in the actual structure, or physiology, of the organ. Something has gone wrong, but the root cause cannot be identified as the working of the organ itself. Schizophrenia is a good example of a functional disorder.

These two types of disorders can look very much alike. An **altered mental status**, or a change in the way a person thinks or behaves, is one indicator of central nervous system diseases. A patient displaying bizarre behavior may turn out to have an acute medical illness that is the cause, or a partial cause, of the behavior. Recognizing this possibility may allow you to save a life.

TABLE 19-1 Safety Guidelines for Behavioral Emergencies

- **Be prepared to spend extra time.** It may take longer to assess, listen to, and prepare the patient for transport.

- **Have a definite plan of action.** Decide who will do what. If restraint is needed, how will it be accomplished?

- **Identify yourself calmly.** Try to gain the patient's confidence. If you begin shouting, the patient is likely to shout louder or become more excited. A low, calm voice is often a quieting influence.

- **Be direct.** State your intentions and what you expect of the patient.

- **Assess the scene.** If the patient is armed or has potentially harmful objects in his or her possession, have these removed by law enforcement personnel before you provide care.

- **Stay with the patient.** *Do not let the patient leave the area, and do not leave yourself unless law enforcement personnel can stay with the patient.* Otherwise, the patient may go to another room and obtain weapons, lock himself or herself in the bathroom, or take pills.

- **Encourage purposeful movement:** Help the patient to get dressed and gather appropriate belongings to take to the hospital.

- **Express interest in the patient's story.** Let the patient tell you what happened or what is going on now in his or her own words. However, do not play along with auditory or visual disturbances.

- **Do not get too close to the patient;** everyone needs personal space. Furthermore, you want to be sure you can move quickly if the patient becomes violent or tries to run away. Do not physically talk down to or directly confront the patient. A squatting, 45° angle approach is usually not confrontational but may hinder your movements. Do not allow the patient to get between you and the exit.

- **Avoid fighting with the patient.** You do not want to get into a power struggle. Remember, the patient is not responding to you in a normal manner; he or she may be wrestling with internal forces over which neither of you has control. You and others may be stimulating these inner forces without knowing it. If you can respond with understanding to the feeling that the patient is expressing, whether this is anger or fear or desperation, you may be able to gain his or her cooperation. If it is necessary to use force, be sure you have adequate help and move toward the patient quietly and with assured firmness.

- **Be honest and reassuring.** If the patient asks whether he or she has to go to the hospital, the answer should be, "Yes, that is where you can receive medical help."

- **Do not judge.** You may see behavior that you dislike. Set those feelings aside and concentrate on providing emergency medical care.

Safe Approach to a Behavioral Emergency

All the regular EMT-B skills—assessment, providing care, patient approach, history taking, and patient communication—are used in behavioral emergencies. However, other management techniques also come into play. There is not room in this chapter for a full discussion of these techniques, but you should follow general guidelines to ensure your safety at the scene of a behavioral emergency (◄ **Table 19-1**).

Assessing a Behavioral Emergency

In evaluating a situation that is considered a behavioral emergency, the first things to consider are your safety and how the patient is responding to the environment (▼ **Table 19-2**). Is the situation unduly dangerous to you and your partner? Do you need immediate law enforcement backup? Does the patient's behavior seem typical or normal in the circumstances? For example, a patient who has just been assaulted has good reason to be fearful of other people, including you. On the other hand, if you ask a person, "Do you know where you are?" and he or she replies, "The planet Venus" (and does not seem to be joking), you may conclude that the person is disoriented, regardless of the cause.

A behavioral crisis puts tremendous stress on a person's coping mechanisms, including natural abilities

---

TABLE 19-2 Questions to Ask in Evaluating a Behavioral Crisis

- How does the patient relate to you?

- Does the patient answer your questions appropriately?

- Is the patient withdrawn or detached?

- Is the patient hostile or friendly? Too friendly?

- Does the patient understand why you are there?

- How is the patient dressed? Is the dress appropriate for the time of year and occasion? Are the clothes clean or dirty?

- Are the patient's movements coordinated or jerky and awkward? Does he or she appear to be agitated?

- Are the patient's movements purposeful? Are the movements helping to accomplish a task, such as sitting down and putting on a pair of shoes, or do they appear to be aimless, such as rocking back and forth in the chair?

- Has the patient harmed himself or herself? Is there damage to the surroundings?

- What are the patient's facial expressions? Are they bland and flat or expressive? Does the patient show joy, fear, or anger as appropriate? To what degree?

- Does the patient appear relaxed, or stiff and guarded?

- Are the patient's vocabulary and expressions what you would expect under the circumstances? Are they in line with the patient's social and educational background?

- Is the patient easily distracted?

- Are the patient's responses to what is going on around him or her appropriate?

- Is the patient's memory intact? Check orientation to time, place, person: Do you know what day/month/year it is? Do you know where you are? Do you know who I am?

- Is the patient alert and able to talk logically and coherently?

- What is the patient's mood? Does he or she seem agitated, elated, abnormally depressed?

- Does the patient appear fearful or worried?

- Does the patient express disordered thoughts, delusions, or hallucinations? That is, does he or she appear to be seeing, hearing, or responding to people or situations that are not present?

Figure 19-1 Making eye contact with a patient can provide useful clues about a patient's emotional state.

and training. The person is actually incapable of responding reasonably to the demands of the environment. This state may be temporary, as in an acute illness, or longer-lived, as in a complex, chronic mental illness. In either case, the patient's perception of reality may be compromised or distorted.

Sometimes a patient in a behavioral or psychiatric emergency will not respond at all to your questions. In those cases, you may be able to tell quite a lot about the patient's emotional state from facial expressions, pulse, and respirations. Tears, sweating, and blushing may be significant indicators of state of mind. Also, make sure that you look at the patient's eyes; a patient who has a blank gaze or rapidly moving eyes may be experiencing CNS depression or some type of extra stress **▲ Figure 19-1** .

In trying to determine the reason for the patient's state, you should consider three major areas as possible contributors:

- Is the patient's central nervous system functioning properly? For example, the patient may be experiencing diabetic problems, particularly hypoglycemia. He or she may have been poisoned or may be responding to a physical trauma of some sort. Any of these situations could cause the patient to behave in an unusual or irrational fashion.

- Are hallucinogens or other drugs or alcohol a factor? Does the patient see strange things? Is everything distorted? Do you smell alcohol on the patient's breath?

- Are **psychogenic** circumstances, symptoms, or illness (caused by mental rather than physical factors) involved? These might include the death of a loved one, severe depression, a history of mental illness, threats of suicide, or some other major interruption of ADL.

Family, friends, and observers may be of great help in answering these questions. Together with your observations and interaction with the patient, they should provide enough data for you to assess the situation. This assessment has two primary goals: recognizing major threats to life, and reducing the stress of the situation as much as possible.

Suicide

The single most significant factor that contributes to suicide is depression. Any time you encounter an emotionally depressed patient, you must consider the possibility of suicide. Risk factors for suicide are listed in **▶ Table 19-3** .

It is a common misconception that people who threaten suicide never commit it. This is not correct. Suicide is a cry for help. Threatening suicide is an indication that someone is in a crisis he or she cannot handle. Immediate intervention is necessary.

Whether or not the patient has any of these risk factors, you must be alert to the following warning signs:

- Does the patient have an air of tearfulness, sadness, deep despair, or hopelessness that suggests depression?

- Does the patient avoid eye contact, speak slowly or haltingly, and project a sense of vacancy, as if he or she really isn't there?

TABLE 19-3 Risk Factors for Suicide

- Depression, any age
- Previous suicide attempt (80% of successful suicides were preceded by at least one attempt.)
- Current expression of wanting to commit suicide or sense of hopelessness
- Family history of suicide
- Age older than 40 years, particularly for single, widowed, divorced, alcoholic, or depressed individuals (Men in this category who are older than age 55 years have an especially high risk.)
- Recent loss of spouse, significant other, family member, or support system
- Chronic debilitating illness or recent diagnosis of serious illness
- Holidays
- Financial setback, loss of job, police arrest, imprisonment, or some sort of social embarrassment
- Substance abuse, particularly with increasing usage
- Children of an alcoholic parent
- Severe mental illness
- Anniversary of death of loved one, job loss, marriage, etc
- Unusual gathering or new acquisition of things that can cause death, such as purchase of a gun, a large volume of pills, or increased use of alcohol

---

- Does the patient seem unable to talk about the future? Ask the patient whether he or she has any vacation plans. Suicidal people consider the future so uninteresting that they do not think about it; people who are seriously depressed consider the future so distant that they may not be able to think about it at all.

- Is there any suggestion of suicide? Even vague suggestions should not be taken lightly, even if presented as a joke. If you think that suicide is a possibility, do not hesitate to bring the subject up. You will not "give the patient ideas" if you ask directly, "Are you considering suicide?"

- Does the patient have any specific plans relating to death? Has the patient recently prepared a will? Given away significant possessions or advised close friends what he or she would like done with them? Arranged for a funeral service? These are critical warning signs.

Consider also the following additional risk factors for suicide:

- Are there any unsafe objects in the patient's hands or nearby (eg, a sharp knife, glass, poisons, a gun)?
- Is the environment unsafe (eg, an open window in a high-rise building, a patient standing on a bridge or precipice)?

- Is there evidence of self-destructive behavior (eg, partially cut wrists, large alcohol or drug intake)?
- Is there an imminent threat to the patient or others?
- Is there an underlying medical problem?

Remember, the suicidal patient may be homicidal as well. Do not jeopardize your life or the lives of your fellow EMT-Bs. If you have reason to believe that you are in danger, you must obtain police intervention. In the meantime, try not to frighten the patient or make him or her suspicious.

Medicolegal Considerations

The medical and legal aspects of emergency medical care become more complicated when the patient is undergoing a behavioral or psychiatric emergency. Nevertheless, legal problems are greatly reduced with the emotionally disturbed patient who consents to care. Gaining that patient's confidence is therefore a critical task for the EMT-B.

Mental incapacity can take many forms: unconsciousness (as a result of hypoxia, alcohol, or drugs), temporary but severe stress, or depression. Once you have determined that a patient has impaired mental capacity, you must decide whether he or she requires

Geriatric Needs

As the population ages, you will begin to see more patients in the over-65 age group. In responding to an increasing number of geriatric patients, you will probably notice some behavioral or mental health problems, including depression, dementia, and delirium. These mental status changes can affect your ability to thoroughly assess and treat the ill or injured geriatric patient. Understanding the causes of altered behavior in the elderly patient will help you in patient care.

Depression is one of the more common mental status problems that you will see in the older population. While a lot of attention has been paid to depression in younger adults, the media has not given much credence to the older adult's mental health challenges. As an EMT, you can recognize a problem and perhaps prevent a suicide in the depressed elderly person.

Depression has a number of causes, some organic, some psychological, and some cultural. Organic causes of depression include an emotional response to a major illness such as cancer or dementia. Furthermore, medications can induce a feeling of depression, especially when interacting with other prescription drugs. Finally, changes in the endocrine system, such as menopause, can elicit depression.

With all the possible causes of depression, an older adult can feel helpless and hopeless. The depressed person can be either argumentative or placid. He or she might trivialize complaints, not wanting to be of a bother to anyone. Someone who sees no way out of his or her situation may turn to suicide. Be alert for a suicide gesture or ideation, even though it may not be obvious.

While depression can create behavioral problems in the elderly patient, dementia is another cause of abnormal behavior. The most common cause of dementia is primary progressive dementia, also known as Alzheimer's dementia. It is estimated that 10% of the population older than age 65 years and 50% of the population older than age 85 years have Alzheimer's dementia. Currently, there is no cure for Alzheimer's, and once it has been diagnosed, the patient's life expectancy can range from 7 to 20 years.

During the progression of the disease, the patient can develop openly hostile behavior, kicking, yelling, pinching, and hitting you, your partner, or the patient's caregiver. You might need to contain the violent patient, but do so gently and only to the point at which the violent behavior stops.

Other causes of altered behavior include diabetic emergencies, heat- and cold-related illnesses, poisoning or overdose, strokes or TIAs, and infection. It is interesting to note that, while the mechanism is not understood, urinary tract infection or constipation can alter an elderly person's behavior.

As the EMT responding to a call for help, you should accept the possibility of depression in the elderly patient. Do not discount the patient's feelings or devalue his or her emotions. Be alert for a suicide gesture, and pay attention to any statements about death. To get the patient's cooperation, you can elicit his or her help in providing care for the acute illness or injury. A smile and a touch can go a long way in alleviating fear in all of your patients, especially the elderly.

---

immediate emergency medical care. A patient who is mentally unstable may resist your attempts to render care. Nevertheless, you must not leave this patient alone. Doing so may expose you to civil action for abandonment or negligence. In such situations, you should request that law enforcement personnel handle the patient. Another reason for seeking law enforcement support is for the patient who resists treatment; such a patient will often threaten EMT-Bs and others.

Consent

When a patient is not mentally competent to grant consent for emergency medical care, the law assumes that there is implied consent. For example, the consent of an unconscious patient is implied if life or health is at risk. The law refers to this as the emergency doctrine: consent is implied because of the necessity for immediate emergency treatment. In a situation that is not immediately life threatening, emergency medical care or transportation may be delayed until the proper consent is obtained.

In cases involving psychiatric emergencies, however, the matter is not always clear-cut. Does a life-threatening emergency exist or not? If you are not sure, you should request the assistance of law enforcement personnel.

Limited Legal Authority

As an EMT-B, you have limited legal authority to require or force a patient to undergo emergency medical care when no life-threatening emergency

> When a patient is not mentally competent to grant consent for emergency medical care, the law assumes that there is implied consent.

exists. Patients have the right to refuse care. However, most states have legal statutes regarding the emergency care of mentally ill and drug-impaired individuals. These statutory provisions permit law enforcement personnel to place such a person in protective custody so that emergency care can be rendered. You should be familiar with your local and state laws regarding these situations.

The typical provision states that "any police officer who has reasonable cause to believe that a person is mentally ill and dangerous to himself, herself, or others or gravely disabled...may take such person into custody and take or cause such person to be taken to a general hospital for emergency examination..." Again, since these provisions vary, you should become familiar with those in your state.

The general rule of law is that a competent adult has the right to refuse treatment, even if lifesaving care is involved. In psychiatric cases, however, a court of law would probably consider your actions in providing lifesaving care to be appropriate, particularly if you have a reasonable belief that the patient would harm himself, herself, or others without your intervention.

Restraint

Ordinarily, restraint of a person must be ordered by a physician, a court order, or a law enforcement officer. If you restrain a person without authority in a nonemergency situation, you expose yourself to a possible lawsuit, as well as to personal danger. Legal actions against the EMT-B can involve charges of assault, battery, false imprisonment, and violation of civil rights. You may use restraints only to protect yourself or others from bodily harm or to prevent the patient from causing injury to himself or herself ▶ **Figure 19-2** . In either case, you may use only reasonable force as necessary to control the patient, something that different courts may define differently. For this reason, you should always consult medical control and contact law enforcement for help before restraining a patient.

In fact, you probably should always involve law enforcement personnel if you are called to assist a patient in a severe behavioral or psychiatric crisis. They will provide physical backup in managing the patient as well as the necessary witness and legal authority to restrain the patient. A patient who is restrained by law enforcement personnel is in their custody.

Always try to transport a disturbed patient without restraints if possible. Once the decision has been made to restrain a patient, however, you should carry it out quickly. Be aware of BSI precautions. If the patient is spitting, place a surgical mask over his or her mouth.

Make sure you have adequate help to restrain a patient safely. At least four people should be present to carry out the restraint, each being responsible for one extremity. Before you begin, discuss the plan of action. As you prepare to restrain the patient, stay outside the patient's range of motion.

In subduing a disturbed patient, use the minimum force necessary. You should avoid acts or physical force that may cause injury to the patient. The level of force will vary, depending on the following factors:

- The degree of force that is necessary to keep the patient from injuring himself or herself, or others

- A patient's gender, size, strength, and mental status

Figure 19-2 You may use restraints only to protect yourself or others, or to prevent a patient from causing injury to himself or herself.

- The type of abnormal behavior the patient is exhibiting. You should use only restraint devices that have been approved by your state's health department for this purpose; soft, wide leather or cloth restraints are preferred to police-type handcuffs.

Acting at the same time, the police officers should secure the patient's extremities with approved equipment. Somebody, preferably you or your partner, should continue to talk to the patient throughout the process. Remember to treat the patient with dignity and respect at all times. Also, monitor the patient for vomiting, airway obstruction, and cardiovascular stability, since the patient cannot fend for himself or herself. Drug or alcohol intoxication may cause violent behavior but then lead to such physical problems as well. To enhance your protection of the patient, you might place the patient face down on a stretcher and secure the patient with multiple straps. Assess the airway even more frequently while the patient is restrained in this manner. You should make frequenct checks of circulation on all restrained extremities, regardless of patient position (▼ **Figure 19-3**). Document the reason for the restraint and the technique that was used. Be especially careful if a combative patient suddenly becomes calm and cooperative. This is the time not to relax but to secure the situation. The patient may suddenly become combative again and injure someone. Keep in mind that you may use reasonable force to defend yourself against an attack by an emotionally disturbed patient. It is extremely helpful to have (and document) witnesses in attendance even

Figure 19-3 Assess circulation frequently while the patient is restrained.

Documentation Tips

After restraining a patient, document the reason for doing so and the method you used. Check pulse, motor, and sensory function in all extremities, make any adjustments needed to ensure adequate function, and record your actions and findings in detail.

during transport to protect against false accusations. EMT-Bs have been accused of sexual misconduct or other physical abuse in such circumstances.

The Potentially Violent Patient

Violent patients make up only a small percentage of those undergoing a behavioral or psychiatric crisis. However, the potential for violence by such a patient is always an important consideration for the EMT-B.

Use the following list of risk factors to assess the level of danger:

- **Past history.** Has the patient previously exhibited hostile, overly aggressive, or violent behavior? Ask individuals at the scene, or request this information from law enforcement personnel or family.

- **Posture.** How is the patient sitting or standing? Is the patient tense, rigid, or sitting on the edge of his or her seat? Such physical tension is often a warning signal of impending hostility.

- **The scene.** Is the patient holding or near potentially lethal objects such as a knife, gun, glass, poker, or bat (or near a window or glass door)?

- **Vocal activity.** What kind of speech is the patient using? Loud, obscene, erratic, and bizarre speech patterns usually indicate emotional distress. Someone using quiet, ordered speech is not as likely to strike out as someone who is yelling and screaming.

- **Physical activity.** The motor activity of a person undergoing a psychiatric crisis may be the most telling factor of all. The patient who has tense muscles, clenched fists, or glaring eyes; is pacing; cannot sit still; or is fiercely protecting personal space requires careful watching. Agitation may predict a quick escalation to violence.

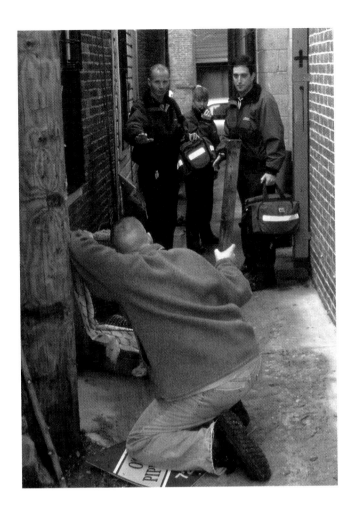

Other factors to consider in assessing a patient's potential for violence include the following:

- Poor impulse control
- A history of truancy, fighting, and uncontrollable temper
- Low socioeconomic status, unstable family structure, or inability to keep a steady job
- Tattoos, especially those with gang identification or statements such as "Born to Kill" or "Born to Lose"
- Substance abuse
- Depression, which accounts for 20% of violent attacks
- Functional disorder (If the patient says that voices are telling him or her to kill, believe it.)

Prep Kit

Ready for Review

Behavioral emergencies can present the EMT-B with great difficulties in patient management. Your major responsibility in these situations is to defuse potentially life-threatening incidents and reduce the impact of the stressful condition without exposing yourself to unnecessary risks. While only a small percentage of individuals with mental health disorders are dangerous to themselves or others, you may be exposed to a higher proportion of violent individuals in your daily activities. There are a number of warning signs of violence, including a past history of hostile behavior, rigidity, loud and erratic speech patterns, agitation, and depression.

A behavioral emergency is any reaction to events that interferes with activities of daily living. A person who is no longer able to respond appropriately to the environment may be having a more serious psychiatric emergency. Not all behavioral emergencies involve a mental health problem, however. Some emergencies are a temporary response to a traumatic event.

Underlying causes of behavioral emergencies fall into two categories: organic brain syndrome and functional disorders.

Assessing a person who may be having a behavioral crisis involves observing the person, talking with the person, and talking with friends, family members, and witnesses to the person's behavior. You are looking for indications that the person's thoughts, feelings, and reactions are inappropriate for the circumstances.

Consider contributing factors in three areas: central nervous system functioning, drug or alcohol use, and psychogenic circumstances such as the death of a loved one or other major interruption of normal life.

The threat of suicide requires immediate intervention. Depression is the most significant risk factor for suicide. Others include personal or family history of suicide attempts, chronic debilitating illness, financial setback, and severe mental illness.

As an EMT-B, you have limited legal authority to require a patient to undergo emergency medical care in the absence of a life-threatening emergency. However, most states have provisions allowing law enforcement personnel to place mentally impaired persons in custody so that such care can be provided. You should always involve law enforcement personnel any time you are called to assist a patient in a severe behavioral or psychiatric crisis. Always consult medical control and contact law enforcement for help before restraining a patient. If restraints are required, use the minimum force necessary. Assess the airway and circulation frequently while the patient is restrained.

In providing emergency medical care for a patient having a behavioral emergency, be direct, honest, and calm; have a definite plan of action; stay with the patient at all times, but don't get too close; express interest in the patient's story, but do not judge his or her behavior. Always treat such patients with respect.

Vital Vocabulary

activities of daily living (ADL) The basic activities a person usually accomplishes during a normal day, such as eating, dressing, and washing.

altered mental status A change in the way a person thinks and behaves that may signal disease in the central nervous system.

behavior How a person functions or acts in response to his or her environment.

behavioral crisis The point at which a person's reactions to events interfere with activities of daily living; a behavioral crisis becomes a psychiatric emergency when it causes a major life interruption, such as attempted suicide.

depression A persistent mood of sadness, despair, and discouragement; depression may be a symptom of many different mental and physical disorders, or it may be a disorder on its own.

functional disorder A disorder in which there is no known physiologic reason for the abnormal functioning of an organ or organ system.

mental disorder An illness with psychological or behavioral symptoms and/or impairment in functioning, caused by a social, psychological, genetic, physical, chemical, or biologic disturbance.

organic brain syndrome Temporary or permanent dysfunction of the brain, caused by a disturbance in the physical or physiologic functioning of brain tissue.

psychogenic A symptom or illness that is caused by mental factors as opposed to physical ones.

Assessment in Action

You are dispatched to a duplex for an "unknown medical emergency." On arrival, you find an unkempt 57-year-old man lying on the couch in a well-furnished living room. He is awake but does not focus on you and seems to be oblivious to what is going on around him. He slowly responds when you speak to him but still seems drowsy as you begin to ask questions.

The woman who met you at the door is apparently his soon-to-be ex-wife. She states that she and the patient have been fighting, and she leaves in a huff. Afterward, the patient tells you that he lost his job 2 months ago and has been unable to find work. He admits that he has probably been drinking too much, and now his wife is telling him that she wants a divorce. He then yells, "I can't take anymore. Enough is enough!"

1. Which of the following characterize this patient's behavior?
   A. A panic attack
   B. An anxiety disorder
   C. Depression
   D. Hallucinations

2. In assessing the patient's potential for violence, which of the following factors concerns you the most?
   A. The patient is talking to you while he is lying on the couch.
   B. The patient yells at you when you ask him about the comment he made.
   C. A family member at the scene reports that the patient has no history of violence.
   D. The patient has a medium physical build and does not appear to have a weapon.

3. This patient may be at risk for suicide. Which of the following are risk factors to assess in determining the probability for suicide?
   A. Does the patient talk about the future in a negative way?
   B. Does the patient challenge you with direct eye contact?
   C. Is the patient unable to talk about the future at all?
   D. Does the patient have a habit of collecting unusual things?

4. An appropriate way to communicate with this patient includes:
   A. using a low, calm voice.
   B. responding to the yelling with a loud voice.
   C. using a commanding tone.
   D. responding with a disinterested, detached voice.

5. Assessment of this patient includes:
   A. taking his shirt off to observe chest rise.
   B. evaluating movement of all four extremities.
   C. listening to lung sounds.
   D. a complete set of vital signs.

6. En route to the emergency department this patient starts screaming at you. While you try and verbally calm him, he turns and physically attacks you. You have the right to:
   A. physically strike him in return.
   B. stop the ambulance and order him out.
   C. use reasonable force to protect yourself.
   D. do whatever it takes to restrain him.

7. With the help of law enforcement, restraints are used on this patient. After the restraints are applied, he suddenly becomes quiet and stops yelling. Which course of action would be appropriate?
   A. Continue to transport.
   B. Assess airway and circulation.
   C. Re-evaluate the security of the restraints.
   D. Document the reasons for the restraints.

8. This patient admits to wanting to end his life and has a plan to do so but he refuses to go to the hospital. When a patient is not mentally competent to grant consent, but he or she is transported anyway, what type of consent is used?
   A. Informed consent
   B. Non-consent
   C. Implied consent
   D. Uninformed consent

Challenging Questions

9. Head injuries, diabetic reactions, and hypoxia can all result in behaviors that appear to be psychotic in nature. What do they all have in common that cause this?

10. When documenting a patient care run for an emotionally disturbed patient, it is helpful to also list the names of those who were in attendance, including police officers, security guards, nurses, etc. Why is this necessary?

Points to Ponder

You arrive at a "domestic dispute" to find that police officers were first on scene and have the husband and wife separated. The husband is in the bedroom and the wife is in the kitchen. They tell you that the wife is bleeding and the husband has been hit in the head. Your partner takes the husband and you find the wife standing at the sink washing a wound on her hand. The husband starts yelling things at the wife and the police officer that was with you goes to help subdue the husband. You open your kit and get out some bandaging material. When you turn back to the wife, she has moved and is now between you and the door. She is holding a knife and claiming that you are on her husband's side. While she is threatening to stab you, she is not moving any closer to you. How would you handle this situation? What would you tell her? Would you hit her if she came toward you? How could this have been prevented?

Issues Safety Concerns, Willingness to Protect Yourself and Your Partner, Legal and Safety Issues of Domestic Disputes, Use of Law Enforcement, Personal Feelings about Spouse Abuse.

Online Outlook

Any time you encounter an emotionally depressed patient, you must consider the possibility of suicide. To learn more about suicide and suicide prevention, complete Exercise 19 at the www.emtb.com.

www.emtb.com

Obstetrics and Gynecological Emergencies

Objectives

Cognitive

1. Identify the following structures: uterus, vagina, fetus, placenta, umbilical cord, amniotic sac, perineum (p 492).
2. Identify and explain the use of the contents of an obstetrics kit (p 496).
3. Identify predelivery emergencies (p 493).
4. State indications of an imminent delivery (p 495).
5. Differentiate the emergency medical care provided to a patient with predelivery emergencies from a normal delivery (p 493).
6. State the steps in the predelivery preparation of the mother (p 495).
7. Establish the relationship between body substance isolation and childbirth (p 496).
8. State the steps to assist in the delivery (p 497).
9. Describe care of the baby as the head appears (p 499).
10. Describe how and when to cut the umbilical cord (p 499).
11. Discuss the steps in the delivery of the placenta (p 501).
12. List the steps in the emergency medical care of the mother postdelivery (p 500).
13. Summarize neonatal resuscitation procedures (p 502).
14. Describe the procedures for the following abnormal deliveries: breech birth, prolapsed cord, limb presentation (p 504).
15. Differentiate the special considerations for multiple births (p 506).
16. Describe special considerations of meconium (p 499).
17. Describe special considerations of a premature baby (p 507).
18. Discuss the emergency medical care of a patient with a gynecological emergency (p 509).

Affective

19. Explain the rationale for understanding the implications of treating two patients (mother and baby) (p 500).

Psychomotor

20. Demonstrate the steps to assist in the normal cephalic delivery (p 497).
21. Demonstrate necessary care procedures of the fetus as the head appears (p 497).
22. Demonstrate infant neonatal procedures (p 497).
23. Demonstrate postdelivery care of infant (p 500).
24. Demonstrate how and when to cut the umbilical cord (p 499).
25. Attend to the steps in the delivery of the placenta (p 501).
26. Demonstrate the postdelivery care of the mother (p 501).
27. Demonstrate the procedures for the following abnormal deliveries: vaginal bleeding, breech birth, prolapsed cord, limb presentation (p 504).
28. Demonstrate the steps in the emergency medical care of the mother with excessive bleeding (p 506).
29. Demonstrate completing a prehospital care report for patients with obstetrical/gynecological emergencies (p 299).

While most births are uneventful and require little or no medical intervention, others may be life threatening to both the mother and baby. This chapter will help prepare you to be an active and positive part of the birthing process and will also help you answer the following questions:

1. What are the most common indicators that birth is imminent?

2. How does the care provided during a normal delivery differ from that provided to an expectant mother experiencing a predelivery emergency?

Obstetrics and Gynecological Emergencies

Most infants in the United States are delivered in a hospital, with doctors and nurses in attendance to care for not only the mother, but also the newborn infant. Occasionally, the birth process will move along faster than the mother expects, and you will find yourself with a decision to make: Should you stay on the scene and deliver the infant or transport the patient to the hospital? This chapter will tell you how to make this decision and how to proceed if on-scene delivery is necessary. It describes the normal process of childbirth and discusses common complications so that you will be prepared to handle both normal and abnormal deliveries. Next, it describes the evaluation and care of the newborn. Finally, the chapter discusses gynecological emergencies unrelated to childbirth.

Anatomy of the Female Reproductive System

The **fetus** is the developing, unborn infant that grows inside the mother's uterus for approximately 9 months. The **uterus**, or womb, is the muscular organ where the fetus grows (▶ **Figure 20-1**). It is responsible for contractions during labor and ultimately helps to push the infant through the birth canal. The **birth canal** is made up of the vagina and the lower one third or neck of the uterus, called the **cervix**. The cervix contains a mucous plug that seals the uterine opening, preventing contamination from the outside world. When the cervix begins to dilate, this plug is discharged as pink-tinged mucus, or a **bloody show**. This "show" may signal the first stage of labor.

The **vagina** is the outermost cavity of a woman's reproductive system and forms the lower part of the

birth canal. It is about 8 to 12 cm in length, begins at the cervix, and ends as an external opening of the body. Essentially, the vagina completes the passageway from the uterus to the outside world for the delivering infant. The **perineum** is the area of skin between the vagina and the anus. During birth, as the infant moves through the birth canal, the perineum will begin to bulge significantly.

As the fetus grows, it requires more and more nourishment. The **placenta**, a disk-shaped structure, is body tissue that attaches to the inner lining of the wall of the uterus and is connected to the fetus by the umbilical cord. After delivery, the placenta, or afterbirth, separates from the uterus and is delivered. The **umbilical cord** is the infant's lifeline, connecting mother and infant through the placenta. The umbilical cord contains two arteries and one vein. These vessels supply blood to the

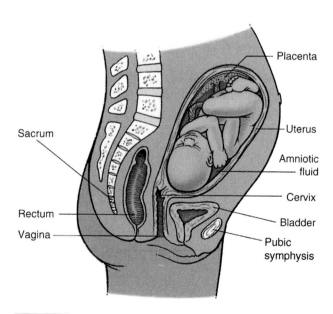

Figure 20-1 Anatomic structures of the pregnant woman.

fetus: the vein carries blood toward the heart (baby) and the arteries carry blood away from the heart (baby). Oxygen and other nutrients cross from the mother's circulation through the placenta and then along the umbilical cord to support the fetus as it grows. Carbon dioxide and waste products travel the same route in the opposite direction. The remarkable thing about this exchange is that the mother's blood and that of the fetus do not mix during the process.

The fetus develops inside a fluid-filled, baglike membrane called the **amniotic sac**, or bag of waters. The sac contains about 500 to 1,000 mL of amniotic fluid, which helps to insulate and protect the floating fetus as it develops. Released in a gush when the sac ruptures, usually at the onset of labor, this fluid helps to lubricate the birth canal and remove bacteria.

A full-term pregnancy is from 36 to 40 weeks, counting from the first day of the last menstrual cycle. The pregnancy is divided into 3 trimesters of about 3 months each. Deliveries before 36 weeks are considered premature. Toward the end of the third trimester, the head of the fetus normally descends through the broad upper inlet of the mother's pelvis, positioning itself for the delivery.

Stages of Labor

There are three stages of labor: dilation of the cervix, expulsion of the baby, and delivery of the placenta. The first stage begins with the onset of contractions and ends when the cervix is fully dilated. Because the cervix has to be stretched thin by uterine contractions until the opening is large enough for the infant to pass through into the vagina, the first stage is usually the longest, lasting an average of 16 hours for a first delivery. You will usually have time to transport the mother during the first stage of labor.

The onset of labor starts with contractions of the uterus. Other signs of the beginning of labor are the bloody show and the rupture of the amniotic sac, called breaking of the water. These events may occur before the first labor pain or later in the first stage of labor. The uterine contractions may not come at regular intervals at first. The mother may think that she simply has a nagging backache. The frequency and intensity of true labor increase with time. The uterine contractions become more regular and last about 30 to 60 seconds each. The length of labor varies greatly. As a general rule, it is longer in a **primigravida**, a woman who is experiencing her first pregnancy, and becomes shorter in a **multigravida**, a woman who has experi-

enced previous pregnancies. (Two similar terms refer to the outcomes of those pregnancies. A **multipara** is a woman who has had more than one baby born alive, and a **primipara** has had one live birth.)

The second stage of labor begins when the cervix is fully dilated and ends when the infant is born. During this stage, you will have to make a decision about helping the mother to deliver on scene or providing transport to the hospital. Because the infant has to move through the birth canal during this stage, the uterine contractions are usually closer together and last longer. Pressure on the rectum may make the mother feel as if she needs to have a bowel movement. Under no circumstances should you let the mother sit on the toilet. She may also have the uncontrollable urge to push down. The perineum will begin to bulge significantly, and the top of the infant's head should begin to appear at the vaginal opening. This is called **crowning** ▼ **Figure 20-2** .

The third stage begins with the birth of the infant and ends with the delivery of the placenta. This may take up to 30 minutes. Usually, you will not transport the mother during that time. It is important that you always follow BSI precautions, to protect yourself, the baby, and the mother from exposure to body fluids. There is a high potential of exposure due to body fluids released during childbirth.

Emergencies Prior to Delivery

Most pregnant women are healthy, but some may be ill when they conceive or become ill during pregnancy. You may safely use oxygen to treat any heart or lung disease in the mother without harm to the fetus.

Figure 20-2 Crowning occurs when the infant's head appears at the vaginal opening.

As the time for delivery nears, certain complications can occur. One of these is **pre-eclampsia**, or **pregnancy-induced hypertension**, a condition that can develop after the 20th week of gestation, most commonly in primigravidas. This condition is characterized by the following signs and symptoms:

- Headache
- Seeing spots
- Swelling in the hands and feet
- Anxiety
- High blood pressure

Another condition is **eclampsia**, convulsions that result from severe hypertension. To treat eclampsia, lay the mother on her side, maintain an airway, and provide supplemental oxygen; if vomiting occurs, suction the airway. Transport a pregnant patient with convulsions promptly. As usual, size up the situation and perform your initial assessment, history, and physical exam, and assess the baseline vital signs. Provide treatment based on signs and symptoms.

If the patient is hypotensive, transport her on the left side. Transporting the mother in this position can prevent **supine hypotensive syndrome**, a problem in which low blood pressure develops when the mother lies supine resulting from compression by the weight of the fetus onto the inferior vena cava.

Hemorrhage from the vagina that occurs before labor begins may be very serious, call for ALS backup. In early pregnancy, it may be a sign of a **spontaneous abortion**, or **miscarriage**. Bleeding may be the sign of an **ectopic pregnancy**, a pregnancy that develops outside the uterus, most often in a fallopian tube. Ectopic pregnancy occurs about once in every 200 pregnancies. The leading cause of maternal death in the first trimester is internal hemorrhage into the abdomen following rupture of an ectopic pregnancy. For this reason, you should consider the possibility of an ectopic pregnancy in women who have missed a menstrual cycle and complain of sudden stabbing and usually unilateral pain in the lower abdomen. A history of pelvic inflammatory disease, tubal ligations, or previous ectopic pregnancies should heighten your suspicions for a possible ectopic pregnancy.

In the later stages of pregnancy, hemorrhage may indicate problems with the placenta. In **placenta abruptio**, the placenta separates prematurely from the wall of the uterus (▼ **Figure 20-3**). In **placenta previa**, the placenta develops over and covers the cervix (▼ **Figure 20-4**).

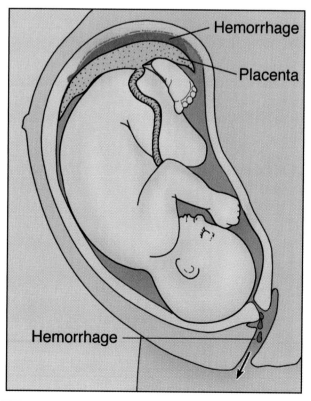

Figure 20-3 In placenta abruptio, the placenta separates prematurely from the wall of the uterus.

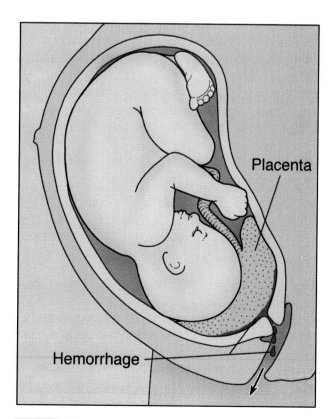

Figure 20-4 In placenta previa, the placenta develops over and covers the cervix.

Any bleeding from the vagina in a pregnant woman is a serious sign and should be treated in the hospital promptly. If the mother shows signs of shock, have her lie on her left side during transportation, and give her high-flow oxygen. Place a sterile pad or sanitary napkin over the vagina, and replace it as often as necessary. Save the pads so that hospital personnel can estimate how much blood she has lost. Also save any tissue that may be passed from the vagina. Do not put anything into the vagina.

When a pregnant woman is involved in an automobile crash, severe hemorrhage may occur from injuries to the pregnant uterus. The resulting oxygen deprivation can cause grave injury to the fetus. Promptly evaluate and transport a pregnant crash victim; support the airway, and if there is any sign of bleeding, administer high-flow oxygen and call for ALS backup. Have the mother lie on her left side rather than on her back; this will relieve the pressure of the uterus on intra-abdominal organs, especially the inferior vena cava and abdominal aorta. Pregnant women have an increased amount of blood volume. Therefore, a pregnant trauma patient may have a significant amount of blood loss before showing signs of shock. However, the infant may be in trouble well before this. Often, if the mother has sustained serious trauma, the blood supply to the fetus is reduced so that the body can supply an adequate amount of blood to the mother. In most cases, the only chance to save the infant is to adequately resuscitate the mother.

Preparing for Delivery

Consider delivering the patient at the scene in the following circumstances:

- When delivery can be expected within a few minutes
- When a natural disaster, bad weather, or some other type of catastrophe makes it impossible to reach the hospital
- When no transportation is available

How do you determine whether delivery is going to occur within a few minutes? First, look for crowning. Second, ask the mother these questions:

- How long have you been pregnant?
- When are you due?
- Is this your first baby?
- Are you having contractions? How far apart are the contractions? How long do the contractions last?

> In the first trimester, the leading cause of maternal death is internal hemorrhage into the abdomen, resulting from a ruptured ectopic pregnancy.

- Do you feel as though you have to strain or move your bowels?
- Have you had any spotting or bleeding?
- Have you had any gushing of fluid from the vagina?
- Were any of your previous children delivered by cesarean section?

Also consider asking the following questions:

- Have you had a complicated pregnancy in the past?
- Do you use drugs, drink alcohol, or take any medications?
- Is there any possibility that this is a multiple birth?
- Does your doctor expect any complications?

If this is not the patient's first child, she may be able to tell you whether she is about to deliver. If she says that she is, make immediate preparations for delivery. Otherwise, does she have a rock-hard abdomen? Does she say that she has to move her bowels or feels the need to push? If so, the infant's head is probably pressing on the rectum, and delivery is about to occur. At this point, you should inspect the vagina to determine whether crowning has occurred; if so, delivery is imminent. Do not touch the vaginal area until you are sure that delivery is, in fact, imminent. In general, do not touch vaginal areas except during delivery (under certain circumstances) and when your partner is present. Spread the mother's legs apart gently, explaining that you are doing so to decide whether the baby should be delivered immediately or if she should be transported to the hospital for the delivery.

Once labor has begun, there is no way it can be slowed down or stopped. Never attempt to hold the mother's legs together. To do so would only complicate the delivery. Do not let her go to the bathroom. Instead, reassure her that the sensation of needing to move her bowels is normal and that it means she is about to deliver.

If you decide to deliver at the scene, remember that you are only *assisting* the mother with the delivery. Your part is to help, guide, and support the infant as it is born. Remember to use BSI precautions at all times. Try to limit distractions for yourself and for the mother. You want to appear calm and reassuring while protecting the mother's modesty. Most important, recognize when the situation is beyond your level of training. If delivery is imminent with crowning, contact medical control for a decision to deliver on scene or to transport. When in doubt, contact medical control for further guidance. Always recognize your own limitations, and when you are unsure about what to do, transport the patient even if delivery must occur during transport.

Your emergency vehicle should always be equipped with a sterile emergency OB kit containing the following items (▼ **Figure 20-5**):

- Surgical scissors or a scalpel
- Umbilical cord clamps
- Umbilical tape
- A small rubber bulb syringe
- Towels
- 4″ × 4″ gauze sponges and/or 2″ × 10″ gauze sponges
- Sterile gloves
- Infant blanket
- Sanitary napkins
- An infant size bag-valve-mask
- Goggles
- A plastic bag

Remember the importance of using BSI precautions at all times.

Remember to size up the situation, perform your initial assessment, focused history, and physical exam, assess baseline vital signs, and provide treatment based on signs and symptoms.

PATIENT POSITION. The mother's clothing should be pushed up to her waist or, if she is wearing trousers and undergarments, removed. Remember to limit the mother's exposure and preserve her modesty as much as you can while helping her to move into a semi-Fowler's position. Place the mother on a firm surface that is padded with blankets, folded sheets, or towels. Put a pillow or blankets beneath her hips to elevate them about 2″ to 4″. It is sometimes better to put a pillow under one hip to allow the mother to turn to one side. This may also make it easier to suction the infant once it is born. Support the mother's head, neck, and upper back with pillows and blankets. If delivery is occurring in an automobile, the patient should lie on the seat, with one foot on the floor and the other on the seat, with the upper knee and hip bent (▼ **Figure 20-6**).

If the emergency delivery is occurring at home, you should move the mother to a sturdy flat surface. You will find it easier to work on a firm surface than on a

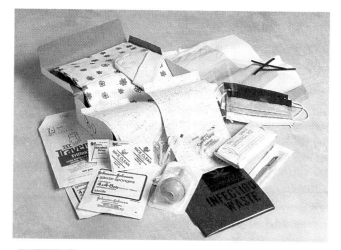
Figure 20-5 Your unit should contain a sterile OB kit. Items usually found in this kit are listed above.

Figure 20-6 For delivery in a car, have the mother lie on the seat with one foot on the floor and the other on the seat. Make sure the upper knee is bent and the upper hip is flexed.

bed. Elevate the mother's hips, and support her head with one or two pillows. Have her keep her legs and hips flexed, with her feet flat on the surface beneath her and her knees spread apart. Track the progression of the delivery closely at all times; you do not want an abrupt delivery, when the crowning head pops out uncontrollably, to occur.

PREPARING THE DELIVERY FIELD. Take the following steps to prepare the area where the infant will be born:

1. As time allows, place towels or sheets on the floor around the delivery area to help soak up the amniotic fluid that will be released when the amniotic sac ruptures ▶ **Figure 20-7A** . Note that the amniotic sac may have ruptured before you arrived. Elevate the mother's hips, and support her head with one or two pillows.

2. Open the OB kit carefully so that its contents remain sterile.

3. Put on the sterile gloves.

4. Use the sterile sheets and towels from the OB kit to make a sterile delivery field. Place one sheet or towel under the mother's buttocks, and unfold it toward her feet. The other sheet should be draped over her abdomen and upper legs. Alternatively, you can use three sheets: (1) folded under the buttocks, (2) placed between the legs, just below the vagina, and (3) placed across the abdomen ▶ **Figure 20-7B** .

Delivering the Baby

Your partner should be at the mother's head to comfort, soothe, and reassure her during the delivery. The mother may want to grip someone's hand. She may yell, cry, or say nothing at all. It is not uncommon for mothers to become nauseated, and some may vomit. If this occurs, have your partner turn the mother's head to the side so that her mouth and airway can be cleared manually or with suction, as needed.

You must continually assess the mother for crowning. Do not allow an abrupt delivery to occur. Position yourself so that you can see the vagina at all times. Time the mother's contractions from the beginning of one to the beginning of the next to determine the frequency of the contractions. In addition, time the duration of each contraction. You do this by feeling the mother's abdomen from the moment the contraction begins (uterus/abdomen tightening) to the moment it ends (uterus/abdomen relaxing). Remind the patient to take quick, short breaths during each contraction but

Figure 20-7 Preparing the delivery field. **A.** Place sheets or towels under the mother, elevate the mother's hips, and support her head with one or two pillows. **B.** Use sterile sheets and towels from the OB kit to make a clean delivery field. Place one sheet under her buttocks, drape the other over her abdomen, and place drapes over the thighs.

not to strain. In between contractions, encourage the mother to rest and breathe deeply through her mouth.

Follow the steps in ▶ **Skill Drill 20-1** to deliver the baby. These steps are described in more detail.

1. Allow the mother to push the head out. Support it as it emerges, **placing your gloved hand over its bony parts. Suction fluid from the mouth first, then the nostrils (Step 1).**

2. **Feel at the neck to see if the cord is wrapped** around it. If it is, gently lift it over the baby's head without pulling hard on the cord.

SkillDrill 20-1 Delivering the Baby

Support the bony parts of the head with your hands as it emerges. Suction fluid from the mouth, then nostrils.

As the upper shoulder appears, guide the head down slightly, if needed to deliver the shoulder.

Support the head and upper body as the lower shoulder delivers, guiding the head up if needed.

Handle the slippery delivered infant firmly but gently, keeping the neck in neutral position to maintain the airway.

Place clamps 2" to 4" apart and cut between them.

Allow the placenta to deliver itself. Do not pull on the cord to speed delivery.

3. Once the head is delivered, the upper shoulder will be visible. **Guide the head down slightly, if needed to help that shoulder deliver (Step 2).**

4. **Support the head and upper body as the shoulders deliver.** You may need to guide the head up slightly to deliver the lower shoulder **(Step 3)**.

5. Once the body is delivered, handle the infant firmly but gently. It will be slippery. **Make sure the baby's neck is in a neutral position to keep the airway open (Step 4).**

6. **Place the clamps about 2″ to 4″ apart,** about four fingerwidths from the infant's body. Once they are firmly in place, cut between the clamps **(Step 5)**.

7. **The placenta delivers itself,** usually within 30 minutes of birth. Never pull on the end of the umbilical cord in an attempt to speed delivery of the placenta **(Step 6)**.

Delivering the Head

Watch the head as it begins to exit the vagina, as it must be supported as it emerges. It may take two, three, or more contractions for the delivery of the head to occur from the time it begins to crown. Once it is obvious that the head is coming out farther with each contraction, you should place your gloved hand over the emerging bony parts of the head and exert very gentle pressure on it, decreasing the pressure slightly between contractions. This will allow the head to come out smoothly and prevent it and the rest of the infant from suddenly popping out during a strong contraction, possibly causing injury. You may want to move the patient's feet so that you are between the patient's legs during the delivery. Be careful that you do not poke your fingers into the infant's eyes or into the two soft spots, called *fontanels,* on the head. One fontanel is located at the front of the head, near the brow, and one is near the back of the head. The brain is covered only by skin and membranes at these spots.

Gentle pressure, exerted horizontally across the perineum with a sterile gauze pad, may reduce the risk of tearing as the infant is emerging ◀ Figure 20-8 . Also be prepared for the possibility that feces may come out because of the pressure on the rectum.

Figure 20-8 Applying gentle pressure on the perineum may reduce the risk of tearing as the infant emerges.

UNRUPTURED AMNIOTIC SAC. Usually, the amniotic sac will break or rupture at the beginning of labor. The sac may also rupture during contractions. If the amniotic sac has not ruptured by this point, it will appear as a fluid-filled sac (like a water balloon) emerging from the vagina. This situation is serious, as the sac will suffocate the baby if it is not removed. If it has not spontaneously ruptured, you may puncture the sac with a clamp, away from the baby's face, only as the head is crowning, not before. As the sac is punctured, amniotic fluid will gush out. Push the ruptured sac away from the infant's face as the head is delivered. Clear the baby's mouth and nose immediately, using the bulb syringe and gauze sponge. If the amniotic fluid is greenish instead of clear or has a foul odor (meconium staining), make note of this in the information you will relay to medical control. Meconium is a sign of two possible problems: a depressed newborn or airway obstruction. Thick meconium can clog the airway of the newborn. Aggressive suctioning of the baby's mouth and oropharynx before delivery of the body may prevent meconium aspiration and respiratory distress. Once the head has been delivered, it usually rotates to one side or the other rather than straight up and down.

UMBILICAL CORD AROUND THE NECK. As soon as the head is delivered, use the index finger of your other hand to feel whether the umbilical cord is wrapped around the neck. This commonly is called a **nuchal cord**. A nuchal cord that is wound tightly around the neck could cause the infant to strangle. It must therefore be released from the neck immediately ▼ Figure 20-9 . Usually, you can slip the cord gently over the infant's delivered head

Figure 20-9 If the umbilical cord is wound tightly around the baby's neck, it must be released immediately by either slipping it gently over the infant's delivered head or, if necessary, by placing two clamps about 2″ apart on the cord and cutting between the clamps.

> A newborn's body temperature can drop very quickly, so dry and wrap the infant as soon as possible. Only then will you clamp and cut the umbilical cord.

EMT-B Tips

As a baby delivers, you must divide your attention between two patients. This can keep two EMT-Bs busy, even when things go well. To ensure that special care needs do not result in neglecting one patient, designate one member of the crew to pay primary attention to each patient. Call for help early if you suspect that both will need special care, or that one will require resuscitation.

(or over the shoulder, if necessary). If not, you must cut it by placing two clamps about 2″ apart on the cord and cutting the cord between the clamps. If the cord is wrapped more than once around the neck, a rare event, you have to clamp and cut only once; then you can unwrap the cord from around the neck. Handle the cord very carefully; it is fragile and easily torn. Do not let the clamps come off until the ends of the cord have been tied. Fortunately, the cord is usually not wrapped around the infant's neck and does not have to be cut until after the entire infant has been delivered. However, you must always check for a nuchal cord.

Now that you have delivered the infant's head and verified that no nuchal cord is present, you will need to suction the amniotic fluids from the infant's airway before the delivery proceeds. You must ask the mother not to push while you are doing this, although her desire to do so will be very strong. While supporting the infant's head with one hand, quickly and efficiently suction the fluid from the mouth first and then the nostrils. If you suction the nostrils first, you may stimulate the infant to aspirate the fluid in the mouth or pharynx; since infants are nose breathers, any stimulation of the nose will cause a gasping response. In suctioning the airway, fully compress the bulb syringe before it is inserted 1″ to 1½″ into the infant's mouth, then release the bulb to suction fluids and mucus into the syringe. Make sure the syringe does not touch the back of the mouth. Discard the fluid into a towel, and repeat the procedure, suctioning the mouth and nostrils two or three times each, or until they are clear.

Delivering the Body

By the time you are finished suctioning, the mother will most likely be pushing again, and the upper shoulder will be visible in the vagina. The infant's head is the largest part of the body. Once it is born, the rest of the infant usually delivers easily. Support the head and upper body as the shoulders deliver. Do not pull the infant from the birth canal. The abdomen and hips will appear; once these deliver, support them with your other hand. Grasp the infant's feet as they are born.

Now the infant is being well supported with both hands. Handle the infant firmly but carefully. It will be slippery with a white, cheesy substance, called vernix caseosa.

Postdelivery Care

As soon as the entire infant is born, dry the baby off and wrap it immediately in a blanket or towel, and place it on one side, with the head slightly lower than the rest of its body. Wrap the baby so that only the face is exposed, making sure that the top of the head is covered. Also make sure that the baby's neck is in a neutral position so the airway remains open. Newborn babies are very sensitive to cold, so if it is at all possible, you should keep the blanket or towel warm before you use it. Use a sterile gauze pad to wipe the infant's mouth, and once again suction the mouth and nose. Suctioning the nose is particularly important, since babies breathe through their noses. If you prefer, you can pick-up and cradle the infant in your arm at the level of the mother's vagina while doing this, but always keep the head slightly downward to help prevent aspiration. After suctioning, keep the infant at the same level as the mother's vagina until the umbilical cord is cut. If the infant is higher than the vagina, blood will be siphoned from the infant through the umbilical cord back into the placenta.

A newborn's body temperature can drop very quickly, so dry and wrap the infant as soon as possible. Only then will you clamp and cut the umbilical cord.

Once the infant is born, the umbilical cord is of no further use to either mother or infant. Postdelivery care of the umbilical cord is important, as infection is easily transmitted through the cord to the baby. Using the two clamps in the OB kit, clamp the cord somewhere between the mother and the infant, preferably four fingers' width from the infant. Place the clamps about 2″ to 4″ apart. Once they are firmly in place, cut the cord between them with the sterile scissors or scalpel, using great care. Remember, the cord is fragile; if handled too roughly, it could be torn from the infant's abdomen, resulting in a fatal hemorrhage. Once the clamps are in place, there is no need to rush.

After you have cut the cord, tie the end coming from the infant. If it was a nuchal cord and cut during delivery, now is the time to tie it. Do not use ordinary string or twine, which will cut through the soft, fragile tissues of the cord. Place a loop of the special "umbilical tape" around the cord about 1″ nearer to the infant than to the clamp. Tighten the tape slowly so that it does not cut the cord, then tie it firmly with a square knot. Cut the ends of the tape, but do not remove either clamp. The part of the cord that is coming out of the mother's vagina is attached to the placenta and will be delivered when the placenta delivers.

By now, the infant should be pink and breathing on its own. Give the infant, wrapped in a warm blanket, to your partner; he or she can monitor the infant and complete its initial care. Alternatively, you can give the infant to the mother if she is alert and in stable condition, if you are allowed to do so by local protocol. The mother may want to begin breastfeeding at this time. You need to return your attention to the mother and the delivery of the placenta.

Delivery of the Placenta

The placenta is attached to the end of the umbilical cord that is coming out of the mother's vagina. Again, you need only assist. Like the infant, the placenta delivers itself, usually within a few minutes of the birth, though it may take as long as 30 minutes. Never pull on the end of the umbilical cord in an attempt to speed delivery of the placenta. You may tear the cord, the placenta, or both and cause serious, perhaps life-threatening, hemorrhage.

The normal placenta is round, about 7″ in diameter and about 1″ thick. One surface is smooth and covered with a shiny membrane; the other surface is rough and divided into lobes ▶ **Figure 20-10** . Wrap the entire placenta and cord in a towel, place them into a plastic bag, and take them to the hospital. Hospital personnel will

examine the placenta and the cord to make certain that the entire placenta has been delivered. If a piece of the placenta has been retained inside the mother, it could cause persistent bleeding or infection.

After delivery of the placenta and before transport, place a sterile pad or sanitary napkin over the vagina and straighten the mother's legs. You can help to slow bleeding by gently massaging the mother's abdomen with a firm, circular motion. The abdominal skin will be wrinkled and very soft. You should be able to feel a firm, grapefruit-sized mass in the lower abdomen. This is called the fundus. As you massage the fundus, the uterus will contract and become firmer. You can also place the infant at the mother's breast to nurse, which stimulates the uterus to contract. Both massaging the uterus and having the baby stimulate the mother's nipples will cause a production of oxytocin, which is a hormone that will help to contract the uterus and slow bleeding. Before taking her, the infant, and the placenta to the hospital, take a minute to congratulate the mother and thank anyone who assisted. In writing your medical report, be sure to record the time of birth for the birth certificate.

Some bleeding, usually less than 500 mL, occurs before the placenta delivers. The following are emergency situations:

- More than 30 minutes elapse, and the placenta has not delivered.
- There is more than 500 mL of bleeding before delivery of the placenta.
- There is significant bleeding after the delivery of the placenta.

Figure 20-10 The normal placenta is round, about 7″ in diameter and 1″ thick. One surface is smooth; the other is rough and divided into lobes.

If one or more of these events occur, transport mother and infant to the hospital promptly. Place a sterile pad or sanitary napkin over the mother's vagina, place her in Trendelenburg's (shock) position, administer oxygen, and monitor her vital signs closely. Never put anything into the vagina.

Neonatal Evaluation and Resuscitation

Remember that before you handle a newborn infant, put on gloves and follow BSI precautions. As soon as the infant is born, you must complete an initial assessment. A newborn infant will usually begin breathing spontaneously within 15 to 20 seconds after birth. If not, gently tap or flick the soles of the feet or rub the baby's back to stimulate breathing. If the baby does not breathe after 10 to 15 seconds, begin resuscitation efforts. You should use the same scoring system that physicians in hospitals use to assess the status of the infant: the <u>Apgar Score</u>. This system assigns a number value (0, 1, or 2) to each of five areas of activity of the newborn infant:

- **A**ppearance. Shortly after birth, the skin of a light-skinned infant and the mucous membranes of a dark-skinned infant should turn pink. Infants often have cyanosis of the extremities for a few minutes after birth, but hands and feet should "pink up" quickly. Blue skin all over or blue mucous membranes signal a central cyanosis.

- **P**ulse. If a stethoscope is unavailable, you can measure pulsations in the umbilical cord with your fingers. Obviously, the infant with no pulse requires immediate CPR.

- **G**rimace or irritability. Grimacing, crying, or withdrawing in response to stimuli is normal in a newborn and indicates that the infant is doing well. The way to test this is to snap a finger against the sole of the infant's foot.

Remember

APGAR scoring system

- Appearance.
- Pulse.
- Grimace or irritability.
- Activity or muscle tone.
- Respirations.

- **A**ctivity or muscle tone. The degree of muscle tone indicates the oxygenation of the infant's tissues. Normally, the hips and knees are flexed at birth, and, to some degree, the infant will resist attempts to straighten them out. A newborn should not be floppy or limp.

- **R**espirations. Normally, the newborn's respirations are regular and rapid, with a good strong cry. If the respirations are slow, shallow, or labored or if the cry is weak, the infant may have respiratory insufficiency and need assistance with ventilations. Complete absence of respirations or crying is obviously a very serious sign; in addition to assisted ventilations, CPR may be necessary.

The total of the five numbers is the **Apgar score**. A perfect score is 10. The Apgar score should be calculated at 1 minute and 5 minutes after birth. Most infants will have a score of 7 or 8 at one minute and a score of 8 to 10 four minutes later. (▶ **Table 20-1**) shows how to calculate an Apgar score.

Consider the following delivery situation. You have assisted a delivery or arrived to find that a delivery has already taken place. You now have two patients who need assessment and care: the mother and the infant. Follow these steps in assessing the infant:

1. **Quickly calculate the Apgar score** to establish a baseline for the infant's vital functions.

2. **Suctioning and stimulation** should result in an immediate increase in respirations. If they do not, you must begin artificial ventilation. Resuscitation efforts should follow the 2000 guidelines established by the American Heart Association (▶ **Figure 20-11**). Unlike adults, who may have a sudden cardiac arrest, infants who get into trouble usually have a respiratory arrest first. Therefore, it is essential to keep the infant ventilating and oxygenating well.

3. **If the infant is breathing well,** you should next check the pulse rate by feeling the brachial pulse or the pulsations in the umbilical cord. The pulse rate should be at least 100 beats/min. If it is not, begin artificial ventilation. This alone may increase the infant's heart rate. Reassess respirations and heart rate at least every 30 seconds to make sure that the pulse rate is increasing and that respirations are becoming spontaneous.

TABLE 20-1 Apgar Scoring System

Area of Activity	Score		
	2	1	0
Appearance	Entire infant is pink.	Body is pink, but hands and feet remain blue.	Entire infant is blue or pale.
Pulse	More than 100 beats/min	Fewer than 100 beats/min	Absent pulse
Grimace or Irritability	Infant cries and tries to move foot away from finger snapped against its sole.	Infant gives a weak cry in response to stimulus.	Infant does not cry or react to stimulus.
Activity or Muscle Tone	Infant resists attempts to straighten out hips and knees.	Infant makes weak attempts to resist straightening.	Infant is completely limp, with no muscle tone.
Respiration	Rapid respirations	Slow respirations	Absent respirations

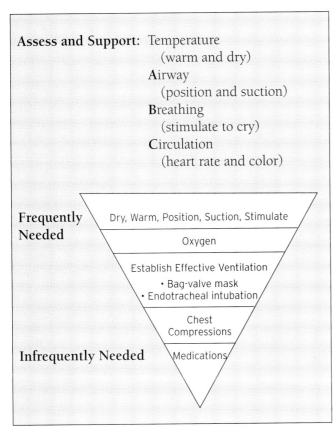

Assess and Support: Temperature
(warm and dry)
Airway
(position and suction)
Breathing
(stimulate to cry)
Circulation
(heart rate and color)

Frequently Needed

Dry, Warm, Position, Suction, Stimulate

Oxygen

Establish Effective Ventilation
• Bag-valve mask
• Endotracheal intubation

Chest Compressions

Medications

Infrequently Needed

Figure 20-11 Guidelines for neonatal resuscitation as recommended by the American Heart Association.

4. **Assess the infant's skin color.** You are looking for the central cyanosis. If you find it, administer high-flow oxygen (10 to 15 L/min) through oxygen tubing held close to the infant's face.

5. **Remember, you now have two patients.** You should request a second unit as soon as possible, if you determine that the infant is having problems.

In situations in which assisted ventilations are needed, you should use an infant BVM device
▼ Figure 20-12). Cover the infant's mouth and nose with the mask and begin ventilations with high-flow oxygen at a rate of 40 to 60 breaths/min. Make sure you have a good mask-to-face seal. Using gentle pressure, make the chest rise with each breath. Initially, it may be necessary to bypass the pop-off valve to accomplish this.

Assisted ventilation has been successful if

Figure 20-12 Use an infant bag and mask, ensuring that you cover both the infant's nose and mouth. Ventilate with high-flow oxygen at a rate of 40 to 60 breaths/min.

SkillDrill 20-2 Giving Chest Compressions to an Infant

1 Find the proper position: just below nipple line, middle of lower third of the sternum.

2 Wrap your hands around the body, with your thumbs resting at that position.

3 Press your thumbs gently against the sternum, compressing ¹/₂″ to ³/₄″ deep.

you see both sides of the chest rise and hear breath sounds. After 15 to 30 seconds of adequate ventilations, assess the heart rate. If the heart rate is at least 100 beats/min and the infant is breathing spontaneously, you can stop the assisted ventilations. Do not stop suddenly. Instead, gradually decrease the rate and pressure of the assisted ventilations to determine whether the infant will continue to breathe adequately on its own. If not, continue assisted ventilations until it does. You may find that gently stimulating the infant by rubbing it will help it to maintain its respirations.

If the heart rate is less than 80 beats/min or between 80 and 100 beats/min and not coming up with ventilations, continue assisted ventilations and start cardiac compressions. Even though this infant has a pulse, the rate and blood output from the heart are not adequate for the needs of a newborn.

There are two ways to give chest compressions to an infant. For the preferred method, follow the steps in **▲ Skill Drill 20-2** :

1. **Find the proper position:** one finger width below an imaginary line drawn between the nipples on the middle third of the sternum **(Step 1)**.

2. On a normal, full-term-sized infant, **place both hands around the infant so that your thumbs are side by side,** resting on the middle third of the sternum, and the rest of your fingers encircle the thorax. In premature or very small infants, you may have to place one thumb over the other to perform chest compressions **(Step 2)**.

3. **Press the two thumbs gently against the sternum.** The newborn's chest is easy to compress. Use only enough force to compress the sternum ¹/₂″ to ³/₄″ **(Step 3)**.

If your hands are too small to encircle the chest, you should use the middle and ring fingers of one hand to provide the compressions while your other hand supports the infant's back.

BVM ventilation is performed during the pause after every third compression. You should deliver a combined total of 120 ventilations and compressions per minute, 90 compressions to 30 ventilations. Keep in mind that ventilation is absolutely crucial to the successful resuscitation of the neonate.

If the infant does not begin breathing on its own or does not have an adequate heart rate, continue CPR on the way to the hospital. Once CPR has been started, do not stop until the infant responds with adequate respirations and heart rates or is pronounced dead by a physician. Do not give up! Many infants have survived without brain damage after prolonged periods of effective CPR. If the infant presents in distress, you should not wait to measure the Apgar score, but begin appropriate care measures immediately.

Abnormal or Complicated Delivery Emergencies

Breech Delivery

The **presentation** is the position in which an infant is born, the part of the body that comes out first. Most infants are born head first, in what is called a vertex presentation. Occasionally, the buttocks come out first. This is called a **breech presentation** (▼ Figure 20-13). With a breech presentation, the infant is at great risk for delivery trauma. In addition, prolapsed cords are more common. Breech deliveries are usually slow, so there is time to get the mother to the hospital. However, if the buttocks have already passed through the vagina, delivery is underway, and you should follow emergency procedures and call for ALS backup. In general, if the mother does not deliver within 10 minutes of the buttocks presentation, provide prompt transport. Have medical control guide you in this difficult situation.

The preparations for a breech delivery are the same as those for a vertex delivery. Position the mother, unwrap the emergency delivery kit, and place yourself and your partner as you would for a normal delivery. Allow the buttocks and legs to deliver spontaneously, supporting them with your hand to prevent rapid expulsion. The buttocks will usually come out easily. Let the legs dangle on either side of your arm while you support the trunk and chest as they are delivered. The head is almost always face down and should be allowed to deliver spontaneously. As the head is delivering, you should keep the infant's airway open: Make a "V" with your gloved fingers, and then place them into the vagina

to keep the walls of the vagina from compressing the airway. *This is one of only two circumstances in which you should put your fingers into the vagina.*

Rare Presentations

On very rare occasions, the presenting part of the infant is neither the head nor buttocks, but a single arm, leg, or foot. This is called a **limb presentation** (▼ Figure 20-14). You cannot successfully deliver such a presentation in the field. These infants usually must be delivered surgically. If you are faced with a limb presentation, you must transport the mother to the hospital immediately. If a limb is protruding, cover it with a sterile towel. Never try to push it back in, and never pull on it. Place the mother on her back, with head down and pelvis elevated. Since both mother and infant are likely to be physically stressed in this situation, remember to place the mother on high-flow oxygen.

Prolapse of the umbilical cord, a situation in which the umbilical cord comes out of the vagina before the infant (▶ Figure 20-15), is another rare presentation that must be handled in the hospital. This situation is very dangerous, because the infant's head will compress the cord during birth and cut off circulation to the infant, depriving it of oxygenated blood. Do not attempt to

Figure 20-13 An infant in a breech presentation presents with the buttocks first. Breech deliveries are usually slow, so you will often have time to transport the mother to the hospital.

Figure 20-14 In very rare instances, an infant's limb, usually a single arm or leg, presents first. This is a very serious situation, and you must provide prompt transport for hospital delivery.

Figure 20-15 A prolapsed umbilical cord, another rare situation, is very dangerous and must be cared for at the hospital.

push the cord back into the vagina. Prolapse of the umbilical cord usually occurs early in labor when the amniotic sac ruptures. As a result, there is time to get the mother to the hospital. Your job is to try to keep the infant's head from compressing the cord.

Place the mother on a backboard in Trendelenburg's position, with her hips elevated on a pillow or folded sheet. Alternatively, the mother may be placed in a knee-chest position: kneeling and bent forward, face down. Either of these positions is meant to help keep the weight of the infant off the prolapsed cord. Carefully insert your sterile gloved hand into the vagina, and gently push the infant's head away from the umbilical cord. *Note that this is the only other occasion on which you should actually place a hand into the vagina.* Wrap a sterile towel, moistened with saline, around the exposed cord. Give the mother high-flow oxygen, and transport her rapidly.

Excessive Bleeding

Some bleeding always occurs with delivery. However, bleeding that exceeds approximately 500 mL is considered excessive. Although up to 500 mL of blood loss is tolerated, you should continue to massage the uterus. Be sure to check the massage technique if bleeding continues. If the mother appears to be in shock, treat her accordingly and transport, massaging the uterus en

route. There are several other possible causes of excessive bleeding, all of which may be serious and require emergency care. Treat this condition by covering the vagina with a sterile pad, changing the pad as often as necessary. Do not discard these blood-soaked pads; hospital personnel will use them to estimate the amount of blood that the mother has lost. Also save any tissue that may have passed from the vagina.

Place the mother in Trendelenburg's position, administer oxygen, monitor vital signs frequently, and transport her immediately to the hospital. Never hold the mother's legs together in an effort to stop the bleeding, and never pack the vagina with gauze pads in an attempt to control bleeding.

Abortion (Miscarriage)

Delivery of the fetus and placenta before 20 weeks is called abortion, or miscarriage. Abortions may be spontaneous, without any obvious known cause, or deliberate. Deliberate abortions may be self-induced, by the mother herself or by someone else, or planned and performed in a hospital or clinic. Regardless of the reasons for the abortion, it may cause complications that you may be called upon to treat.

The most serious complications of abortion are bleeding and infection. Bleeding can result from portions of the fetus or placenta being left in the uterus (incomplete abortion) or from injury to the wall of the uterus (perforation of the uterus and possibly the adjacent bowel or bladder). Infection can result from such perforation, as well as from the use of nonsterile instruments. If the mother is in shock, treat and transport her promptly to the hospital. Collect and bring to the hospital any tissue that passes through the vagina. Never try to pull tissue out of the vagina; instead, cover it with a sterile pad.

Again, as you encounter a patient who is in shock as a result of complications of abortion, be sure to size up the situation, perform your initial assessment, focused history and physical exam, and assess baseline vital signs.

In rare instances of abortion, massive bleeding may occur and cause severe hypovolemic or hemorrhagic shock. In these instances, provide immediate transport to the emergency department.

Twins

Twins occur about once in every 80 births. Sometimes, there is a family history of twins. The mother may suspect that she is having twins because she has an unusually large abdomen. Usually, however, twins are diagnosed early in pregnancy with modern ultrasound

Twins occur about once in every 80 births. With twins, always be prepared for more than one resuscitation, and call for assistance.

techniques. With twins, always be prepared for more than one resuscitation, and call for assistance.

Twins are smaller than single infants, and delivery is typically not difficult. Consider the possibility that you are dealing with twins any time the first infant is small or the mother's abdomen remains fairly large after the birth. If twins are present, the second one will usually be born within 45 minutes of the first. About 10 minutes after the first birth, contractions will begin again, and the birth process will repeat itself.

The procedure for delivering twins is the same as that for single infants. Clamp and cut the cord of the first infant as soon as it has been born and before the second infant is delivered. The second infant may deliver before or after the first placenta. There may be only one placenta, or there may be two. When the placenta has been delivered, check whether there is one umbilical cord or two. If two cords are coming out of one placenta, the twins are called identical. If only one cord is coming out of the placenta, then the twins are called fraternal, and there will be two placentas. Occasionally, the two placentas of fraternal twins are fused, so you might think that you are dealing with identical twins. Remember, if you see only one umbilical cord coming out of the first placenta, there is still another placenta to be delivered. However, if both cords are attached to one placenta, the delivery is over. Identical twins are of the same gender; fraternal twins may be of different genders, or they may be the same.

Record the time of birth of each twin separately. Twins may be so small in weight that they look premature; handle them very carefully and keep them warm.

Delivering an Infant of an Addicted Mother

Unfortunately, more and more infants are being born to mothers who are addicted to medications or alcohol. These mothers often have had little or no prenatal care. The effects of the addiction on the infants include prematurity, low birth weight, and severe respiratory depression. Some of these infants will die. **Fetal alcohol syndrome** is the term used to describe the condition of infants born to mothers who have abused alcohol.

If you are called to handle a delivery of a drug- or alcohol-addicted mother, pay special attention to your own safety. As with all other cases, follow BSI precautions. Wear goggles and sterile gloves at all times. Clues that you are dealing with an addicted mother may include the presence of drug paraphernalia, empty wine or liquor bottles, and statements made by neighbors or by the mother herself. The newborn infant of an addicted mother will probably need immediate hospital care. Carry out the delivery as outlined earlier, but be prepared to support the infant's respirations and administer oxygen during transport. Do not judge or lecture the mother. Your job is to help deliver the infant as best you can and to get both infant and mother to the hospital.

Premature Infant

The usual *gestational period*, the period of prenatal development, is 9 calendar months, or 40 weeks. A normal, single infant will weigh approximately 7 lb at birth. Any infant that delivers before 8 months (36 weeks of gestation) or weighs less than 5 lb at birth is considered *premature*. This determination is not always easy to make. Often, the exact gestation time cannot be determined. Since you probably have no scale to weigh the infant, you will have to use physical guidelines. A premature infant is smaller and thinner than a full-term infant, and its head is proportionately larger in comparison with the rest of its body (▼ **Figure 20-16**). The *vernix caseosa*, a cheesy white coating on the skin that is found on the full-term infant, will be missing on the premature infant or will be very minimal. There will also be less body hair.

Premature infants need special care to survive. Often, they require resuscitation, which should be done unless it is physically impossible. With such care, infants as

Figure 20-16 Premature infants (right) are smaller and thinner than full-term infants (left).

small as 1 lb have survived and developed normally. Follow these procedures when you are handling a premature infant:

1. **Keep the infant warm.** Dry the infant as soon as it is born, and then remove the wet towels. Wrap it in a warm blanket, exposing the face but covering the head. Keep the infant in a place where the temperature is between 90°F and 95°F (between 32.2°C and 35°C).

2. **Keep the mouth and nose clear of mucus.** Like all newborn infants, premature ones are nose breathers, and the small nasal passages can easily be obstructed. Use the bulb syringe to suction the mouth and nostrils frequently. Handle the infant very gently.

3. **Carefully observe** the cut end of the cord attached to the infant, and be sure that it is not bleeding. The loss of even a few drops of blood can be very serious.

4. **Give oxygen.** Open the valve on your oxygen cylinder slowly to give a steady stream of oxygen (about 70 to 100 bubbles per minute through the water bottle that is attached to the oxygen tank). Direct the stream of oxygen not into the infant's mouth, but into a small tent over the infant's head; you can use a blanket or a piece of aluminum foil to make the tent. Although there is some danger to a premature infant from receiving very high concentrations of oxygen, there is no danger if it is given over a short period of time in this manner.

5. **Do not infect the infant.** Premature infants are very susceptible to infection. Protect them from contamination. Do not breathe directly into the infant's face. Your mask will help to create a barrier. Keep everyone else as far away from the infant as possible.

6. **Notify the hospital.** Does your system have a neonatal (newborn) transport team with specialized personnel and equipment for the care of premature and sick newborn infants? If so, be sure to contact the hospital before leaving the scene so that medical control can decide whether to call in the team. If not, you should still notify the hospital as soon as possible so that staff can be ready to receive the premature infant and mother. Avoid unnecessary on-scene delays.

You may have access to a specialized premature infant carrier, which can be used for immediate care as well as transport. Carrier supplies may include a quilted pad, infant blanket, diaper, thermometer, suction tube and suction bulb, sterile Kelly clamp, and, most important, hot water bottles and an oxygen cylinder with the necessary attachments. Fill the hot water bottles, and pad them well so that they do not come into direct contact with the infant's skin. Place one on the bottom of the carrier and one on each side of the space for the infant. Once you have wrapped the infant in a blanket and placed it inside the carrier, secure the carrier inside the vehicle.

Keep the temperature of the vehicle at 90°F to 95°F (32.2°C to 35°C) while the infant and mother are being transported to the hospital. If a special carrier is not available, you must keep the premature infant warm with additional blankets, thermal packets, and warmed patient compartments. Any delays will lower the infant's body temperature.

Fetal Demise

Unfortunately, you may find yourself delivering an infant that has died in the mother's uterus before labor. This will be a true test of your medical, emotional, and social abilities. Grieving parents will be emotionally distraught and perhaps even hostile, requiring all your professionalism and support skills.

The onset of labor may be premature, but labor will otherwise progress normally in most cases. If an intrauterine infection has caused the demise, you may note an extremely foul odor. The delivered infant may have skin blisters, skin sloughing, and a dark discoloration, depending on the stage of decomposition. The head will be soft and perhaps grossly deformed.

Do not attempt to resuscitate an obviously dead infant. However, do not confuse such an infant with those who have had a cardiopulmonary arrest as a complication of the birthing process. You must attempt to resuscitate normal-appearing infants.

Delivery Without Sterile Supplies

On rare occasions, you may have to deliver an infant without a sterile OB kit. Even if you do not have a sterile kit, you should always have goggles and sterile gloves with you. These are for your own protection as well as that of the mother and infant. Carry out the delivery as if sterile supplies were on hand. If you can, use clean sheets and towels that have not been used since they were laundered. As soon as the infant is born, wipe the inside of its mouth with your finger to clear away blood and mucus. Without the OB kit, you should not cut or tie the umbilical cord. Instead, as soon as the placenta delivers, wrap it in a clean towel or put it in a plastic bag and transport it with the infant and mother to the hospital. Always keep the placenta and the infant at the same level so that blood does not drain from the infant into the placenta. Be sure to keep the infant warm. As in the case of other deliveries, note the presence of green-tinged fluid or secretions (meconium staining).

Gynecological Emergencies

Occasionally, women who are not pregnant will have major gynecological problems requiring urgent medical care. These include excessive bleeding and soft-tissue injuries to the external genitalia. These genital parts have a rich nerve supply, making injuries very painful.

Treat lacerations, abrasions, and tears with moist, sterile compresses, using local pressure to control bleeding and a diaper-type bandage to hold the dressings in place. Leave any foreign bodies in place after stabilizing them with bandages. Under no circumstances should you ever pack or place dressings in the vagina. Continue to assess these patients while transporting them to the emergency department. Contusions and other blunt trauma will require careful in-hospital evaluation.

Although you might not know the exact cause of a gynecological emergency, you should treat these individuals as you would any other victim of blood loss: Observe BSI precautions, ensure maintenance of the airway, give oxygen, take and document vital signs, and treat for shock while arranging for prompt transport.

Sexual Assault

Sexual assault and rape are all too common. Although most victims are women, men and children are also victims. Often, you can do little beyond providing compassion and transportation to the emergency department. On some occasions, these patients will have suffered multiple-system trauma and will also need treatment for shock.

Do not examine the genitalia of a victim of sexual assault unless obvious bleeding requires you to apply a dressing. Advise the patient not to wash, douche, urinate, or defecate until after a physician has examined him or her; this will help to preserve any evidence of a crime. If oral penetration has occurred, advise the patient not to eat, drink, brush the teeth, or use mouthwash until he or she has been examined.

Treat all other injuries according to appropriate procedures and protocols for your EMS system. Observe BSI precautions. Take the patient's history, perform a limited physical exam, and provide treatment as quickly, quietly, and calmly as possible. Take care to shield the patient from curious onlookers.

The patient may refuse assistance or transport, often because he or she wants to maintain privacy and thus avoid public exposure. For adults, this is the patient's right. In such cases, you should follow your system's refusal of treatment policy or procedure for sexual assault victims without judging or being condescending to the patient. Your compassion is the best tool to gain the patient's confidence to get further help.

Offer to call the local rape crisis center for the patient. The center will have an advocate meet the patient at the hospital and provide support through the rape exam.

In addition to the usual treatment principles that apply to all victims of trauma, you should follow these special steps with patients who have been sexually assaulted:

1. Since you may have to appear in court as much as 2 or 3 years later, you must document the patient's history, assessment, treatment, and response to treatment *in detail*. Do not speculate. Record only the facts.

2. Make airway maintenance a major priority.

3. Complete the SAMPLE history in an objective and nonjudgmental fashion.

4. Follow any crime scene policy established by your system to protect the scene and any potential evidence for police, particularly that for evidence collection. If the patient will tolerate being wrapped in a sterile burn sheet, this may help investigators to find any hair, fluid, or fiber from the alleged offender.

5. Do not examine the genitalia unless there is major bleeding. If an object has been inserted into the vagina or rectum, do not attempt to remove it.

6. To reduce the patient's anxiety, make sure the EMT-B is the same gender as the patient whenever possible.

7. Discourage the patient from bathing, voiding, or cleaning any wounds until hospital staff have completed an assessment. Handle the patient's clothes as little as possible, placing articles and any other evidence in paper bags. Do not use plastic bags. If the female patient insists on urinating, have her do so in a sterile urine container (if available). Also, have her deposit the toilet paper in a paper bag. Seal and mark the bag for the police. This can be critical evidence.

Prep Kit

Ready for Review

Inside the uterus, the developing fetus floats in the amniotic sac. The umbilical cord connects mother and infant through the placenta. Eventually, the uterus will propel the infant through the birth canal. The first stage of labor, dilation, begins with the onset of contractions and ends when the cervix is fully dilated. The second stage, expulsion of the baby, begins when the cervix is fully dilated and ends when the infant is born. The third stage, delivery of the placenta, begins with the birth of the infant and ends with the delivery of the placenta.

Once labor has begun, it cannot be slowed or stopped; however, there is usually time to transport the patient to the hospital during the first stage. During the second stage, you must decide whether to deliver the baby at the scene or transport the mother. During the third stage, once the infant has been born, you will probably not transport until the placenta has delivered.

Use an infant BVM device to assist ventilations, starting with high-flow oxygen at a rate of 40 to 60 breaths/min. If the infant starts to breathe on its own, attach an oxygen tubing mask and watch for signs of adequate oxygenation. If the heart rate is less than 80 beats/min, start cardiac compressions, using only enough force to compress the sternum 1/2" to 3/4". Perform a combined total of 120 ventilations and compressions per minute, 90 compressions to 30 ventilations.

Abnormal or complicated deliveries include breech deliveries (buttocks first), limb presentations (arm, leg, or foot first), and prolapse of the umbilical cord (umbilical cord first). Quickly transport the patient with a limb presentation or prolapsed umbilical cord to the hospital. The only times you should place a finger or hand into the vagina are to keep the walls of the vagina from compressing the infant's airway during a face-down breech presentation or to push the infant's head away from the cord in a prolapse situation.

Excessive bleeding is a serious emergency. Cover the vagina with a sterile pad; change the pad as often as necessary, and take all used pads to the hospital for examination. Be prepared to support respirations during transport in an infant delivered by a drug- or alcohol-addicted mother. Also use oxygen with premature infants, and keep the temperature of the ambulance at 90°F (32.2°C) or more during transport.

Use local pressure and a diaper-type bandage to hold dressings in place when treating nonobstetric injuries to the external genitalia. Never place dressings in the vagina. Treat patients with these injuries as you would any other victim of blood loss. In the case of sexual assault or rape, treat for shock if necessary, and record all the facts in detail. Follow any crime scene policy established by your system to protect the scene and any potential evidence. Advise the patient not to wash, douche, or void until after a physician has examined him or her.

Vital Vocabulary

abortion Delivery of the fetus and placenta before 20 weeks; miscarriage.

amniotic sac The fluid-filled, baglike membrane in which the fetus develops.

apgar score A scoring system for assessing the status of a newborn that assigns a number value to each of five areas of assessment.

birth canal The vagina and cervix.

bloody show A plug of pink-tinged mucus that is discharged when the cervix begins to dilate.

breech presentation Delivery in which the buttocks come out first.

cervix The lower one-third, or neck, of the uterus.

crowning The appearance of the infant's head at the vaginal opening during labor.

eclampsia Convulsions (seizures) resulting from severe hypertension in the pregnant woman.

ectopic pregnancy A pregnancy that develops outside the uterus, typically in a fallopian tube.

fetal alcohol syndrome A condition of infants who are born to alcoholic mothers; characterized by physical and mental retardation and a variety of congenital abnormalities.

fetus The developing, unborn infant inside the uterus.

limb presentation A delivery in which the presenting part is a single arm, leg, or foot.

multigravida A woman who has had previous pregnancies.

multipara A woman who has had more than one live birth.

nuchal cord An umbilical cord that is wrapped around the infant's neck.

perineum The area of skin between the vagina and the anus.

placenta Tissue attached to the uterine wall that nourishes the fetus through the umbilical cord.

placenta abruptio Premature separation of the placenta from the wall of the uterus.

placenta previa A condition in which the placenta develops over and covers the cervix.

pregnancy-induced hypertension A condition of late pregnancy that also involves headache, visual changes, and swelling of the hands and feet; also called pre-eclampsia.

presentation The position in which an infant is born; the part of the infant that appears first.

primigravida A woman who is experiencing her first pregnancy.

prolapse of the umbilical cord A situation in which the umbilical cord comes out of the vagina before the infant.

primipara A woman who has had one live birth.

supine hypotensive syndrome Low blood pressure resulting from compression of the inferior vena cava by the weight of the fetus when the mother is supine.

umbilical cord The conduit connecting mother to infant via the placenta; contains two arteries and one vein.

uterus The muscular organ where the fetus grows, also called the womb; responsible for contractions during labor.

vagina The outermost cavity of a woman's reproductive system; the lower part of the birth canal.

www.emtb.com

Assessment in Action

You are dispatched to a woman having a baby. Upon arrival at a private residence, you find a 22-year-old woman lying on the bathroom floor with a small puddle of blood under her buttocks. A 2-year-old child is crying in a playpen across the hall.

The patient tells you that she has been having contractions for the last hour but thought that she and her husband could get to the hospital in time. However, she states that her water "broke," and she estimates that her contractions are now only 2 to 3 minutes apart. She also says that because of financial difficulties, she has not seen a physician since she first found out that she was pregnant again. You check and find the baby's head at the vaginal opening. While you are getting the history and checking the patient, your partner obtains baseline vital signs, including a pulse of 138 beats/min, respirations of 32 breaths/min, and a blood pressure of 118/68 mm Hg. The closest hospital is 20 minutes away.

1. The most important assessment finding for this patient at this time is:
   A. vital signs.
   B. visualizing the presenting part.
   C. absence of prenatal care.
   D. presence of contractions.

2. This patient states her "bag of waters" has broken. What is the medical term for the "bag of waters"?
   A. Uterus
   B. Amniotic sac
   C. Cervix
   D. Placenta

3. This patient was found lying in a puddle of blood under her buttocks. Some of that was from the amniotic fluid and some was blood from capillaries breaking. What is a normal amount of blood that can be expected prior to delivery of the placenta? About
   A. 250 mL
   B. 500 mL
   C. 750 mL
   D. 1,000 mL

4. From the assessment findings of this patient, what is her stage of labor?
   A. First stage
   B. Transition from first to second stage
   C. Second stage
   D. Third stage

5. As you prepare for the birth of this infant, it is very important to find out which one of the following?
   A. Do you feel as though you have to have a bowel movement?
   B. Do you feel pressure in the small of your back?
   C. When is your due date or how long have you been pregnant?
   D. Have you had any gushing of fluid or spotting?

6. She tells you that she didn't think the baby was due for another month. How does this change what you will be doing?
   A. The mother will need more oxygen.
   B. There is more likelihood of bleeding.
   C. The baby will be easier to care for.
   D. The baby may need more resuscitation.

7. When should the baby be suctioned? As soon as the:
   A. baby is completely out of the vagina.
   B. baby begins to cry.
   C. head emerges from the vagina.
   D. umbilical cord is clamped.

8. As the baby is being delivered, you discover the cord is wrapped around the baby's neck. What should you do?
   A. Nothing, delivery of the baby will straighten it out.
   B. Try to ease the cord over the baby's head or shoulders.
   C. Stop the delivery and immediately transport.
   D. Attempt to reinsert the baby to loosen the cord.

Challenging Questions

9. Why is it important to find out how many times this mother has been pregnant?

10. Resuscitating a newborn includes drying, warming, suctioning, and stimulating. Why are these so important?

Points to Ponder

You are dispatched to the dorms at a local college. You find a 19-year-old woman in the bathroom. She is crying and appears hysterical. Her boyfriend is there talking to her through the door and trying to calm her down. It becomes apparent that the more he tries to calm her, the worse she gets, so your partner takes him into the hall to talk with him. Once he is gone, the woman unlocks the door and allows you in. You find her sitting on the floor in a pool of blood and you see a fetus in the toilet. You find that she has had a spontaneous abortion. She explains that her boyfriend is not the father and did not know she was pregnant. She asks you not to tell him what is wrong, but she wants him to stay and to go to the hospital with her. What are you going to tell the boyfriend? Would you lie to keep the patient's confidence? As her dorm friends begin to appear and ask what happened, how will you handle them and what will you tell them?

Issues Dealing with Bystanders, Patient Confidentiality, Personal Feelings about Unmarried Sexuality, Personal Feelings about Miscarriage, Optional Answers to Difficult Questions.

Online Outlook

Watch how the fetus grows from conception through delivery from actual ultrasound images and review postdelivery care by completing Exercise 20 at **www.emtb.com**.

www.emtb.com

Trauma

5

Section

Kinematics of Trauma

Objectives*

Cognitive

1. Describe the "three collisions" associated with motor vehicle crashes (p 517).
2. Relate how the fundamental principles of physics apply to motor vehicle crashes and other types of accidents (p 516).
3. State Newton's three laws (p 525).

Affective

None

Psychomotor

4. Observe various high-energy injuries and identify potential damage to the patient (p 524).

* All of the objectives in this chapter are noncurriculum objectives.

www.emtb.com

Online Chapter Pretest
Interactivities
Vocabulary Explorer
Anatomy Review
Web Links
Online Review Manual
Distance Learning

TECHNOLOGY

Skill Drills
Vital Vocabulary
Pediatric Needs
Geriatric Needs
EMT-B Safety
EMT-B Tips
Documentation Tips
Remember
Prep Kit

Chapter FEATURES

Dispatch receives a call from a driver on the interstate who just saw a car go off the road and roll over. You arrive to find both occupants still in the upside-down car, seat-belted in.

Trauma takes many lives each year, often young persons with their whole lives ahead of them. This chapter will help you understand what events occur during common traumatic situations, focusing primarily on your assessment skills. It will also help you answer the following questions:

1. How does a basic understanding of physics as it relates to "kinetic energy" contribute to improving the care you provide to trauma patients?

2. What are the so-called three collisions that occur during a motor vehicle crash?

Kinematics of Trauma

Injuries are the leading cause of death and disability in the United States among children and young adults (ages 1 to 34), claiming 140,000 lives annually—more than all other diseases combined. Each year, one person in three sustains an injury that requires medical treatment. Proper prehospital evaluation and care can do much to minimize suffering, long-term disability, and death from trauma.

This chapter introduces the basic physical concepts that dictate how injuries occur and affect the human body. When you understand these concepts, you will be better able to size up a crash scene and use that information as a vital part of patient assessment. The chapter begins with a basic discussion of energy and trauma. Next, different types of crashes and their impact on the body are explained. By assessing the body of a vehicle that has crashed, you can often determine what happened to the passengers at the time of impact, which may allow you to predict what injuries the passengers sustained at the time of impact. Certain injury patterns occur with certain types of injury events. Answers to simple questions will provide you with information on how to identify both life-threatening and other serious injuries. The chapter concludes with a brief discussion of falls and penetrating trauma. A brief section on Newton's laws is also presented.

Energy and Trauma

Traumatic injury occurs to the body when the body's tissues are exposed to energy levels beyond their tolerance. Three concepts of energy are typically associated with injury (not including thermal energy, which causes burns): potential energy, kinetic energy, and work. In considering the effects of energy on the human body, it is important to remember that energy can be neither created nor destroyed, but can only be converted or transformed. It is not the objective of this section to help you to reconstruct the scene of a motor vehicle crash. Rather, you should have a sense of the effects of work on the body and understand, in a broad sense, how that work is related to potential and kinetic energy. For example, when you are assessing a patient who fell, you need not calculate the speed at which the person hit the ground. However, it is important to estimate the height from which he or she fell and to appreciate the injury potential of the fall.

Work is defined as *force* acting over a distance. For example, the force needed to bend metal multiplied by the distance over which the metal is bent is the work that crushes the front end of an automobile that is involved in a frontal impact. Similarly, forces that bend, pull, or compress tissues beyond their inherent limits result in the work that causes injury.

The energy of a moving object is called **kinetic energy** and is calculated as follows: kinetic energy = $\frac{1}{2}mv^2$, where m = mass (weight) and v = velocity (speed). Remember that energy cannot be created or destroyed, only converted. In the case of a motor vehicle crash, the kinetic energy of the speeding car is converted into the work of stopping the car, usually by crushing the car's exterior ▶ **Figure 21-1** . Similarly, the passengers of the car have kinetic energy because they were traveling at the same speed as the car. Their kinetic energy is converted to the work of bringing them to a stop. It is this work on the passengers that results in injury. Notice that, according to the equation

EMT-B Tips

Do a "vehicle assessment" if circumstances at the scene allow it. There may be time for one EMT-B to circle the vehicle and assess damage while the other EMT-B begins patient assessment.

for kinetic energy, the energy that is available to cause injury doubles when an object's weight doubles but quadruples when its speed doubles. Consider the debate over raising the speed limit. Increasing a car's speed from 50 mph to 70 mph doubles the energy that is available to cause injury. This point will be even clearer in considering gunshot wounds. The speed of the bullet (high-velocity compared with low-velocity) has a greater impact on producing injury than the mass (size) of the bullet. As has already been noted, this is why it is so important to report to the hospital the type of firearm that was used in a shooting. The amount of kinetic energy that is converted to do work on the body dictates the severity of the injury. High-energy injuries often produce such severe damage that patients can be saved only by immediate transport to an appropriate facility.

<u>Potential energy</u> is the product of mass (weight), force of gravity, and height and is mostly associated with the energy of falling objects. A worker on a scaffold has some potential energy because he or she is some height above the ground. When the worker falls, potential energy is converted into kinetic energy. As the worker hits the ground, the kinetic energy is converted into work—that is, the work of bringing the body to a stop and thereby breaking bones and damaging tissues.

Blunt Trauma: Vehicular Collisions

Motor vehicle crashes, one of the most common sources of <u>**blunt trauma**</u>, are classified traditionally as frontal (head-on), lateral (T-bone), rear-end, rotational (spins), and rollovers. The principal difference among these collision types is the direction of the force of impact; also, with spins and rollovers, there is the possibility of multiple impacts. Motor vehicle crashes typically consist of a series of three collisions. Understanding the events that occur during each collision will help you be alert for certain types of injury patterns. The three collisions in a frontal impact are as follows:

1. **The collision of the car against another car, a tree, or some other object.** Damage to the car

Figure 21-1 The kinetic energy of a speeding car is converted into the work of stopping the car, usually by crushing the car's exterior.

Figure 21-2 The first collision in a frontal impact is that of the car against another object (in this case, a utility pole). The appearance of the car can provide you with critical information about the severity of the crash. The greater the damage to the car, the greater is the energy that was involved.

is perhaps the most dramatic part of the collision, but it does not directly affect patient care, except possibly to make extrication difficult ▲ **Figure 21-2** . However, it does provide information about the severity of the collision and therefore has an indirect effect on patient care. The greater the damage to the car, the greater is the energy that was involved and therefore the greater the potential to cause injury to the patient. By assessing the body of a vehicle that has crashed, you can often determine the <u>**mechanism of injury**</u>, which may allow you to predict what injuries may have happened to the passengers at the time of impact according to forces that acted on their bodies. When you arrive at the crash scene and perform your scene size-up, quickly inspect the severity of damage to the vehicle(s). If there is significant damage to a vehicle, your index of suspicion for the presence of life-threatening injuries should automatically increase. A great amount of force is required to crush and deform a vehicle, cause intrusion into the passenger compartment, tear seats from their mountings, and collapse steering wheels. Such damage suggests the presence of high-energy trauma.

2. **The collision of the passenger against the interior of the car.** Just as the kinetic energy produced by the car's mass and velocity is converted into the work of bringing the car to a stop, the kinetic energy produced by the passenger's mass and velocity is converted into the work of stopping his or her body ▼ Figure 21-3 . Just like the obvious damage to the exterior of the car, the injuries that result are often dramatic and usually immediately apparent during your initial assessment. Common injuries include lower extremity fractures (knees into the dashboard), flail chest (rib cage into the steering wheel), and head trauma (head into the windshield). Such injuries occur more frequently if the passenger is not restrained. But even when the passenger is restrained with a properly adjusted seat belt, injuries can occur, especially in lateral and rollover impacts.

3. **The collision of the passenger's internal organs against the solid structures of the body.** The injuries that occur during the third collision may not be as obvious as external injuries, but they are often the most life-threatening. For example, as the passenger's head hits the windshield, the brain continues to move forward until it comes to rest by striking the inside of the skull. This results in compression injury (or bruising) to the anterior portion of the brain and stretching (or tearing) of the posterior portion of the brain ▼ Figure 21-4 . Similarly, in the thoracic cage, the heart may slam into the sternum, occasionally rupturing the aorta and causing fatal bleeding.

Understanding the relationship between the three collisions will help you to make the connections between the amount of damage to the exterior of the car and potential injury to the passenger. For example, in a high-speed collision that results in massive damage to the car, you should suspect serious injuries to the passengers, even if the injuries are not readily apparent. A number of potential physical problems may develop as a result of traumatic injuries. Your quick initial assessment of the patient and the evaluation of the mechanism of injury can help to direct lifesaving care and provide critical information to the hospital staff ▶ Table 21-1 . Therefore, if you see a contusion on the patient's forehead and the windshield is starred and pushed out, you should strongly suspect an injury to the brain. After you inform medical control about the

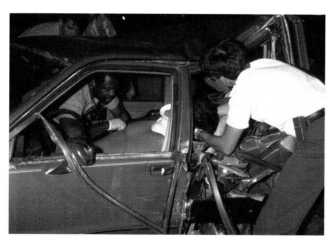

Figure 21-3 The second collision in a frontal impact is that of the passenger against the interior of the car. The appearance of the interior of the car can provide you with information about the severity of the patient's injuries.

Figure 21-4 The third collision in a frontal impact is that of the passenger's internal organs against the solid structures of the body. In this illustration, the brain continues its forward motion and strikes the inside of the skull, resulting in a compression injury to the anterior portion of the brain and stretching of the posterior portion.

Table 21-1 Recognizing Developing Problems in Trauma Patients	
Problem	**Signs and Symptoms or Mechanism of Injury**
Airway Obstruction	Noisy or labored respirations may indicate one or more of the following:
	Significant bleeding into the mouth, back of the throat, or nose
	Swelling or bleeding following blunt or penetrating trauma to the face
	Swelling about the neck (may compress the airway) following blunt or penetrating trauma to the neck
	Inability to swallow, resulting in possible choking on secretions
	Partial airway obstruction secondary to teeth or blood clots
Breathing Problems	Significant chest pain following blunt trauma
	Any penetrating trauma to the chest, unless it is a superficial cut (Remember to check the back too.)
	Bent or crushed steering wheel or deployed air bag, indicating blunt trauma to the chest
Hidden Blood Loss	Bruising, redness, abrasions, or obvious trauma to the upper abdomen
	Abdominal distention or rigidity
	Significant mechanism of injury, including blunt and penetrating trauma
	Obvious bruising, redness, or abrasions in the area of the pelvis
	Tenderness on gentle palpation of the pelvis
Damage to Major Vessels	Blunt or penetrating trauma to the neck, chest, or groin area (which could tear the major vessels in these areas)
	Bent or crushed steering wheel, indicating blunt trauma to the chest
Damage to the Heart	Bent or crushed steering wheel, indicating blunt trauma to the chest
Brain Injury	History of losing consciousness, inability to recall what happened, dazed appearance, confusion, disorientation, combativeness after the traumatic incident
	Slurred speech
	Difficulty moving the extremities
	Severe headache, especially if accompanied by nausea and vomiting
	Obvious blunt or penetrating trauma to the head, other than superficial cuts
	Appearance of intoxication, as signs and symptoms (especially head trauma) may be masked by the effects of alcohol
	Starred windshield, indicating that the patient's head flexed forward and struck the windshield with significant force
Possible Spinal Injury	Severe neck or back pain
	History of difficulty moving or feeling the extremities
	Starred windshield, indicating that the patient's head flexed forward and struck the windshield with significant force

Documentation Tips

In trauma, mechanism of injury is a crucial element of patient history. Combine your knowledge of kinematics with observations at the scene to paint a verbal picture for later caregivers in the History section of your written report.

windshield, hospital staff can prepare the patient by ordering a CT scan of the brain. Without your input, the physician might have found the brain injury anyway, but it might have not been detected until the brain had swollen sufficiently to cause clinical signs of the injury.

The amount of damage that is considered significant varies, depending on the type of collision, but any substantial deformity of the vehicle should be enough cause for you to consider transporting the patient to a trauma center. Significant mechanisms of injury include the following:

- Severe deformities of the frontal part of a vehicle, with or without intrusion to the passenger compartment
- Moderate intrusions from a lateral (T-bone) type of accident
- Severe damage from the rear
- Collisions in which rotation is involved (rollover and spins)

Damage to the vehicle that was involved and information obtained from patient assessment are not the only clues to crash severity. Clearly, if one or more of the passengers are dead, you should suspect that the other passengers have sustained serious injuries, even if the injuries are not obvious. Therefore, you should focus on treating life-threatening injuries and providing transport to a trauma center, because these passengers have likely experienced the same amount of force that caused the death of the others. Polaroids of the crash scene may provide valuable information to the staff and treating physicians of the trauma center.

Frontal Collisions

Understanding the mechanism of injury after a frontal collision first involves evaluation of the supplemental restraint system, including seat belts and air bags. You should determine whether the passenger was restrained by a full and properly applied three-point restraint. In addition, you should determine whether the air bag was deployed. Identifying the types of restraints used

and whether air bags were deployed will help you to identify injury patterns that occur related to the supplemental restraint systems.

When properly applied, seat belts are successful in restraining the passengers in a vehicle and preventing a second collision inside the motor vehicle. In addition, they may decrease the severity of the third collision, that of the passenger's organs with the chest or abdominal wall. The very presence of air bags allows seat belts to provide even more "ride down," or the gentle cushioning of the occupant as the body slows, or decelerates. Air bags provide the final capture point of the passengers and again decrease the severity of **deceleration** injuries by allowing seat belts to be more compliant and by cushioning the occupant as he or she moves forward.

Remember that air bags decrease injury to the chest, face, and head very effectively. However, you should still suspect that other serious injuries to the extremities (resulting from the second collision) and to internal organs (resulting from the third collision) have occurred. In addition, individuals with short statures (including children) are more likely to suffer from airbag injuries even if properly restrained.

You should also remember that supplemental restraint systems can cause harm whether they are used properly or improperly. For example, seat belts that buckle automatically at the shoulder but require the passengers to buckle the lap portion can result in the body "submarining" forward underneath the shoulder restraint when the lap portion is not attached. This movement of the body can cause the lower extremities and the pelvis to crash into the dashboard, as that part of the body is unrestrained. In addition, individuals of short stature can sustain significant neck and facial injuries caused by the belting systems when their lower torso is unrestrained.

When passengers are riding in vehicles equipped with air bags but are not restrained by seat belts, they are often thrown forward in the act of emergency braking. As a result, they come into contact with the air bag and/or the doors at the time of deployment. This mechanism of injury is also responsible for some severe injuries to children who are riding unrestrained in the front seats of vehicles. In addition, some passengers may pass out before impact, and you may find them lying against the air bag when it deploys. You should look for abrasions and/or traction-type injuries on the face, lower part of the neck, and chest ▶ Figure 21-5 .

Contact points are often obvious from a simple quick evaluation of the interior of the vehicle. If there is no intrusion, you might see that an unrestrained front-seat passenger in a frontal collision will come into contact with the dashboard or instrument panel at the knees and transfer loads from the knees through the femur to the pelvis and hip joint (▼ **Figure 21-6A**). The chest and/or abdomen may also hit the steering wheel (▼ **Figure 21-6B**). In addition, the passenger's face often hits the steering wheel or may launch forward and up, hitting the windshield and/or the roof header in the area of the visors (▼ **Figure 21-6C**). Signs of most of these injuries can be found by simply inspecting the interior of the vehicle during extrication of the patient.

Figure 21-5 Air bags can cause injury in frontal collisions, specifically, abrasions and traction-type injuries to the face, neck, and chest.

Figure 21-6 Mechanism of injury and condition of the vehicle interior suggest likely areas of injury. **A.** The knee can strike the dashboard, resulting in a hip fracture or dislocation. **B.** Serious chest and abdominal injuries can result from striking the steering wheel. **C.** Head and spinal injuries can result when the face and head strike the windshield.

Rear-End Collisions

Rear-end impacts are known to cause whiplash-type injuries, particularly when the head and/or neck is not restrained by an appropriately placed headrest ▼ Figure 21-7 . Upon impact, the body and torso move forward. As the body is propelled forward, the head and neck are left behind because they are not restrained by a headrest, and they appear to be whipped back relative to the torso. As the vehicle comes to rest, the unrestrained passenger moves forward, striking the dashboard. In this type of collision, the cervical spine and surrounding area may be injured. The cervical spine is less tolerant of damage when it is bent back (in extension). Other parts of the spine and the pelvis may also be at risk for injury. In addition, the patient may sustain an acceleration-type injury to the brain, that is, the third collision of the brain within the skull. Passengers in the back seat wearing only a lap belt might have a higher incidence of injuries to the thoracic and lumbar spine.

Figure 21-7 Rear-end impacts often cause whiplash-type injuries, particularly when the head and/or neck is not restrained by a headrest.

Figure 21-8 In a lateral collision, the car is typically struck above its center of gravity and begins to rock away from the side of impact. This causes a type of lateral whiplash in which the passenger's shoulders and head whip toward the intruding vehicle.

Lateral Collisions

Lateral impacts are probably now the number one cause of death associated with motor vehicle crashes. When a vehicle is struck from the side, it is typically struck above its center of gravity and begins to rock away from the side of the impact. This results in a lateral whiplash injury ▼ Figure 21-8 . The movement is to the side, and the passenger's shoulders and head whip toward the intruding vehicle. This action may thrust the shoulder, thorax, and upper extremity and, more important, the skull against the doorpost or the window. The cervical spine has little tolerance for lateral bending.

If there is substantial intrusion into the passenger compartment, you should suspect lateral chest and abdomen injuries on the side of the impact, as well as possible fractures of the lower extremities, pelvis, and ribs. In addition, the organs within the abdomen are at risk because of a possible third collision. Approximately 25% of all severe injuries to the aorta that occur in motor vehicle crashes are a result of lateral collisions.

Rollover Crashes

Injury patterns that are commonly associated with rollover crashes differ, depending on whether the passenger was restrained. The most unpredictable are rollover crashes in which an unrestrained passenger may have sustained multiple strikes within the interior of the vehicle as it rolled one or more times. The most common life-threatening event in a rollover is ejection or partial ejection of the passenger from the vehicle ▼ Figure 21-9 . Passengers who have been ejected may have struck the interior of the vehicle many times before ejection. The passenger may also

Figure 21-9 Passengers who have been ejected or partially ejected may have struck the interior of the car many times before ejection.

have struck several objects, such as trees, a guardrail, or the vehicle's exterior, before landing. Passengers who have been partially ejected may have struck both the interior and exterior of the vehicle and may have been sandwiched between the exterior of the vehicle and the environment as the vehicle rolled. Ejection and partial ejection are significant mechanisms of injury; in these instances, you should prepare to care for life-threatening injuries.

Even when restrained, passengers can sustain severe injuries during a rollover crash, although the patterns of injury tend to be more predictable, and when properly used, the restraint system will prevent ejection from the vehicle. A passenger on the outboard side of a vehicle that rolls over is at high risk for injury because of the centrifugal force (the patient is pinned against the door of the vehicle). When the roof hits the ground during a rollover, a passenger who is restrained can still move far enough toward the roof to make contact and sustain a spinal cord injury. Therefore, rollover crashes are particularly dangerous for both restrained and, to a greater degree, unrestrained passengers because these crashes provide multiple opportunities for second and third collisions.

Spins

Spins are conceptually similar to rollovers. The rotation of the vehicle as it spins provides opportunities for the vehicle to strike objects such as utility poles. For example, as a vehicle spins and strikes a pole, the passengers experience not only the rotational motion, but also a lateral impact.

Falls

The injury potential of a fall is related to the height from which the patient fell. The greater the height of the fall, the greater the potential for injury. A fall from more than 15' or 3 times the patient's height is considered to be significant. The patient lands on the surface just as an unrestrained passenger smashes into the interior of a vehicle. The internal organs travel at the speed of the patient's body before it hits the ground and stop by smashing into the interior of the body. Again, as in a motor vehicle crash, it is these internal injuries that are the least obvious on assessment but pose the gravest threat to life. Therefore, you should suspect internal injuries in a patient who has fallen from a significant height, just as you would in a patient who has been in a high-speed motor vehicle crash. Always consider syncope or other underlying medical causes of the fall.

Pediatric Needs

To evaluate the MOI when your patient is a child, remember this:

Falls greater than 3 times the child's height = a significant MOI

Patients who fall and land on their feet may have less severe internal injuries because their legs may have absorbed much of the energy of the fall ▼ Figure 21-10 . Of course, as a result, they may have very serious injuries to the lower extremities, as well as pelvic and spinal injuries from energy that the legs do not absorb. Patients who fall onto their heads, as do victims of diving accidents, will likely have serious head and/or spinal injuries. In either case, a fall from a significant height is a serious event with great injury potential, and the patient should be evaluated thoroughly. Take the following factors into account:

- The height of the fall
- The surface struck
- The part of the body that hit first, followed by the path of energy displacement

Figure 21-10 When a patient falls and lands on his or her feet, the energy is transmitted to the spine, sometimes producing a spine injury as well as injuries to the legs and pelvis.

Calcaneus

Some texts consider falls to be the most common form of trauma. Many falls, especially those by the elderly, are not considered "true" trauma, even though bones may be broken. Often, these falls occur as a result of a fracture. Elderly patients often have osteoporosis, a condition in which their musculoskeletal system can fail under relatively low stress. Because of this condition, an elderly patient can sustain a fracture while in a standing position and then fall as a result. Therefore, an elderly patient may have actually sustained a fracture before the fall. These instances do not constitute true high-energy trauma unless the patient fell from a significant height.

Penetrating Trauma

Penetrating trauma is the second largest cause of death in the United States after blunt trauma. Low-energy penetrating trauma may be caused accidentally by impalement or intentionally by a knife, ice pick, or other weapon (▼ **Figure 21-11**). Once you have identified the entrance wound and the exit wound (if one exists), you know some important things about the path of the penetrating object. With low-energy penetrations, injuries are caused by the sharp edges of the object moving through the body and are therefore close to the object's path. Weapons such as knives, however, may have been deliberately moved around internally, causing more damage than the external wound might suggest.

In medium-velocity and high-velocity penetrating trauma, the path of the object (usually a bullet) may not be as easy to predict. This is because the bullet may flatten out, tumble, or even ricochet within the body before exiting. Also, because of its speed,

> Penetrating trauma is the second largest cause of death in the United States after blunt trauma.

pressure waves emanate from the bullet, causing damage remote from its path. This phenomenon, called **cavitation**, can result in serious injury to internal organs distant to the actual path of the bullet. Much like a boat moving through water, the bullet disrupts not only the tissues that are directly in its path but also those in its wake. Therefore, the area that is damaged by medium- and high-velocity projectiles can be many times larger than the diameter of the projectile itself (▼ **Figure 21-12**). This is one reason that exit wounds are often many times larger than entrance wounds. As with motor vehicle crashes, the energy available for a bullet to cause damage is more a function of its speed than its mass (weight). If the mass of the bullet is doubled, the energy that is available to cause injury is doubled. If the speed (velocity) of the bullet is doubled, the energy that is available to cause injury is quadrupled. For this reason, it is important for you to try to determine the type of weapon that was used. Although it is not necessary (or always possible) for you to distinguish between medium- and high-velocity injuries, any information regarding the type of weapon that was used should be relayed to medical control. Police at the scene may be a useful source of information regarding the caliber of weapon.

Figure 21-11   Injuries from low-energy penetrations, such as a stab wound, are caused by the sharp edges of the object moving through the body.

Figure 21-12   The area damaged by high-velocity projectiles, such as bullets, can be many times larger than the diameter of the projectile itself.

Newton's Laws

Newton's First Law

Newton's first law states that objects at rest tend to stay at rest and objects in motion tend to stay in motion unless acted upon by some force. The first part of the law is fairly clear. An object such as an empty soda can will not move spontaneously unless some force, such as a gust of wind, acts on it. An example will help to illustrate the second part. In a car going 30 mph, the passengers as well as the car are moving at 30 mph. The passengers do not feel as though they are moving because they are not moving relative to the car. However, when the car strikes a concrete barrier and comes to a sudden stop, the passengers continue to travel at 30 mph. They stay in motion until they are acted on by an external force—most likely the windshield, steering wheel, or dashboard. To appreciate the severity of the impact, think of the driver as sitting motionless while a steering wheel rams into his or her chest at 30 mph. Now consider that the same thing happens to the driver's internal organs. They also are in motion, traveling at 30 mph relative to the ground, until they are acted on by an external force, in this case the sternum, rib cage, or other body structure. This scenario illustrates the three collisions that are associated with blunt trauma.

Newton's Second Law

Newton's second law states that force (F) equals mass (M) times acceleration (A), that is, F = MA, in which acceleration is the change in velocity (speed) that occurs over time. Therefore, it is not so much that "speed kills" but that the change in velocity with respect to time generates the forces that cause injury. Simply put, it is not the fall, but the sudden stop at the bottom, that hurts.

In the example of the car traveling at 30 mph, it takes about 3 seconds for the car to decrease its speed from 30 mph to 0 mph when the driver applies the brakes smoothly. If he or she is properly restrained by well-adjusted seat belts, the driver slows, or decelerates, at the same rate as the car. But if the car is stopped not by braking but by hitting a large tree and the driver is not restrained, his or her body will continue to stay in motion at 30 mph until it is stopped by an external force—in this case, the steering wheel. Although the change in the body's velocity is the same as when the car was braking smoothly over 3 seconds (30 to 0 mph), that change now takes place in about 0.01 second. Because the time period of deceleration is 300 times less, the average force of impact is 300 times greater. This means that the force is approximately 150 times the force of gravity. Imagine a force 150 times your body weight slamming into your chest.

Now consider the same car striking the same tree, but this time, the driver is restrained with a shoulder and lap belt. The driver is essentially tied to the car and stops during the same period the car stops. It takes some time, although brief,

to crush the front of the car and bring it to a halt. The car comes to a stop in approximately 0.05 second. The change in the driver's velocity is the same (30 to 0 mph), but the longer period of deceleration results in a g-force of only 30 times that of gravity. This is still a substantial force, but it is much less than the force that is experienced by the unrestrained driver. More to the point, it is survivable.

In a final example, the car and driver, as before, are traveling at 30 mph, and the driver is properly restrained with a 3-point belt. In this case, however, the car is also equipped with an air bag. When the car hits the tree and suddenly stops, the driver's upper body initially continues forward at 30 mph. The body is partially slowed by the lap and shoulder belts but is finally brought to rest by the air bag. The upper body compresses the air bag, which stops the body's forward motion in about 0.1 second. Thus, the air bag stretches the duration of impact by 0.05 second, buying the body even more time, and the force on the upper body drops to approximately 15 times that of gravity.

The air bag has another advantage. The force of its impact is applied over a much larger area than the area that is affected by the steering wheel or the shoulder belt, shrinking the force per unit area. This point can be illustrated by an analogy. A person standing on one toe on a sheet of ice applies a concentrated load in a very small area, thus breaking the ice and falling through. If the person lies flat on the ice, he or she greatly expands the contact area and reduces the stress on the ice, which, depending on conditions, should not break. The dual action of the air bag (distributing the force of impact over a greater area and increasing the duration of impact) results in less severe injuries.

Newton's Third Law

Newton's third law states that for every action, there is an equal and opposite reaction. Therefore, if you push on a door, the door pushes back (reacts) with an equal force but in the opposite direction. In the case of a dented A-pillar, the force of the driver's head was sufficient to dent the strong metal. But in terms of patient assessment, the more important point is the reaction force of the pillar on the head. Newton's third law states that the two forces are equal but occur in opposite directions. In other words, the head was essentially hit by an A-pillar traveling at 30 mph. Similarly, it takes a substantial force to collapse a steering wheel. When you notice a collapsed steering wheel during scene size-up, you should suspect serious chest injuries even if the driver initially has no visible signs of chest injury. Often, reading the scene and understanding the basic principles of energy transfer will give you as clear a picture of the patient's potential injuries and injury severity as the actual physical patient assessment.

Prep Kit

Ready for Review

Obtaining information about the mechanism of injury—that is, how the injuries occurred and what forces were likely involved—can be just as important as obtaining vital signs in assessing the patient. This information can help hospital staff to focus their attention on damage that may not be immediately obvious. Motor vehicle crashes are the leading cause of unintentional injury. In every crash, there are really three collisions: the collision of the car against another car or some other object, the collision of the passenger against the interior of the car, and the collision of the passenger's internal organs against the solid structures of the body. You should suspect serious injuries in passengers who have been involved in a high-speed collision that results in massive damage to the car. The same is true of a patient who has fallen from a significant height or sustained a high-velocity penetrating injury.

Vital Vocabulary

blunt trauma Impact on the body by objects that cause injury without penetrating soft tissues or internal organs and cavities.

cavitation A phenomenon in which speed causes a bullet to generate pressure waves, which cause damage distant from the bullet's path.

deceleration The slowing of an object.

kinetic energy The energy of a moving object.

mechanism of injury The way in which traumatic injuries occur; the forces that act on the body to cause damage.

penetrating trauma Injury caused by objects that pierce the surface of the body and damage internal tissues and organs, such as knives and bullets.

potential energy The product of mass, gravity, and height, which is converted into kinetic energy and results in injury, such as from a fall.

Points to Ponder

You respond to an accident where a 6-year-old girl has been struck by an automobile. The girl is very seriously injured. A rather large crowd begins to form and a TV news crew begins filming. As you are going for the backboard the TV reporter steps in front of you and with camera running asks, "What happened?" and follows quickly with "Is the girl going to be ok?" What would you tell the reporter about the accident and the girl's condition? How would you deal with them filming your care? Is this an infringement on the girl's privacy?

Issues Dealing with the Press, Local Laws Regarding Privacy, Concerns for the Patient's Family, Others Watching and Critiquing Your Care.

Online Outlook

Injuries are the leading cause of death and disability in the United States among children and young adults (ages 1 to 34). To learn more about the specific injuries and their frequencies, complete Exercise 21 at www.emtb.com.

www.emtb.com

Assessment in Action

About 2:30 AM on a foggy Sunday morning, you and your partner are dispatched to a motor vehicle crash on Mountain View Road. You have been called several times to this stretch of two-lane highway. Because of the many curves and high rates of speed, it is the site of many collisions.

As you pull up you see that a pickup truck is lying on its roof partway down a shallow embankment. A second vehicle, a late-model Ford, is across the road facing the opposite direction, with the front grill caved in on the driver's side and a bull's eye impact on the driver's side of the windshield. The county sheriff has secured the scene and tells you that there are two patients. One is lying approximately 30' from the truck, after he was apparently ejected from the vehicle. The other is still in the Ford. Your partner goes to check on the victim that was apparently ejected while you check on the driver of the Ford.

1. Given the fact that this was a collision between two vehicles, which of the following would be of greatest importance in determining the severity of injury?
   A. The number of vehicles involved
   B. The speed of the vehicles
   C. The weight of the vehicles
   D. Hitting a moving object versus a fixed object

2. Of the impacts that occur during a motor vehicle collision, which one has the greatest potential to result in life-threatening injury?
   A. The first impact
   B. The second impact
   C. The third impact
   D. Both second and third impacts

3. Given the mechanism of injury, the ejected driver of the truck is at greatest risk for which of the following injuries?
   A. Sternal bruising
   B. Hollow organ rupture
   C. Head and spine injury
   D. It depends on the landing surface

4. The bull's eye impact on the driver's side of the Ford should lead you to suspect that the driver of the vehicle may have suffered a head injury as well as trauma to his:
   A. clavicles.
   B. scapula.
   C. chest.
   D. radius/ulna.

5. The head striking the windshield may also suggest lower extremity injury. Which of the following is most likely?
   A. Injury to the knee and femur
   B. Injury to the knee and tibia
   C. Injury to the feet and ankle
   D. Injury to the knee and ankle

6. Wearing seat belts saves lives but does not guarantee that motor vehicle crash victims will not be injured. Which of the following impacts will likely cause injury even if the patient is wearing a seat belt?
   A. Frontal impact
   B. Lateral impact
   C. Rear impact
   D. Multiple-vehicle impact

7. A brief look inside the truck reveals bilateral dents in the dash on either side of the steering wheel. This should alert you to which of the following potential injuries:
   A. Spine injury
   B. Abdominal organ rupture
   C. Flail chest
   D. Pelvic fracture

Challenging Questions

8. Your adult patient jumped approximately 20' from a tree, landing feet first then falling forward on his hands. Which bones/joints may be injured?

9. Your patient has been shot at close range three times. What would be most important to assess for in this patient that a victim of a fall off a curb would not require?
   A. Vital signs
   B. Mental status
   C. Find all the holes
   D. Determine chief complaint

10. Your 24-year-old patient was shot once in the lower right side of his back with an exit wound located in the upper left side of his abdomen. He is complaining of difficulty breathing. At the hospital the physician tells you this patient sustained a collapsed lung. How did that happen?

Bleeding

Objectives

Cognitive

1. List the structure and function of the circulatory system (p 530).
2. Differentiate between arterial, venous, and capillary bleeding (p 531).
3. State methods of emergency medical care of external bleeding (p 535).
4. Establish the relationship between body substance isolation and bleeding (p 533).
5. Establish the relationship between airway management and the trauma patient (p 534).
6. Establish the relationship between mechanism of injury and internal bleeding (p 542).
7. List the signs of internal bleeding (p 542).
8. List the steps in the emergency medical care of the patient with signs and symptoms of internal bleeding (p 543).

Affective

9. Explain the sense of urgency to transport patients who are bleeding and show signs of shock (hypoperfusion) (p 534).

Psychomotor

10. Demonstrate direct pressure as a method of emergency medical care of external bleeding (p 535).
11. Demonstrate the use of diffuse pressure as a method of emergency medical care of external bleeding (p 537).
12. Demonstrate the use of pressure points and tourniquets as a method of emergency medical care of external bleeding (p 536).
13. Demonstrate the care of the patient exhibiting signs and symptoms of internal bleeding (p 543).

www.emtb.com

Online Chapter Pretest

Interactivities

Vocabulary Explorer

Anatomy Review

Web Links

Online Review Manual

Distance Learning

TECHNOLOGY

Skill Drills

Vital Vocabulary

Pediatric Needs

Geriatric Needs

EMT-B Safety

EMT-B Tips

Documentation Tips

Remember

Prep Kit

Chapter FEATURES

While waiting for a light to change, you and your partner hear the unmistakable sound of gunshots. Moments later, dispatch sends you to the Jacks or Better pub for a shooting.

Penetrating trauma can produce injuries ranging from minor soft-tissue wounds to fatalities, either of which can present with little visible outward signs indicating the severity of the injury. This chapter will provide information on the methods recommended to control bleeding along with helping you answer the following questions:

1. Why does internal bleeding often go unnoticed until the patient "crashes"?

2. Under what circumstances might the rarely used tourniquet be the best choice for bleeding control?

Bleeding

After managing the airway, recognizing bleeding and understanding how it affects the body are perhaps the most important skills you will learn as an EMT-B. Bleeding can be external and obvious or internal and hidden. Either way, it is potentially dangerous, causing first weakness and, if left uncontrolled, eventually shock and death. The most common cause of shock after trauma is bleeding.

The purpose of this chapter is to help you understand how the cardiovascular system reacts to blood loss. The chapter begins with a brief review of the anatomy and function of the cardiovascular system. It then describes the signs, symptoms, and emergency medical care of both external and internal bleeding. The chapter concludes with a discussion on the relationship between bleeding and hypovolemic shock.

Anatomy and Physiology of the Cardiovascular System

The cardiovascular system circulates blood to all of the body's cells and tissues, delivering oxygen and nutrients and carrying away metabolic waste products ▶ **Figure 22-1** . Certain parts of the body, such as the brain, spinal cord, and heart, require a constant flow of blood to live. The cells in these organs cannot tolerate a lack of blood for more than a few minutes. Other organs, such as the lungs and kidneys, can survive for short periods of time without adequate blood flow. After that, their cells begin to die. This can lead to a permanent loss of function or, if enough cells die, death.

The cardiovascular system, the main system responsible for supplying and maintaining adequate blood flow, consists of three parts:

- The pump (the heart)
- A container (the blood vessels that reach every cell in the body)
- The fluid (blood and body fluids)

The Heart

The heart is a hollow muscular organ about the size of a clenched fist. It is an involuntary muscle that is under the control of the autonomic nervous system, but it has its own regulatory system. Thus, it can function even if the nervous system shuts down.

The heart is always working; all other organs depend on it to provide a rich blood supply. For this reason, it has a number of special features that other muscles do not. First, because the heart can tolerate a serious interruption of its blood supply for only a few seconds, its blood supply is as rich and well distributed as possible. Second, the heart works as two paired pumps ▶ **Figure 22-2** . Each side of the heart has an upper chamber (atrium) and a lower chamber (ventricle), both of which pump blood. Blood leaves each chamber of a normal heart through a one-way valve, which keeps the blood moving in the proper direction by preventing a backflow.

The right side of the heart receives oxygen-poor (deoxygenated) blood from the veins of the body. Blood enters into the right atrium from the vena cava, then fills the right ventricle. After the right ventricle contracts, blood flows into the pulmonary artery and the pulmonary circulation. The now oxygen-rich (oxygenated) blood returns to the left side of the heart from the lungs through the pulmonary veins. Blood enters the left atrium, then passes into the left ventricle. This side of

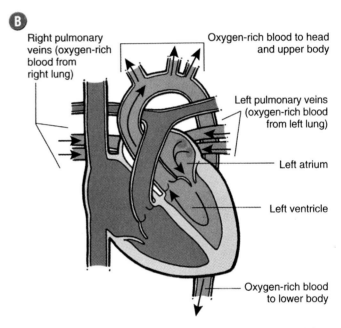

Figure 22-1 The cardiovascular system includes the heart, arteries, veins, and interconnecting capillaries. The exchange of nutrients and waste products that occurs in the capillaries is shown.

Figure 22-2 **A.** The left side of the heart circulates oxygen-rich blood to all parts of the body. It is the more muscular of the two pumps, as it must pump blood into the aorta and into the arteries. **B.** The right side of the heart circulates blood from the body to the lungs.

the heart is more muscular than the other because it must pump blood into the aorta and on to the arteries throughout the body.

Blood Vessels and Blood

There are five types of blood vessels:

- Arteries
- Arterioles
- Capillaries
- Venules
- Veins

As blood flows out of the heart, it passes into the **aorta**, the largest **artery** in the body. The arteries become smaller as they move away from the heart. The smaller vessels that connect the arteries and capillaries are called **arterioles**. **Capillaries** are small tubes, with

the diameter of a single red blood cell, that pass among all the cells in the body, linking the arterioles and the venules. Blood leaving the distal side of the capillaries flows into the venules. These small, thin-walled vessels empty into the **veins**, which return the blood to the heart. Oxygen and nutrients easily pass from the capillaries into the cells, and waste and carbon dioxide move

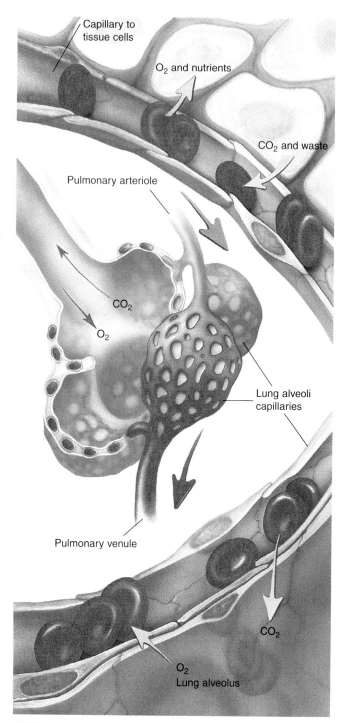

Figure 22-3 Oxygen and nutrients pass easily from the capillaries into the cells, and waste and carbon dioxide move out of the cells into the capillaries (top). Oxygen and carbon dioxide pass freely between the lungs and the capillaries (bottom).

out of the cells and into the capillaries ▲ Figure 22-3 . This transportation system allows the body to rid itself of waste products.

At the arterial ends of the capillaries and in the arteries themselves are circular muscular walls, which

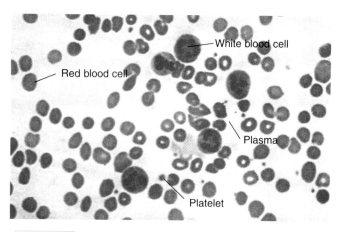

Figure 22-4 The microscopic appearance of the three major elements in blood: red blood cells, white blood cells, and platelets.

constrict and dilate automatically under the control of the autonomic nervous system. When these muscles open (dilate), blood passes into the capillaries into close proximity to each cell of the surrounding tissue; when the muscles are closed (constricted), there is no capillary blood flow. The muscles dilate and constrict in response to conditions such as fright, heat, cold, a specific need for oxygen, and the need to dispose of metabolic waste. In a healthy individual, all the vessels are never fully dilated or fully constricted at the same time.

The last part of the cardiovascular system is the contents of the container, or the blood. Blood contains red cells, white cells, platelets, and a liquid called plasma ▲ Figure 22-4 .

Physiology and Perfusion

Perfusion is the circulation of blood within an organ or tissue in adequate amounts to meet the cells' current needs for oxygen, nutrients, and waste removal. Blood enters an organ or tissue first through the arteries, then the arterioles, and finally the capillary beds ▶ Figure 22-5 . While passing through the capillaries, the blood delivers nutrients and oxygen to the surrounding cells and picks up the wastes they have generated. Then the blood leaves the capillary beds through the venules and finally reaches the veins, which take the blood back to the heart. Oxygen and carbon dioxide exchange takes place in the lungs.

Blood must pass through the cardiovascular system at a speed that is fast enough to maintain adequate circulation throughout the body and slow enough to allow each cell time to exchange oxygen and nutrients for carbon dioxide and other waste products. While some tissues, such as the lungs and kidneys, never rest and require a constant blood supply, most require circulating

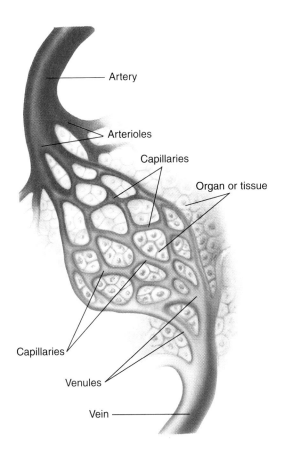

Artery

Arterioles

Capillaries

Organ or tissue

Capillaries

Venules

Vein

Figure 22-5   Perfusion occurs when blood circulates through tissues or an organ to provide the necessary oxygen and nutrients and remove waste products.

EMT-B Safety

Remember that a bleeding patient may expose you to potentially infectious body fluids; therefore, you must always follow BSI precautions in treating patients with external bleeding. Wear gloves and eye protection in all situations, and wear a gown and mask if there is a risk of blood splatter (▼ **Figure 22-6**). Avoid direct contact with body fluids if possible. Take special care if you have an open sore, cut, scratch, or ulcer. Also remember that frequent, thorough handwashing between patients and after every run is a simple yet important protective measure.

Figure 22-6   Your safety is paramount; therefore, you should always wear proper protective equipment when caring for a patient who is bleeding.

blood only intermittently, especially when active. Muscles are a good example. When you sleep, they are at rest and require a minimal blood supply. However, during exercise, they need a very large blood supply. The gastrointestinal tract requires a high flow of blood after a meal. After digestion is completed, it can do quite well with a small fraction of that flow.

The autonomic nervous system monitors the body's needs from moment to moment and adjusts the blood flow as required. During emergencies, the autonomic nervous system automatically redirects blood away from other organs to the heart, brain, lungs, and kidneys. Thus, the cardiovascular system is dynamic, constantly adapting to changing conditions. At times, the system fails to provide sufficient circulation for every body part to perform its function. This condition is called hypoperfusion, or **shock**.

Knowing which organs need adequate perfusion is the foundation on which your treatment of patients is based. Emergency medical care is designed to support the following systems:

- The heart (cardiovascular system)
- The brain (central nervous system)
- The lungs (respiratory system)
- The kidneys (renal system)

The heart requires constant perfusion, or it will not function properly. The brain and spinal cord cannot go for more than 4 to 6 minutes without perfusion, or the nerve cells will be permanently damaged. It is important to remember that cells of the central nervous system do not have the capacity to regenerate. The kidneys will be permanently damaged after 45 minutes of inadequate perfusion. Skeletal muscles cannot tolerate more than 2 hours of inadequate perfusion. The gastrointestinal tract can exist with limited (but not absent) perfusion for several hours. These times are based on a normal body temperature (98.6°F [37.0°C]). An organ or tissue that is considerably colder is much better able to resist damage from hypoperfusion.

External Bleeding

Hemorrhage means "bleeding." External bleeding is a visible hemorrhage. Examples include nosebleeds and bleeding from open wounds. As an EMT-B, you must understand how to control external bleeding.

The Significance of Bleeding

The body will not tolerate an acute blood loss of greater than 20% of blood volume ▼ **Figure 22-7** . The typical adult has approximately 70 mL of blood per kilogram of body weight, or 6 L (10 to 12 pints) in a body weighing 80 kg (175 lb). If the typical adult loses more than 1 L of blood (about 2 pints), significant changes in vital signs will occur, including increasing heart and respiratory rates and decreasing blood pressure. Because infants and children have less blood volume to begin with, the same effect is seen with smaller amounts of blood loss. For example, a 1-year-old infant has a total blood volume of about 800 mL. Significant symptoms of blood loss will occur after only 100 to 200 mL of blood loss. To put this in perspective, a soft drink can holds roughly 345 mL of liquid.

How well people compensate for blood loss is related to how rapidly they bleed. A normal, healthy adult can comfortably donate 1 unit (500 mL) of blood over a period of 15 to 20 minutes, adapting well to this decrease in blood volume. However, if a similar blood loss occurs in a much shorter period of time, the person may rapidly develop **hypovolemic shock**, a condition in which low blood volume results in inadequate perfusion and even death. The body simply cannot compensate for such a rapid blood loss.

Figure 22-7   Loss of approximately 1 L of blood will cause significant changes in an adult; a much smaller blood loss will result in shock in a child or infant.

Signs and Symptoms of Hypovolemic Shock

Rapid, weak pulse

Low blood pressure (late sign)

Mental status changes

Cool, clammy skin

Cyanosis (lips, under nails)

You should consider bleeding to be serious if the following conditions are present:

- It is associated with a significant mechanism of injury.
- The patient has a poor general appearance.
- Assessment reveals signs and symptoms of shock (hypoperfusion).
- You note a significant amount of blood loss.
- The blood loss is rapid.
- You cannot control the bleeding.

In any situation, blood loss is an extremely serious problem. It demands your immediate attention as soon as you have cleared the airway and managed the patient's breathing.

Characteristics of Bleeding

Injuries and some illnesses can disrupt blood vessels and cause bleeding. Typically, bleeding from an open artery is bright red (high in oxygen) and spurts in time with the pulse. The pressure that causes the blood to spurt also makes this type of bleeding difficult to control. As the amount of blood circulating in the body drops, so does the patient's blood pressure and, eventually, the arterial spurting.

Blood from an open vein is much darker (low in oxygen) and flows steadily. Because it is under less pressure, most venous blood does not spurt and is easier to manage. Bleeding from damaged capillary vessels is dark red and oozes from a wound steadily but slowly. It may clot spontaneously ▶ **Figure 22-8** .

On its own, bleeding tends to stop rather quickly, within about 10 minutes, in response to internal mechanisms and exposure to air. When we are cut, blood flows rapidly from the open vessel. Soon afterward, the cut ends of the vessel begin to narrow, reducing the amount of bleeding. Then a clot forms, plugging the hole and sealing the injured portions of the vessel. This process is called <u>coagulation</u>. Bleeding will never stop if a clot does not form, unless the injured vessel is completely cut off from the main blood supply. Direct contact with body tissues and fluids or the external environment commonly triggers the blood's clotting factors.

Despite the efficiency of this system, it may fail in certain situations. A number of medications, including aspirin, interfere with normal clotting. With a severe injury, the damage to the vessel may be so large that a clot cannot completely block the hole. Sometimes, only part of the vessel wall is cut, preventing it from constricting. In these cases, bleeding will continue unless it is stopped by external means. Occasionally, blood loss occurs very rapidly. In these instances, the patient might die before the body's defenses, such as clotting, could help.

A very small portion of the population lacks one or more of the blood's clotting factors. This condition is called <u>hemophilia</u>. There are several forms of hemophilia, most of which are hereditary and some of which are severe. Sometimes, bleeding may occur spontaneously in hemophilia. Because the patient's blood does not clot, all injuries, no matter how trivial, are potentially serious. A patient with hemophilia should be transported immediately.

Emergency Medical Care

As you begin to care for a patient with obvious external bleeding, remember to follow BSI precautions. As with all patient care, make sure that the patient has an open airway and is breathing ade-

quately. Provide oxygen if it is needed. You may then concentrate on controlling the bleeding.

Several methods are available to control external bleeding. Starting with the most commonly used, these include the following:

- Direct pressure and elevation
- Pressure dressings
- Pressure points (for upper and lower extremities)
- Splints
- Air splints
- Pneumatic antishock garment
- Tourniquets (last resort)

Basic methods. It will often be useful to combine these methods. ▶ **Skill Drill 22-1** illustrates the basic techniques that do not require special equipment:

1. Almost all instances of external bleeding can be controlled simply by **applying direct local pressure to the bleeding site.** This method is by far the most effective way to control external bleeding. Pressure stops the flow of blood and permits normal coagulation to occur. You may apply pressure with your gloved fingertip or hand, over the top of a sterile dressing if one is immediately available.

2. **Elevating a bleeding extremity** by as little as 6″ often stops venous bleeding. Whenever possible, use both techniques: direct pressure and elevation. In most cases, this will stop the bleeding. However, if it does not, you still have several options **(Step 1)**.

Figure 22-8 **A.** Bleeding from capillary vessels is dark red and oozes from the wound slowly but steadily. **B.** Venous bleeding is darker than arterial bleeding and flows steadily. **C.** Arterial bleeding is characteristically bright red and spurts in time with the pulse.

SkillDrill 22-1 Controlling External Bleeding

Apply direct pressure over the wound. Elevate the injury above the level of the heart if no fracture is suspected.

Apply a pressure dressing.

Apply pressure at the appropriate pressure point while continuing to hold direct pressure and elevation.

3. **Once you have applied a dressing and controlled the bleeding,** you can create a pressure dressing to maintain the pressure by firmly wrapping a sterile, self-adhering roller bandage around the entire wound. Use 4″ × 4″ or 4″ × 8″ sterile gauze pads for small wounds, and sterile universal dressings for larger wounds. If sterile gauze pads are not immediately available, use a clean handkerchief, sanitary napkin, or clean cloth. If no material is available, use your gloved hand to continue to provide the necessary pressure.

Cover the entire dressing, above and below the wound. Stretch the bandage tight enough to control bleeding but not so tight as to decrease blood flow to the extremity. You should still be able to palpate a distal pulse on the injured extremity after applying the pressure dressing. If bleeding continues, the dressing is probably not tight enough. Do not remove a dressing until a physician has evaluated the patient. Instead, apply additional manual pressure through the dressing. Then add more gauze pads over the first dressing, and secure them both with a second, tighter, roller bandage.

Bleeding will almost always stop when the pressure of the dressing exceeds arterial pressure. On those rare occasions when direct pressure fails to stop bleeding from a large gaping wound, you may need to pack the wound with sterile gauze pads, in addition to direct hand pressure. Applying ice may help control bleeding and reduce the pain **(Step 2)**.

4. **If a wound continues to bleed** despite use of direct pressure, elevate the extremity and try placing additional pressure over a proximal **pressure point**, or pulse point. A pressure point is a spot where a blood vessel lies near a bone. This technique is also useful if you have no material on hand to use for a dressing. Because a wound usually draws blood from more than one major artery, proximal compression of a major artery rarely stops bleeding completely, but it helps to slow the loss of blood. You must be thoroughly familiar with the location of the pulse points for this to work ▶ **Figure 22-9** **(Step 3)**.

SPECIAL TECHNIQUES. Much of the bleeding associated with broken bones occurs because the sharp ends of the bones cut muscles and other tissues. As long as a fracture remains unstable, the bone ends will move and continue to injure partially clotted vessels. Therefore, stabilizing a fracture and decreasing movement is a high priority in the prompt control of bleeding. Often, simple splints will quickly control bleeding associated with a fracture ▶ **Figure 22-10**. If not, you may need to use another splinting device.

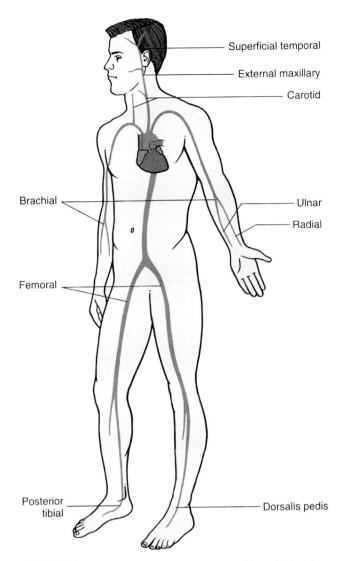

Figure 22-9 You should be familiar with the locations of arterial pressure points.

Figure 22-10 Use of a simple splint will often quickly control bleeding associated with a fracture. As long as a fracture is not immobilized, the bone ends are free to move and may continue to injure partially clotted vessels.

Figure 22-11 Air splints can also be used to control bleeding as they act as a pressure bandage for the entire extremity.

- **Air splints.** Air splints can control the bleeding associated with severe soft-tissue injuries, such as massive or complex lacerations, or fractures ◢ **Figure 22-11**. They also stabilize the fracture itself. An air splint acts like a pressure dressing applied to an entire extremity rather than to a small, local area. Once you have applied an air splint, be sure to monitor circulation in the distal extremity. Use only BSI-approved, clean, or disposable valve stems when orally inflating air splints.
- **Pneumatic antishock garments.** If a patient has injuries to the lower extremities and/or pelvis, you may be able to use a **pneumatic antishock garment (PASG)** as a splinting device, if local protocol allows. Situations in which use of a PASG is allowed vary widely by locale. Be sure to check with medical control in every case.

Following are the few, very specific instances in which a PASG may be effective:

- To stabilize fractures of the pelvis and proximal femurs
- To control significant internal bleeding associated with fractures of the pelvis and proximal femurs
- To control massive soft-tissue bleeding of the lower extremities when direct pressure is not effective

Do not use the PASG if any of the following conditions exist:

- Pregnancy
- Pulmonary edema of a cardiac origin

- Acute heart failure
- Penetrating chest injuries
- Groin injuries
- Major head injuries
- A transport time of less than 30 minutes

In these situations, the PASG may worsen or complicate the patient's condition. Consult with medical control if you think prolonged use or use in unusual circumstances may be necessary. The PASG works by compressing the abdomen and lower extremities, increasing peripheral resistance in the circulatory system. This increases the amount of blood that is available to perfuse the vital organs. In applying the PASG, you should carefully inflate the device in increments. As a general rule, gradually inflate the legs of the PASG before inflating the abdominal portion. If you are using the device to stabilize a possible pelvic fracture, you must inflate all compartments. Always document all obvious injuries or deformities prior to application of the PASG. Follow these steps to apply the PASG for bleeding control (▶ **Skill Drill 22-2**):

1. **Apply the garment.** If you will immobilize or move the patient on a backboard, lay the PASG out on the board before rolling the patient onto it. Position the top of the abdominal section of the PASG below the lowest rib to ensure that it does not compromise chest expansion **(Step 1)**.

2. **Close and fasten both leg compartments** and the abdominal compartment **(Step 2)**.

3. **Open the stopcocks** (valves) to the compartments you are preparing to inflate. You will inflate either both legs (lower extremity bleeding), or all three compartments together (internal pelvic or abdominal bleeding) **(Step 3)**.

4. **Inflate the compartments** with the foot pump. Do not increase the garment's pressure any more

than necessary. A PASG is adequately inflated when the Velcro crackles. Higher pressures may cause local tissue damage. Always stop inflating the PASG once the patient's systolic blood pressure exceeds 100 mm Hg **(Step 4)**.

5. **Check the patient's blood pressure** during inflation, and continue to monitor vital signs at least every 5 minutes afterward. Remember that the pressure gauges of the PASG measure the air pressure in the device. They in no way reflect the patient's blood pressure. Be aware of temperature extremes or external pressure changes that can significantly affect the pressure exerted by the PASG, thus requiring frequent monitoring and adjustment **(Step 5)**.

You will know that the device has worked if the patient's blood pressure increases.

Do not remove a PASG in the field. It must be deflated gradually in the hospital under careful supervision by a physician and only after appropriate IV solutions have been given. Before turning your patient over to hospital personnel, report the patient's blood pressure, the time you applied the PASG, and the results.

- **Tourniquets.** A **tourniquet** is rarely needed to control bleeding. Applying a tourniquet is considered a last resort, because it is rarely necessary and is effective for only a very limited number of injuries. Thus, a tourniquet often creates, rather than solves, problems. Application of a tourniquet can cause permanent damage to nerves, muscles, and blood vessels, resulting in the loss of an extremity. In addition, tourniquets are often improperly applied.

If you cannot control bleeding from the major vessel in an extremity *in any other way*, a properly applied tourniquet may save a patient's life. Specifically, the tourniquet is useful if a patient is bleeding severely from a partial or complete amputation.

Follow these steps to apply a tourniquet (▶ **Skill Drill 22-3**):

1. **Fold a triangular bandage** until it is 4" wide and six to eight layers thick.

2. **Wrap the bandage** around the extremity twice. Choose an area only slightly proximal to the bleeding, to reduce the amount of tissue damage to the extremity **(Step 1)**.

Skill Drill 22-2   Applying a Pneumatic Antishock Garment (PASG)

Apply the garment so that the top is below the lowest rib.

Enclose both legs and the abdomen.

Open the stopcocks.

Inflate with the foot pump, and close the stop-cocks either when the patient's systolic blood pressure reaches 100 mm Hg or the Velcro crackles.

Check the patient's blood pressure again. Monitor the vital signs.

3. **Tie one knot** in the bandage. Then place a stick or rod on top of the knot, and tie the ends of the bandage over the stick in a square knot **(Step 2)**.

4. **Use the stick as a handle,** and twist it to tighten the tourniquet until the bleeding has stopped; then stop twisting **(Step 3)**.

5. **Secure the stick in place,** and make the wrapping neat and smooth.

6. **Write "TK"** and the exact time (hour and minute) that you applied the tourniquet on a piece of adhesive tape. Use the phrase "time applied." Securely fasten the tape to the patient's forehead. Notify hospital personnel on your arrival that your patient has a tourniquet in place. Record this same information on the ambulance run report form **(Step 4)**.

7. **As an alternative method,** you can use a blood pressure cuff as an effective tourniquet. Position the cuff proximal to the bleeding point, and inflate it just enough to stop the bleeding. Leave the cuff inflated. If you use a blood pressure cuff, monitor the gauge continuously to make sure that the pressure is not gradually dropping. You may have to clamp the tube with a hemostat leading from the cuff to the inflating bulb to prevent loss of pressure **(Step 5)**.

SkillDrill 22-3 Applying a Tourniquet

①

Create a 4"-wide, multilayered bandage. Wrap the bandage twice around the extremity, just above the bleeding site.

②

Tie a single knot, and place a stick on the top of it.

③

Tie a square knot over the stick, and then twist the stick until the bleeding stops.

④

Secure the stick so that it will not unwind. Write "TK" and the exact time you applied the tourniquet on a piece of adhesive tape, fasten the tape to the patient's forehead, and notify hospital personnel on arrival.

⑤

You can also use a blood pressure cuff as an effective tourniquet.

Whenever you apply a tourniquet, make sure you observe the following precautions:

- Do not apply a tourniquet directly over any joint. Keep it as close to the injury as possible.
- Use the widest bandage possible. Make sure that it is tightened securely.
- Never use wire, rope, a belt, or any other narrow material. It could cut into the skin.
- Use wide padding under the tourniquet if possible. This will protect the tissues and help with arterial compression.
- Never cover a tourniquet with a bandage. Leave it open and in full view.
- Do not loosen the tourniquet after you have applied it. Hospital personnel will loosen it once they are prepared to manage the bleeding.

Bleeding from the Nose, Ears, and Mouth

Several conditions can result in bleeding from the nose, ears, and/or mouth, including the following:

- Skull fracture
- Facial injuries, including those caused by a direct blow to the nose
- Sinusitis, infections, nose drop use and abuse, dried or cracked nasal mucosa, or other abnormalities
- High blood pressure
- Coagulation disorders
- Digital trauma (nose picking)

Epistaxis, or nosebleed, is a common emergency. Occasionally, it can cause enough of a blood loss to send a patient into shock. Keep in mind that the blood you

SkillDrill 22-4   Controlling Epistaxis

Use BSI precautions. Position the patient: sitting, leaning forward. Apply direct pressure, pinching the fleshy part of the nostrils.

Alternate method: Use pressure with a rolled gauze bandage between the upper lip and gum. Calm the patient.

Apply ice over the nose. Maintain pressure until bleeding is controlled. Provide prompt transport after bleeding stops.
Transport immediately if indicated. Assess and treat for shock, including oxygen, as needed.

see may be only a small part of the total blood loss. Much of the blood may pass down the throat into the stomach as the patient swallows. A person who swallows a large amount of blood may become nauseated and start vomiting the blood, which is sometimes confused with internal bleeding. Most nontraumatic nosebleeds occur from sites in the septum, the tissue dividing the nostrils. You can usually handle this type of bleeding effectively by pinching the nostrils together.

Follow these steps to treat a patient with epistaxis **▲ Skill Drill 22-4** :

1. **Follow BSI precautions.**

2. **Help the patient to sit,** leaning forward, with the head tilted forward. This position stops the blood from trickling down the throat or being aspirated into the lungs.

3. **Apply direct pressure** for at least 15 minutes by pinching the fleshy part of the nostrils together. This is the preferred method. This technique may also be self-administered by the patient if he or she is capable and bleeding is severe **(Step 1)**.

4. **Placing a rolled 4″ × 4″ gauze bandage** between the upper lip and the gum is another option. Have the patient apply pressure by stretching the upper lip tightly against the rolled bandage and pushing it up into and against the nose. If the

patient is unable to do this effectively, use your gloved fingers to press the gauze against the gum.

5. **Keep the patient calm and quiet,** especially if he or she has high blood pressure or is anxious. Anxiety tends to increase blood pressure, which could worsen the nosebleed **(Step 2)**.

6. **Apply ice over the nose.**

7. **Maintain the pressure** until the bleeding is completely controlled, usually no more than 15 minutes (assuming that this is the patient's only problem). Most often, failure to stop a nosebleed is the result of releasing the pressure too soon.

8. **Provide prompt transport** once the bleeding has stopped.

9. **If you cannot control the bleeding,** if the patient has a history of frequent nosebleeds, or if there is a significant amount of blood loss, transport the patient immediately. Assess the patient for signs and symptoms of shock. Treat appropriately for shock and administer oxygen via mask, if necessary **(Step 3)**.

Bleeding from the nose or ears following a head injury may indicate a skull fracture. In these instances, you should not attempt to stop the blood flow. This bleeding may be difficult to control. Second, applying excessive pressure to the injury may force the blood leaking through the ear or nose to collect within the head. This could increase the pressure on the brain and possibly cause permanent damage. If you suspect a skull fracture, loosely cover the bleeding site with a sterile gauze pad to collect the blood and help keep contaminants away from the site. There is always a risk of infection to the brain. Apply light compression by wrapping the dressing loosely around the head (▶ **Figure 22-12**). If blood or drainage contains cerebrospinal fluid, a characteristic staining of the dressing, much like a target, will occur.

Internal Bleeding

Internal bleeding can be very serious, especially because you might not be aware that it is happening. Injury or damage to internal organs commonly results in extensive internal bleeding, which can cause hypovolemic shock before you realize the extent of blood loss. A person with a bleeding stomach ulcer may lose a large amount of blood very quickly. Similarly, a person who has a lacerated liver or a ruptured spleen may lose a considerable amount of blood within the abdomen. Yet the patient has no outward signs of bleeding.

Broken bones, especially broken ribs, also may cause serious internal blood loss. Sometimes this bleeding extends into the chest cavity and the soft tissues of the chest wall. A broken femur can easily result in the loss of 1 L or more of blood into the soft tissues of the thigh. Often, the only signs of such bleeding are local swelling and bruising due to the accumulation of blood around the ends of the broken bone. Severe pelvic fractures may result in life-threatening hemorrhage.

You must always be alert to the possibility of internal bleeding and assess the patient for related signs and symptoms, particularly if the mechanism of injury is severe. If you suspect that a patient is bleeding internally, you should promptly transport him or her to the hospital.

Mechanism of Injury

Internal bleeding is possible whenever the mechanism of injury suggests that severe forces affected the abdomen and/or the chest. These forces include blunt and penetrating trauma. Internal bleeding commonly occurs as a result of falls, blast injuries, and automobile or motorcycle crashes.

As you assess a patient, look for signs of injury over the chest or abdomen, including contusions, abrasions, lacerations, or other signs of injury or deformity. You should always suspect internal bleeding in a patient who has penetrating injury or blunt trauma.

Figure 22-12 Bleeding from the ear after a head injury may indicate a skull fracture. Loosely cover the bleeding site with a sterile gauze pad, and apply light compression by wrapping the dressing loosely around the head.

Nature of Illness

Nontraumatic internal bleeding can lead to shock just as easily as bleeding caused by injury. Usually, internal bleeding occurs in the abdomen as a result of irritable bowel syndrome, an aneurysm, an ulcer, a ruptured ectopic pregnancy, or another condition. Abdominal pain and distention are frequent in these situations but are not always present. In older patients, dizziness, faintness, or weakness may be the first sign of nontraumatic internal bleeding. Ulcers or other gastrointestinal problems may cause vomiting of blood or bloody diarrhea.

It is not as important for you to know the specific organ involved as it is to recognize that the patient is in shock and *respond appropriately.*

Signs and Symptoms

The most common symptom of internal abdominal bleeding is acute abdominal pain. Another common sign is bruising around the abdomen. This can occur with or without trauma. Bruising is also called **contusion**, or **ecchymosis**. A **hematoma**, a mass of blood in the soft tissues beneath the skin, indicates bleeding into soft tissues and may be the result of either a minor or a severe injury. Bruising or ecchymosis may not be present initially, however, and the only sign of severe pelvic or abdominal trauma may be redness or skin abrasions acutely.

Bleeding, however slight, from any body opening is serious. It usually indicates internal bleeding that is not easy to see or control. Bright red bleeding from the mouth or rectum (hematochezia) or blood in the urine (hematuria) may suggest serious internal injury or disease. Nonmenstrual vaginal bleeding is always significant.

Other signs and symptoms of internal bleeding in both trauma and medical patients include the following:

- **Hematemesis.** This is vomited blood. It may be bright red or dark red, or if the blood has been partially digested, it may look like coffee ground vomitus.
- **Melena.** This is a black, foul-smelling, tarry stool that contains digested blood.
- **Hemoptysis.** This is bright red blood that is coughed up by the patient.
- **Pain, tenderness, bruising, guarding, or swelling.** These signs and symptoms may mean that a closed fracture is bleeding.
- **Broken ribs, bruises over the lower chest, or a rigid, distended abdomen.** These signs and symptoms may indicate a lacerated spleen or liver. Patients with an injury to either organ may have referred pain in the right shoulder (liver) or left shoulder (spleen). You should suspect internal abdominal bleeding in a patient with referred pain.

The first sign of hypovolemic shock (hypoperfusion) is a change in mental status, such as anxiety, restlessness, or combativeness. In nontrauma patients, weakness, faintness, or dizziness on standing is another early sign. Changes in skin color, or pallor, are seen often in both trauma and medical patients. Later signs of hypoperfusion suggesting internal bleeding include the following:

- Tachycardia
- Weakness, fainting, or dizziness at rest
- Thirst
- Nausea and vomiting
- Cold, moist (clammy) skin
- Shallow, rapid breathing
- Dull eyes
- Slightly dilated pupils that are slow to respond to light
- Capillary refill in infants and children of more than 2 seconds
- Weak, rapid (thready) pulse
- Decreasing blood pressure
- Altered level of consciousness

Patients with these signs and symptoms are at risk. Some may be in danger. Even if their bleeding stops, it could begin again at any moment. Therefore, prompt transport is necessary.

Emergency Medical Care

Controlling internal bleeding or bleeding from major organs usually requires surgery or other procedures that must be done in the hospital. Your role as an EMT-B in these cases is to keep the patient still to promote clot formation and to provide high-flow oxygen and prompt transport. However, you can usually control internal bleeding into the extremities quite well in the field simply by splinting the extremity, usually most effectively with an air splint. You will rarely need to use PASG, and you should never use a tourniquet to control the bleeding from closed, internal, soft-tissue injuries.

Follow these steps to care for patients with possible internal bleeding:

1. **Follow BSI precautions.**

2. **Maintain the airway** with cervical spine immobilization if the mechanism of injury suggests the possibility of spinal injury.

3. **Administer high-flow oxygen** and provide artificial ventilation as necessary.

4. **Control all obvious external bleeding.**

5. **Treat suspected internal bleeding** in an extremity by applying a splint.

6. **Monitor and record the vital signs** at least every 5 minutes.

7. **Give the patient nothing** (not even small sips of water) by mouth.

8. **Elevate the patient's legs 6″ to 12″ in nontrauma patients** to help the blood return to the vital organs.

9. **Keep the patient warm.**

10. **Provide immediate transport** for all patients with signs and symptoms of shock (hypoperfusion). Report any changes in the patient's condition to emergency department personnel.

Prep Kit

Ready for Review

Perfusion is the circulation of blood in adequate amounts to meet each cell's current needs for oxygen, nutrients, and waste removal. Hypoperfusion, or shock, occurs when the cardiovascular system fails to provide adequate perfusion. Both internal and external bleeding can cause shock. You must know how to recognize and control both.

In the order of preference, the six methods for controlling external bleeding are direct local pressure and elevation, pressure dressings, pressure points, splints, air splints, pneumatic antishock garment (PASG), and tourniquets. Do not remove a dressing until a physician has evaluated the patient; instead, apply additional dressings as needed. Stabilizing a serious fracture has a high priority in the control of bleeding. Use a PASG to prevent or minimize hypovolemic shock only when there is internal bleeding, massive soft-tissue bleeding of the lower extremities that cannot be otherwise controlled, or bleeding associated with fractures of the pelvis and proximal femurs. Use a tourniquet only as a last resort, typically with amputations.

Bleeding from the nose, ears, and/or mouth may result from skull fracture, facial injuries, sinusitis, high blood pressure, and coagulation disorders. To treat epistaxis, apply direct pressure for at least 15 minutes by pinching the nostrils together or using gauze between the upper lip and gum. Do not attempt to stop bleeding from the nose or ears. If you suspect a skull fracture, cover the bleeding site loosely with a sterile gauze pad.

You should assess and promptly transport any patient who may have internal bleeding, particularly if the mechanism of injury is severe and has affected the abdomen and/or the chest. The most common sign of internal abdominal bleeding is acute abdominal pain. Bleeding from any body opening is serious. Signs of internal bleeding include hematemesis, melena, hemoptysis, broken ribs, bruised chest, distended abdomen, and referred pain. Signs of shock that suggest internal bleeding include change in mental status, pallor, weakness and dizziness, tachycardia, thirst, nausea and vomiting, and shallow, rapid breathing. If you suspect that a patient is bleeding internally, maintain the airway, administer high-flow oxygen, keep the patient still, apply a splint to the affected extremity, monitor vital signs at least every 5 minutes, and, in nontrauma patients, elevate the legs.

Vital Vocabulary

aorta The main artery, which receives blood from the left ventricle and delivers it to all the other arteries that carry blood to the tissues of the body.

arterioles The smallest branch of an artery leading to the vast network of capillaries.

artery A blood vessel, consisting of three layers of tissue and smooth muscle that carries blood away from the heart.

capillary Any one of the small blood vessels that connect arteriole and venule and through whose walls various substances pass into and out of the interstitial tissues and then on to the cells.

coagulation Formation of clots to plug openings in injured blood vessels and stop blood flow.

contusion Bruising, or ecchymosis.

ecchymosis Discoloration of the skin associated with a closed wound; bruising.

epistaxis Nosebleed.

hematoma Mass of blood in the soft tissues beneath the skin.

hemophilia A congenital condition in which the patient lacks one or more of the blood's normal clotting factors.

hemorrhage Bleeding.

hypovolemic shock A condition in which low blood volume, due to either massive internal or external bleeding or extensive loss of body water, results in inadequate perfusion.

perfusion Circulation of blood within an organ or tissue in adequate amounts to meet the cells' current needs.

pneumatic antishock garment (PASG) An inflatable device that covers the legs and abdomen; used to splint the lower extremities or pelvis, or to control bleeding in the lower extremities, pelvis, or abdominal cavity.

pressure point A point where a blood vessel lies near a bone; useful when direct pressure and elevation do not control bleeding.

shock A condition in which the circulatory system fails to provide sufficient circulation so that every body part can perform its function; also called hypoperfusion.

tourniquet The bleeding control method of last resort that occludes arterial flow; used only when all other methods have failed and the patient's life is in danger.

vein Any blood vessel that carries blood from the tissues to the heart.

Assessment in Action

You are dispatched to a local machine shop for "a man with his arm caught in a machine." On arrival, a security guard leads you to the fabrication department where coworkers have dismantled a wiring machine. You find a 27-year-old man lying in the aisle, next to the dismantled machine. The patient is conscious and answering questions, though he appears somewhat disoriented.

Given what he has just been through, you consider that normal. A coworker is kneeling in a puddle of blood as he holds a shop towel around the injured man's upper arm. You look quickly under the towel and see a 5" laceration from which bright red blood immediately spurts. The patient appears pale and has multiple small cuts on his face and arms. His safety glasses have protected his eyes, and his shop apron seems to have done the same for his chest and abdominal area.

1. Your first priority on this call is to:
   A. evaluate the patient's level of consciousness.
   B. quickly open and maintain the patient's airway.
   C. ensure that the scene is safe and secured.
   D. call for law enforcement officers to respond.

2. In this case, the patient's bright red blood spurting from his laceration is most likely from a/an:
   A. vein.
   B. capillary.
   C. arteriole.
   D. artery.

3. Why does blood continue to spurt from the laceration on his arm?
   A. Profuse bleeding is common when the patient is young.
   B. Muscle spasms in the arm are forcing the blood out.
   C. There is a surge in arterial pressure with each heart contraction.
   D. Any injury in which the patient goes into shock causes bleeding.

4. Which artery in the patient's arm may have been lacerated?
   A. Jugular
   B. Carotid
   C. Brachial
   D. Femoral

5. When obtaining a blood pressure on this patient, you are measuring the pressure that the circulating blood is exerting on the walls of the:
   A. veins when the right atrium contracts.
   B. veins when the right ventricle contracts.
   C. arteries when the left ventricle contracts.
   D. arteries when the left atrium contracts.

6. If the patient's blood pressure is low, due to blood loss, other signs that should be apparent include pale, cold, clammy skin and:
   A. tachycardia.
   B. bradycardia.
   C. slower breathing.
   D. bounding pulse.

7. Immediate treatment for this type of bleeding includes:
   A. a tourniquet.
   B. compression dressing.
   C. elevation.
   D. direct pressure.

8. Further assessment of this patient reveals continued disorientation. What might his disorientation be indicating?
   A. Head injury
   B. Shock
   C. Intoxication
   D. Psychological impact of what happened

Challenging Questions

9. Why does direct pressure work?

10. Of the signs of shock, which will occur first?

Points to Ponder

You respond to a motor vehicle crash and you and your partner each choose a car. When you approach the driver of your vehicle you find her unconscious, breathing loudly, and bleeding severely from a large wound on her head. You grab a large dressing and reach through a broken window to place it on her wound. You hold the dressing in place with one hand as you survey the woman for other injuries. The woman's blood has soaked through and when you reach for another, you realize that your glove is split and you have cut your hand as you reached through the window. Based on the amount of blood on the dressing, you are sure you have "mixed blood" with the woman. When do you take time to put on

new gloves? When do you take time to wash your hands and clean the wound? Who would you report this to? When would you seek testing and treatment for blood-borne exposures?

Issues BSI Precautions, HIV Testing, HIV Risks, Exposure Reporting, Workers' Compensation.

Online Outlook

Six ways to control external bleeding are presented in this chapter. Test your ability to choose the appropriate way to control bleeding for different situations by completing Exercise 22 at www.emtb.com.

www.emtb.com

Shock

TECHNOLOGY

www.emtb.com

- Online Chapter Pretest
- Interactivities
- Vocabulary Explorer
- Anatomy Review
- Web Links
- Online Review Manual
- Distance Learning

Chapter FEATURES

- Skill Drills
- Vital Vocabulary
- Pediatric Needs
- Geriatric Needs
- EMT-B Safety
- EMT-B Tips
- Documentation Tips
- Remember
- Prep Kit

Rescue 21, respond to the Archer Hotel for a "man down" in the lobby. On arrival you find a 58-year-old man lying on the floor in a large puddle of emesis the color of coffee grounds.

A critical part of the EMT-B's job is having an understanding of shock and shock management. This chapter will present valuable information on the topic of shock in addition to helping you answer the following questions:

1. How does compensated shock differ from decompensated shock? Does your care differ as well?

2. Is there a difference in how children and adults compensate for severe traumatic injuries?

Shock

Shock has a number of meanings. For example, we often say that a person who has received a fright or a piece of bad news is in shock. An electric current passing through the body delivers a shock. In this chapter, shock describes a state of collapse and failure of the cardiovascular system in which blood circulation slows and eventually ceases. If not treated promptly, shock can be fatal.

Shock often accompanies the events, such as heart attacks and automobile crashes, to which you will respond as an EMT-B. Therefore, you should always be able to anticipate, recognize, and treat shock in order to manage patients effectively.

This chapter begins with a close-up look at perfusion, the function that fails in shock. Next it looks at the physiologic causes of shock, describing each of its major forms. Finally, it discusses the emergency treatment of shock in general and of each kind of shock in particular.

Perfusion

Shock, or hypoperfusion, refers to a state of collapse and failure of the cardiovascular system that leads to inadequate circulation. Like internal bleeding, shock cannot be seen. It is not a specific disease or injury. However, it is a dangerous condition that results in the inadequate flow of blood to the body's cells and failure to rid cells of metabolic wastes. As the cells begin to die, the body attempts to compensate by redirecting blood flow from nonessential organs (skin and intestines) to essential organs (heart, lungs, and brain). If the conditions causing shock are not promptly addressed, the patient will soon die.

As we have seen, the cardiovascular system consists of three parts: a pump (heart), a container (vessels), and the container's contents (blood) ▶ **Figure 23-1** . Blood is the vehicle for carrying oxygen and nutrients through the vessels to the capillary beds, where these supplies are exchanged for waste products. The blood keeps moving as a result of pressure that is generated by the contractions of the heart and affected by the dilating and constricting of the vessels. This pressure, which we call blood pressure, is usually carefully controlled by the body so that there is always sufficient circulation, or **perfusion**, in the various tissues and organs. Blood pressure is, in fact, a rough measure of perfusion. It tells us how well the body's oxygen, nutrient, and waste removal needs are being met.

Remember that blood pressure is really the pressure of blood within the vessels at any one time. The systolic pressure is the arterial pressure, or pressure generated every time the heart contracts; the diastolic pressure is the pressure maintained within the system.

Blood flow through the capillary beds is regulated by the capillary sphincters, circular muscular walls that constrict and dilate. These **sphincters** are under the control of the **autonomic nervous system**, which regulates involuntary functions such as sweating and digestion. Capillary sphincters also respond to other stimuli such as heat, cold, the need for oxygen, and the need for waste removal. Keep in mind that, under normal circumstances, not all cells have the same needs at the same time. For example, the stomach and intestines have a high need for blood flow during and shortly after eating, when digestion is at a peak. Between meals, blood flow is lessened, and blood is diverted to other areas. The brain, by contrast, needs a constant and consistent supply of blood to function.

Thus, regulation of blood flow is determined by cellular need and is accomplished by vessel constriction or dilation, together with sphincter constriction or dilation.

Maintenance of blood flow, or perfusion, is accomplished by the heart, blood vessels, and blood, working together.

Perfusion requires more than just having a working cardiovascular system, however. It also requires adequate oxygen exchange in the lungs, adequate nutrients in the form of glucose in the blood, and adequate waste removal, primarily through the lungs. Therefore, the respiratory system is also a major contributor to maintaining adequate perfusion.

In addition, the body also has mechanisms in place to help support the respiratory and cardiovascular systems when the need for perfusion of vital organs is increased. These mechanisms, including the autonomic nervous system and certain chemicals called hormones, are triggered when the body senses that the pressure in the system is falling. The action of the hormones stimulates an increase in heart rate and in the strength of cardiac contractions and vasoconstriction in nonessential areas, primarily in the skin and gastrointestinal tract (peripheral vasoconstriction). Together, these actions are designed to maintain pressure in the system and, as a result, perfusion of all vital organs.

Eventually, there is also a shifting of body fluids to help maintain pressure within the system. However, the response of the autonomic nervous system and hormones comes within seconds. It is this response that causes all the signs and symptoms of a patient in shock.

Causes of Shock

Shock can result from many different conditions, including respiratory failure, acute allergic reactions, and overwhelming infection. In all cases, however, the damage occurs because of insufficient perfusion of organs and tissues. As soon as perfusion stops or becomes impaired, tissues start to die, affecting all local body processes. If the conditions causing shock are not promptly arrested and reversed, death soon follows.

Understanding the basic physiologic causes of shock will better prepare you to treat it (▼ **Figure 23-2**).

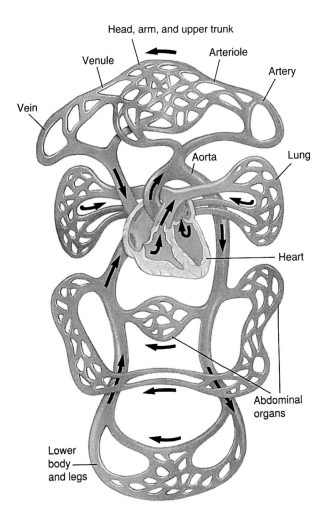

Head, arm, and upper trunk
Venule
Arteriole
Artery
Vein
Aorta
Lung
Heart
Abdominal organs
Lower body and legs

Figure 23-1 The cardiovascular system consists of three parts: the pump (heart), the container (vessels), and the contents (blood). The blood carries oxygen and nutrients through the vessels to the capillary beds, where they are exchanged for waste products.

A **Poor pump function**
Causes: Heart attack, trauma to heart

B **Blood or fluid loss from blood vessels**
Causes: Trauma to vessels or tissues, fluid loss from GI tract (vomiting/diarrhea can also lower the fluid component of blood)

C **Blood vessels dilate**
Causes: Infection, drug overdose (narcotic), spinal cord injury

Figure 23-2 There are three basic causes of shock and impaired tissue perfusion. **A.** Pump failure occurs when the heart is damaged by disease or injury. The heart does not generate enough energy to move the blood through the system. **B.** Decreased blood volume, usually a result of bleeding, results in inadequate perfusion. **C.** The blood vessels can dilate enough that the blood within them, even though it is of normal volume, is inadequate to fill the system and provide efficient perfusion.

There are both cardiovascular and noncardiovascular causes of shock. The three major cardiovascular causes of shock are as follows:

- **Poor pump function.** The heart, if damaged by muscular disease or injury, may fail to perform properly as a pump. That is, it does not generate sufficient energy to move blood through the system.

- **Blood or fluid loss from blood vessels.** If enough blood or plasma is lost, the volume of fluid contained within the vascular system is insufficient to perfuse all tissues and organs.

- **Poor vessel function.** If all the blood vessels dilate at once, the normal volume of blood will be insufficient to fill the system and provide efficient perfusion.

The noncardiovascular causes of shock are respiratory insufficiency and **anaphylaxis**, an unusual or exaggerated allergic reaction to foreign protein or other substances.

Cardiovascular Causes of Shock

PUMP FAILURE. **Cardiogenic shock** is caused by inadequate function of the heart, or pump failure. Circulation of blood throughout the vascular system requires the constant pumping action of a normal and vigorous heart muscle. Many diseases can cause destruction or inflammation of this muscle. Within certain limits, the heart can adapt to these problems. If too much muscular damage occurs, however, as sometimes happens after a heart attack, the heart no longer functions well. A major effect is the backup of blood into the lungs. The resulting buildup of fluid within the pulmonary tissue is called pulmonary edema. **Edema** is the presence of abnormally large amounts of fluid between cells in body tissues, causing swelling of the affected area ▶ **Figure 23-3** . Pulmonary edema leads to impaired ventilation, which may be manifested by an increased respiratory rate and abnormal lung sounds.

The muscular contraction of the heart moves blood through the vessels at distinct pressures. For blood to circulate efficiently throughout the entire system, there must be both the right amount of pressure and an adequate number of heartbeats. For this reason, the heart has its own electrical system that initiates and regulates its beating. Disease or injury can damage or destroy this system, causing irregular and uncoordinated beats, beats that are too slow (fewer than 60/min), or beats that are too fast (greater than 150/min).

Cardiogenic shock develops when the heart muscle can no longer generate enough pressure to circulate the blood to all organs or when the regularity of the heartbeat is so disrupted that the volume of blood within the system can no longer be handled efficiently. In either case, direct pump failure is the cause of shock.

POOR VESSEL FUNCTION. Damage to the spinal cord, particularly at the upper cervical levels, may cause significant injury to the part of the nervous system that controls the size and muscular tone of the blood

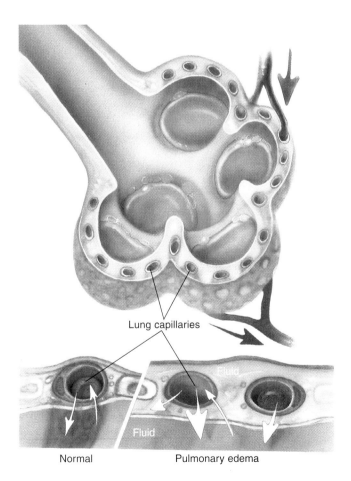

Lung capillaries

Normal   Pulmonary edema

Figure 23-3 Pulmonary edema develops as a result of fluid buildup within the pulmonary tissue. The edema causes swelling and leads to impaired ventilation.

vessels. <u>**Neurogenic shock**</u> is usually the result. Although not as common, there are medical causes as well. These include brain conditions, tumors, pressure on the spinal cord, or spina bifida. In this condition, the muscles in the walls of the blood vessels are cut off from the nerve impulses that cause them to contract. Therefore, all the vessels below the level of the spinal injury dilate widely, increasing the size and capacity of the vascular system (▼ **Figure 23-4**), and causing blood to pool. The available 6 L of blood in the body can no longer fill the enlarged vascular system. Even though no blood or fluid has been lost, perfusion of organs and tissues becomes inadequate, and shock occurs. In this condition, a radical change in the size of the vascular system has caused shock. A characteristic sign of this type of shock is the absence of sweating below the level of injury.

With this type of injury, many other functions that are under the control of the same part of the nervous system are also lost. The most important of them, in an acute injury setting, is the ability to control body temperature. Body temperature in the patient with neurogenic shock can rapidly fall to match that of the environment. In many situations, significant hypothermia occurs, severely complicating the situation. <u>**Hypothermia**</u> is a condition in which the internal body temperature falls below 95°F (35°C), usually after prolonged exposure to cool or freezing temperatures.

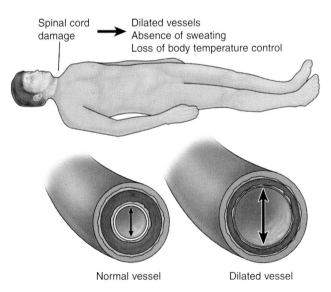

Figure 23-4 Damage to the spinal cord can cause significant injury to the part of the nervous system that controls the size and muscle tone of blood vessels. If the muscles in the blood vessels are cut off from their impulses to contract, then the vessels dilate widely, increasing the size and capacity of the vascular system. The blood in the body can no longer fill the enlarged vessels, resulting in inadequate perfusion.

Maintenance of body temperature is always an important element of treatment for a patient in shock.

CONTENT FAILURE. Following injury, shock is often a result of fluid or blood loss. This type of shock is called <u>**hypovolemic**</u> (low-volume) <u>**shock**</u> or, when caused by blood loss, hemorrhagic shock. The loss may be due to external bleeding, which is common in patients who have suffered severe lacerations or fractures. Or it may be due to internal bleeding, which follows a variety of injuries or diseases, such as rupture of the liver or the spleen, lacerations of the great vessels within the abdomen or the chest, bleeding peptic ulcers, and tumors, among others.

Hypovolemic shock also occurs with severe thermal burns. In this case, it is intravascular plasma (the colorless part of the blood) that is lost, leaking from the circulatory system into the burned tissues that lie adjacent to the injury. Likewise, crushing injuries may result in the loss of blood and plasma from damaged vessels into injured tissues. <u>**Dehydration**</u>, the loss of water from body tissues, aggravates shock.

In these circumstances, the common factor is an insufficient volume of blood within the vascular system to provide adequate circulation to the organs of the body.

COMBINED VESSEL AND CONTENT FAILURE. In some patients who have severe bacterial infections, toxins (poisons) generated by the bacteria or by infected body tissues produce a condition called <u>**septic shock**</u>. In this condition, the toxins damage the vessel walls, causing them to become leaky and unable to contract well. Widespread dilation of vessels, in combination with plasma loss through the injured vessel walls, results in shock.

Septic shock is a complex problem. First, there is an insufficient volume of fluid in the container, because much of the blood has leaked out of the vascular system (hypovolemia). Second, the fluid that has leaked out often collects in the respiratory system, interfering with ventilation. Third, there is a larger-than-normal vascular bed to contain the smaller-than-normal volume of intravascular fluid.

Septic shock is almost always a complication of some very serious illness, injury, or surgery.

Noncardiovascular Causes of Shock

There are two causes of shock that do not result from disturbances of the cardiovascular system: respiratory insufficiency and anaphylaxis.

RESPIRATORY INSUFFICIENCY. A patient with a severe chest injury or obstruction of the airway may be unable to breathe in an adequate amount of oxygen.

An insufficient concentration of oxygen in the blood can produce shock as rapidly as vascular causes, even if the volume of blood, the volume of the vessels, and the action of the heart are all normal. Without oxygen, the organs in the body cannot survive, and their cells promptly start to deteriorate.

This is why the first two steps in resuscitation are always securing an airway and restoring respirations. Circulation of nonoxygenated blood will not benefit the patient.

ANAPHYLACTIC SHOCK. Anaphylaxis, or **anaphylactic shock**, occurs when a person reacts violently to a substance to which he or she has been sensitized. **Sensitization** means becoming sensitive to a substance that did not initially cause a reaction. Do not be misled by a patient who reports no history of allergic reaction to a substance on first or second exposure. Each subsequent exposure after sensitization tends to produce a more severe reaction.

Instances that cause severe allergic reactions commonly fall into the following four categories:

- Injections (tetanus antitoxin, penicillin)
- Stings (honeybee, wasp, yellow jacket, hornet)
- Ingestion (shellfish, oral penicillin)
- Inhalation (dusts, pollens)

Anaphylactic reactions can develop in minutes or even seconds after contact with the substance to which the patient is allergic. The signs of such allergic reactions are very distinct and not seen with other forms of shock. ▶ **Table 23-1** shows the signs of anaphylactic shock in the order in which they typically occur.

In anaphylactic shock, there is no loss of blood, no vascular damage, and only a slight possibility of direct cardiac muscular injury. Instead, there is widespread vascular dilation. The combination of poor oxygenation and poor perfusion in anaphylactic shock may easily prove fatal.

PSYCHOGENIC SHOCK. A patient in **psychogenic shock** has had a sudden reaction of the nervous system that produces a temporary, generalized vascular dilation, resulting in fainting or **syncope**. Blood pools in the dilated vessels, reducing the blood supply to the brain; as a result, the brain ceases to function normally, and the patient faints. Causes of syncope range from fear, bad news, or unpleasant sights (often the sight of blood) to life-threatening cardiac arrhythmias or **aneurysms**.

TABLE 23-1 Signs of Anaphylactic Shock

Skin

- Flushing, itching, or burning, especially over the face and upper chest
- Urticaria (hives), which may spread over large areas of the body
- Edema, especially of the face, tongue, and lips
- **Cyanosis** (a bluish cast to the skin resulting from poor oxygenation of circulating blood) about the lips

Circulatory System

- Dilation of peripheral blood vessels
- A drop in blood pressure
- A weak, barely palpable pulse
- Pallor
- Dizziness
- Fainting and coma

Respiratory System

- Sneezing or itching in the nasal passages
- Tightness in the chest, with a persistent dry cough
- Wheezing and **dyspnea**, or difficulty in breathing
- Secretions of fluid and mucus into the bronchial passages, alveoli, and lung tissue, causing coughing
- Constriction of the bronchi; difficulty drawing air into the lungs
- Forced expiration, requiring exertion and accompanied by wheezing
- Cessation of breathing

The Progression of Shock

Although you cannot see shock, you can see its signs and symptoms (▶ **Table 23-2**). The early stage of shock, while the body can still compensate for blood loss, is called **compensated shock**. The late stage, when blood pressure is falling, is called **decompensated shock**. The last stage, when shock has progressed to a terminal stage, is called **irreversible shock**. A transfusion of any type at this point will not save the patient's life.

Remember that blood pressure may be the last measurable factor to change in shock. As we have seen, the body has several automatic mechanisms to compensate for initial blood loss and to help maintain blood pressure. Thus, by the time you detect a drop in blood pressure, shock is well developed. This is particularly true of infants and children, who can maintain their blood pressure until they have lost more than half their blood volume. By the time blood pressure drops in infants and children who are in shock, they are close to death.

You should expect shock in many emergency medical situations. For example, you would expect shock to accompany massive external or internal bleeding. You should also expect shock if a patient has any one of the following conditions:

- Multiple severe fractures
- Abdominal or chest injury
- Spinal injury
- A severe infection
- A major heart attack
- Anaphylaxis

Emergency Medical Care

You must begin immediate treatment for shock as soon as you realize that the condition may exist. Follow the steps in (▶ **Skill Drill 23-1**):

1. As with any type of patient care, you should **begin by following BSI precautions,** making sure the patient has an open airway, and checking breathing and pulse. In general, keep the patient in a supine position. Patients who have had a severe heart attack or who have lung disease may find it easier to breathe in a sitting or semi-sitting position **(Step 1)**.

TABLE 23-2 Progression of Shock

Compensated Shock

Agitation

Anxiety

Restlessness

Feeling of impending doom

Altered mental status

Weak, rapid (thready), or absent pulse

Clammy (pale, cool, moist) skin

Pallor, with cyanosis about the lips

Shallow, rapid breathing

Air hunger (shortness of breath), especially if there is a chest injury

Nausea or vomiting

Capillary refill in infants and children of longer than 2 seconds

Marked thirst

Decompensated Shock

Falling blood pressure (systolic blood pressure of 90 mm Hg or lower in an adult)

Labored or irregular breathing

Ashen, mottled, or cyanotic skin

Thready or absent peripheral pulses

Dull eyes, dilated pupils

Poor urinary output

SkillDrill 23-1 Treating Shock

Keep the patient supine, open the airway, and check breathing and pulse.

Control obvious external bleeding.

Splint any broken bones or joint injuries.

Give high-flow oxygen if you have not already done so, and place blankets under and over the patient.

If no fractures are suspected, elevate the legs 6" to 12".

2. **Next, control all obvious external bleeding.** Place dry, sterile dressings over the bleeding sites, and secure with bandages **(Step 2)**.

3. **Splint any bone or joint injuries.** This minimizes pain, bleeding, and discomfort, all of which can aggravate shock. It also prevents the broken bone ends from further damaging adjacent soft tissue. In general, splinting also makes it easier to move the patient. Handle the patient gently and no more than is necessary **(Step 3)**.

There is some controversy surrounding the use of the pneumatic antishock garment (PASG). Used improperly, the device can increase bleeding from chest injuries, interfere with adequate air exchange, and promote cardiovascular collapse. Used properly, it can effectively control bleeding from fractures and massive soft-tissue wounds. In general, the PASG should not be used without the approval of medical control or established local protocols.

4. **Remember that inadequate ventilation** may be the primary cause of shock or a major factor in its development. Always provide oxygen, assist with ventilations as needed, and continue to monitor the patient's breathing. To prevent the loss of body heat, place blankets under and over the patient. Be careful not to overload the patient with covers or attempt to warm the body too much. It is better for the patient to be slightly cool rather than too hot. Do not use any external heat sources, such as hot water bottles or heating pads. They may harm a patient in shock by causing vasodilation and decreasing blood pressure even more **(Step 4)**.

5. **If there are no broken bones,** elevate the lower extremities 6″ to 12″. This not only stops venous bleeding in an extremity, it allows blood in the legs to return to the heart more rapidly **(Step 5)**.

Do not give the patient anything by mouth, no matter how urgently you are asked. To relieve the intense thirst that often accompanies shock, give the patient a moistened piece of gauze to chew or suck. Never give a patient in shock an alcoholic drink or other depressant. A stimulant, such as coffee, also has little value in treating shock.

> Early resuscitation and treatment of a patient in shock or with severe injuries is critically important during the Golden Hour immediately after injury.

Accurately record the patient's vital signs approximately every 5 minutes throughout treatment and transport. It is essential to transport the trauma patient to the hospital as rapidly as possible for definitive treatment. The Golden Hour refers to the first 60 minutes after injury, which is felt to be a critically important period for the early resuscitation and treatment of severely injured trauma patients. This concept underscores the importance of rapid evaluation, stabilization, and transport. The goal of EMS is to limit on-scene time (time on-scene until transport to hospital is started) to ten minutes or less. Remember to speak calmly and reassuringly to a conscious patient throughout assessment, care, and transport.

▶ **Table 23-3** lists the general supportive measures for the major types of shock. Not every measure is used for every type of shock.

Treating Cardiogenic Shock

The patient who is in shock as a result of a heart attack does not require a transfusion of blood, IV fluids, elevation of the legs, or PASG. There is already a greater volume of blood in circulation than the heart can handle. The damaged heart muscle simply cannot generate the necessary power to pump blood throughout the circulatory system.

Keep in mind that chronic lung disease will aggravate cardiogenic shock. If the patient has COPD, as well as heart disease, oxygenation of the blood passing through the lungs is impaired. Because fluid is collecting in the lungs, this patient is often able to breathe better in a sitting or semi-sitting position and may tell you so.

Usually, patients with cardiogenic shock do not have any injury, but they may be having chest pain. Such a patient may have taken nitroglycerin before your arrival and may want to take more. Before helping the patient self-administer nitroglycerin, be sure to consult with medical control for instructions. You will also need to perform an accurate assessment and to ensure that the

TABLE 23-3 Types of Shock

Types of Shock	Examples of Potential Causes	Signs/Symptoms
Anaphylactic	Allergic reaction	Can develop within seconds Mild itching/rash Burning skin Vascular dilation Generalized edema Profound coma Rapid death
Cardiogenic	Inadequate heart function Disease of muscle tissue Impaired electrical system Disease or injury	Chest pains Irregular pulse Weak pulse Low blood pressure Cyanosis (lips, under nails) Anxiety
Hypovolemic	Loss of blood or fluid	Rapid, weak pulse Low blood pressure Change in mental status Cyanosis (lips, under nails) Cool, clammy skin Increased respiratory rate
Metabolic	Excessive loss of fluid and electrolytes due to vomiting, urination, or diarrhea	Rapid, weak pulse Low blood pressure Change in mental status Cyanosis (lips, under nails) Cool, clammy skin Increased respiratory rate
Neurogenic	Damaged cervical spine, which causes widespread blood vessel dilation	Bradycardia (slow pulse) Low blood pressure Signs of neck injury
Psychogenic (fainting)	Temporary, generalized vascular dilation Anxiety, bad news, sight of injury/blood, prospect of medical treatment, severe pain, illness, tiredness	Rapid pulse Normal or low blood pressure
Septic	Severe bacterial infection	Warm skin Tachycardia Low blood pressure

Treatment

Manage the airway
Assist ventilations
Administer high-flow oxygen
Determine cause
Assist with administration of epinephrine
Transport promptly

Position comfortably
Administer oxygen
Assist ventilations
Transport promptly

Secure airway
Assist ventilations
Administer high-flow oxygen
Control external bleeding
Elevate legs
Keep warm
Transport promptly

Secure airway
Assist ventilations
Administer high-flow oxygen
Determine illness
Transport promptly

Secure airway
Spinal immobilization
Assist ventilations
Administer high-flow oxygen
Transport promptly

Determine duration of unconsciousness
Record initial vital signs and mental status
Suspect head injury if patient is confused or
    slow to regain consciousness
Transport promptly

Transport promptly
Administer oxygen en route
Provide full ventilatory support
Elevate legs
Keep patient warm

patient's blood pressure meets the criteria for this medication. If the blood pressure is too low, nitroglycerin may increase the problem. Remember that patients in cardiogenic shock usually have a low blood pressure. Other signs include a weak, irregular pulse, cyanosis about the lips and underneath the fingernails, anxiety, and nausea.

Treatment of cardiogenic shock should begin by placing the patient in the position in which breathing is easiest as you give high-flow oxygen. Be ready to assist ventilations as necessary, and have suction nearby in case the patient vomits. Provide prompt transport to the emergency department. Remember also to approach a patient who has had a suspected heart attack with calm reassurance.

Treating Neurogenic Shock

Shock that accompanies spinal cord injury is best treated by a combination of all the known supportive measures. The patient who has sustained this kind of injury usually will require hospitalization for a long time. Emergency treatment must be directed at obtaining and maintaining a proper airway, providing spinal immobilization, assisting inadequate breathing as needed, conserving body heat, and providing the most effective circulation possible.

This patient usually is not losing blood. However, the capacity of his or her blood vessels has become significantly larger than the volume of blood they contain. Supplemental oxygen will boost the concentration of oxygen in the blood. If respirations are weak or inadequate, provide assisted ventilations. Keep the patient as warm as possible with blankets, because the injury may have disabled the body's normal temperature controls. Transport promptly.

Treating Hypovolemic Shock

The emergency treatment of hypovolemic or hemorrhagic shock includes the control of all obvious external bleeding. To prevent continued bleeding, must apply sufficient pressure to control obvious external bleeding, splint any bone and joint injuries, and ensure that you use great care to handle the patient gently. If there are no fractured extremities, you should raise the legs 6″ to 12″, keeping the torso in a horizontal position. This will increase blood flow to the heart from the lower body and keep unwanted pressure off the diaphragm. This method combats shock by using the patient's own blood to its best advantage.

> Although you cannot control internal bleeding in the field, you must recognize its existence and provide aggressive general support.

Although you cannot control internal bleeding in the field, you must recognize its existence and provide aggressive general support. Secure and maintain an airway, and provide respiratory support, including supplemental oxygen and, if needed, assisted ventilations. Start the oxygen as soon as you suspect shock, and continue it during transport; with too little circulating blood, additional oxygen may be lifesaving. Be sure the patient does not aspirate blood or vomitus. Most important, you must transport the patient as rapidly as possible to the emergency department.

Treating Septic Shock

The proper treatment of septic shock requires complex hospital management. If you suspect that a patient has septic shock, you must transport him or her as promptly as possible. Use high-flow oxygen during transport. Ventilatory support may be necessary to maintain adequate tidal volume in this patient. Use blankets to conserve body heat.

Treating Respiratory Insufficiency

In treating the patient who is in shock as a result of inadequate respiration, you must immediately secure and maintain the airway. Clear the mouth and throat of anything obstructing the air passages, including mucus, vomitus, and foreign material. If necessary, provide ventilations with a BVM. Give supplemental oxygen, and transport the patient promptly.

Treating Anaphylactic Shock

The only really effective treatment for a severe, acute allergic reaction is to administer epinephrine by way of subcutaneous, intramuscular, or intravenous injection. For more information on the emergency care for allergic reactions, see Chapter 16. A patient who is aware of having a specific sensitivity may carry a bee sting kit containing epinephrine (▼ **Figure 23-5**). If he or she is unable to inject the medication, you may have to do so if you are allowed by local protocol. If the patient's signs and symptoms recur or deteriorate, you should repeat the injection after consulting with medical control.

Promptly transport the patient to the emergency department while providing all possible support, prima-

Figure 23-5 Patients who are allergic to bee stings often carry commercial bee sting kits, such as an IM injector or autoinjector, containing epinephrine.

rily supplemental oxygen and ventilatory assistance. You should also try to find out what agent caused the reaction (eg, a drug, an insect bite or sting, a food item) and how it was received (eg, by mouth, by inhalation, or by injection). The severity of allergic reactions can vary greatly, with symptoms ranging from mild itching to profound coma and rapid death. Keep in mind that a mild reaction may worsen suddenly or over time. Consider requesting advanced life support backup, if available.

Treating Psychogenic Shock

In an uncomplicated case of fainting, once the patient collapses and becomes supine, circulation to the brain is usually restored, and with it a normal state of functioning. If the attack has caused the patient to fall, you must check for injuries, especially in older patients. However, you should also assess the patient thoroughly for any other abnormality. If, after regaining consciousness, the patient is unable to walk without weakness, dizziness, or pain, you should suspect another problem, such as head injury. You should transport this patient promptly.

Be sure to record your initial observations of vital signs and level of consciousness. In addition, try to learn from bystanders whether the patient complained of anything before fainting and how long he or she had been unconscious.

Prep Kit

Ready for Review

Shock (hypoperfusion) is the collapse and failure of the cardiovascular system, in which blood circulation slows and eventually ceases. Perfusion requires a cardiovascular system with all three parts (the pump, container, and contents) working, but it also requires a functioning respiratory system. The signs and symptoms of shock are caused by the actions of the autonomic nervous system and of hormones responding to the need for additional perfusion.

The cardiovascular causes of shock include poor pump function (cardiogenic shock), blood or fluid loss from blood vessels (hypovolemic shock), and/or poor vessel function (neurogenic shock), as when all vessels dilate at once. Septic shock is a combination of vessel and content failure; it is the result of a serious infection. The noncardiovascular causes of shock are respiratory insufficiency and anaphylaxis.

Signs of compensated shock include agitation or anxiety, a weak, rapid pulse, clammy skin, air hunger, nausea or vomiting, slow capillary refill in children and infants, and marked thirst. Signs of decompensated shock include labored or irregular breathing, ashen or cyanotic skin, thready or absent peripheral pulses, dilated pupils, poor urinary output, and, finally, falling blood pressure. By the time you detect a drop in blood pressure, shock is well developed. Expect shock in cases of massive internal or external bleeding, multiple severe fractures, abdominal or chest injury, spinal injury, severe infection, a major heart attack, and anaphylaxis.

Treat patients with shock by (1) opening and maintaining the airway; (2) providing oxygen and, if necessary, assisting ventilations; (3) controlling all obvious external bleeding; (4) conserving body heat with blankets; and (5) transporting promptly. Use high-flow oxygen to all patients in shock.

Vital Vocabulary

anaphylactic shock Severe shock caused by allergic reactions.

anaphylaxis An unusual or exaggerated allergic reaction to foreign protein or other substances.

aneurysms A swelling or enlargement of a part of an artery, resulting from weakening of the arterial wall.

autonomic nervous system The part of the nervous system that regulates involuntary functions, such as digestion and sweating.

cardiogenic shock Shock caused by inadequate function of the heart, or pump failure.

compensated shock The early stage of shock, in which the body can still compensate for blood loss.

cyanosis Bluish color of the skin resulting from poor oxygenation of the circulating blood.

decompensated shock The late stage of shock, when blood pressure is falling.

dehydration Loss of water from the tissues of the body.

dyspnea Difficulty in breathing.

edema The presence of abnormally large amounts of fluid between cells in body tissues, causing swelling of the affected area.

hypothermia A condition in which the internal body temperature falls below 95°F (35°C), usually as a result of prolonged exposure to cool or freezing temperatures.

hypovolemic shock Shock caused by fluid or blood loss.

irreversible shock The final stage of shock, resulting in death.

neurogenic shock Circulatory failure caused by paralysis of the nerves that control the size of the blood vessels, leading to widespread dilation; seen in spinal cord injuries.

perfusion Circulation of blood within an organ or tissue in adequate amounts to meet the cells' current needs.

psychogenic shock Shock caused by a sudden, temporary reduction in blood supply to the brain that causes fainting (syncope).

sensitization Developing a sensitivity to a substance that initially caused no allergic reaction.

septic shock Shock caused by severe bacterial infection.

shock A condition in which the circulatory system fails to provide sufficient circulation to enable every body part to perform its function; also called hypoperfusion.

sphincters Circular muscles that encircle and, by contracting, constrict a duct, tube, or opening.

syncope Fainting.

Assessment in Action

You and your partner are dispatched to a car crash. On arrival, you see a small sports car crushed against a concrete bridge support. As the rescue team is working on gaining access, you look in to see the unbelted patient, who has gone down and under the steering wheel.

The patient has a laceration to his forehead, just barely responds to voice, and appears pale. The door is finally torn loose, and as you get your first close look at the patient, you see two obviously fractured legs with extensive soft-tissue injuries to both extremities. Your patient has no radial pulse but does have a weak carotid pulse of 138 beats/min, with shallow respirations of 28 breaths/min. His skin is cool and moist to the touch, and he is moving both arms.

1. Which of the following action plans would be most appropriate for this patient?
   A. Rapidly extricate the patient, splint the fractured legs, dress the wounds, immobilize the patient to a long backboard, and then transport.
   B. Completely immobilize the patient, extricate, initiate transport, and then dress the wounds and splint the fractured legs en route to the hospital.
   C. Rapidly extricate and then completely immobilize the patient to a long backboard, initiate transport, and then dress the wounds and splint the fractures en route to the hospital.
   D. Splint the fractures and dress the wounds while the patient is still in the car, immobilize the patient, and then extricate and initiate transport to the hospital.

2. Once the extrication is complete and the patient is accessible, scene time before initiating transport should be limited to no more than how many minutes?
   A. 10   B. 20
   C. 30   D. 40

3. On the basis of this patient's signs and symptoms, you should prepare to care for:
   A. a diabetic emergency.   B. hypovolemic shock.
   C. neurogenic shock.   D. hyperventilation syndrome.

4. On the basis of the patient's vital signs, you would expect capillary refill to be:
   A. almost instantaneous.   B. less than 2 seconds.
   C. greater than 2 seconds.   D. virtually nonexistent.

5. The patient's respirations increase to about 40/min and they become more shallow. To ensure adequate ventilation, you should:
   A. apply a nasal cannula with oxygen at 4 to 6 L/min.
   B. insert a nasopharyngeal airway.
   C. administer a breathing treatment immediately.
   D. assist ventilations with a BVM device at 15 L/min.

6. After splinting the fractures, your partner prepares to elevate this patient's legs. Your best course of action is to:
   A. elevate 6" to 12" with towels/blankets.
   B. tell him to keep the legs supine.
   C. elevate the foot of the backboard 6" to 12".
   D. elevate the head of the stretcher 6" to 12".

7. The patient complains of extreme thirst. To alleviate his complaint, your best course of action would be to provide:
   A. water.   B. saline.
   C. moistened gauze.   D. juice.

Challenging Questions

8. Why are patients who have suffered neurogenic shock prone to hypothermia?

9. Victims of cardiogenic shock and hypovolemic shock look alike. How can you tell the difference?

10. What are some differences between anaphylaxis and other types of shock?

Points to Ponder

You have been feeling very tired for almost a month and decide you should have a "check-up." You do not have a physician and upon advice from your agency you go to the doctor that they use for "workers' comp" claims. You return to the clinic a week later for a follow-up on the tests that were run. The physician informs you that you have a hepatitis C infection. The physician asks you many questions about your work-related body substance exposures, explaining that treatment can be very expensive and if they can document a workplace exposure, workers compensation will cover it. You ask the physician not to do anything for a week while you think about things. During the week you realize that in your agency, this will end your patient care career and will significantly affect your ultimate goal of becoming a surgeon.

Who would you report this to? Would you file a workers' compensation claim? How much risk are you putting your patients at? Is this a reasonable risk? How else may you have been infected?

Issues BSI Precautions, Long-Term Effects of Infectious Disease, Reporting Requirements, Reasonable Risk, Responsibility to Patients and Employers.

Online Outlook

The signs and symptoms of shock are presented in this chapter. Test your ability to recognize shock by completing Exercise 23 at <u>www.emtb.com.</u>

www.emtb.com

Soft-Tissue Injuries

Objectives

Cognitive

1. State the major functions of the skin (p 565).

2. List the layers of the skin (p 564).

3. Establish the relationship between body substance isolation (BSI) and soft-tissue injuries (p 565).

4. List the types of closed soft-tissue injuries (p 566).

5. Describe the emergency medical care of the patient with a closed soft-tissue injury (p 567).

6. State the types of open soft-tissue injuries (p 567).

7. Describe the emergency medical care of the patient with an open soft-tissue injury (p 570).

8. Discuss the emergency medical care considerations for a patient with a penetrating chest injury (p 571).

9. State the emergency medical care considerations for a patient with an open wound to the abdomen (p 572).

10. Differentiate the care of an open wound to the chest from an open wound to the abdomen (p 571).

11. List the classification of burns (p 575).

12. Define superficial burn (p 576).

13. List the characteristics of a superficial burn (p 576).

14. Define partial-thickness burn (p 576).

15. List the characteristics of a partial-thickness burn (p 576).

16. Define full-thickness burn (p 576).

17. List the characteristics of a full-thickness burn (p 576).

18. Describe the emergency medical care of the patient with a superficial burn (p 577).

19. Describe the emergency medical care of the patient with a partial-thickness burn (p 577).

20. Describe the emergency medical care of the patient with a full-thickness burn (p 577).

21. List the functions of dressing and bandaging (p 582).

22. Describe the purpose of a bandage (p 582).

23. Describe the steps in applying a pressure bandage (p 570).

24. Establish the relationship between airway management and the patient with chest injury, burns, and blunt and penetrating injuries (p 571).

25. Describe the effects of improperly applied dressings, splints, and tourniquets (p 583).

26. Describe the emergency medical care of a patient with an impaled object (p 573).

27. Describe the emergency medical care of a patient with an amputation (p 574).*

28. Describe the emergency care for a chemical burn (p 578).

29. Describe the emergency care for an electrical burn (p 580).

* These are noncurriculum objectives.

Affective

None

Psychomotor

30. Demonstrate the steps in the emergency medical care of closed soft-tissue injuries (p 567).

31. Demonstrate the steps in the emergency medical care of open soft-tissue injuries (p 570).

32. Demonstrate the steps in the emergency medical care of a patient with an open chest wound (p 571).

33. Demonstrate the steps in the emergency medical care of a patient with open abdominal wounds (p 572).

34. Demonstrate the steps in the emergency medical care of a patient with an impaled object (p 573).

35. Demonstrate the steps in the emergency medical care of a patient with an amputation (p 574).

36. Demonstrate the steps in the emergency medical care of an amputated part (p 574).

37. Demonstrate the steps in the emergency medical care of a patient with superficial burns (p 577).

38. Demonstrate the steps in the emergency medical care of a patient with partial-thickness burns (p 577).

39. Demonstrate the steps in the emergency medical care of a patient with full-thickness burns (p 577).

40. Demonstrate the steps in the emergency medical care of a patient with a chemical burn (p 578).

41. Demonstrate completing a prehospital care report for patients with soft-tissue injuries (p 299).

"Medic One, Highway Patrol is requesting an ambulance be sent to the Southbound I-5 exit at 72nd Street for a 'motorcyclist down.'" Motorcycle trauma often produces devastating soft-tissue injuries.

This chapter will help prepare you to properly care for these injuries as well as help you answer the following questions:

1. What is the difference between a dressing and a bandage?

2. Is there a difference in the care for chemical burns and electrical burns? Please describe it.

Soft-Tissue Injuries

The skin is our first line of defense against external forces. And although it is relatively tough, skin is still quite susceptible to injury. Injuries to soft tissues range from simple bruises and abrasions to serious lacerations and amputations. Soft-tissue injury may result in loss of soft tissue, exposing deep structures such as blood vessels, nerves, and bones. In all instances, you must control bleeding, prevent further contamination, and protect the wound from further damage. Therefore, you must know how to apply dressings and bandages to various parts of the body.

The Anatomy and Function of the Skin

The skin is the largest organ in the body. It varies in thickness, depending on age and its location. The skin of the very young and very old is thinner than the skin of a young adult. The skin covering your scalp, your back, and the soles of your feet is quite thick, while the skin of your eyelids, lips, and ears is very thin. Thin skin is more easily damaged than thick skin.

Anatomy of the Skin

The skin has two principal layers: the **epidermis** and the **dermis** (► Figure 24-1). The epidermis is the tough, external layer that forms a watertight covering for the body. The epidermis is itself composed of several layers. The cells on the surface layer of the epidermis are constantly worn away. They are replaced by cells that are pushed to the surface when new cells form in the germinal layer at the base of the epidermis. Deeper cells in the germinal layer contain pigment granules. Along with blood vessels in the dermis, these granules produce skin color.

The dermis is the inner layer of the skin. It lies below the germinal cells of the epidermis. The dermis

EMT-B Tips

Although it may be tempting to think of skin injuries as unimportant, the skin plays several crucial protective and regulatory roles. When dealing with skin injuries, remember the importance of this organ in protecting against infection and maintaining internal temperature and fluid balance. The skin can also be very important emotionally to the patient; concerns about how bruising and scarring will look later may require your attention and communication skills during a response.

contains the structures that give the skin its characteristic appearance: hair follicles, sweat glands, and sebaceous glands. The sweat glands act to cool the body. They discharge sweat onto the surface of the skin through small pores, or ducts, that pass through the epidermis. Sebaceous glands produce sebum, the oily material that waterproofs the skin and keeps it supple. Sebum travels to the skin's surface along the shaft of adjacent hair follicles. Hair follicles are small organs that produce hair. There is one follicle for each hair, each connected with a sebaceous gland and a tiny muscle. This muscle pulls the hair erect whenever you are cold or frightened.

Blood vessels in the dermis provide the skin with nutrients and oxygen. Small branches reach up to the germinal cells, but no blood vessels penetrate farther into the epidermis. There are also specialized nerve endings within the dermis.

The skin covers all external surfaces of the body. The various openings in our body, including the mouth, nose, anus, and vagina, are not covered by skin. Instead, these openings are lined with **mucous membranes**. These membranes are similar to skin in that they, too, provide a protective barrier against bacterial invasion. But mucous membranes differ from skin in that they secrete a watery substance that lubricates the openings. Therefore, mucous membranes are moist, while skin is dry.

Functions of the Skin

The skin serves many functions. It protects the body by keeping bacteria out and water in. The nerves in the skin report to the brain on the environment and on many sensations.

The skin is also the body's major organ for regulating temperature. In a cold environment, the blood vessels in the skin constrict, diverting blood away from the skin and decreasing the amount of heat that is radiated from the body's surface. In hot environments, the vessels in the skin dilate. The skin becomes flushed or red, and heat radiates from the body's surface. Also, sweat glands secrete sweat. As the sweat evaporates from the skin's surface, your body temperature drops, and you begin to cool down.

Any break in the skin allows bacteria to enter and raises the possibilities of infection, fluid loss, and loss of temperature control. Any one of these problems can cause serious illness and even death.

> The skin is our first line of defense against external forces. And although it is relatively tough, skin is still quite susceptible to injury.

Types of Soft-Tissue Injuries

Soft tissues are often injured because they are exposed to the environment. There are three types of soft-tissue injuries:

- **Closed injuries**, in which soft-tissue damage occurs beneath the skin or mucous membrane but the surface remains intact.

- **Open injuries**, in which there is a break in the surface of the skin or the mucous membrane, exposing deeper tissue to potential contamination.

- **Burns**, in which the soft tissue receives more energy than it can absorb without injury. The source of this energy can be thermal heat, frictional heat, toxic chemicals, electricity, or nuclear radiation.

EPIDERMIS

DERMIS

SUBCUTANEOUS TISSUE

Hair

Pore

Germinal layer of epidermis

Sebaceous gland

Nerve (sensory)

Sweat gland

Hair follicle

Blood vessel

Subcutaneous fat

Fascia

Muscle

Figure 24-1 The skin is composed of a tough external layer called the epidermis and a vascular inner layer called the dermis.

Closed Injuries

Closed soft-tissue injuries are characterized by a history of blunt trauma, pain at the site of injury, swelling beneath the skin, and discoloration. Such injuries can vary from mild to quite severe.

A <u>contusion</u>, or bruise, results from blunt force striking the body. The epidermis remains intact, but cells within the dermis are damaged, and small blood vessels are usually torn. The depth of the injury varies, depending on the amount of energy absorbed. As fluid and blood leak into the damaged area, the patient may have swelling and pain. The buildup of blood produces a characteristic blue or black discoloration called <u>ecchymosis</u> (▼ Figure 24-2).

A <u>hematoma</u> is a pool of blood that has collected within damaged tissue or in a body cavity (▼ Figure 24-3). It occurs whenever a large blood vessel is damaged and bleeds rapidly. It is usually associated with extensive tissue damage. A hematoma can result from a soft-tissue injury, a fracture, or any injury to a large blood vessel. In severe cases, the hematoma may contain more than a liter of blood.

A crushing injury occurs when a great amount of force is applied to the body for a long period of time (▼ Figure 24-4). The extent of the damage depends on just how long that period is. In addition to causing some direct soft-tissue damage, continued compression of the soft tissues will cut off their circulation, producing further tissue destruction. For example, if a patient's legs are trapped under a collapsed pile of rocks, damage to the leg tissues will continue until the rocks are removed.

Another form of compression can result from the swelling that occurs whenever tissues are injured. The cells that are injured leak watery fluid into the spaces between the cells. If swelling is excessive or occurs in a confined space such as the skull, the tissue pressure will increase to dangerous levels. The pressure of the fluid may become great enough to compress the tissue and cause further damage. This is especially true if the blood vessels become compressed, cutting off blood flow to the tissue. This condition is called <u>compartment syndrome</u>. Excessive swelling often follows injury of the brain, the spinal cord, and the extremities.

Figure 24-2 Contusions, more commonly known as bruises, occur as a result of a blunt force striking the body. The buildup of blood produces a characteristic blue or black discoloration (ecchymosis).

Figure 24-3 A hematoma develops whenever a large blood vessel is damaged and bleeds rapidly.

Figure 24-4 The damage associated with a crush or compression injury varies depending on the direct damage to the soft tissues and on how long the tissue was cut off from circulation.

Severe closed injuries can also damage internal organs. The greater the amount of energy absorbed from the blunt force, the greater is the risk of injury to deeper structures. Therefore, you must assess all patients with closed injuries for more serious hidden injuries. Remain alert for signs of shock or internal bleeding, and begin treatment of these conditions if necessary.

Emergency Medical Care

Small contusions require no special emergency medical care. More extensive closed injuries may involve significant swelling and bleeding beneath the skin, which could lead to hypovolemic shock. Before treating a closed injury, make sure to follow BSI precautions. Wear gloves as you work with the patient.

Soft-tissue injuries may look rather dramatic. However, you must still focus on airway and breathing first. Always provide oxygen and maintain the airway in patients who need it. If the patient has difficulty breathing, you may have to assist ventilations.

Treat a closed soft-tissue injury by applying the acronym ICES:

- **Ice** (or a cold pack) slows bleeding by causing blood vessels to constrict and also reduces pain.

- **Compression** over the injury site slows bleeding by compressing the blood vessels.

- **Elevation** of the injured part just above the level of the patient's heart decreases swelling.

- **Splinting** decreases bleeding and also reduces pain by immobilizing a soft-tissue injury or an injured extremity.

In addition to using these measures to control bleeding and swelling, you should also be alert for signs of developing shock, including increased heart rate, increased respiratory rate, cool or clammy skin, and decreased blood pressure. Any or all of these signs may indicate internal bleeding, resulting from injuries to internal organs. If the patient appears to be in shock, you should elevate his or her legs, give supplemental oxygen, and provide prompt transport to the hospital.

Open Injuries

Open injuries differ from closed injuries in that the protective layer of skin is damaged. This can produce more extensive bleeding. More important, however, a break in the protective skin layer or mucous membrane means that the wound is contaminated and may become infected. **Contamination** means that infective organisms or foreign bodies, such as dirt, gravel, or

metal, are present. You must address these two problems in your treatment of open soft-tissue wounds. There are four types of open soft-tissue wounds that you must be prepared to manage: abrasions, lacerations, avulsions, and penetrating wounds.

An **abrasion** is a wound of the superficial layer of the skin, caused by friction when a body part rubs or scrapes across a rough or hard surface. An abrasion usually does not penetrate completely through the dermis, but blood may ooze from the injured capillaries in the dermis. Known by a variety of names, including road rash, road burn, strawberry, and mat burn, abrasions can be extremely painful (▼ **Figure 24-5**).

Figure 24-5 Abrasions usually do not penetrate completely through the dermis, but blood may ooze from the capillaries. These wounds are typically superficial and result from rubbing or scraping across a hard surface.

A <u>laceration</u> is a smooth or jagged cut caused by a sharp object or a blunt force that tears the tissue. The depth of the injury can vary, extending through the skin and subcutaneous tissue even into the underlying muscles and adjacent nerves and blood vessels (▼ **Figure 24-6**). A laceration may appear linear (regular) or stellate (irregular) and may occur along with other types of soft-tissue injury. Lacerations that involve cut arteries may result in severe bleeding.

An <u>avulsion</u> is an injury that separates various layers of soft tissue (usually between the subcutaneous layer and fascia) so that they are either completely unattached or hanging as a flap (▼ **Figure 24-7**). Usually, there is significant bleeding. If the avulsed tissue is hanging from a small piece of skin, the circulation through the flap may be at risk. If you can, replace the avulsed flap in its original position. If an avulsion is complete, you should wrap the separated tissue in sterile gauze and bring it with you to the emergency department.

We usually think of amputations as involving the upper and lower extremities. But other body parts, such as the scalp, ear, nose, penis, or lips, may also be totally avulsed, or amputated. You can easily control the bleeding from some amputations, such as the fingers, with pressure dressings. But if an avulsion involves a large area of muscle mass, such as a thigh, there may be massive bleeding. In this situation, you need to treat the patient for hypovolemic shock. The use of pressure points may also be necessary to control bleeding not controlled with a pressure dressing (see Skill Drill 22-1 in Chapter 22).

Figure 24-6 Lacerations vary in depth and can extend through the skin and subcutaneous tissue to the underlying muscles, nerves, and blood vessels. These wounds can be smooth or jagged as a result of a cut by a sharp object or a blunt force that tears the tissue.

Figure 24-7 Avulsions are injuries characterized by either complete separation of tissue or tissue hanging as a flap. Significant bleeding is common.

A **penetrating wound** is an injury resulting from a sharp, pointed object, such as a knife, ice pick, splinter, or bullet. Such objects leave relatively small entrance wounds, so there may be little external bleeding . However, these objects can damage structures deep within the body. If the wound is in the chest or abdomen, the injury can cause rapid, fatal bleeding. Assessing the amount of damage a puncture wound has created is very difficult.

Stabbings and shootings often result in multiple penetrating injuries. You must assess these patients carefully to identify all wounds. Since a penetrating object can pass completely through the body, always look for both entrance and exit wounds, especially with gunshot wounds. An entrance wound is usually smaller than an exit wound. A gun shot at close range will leave an

entrance wound with powder burns around the edges **▼ Figure 24-9**. Because of its larger size, an exit wound may bleed excessively.

Gunshot wounds have some unique characteristics that require special care. The amount of damage from a gunshot wound is directly related to the speed of the bullet. Thus, it is important to find out the type of gun that was used in the shooting. Sometimes, the patient or bystanders can tell you how many rounds were fired. This information can help hospital personnel to better care for the patient. Shotgun wounds create multiple paths of missiles (shot) and create a larger surface area and volume of tissue damage.

Most shootings end up in court at some point, and you may be called to testify. For this reason, you must carefully document the circumstances surrounding any gunshot injury, the patient's condition, and the treatment you give.

As with closed wounds caused by crushing, open wounds caused by crushing may involve damaged

Figure 24-8   Penetrating wounds often cause very little external bleeding but can damage structures deep within the body.

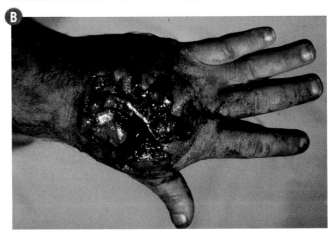

Figure 24-9   **A.** An entrance wound from a gunshot may have burns around the edges. **B.** An exit wound is larger and results in greater damage to soft tissues.

All open wounds are assumed
to be contaminated and present
a risk of infection.

internal organs or broken bones, as well as extensive soft-tissue damage (▼ **Figure 24-10**). While external bleeding may be minimal, internal bleeding may be severe, even life-threatening. The crushing force damages soft tissues, as well as vessels and nerves. This frequently results in a painful, swollen, deformed area.

Emergency Medical Care

Before you begin caring for a patient with an open wound, you should be sure to protect yourself by following BSI precautions. Wear gloves, eye protection, and, if necessary, a gown. Remember that you must be sure the patient has an open airway and administer oxygen if necessary before caring for the wound. Then assess the severity of the wound, removing any clothing that may be covering it.

Your treatment priority is ABC, including controlling the bleeding, which can be extensive and severe. Follow the steps in (▶ **Skill Drill 24-1**):

1. **Apply a dry, sterile dressing** over the entire wound. Apply pressure to the dressing with your gloved hand **(Step 1)**.

Figure 24-10 A crushing open wound is characterized by extensive tissue damage and deformity that is often accompanied by swelling and extreme pain.

2. **Maintain the pressure** and secure the dressing with a roller bandage **(Step 2)**.

3. **If bleeding continues or recurs, leave the original dressing in place.** Apply a second dressing on top of the first, and secure it with another roller bandage **(Step 3)**.

4. **Splint the extremity** to stabilize the injury even if there is no suspected fracture, to help minimize movement, further control the bleeding, and keep the dressing in place **(Step 4)**.

Assessment of the patient for further signs of injury follows the DCAP-BTLS method: inspect and palpate for Deformities, Contusions, Abrasions, Punctures/ Penetrations, Burns, Tenderness, Lacerations, Swelling, and Crepitation. It is important not to focus all of your attention on the obvious open wound and neglect a systematic evaluation of the entire patient in this manner. If you follow this systematic approach, you are unlikely to miss other significant injuries that the patient may have sustained.

All open wounds are assumed to be contaminated and present a risk of infection. By applying a sterile dressing, you are reducing the risk of further contamination. This keeps foreign material, such as hair, clothing, and dirt, out of the wound and decreases the risk of secondary infection. However, do not try to remove material from an open wound, no matter how dirty the wound is. Rubbing, brushing, or washing an open wound will only cause additional bleeding. Only hospital personnel should clean out an open wound. To prevent the wound from drying, you may apply moistened sterile dressings with sterile saline solution, if possible, then cover the wound with a dry, sterile dressing.

Often, you can better control bleeding from open soft-tissue wounds by splinting the extremity, even if there is no fracture. Splinting can also help you to keep the patient calm and quiet, as it typically reduces pain. In addition, splinting keeps sterile dressings in place, minimizes damage to an already injured extremity, and makes moving the patient easier.

Keep in mind that a patient who is bleeding significantly from an open wound is at risk for hypovolemic shock. You must be alert for this possibility and provide treatment, as needed.

Skill Drill 24-1   Controlling Bleeding from a Soft-Tissue Injury

1

Apply direct pressure with a sterile bandage.

2

Maintain pressure with a roller bandage.

3

If bleeding continues, apply a second dressing and roller bandage over the first.

4

Splint the extremity.

Chest Wounds

A penetrating wound to the chest may cause air to enter the pleural space (**pneumothorax**) or blood to collect in the chest (**hemothorax**) (▶ **Figure 24-11**). Ordinarily, the pressure inside the chest cavity is slightly lower than the pressure of the atmosphere. Inhalation further reduces this pressure, so air will move through a wound just as easily as it moves through the nose and mouth during normal breathing. The air that enters through the wound remains in the pleural space, and the lung does not expand; when the patient exhales, air passes back through the wound. Such "sucking chest wounds" reduce the ability of the lungs to provide fresh oxygen to the blood.

Initial emergency care should include giving supplemental oxygen, sealing the wound, and transporting the patient promptly to the nearest hospital. Follow the steps in (▶ **Skill Drill 24-2**):

1. **Keep the patient supine and administer oxygen.** The buildup of blood in the chest can result in difficulty breathing and shock. The patient may be placed in a position of comfort if no spinal injury is suspected **(Step 1)**.

2. **Seal the wound** with an <u>occlusive dressing</u> large enough that it is not pulled or sucked into the chest cavity. An occlusive dressing prevents air from being sucked into the chest through the wound. Several sterile materials, including aluminum foil, Vaseline gauze, or a folded universal dressing, may be used for this purpose **(Step 2)**.

3. **Depending on your local protocol, you may seal the dressing on all four sides,** or you may seal only three sides to create a flutter valve, which is a one-way valve that allows air to leave the chest cavity but not return **(Step 3)**.

Skill Drill 24-2 Sealing a Sucking Chest Wound

① Keep the patient supine and give oxygen.

② Seal the wound with an occlusive dressing.

③ Follow local protocol regarding sealing or leaving open the dressing's fourth side.

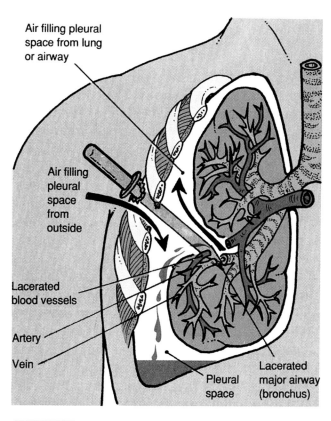

Air filling pleural space from lung or airway

Air filling pleural space from outside

Lacerated blood vessels

Artery

Vein

Pleural space

Lacerated major airway (bronchus)

Figure 24-11 Penetrating wounds can cause air to enter the chest or blood to collect in the chest.

Abdominal Wounds

An open wound in the abdominal cavity may expose internal organs. In some cases, the organs may even protrude through the wound, an injury called an **evisceration** ▶ **Figure 24-12** . Do not touch or move the exposed organs. Rather, cover the wound with sterile gauze compresses moistened with sterile saline solution and secured with a sterile dressing ▶ **Figure 24-13** . Because the open abdomen radiates body heat very effectively, and because exposed organs lose fluid rapidly, you must keep the organs moist and warm. If you do not have gauze compresses, you may use moist sterile dressings, covered and secured in place with a bandage and tape. Do not use any material that is adherent or loses its substance when wet, such as toilet paper, facial tissue, paper towels, or absorbent cotton. If the patient's legs and knees are uninjured, flex them to relieve pressure on the abdomen. Most patients with abdominal wounds require immediate transport to a trauma center, depending upon the local protocol.

Figure 24-12 An abdominal evisceration is an open wound to the abdomen in which organs protrude through the wound.

Skill Drill 24-3   Stabilizing an Impaled Object

Do not attempt to move or remove the object.

Control bleeding and stabilize the object in place using soft dressings, gauze, and/or tape.

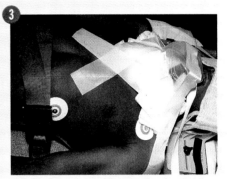
Tape a rigid item over the stabilized object to protect it from movement during transport.

Figure 24-13   **A.** Cover exposed organs with sterile gauze compresses moistened with sterile saline solution. **B.** Place a dressing over the compresses, and secure it in place by taping all four sides.

Impaled Objects

Occasionally, a patient will have an object, such as a knife, fishhook, wood splinter, or piece of glass, impaled in his or her body. To treat this, follow the steps in (▲ **Skill Drill 24-3**):

1. **Do not attempt to move or remove the object** unless it is impaled through the cheek or if the object is in the chest and interferes with CPR. In most cases, a surgeon will have to remove the object; moving it in the field may damage nerves, blood vessels, or muscles within the wound **(Step 1)**.

2. **Remove any clothing covering the injury. Control bleeding, and apply a bulky dressing** to stabilize the object. Some combination of soft dressings, gauze, and tape may be effective, depending on the location and size of the object. To prevent further injury, manually secure the object by incorporating it into the dressing **(Step 2)**.

3. **Protect the impaled object** from being bumped or moved during transport by taping a rigid item such as a plastic cup, a section of a plastic water bottle, or a supply container over the stabilized object and its bandaging **(Step 3)**.

The only exception to the rule of not removing an impaled object is an object in the cheek that obstructs breathing. In this situation, restoring the airway takes priority. If the object is very long, cut off (shorten) the exposed portion, first securing it to minimize motion

Figure 24-14 Amputated parts can often be reimplanted, so you should make every attempt to find the part and transport it to the emergency department along with the patient.

Figure 24-15 Open injuries to the neck can be very dangerous. If veins are open to the environment, they can suck in air, resulting in a potentially fatal condition called air embolism.

Figure 24-16 Cover neck wounds with an airtight dressing, and apply manual pressure. Be sure that you do not compress both carotid arteries at the same time, as this may impair circulation to the brain.

and thus internal damage and pain. Once the object is secured and the bleeding is under control, provide prompt transport.

Amputations

Surgeons today can often reimplant an amputated part ◀ **Figure 24-14** . However, correct prehospital care of the amputated part is vital to successful reattachment. With partial amputations, make sure to immobilize the part with bulky compression dressings and a splint to prevent further injury. Do not sever any partial amputations; this may make it impossible to reimplant the part.

With a complete amputation, make sure to wrap the part in a sterile dressing and place it in a plastic bag. Follow your local protocols regarding how to preserve amputated parts. In some areas, dry sterile dressings are recommended for wrapping amputated parts; in other areas, dressings moistened with sterile saline are recommended. Put the bag in a cool container filled with ice. The goal is to keep the part cool without allowing it to freeze or develop frostbite. The amputated part should be transported with the patient.

Neck Injuries

An open neck injury can be life-threatening. If the veins of the neck are open to the environment, they may suck in air ◀ **Figure 24-15** . If enough air is sucked into a blood vessel, it can actually block the flow of blood in the lungs, sending the patient into cardiac arrest. This condition is called air embolism. To control bleeding and prevent the possibility of air embolism, cover the wound with an occlusive dressing. Apply manual pressure, but do not compress both carotid vessels at the same time; if you do, this may impair circulation to the brain ◀ **Figure 24-16** . Secure a pressure dressing over the wound by wrapping roller gauze loosely around the neck and then firmly through the opposite axilla.

Burns

As an EMT-B, you will often provide care to patients who have been burned. Burns account for over 10,000 deaths a year. Burns are also among the most serious and painful of all injuries. A burn occurs when the body, or a body part, receives more energy than it can absorb without injury. Potential sources of this energy include heat, toxic chemicals, and electricity. The proper emergency care of a burn may increase a patient's chances of survival and decrease the risk or duration of a long-term disability. Although a burn may be the patient's most obvious injury, you should always perform a complete assessment to determine whether there are other serious injuries.

Burn Severity

The seriousness of a burn may influence medical control's choice of a treatment facility. Five factors will help you to determine the severity of a burn:

1. What is the depth of the burn?

2. What is the extent of the burn?

These first two factors are the most important. After gauging these, ask yourself the remaining questions:

3. Are any critical areas (face, upper airway, hands, feet, genitalia) involved?

4. Are there any preexisting medical conditions or other injuries?

5. Is the patient younger than age 5 years or older than age 55 years?

If the answer to any of these last three questions is yes, you should upgrade the burn's classification ► **Table 24-1** .

Geriatric Needs

When treating elderly patients with burns, it is important to be vigilant for the possibility of elderly abuse. Elderly patients who are institutionalized, disoriented, or incapable of clear communication are particularly susceptible to abuse.

Signs of abuse in the elderly include evidence of multiple injuries in various stages of healing (ie, multiple bruises of different colors, new and old fractures involving more than one extremity), injuries that do not seem to correspond to the history provided by caregivers, and burns with a suspicious history of the incident.

Burns that appear in a "pattern" are suspicious for intentional injuries. Multiple, small circular burns may be indicative of cigarette or cigar injuries. Other patterns may indicate irons, stovetops, or other hot surfaces not easily encountered accidentally. Scalding injuries to hands or feet may also be indicative of abuse. It is important to remember that these injuries are often inflicted in areas not readily seen. If the situation is suspicious for elderly abuse, be sure to fully examine the patient under his or her clothing for signs of abuse. As always, appropriate support and transport of the patient in timely fashion remain a priority.

Table 24-1 Classification of Burns in Adults

Critical Burns

- Full-thickness burns involving the hands, feet, face, upper airway, or genitalia

- Full-thickness burns covering more than 10% of the body's total surface area

- Partial-thickness burns covering more than 30% of the body's total surface area

- Burns associated with respiratory injury (smoke inhalation)

- Burns complicated by fractures

- Burns on patients younger than age 5 years or older than age 55 years that would be classified as "moderate" on young adults

Moderate Burns

- Full-thickness burns involving 2% to 10% of the body's total surface area (excluding hands, feet, face, genitalia, or upper airway)

- Partial-thickness burns covering 15% to 30% of the body's total surface area

- Superficial burns covering more than 50% of the body's total surface area

Minor Burns

- Full-thickness burns covering less than 2% of the body's total surface area

- Partial-thickness burns covering less than 15% of the body's total surface area

- Superficial burns covering less than 50% of the body's total surface area

DEPTH. Burns are first classified according to their depth (▼ Figure 24-17). You must be able to identify the following three types of burns:

- **Superficial (first-degree) burns** involve only the top layer of skin, the epidermis. The skin turns red but does not blister or actually burn through. The burn site is painful. A sunburn is a good example of a superficial burn.

- **Partial-thickness (second-degree)** burns involve the epidermis and some portion of the dermis. These burns do not destroy the entire thickness of the skin, nor is the subcutaneous tissue injured. Typically, the skin is moist, mottled, and white to red. Blisters are common. Partial-thickness burns cause intense pain.

- **Full-thickness (third-degree) burns** extend through all skin layers and may involve subcutaneous layers, muscle, bone, or internal organs. The burned area is dry and leathery and may appear white, dark brown, or even charred. Some full-thickness burns feel hard to the touch. Clotted blood vessels or subcutaneous tissue may be visible under the burned skin. If the nerve endings have been destroyed, a severely burned area may have no feeling. However, the surrounding, less severely burned areas may be extremely painful.

A pure full-thickness burn is unusual. Severe burns are typically a combination of superficial, partial-thickness, and full-thickness burns. Superficial burns heal well without scarring.

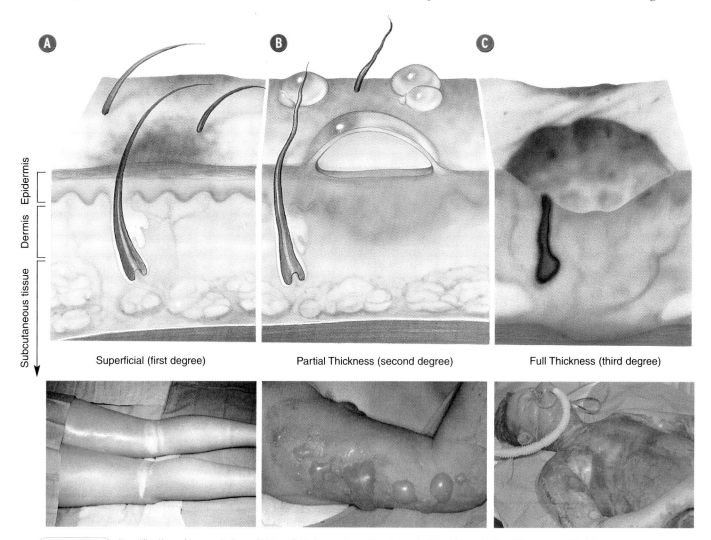

Superficial (first degree)   Partial Thickness (second degree)   Full Thickness (third degree)

Figure 24-17 Classification of burns. **A.** Superficial or first-degree burns involve only the epidermis. The skin turns red but does not blister or actually burn through. **B.** Partial-thickness or second-degree burns involve some of the dermis, but they do not destroy the entire thickness of the skin. The skin is mottled, white to red, and is often blistered. **C.** Full-thickness or third-degree burns extend through all layers of the skin and may involve subcutaneous tissue and muscle. The skin is dry, leathery, and often either white or charred.

Documentation Tips

Burn patterns often require description beyond calculating the amount of body surface involved. If you find written description difficult or too lengthy, try drawing in the affected areas on two outlines of the body, front and back. Your report form may include an area with the outlines provided; if not, don't hesitate to draw them in yourself. One picture can be worth many words.

Pediatric Needs

Burns to children are generally considered more serious than burns to adults (▼ **Table 24-2**). This is because infants and children have more surface area relative to total body mass, which means greater fluid and heat loss. In addition, children do not tolerate burns as well as adults do. Children are also more likely to go into shock, develop hypothermia, and experience airway problems.

Many burns in infants and children result from child abuse. The classic burn resulting from deliberate immersion involves the hands and wrists, as well as the feet, lower legs, and buttocks. Similarly, burns around the genitals and multiple cigarette burns should be viewed as possible abuse. You should report all suspected cases of abuse to the proper authorities (Chapter 33).

TABLE 24-2 Classification of Burns in Infants and Children

Critical Burns

- Full-thickness or partial-thickness burns covering more than 20% of the body's total surface area
- Burns involving the hands, feet, face, airway, or genitalia

Moderate Burns

- Partial-thickness burns covering 10% to 20% of the body's total surface area

Minor Burns

- Partial-thickness burns covering less than 10% of the body's total surface area

Small partial-thickness burns also heal without scarring. However, deep partial-thickness burns and all full-thickness burns are best managed surgically.

- Significant airway burns, which may be associated with singeing of the hair within the nostrils, soot around the nose and mouth, hoarseness, or hypoxia.

It may be impossible to accurately estimate the depth of a particular burn. Even experienced burn surgeons sometimes underestimate or, more commonly, overestimate the extent of a particular burn.

EXTENT. One quick way to estimate the surface area that has been burned is to compare it to the size of the patient's palm, which is roughly equal to 1% of the patient's total body surface area. Another useful measurement system is the **Rule of Nines**, which divides the body into sections, each of which is approximately 9% of the total surface area (▶ **Figure 24-18**). Remember that the head of an infant or child is relatively larger than the head of an adult, and the legs are relatively smaller.

Emergency Medical Care

Your first responsibility in caring for a patient with a burn is to stop the burning process and prevent additional injury. (▶ **Skill Drill 24-4**) presents the steps in caring for a burn patient:

1. **Follow BSI precautions.** Because a burn destroys the patient's protective skin layer, always wear gloves and eye protection when treating a burn patient.

2. **Move the patient away from the burning area.** If any clothing is on fire, wrap the patient in a blanket or follow specific guidelines outlined by your local fire department protocol to put out the flames, then remove any smoldering clothing and/or jewelry.

3. **Immerse the area in cool, sterile water or saline solution,** or cover with a clean, wet, cool dressing, if the skin or clothing is hot. This not only stops the burning, it also relieves pain. However, immersion increases the risk of infection and hypothermia. For this reason, you should not keep the affected part under water for more than 10 minutes. If the burning has stopped before you arrive, *do not immerse it at all.* As an alternative to immersion, irrigation of the burned area until the burning stops may also be used, followed by the application of a sterile dressing **(Step 1)**.

4. **Give oxygen if the patient has a critical burn.** Also remember that more fire victims die from

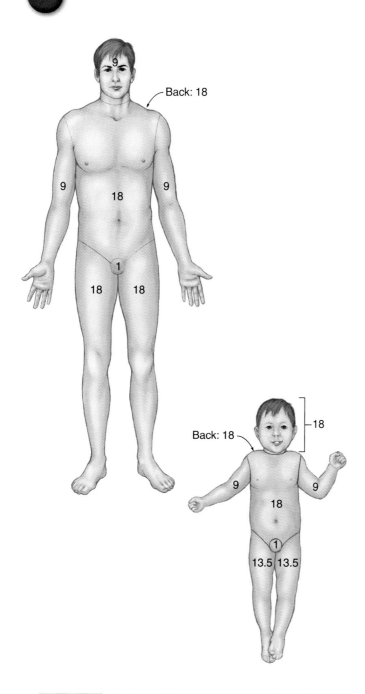

Figure 24-18 The Rule of Nines is a quick way to estimate the amount of surface area that has been burned. It divides the body into sections, each approximately 9% of the total body surface area.

smoke inhalation than from skin burns. A patient who has burns about the face or has inhaled smoke or fumes may develop respiratory distress. Therefore, you should give oxygen to these patients as well. Keep in mind that a patient who appears to be breathing well at first may suddenly develop severe respiratory distress. Therefore, you must continually assess the airway for possible problems **(Step 2)**.

EMT-B Tips

General emergency medical care of burns

1. Follow BSI precautions.
2. Move the patient away from the burning area.
3. Immerse the burned skin in cool sterile water.
4. Give oxygen.
5. An extensive burn can produce hypothermia.
6. Rapidly estimate the burn's severity.
7. Check for traumatic injuries.
8. Treat the patient for shock.
9. Provide prompt transport.

5. **Rapidly estimate the burn's severity.** Then cover the burned area with a dry, sterile dressing to prevent further contamination. Sterile gauze is best if the area is not too large. You may cover larger areas with a clean, white sheet. Most important, do not put anything else on the burned area. Use only a dry, sterile dressing, sterile burn sheet, or clean, white sheet. Never use ointments, lotions, or antiseptics of any kind. In addition, do not intentionally break any blisters.

6. **Check for traumatic injurie**s or other medical conditions that may be more immediately life-threatening. Most patients who have been burned have normal vital signs and can communicate at first, which will make your assessment easier **(Step 3)**.

7. **Treat the patient for shock** if necessary **(Step 4)**.

8. **An extensive burn can produce hypothermia** (loss of body heat). Prevent further heat loss by covering the patient with warm blankets.

9. **Provide prompt transport** by local protocol. Do not delay transport to do a prolonged assessment or to apply coverings to burns in a critical patient **(Step 5)**.

Chemical Burns

A chemical burn can occur whenever a toxic substance contacts the body. Most chemical burns are caused by strong acids or strong alkalis. The eyes are particularly vulnerable to chemical burns ▶ **Figure 24-19**.

SkillDrill 24-4   Caring for Burns

1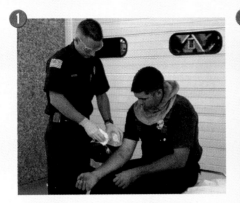

Follow BSI precautions to help prevent infection.

Remove the patient from the burning area; extinguish or remove hot clothing and jewelry as needed.

If the wound(s) is still burning or hot, immerse the hot area in cool, sterile water, or cover with a wet, cool dressing.

2

Give supplemental oxygen and continue to assess the airway.

3

Estimate the severity of the burn, then cover the area with a dry, sterile dressing or clean sheet.

Assess and treat the patient for any other injuries.

4

Prepare for transport.
Treat for shock if needed.

5

Cover the patient with blankets to prevent loss of body heat.
Transport promptly.

Sometimes, simply the fumes of strong chemicals can cause burns, especially to the respiratory tract.

To prevent exposure to hazardous materials, you must wear the appropriate gloves and eye protection whenever you are caring for a patient with a chemical burn. Be particularly careful not to get any chemical, dry or liquid, on yourself or on your uniform; consider wearing a protective gown when this is a possibility. Remember that exposure risk is also present when you are cleaning up after the call. In cases of severe chemical burns or exposure, consider mobilization of the HazMat team, if appropriate.

The emergency care of a chemical burn is basically the same as that for a thermal burn. To stop the burning

Figure 24-19 The eyes are particularly vulnerable to chemical burns.

process, remove any chemical from the patient. A dry chemical that is activated by contact with water may damage the skin more when it is wet than when it is dry. Therefore, always brush dry chemicals off the skin and clothing before flushing the patient with water ▼ Figure 24-20 . Remove the patient's clothing, including shoes, stockings, and gloves, because there may be small amounts of chemicals in the creases.

Immediately begin to flush the burned area with large amounts of water ▶ Figure 24-21 , taking care not to contaminate uninjured areas or make the patient hypothermic. Never direct a forceful stream of water from a hose at the patient; the extreme water pressure may mechanically injure the burned skin. Continue flooding the area with gallons of water for 15 to 20 minutes after the patient says the burning pain has stopped. If an eye has been burned, hold the eyelid open while flooding the eye with a gentle stream of water ▼ Figure 24-22 . Continue flushing the contaminated area on the way to the hospital.

Electrical Burns

Electrical burns may be the result of contact with high- or low-voltage electricity. High-voltage burns may occur when utility workers make direct contact with power lines. However, ordinary household current is powerful enough to cause severe burns.

For electricity to flow, there must be a complete circuit between the electrical source and the ground. Any substance that prevents this circuit from being

Figure 24-21 Flush the burned area with large amounts of water for 15 to 20 minutes after the patient says that the burning pain has stopped. Be careful to avoid contaminating uninjured areas.

Figure 24-20 Brush dry chemicals off the patient before you flush the burned area with water.

Figure 24-22 Flood the affected eye with a gentle stream of water. Hold the eyelids open, a challenging task because the patient's reflex is to keep the eye shut. Take care to prevent any of the chemical from getting into the other eye during flushing.

EMT-B Safety

Your safety is the first priority when an electrical hazard may be involved. Do not try to remove someone from an electrical source or move a downed power line unless you are specially trained and equipped to do so. Before approaching someone who may still be in contact with a power line or electrical appliance, ensure that all power is turned off.

completed, such as rubber, is called an insulator. Any substance that allows a current to flow through it is called a conductor. The human body, which is primarily water, is a good conductor. Thus, electrical burns occur when the body, or a part of it, completes a circuit connecting a power source to the ground ▼ **Figure 24-23** .

Your safety is of particular importance when you are called to the scene of an emergency involving electricity. Obviously, you can be fatally injured by coming into contact with power lines. But you can also be fatally injured by touching a patient who is still in contact with a live power line or any other electrical source. For this reason, you must never attempt to remove someone from an electrical source unless you are specially trained to do so. Likewise, you should never move a downed power line unless you have the special training and equipment necessary for the job or unless you are absolutely certain that the line is not live. Before even approaching someone who may still be in contact with a power line or an electrical appliance, make certain that the power is turned off. Always assume that any downed power line is live.

There is always a burn injury where the electricity entered the body (an entrance wound) and another where it exited (an exit wound). The entrance wound may be quite small ▼ **Figure 24-24A** , but the exit wound can be extensive and deep ▼ **Figure 24-24B** . Always look for both entrance and exit wounds. There are two dangers specifically associated with electrical burns. First, there may be a large amount of deep tissue injury. Electrical burns are always more severe than the external signs indicate. The patient may have only a small burn to the skin but have massive damage to the

Figure 24-23 The human body is a good conductor of electricity. An electrical burn usually occurs when the body, acting as a conductor, completes a circuit.

Figure 24-24 Electrical burns, like gunshot wounds, have entrance and exit wounds. **A.** An entrance wound is often quite small. **B.** The exit wound can be extensive and deep.

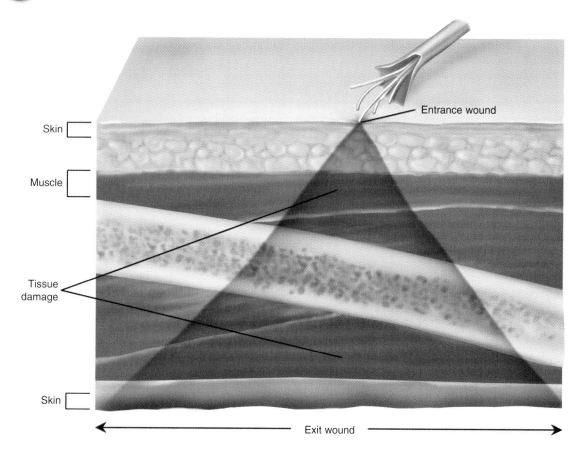

Skin

Muscle

Tissue
damage

Skin

Entrance wound

Exit wound

Figure 24-25   External signs of an electrical burn may be deceiving. The entrance wound may be a small burn, while the damage to deeper tissue may be massive.

deeper tissues (▲ **Figure 24-25**). Second, the patient may go into cardiac arrest from the electric shock.

If indicated, begin CPR and apply the AED. Although CPR may need to be quite prolonged in electrical burn cases, it has a high success rate if started promptly. You should be prepared to defibrillate if necessary. If neither CPR nor defibrillation is indicated, give supplemental oxygen, and monitor the patient closely for respiratory and cardiac arrest. Treat the soft-tissue injuries by placing dry, sterile dressings on all burn wounds and splinting suspected fractures. Provide prompt transport; all electrical burns are potentially severe injuries that require further treatment in the hospital.

Dressing and Bandaging

All wounds require bandaging. In most instances, splints help to control bleeding and provide firm support for the dressing. There are many different types of dressings

and bandages (▶ **Figure 24-26**). You should be familiar with the function and proper application of each.

In general, dressings and bandages have three primary functions:

- To control bleeding
- To protect the wound from further damage
- To prevent further contamination and infection

Sterile Dressings

Universal dressings, conventional 4" × 4" and 4" × 8" gauze pads, and assorted small adhesive-type dressings and soft self-adherent roller dressings will cover most wounds.

Measuring 9" × 36" and made of thick, absorbent material, the universal dressing is ideal for covering large open wounds. It also makes an efficient pad for rigid splints. These dressings are available in compact,

Figure 24-26 **A.** Many types of sterile dressings are used for covering open wounds, including universal dressings, gauze pads, adhesive dressings, and occlusive dressings. **B.** Bandages keep dressings in place and include soft roller bandages, triangular bandages, and adhesive tape. Splints may also be used to hold dressings in place.

commercially sterilized packages. The universal dressing material is also available in 20-yard rolls, which some EMS personnel cut into 3-foot lengths, package, and sterilize themselves.

Gauze pads are appropriate for smaller wounds, and adhesive-type dressings are useful for minor wounds. Occlusive dressings, made of Vaseline gauze, aluminum foil, or plastic, prevent air and liquids from entering (or exiting) the wound. They are used to cover sucking chest wounds, abdominal eviscerations, and neck injuries.

Bandages

To keep dressings in place during transport, you can use soft roller bandages, rolls of gauze, triangular bandages, or adhesive tape. The self-adherent, soft roller bandages are probably easiest to use. They are slightly elastic, which makes them easy to apply, and you can tuck the end of the roll into a deeper layer to secure it in place. The layers adhere somewhat but should not be applied too tightly to one another.

Adhesive tape holds small dressings in place and helps to secure larger dressings. Some people, however, are allergic to adhesive tape. If you know that a patient has this problem, use paper or plastic tape instead.

Do not use elastic bandages to secure dressings. If the injury swells, the bandage may become a tourniquet and cause further damage. Any improperly applied bandage that impairs circulation can result in additional tissue damage or even the loss of a limb. For this reason, you should always check a limb distal to a bandage for signs of impaired circulation or loss of sensation. Air splints are useful in stabilizing broken extremities, and they can be used with dressings to help control bleeding from soft-tissue injuries.

Prep Kit

Ready for Review

The skin has two principal layers: the tough outer layer, called the epidermis, and the inner layer, called the dermis, which contains the hair follicles, sweat glands, and sebaceous glands. The functions of the skin are to keep bacteria out and water in, to report to the brain on the environment, and to regulate body temperature.

There are three types of soft-tissue injuries: closed injuries, open injuries, and burns. Closed injuries include contusions, hematomas, and crushing injuries. They can be treated by applying ICES (ice, compression, elevation of the injured part, and splinting). Open injuries produce more extensive bleeding and may become infected. There are four types of open injuries: abrasions, lacerations, avulsions, and penetrating wounds. In treating these injuries, you must first control bleeding. Use a dry, sterile dressing, covered by a roller bandage, a second pressure dressing (if necessary), and a splint. Do not try to clean out an open wound.

Burns are one of the most serious and painful of soft-tissue injuries. They can occur from heat (thermal), chemicals, electricity, and radiation. Burns are classified primarily by the depth and extent of the burn, the body area involved, and are either superficial, partial-thickness, or full-thickness.

Treatment for burns includes BSI precautions, stopping the burning process, caring for the burn wounds, and treating the patient for shock (oxygen and prevention of further heat loss).

Dressings and bandages are designed to control bleeding, protect the wound from further damage, and prevent further contamination and infection. Use universal dressings for large open wounds, gauze pads for smaller wounds, adhesive-type dressings for minor wounds, and occlusive dressings for sucking chest wounds and abdominal eviscerations. Use soft roller bandages, rolls of gauze, triangular bandages, or adhesive tape to keep dressings in place. Do not use elastic bandages. Always check a limb distal to a bandage for signs of impaired circulation.

Vital Vocabulary

abrasion Loss or damage of the superficial layer of skin as a result of a body part rubbing or scraping across a rough or hard surface.

avulsion An injury in which soft tissue either is torn completely loose or is hanging as a flap.

burns An injury in which the soft tissue receives more energy than it can absorb without injury, from thermal heat, frictional heat, toxic chemicals, electricity, or nuclear radiation.

closed injury Injury in which damage occurs beneath the skin or mucous membrane but the surface remains intact.

compartment syndrome Swelling in a confined space that produces dangerous pressure; may cut off blood flow or damage sensitive tissue.

contamination The presence of infective organisms or foreign bodies such as dirt, gravel, or metal.

contusion A bruise without a break in the skin.

dermis The inner layer of the skin, containing hair follicles, sweat glands, nerve endings, and blood vessels.

ecchymosis Discoloration associated with a closed wound; signifies bleeding.

epidermis The outer layer of skin that acts as a watertight protective covering.

evisceration The displacement of organs outside the body.

full-thickness burn A burn that affects all skin layers and may affect the subcutaneous layers, muscle, bone, and internal organs, leaving the area dry, leathery, and white, dark brown, or charred; traditionally called a third-degree burn.

hematoma Blood collected within the body's tissues or in a body cavity.

hemothorax Collection of blood in the chest.

laceration A smooth or jagged open wound.

mucous membrane The lining of body cavities and passages that are in direct contact with the outside environment.

occlusive dressing Dressing made of Vaseline gauze, aluminum foil, or plastic, that prevents air and liquids from entering or exiting a wound.

open injury An injury in which there is a break in the surface of the skin or the mucous membrane, exposing deeper tissue to potential contamination.

partial-thickness burn A burn affecting the epidermis and some portion of the dermis but not the subcutaneous tissue, characterized by blisters and skin that is white to red, moist, and mottled; traditionally called a second-degree burn.

penetrating wound An injury resulting from a sharp, pointed object.

pneumothorax Entry of air into the pleural space.

Rule of Nines A system that assigns percentages to sections of the body, allowing calculation of the amount of skin surface involved in the burn area.

superficial burn A burn affecting only the epidermis, characterized by skin that is red but not blistered or actually burned through; traditionally called a first-degree burn.

Points to Ponder

You are working at a high school wrestling meet and notice a wrestler twists his knee during a match. His coach has evaluated the knee and when the wrestler stands, his knee collapses. His parents wave for you to come over. You find that the wrestler and the coach believe he can still wrestle, but the parents want your opinion. You have recently completed the EMT class and were not trained in evaluating sports injuries. Your protocol would be to splint and transport. The referee is pushing for an answer to whether he can wrestle or to end the match. Would you evaluate the wrestler? Would you make a decision to allow him to continue? What would you tell the parents? Once the parents call you over, can you NOT treat the patient?

Issues Legal Liability, Training Standards and Protocols, Refusing Treatment, Use of Non-EMT Skills and Outside Knowledge.

www.emtb.com

Assessment in Action

It's a beautiful summer Saturday at the state park, and a group of teens has been canoeing down a small river. They stopped at a popular small waterfall to take a break. When one teen dares another to jump across the top of the waterfall, another teen immediately accepts the challenge. A mighty leap later, he almost makes it to the other side, but he comes up short on the landing. His feet go out from under him, and he crashes down the bank and falls about 10 feet. He slides into a rock, and rolls off into the remains of a downed tree.

The broken end of a branch leaves a 1" hole under his right scapula. The wound is still bubbling with each breath when you arrive. The patient is alert and articulate and appears pale. He tells you that the reason he stayed motionless by the creek edge was because it "hurt too bad" to move. He has numerous contusions and abrasions, primarily to his right side. He also has a large avulsion to his right calf that is bleeding freely. Vital signs include a pulse of 126 beats/min, shallow respirations of 40 breaths/min, and a blood pressure of 134/70 mm Hg.

1. Your first step in caring for this patient is to:
   A. check his pulse, sensation, and function in all four extremities.
   B. apply oxygen and cover the open chest wound and stop the bleeding.
   C. ask him to identify what he thinks is the biggest problem.
   D. ask him if he has any allergies or is on any medication.

2. The most appropriate method to manage bleeding from his avulsion is to:
   A. separate the layers of tissue with sterile gauze and bandage.
   B. apply a wide-band tourniquet and loosen regularly.
   C. apply sterile gauze over the injury with an elastic bandage.
   D. replace the tissue and apply direct pressure over the bleeding site.

3. The patient's right shoulder and upper arm are both quite swollen with an extensive contusion. This is an indicator of which of the following?
   A. Nerve damage
   B. Systemic infection
   C. Internal bleeding
   D. Allergic reaction

4. If this patient were to survive his first couple of days, because of the nature of his injuries, he would still be at high risk for:
   A. infection.
   B. infarction.
   C. malnutrition.
   D. hypertension.

5. During your care you note that this patient is becoming confused. Which of the following must you immediately assess?
   A. Ability to obey commands
   B. Movement, pulse, and sensation of the distal extremity
   C. Respirations, pulse, and BP
   D. Pupil reaction

6. It is important to continue to assess vital signs and assess for hypoperfusion because of this patient's penetrating injury. Which of the following explanations for this is most correct?
   A. The spleen is located in that area.
   B. The liver is located in that area.
   C. The heart is located in that area.
   D. The pancreas is located in that area.

Later that same day, you are called to another incident at the same park. This time a camper tried to light a campfire with lighter fluid. He has suffered burns to the anterior surface of both of his arms, face, and upper chest to his nipple line. He is screaming in pain. The burned areas are bright red with some blistering of his hands and lower arms. His eyebrows have been singed and blisters are forming on his chin. The following questions apply to this patient.

7. What do you know about this patient's airway?
   A. Nothing until you check his respiratory rate.
   B. His airway is intact because he is screaming.
   C. His respirations are inadequate because he is screaming.
   D. Nothing until you check his mucous membranes and tongue.

8. This patient has signs of possible respiratory involvement. Without looking at his mucous membranes and tongue, how can you tell?
   A. His mental status
   B. His pulse
   C. The blisters on his face
   D. His respiratory rate

9. This patient has burns over the anterior surface of both his arms, upper chest to the nipple line, and face. What percentage of body surface area burn should you report to the receiving hospital? Approximately:
   A. 18%
   B. 23%
   C. 27%
   D. 32%

Challenging Question

10. If both arms of your patient are burned, how can you obtain a blood pressure?

Online Outlook

Because the soft tissues are exposed to the environment, they are often injured. Test your ability to identify different soft-tissue injuries by completing Exercise 24 at www.emtb.com.

www.emtb.com

Eye Injuries

Objectives*

Cognitive

1. List the main anatomical features of the eye (p 588).
2. Describe the principal functions of the eye (p 588).
3. Describe the signs and symptoms of eye injuries (p 589).
4. List the steps necessary to assess eye injuries (p 589).
5. Describe the steps for managing foreign objects in the eye (p 590).
6. Describe the steps for managing puncture wounds to the eye (p 590).
7. Describe how to manage burns to the eye (p 592).
8. Describe how to remove contact lenses from the eye (p 597).
9. Recognize abnormalities of the eyes that may indicate underlying head injury (p 595).
10. Recognize and manage a patient with an artificial eye (p 597).

Affective

None

Psychomotor

11. Demonstrate the use of irrigation to flush out foreign bodies lying on the surface of the eye (p 590).
12. Demonstrate the care of the patient with chemical burns to the eye (p 592).
13. Demonstrate the steps in the emergency care of the patient with lacerations of the eyelids (p 594).

* All of the objectives in this chapter are noncurriculum objectives.

TECHNOLOGY

www.emtb.com

- Online Chapter Pretest
- Interactivities
- Vocabulary Explorer
- Anatomy Review
- Web Links
- Online Review Manual
- Distance Learning

Chapter FEATURES

- Skill Drills
- Vital Vocabulary
- Pediatric Needs
- Geriatric Needs
- EMT-B Safety
- EMT-B Tips
- Documentation Tips
- Remember
- Prep Kit

"Engine 6 and Squad 3, respond to 181 Madison Street for an explosion." You arrive to find a machinist and his assistant both covered in blood with suspected eye injuries.

The possible loss of sight is a frightening event, making calls involving eye injuries very stressful for both patients and care providers. This chapter will present practical information about caring for these fragile organs and will also help you answer the following questions:

1. Why is it important to bandage both eyes in cases where only one eye is injured?

2. When is it appropriate to remove contact lenses from your patient's eyes?

Eye Injuries

Injuries to the eye are very common, and you will encounter many in your work as an EMT-B. Proper emergency medical care for these injuries can minimize damage, which can often be severe. Fortunately, most eye injuries are relatively minor, such as foreign objects in the eye, corneal abrasions, and contusions. Some injuries are more serious, such as rupture of the globe, which requires immediate expert management. This chapter first reviews the structure and function of the eye and then looks at the different types of eye injuries, describing the emergency management of each. The handling of contact lenses and artificial eyes is also discussed.

Anatomy and Physiology of the Eye

The eye is globe-shaped, approximately 1" in diameter, and located within a bony socket in the skull called the **orbit** (▶ **Figure 25-1**). The orbit is composed of the adjacent bones of the face and skull; the orbit forms the base of the floor of the cranial cavity, and directly above it are the frontal lobes of the brain. In the adult, more than 80% of the eyeball is protected within this bony orbit. Between and below the orbits are the nasal bones and the sinuses, respectively. Therefore, any severe injury to the face or head can potentially damage the eyeball or the muscles attached to the eyeball that cause the eye to move.

The eyeball, or **globe**, keeps its global shape as a result of the pressure of the fluid contained within its two chambers. The clear, jellylike fluid near the back of the eye is called the vitreous humor. If the globe is ruptured and this gel leaks out, it cannot be replaced. In front of the lens is a clear fluid called the aqueous humor, named for its watery appearance; in Latin,

aqua means "water." In penetrating injuries of the eye, aqueous humor can also leak out, but with time and good medical treatment, the body can make more.

The inner surface of the eyelids and the exposed surface of the eye itself, which are covered by a delicate membrane, the **conjunctiva**, are kept moist by fluid produced by the **lacrimal glands**, often called tear glands (▶ **Figure 25-2**). Humans blink unconsciously many times per minute. This action sweeps fluid from the lacrimal glands over the surface of the eye, cleaning it. The tears drain on the inner side of the eye through two lacrimal (tear) ducts into the nasal cavity. This is why, when people cry, they sometimes need to blow their nose.

The white of the eye, called the **sclera**, extends over the surface of the globe. This is extremely tough, fibrous tissue that helps to maintain the eye's globular shape

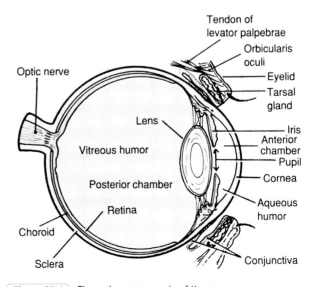

Figure 25-1 The major components of the eye.

and protect the more delicate inner structures. On the front of the eye, the sclera is replaced by a clear, transparent membrane called the <u>cornea</u>, which allows light to enter the eye. A circular muscle lies behind the cornea with an opening in its center. Like the shutter in a camera, this muscle adjusts the size of the opening to regulate the amount of light that enters the eye. This circular muscle and surrounding tissue are called the <u>iris</u>. The iris is pigmented, giving the eye its characteristic brown, green, or blue color.

The opening in the center of the iris, which allows light to move to the back of the eye, is called the <u>pupil</u>. Normally, the pupil appears black. Like the aperture in a camera, the pupil becomes smaller in bright light and larger in dim light. The pupil also becomes smaller and larger when the person is looking at objects near at hand and farther away; these adjustments occur almost instantaneously. Normally, the pupils in both eyes are equal in size. A difference between them may indicate injury to the eye or to the brain.

Behind the iris is the <u>lens</u>. Like the lens of a camera, this lens focuses an image on the light-sensitive area at the back of the globe, called the <u>retina</u>. You can think of the retina as the film in the camera. Within the retina are numerous nerve endings, which respond to light by transmitting nerve impulses through the <u>optic nerve</u> to the brain. In the brain, the impulses are interpreted as vision.

The retina is nourished by a layer of blood vessels between it and the sclera at the back of the globe. This layer is called the choroid. If, as sometimes happens, the retina detaches from the underlying choroid and sclera, the nerve endings are not nourished, and the patient then experiences blindness. This may be partial blindness, depending on how much of the retina is separated. This condition is called <u>retinal detachment</u>.

Common Eye Injuries

Eye injuries are common, particularly in sports. An eye injury can produce severe complications, including blindness. Proper emergency treatment will minimize pain and may very well help to prevent permanent loss of vision.

Treatment starts with a thorough examination to determine the extent and nature of any damage. Always perform your examination using BSI precautions, taking great care to avoid aggravating the problem. You are looking for specific abnormalities or conditions that may suggest the nature of the problem ▼ **Figure 25-3** . For example, blunt or penetrating injuries can produce swollen or lacerated eyelids. Bleeding soon after irritation or injury can result in a bright red conjunctiva. A damaged cornea quickly loses its smooth, wet appearance.

In a normal, uninjured eye, the entire circle of the iris is visible. The pupils are round, equal in size, and react equally when exposed to light ▶ **Figure 25-4** . Both eyes move together in the same direction when following your moving finger. After an injury, pupil reaction or shape and eye movement are often disturbed. Any of these conditions should cause you to suspect an injury of the globe or its associated tissues. Remember, though, that abnormal pupil reactions sometimes are a sign of brain injury rather than eye injury.

Figure 25-2 The lacrimal system consists of tear glands and ducts. Tears act as lubricants and keep the front of the eye from drying out.

Figure 25-3 Injuries to the eyes are easily detected by **A.** Swelling, **B.** Bleeding, and **C.** The presence of foreign objects in the eye.

Figure 25-4 Normally, the pupils are round, equal in size, and equally reactive when exposed to light.

Figure 25-5 Conjunctivitis is often associated with the presence of a foreign object in the eye.

Figure 25-6 One method of irrigation is to direct saline into the injured eye using a round nasal airway or cannula. Always flush from the nose side of the eye toward the outside to avoid flushing material into the other eye.

Certain elements of the patient's history are particularly important. Therefore, as you perform your assessment, always note and record the patient's signs and symptoms, including their severity and duration, the details of how the injury occurred, any reported changes in vision, the use of any eye medications, and any history of eye surgery.

Foreign Objects

Large objects are prevented from penetrating the eye by the protective orbit that surrounds it. However, moderate-sized and smaller foreign objects of many different types can enter the eye and cause significant damage. Even a very small foreign object, such as a grain of sand lying on the surface of the conjunctiva, may produce severe irritation (▲ **Figure 25-5**). The conjunctiva becomes inflamed and red—a condition known as <u>conjunctivitis</u>—almost immediately, and the eye begins to produce tears in an attempt to flush out the object. Irritation of the cornea or conjunctiva causes intense pain. The patient may have difficulty keeping the eyelids open, because the irritation is further aggravated by bright light.

If a small foreign object is lying on the surface of the patient's eye, you should use a normal saline solution to gently irrigate the eye. Irrigation with 500 to 1,000 mL of sterile saline solution will frequently flush away loose, small particles. If a small bulb syringe is at hand, you

can use this, or a nasal airway or cannula, to direct the saline into the affected eye (▲ **Figure 25-6**). Always flush from the nose side of the eye toward the outside to avoid flushing material into the other eye. After it is flushed away, a foreign body will often leave a small abrasion on the surface of the conjunctiva. For this reason, the patient will complain of irritation even when the particle itself is gone.

Gentle irrigation usually will not wash out foreign bodies that are stuck to the cornea or lying under the upper eyelid. To examine the undersurface of the upper eyelid, pull the lid upward and forward. If you spot a foreign object, you may be able to remove it with a moist, sterile, cotton-tipped applicator. (Never attempt to remove a foreign body that is stuck to the cornea.)

▶ **Skill Drill 25-1**

1. **Tell the patient to look down** while you grasp the lashes of the upper eyelid with your thumb and index finger. Gently pull the eyelid away from the eyeball **(Step 1)**.

2. **Gently place a cotton-tipped applicator** horizontally along the center of the outer surface of the upper eyelid **(Step 2)**.

3. **Pull the eyelid forward and up,** which causes it to roll or fold back over the applicator, exposing the undersurface of the eyelid **(Step 3)**.

Figure 25-7 Any number of objects can become impaled in the eye. **A.** Fishhook. **B.** Sharp, metal sliver. **C.** Knife blade.

SkillDrill 25-1 **Removing a Foreign Object from Under the Upper Eyelid**

Have the patient look down, grasp the upper lashes, and gently pull the lid away from the eye.

Place a cotton-tipped applicator on the upper lid.

Pull the lid forward and up, folding it back over the applicator.

Gently remove the foreign object with a moistened, sterile applicator.

4. **If you see a foreign object, gently remove it** with a moistened, sterile, cotton-tipped applicator **(Step 4)**.

Foreign bodies ranging in size from a pencil to a sliver of metal may be impaled in the eye (◄ **Figure 25-7**). These objects must be removed by a physician. Your care involves stabilizing the object and preparing the patient for transport to definitive care. The greater the length of foreign object you can see sticking out of the eye, the more important stabilization becomes in avoiding further damage. Bandage the object in place to support it. Cover the eye itself with a moist, sterile dressing, and then surround the object with a doughnut-shaped collar made from roller gauze or a small gauze pack. Follow the steps in ► **Skill Drill 25-2** :

1. **Begin to prepare the doughnut ring** by wrapping a 2″ gauze roll around your fingers and thumb enough times to make a thick

dressing layer. You can adjust the inner diameter of what will become the ring by spreading your fingers or squeezing them together **(Step 1)**.

2. **Remove the gauze** from your hands and start wrapping the remainder of the gauze roll around this ring that you have created **(Step 2)**.

3. **Work your way around the ring** until you have wrapped all the way around it and finished the "doughnut" **(Step 3)**.

4. **Carefully place the ring over the eye** and impaled object, without bumping the object. You can then stabilize the object and the gauze collar with a roller bandage surrounding the head. Bandage both the injured and uninjured eyes to minimize eye movement and prevent further damage to the globe, since both eyes move in concert **(Step 4)**.

Skill Drill 25-2 Stabilizing a Foreign Object Impaled in the Eye

To prepare a doughnut ring, wrap a 2" roll around your fingers and thumb seven or eight times. Adjust the diameter by spreading your fingers.

Wrap the remainder of the roll, . . .

. . . working around the ring.

Place the dressing over the eye to hold the impaled object in place, then secure it with a gauze dressing.

Sometimes, foreign bodies, particularly small metal fragments, become completely embedded within the eye itself. The patient may not even be aware of the cause of the problem. Suspect such an injury when the history includes metal work (eg, hammering, exposure to splinters, vigorous filing) and when there are other signs of ocular injury. This type of injury must be handled by an ophthalmologist on an urgent basis. It may require X-rays and special equipment to find the foreign body.

Burns of the Eye

Chemicals, heat, and light rays all can burn the delicate tissues of the eye, often causing permanent damage. Your role is to stop the burn and prevent further damage.

CHEMICAL BURNS. Chemical burns, usually caused by acid or alkaline solutions, require immediate emergency care ▶ **Figure 25-8** . This consists of flushing the eye with water or a sterile saline irrigation solution. If sterile saline is not available, you can use any clean water.

The idea is to direct the greatest amount of solution or water into the eye as gently as possible ▶ **Figure 25-9** . Because opening the eye spontaneously may cause the patient pain, you may have to force the lids open to irrigate the eye adequately. Ideally, you will use a bulb or irrigation syringe, a nasal cannula, or some other device that will allow you to control the flow. In some circumstances, you may have to resort to pouring water into the eye by holding the patient's head under a gently

Figure 25-8 **A.** Chemical burns typically occur when an acid or alkali is splashed into the eye. **B.** This figure shows a chemical burn from lye, an alkaline solution. Because lye can continue to damage the eye even when diluted, fast action is needed.

Figure 25-9 The following are four ways to effectively irrigate the eye. **A.** Nasal cannula. **B.** Shower. **C.** Bottle. **D.** Basin. Remember, you must protect the uninjured eye from the irrigating solution.

running faucet. You can even have the patient immerse his or her face in a large pan or basin of water and rapidly blink the affected eyelid. If only one eye is affected, care must be taken to avoid contaminated water from getting into the unaffected eye.

Irrigate the eye for at least 5 minutes. If the burn was caused by an alkali or a strong acid, you should irrigate the eye for 20 minutes. Strong acids and all alkaline solutions can penetrate deeply, requiring a prolonged flush. Again, always take care to protect the uninjured eye and prevent irrigation fluid from running into it.

After you have completed irrigation, apply a clean, dry dressing to cover the eye, and transport the patient

Figure 25-10 Apply a clean, dry dressing to cover the eye after you have finished irrigation.

Figure 25-11 Thermal burns occasionally cause significant damage to the eyelids. **A.** Arrows show some full-thickness burns. **B.** Burns of the eyelids require immediate hospital care.

promptly to the hospital for further care (▲ **Figure 25-10**). If the irrigation can be carried out satisfactorily in the ambulance, it should be done during transport to save time.

THERMAL BURNS. When a patient is burned in the face during a fire, the eyes usually close rapidly because of the heat. This reaction is a natural reflex to protect the eye from further injury. However, the eyelids remain exposed and are frequently burned (▶ **Figure 25-11**). Burns of the eyelids require very specialized care. It is best to provide prompt transport for these patients without further examination. First, however, you should cover both eyes with a sterile dressing moistened with sterile saline. You may apply eye shields over the dressing.

LIGHT BURNS. Infrared rays, eclipse light (if the patient has looked directly at the sun), and laser burns all can cause significant damage to the sensory cells of the eye when rays of light become focused on the retina. Retinal injuries that are caused by exposure to extremes of light are generally not painful but may result in permanent damage to vision.

Superficial burns of the eye can result from ultraviolet rays from an arc welding unit, light from prolonged exposure to a sunlamp, or reflected light from a bright snow-covered area (snow blindness). This kind of burn often is not painful at first but may become so 3 to 5 hours later, as the damaged cornea responds to the injury. The patient usually develops a severe conjunctivitis with redness, swelling, and excessive tear production. You can ease the pain from these corneal burns by covering each eye with a sterile, moist pad

and an eye shield. Have the patient lie down during transport to the hospital, and protect him or her from further exposure to bright light. This patient should be examined by a physician as soon as possible.

Lacerations

Lacerations of the eyelids require very careful repair to restore both appearance and function (▶ **Figure 25-12**). Bleeding may be heavy, but it usually can be controlled by gentle, manual pressure. If there is a laceration of the globe itself, apply no pressure to the eye; compression can interfere with the blood supply to the back of the eye and result in loss of vision from damage to the retina. Furthermore, pressure may squeeze the vitreous humor, iris, lens, or even the retina out of the eye and cause irreparable damage or blindness.

Follow these three important guidelines in treating penetrating injuries of the eye:

Figure 25-12 Lacerations are serious injuries that require prompt transport. **A.** While bleeding can be heavy, never exert pressure on the eye. **B.** Pressure may squeeze the vitreous humor, iris, lens, or even the retina out of the eye.

Figure 25-13 The typical "black eye" is caused by bleeding into the tissue around the orbit.

1. **Never exert pressure** on or manipulate the injured eye (globe) in any way.

2. **If part of the eyeball is exposed,** gently apply a moist, sterile dressing to prevent drying.

3. **Cover the injured eye** with a protective metal eye shield or sterile dressing.

On rare occasions following a serious injury, the eyeball may be displaced out of its socket. Do not attempt to reposition it. Simply cover the eye, and stabilize it with a moist, sterile dressing. Have the patient lie in a supine position while en route to the hospital.

Blunt Trauma

Blunt trauma can cause a number of serious injuries of the eye. These range from the ordinary "black eye," a result of bleeding into the tissue around the orbit

Hyphema

Figure 25-14 A hyphema, characterized by bleeding into the anterior chamber of the eye, is common following blunt trauma to the eye. This condition may seriously impair vision.

▲ **Figure 25-13** , to a severely damaged globe. You may see an injury called <u>hyphema</u>, or bleeding into the anterior chamber of the eye, that obscures part or all of the iris ▲ **Figure 25-14** . This injury is common in blunt trauma and may seriously impair vision. It may also be a sign of a more serious injury to the globe.

Figure 25-15 A patient with a blowout fracture will not move his or her eyes together because of muscle entrapment. The patient therefore sees double images of any object.

Figure 25-16 Variation of pupil size may indicate a head injury.

Blunt trauma can also cause a fracture of the orbit, particularly of the bones that form its floor and support the globe. This injury is called a **blowout fracture**. The fragments of fractured bone can entrap some of the muscles that control eye movement, causing double vision (▲ **Figure 25-15**). Any patient who reports pain, double vision, or decreased vision following a blunt injury about the eye should be placed on a stretcher and transported promptly to the emergency department. Protect the eye from further injury with a metal shield; cover the other eye to minimize movement on the injured side.

Another possible result of blunt eye injury is retinal detachment. This injury is often seen in sports, especially boxing. It is painless but produces flashing lights, specks, or "floaters" in the field of vision and a cloud or shade over the patient's vision. Because the retina is separated from the nourishing choroid, this injury requires prompt medical attention to preserve vision in that eye.

Eye Injuries Following Head Injury

Abnormalities in the appearance or function of the eyes often occur following a closed head injury. Any of the following eye findings should alert you to the possibility of a head injury:

- One pupil larger than the other (▲ **Figure 25-16**)
- The eyes not moving together or pointing in different directions
- Failure of the eyes to follow the movement of your finger as instructed
- Bleeding under the conjunctiva, which obscures the sclera (white portion) of the eye
- Protrusion or bulging of one eye

Record any of these observations, along with the time that you make them. For an unconscious patient, remember to keep the eyelids closed; drying of the ocular tissue can cause permanent injury and may result in blindness. Cover the lids with moist gauze, or hold them closed with clear tape. Normal tears will then keep the tissues moist.

Contact Lenses and Artificial Eyes

Small, hard contact lenses usually are tinted, making them relatively easy to see. Large, soft ones are clear and can be very difficult to see. In general, you should not attempt to remove either kind of lens from a patient. You should never attempt to remove a lens from an eye that has been—or may have been—injured, since manipulating the lens can aggravate the problem. The only time that contact lenses should be removed immediately in the field is in the case of a chemical burn of the eye. In this situation, the lens can trap the chemical and make irrigation difficult.

If it is necessary to remove a hard contact lens, use a small suction cup, moistening the end with saline (▶ **Figure 25-17A**). To remove soft lenses, place one to two drops of saline onto the lens (▶ **Figure 25-17B**), gently pinch it between your thumb and index finger, and lift it off the surface of the eye (▶ **Figure 25-17C**).

Always advise emergency department staff if a patient is wearing contact lenses so that the patient can be properly cared for at the hospital.

Occasionally, you may find yourself caring for a patient who is wearing an eye prosthesis, an artificial eye. Many people are surprised to find that it can be difficult to distinguish a prosthesis from a natural eye. You should suspect an eye of being artificial when it does not respond to light, move in concert with the opposite eye, or appear quite the same as its mate. If you think that a patient may have an artificial eye but you are not sure, go ahead and ask about it. Although no harm will be done if you care for an artificial eye as you would a normal one, you need to be totally clear about the patient's eye function.

Figure 25-17 Removing contact lenses should be limited to patients with burn injuries. **A.** To remove hard contact lenses, use a specialized suction cup moistened with sterile saline solution. **B.** To remove soft contact lenses, instill one or two drops of saline or irrigating solution. **C.** Next, pinch off the lens with your thumb and index finger.

Prep Kit

Ready for Review

The eye is globe-shaped, about 1" in diameter, and located within a bony socket called the orbit, which is actually part of the skull. Any severe injury to the face or head can potentially damage the eyeball or eye muscles. The fluid in the back of the eye is called the vitreous humor and cannot be replaced; the fluid in the front of the eye is called the aqueous humor and can be replaced. The eye works like a camera, with the iris and pupil making adjustments to light and the retina acting like film. Nerve endings in the retina send impulses through the optic nerve to the brain, which interprets them as vision.

In assessing a patient with a possible eye injury, look for swollen or lacerated eyelids, a bright red conjunctiva, irregular pupil reactions or eye movements, and a cornea that no longer appears wet and smooth. Foreign bodies on the surface of the eye should be irrigated gently with a normal saline solution; always flush from the nose side of the eye toward the outside. If a foreign body is on the undersurface of the lid, remove it with a moist, cotton-tipped applicator. Do not remove foreign bodies that are stuck to the cornea. If a foreign body is impaled in the eye, bandage the object in place, using roller gauze to create a collar around it, until it can be removed by a physician. Small metal fragments that are entirely embedded within the eye must be treated by an ophthalmologist.

Chemicals, heat, and light rays can all burn the eyes, causing permanent damage. Irrigate chemical burns with saline solution or clean water for at least 5 minutes, then apply a clean, dry dressing to the eye and transport the patient promptly. Transport the patient with heat burns of the eyelid immediately, covering both eyes with a sterile, moist dressing. Superficial burns of the eye resulting from exposure to ultraviolet rays or a sunlamp can become very painful after several hours. You can ease the pain from these corneal burns by covering the eyes with a sterile, moist pad and eye shield; the patient should lie down during transport.

Use gentle manual pressure to control bleeding from a lacerated eyelid, but do not apply pressure to a laceration of the globe itself. Instead, apply a moist, sterile dressing to prevent drying, cover the injured eye with a protective metal shield, cover the opposite eye, and transport the patient. Never attempt to reposition a displaced eyeball. Blunt trauma can cause a range of injuries, including hyphema, retinal detachment, and blowout fractures. Any patient who complains of pain, double vision, or decreased vision following a blunt injury about the eye should be placed on a stretcher and transported promptly to the emergency department.

Suspect a head injury if the patient has one pupil larger than the other, eyes not moving together, bleeding under the conjunctiva, or protrusion or bulging of one eye. Keep the eyelids closed if the patient is unconscious so that the eyes do not dry out.

Never remove contact lenses from an injured eye unless the injury is a chemical burn.

Vital Vocabulary

blowout fracture Fracture of the orbit or of the bones that support the floor of the orbit.

conjunctiva The delicate membrane that lines the eyelids and covers the exposed surface of the eye.

conjunctivitis Inflammation of the conjunctiva.

cornea The transparent tissue layer in front of the pupil and iris of the eye.

globe The eyeball.

hyphema Bleeding into the anterior chamber of the eye, obscuring the iris.

iris The muscle and surrounding tissue behind the cornea that dilate and constrict the pupil, regulating the amount of light that enters the eye; pigment in this tissue gives the eye its color.

lacrimal glands The glands that produce fluids to keep the eye moist; also called tear glands.

lens The transparent part of the eye through which images are focused on the retina.

optic nerve A cranial nerve that transmits visual information to the brain.

orbit The bony eye socket.

pupil The circular opening in the middle of the iris that admits light to the back of the eye.

retina The light-sensitive area of the eye where images are projected; a layer of cells at the back of the eye that changes the light image into electrical impulses, which are carried by the optic nerve to the brain.

retinal detachment Separation of the retina from its attachments at the back of the eye.

sclera The tough, fibrous white portion of the eye that protects the more delicate inner structures.

Assessment in Action

You are dispatched to a "fireworks incident, child injured." You arrive at a private residence to find an alert, oriented, screaming 10-year-old boy who, according to his parents, was coming around the corner of the house when a cherry bomb was thrown in that direction. Apparently, the cherry bomb exploded in his face. The parents state that the child did not lose consciousness.

Assessment reveals superficial and partial-thickness burns on the left side of his face involving his ear, left cheek, nose, and lips. His left eye appears swollen, with bruising appearing on both his upper and lower eyelids. His left eye appears to be tearing; the tears appear clear. A section of his hair is singed as is his left eyebrow and eyelashes. He also has smoke and powder residue on the left side of his face. As you progress through your assessment, you cannot convince the patient to open his eye because "it hurts too much." He does not know if he could see out of that eye immediately after the incident. Vital signs include a pulse of 134 beats/min, respirations of 26 breaths/min, and a blood pressure of 124/82 mm Hg.

1. Excessive tearing from his left eye may indicate which of the following?
   A. The eye is irritated.
   B. He has lacerated the globe.
   C. A hyphema is present.
   D. The lens has ruptured.

2. The purpose of tearing is to:
   A. express emotions such as sadness or happiness.
   B. flush the eye of any foreign material.
   C. prevent any mucus from clouding the eye.
   D. provide nourishment to the conjunctiva.

3. Which of the following should be done for this patient's eyes immediately?
   A. Patching both eyes to prevent any unnecessary movement of the eye itself
   B. Attempting to visualize his eye to determine appropriate treatment
   C. Irrigating his eyes immediately; visualization is not necessary
   D. Applying direct pressure with dry, sterile dressings for 3 to 5 minutes

4. You attempt to look at the patient's eye and discover that the conjunctiva of his eye is extremely red and irritated. You notice black powder located on the right half of his globe. You also note a hyphema is present. Appropriate treatment includes which of the following?
   A. Immediate patching of both eyes
   B. Applying a moist, sterile dressing over the injured eye
   C. Covering the injured eye with a protective metal eye shield
   D. Irrigating the eye to remove the powder

5. Which of the following is the appropriate method to use to irrigate this patient's eye?
   A. Running water from the right eye to the left eye
   B. Running water from the left eye to the right eye
   C. Squirting water under high pressure into the left eye
   D. Flushing from the nasal side of the eye to the lateral side

6. Your patient is complaining of seeing a very bright light prior to the explosion and now has pain and excessive tearing. After irrigating his eye, the best method of treatment en route to the hospital includes:
   A. shutting off all interior lights and maintaining a calm atmosphere.
   B. patching both eyes with sterile, moist pads and transport supine.
   C. transporting in a sitting position and keep him warm en route.
   D. patching the eyes is not necessary but you should protect them from bright lights.

7. Because this was an explosion from a firecracker that occurred in close proximity to the patient, what other injuries should you suspect?
   A. Ruptured eardrums
   B. Lung damage
   C. Ruptured abdominal hollow organs
   D. Ruptured abdominal solid organs

Challenging Questions

8. On arrival at the hospital, your patient starts to have a nosebleed. The physician tells you the bleeding is coming from the patient's eye. How could this be?

9. Why should patients with traumatic eye injuries be transported in a supine position?

10. What is the advantage of having both eyes patched?

Points to Ponder

You are dispatched to chemical burn at a local manufacturing plant. You arrive to find an employee standing at an eye wash station, flushing her eyes. Other employees are watching and encouraging her to keep flushing. You find out that she has spilled sulfuric acid in her eyes and that she has been flushing them for about 20 minutes. You decide to stop flushing long enough to assess the injury. You find her left eye to be surprisingly unaffected considering the amount of burns around the eyelid. Her right eye appears to be burned quite badly. The patient tells you that her left eye is "fake," she lost it in a childhood accident and wants to know how bad her right eye is. She keeps asking if she is going to be blind. What would you tell the woman?

How would you treat this differently knowing that she has lost one eye already? How would you comfort her?

Issues Dealing with Disabling Injuries, Comforting Patients, Honesty vs Comfort, Affects of Disabling Injuries on Care Providers, Critical Incident Stress Teams.

Online Outlook

Injuries to the eye are very common, and you will encounter many in your work as an EMT-B. Proper emergency medical care for these injuries can minimize damage, which can often be severe. Review your knowledge of different types of eye injuries by completing Exercise 25 at www.emtb.com.

www.emtb.com

Face and Throat Injuries

Cognitive

1. Describe the causes of upper airway obstruction in facial injuries (p 604).
2. List the steps in the emergency medical care of the patient with soft-tissue wounds of the face and neck (p 604).
3. List the steps in the emergency medical care of the patient with injuries of the nose and ear (p 606).
4. List the physical findings of a patient with a facial fracture (p 608).
5. List the steps in the emergency medical care of the patient with a penetrating injury to the neck (p 609).
6. List the steps in the emergency medical care of the patient with an upper airway injury (p 609).
7. List the steps in the emergency medical care of the patient with dental injuries (p 608).

Affective

None

Psychomotor

8. Demonstrate the care of a patient with soft-tissue wounds of the face and neck (p 605).
9. Demonstrate the care of a patient with injuries of the nose and ear (p 606).
10. Demonstrate the care of a patient with a penetrating injury to the neck (p 609).
11. Demonstrate the care of a patient with an upper airway injury (p 609).
12. Demonstrate the care of a patient with dental injuries (p 608).

* All of the objectives in this chapter are noncurriculum objectives.

You are the EMT

You are dispatched to the North End Karate School for a 19-year-old female patient who is having difficulty breathing after being kicked in the throat.

Because of the associated airway management implications, injuries to the face and/or throat must be carefully assessed and managed. This chapter offers information that you will need to know to manage these injuries appropriately. It will also help you answer the following questions:

1. What are some of the physical findings you'd expect when caring for a patient with a suspected facial fracture?

2. Can you list at least two possible causes of airway obstruction for a patient with facial injuries?

Face and Throat Injuries

T he face and neck are particularly vulnerable to injury because of their relatively unprotected positions on the body. Soft-tissue injuries and fractures to the bones of the face are common and vary greatly in severity. Some are potentially life-threatening, and many leave disfiguring scars if not treated properly. With appropriate prehospital and hospital care, what may at first seem to be a devastating injury can have a surprisingly good outcome.

As an EMT-B, your objective is to prevent further injury, particularly to the cervical spine, to manage any acute airway problems, and to control bleeding. This chapter first reviews the anatomy of the head and neck, then examines the factors that can produce upper airway obstruction. A discussion of emergency medical care of soft-tissue wounds of the face, nose, and ear; facial fractures; penetrating injuries of the neck; and dental injuries follows.

Anatomy of the Head and Neck

The head is divided into two parts: the cranium and the face. The **cranium**, or skull, contains the brain, which connects to the spinal cord through the **foramen magnum**, a large opening at the base of the skull. The most posterior portion of the cranium is called the **occiput**. On each side of the cranium, the lateral portions are called the temples or temporal regions. Between the temporal regions and the occiput lie the parietal regions. The forehead is called the frontal region. Just anterior to the ear, in the temporal region, you can feel the pulse of the superficial temporal artery. The thick skin covering the cranium, which usually bears hair, is called the scalp.

The face is composed of the eyes, ears, nose, mouth, cheeks, and jowls. Six bones—the nasal bone, the two **maxillae** (upper jawbones), the two zygomas (cheekbones), and the mandible (jawbone)—are the major bones of the face (► **Figure 26-1**).

The orbit of the eye is composed of the lower edge of the frontal bone of the skull, the zygoma, the maxilla, and the nasal bone. The bony orbit protects the eye from injury. By viewing the face from the side, you can see the eyeball recessed in the orbit. Only the proximal one-third of the nose—the bridge—is formed by bone. The remaining two-thirds are composed of cartilage. Unlike the nose, the exposed portion of the ear is composed entirely of cartilage that is covered by skin. The external, visible part of the ear is called the **pinna** (► **Figure 26-2**). The earlobes are the fleshy portions at the bottom of each ear. The **tragus** is a small, rounded, fleshy bulge immediately anterior to the ear canal. The superficial temporal artery can be palpated just anterior to the tragus. About 1″ posterior to the external opening of the ear is a prominent bony mass at the base of the skull called the **mastoid process**.

The **mandible** forms the jaw and chin. Motion of the mandible occurs at the **temporomandibular joint (TMJ)**, which lies just in front of the ear on either side of the face. Below the ear and anterior to the mastoid process, the angle of the mandible is easily palpated.

The neck also contains many important structures. It is supported by the cervical spine, or the first seven vertebrae in the spinal column (C1 through C7). The spinal cord exits from the foramen magnum and lies within the spinal canal formed by the vertebrae. The upper part of the esophagus and the trachea lie deep in the midline of the neck. The carotid arteries may be

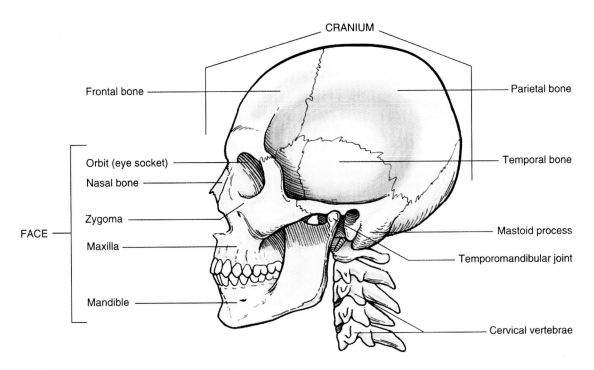

CRANIUM

Frontal bone

Parietal bone

Temporal bone

Orbit (eye socket)

Nasal bone

Zygoma

FACE

Maxilla

Mastoid process

Temporomandibular joint

Mandible

Cervical vertebrae

Figure 26-1 The face is composed of six bones: the nasal bone, two maxillae, two zygomas, and the mandible.

Figure 26-2 Principal features of the head and neck include the pinna, the tragus, the mastoid process, the occiput, the seventh cervical vertebra, and the temporomandibular joint.

Thyroid cartilage

Carotid arteries

Sternocleido-mastoid muscle

Cricoid cartilage

Cricothyroid membrane

Trachea

Figure 26-3 Important landmarks in the neck include the cricoid cartilage, the thyroid cartilage, the carotid arteries, the cricothyroid membrane, and the sternocleidomastoid muscles.

found on either side of the trachea, along with the jugular veins and several nerves.

Several useful landmarks can be palpated and seen in the neck ▲ **Figure 26-3**. The most obvious is the firm prominence in the center of the anterior surface commonly known as the **Adam's apple**. Specifically, this prominence is the upper part of the larynx, formed by the thyroid cartilage. It is more prominent in men than in women. The other portion of the larynx is the cricoid cartilage, a firm ridge of cartilage inferior to the thyroid cartilage, which is somewhat more difficult to palpate. Between the thyroid cartilage and the cricoid cartilage in the midline of the neck is a soft depression, the cricothyroid membrane. This is a thin sheet of connective tissue (fascia) that joins the two cartilages. The cricothyroid membrane is covered at this point only by skin.

Inferior to the larynx, several additional firm ridges are palpable in the anterior midline. These ridges are the cartilage rings of the trachea. The trachea connects the larynx with the main air passages of the lungs (the bronchi). On either side of the lower larynx and the upper trachea lies the thyroid gland. Unless it is enlarged, this gland is usually not palpable.

Pulsations of the carotid arteries are easily palpable in a groove 1 to 2 cm lateral to the larynx. Lying immediately adjacent to these arteries, but not palpable, are the internal jugular veins and several important nerves. Lateral to these vessels and nerves lie the **sternocleidomastoid muscles**. These muscles originate from the mastoid process of the cranium and insert into the medial border of each collarbone and the sternum at the base of the neck. They allow movement of the head.

A series of bony prominences lie posteriorly, in the midline of the neck. They are the spines of the cervical vertebrae. The lower cervical spines are more prominent than the upper ones. They are more easily palpable when the neck is in flexion. At the base of the neck posteriorly, the most prominent spine is the seventh cervical vertebra.

Injuries of the Face

Injuries about the face often lead to partial or complete obstruction of the upper airway. Several factors may contribute to the obstruction. Bleeding from facial injuries can be very heavy, producing large blood clots in the upper airway. These clots can lead to complete obstruction, particularly in a patient who is not fully conscious. In particular, direct injuries to the nose and mouth, the larynx, or the trachea are often the source of significant bleeding. In addition, as a result of an injury, loosened teeth or dentures may become dislodged into the throat, where they may be swallowed or aspirated. The swelling that often accompanies injury to the soft tissues in these areas can also contribute to the obstruction.

The airway may also be affected when the patient's head is turned to the side, as so often is the case with a patient who has an altered level of consciousness or is unconscious. Other factors that interfere with normal respirations include possible injuries to the brain and/or

cervical spine that may be associated with facial injuries. If the great vessels in the neck are injured, significant bleeding and pressure on the upper airway are common; these result in airway obstruction as well.

Soft-Tissue Injuries

Soft-tissue injuries of the face and scalp are very common. The skin and underlying tissues in these areas have a rich blood supply, so bleeding from penetrating injuries may be heavy. Indeed, even minor soft-tissue wounds of the face and scalp may bleed a great deal. A blunt injury that does not break the skin may cause a break in a blood vessel wall, leading blood to collect under the skin; this is called a **hematoma** (▼ **Figure 26-4**). Often, a flap of skin is peeled back, or **avulsed**, from the underlying muscle and fascia (▼ **Figure 26-5**).

Figure 26-4 Facial hematoma. These injuries are often caused by interpersonal altercations.

Figure 26-5 A major avulsion injury is characterized by a large flap of skin that is peeled back from the underlying muscle and tissue.

The emergency care of soft-tissue injuries to the face and scalp is the same as treatment of soft-tissue injuries elsewhere on the body. You should assess the ABCs and care for any life threats first. Remember also to follow BSI precautions in all cases.

Your first step is to open and clear the airway. Remember that blood draining into the throat can produce vomiting and airway obstruction. Take appropriate precautions if you suspect that the patient has sustained a cervical spine injury; be sure to avoid moving the neck. Use the jaw-thrust to open the patient's airway, and then suction the mouth. Once the patient is immobilized in a cervical collar and on a backboard, you can turn the backboard to one side to allow any blood or vomitus to drain out of the mouth rather than pool in the pharynx and obstruct the airway.

Control bleeding by applying direct manual pressure with a dry, sterile dressing. Use roller gauze, wrapped around the circumference of the head, to hold a pressure dressing in place ▼ Figure 26-6 . Do not apply excessive pressure if there is a possibility of underlying skull fracture. When an injury exposes the brain, eye, or other structures, cover the exposed parts with a moist, sterile dressing to protect them from further damage ▶ Figure 26-7 . For injuries in which the skin is not broken, apply ice locally to help control the swelling of bruised tissues.

For soft-tissue injuries around the mouth, you should always check for bleeding inside the mouth. Broken teeth and lacerations to the tongue may cause profuse bleeding and obstruction of the upper airway ▼ Figure 26-8 . Often, the patient will swallow the blood from lacerations inside the mouth, so the hemorrhage may not be apparent. You should also inspect the

Figure 26-7   An injury that exposes the brain, eye, or other structures (A) should be covered with a moist, sterile dressing to prevent further damage (B).

Figure 26-6   Use roller gauze, wrapped around the circumference of the head, to hold a pressure dressing in place.

Figure 26-8   Soft-tissue injuries around the mouth can be associated with profuse bleeding inside the mouth and obstruction of the airway.

inside of the mouth for bleeding and hidden injuries in patients who have sustained facial trauma. Remember that patients who swallow blood are prone to vomiting.

Often, physicians will be able to graft a piece of avulsed skin back into the appropriate position. For this reason, if you find portions of avulsed skin that have become separated, you should wrap them in a sterile dressing, place them in a plastic bag, and keep them cool. Deliver the bag to the emergency department along with the patient. In many avulsion injuries, the skin will still be attached in a loose flap (▼ **Figure 26-9**). Place the flap in a position that is as close to normal as possible, and hold it in place with a dry, sterile dressing. These steps will help to increase the patient's chances of being restored to normal appearance.

Injuries of the Nose

The nose often takes the brunt of deliberate physical assaults and car crashes. Blunt injuries to the nose caused by a fist or a dashboard may be associated with fractures and soft-tissue injuries of the face, head injuries, and/or injuries to the cervical spine.

In assessing injuries involving the nose, it helps to picture the inside of the nose itself (▶ **Figure 26-10**). The nasal cavity is divided into two sections or chambers by the nasal septum, which is made of cartilage. Within each nasal chamber, there are layers of bone called the **turbinates**, which are covered with a moist lining. Both chambers have a superior turbinate, a middle turbinate, and an inferior turbinate. As we breathe, the air moves through the nasal chambers and is humidified as it passes over the turbinates. Directly above the nose are the frontal sinuses and, on either side, the orbit of the eye.

All these structures should be assessed for injury. In cases of severe injury, there may also be injury to the

cervical spine. Keep in mind that cerebrospinal fluid (CSF) may escape down through the nose (or ears) following a fracture at the base of the skull. If blood or drainage contains CSF, a characteristic staining of the dressing will occur.

You can control bleeding from abrasions and lacerations to the nose by applying a sterile dressing. If the patient is bleeding heavily from the nose, place the patient in a sitting position, leaning forward, and pinch the nostrils together (▼ **Figure 26-11**). For a detailed

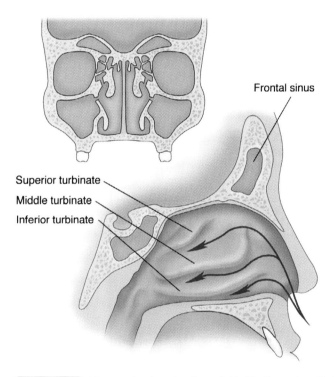

Figure 26-10 The nose has two chambers, divided by the septum. Each chamber is composed of layers of bone called turbinates. Above the nose are the frontal sinuses and, on either side, the orbit of the eye.

Figure 26-9 If avulsed skin is still attached, place the flap in a position that is as close to normal as possible, and hold it in place with a dry, sterile dressing.

Figure 26-11 Control bleeding from the nose by pinching the nostrils together.

discussion of the care for epistaxis, see *Skill Drill 22-4* in the Bleeding chapter.

Injuries of the Ear

The ear is a complex organ that is associated with both hearing and balance. The ear is divided into three parts ▼**Figure 26-12** . The external ear is composed of the pinna, or auricle, which is the part lying outside of the head, and the **external auditory canal**, which leads in toward the **tympanic membrane**, or eardrum. The middle ear contains three small bones (the hammer, anvil, and stirrup) that move in response to sound waves hitting the tympanic membrane. This is the mechanism by which we appreciate sounds. The middle ear is connected to the nasal cavity by the **eustachian tube**, which is the internal auditory canal. This connection permits equalization of pressure in the middle ear when external atmospheric pressure changes. The inner ear is composed of bony chambers filled with fluid. As the head moves, so does the fluid. In response, fine nerve endings within the fluid send impulses to the brain indicating both the position of the head and the rate of change of position.

Ears are often injured, but they usually do not bleed very much. If local pressure does not control the bleeding, you can apply a roller dressing ▶**Figure 26-13** . First, however, you should place a soft, padded dressing

between the ear and the scalp, as bandaging the ear against the tender underlying scalp is extremely painful. In the case of an ear avulsion, you should wrap the avulsed part in a moist sterile dressing and put it in a plastic bag. Often, avulsed tissue from the ear can be reattached.

The external auditory canal is a favorite place for children to place foreign bodies such as peanuts or candy. All such items should be removed by a physician in the emergency department. Never try to manipulate the foreign body, as you may press it further into the auditory canal and cause permanent damage to the tympanic membrane.

Again, you should note any clear fluid coming from the ear of a severely injured patient, since this may indicate a fracture at the base of the skull.

Figure 26-12 The ear has three principal parts: the external ear, composed of the pinna, external auditory canal, and tympanic membrane; the middle ear, including the hammer, anvil, and stirrup; and the inner ear, composed of bony chambers filled with fluid.

Figure 26-13 **A.** A major laceration of the ear is shown. **B.** Proper treatment includes use of a soft, sterile pad behind the ear, between it and the scalp. Then wrap a roller gauze dressing around the head to include the entire ear.

Facial Fractures

Fractures of the facial bones typically result from blunt impact. For example, the patient's head collides with a steering wheel or windshield in an automobile crash or is hit by a baseball bat or pipe in an assault. You should assume that any patient who has sustained a direct blow to the mouth or nose has a facial fracture. Other clues to the possibility of fracture include bleeding in the mouth, inability to swallow or talk, absent or loose teeth, and/or loose or movable bone fragments. Patients may also report that "it doesn't feel right" when they close their jaw, signaling an irregularity of bite.

Facial fractures alone are not acute emergencies unless there is serious bleeding ▶ **Figure 26-14** . Such bleeding can be life-threatening. In addition to external hemorrhage, there is the danger of blood clots in the upper airway, leading to obstruction of the upper airway. Fractures around the face and mouth can also produce deformity and loose bone fragments. However, plastic surgeons can repair the damage perfectly as long as 7 to 10 days after the injury. Be sure to remove and save loose teeth or bone fragments from the mouth; it is often possible to reimplant them ▶ **Figure 26-15** . Remove dentures and dental bridges to protect against airway obstruction.

Another source of potential airway obstruction is swelling, which can be extreme within the first 24 hours after injury. If you notice swelling during assessment or at any time while the patient is under your care, you should check for airway obstruction.

Dislodged teeth which are not causing airway obstruction should be transported with the patient, either in a container of the patient's saliva or milk, if possible.

Injuries of the Neck

The neck contains many structures that are vulnerable to injury either by blunt trauma, such as from a steering wheel in a car crash, or by penetrating injury, such as a stab or gunshot wound. These structures include the upper airway, the esophagus, the carotid arteries and jugular veins, the thyroid cartilage or Adam's apple, the cricoid cartilage, and the upper trachea. Any injury to the neck is serious and should be considered life-threatening until proven otherwise in the emergency department.

Blunt Injuries

Any crushing injury of the upper part of the neck is likely to involve the larynx or trachea. Examples include a collision with a steering wheel, an attempted suicide by hanging, and a clothesline injury sustained while riding a bicycle. Once the cartilages of the upper airway and larynx are fractured, they do not spring

Figure 26-14 Bleeding following a crush injury to the face can be life-threatening because, in addition to the external hemorrhage, blood clots in the airway can cause a complete obstruction.

Figure 26-15 **A.** Save any lost teeth or bone fragments following an injury to the mouth. **B.** Even with traumatic loss of a tooth, the possibility of successful reimplantation is very good.

back to their normal position. Such a fracture can lead to loss of voice, severe and sometimes fatal airway obstruction, and leakage of air into the soft tissues of the neck ▶ **Figure 26-16** . The presence of air in the soft tissues produces a characteristic crackling sensation called **subcutaneous emphysema**. If you feel this sensation when you palpate the neck, you should maintain the airway as best you can and provide immediate transport. Be aware that complete airway obstruction can develop very rapidly in these patients as a result of

Skill Drill 26-1   Controlling Bleeding from a Neck Injury

Apply direct pressure to control bleeding.

Use a roller gauze to secure a dressing in place.

Wrap the bandage around and under the patient's shoulder.

swelling or bleeding into underlying tissues. It may be very difficult to manage the airway in patients; some will require a surgical airway at the hospital. You should also keep in mind that an incident involving an injury to the throat may also have caused a c-spine injury.

Figure 26-16 Fractures of the larynx or trachea can cause air to leak from the airway into the subcutaneous tissues. The presence of air in the soft tissues produces a crackling sensation called subcutaneous emphysema.

Figure 26-17 Penetrating injuries to the neck can result in profuse bleeding if the carotid artery or the jugular vein is damaged.

Penetrating Injuries

Penetrating injuries to the neck can cause profuse bleeding from laceration of the great vessels in the neck, either the carotid artery or the jugular veins **▼ Figure 26-17** . The airway, the esophagus, and even the spinal cord can also be damaged by a penetrating injury.

Direct pressure over the bleeding site will control most neck bleeding. Follow the steps in **▲ Skill Drill 26-1** :

1. **Apply direct pressure** to the bleeding site using your gloved fingertips and a sterile dressing **(Step 1)**.
2. **Secure the dressing in place** with roller gauze adding more dressing if needed **(Step 2)**.
3. **Wrap the gauze around and under the patient's shoulder.** Do not wrap the gauze around the neck to avoid possible airway and circulation problems **(Step 3)**.

However, the tissues within the neck may still bleed and compress the upper airway, so you should look for signs of airway obstruction. If a vein has been opened, air may be sucked through it to the heart, a clinical situation called **air embolism**. A large amount of air in the right atrium and right ventricle can lead to cardiac arrest.

You might find it necessary to apply pressure both above and below the penetrating wound to control life-threatening bleeding from the carotid artery (above) and the jugular vein (below). You may also need to treat the patient for shock.

Always maintain cervical spine immobilization, and with the patient fully immobilized to a backboard, provide prompt transport. Ensure that the airway remains open en route and apply high-flow oxygen.

Prep Kit

Ready for Review

Soft-tissue injuries and fractures to the bones of the face and neck are common and vary in severity. Proper emergency care can improve the patient's chances of making a complete recovery in health and appearance. Your priorities are to prevent further injury, especially to the cervical spine, and to manage any acute airway problems. These problems can result from heavy bleeding, swelling, and injuries to the brain or cervical spine that interfere with normal respiration.

To control the often heavy bleeding from soft-tissue injuries to the face and scalp, use direct manual pressure with a dry sterile dressing, unless you suspect a skull fracture. Use a moist sterile dressing for exposed parts of the brain or eye. Always check for bleeding inside the mouth. Open and clear the airway in all patients with facial injuries. Save any pieces of avulsed skin for possible attachment later; hold any avulsed flaps in place with a dry sterile dressing. If the patient is bleeding heavily from an injury to the nose, apply a sterile dressing.

Injuries to the ear usually do not bleed very much. If local pressure does not control the bleeding, you can apply a roller dressing. Remember to place padding between the ear and the scalp, as bandaging the ear against the tender underlying scalp is extremely painful. Often, avulsed tissue from the ear can be reattached, so save any avulsed tissue. Always leave foreign bodies in the ear for a physician to remove. Watch for clear fluid coming from the ear or nose; this may indicate a basal skull fracture.

Assume that any patient who has sustained a direct blow to the nose or mouth has a facial fracture. Signs of fracture include irregularity of bite, inability to swallow or talk, and bleeding in the mouth. Check for airway obstruction if you notice swelling or if there is serious bleeding.

Both blunt and penetrating injuries to the neck can be life-threatening. With blunt injuries, you should palpate the neck and feel for the characteristic crackling called subcutaneous emphysema; patients with this sign may be in danger of complete airway obstruction within minutes. Direct pressure over the bleeding site will control most neck bleeding. However, bleeding may still occur within the tissues of the neck and compress the upper airway. If a vein has been lacerated, be alert for the possibility of air embolism. You may have to apply pressure both above and below the penetrating wound to control life-threatening bleeding from the carotid artery and jugular vein. Patients with a neck injury require spinal immobilization and prompt transport.

Vital Vocabulary

Adam's apple The firm prominence in the upper part of the larynx formed by the thyroid cartilage.

air embolism The presence of air in the veins, which can lead to cardiac arrest if it enters the heart.

avulse To pull or tear away.

cranium The skull.

eustachian tube The internal auditory canal that connects the middle ear to the nasal cavity.

external auditory canal The ear canal; leads to the tympanic membrane.

foramen magnum The large opening at the base of the skull through which the brain connects to the spinal cord.

hematoma The collection of blood in a space, tissue, or organ due to a break in the wall of a blood vessel.

mandible The bone of the lower jaw.

mastoid process The prominent bony mass at the base of the skull about 1" posterior to the external opening of the ear.

maxilla The bone that forms the upper jaw on either side of the face and contains the upper teeth, the orbit of the eye, the nasal cavity, and the palate.

occiput The most posterior portion of the skull.

pinna The external, visible part of the ear.

sternocleidomastoid muscles Muscles on either side of the neck that allow movement of the head.

subcutaneous emphysema A characteristic crackling sensation on palpation, caused by the presence of air in soft tissues.

temporomandibular joint (TMJ) The joint formed where the mandible and cranium meet, just in front of the ear.

tragus The small, rounded, fleshy bulge that lies immediately anterior to the ear canal.

turbinates Layers of bone within the nasal cavity.

tympanic membrane The eardrum, which lies between the external and middle ear.

Assessment in Action

Thirty minutes before shift change, you and your partner are dispatched to a duplex for a "man hemorrhaging." When you arrive you find a 31-year-old man lying on the floor next to a shattered glass coffee table. According to his wife, your patient tripped over a rug and fell onto the glass coffee table. The wife stated that she heard a crash and ran into the room to see what happened.

When she saw her husband bleeding on the floor, she called EMS. She stated that he did not lose consciousness. However, she admitted that she was only focusing on controlling the bleeding from her husband's neck wound. Your assessment reveals that the man is alert and oriented. He is talking in complete sentences but is spitting blood. He has suffered multiple lacerations to the face and neck. He has a laceration to the right cheek about 2" long and a 4"-long laceration to the right side of his neck, just below the ear, and down the shoulder. The bleeding from the neck appears to be controlled, but there is a significant amount of blood on the towel that the wife used to apply pressure to the wound. Vital signs include a pulse of 110 beats/min, respirations of 22 breaths/min, and a blood pressure of 132/82 mm Hg.

1. What is the highest priority in caring for this patient?
   - **A.** Administering low concentrations of oxygen.
   - **B.** Treating potential or actual airway obstruction.
   - **C.** Applying sterile dressings and bandaging the wound.
   - **D.** Providing complete immobilization to a long spine board.

2. Which of the following interventions is acceptable for controlling bleeding of his neck injury?
   - **A.** A wide band as a tourniquet
   - **B.** A circumferential pressure dressing
   - **C.** Direct pressure with a sterile dressing
   - **D.** A pressure point

3. In most cases, a patient who sustains trauma to the face or throat should be placed in which of the following positions?
   - **A.** Prone
   - **B.** Supine
   - **C.** Sitting up
   - **D.** Turned to the side

4. Which of the following tools is considered an essential treatment adjunct for this patient, who has sustained face and neck trauma and is spontaneously breathing?

   - **A.** PASG
   - **B.** BVM device
   - **C.** Portable suction
   - **D.** Hemostats

5. Which of the following statements about airway obstruction related to blunt trauma to the neck is true in this patient situation?
   - **A.** Immediate transport is necessary because of the danger of possible obstruction.
   - **B.** Airway obstruction is not likely to develop for at least 2 to 3 hours after the injury.
   - **C.** Complete airway obstruction secondary to trauma is easily managed in the field by EMT-Bs.
   - **D.** Airway obstruction rarely occurs as a complication of blunt trauma to the neck.

6. Additional injuries that you should suspect in this patient include:
   - **A.** internal abdominal injuries.
   - **B.** head and spinal injuries.
   - **C.** injury to the respiratory system.
   - **D.** disturbance with hearing and sight.

7. Assessment of this patient's neck should involve which of the following?
   - **A.** Palpation for subcutaneous emphysema
   - **B.** Palpation of the anterior cervical vertebra
   - **C.** Listening over the carotid artery for abnormal sounds
   - **D.** Listening over the wound site for subcutaneous emphysema

Challenging Questions

8. Every effort should be taken to prevent this patient from swallowing blood. Why is this important?

9. This patient is at risk for an air embolism if a major vein has been lacerated. How would you know if an air embolism occurred?

10. How would you appropriately bandage this patient's neck wound?

Points to Ponder

You work in a system where paramedics are dispatched through the fire system and cannot transport. EMT-Bs staff a private ambulance and transport patients. You are first on scene at a softball game where a player was hit in the throat by a ball. The patient is unresponsive and rapidly losing the ability to breathe. You insert an nasopaharyngeal airway and there is no improvement. You start oxygen. The paramedics arrive shortly after your patient assessment. You provide a hand-off report emphasizing the decreased ability to breathe. By this time the patient is unable to exchange air. The paramedics argue briefly about whether to intubate or to "load and go." They decide to transport and intubate on the way. You are in the back with the paramedic and your partner is driving. In the ambulance, the paramedic is unable to intubate the patient. Shortly after reaching the hospital the patient arrests and dies. You hear the physician ask why they did not intubate on-scene and the paramedic says that the patient had an airway until just before they arrived at the hospital. Would you report this and if so, to whom? Would you tell the family what happened? How would reporting this affect your relationship with other paramedics?

Issues Advanced Airway Management, EMT/Paramedic Relationships, Reporting Procedures, Impact of Reporting Treatment Issues.

Online Outlook

Soft-tissue injuries and fractures to the bones of the face and neck are common and vary in severity. Your priorities are to prevent further injury, especially to the cervical spine, and to manage any acute airway problems. Review your knowledge of these priorities by completing Exercise 26 at www.emtb.com.

www.emtb.com

Chest Injuries

www.emtb.com

Online Chapter Pretest	◄
Interactivities	
Vocabulary Explorer	
Anatomy Review	
Web Links	
Online Review Manual	
Distance Learning	

Skill Drills	◄
Vital Vocabulary	
Pediatric Needs	
Geriatric Needs	
EMT-B Safety	
EMT-B Tips	
Documentation Tips	
Remember	
Prep Kit	

You are the EMT

"Squad 4, respond to Nelling College behind the gymnasium for a student shot in the chest with an arrow."

Many of the organs essential for life itself are found in the chest cavity. Injuries to this area of the body are therefore challenging. This chapter will provide you with the knowledge you'll need to care for these injuries, along with helping you answer the following questions:

1. Why is it important to seal open chest wounds as quickly as possible?

2. What are some of the possible consequences of a blunt injury to the heart? A penetrating injury?

Chest Injuries

Chest injuries are both very common and, given the likelihood of damage to the heart, lungs, or great blood vessels, potentially very serious. Any injury that interferes with normal breathing must be treated without delay to prevent permanent damage to tissues that depend on a continuous supply of oxygen. Another major problem with chest injuries may be internal bleeding. Blood from lacerations of the thoracic organs or major blood vessels can collect in the chest cavity, compressing the lungs. Also, air can collect in the chest and prevent the lungs from expanding. Your ability to act quickly to care for patients with these injuries can make the difference between a successful outcome and death.

This chapter begins with a review of the anatomy of the chest and the physiology of respiration. It then describes the common signs and symptoms of chest injuries and the proper emergency medical treatment for specific injuries.

Anatomy and Physiology of the Chest

To understand and evaluate chest injuries in the pre-hospital setting, you must first understand the anatomy of the chest and the mechanism by which gases are exchanged during breathing. A quick review will help you to appreciate the logic in both the emergency treatment of chest injuries and the potential complications of that treatment.

The chest (thoracic cage) extends from the lower end of the neck to the diaphragm ▶ **Figure 27-1** . In an individual who is lying down or who has just completed exhalation, the diaphragm may rise as high as the nipple line. Thus, a penetrating injury to the chest, such as a gunshot or stab wound, may penetrate the lung and diaphragm and injure the liver or stomach.

The contents of the chest are partially protected by the ribs, which are connected in the back to the vertebrae and in the front, through the costal cartilages, to the sternum ▶ **Figure 27-2** . The trachea, which is in the middle of the neck, divides into the left and right mainstem bronchi, which supply air to the lungs. Of course, the thoracic cage also contains the heart and the great vessels: the aorta, the right innominate and left subclavian arteries and their branches, and the superior and inferior venae cavae. The esophagus runs through the back of the chest, connecting the pharynx above with the stomach and the abdomen. At the bottom of the chest, the diaphragm is a muscle that separates the thoracic cavity from the abdominal cavity.

When you inhale, the intercostal muscles between the ribs contract, elevating the rib cage. At the same time, the diaphragm contracts and pushes the contents of the abdomen down. The pressure inside the chest decreases, and air enters the lungs through the nose and mouth. When you exhale, the intercostal muscles and diaphragm relax, and the tissues move back to their normal positions, allowing air to be exhaled. Note that the nerves supplying the diaphragm (the phrenic nerves) exit the spinal cord at C3, C4, and C5. A patient whose spinal cord is injured at the C5 level or below will lose the power to move his or her intercostal muscles, but the diaphragm will still contract. The patient will still be able to breathe because the phrenic nerves remain intact. Patients with spinal cord injuries at C3 or above can lose their ability to breathe entirely ▶ **Figure 27-3** .

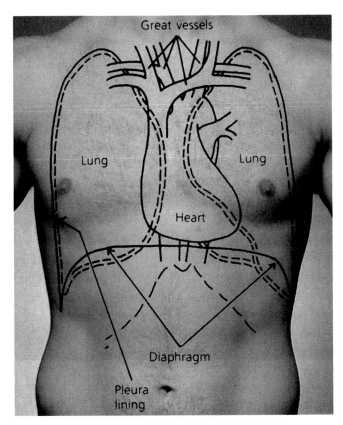

Figure 27-1 A view of the anterior aspect of the chest shows the major organs beneath the surface.

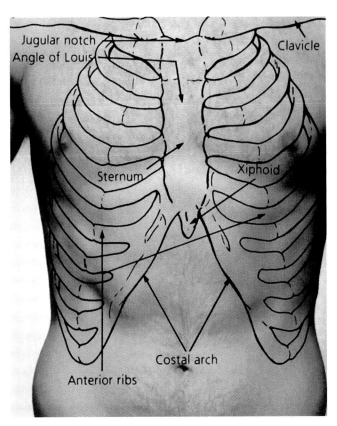

Figure 27-2 The organs within the chest are protected by the ribs, which are connected in back to the vertebrae and in the front, through the costal cartilages, to the sternum.

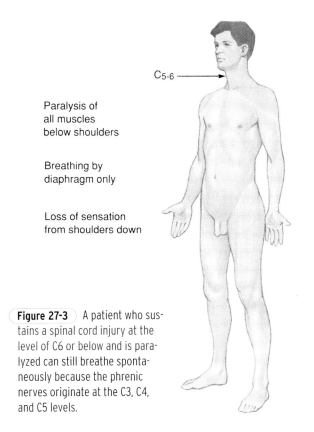

C_{5-6}

Paralysis of all muscles below shoulders

Breathing by diaphragm only

Loss of sensation from shoulders down

Figure 27-3 A patient who sustains a spinal cord injury at the level of C6 or below and is paralyzed can still breathe spontaneously because the phrenic nerves originate at the C3, C4, and C5 levels.

Injuries of the Chest

There are two basic types of chest injuries: open or closed. As the name implies, a **closed chest injury** is one in which the skin is not broken. This type of injury is generally caused by blunt trauma, such as when a driver strikes a steering wheel in a motor vehicle crash or is struck by a falling object ▶ **Figure 27-4** . In **open chest injuries**, the chest wall itself is penetrated by some object such as a knife, a bullet, a piece of metal, or the broken end of a fractured rib ▶ **Figure 27-5** .

In blunt trauma, a blow to the chest may fracture the ribs, the sternum, or whole areas of the chest wall, bruise the lungs and the heart, and even damage the aorta. Almost one-third of people who are killed immediately in car crashes die as a result of traumatic rupture of the aorta. Although the skin and chest wall are not penetrated in a closed injury, the contents of the chest may be lacerated by broken ribs. Indeed, vital organs can actually be torn from their attachment in the chest cavity without any break in the skin.

Figure 27-4 Closed injuries usually result from blunt trauma, such as when a patient strikes the steering wheel in a motor vehicle crash or is struck by a falling object.

Figure 27-5 Open injuries occur when the chest wall is penetrated by some type of object or the broken end of a fractured rib.

Signs and Symptoms

Important signs and symptoms of chest injury include the following:

- Pain at the site of injury
- Pain localized at the site of injury that is aggravated by or increased with breathing
- Dyspnea (difficulty breathing, shortness of breath)
- Hemoptysis (coughing up blood)
- Failure of one or both sides of the chest to expand normally with inspiration
- Rapid, weak pulse and low blood pressure
- Cyanosis around the lips or fingernails

After a chest injury, any change in normal breathing is a particularly important sign. A healthy, uninjured adult usually breathes from 12 to 20 times per minute without difficulty and without pain. Respirations of fewer than 8/min or more than 24/min may indicate inadequate breathing. Patients with chest injuries often have __tachypnea__ (rapid respirations) and shallow respirations because it hurts to take a deep breath.

As with any other injury, pain and tenderness are common at the point of impact as a result of a bruise or fracture. Pain is usually aggravated by the normal process of breathing. Irritation of or damage to the pleural surfaces causes a characteristic sharp or sticking pain with each breath when these normally smooth surfaces slide on one another. This sharp pain is called *pleuritic pain* or *pleurisy*.

In an injured patient, __dyspnea__ (difficulty with breathing) has many causes, including airway obstruction, damage to the chest wall, improper chest expansion due to the loss of normal control of breathing, or lung compression because of accumulated blood or air. Dyspnea in an injured patient indicates significant compromise of lung function; prompt, vigorous support and transport are required.

Patient Assessment

After your initial assessment, in which you quickly evaluate the patient's ABCs and treat potential life threats, carefully observe the patient's chest wall. If the chest wall does not expand on each side when the patient inhales, the chest muscles may have lost their ability to work appropriately. Loss of muscle function may be the result of a direct injury to the chest wall, or it may be related to an injury of the nerves that control those muscles. Check also for paradoxical motion, an abnormality associated with multiple fractured ribs, in which one segment of the chest wall moves opposite of the remainder of the chest, ie, out with expiration and in with inspiration.

Rapid assessment using DCAP-BTLS is mandatory to determine the nature and extent of thoracic injury. Inspection for Deformities, such as asymmetry of the left versus right chest or shoulder girdle, may reveal the presence of multiple rib fractures, crush injuries, or significant chest wall injury. Identification of discrete areas of Contusion or Abrasion may pinpoint a specific point of impact. The presence of Puncture wounds or other penetrating injuries indicates a possible open chest injury which should be managed accordingly. Be alert for associated Burns, which may alter respiratory mechanics. Palpate for Tenderness to localize the injury and the presence of fractures. Look for Lacerations and local Swelling. Application of this systematic approach to patient assessment minimizes the chance of missing significant injury.

Hemoptysis, the spitting or coughing up of blood, usually indicates that the lung itself or the air passages have been damaged. With a laceration of the lung, blood can enter the bronchial passages and is coughed up as the patient tries to clear the airway.

A rapid, weak pulse and low blood pressure are the principal signs of hypovolemic shock, which can result from extensive bleeding from lacerated structures within the chest cavity. Shock following a chest injury may also result from insufficient oxygenation of the blood by the poorly functioning lungs.

Cyanosis in a patient with a chest injury is a sign of inadequate respiration. The classic blue appearance around the lips and fingernails indicates that blood is not being oxygenated sufficiently. Patients with cyanosis are unable to provide a sufficient supply of oxygen to the blood through the lungs and require immediate respiratory support and supplemental oxygen.

Many of these signs and symptoms occur simultaneously. When any one of them develops as a result of a chest injury, the patient requires prompt hospital care. Remember that the principal reason for concern about a patient who has a chest injury is that his or her body has no means of storing oxygen; it is supplied and used continuously, even during sleep. Any interruption in this supply can be rapidly lethal and must be treated aggressively.

Complications of Chest Injuries

Pneumothorax

In any chest injury, damage to the heart, lungs, great vessels, and other organs in the chest can be complicated by the accumulation of air in the pleural space. This is a dangerous condition called a **pneumothorax**. In this condition, air enters through a hole in the chest wall or the surface of the lung as the patient attempts to breathe, causing the lung on that side to collapse ▲ **Figure 27-6** . As a result, any blood that passes through the lung is not oxygenated, and hypoxia will develop. Depending on the size of the hole and

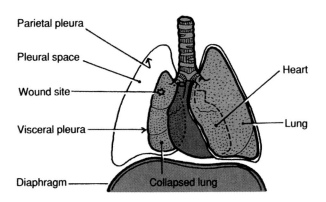

Figure 27-6 Pneumothorax occurs when air leaks into the space between the pleural surfaces from an opening in the chest wall or the surface of the lung. The lung collapses as air fills the pleural space.

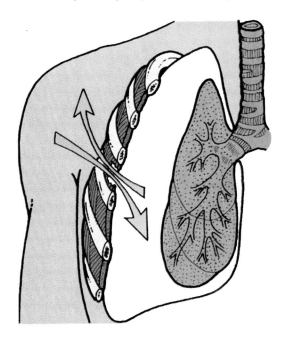

Figure 27-7 With a sucking chest wound, air passes from the outside into the pleural space and back out with each breath, creating the sucking sound.

the rate at which air fills the cavity, the lung may collapse in a few seconds or a few hours. If the hole is in the chest wall, you can actually hear this condition in the form of a sucking sound as the patient inhales and the sound of rushing air as he or she exhales. For this reason, an open or penetrating wound to the chest wall is often called a **sucking chest wound** ▲ **Figure 27-7** .

This type of open pneumothorax is a true emergency requiring immediate emergency medical care and transport. Initial emergency care, after clearing and maintaining the airway and then providing

Figure 27-8 A sucking chest wound can be sealed with a large airtight dressing that either seals all four sides (**A**), or seals three sides with the fourth left open as a flutter valve (**B**). Your local protocol will dictate the way you are to care for this injury.

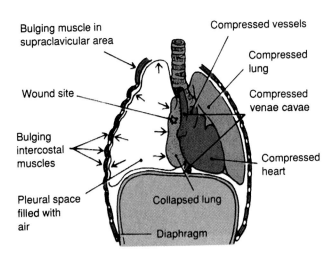

Figure 27-9 A tension pneumothorax can develop if a penetrating chest wound is bandaged tightly and air from a damaged lung cannot escape. The air then accumulates in the pleural space.

oxygen, is to rapidly seal the open wound with a sterile <u>occlusive dressing</u> ▲ Figure 27-8 . The purpose of the dressing is to seal the wound and prevent air from being sucked into the chest through the wound. Several sterile materials, including Vaseline gauze, aluminum foil, or a folded universal dressing, may be used to seal the wound. Use a large enough dressing so that it is not pulled or sucked into the chest cavity. Depending on your local protocol, you may tape the dressing down on all four sides, or you may create a <u>flutter valve</u>, a oneway valve that allows air to leave the chest cavity but not return, by taping only three sides of the dressing.

SPONTANEOUS PNEUMOTHORAX. Some individuals are born with or develop weak areas on the surface of the lungs. Occasionally, such a weak area will rupture spontaneously, allowing air to leak into the pleural space. Usually, this event, called <u>spontaneous pneumothorax</u>, is not related to any major injury but

simply happens with normal breathing. The patient experiences sudden sharp chest pain and increasing difficulty in breathing. The affected lung collapses, losing its ability to expand normally. The amount of pneumothorax that develops varies, as does the amount of respiratory distress the patient experiences.

You should suspect a spontaneous pneumothorax in a patient who experiences sudden chest pain and shortness of breath without a specific known cause. The prehospital treatment that you can provide for this type of pneumothorax is the same as that for a traumatic pneumothorax.

TENSION PNEUMOTHORAX. A potential complication that may develop if your local protocol calls for you to seal all four sides of the dressing is a <u>tension pneumothorax</u> ▲ Figure 27-9 . This can occur when there is significant ongoing air accumulation in the pleural space. In sealing a wound in the chest wall, you have effectively cut off the only escape route for air leaking into the pleural space from a lung laceration. This air gradually increases the pressure in the chest, first causing the complete collapse of the affected lung and then pushing the mediastinum (the central part of the chest containing the heart and great vessels) into the opposite pleural cavity. This prevents blood from returning through the venae cavae to the heart and can cause shock and cardiac arrest.

If signs and symptoms of a tension pneumothorax develop after sealing an open chest wound, you should partly remove the dressing to relieve the tension. As you do so, you may hear a rush of air out of the chest cavity, although this does not occur in all cases.

A tension pneumothorax can also occur as a result of closed, blunt injury of the chest in which a fractured rib lacerates a lung or bronchus. Very rarely, a tension pneumothorax may arise spontaneously. This might happen in a young adult as a result of a spontaneous pneumothorax.

The common signs and symptoms of tension pneumothorax include increasing respiratory distress, distended neck veins, deviation of the trachea to the side of the chest opposite from the tension pneumothorax, tachycardia, low blood pressure, cyanosis, and decreased breath sounds on the side of the pneumothorax.

Relieving a tension pneumothorax due to a blunt trauma in a patient is often done by inserting a needle through the rib cage into the pleural space; however, this procedure must be performed by ALS personnel or emergency department staff depending on the local protocol.

Hemothorax

In both blunt and penetrating chest injury, blood can collect in the pleural space from a bleeding rib cage, lung, or great vessel. This condition is called a **hemothorax** (▲ **Figure 27-10**). You should suspect a hemothorax if the patient has signs and symptoms of shock or decreased breath sounds on the affected side, an indication that the lung is being compressed by the blood. The presence of both air and blood in the pleural space is known as a hemopneumothorax.

Rib Fractures

Rib fractures are very common in the elderly, whose bones are brittle, but relatively uncommon in the very young, whose bones are much more supple.

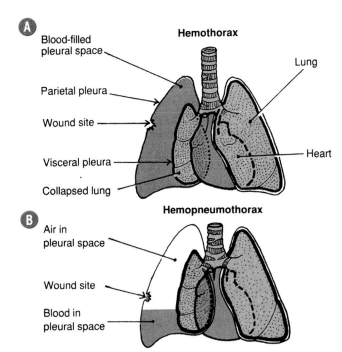

Figure 27-10 **A.** A hemothorax is a collection of blood in the pleural space produced by bleeding within the chest. **B.** When both blood and air are present, the condition is a hemopneumothorax.

Because the upper four ribs are well protected by the bony girdle of the clavicle and scapula, a fracture of one of these upper ribs is a sign of a very severe mechanism of injury.

Be aware that a fractured rib that penetrates into the pleural space may lacerate the surface of the lung, causing a pneumothorax, a tension pneumothorax, a hemothorax, or a hemopneumothorax. One sign of this development can be a crackly feeling to the skin in the area (also called *crepitus*), which indicates that air escaping from a lacerated lung is leaking into the chest wall. Be sure to relay this finding to the hospital.

Patients with one or more cracked ribs will report localized tenderness and pain on breathing. The pain is the result of broken ends of the fracture rubbing against each other with each inspiration and expiration. Patients will tend to avoid taking deep breaths, breathing rapid and shallow instead. They will often hold the affected portion of the rib cage in an effort to minimize the discomfort. These patients should receive supplemental O_2 during assessment and transport.

Flail Chest

Ribs may be fractured in more than one place. If three or more ribs are fractured in two or more places, or if the sternum is fractured along with several ribs, a segment of chest wall may be detached from the rest of the thoracic cage ▶ **Figure 27-11** . This condition is known as <u>flail chest</u>. In what is called <u>paradoxical motion</u>, the detached portion of the chest wall moves opposite of normal: in instead of out during inhalation, out instead of in during expiration. This occurs because of negative pressure that has built up in the thorax. Breathing with a flail chest can be extremely painful and often does not allow for adequate oxygenation.

Your treatment of a patient with a flail chest should include maintaining the airway, providing respiratory support if necessary, giving supplemental oxygen, and performing ongoing assessments for possible pneumothorax or other respiratory complications. Treatment may also include positive pressure ventilation with a BVM device.

The patient may find it easier and less painful to breathe if the flail segment is immobilized. You can tape a bulky pad against that segment of the chest for this purpose, although taping too tightly will also prevent adequate ventilation ▶ **Figure 27-12** . Keep in mind that while flail chest is itself a serious condition, it suggests an injury that was forceful enough to cause other serious internal damage as well.

Other Chest Injuries

Pulmonary Contusion

In addition to fracturing ribs, any severe blunt trauma to the chest can also injure the lung. The pulmonary alveoli become filled with blood, and fluid accumulates in the injured area, leaving the patient hypoxic. Severe <u>pulmonary contusion</u>, bruising of the lung, should always be suspected in patients with a flail chest and usually develops over a period of hours. If you believe that a patient may have a pulmonary contusion, you should provide respiratory support and supplemental oxygen to ensure adequate ventilation.

Traumatic Asphyxia

Sometimes, a patient will experience a sudden, severe compression of the chest, which produces a rapid increase in pressure within the chest. This may occur in an unrestrained driver who hits a steering wheel or a pedestrian who is compressed between a vehicle and a wall. The sudden increase in intrathoracic pressure results in a very characteristic appearance, including distended neck veins, cyanosis in the face and neck, and

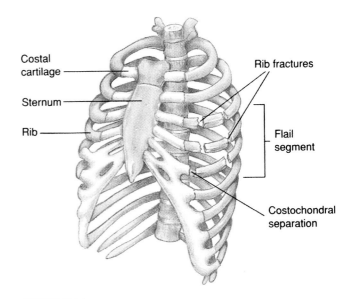

Figure 27-11 When three or more adjacent ribs are fractured in two or more places, a flail chest results. A flail segment will move paradoxically when the patient breathes.

Figure 27-12 A flail anterior chest wall segment can be stabilized by securing (or having the patient hold) a pillow firmly against the chest wall.

hemorrhage into the sclera of the eye, signaling the bursting of small blood vessels in the skin. These findings suggest an underlying injury to the heart and pulmonary contusions. You should provide ventilatory support with supplemental oxygen and monitor the patient's vital signs, as you provide immediate transport.

Blunt Myocardial Injury

Blunt trauma to the chest may injure the heart itself, making it unable to maintain adequate blood pressure. There is much debate in the medical literature over how to assess <u>myocardial contusion</u>, or bruising of the heart muscle. Often, the pulse rate is irregular, but dangerous rhythms such as ventricular tachycardia and ventricular fibrillation are uncommon. There is no specific diagnostic test at this time, and there is no prehospital treatment for the condition. Still, you should suspect myocardial contusion in all cases of severe, blunt injury to the chest. Check the patient's pulse carefully, and note any irregularities. Provide supplemental oxygen and transport immediately.

Pericardial Tamponade

In <u>pericardial tamponade</u>, blood or other fluid collects in the <u>pericardium</u>, the fibrous sac surrounding the heart (▼ **Figure 27-13**). This prevents the heart from filling during the diastolic phase, causing a decrease in the amount of blood pumped to the body and decreased blood pressure. Ultimately, as blood accumulates within the pericardial cavity, it compresses the heart until it can no longer function and the patient goes into cardiac arrest. Signs and symptoms of pericardial tamponade include very soft and faint heart tones, often called muffled heart sounds, a weak pulse, low blood pressure, a decrease in the difference between the systolic and the diastolic blood pressure, and jugular vein distention (JVD).

In a trauma situation, even a small amount of fluid in the pericardial sac is enough to cause fatal pericardial tamponade. (Occasionally, fluid in surprisingly large amounts may collect in the pericardial sac as a chronic condition.) Pericardial tamponade is relatively uncommon, seen more often with penetrating injuries to the heart itself than with blunt injuries to the chest. If you suspect this life-threatening condition, provide

> A healthy, uninjured adult usually breathes from 12 to 20 times per minute without difficulty and without pain.

appropriate respiratory support, supplemental oxygen, and prompt transport. Be sure to notify the hospital of your suspicions so that preparations can be made for immediate treatment.

Laceration of the Great Vessels

The chest contains several large blood vessels: the superior vena cava, the inferior vena cava, the pulmonary arteries, four main pulmonary veins, and the aorta, with its major branches distributing blood throughout the body. Injury to any of these vessels may be accompanied by massive, rapidly fatal hemorrhage. Any patient with a chest wound who shows signs of shock may have an injury to one or more of these vessels. Frequently, blood loss is not obvious, because it remains within the chest cavity.

Emergency treatment for these patients includes CPR, if appropriate, ventilatory support, and supplemental oxygen. Here, particularly, immediate transport to the hospital may be critical. For some of these patients, a few minutes can mean the difference between life and death.

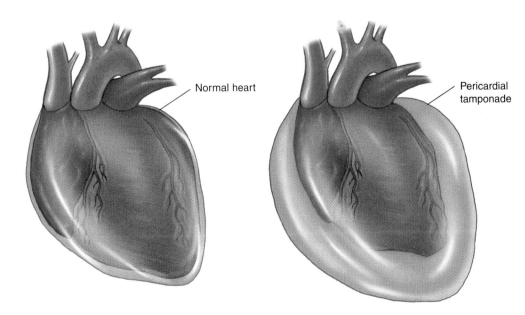

Figure 27-13 Pericardial tamponade is a potentially fatal condition in which fluid builds up within the pericardial sac, causing compression of the heart's chambers and dramatically impairing its ability to pump blood to the body.

Normal heart

Pericardial tamponade

Prep Kit

Ready for Review

There are two types of chest injuries: penetrating, or open, injuries and blunt, or closed, injuries. In blunt trauma, a blow to the chest may fracture the ribs, the sternum, or whole areas of the chest wall. Other problems include bruising of the lungs and the heart and possible damage to the aorta. Even if the skin and chest wall are not broken, the contents of the chest may be injured.

A sucking chest wound can result in an open pneumothorax, in which air entering through the wound accumulates in the pleural space, causing the lung to collapse. You should seal the wound with a sterile dressing, either taping it down on all four sides or creating a flutter valve by sealing only three sides. Sealing all four sides may create a tension pneumothorax, in which air leaking from a lacerated lung is unable to escape and the lung collapses. Eventually, this air may push the mediastinum into the opposite pleural cavity and prevent blood from returning to the heart. Cardiac arrest results. A tension pneumothorax can also occur in a closed, blunt injury of the chest in which a fractured rib lacerates the surface of the lung. Look for increasing respiratory distress, shock, and decreased breath sounds on one side. You may need to partly remove the dressing to relieve the underlying tension in the chest. The accumulation of blood in the chest is called a hemothorax; the collection of both blood and air is called a hemopneumothorax.

A fractured rib may lacerate the surface of the lung, causing some type of pneumothorax. One sign of this is a crackly feeling to the skin in the area. Multiple rib fractures, with or without a fracture of the sternum, often result in a condition called flail chest, in which a portion of the chest wall is detached from the thoracic cage and moves during respiration in a fashion that is the opposite of normal. A flail chest causes very painful breathing and requires respiratory support and supplemental oxygen. It may help to immobilize the flail segment with a pad.

Other chest injuries include contusions of the lungs and heart and traumatic asphyxia, in which a sudden, severe compression of the chest produces a rapid increase in intrathoracic pressure. Signs of this condition include distended neck veins, cyanosis in the face, and hemorrhage in the sclera. Provide ventilatory support, monitor vital signs, and provide immediate transport. In pericardial tamponade, blood collects in the pericardium, preventing the heart from filling during the diastolic phase and eventually causing cardiac arrest. Signs include muffled heart sounds, a weak pulse, low blood pressure, and distended neck veins. Here as well, you should provide vigorous respiratory support and immediate transport. Laceration of the large blood vessels in the chest can cause a fatal hemorrhage. Suspect such a wound in any patient with a chest wound who shows signs of shock, even if you see little blood; it may be collecting within the chest cavity. This person needs ventilatory support, supplemental oxygen, immediate transport, and possibly CPR.

Vital Vocabulary

closed chest injury Injury to the chest in which the skin is not broken, usually due to blunt trauma.

dyspnea Difficulty with breathing.

flail chest A condition in which three or more ribs are fractured in two or more places, or in association with a fracture of the sternum, so that a segment of chest wall is effectively detached from the rest of the thoracic cage.

flutter valve A one-way valve that allows air to leave the chest cavity but not return. Formed by taping three sides of an occlusive dressing to the chest wall, leaving the fourth open as the valve.

hemoptysis The spitting or coughing up of blood.

hemothorax A collection of blood in the pleural cavity.

myocardial contusion A bruise of the heart muscle.

occlusive dressing Dressing made of Vaseline gauze, aluminum foil, or plastic that prevents air and liquids from entering or exiting a wound.

open chest injury Injury to the chest in which the chest wall itself is penetrated by a fractured rib or some external object.

paradoxical motion The motion of the portion of the chest wall that is detached in a flail chest; the motion—in during inhalation, out during exhalation—is exactly the opposite of normal chest wall motion during breathing.

pericardial tamponade Compression of the heart due to a buildup of blood or other fluid in the pericardial sac.

pericardium The fibrous sac that surrounds the heart.

pneumothorax An accumulation of air or gas in the pleural cavity.

pulmonary contusion A bruise of the lung.

spontaneous pneumothorax Pneumothorax that occurs when a weak area on the lung ruptures in the absence of major injury, allowing air to leak into the pleural space.

sucking chest wound An open or penetrating chest wall wound through which air passes during inspiration and expiration, creating a sucking sound.

tachypnea Rapid respirations.

tension pneumothorax An accumulation of air or gas in the pleural cavity that progressively increases the pressure in the chest with potentially fatal results.

Assessment in Action

You and your partner are dispatched to a local liquor store for a shooting. You learn upon arrival that the storeowner had purchased a handgun and shot the robber twice in the chest. You find the 22-year-old patient lying on the floor in a large puddle of blood. He has one entrance wound in the left shoulder and a second wound just under the left clavicle, which is bleeding profusely.

During your initial assessment, you are unable to palpate a radial pulse, but you manage to find a fast, weak carotid pulse. Between the patient's moaning and crying, you determine that he has respirations of more than 40 breaths/min.

1. From this information, you know that the patient has:
   A. normal air exchange.
   B. an open and clear airway.
   C. adequate circulation.
   D. adequate perfusion.

2. Your first step in caring for this patient is to:
   A. apply and quickly inflate all three compartments of the PASG.
   B. cover the wounds, give oxygen, and prepare to transport.
   C. obtain a complete set of vital signs and then check breath sounds.
   D. complete a detailed physical examination and prepare to transport.

3. One additional step that is most important in this situation is to:
   A. quickly check for exit wounds.
   B. palpate his abdomen for internal bleeding.
   C. check his pupil reaction.
   D. determine extremity movement and sensation.

4. Appropriate care for his chest wounds includes:
   A. leaving them open to drain freely.
   B. packing them with gauze to control bleeding.
   C. covering them with an airtight dressing.
   D. inserting a drain to aid removal of body fluids.

5. Appropriate materials to use for an airtight dressing include Vaseline gauze, aluminum foil, or:
   A. a 4" x 4" piece of gauze.
   B. a washcloth.
   C. part of a sheet.
   D. a piece of plastic.

6. The patient has no breath sounds on the left side, appears to be very anxious, and seems to be struggling to breathe. He is becoming cyanotic despite administration of oxygen. His neck veins are distended, and his pulse is so fast and weak that it is almost imperceptible. These signs and symptoms suggest:
   A. a pneumothorax.
   B. an abdominal injury.
   C. a tension pneumothorax.
   D. pericardial tamponade.

7. At this point, the best treatment for this patient is to communicate your findings to the hospital and:
   A. expedite transport.
   B. keep the patient warm.
   C. loosen the dressings over his wounds.
   D. begin positive-pressure ventilation.

Challenging Questions

8. A deviated trachea is listed as one of the signs of a tension pneumothorax. But it is rarely seen in the field. Why?

9. A flail chest is an extremely painful injury for a patient. How can you effectively manage the pain of a flail segment in a conscious patient?

10. The most serious damage from a flail segment is not the broken ribs. What is it?

Points to Ponder

You are dispatched to a suicide attempt and find a patient who is in the end stages of AIDS and confined to his bed. He has a knife stuck in his chest. While he is weak from his illness, the knife wound seems to have caused minimal damage. His partner is very upset because he had given the patient the knife, not knowing what he was going to do. The patient complains of "just wanting to have it over" and asks if you could help him "end it." His partner becomes extremely upset and starts yelling at you to not "kill" his partner. How would you deal with both the patient and his partner?

Issues Terminal Illnesses, Right to Die, Personal Biases and Prejudices, Suicide, Mental Health.

Online Outlook

Chest injuries are both very common and, given the likelihood of damage to the heart, lungs, or great blood vessels, very serious. Test your ability to anticipate and identify different chest injuries by completing Exercise 27 at www.emtb.com.

www.emtb.com

Abdomen and Genitalia Injuries

Objectives*

Cognitive

1. State the steps in the emergency medical care of a patient with a blunt or penetrating abdominal injury (p 629).
2. Describe how solid and hollow organs can be injured (p 626).
3. State the steps in the emergency medical care of a patient with an object impaled in the abdomen (p 629).
4. State the steps in the emergency medical care of a patient with an abdominal evisceration wound (p 631).
5. State the steps in the emergency medical care of the patient with a genitourinary injury (p 632).

Affective

None

Psychomotor

6. Demonstrate proper treatment of a patient who has an object impaled in the abdomen (p 629).
7. Demonstrate how to apply a dressing to an abdominal evisceration wound (p 631).

   * All of the objectives in this chapter are noncurriculum objectives.

TECHNOLOGY

www.emtb.com

Online Chapter Pretest
Interactivities
Vocabulary Explorer
Anatomy Review
Web Links
Online Review Manual
Distance Learning

You and your partner are just leaving a Base Station meeting when you are dispatched to a downtown construction site. You arrive to find a 36-year-old carpenter who fell two stories down an elevator shaft, striking a 2 × 4 board in the groin.

Injuries to the genitalia, while rarely life-threatening, can be painful and stressful nonetheless. This chapter will present content relative to both abdominal and genitalia injuries and will also help you answer the following questions:

1. How would you manage a patient who has suffered a laceration to the abdomen that has left approximately 14" of intestine exposed?

2. What would be the appropriate care for a patient with a knife impaled in the abdomen?

Abdomen and Genitalia Injuries

The abdomen is the lower of the two major body cavities, extending from the diaphragm to the pelvis. It contains several organs that make up the digestive, urinary, and genitourinary systems. Although any of these organs may be injured, some are better protected than others. You must know where these organs are located within the abdominal or pelvic cavities. You must also understand their functions so that when an illness or injury occurs, you can assess its seriousness.

This chapter begins with a brief review of the anatomy of the abdomen, followed by a discussion of common types of abdominal injuries. Next, patient assessment strategies are discussed, followed by a description of specific abdominal injuries that you are likely to encounter and how to treat each. The genitourinary system is then described, and common injuries and treatment are discussed.

The Anatomy of the Abdomen

The abdomen contains both hollow and solid organs, any of which may be damaged. **Hollow organs**, including the stomach, intestines, ureters, and bladder, are actually structures through which materials pass (▶ **Figure 28-1**). They usually contain food that is in the process of being digested, urine that is being passed to the bladder for release, or bile. When ruptured or lacerated, these organs spill their contents into the **peritoneal cavity** (the abdominal cavity), causing an intense inflammatory reaction called **peritonitis**. The first signs of peritonitis are severe abdominal pain, tenderness, and muscular spasm. Later, normal bowel sounds diminish or disappear

as the bowel stops functioning. A patient may feel nauseous and may vomit; the abdomen may become distended and firm to touch.

The **solid organs**, as their name suggests, are solid masses of tissue. They include the liver, spleen, pancreas, and kidneys (▶ **Figure 28-2**). It is here that much of the chemical work of the body—digestion, excretion, and energy production—takes place. Solid organs have

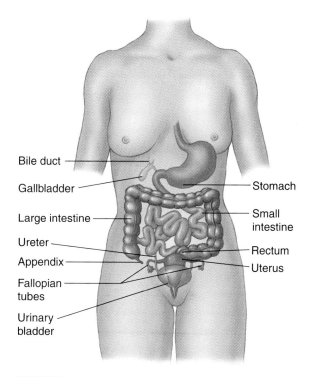

Bile duct

Gallbladder

Large intestine

Ureter

Appendix

Fallopian tubes

Urinary bladder

Stomach

Small intestine

Rectum

Uterus

Figure 28-1 The hollow organs in the abdominal cavity are structures through which materials pass.

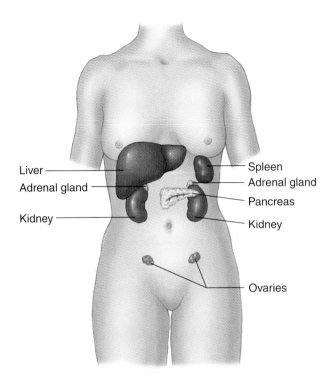

Figure 28-2 The solid organs are solid masses of tissue that do much of the chemical work in the body.

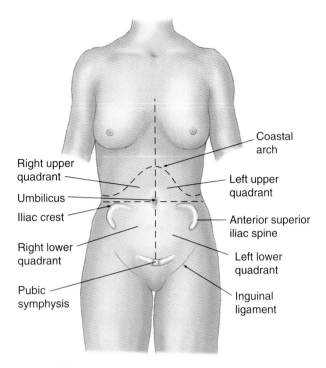

Figure 28-3 The abdominal cavity is divided into four quadrants, which serve as your means of identifying and reporting problems in the abdomen.

a rich blood supply, so injury can cause severe hemorrhage. The same is true of the aorta or inferior vena cava, whether the injury is open or closed. Unlike gastric juices and bacteria, blood within the peritoneal cavity does not provoke an inflammatory response. Therefore, the absence of pain and tenderness does not necessarily mean the absence of major bleeding in the abdomen.

The bony landmarks in the abdomen include the pubic symphysis, the costal arch, the iliac crests, and the anterior superior iliac spines. The major soft-tissue landmark is the umbilicus, which overlies the fourth lumbar vertebra. The abdomen is divided arbitrarily into quadrants by two perpendicular lines that intersect at the umbilicus ▲ **Figure 28-3** . These quadrants provide a frame of reference for identifying and reporting abdominal signs and symptoms.

Injuries of the Abdomen

Abdominal injuries may be as obvious as loops of intestines protruding from a stab wound or as subtle as a laceration to the liver or spleen. Remember to follow BSI precautions as you begin your initial assessment; these injuries often bleed profusely, and even if they do not, some blood or other body fluid is likely to be present. Injuries of the abdomen are considered open

Figure 28-4 Blunt trauma to the abdomen can occur when a patient strikes the steering wheel of an automobile as a result of a crash.

or closed and can involve hollow and/or solid organs. <u>Closed abdominal injuries</u> are those in which a severe blow damages the abdomen without breaking the skin; these are also known as blunt injuries. Such a blow might come from the patient's striking the handlebar of a bicycle or the steering wheel of a car ▲ **Figure 28-4** . <u>Open abdominal injuries</u> are those in which a foreign object enters the abdomen and opens the peritoneal cavity to the outside; these are also known as penetrating injuries (▶ Figure 28-5). Open injuries might not go deeper than the wall of the abdomen, but this is difficult to determine. Therefore, you must assume the worst—that organs have been damaged—and provide prompt transport. Stab wounds and gunshot wounds are examples of open injuries.

Signs and Symptoms

Patients with abdominal injuries generally have one principal complaint: pain. But other significant injuries may mask the pain at first, and some patients may not be able to tell you about pain because they are unconscious or unresponsive, such as after a head injury or drug or alcohol overdose. The most common sign of significant abdominal injury is tachycardia. Later signs are those of shock: decreased blood pressure and pale, cool, moist skin. In some cases, the abdomen may become distended from the accumulation of blood and fluid. As an EMT-B, you must look for other clues. Blunt injuries include bruises or other visible marks, whose location should guide your attention to underlying structures (▶ Figure 28-6). For example, bruises in the right upper quadrant, left upper quadrant, or flank might suggest an injury to the liver, spleen, or kidney, respectively.

The signs of abdominal injury are usually more definite than the symptoms, including firmness on palpation of the abdomen, obvious entry and exit wounds, bruises, and altered vital signs such as increased pulse rate, increased respiratory rate, decreased blood pressure, and shallow respirations (although this might not appear until later). Common symptoms include abdominal tenderness, particularly localized tenderness, and difficulty with movement because of pain.

Evaluating Abdominal Injuries

Your goal in initial assessment is to evaluate the patient's ABCs and then immediately care for any life threats. You should then begin the focused history and physical exam to determine the type of abdominal injury (open or closed), the extent of the damage, and the presence of shock. Note that patients may or may not be able to tell you about the severity and location of their pain. However, they may report that they feel nauseous, and they may vomit. Remember to keep the airway clear of vomitus so that it is not aspirated into the lungs, especially in a patient who is unconscious or

has an altered level of consciousness. Turn the patient to one side, using spinal precautions if necessary, and try to clear any material from the throat and mouth. Note the nature of the vomitus: undigested food, blood, mucus, or bile.

Normally, you will evaluate all patients with abdominal injuries in the same manner. First, you should place

Figure 28-5 Because it is difficult to know how deep a penetrating injury is, assume organ damage and transport promptly.

Figure 28-6 Bruising on the abdomen can provide clues to the possible injury of underlying organs.

the patient in a supine position with the knees slightly flexed and supported (▼ **Figure 28-7**). Remove or loosen clothes. Then, before you do anything else, assess and record baseline vital signs. Many abdominal emergencies, aside from those that cause severe bleeding, can cause a rapid pulse and low blood pressure. Your record of vital signs, made as early as possible and periodically thereafter, will be of tremendous help to physicians in evaluating the problem when the patient arrives in the emergency department.

Further assessment follows the DCAP-BTLS sequence: Inspect and palpate the abdomen for the presence of **D**eformity, which may be subtle in abdominal injuries. Look for the presence of **C**ontusions and **A**brasions, which can help localize focal points of impact and may indicate significant internal injury. Puncture wounds and other **P**enetrating injuries must not be overlooked, as the intra-abdominal extent of these injuries may be life-threatening. The presence of **B**urns must be noted and managed appropriately. Palpate for **T**enderness and attempt to localize to a specific quadrant of the abdomen. Identify and treat any **L**acerations with appropriate dressings. **S**welling may involve the abdomen globally and indicate significant intra-abdominal injury.

Quickly assess the patient's condition with a simple inspection, noting the manner in which he or she is lying. Movement of the body or the abdominal organs irritates the inflamed peritoneum, causing additional pain. To minimize this pain, patients will lie still, usually with the knees drawn up, and breathe rapid and shallow. For the same reason, they will contract their abdominal muscles, a sign called **guarding**.

Figure 28-7 Patients with abdominal injuries should be placed in a supine position with the knees slightly flexed and supported.

Next, inspect the skin of the abdomen for holes through which bullets, knives, or other missile-type foreign bodies may have passed. Keep in mind that the size of the wound does not necessarily indicate the extent of underlying injuries. If you find an entry wound, you must always check for a corresponding exit hole in the patient's back or sides. If the injury was caused by a very high-velocity missile from a rifle, you may see a small, harmless-looking entrance wound with a large, gaping exit wound. Do not attempt to remove a knife or other object that is impaled in the patient. Instead, stabilize the object with supportive bandaging. Bruises or other visible marks are important clues to the cause and severity of any blunt injury. Steering wheels and seat belts produce characteristic patterns of bruising on the abdomen or chest.

Types of Abdominal Injuries

Blunt Abdominal Wounds

A patient with a blunt abdominal wound may have one or some combination of the following:

- Severe bruises of the abdominal wall
- Laceration of the liver and spleen
- Rupture of the intestine
- Tears in the mesentery, membranous folds that attach the intestines to the walls of the body, and injury to blood vessels within them
- Rupture of the kidneys, or tearing of the kidneys from their arteries and veins
- Rupture of the bladder, especially in a patient who had been drinking and therefore had a full and distended bladder at the time of the crash
- Severe intra-abdominal hemorrhage
- Peritoneal irritation and inflammation in response to the rupture of hollow organs

A patient who has sustained a blunt abdominal injury should be log rolled to a supine position on a backboard.

Incorrect position

Correct position

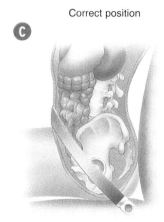

Figure 28-8 The proper position for a seat belt is below the anterior superior iliac spines of the pelvis and against the hip joints, as shown in diagram C. Diagrams A and B show improper positioning of seat belts.

Ensure that you protect the spine as you do so. If the patient vomits, turn him or her to one side and clear the mouth and throat of vomitus. Monitor the patient's vital signs for any indication of shock such as pallor; cold sweat; rapid, thready pulse; or low blood pressure. If you see any of these signs, administer supplemental oxygen via nonrebreathing mask, and take all the appropriate measures to treat for shock. Keep the patient warm with blankets, and provide prompt transport to the emergency department.

Injuries from Seat Belts and Airbags

Seat belts have prevented many thousands of injuries and saved many lives, including those of people who otherwise would have been ejected from a smashed car. However, seat belts occasionally cause blunt injuries of the abdominal organs. When worn properly, a seat belt lies below the anterior superior iliac spines of the pelvis

and against the hip joints. If the belt lies too high, it can squeeze abdominal organs or great vessels against the spine when the car suddenly decelerates or stops ◄ **Figure 28-8** . Occasionally, fractures of the lumbar spine have been reported. If you are called to the scene of such an accident, keep in mind that the use of seat belts in many cases turns what could have been a fatal injury into a manageable one.

In all current-model automobiles, the lap and diagonal (shoulder) safety belts are combined into one so that they may not be used independently. Of course, people can still place the diagonal portion of the belt behind the back, significantly reducing the effectiveness of this design. In some older cars, only lap belts or two separate belts are provided. Used alone, diagonal shoulder safety belts can cause injuries of the upper part of the trunk, such as a bruised chest, fractured ribs, lacerated liver, or even decapitation. Far fewer head and neck injuries are seen when this belt is used in combination with a lap belt and a head rest.

The airbag, which is standard in today's vehicles, is a great advance in automotive safety. In head-on collisions, it can be a genuine lifesaver. However, because frontal airbags provide no protection in a side impact or rollover, they must be used in combination with safety belts. Small children and short individuals who are in the front seat of the automobile may be at risk of injury when the airbag is deployed. Special attention should be used in evaluating these patients when a deployed airbag is noted. Remember to inspect beneath the airbag for signs of damage to the steering column.

Penetrating Abdominal Injuries

Patients with penetrating injuries generally have obvious wounds and external bleeding ► **Figure 28-9A** . A large wound may have bowel, fat, or a fold of peritoneum protruding from it. In addition to pain, these patients often report nausea and vomiting. Patients with peritonitis generally prefer to lie very still with

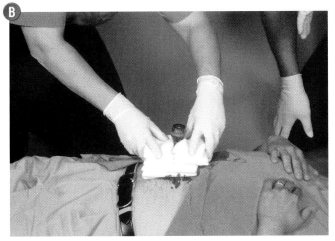

Figure 28-9 **A.** Penetrating injuries have obvious wounds and may also have external bleeding. **B.** If the penetrating object is still in place, use a roller bandage to stabilize the object and to control bleeding.

Figure 28-10 An abdominal evisceration is an open abdominal wound from which internal organs or fat protrude.

their legs drawn up because it hurts to move or straighten their legs. They may complain about every bump in the road during transport.

Some penetrating injuries go no deeper than the abdominal wall, but the severity of the injury can be hard to determine. Only a surgeon can accurately assess the damage. Therefore, as you care for a patient with this type of wound, you should assume that the object has penetrated the peritoneum, entered the abdominal cavity, and possibly injured one or more organs even if there are no immediate obvious signs.

If major blood vessels are cut or solid organs are lacerated, bleeding may be rapid and severe. Other signs of intra-abdominal injuries may develop slowly, particularly in penetrating wounds to hollow organs. Once such an organ is punctured and its contents are discharged into the abdominal cavity, peritonitis may develop, but this may take several hours.

In caring for a patient with a penetrating wound of the abdomen, follow the general procedures described above for care of a blunt abdominal wound, as well as the following specific steps for the penetrating wound. Inspect the patient's back and sides for exit wounds, and apply a dry, sterile dressing to all open wounds. If the penetrating object is still in place, apply a stabilizing bandage around it to control external bleeding and minimize movement of the object ◄ **Figure 28-9B** .

Abdominal Evisceration

Severe lacerations of the abdominal wall may result in an <u>evisceration</u>, in which internal organs or fat protrude through the wound ▲ **Figure 28-10** . Never try to replace an organ that is protruding from an abdominal laceration, whether it is a small fold of peritoneum or nearly all of the intestines. Instead, cover it with sterile gauze compresses moistened with sterile saline solution, and secure them with a sterile dressing. (Protocols in some EMS systems call for an occlusive dressing over the organs, secured by trauma dressings.) Because the open abdomen radiates body heat very effectively, and because exposed organs lose fluid rapidly, you must keep the organs moist and warm. If you do not have gauze compresses, you may use moist, sterile dressings, covered and secured in place with a bandage and tape ► **Figure 28-11** . Do not use any material that is adherent or loses its substance when wet, such as toilet paper, facial tissue, paper towels, or absorbent cotton.

Once you have covered the extruding organ, you should provide other emergency care as necessary and provide prompt transport to the emergency department.

Figure 28-11 **A.** The open abdomen radiates body heat rapidly and must be covered. **B.** Cover the wound with moistened sterile gauze, or with an occlusive dressing, depending on local protocol. **C.** Secure the dressing with a bandage. **D.** Secure the bandage with tape.

Anatomy of the Genitourinary System

The genitourinary system controls both the reproductive functions and the waste discharge system, which are generally considered together.

The urinary system controls the discharge of certain waste materials filtered from the blood by the kidneys. In the urinary system, the kidneys are solid organs; the ureters, bladder, and urethra are hollow organs ▶ **Figure 28-12** .

The genital system controls the reproductive processes from which life is created. The male genitalia, except for the prostate gland and the seminal vesicles, lie outside the pelvic cavity ▶ **Figure 28-13** . The female genitalia, except for the vulva, clitoris, and labia,

are contained entirely within the pelvis ▶ **Figure 28-14** . The male and female reproductive organs have certain similarities and, of course, basic differences. They allow for the production of sperm and egg cells and appropriate hormones, the act of intercourse, and, ultimately, reproduction.

Injuries of the Genitourinary System

Injuries of the Kidney

Injuries of the kidney are not unusual and rarely occur in isolation. This is because the kidneys lie in such a well-protected area of the body. A penetrating wound that reaches the kidneys almost always involves other organs. The same is true with blunt injuries. A blow

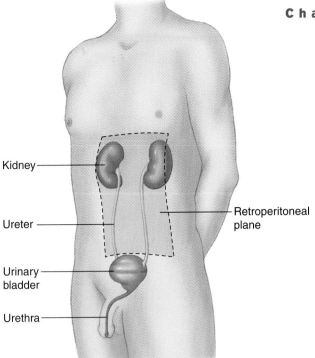

Figure 28-12   The urinary system lies in the retroperitoneal space behind the digestive tract. The kidneys are solid organs; the ureter, bladder, and urethra are hollow organs.

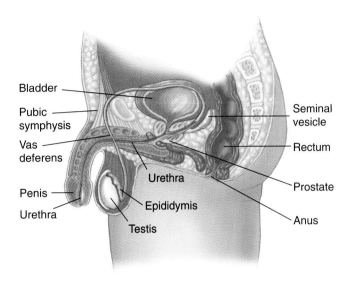

Figure 28-13   The male reproductive system includes the testicles, vasa deferentia, seminal vesicles, prostate gland, urethra, and penis.

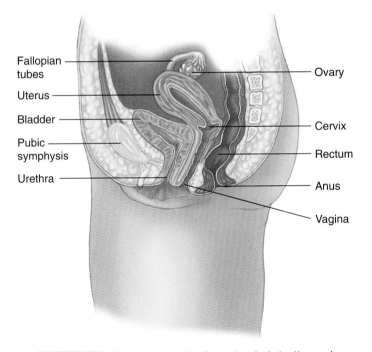

Figure 28-14   The female reproductive system includes the ovaries, fallopian tubes, uterus, cervix, and vagina.

Figure 28-15   A tackle in football that results in blunt trauma to the lower rib cage or the flank can cause kidney injury.

- An abrasion, laceration, or contusion in the flank
- A penetrating wound in the region of the lower rib cage (the flank) or the upper abdomen
- Fractures on either side of the lower rib cage or of the lower thoracic or upper lumbar vertebrae

Damage to the kidneys may not be obvious on inspection of the patient. You may or may not see bruises or lacerations on the overlying skin. However, you will see signs of shock if the injury is associated with significant blood loss. Because one of the functions

that is forceful enough to cause significant kidney damage almost always damages other intra-abdominal organs, often fracturing a rib as well. Less significant injuries to the kidneys may result from a direct blow or even from a tackle in football ▶ **Figure 28-15** . Suspect kidney damage if the patient has a history or physical evidence of any of the following findings:

of the kidney is the formation of urine, another sign of kidney damage is blood in the urine, called **hematuria**. Treat shock and associated injuries in the appropriate manner. Provide prompt transport to the hospital, monitoring the patient's vital signs carefully en route.

Injuries of the Urinary Bladder

Injury of the urinary bladder, either blunt or penetrating, may result in its rupture. When this happens, urine spills into the surrounding tissues, and any urine that passes through the urethra is likely to be bloody. Blunt injuries of the lower abdomen or pelvis often cause rupture of the urinary bladder, particularly when the bladder is full and distended. Sharp, bony fragments from a fracture of the pelvis often perforate the urinary bladder ▶ **Figure 28-16** . Penetrating wounds of the lower midabdomen or the perineum (the pelvic floor and associated structures that occupy the pelvic outlet) can directly involve the bladder. In the male, sudden deceleration from a motor vehicle or motorcycle crash can literally shear the bladder from the urethra.

Suspect a possible injury of the urinary bladder if you see blood at the urethral opening or physical signs of trauma on the lower abdomen, pelvis, or perineum. There may be blood at the tip of the penis or a stain on the patient's underwear.

The presence of associated injuries or of shock will dictate the urgency of transport. In most instances, provide prompt transport, and monitor the patient's vital signs en route.

Injuries of the External Male Genitalia

Injuries of the external male genitalia include all types of soft-tissue wounds. Although these injuries are uniformly painful and generally a source of great concern to the patient, they are rarely life-threatening. Especially in industrial accidents, avulsion (tearing away) of the skin of the penis can occur, particularly in the uncircumcised male. If you encounter a patient with such an injury, wrap the penis in a soft, sterile dressing moistened with sterile saline solution, and transport the patient promptly. Use direct pressure to control any bleeding. You should try to save and preserve the avulsed skin, but do not delay treatment or transport for more than a few minutes to do so.

Managing blood loss is your top priority in amputation of the penile shaft, whether partial or complete.

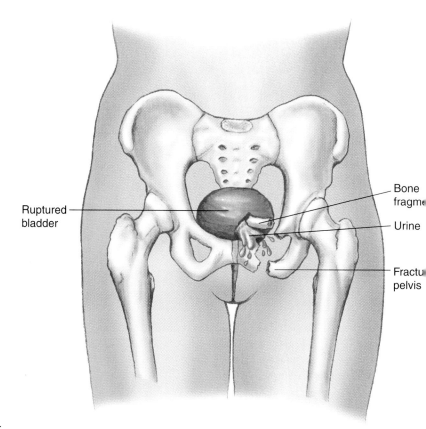

Figure 28-16 Fracture of the pelvis can result in a laceration of the bladder by the bony fragments. Urine then leaks into the pelvis.

You should use local pressure with a sterile dressing on the remaining stump. Never apply a constricting device to the penis to control bleeding. Surgical reconstruction of even a completely amputated penis is possible if you can locate the amputated part. Wrap it in a moist, sterile dressing; place it in a plastic bag; and transport it in a cooled container without allowing it to come in direct contact with ice.

If the connective tissue surrounding the erectile tissue in the penis is severely damaged, the shaft of the penis can be fractured or severely angled, sometimes requiring surgical repair. The injury may occur during particularly active sexual intercourse. It is associated with intense pain, bleeding into the tissues, and fear. Provide prompt transport to the emergency department.

Accidental laceration of the skin about the head of the penis usually occurs when the penis is erect and is associated with heavy bleeding. The injury usually appears worse than it actually is; once the penis becomes flaccid, the size of the laceration decreases. Local pressure with a sterile dressing is usually sufficient to stop the hemorrhage.

It is not uncommon for the skin of the shaft of the penis or the foreskin to get caught in the zipper of pants. If a small segment of the zipper is involved (one or two teeth), you can try to unzip the pants. If a longer segment is involved or the patient is agitated, use heavy scissors to cut the zipper out of the pants to make the patient more comfortable during transport. Be sure to explain what the scissors are for before you begin cutting.

Urethral injuries in the male are uncommon. Lacerations of the urethra can result from straddle injuries, pelvic fractures, or penetrating wounds of the perineum. These injuries may bleed quite a lot, although this may not be evident externally. Direct pressure with a dry, sterile dressing usually controls any external hemorrhage. Because the urethra is the channel for urine, it is very important to know whether the patient can urinate and whether hematuria is present. For this reason, you should save any voided urine for later examination at the hospital. Any foreign bodies that may be protruding from the urethra will have to be removed in a surgical setting.

Avulsion of the skin of the scrotum may damage the scrotal contents. If possible, preserve the avulsed skin in a moist, sterile dressing for possible use in reconstruction. Wrap the scrotal contents or the perineal area with a sterile, moist compress, and use a local pressure dressing to control bleeding. Transport this patient promptly to the emergency department.

Direct blows to the scrotum can result in the rupture of a testicle or significant accumulation of blood around the testes. In either case, you should apply an ice pack to the scrotal area while transporting the patient.

A few general rules apply to the treatment of injuries involving the external male genitalia:

- These injuries are very painful. Make the patient as comfortable as possible.

- Use sterile, moist compresses to cover areas that have been stripped of skin.

- Apply direct pressure with dry, sterile gauze dressings to control bleeding.

- Never move or manipulate impaled instruments or foreign bodies in the urethra.

- If possible, always identify and bring avulsed parts to the hospital with the patient.

Remember, these are rarely life-threatening injuries and should not be given priority over other, more severe wounds.

Injuries of the Female Genitalia

Internal female genitalia. The uterus, ovaries, and fallopian tubes are subject to the same kinds of injuries as any other internal organ. However, they are rarely damaged because they are small, deep in the pelvis, and well protected by the pelvic bones. Unlike the bladder, which lies adjacent to the bony pelvis, they are usually not injured in a pelvic fracture.

An exception is the pregnant uterus. As pregnancy progresses, the uterus enlarges substantially and rises out of the pelvis, becoming vulnerable to both penetrating and blunt injuries. These injuries can be particularly severe because the uterus has a rich blood supply during pregnancy. You must also keep in mind that another life—that of the unborn child—is at risk. You can expect to see the signs and symptoms of shock with these patients; be prepared to provide all necessary support and prompt transport. Note that contractions may begin as well. If possible, ask the patient when she is due, and report this information to the hospital.

In the last trimester of pregnancy, the uterus is large and may obstruct the vena cava, decreasing the amount of blood returning to the heart, if the patient is placed in a supine position (**supine hypotensive syndrome**). As a result, blood pressure may decrease. The patient should be carefully placed on her left side so that the uterus will not lie on the vena cava. If the patient is secured to a backboard, tilt the board to the left.

External female genitalia. The external female genitalia include the vulva, the clitoris, and the major and minor labia (lips) at the entrance of the vagina. Injuries of the external female genitalia can include all types of soft-tissue injuries. Because these genital parts have a rich nerve supply, injuries are very painful. Lacerations, abrasions, and avulsions should be treated with moist, sterile compresses. Use local pressure to control bleeding and a diaper-type bandage to hold dressings in place. Under no circumstances should you pack or place dressings into the vagina. Leave any foreign bodies in place after you stabilize them with bandages.

In general, although these injuries are painful, they are not life-threatening. Bleeding may be heavy, but it can usually be controlled by local compression. Contusions and other blunt injuries all require careful in-hospital evaluation. However, the urgency of the need for transport will be determined by associated injuries, the amount of hemorrhage, and the presence of shock.

Remember that victims of sexual assault, whether they are male or female, need medical assistance. In these cases, you must treat the medical injuries but also provide privacy, support, and reassurance.

Prep Kit

Ready for Review

Abdominal injuries are classified as either open (penetrating) or closed (blunt) in origin. Either type can damage both hollow organs, such as the stomach and ureters; and solid organs, such as the liver, spleen, and kidneys. Penetrating injuries are most frequently caused by knives or handguns; blunt injuries are often the result of a collision with a steering wheel. Both types of injury cause pain, although this may be masked at first.

These injuries are evaluated in a similar fashion. Place the patient in a supine position, assess and record vital signs, and perform a visual inspection. Always assume that major damage has occurred to abdominal organs, even if there are no obvious signs. Look for bruises or other marks that may point you toward underlying damage: a firm abdomen, difficulty in moving, abdominal tenderness and guarding, obvious entry and exit wounds, and altered vital signs. If hollow organs have spilled their contents into the peritoneal cavity, peritonitis will develop. In an effort to minimize the pain of this condition, patients will want to lie still with their knees drawn up. Treat for shock as necessary, keep the throat clear of vomitus, keep the patient warm, and promptly transport him or her to the emergency department.

Never try to replace an eviscerated organ; keep it warm and moist with sterile gauze compresses. Injuries to the kidneys or bladder will not have obvious external signs, but there are usually more subtle clues such as lower rib pain or a possible pelvic fracture. The external genitalia in both males and females can sustain injuries that can be extremely painful, but these are rarely life-threatening.

Vital Vocabulary

closed abdominal injury Any injury of the abdomen caused by a nonpenetrating instrument or force, in which the skin remains intact; also called blunt abdominal injury.

evisceration The displacement of organs outside of the body.

guarding Contracting the stomach muscles to minimize the pain of abdominal movement; a sign of peritonitis.

hematuria The presence of blood in the urine.

hollow organs Structures through which materials pass, such as the stomach, small intestines, large intestines, ureters, and bladder.

open abdominal injury An injury of the abdomen caused by a penetrating or piercing instrument or force, in which the skin is lacerated or perforated and the cavity is opened to the atmosphere; also called penetrating injury.

peritoneal cavity The abdominal cavity.

peritonitis Inflammation of the peritoneum.

solid organs Solid masses of tissue where much of the chemical work of the body takes place (eg, the liver, spleen, pancreas, and kidneys).

supine hypotensive syndrome A drop in blood pressure caused when the heavy uterus of a supine, third-trimester pregnant patient obstructs the vena cava, lowering blood return to the heart.

Assessment in Action

It's a hot, humid July evening, and you and your partner are covering the local rodeo. The bull-riding competition begins and the bull twists and turns out of the chute, launching the rider into the air and tossing him onto a fence. The 27-year-old cowboy falls on the other side of the fence, well away from the bull.

Assessment reveals a large bruise developing across his abdomen. He states that, while he is having difficulty breathing, his chief complaint is abdominal pain. Vital signs include a pulse of 140 beats/min, respirations of 32 breaths/min, and a blood pressure of 138/92 mm Hg. His skin is flushed and moist, and his pupils are equal and reactive to light.

1. Given the patient's mechanism of injury, manual immobilization of the cervical spine should be applied:
   A. immediately after the airway is secured.
   B. after the detailed physical examination is completed.
   C. when the patient is being loaded into the ambulance.
   D. after the patient is in the ambulance and ready to transport.

2. Which of the following steps is the most important part of your examination of the patient's abdomen?
   A. Flexion
   B. Inspection
   C. Massage
   D. Auscultation

3. This patient needs to have breath sounds evaluated. In this situation, when should this be done?
   A. Immediately after scene size-up
   B. As soon as the airway is open
   C. After your initial assessment
   D. Once you have immobilized the patient

4. The bruising over his abdomen is becoming more prominent, and the abdomen is beginning to feel tight, suggesting:
   A. a punctured lung.
   B. rapidly spreading infection.
   C. decreasing oxygen levels.
   D. continued internal bleeding.

5. Appropriate care for this patient includes oxygen, immobilization, and:
   A. keeping him warm.
   B. elevating his head.
   C. elevating his feet.
   D. turning him on his side.

6. En route to the hospital, your patient becomes restless. His skin is cool and moist. Repeat vital signs show a pulse of 146 beats/min, respirations of 32 breaths/min, and a blood pressure of 116/76 mm Hg. You suspect that the patient may:
   A. have a head injury with increasing intracranial pressure.
   B. have a pneumothorax with a buildup of pressure on that side.
   C. be developing another problem unrelated to his injury.
   D. be developing progressive shock as a result of his injuries.

7. Why is a ruptured solid organ more easily recognized in the field?
   A. Ruptured solid organs bleed and shock is more easily recognized.
   B. Ruptured solid organs have more pain than ruptured hollow organs.
   C. Ruptured hollow organs do not cause much of a problem in the field.
   D. Solid organs swell more than hollow organs, so they can be seen more easily.

Challenging Questions

8. Why should an evisceration be covered immediately?

9. Why should one suspect that a trauma patient with unexplained signs of shock and good lung sounds has an abdominal bleed?

10. Patients who have an inflamed peritoneum will prefer to lie on their side with their knees drawn up. Why does this reduce pain?

Points to Ponder

As soon as you hear the address, you know exactly where you are going. It is a vacant lot that kids have built a series of jumps and bumps to ride their bikes over. It seems at least once a week someone gets a fracture or head injury, but because it is private property no one has shut it down. On this run you find a teenage girl who tells you that her feet slipped of the pedals and she straddled the bar between the seat and the handlebars. She is in a great deal of pain and says that it feels like it may be bleeding. She does not think she can stand or walk. She is wearing heavy pants and has told you that she is menstruating and wearing a feminine napkin. You are unable to see any external bleeding. She refuses to remove her pants to allow for visual inspection of the injury. Your partner is of the opposite sex from you. How would you deal with this situation?

Issues Gender Issues of Patient Care, Modesty, Treating Minors Who Refuse Care, Effects of Menstruation on Patient Care, Genital Injuries.

Online Outlook

The abdomen is the lower of the two major body cavities, extending from the diaphragm to the pelvis. You must know where the organs are located within the abdominal or pelvic cavities. Review your knowledge by completing Exercise 28 at www.emtb.com.

www.emtb.com

Musculoskeletal Care

Objectives

Cognitive

1. Describe the function of the muscular system (p 640).
2. Describe the function of the skeletal system (p 640).
3. List the major bones or bone groupings of the spinal column, the thorax, the upper extremities, and the lower extremities (p 640).
4. Differentiate between an open and closed painful, swollen, deformed extremity (fracture) (p 644).
5. State the reasons for splinting (p 651).
6. List the general rules of splinting (p 653).
7. List the complications of splinting (p 653).
8. List the emergency medical care for a patient with a swollen, painful, deformed extremity (fracture) (p 647).

Affective

9. Explain the rationale for splinting at the scene versus load and go (p 652).
10. Explain the rationale for immobilization of the painful, swollen, deformed extremity (fracture) (p 644).

Psychomotor

11. Demonstrate the emergency medical care of a patient with a painful, swollen, deformed extremity (fracture) (p 649).
12. Demonstrate completing a prehospital care report for patients with musculoskeletal injuries (p 299).

www.emtb.com

Online Chapter Pretest
Interactivities
Vocabulary Explorer
Anatomy Review
Web Links
Online Review Manual
Distance Learning

Skill Drills
Vital Vocabulary
Pediatric Needs
Geriatric Needs
EMT-B Safety
EMT-B Tips
Documentation Tips
Remember
Prep Kit

A quick stop at the hospital to pick up a long backboard left from your last call is interrupted as dispatch sends you to American Park for an injured skateboarder.

With the increasing popularity of this sport has come an increase in musculoskeletal injuries, many of which produce extreme pain. This chapter will present the fundamentals of care relative to musculoskeletal injuries in addition to helping you answer the following questions:

1. What is the difference in prehospital care when caring for a suspected fracture versus a dislocation?

2. Why is an open fracture more complicated to care for than a closed one?

Musculoskeletal Care

The human body is a well-designed system whose form, upright posture, and movement are provided by the musculoskeletal system, which also protects the vital internal organs of the body. As its combination form suggests, the term "musculoskeletal" refers to the bones and voluntary muscles of the body. However, the bones and muscles themselves are susceptible to external forces that can cause injury. Also at risk are the tendons that attach muscles to bones, the joints that form wherever two bones come into contact, and the ligaments that hold the bone ends of a joint together.

As an EMT-B, you must be familiar with the basic anatomy of the body's musculoskeletal system. Although muscles are technically soft tissue, they are discussed in this chapter because of their close relationship to the skeleton. Therefore, the chapter begins with a review of the musculoskeletal anatomy. Various types and causes of musculoskeletal injuries in general are identified, and the assessment and treatment process for each is explained, followed by a detailed discussion of splinting. The chapter then focuses on specific musculoskeletal injuries, beginning at the clavicle and ending at the feet.

Anatomy and Physiology of the Musculoskeletal System

Muscles

The musculoskeletal system is composed of three types of muscles: skeletal, smooth, and cardiac ▶ Figure 29-1 . <u>Skeletal muscle</u>, also called striated muscle because of its characteristic stripes, attaches to the bones and usually crosses at least one joint, forming the major muscle mass of the body. This type of muscle is also called voluntary muscle, because it is under direct voluntary control of the brain, responding to commands to move specific body parts. Usually, movement is the result of several muscles contracting and relaxing simultaneously.

All skeletal muscles are supplied with arteries, veins, and nerves. Blood from the arteries brings oxygen and nutrients to the muscles ▶ Figure 29-2 . Waste products, including carbon dioxide and lactic acid, are carried away in the veins. Either disease or trauma can result in the loss of a muscle's nervous energy; this, in turn, can lead to *atrophy*, or a wasting of the muscle. Muscle tissue is directly attached to the bone by tough, ropelike fibrous structures known as <u>tendons</u>, which are extensions of the fascia that covers all skeletal muscle.

Smooth muscle, also called involuntary muscle, performs much of the automatic work of the body. This type of muscle is found in the walls of most tubular structures of the body, such as the gastrointestinal tract and the blood vessels. Smooth muscle contracts and relaxes to control the movement of the contents of these structures ▶ Figure 29-3 .

The heart neither looks nor acts like skeletal or smooth muscle. It is a specially adapted involuntary muscle with its own regulatory system.

The remainder of this chapter is concerned exclusively with skeletal muscle.

The Skeleton

The skeleton, which gives us our recognizable human form, protects our vital internal organs, and allows us

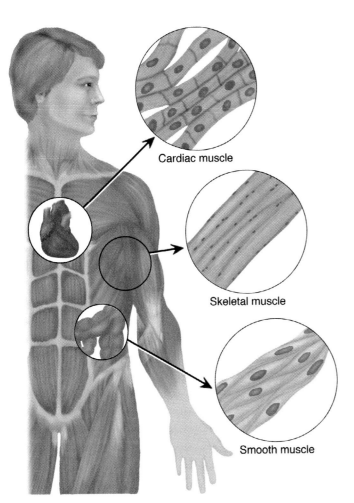

Figure 29-1 The musculoskeletal system includes three types of muscle: skeletal or voluntary muscles, smooth or involuntary muscles, and cardiac muscle.

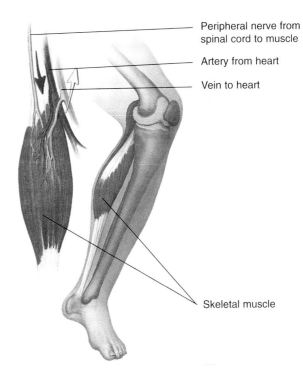

Figure 29-2 Skeletal muscles are supplied with arteries, veins, and nerves that bring oxygen and nutrients, carry away waste products, and supply nervous stimuli.

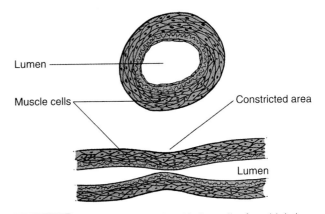

Figure 29-3 Smooth muscle is found in the walls of most tubular structures in the body. These muscles contract and relax to control the movement of the contents of these structures.

to move, is made up of approximately 206 bones ▶ **Figure 29-4** . The bones in the skeleton also produce blood cells (in the bone marrow) and serve as a reservoir for important minerals and electrolytes.

The skull surrounds and protects the brain. The thoracic cage protects the heart, lungs, and great vessels; the lower ribs protect the liver and spleen. The bony spinal canal encases the spinal cord. The upper extremity extends from the shoulder to the fingertips and is composed of the arm, elbow, forearm, wrist, hand, and fingers. The arm extends from the shoulder to the elbow. The pelvis supports the body weight and protects the structures within the pelvis: the bladder, rectum, and female reproductive organs. The lower extremity consists of the thigh, leg, and foot. The joint between the pelvis and the thigh is the hip; the joint between the thigh and lower leg is the knee, and the joint between the lower leg and foot is the ankle.

The bones of the skeleton provide a framework to which the muscles and tendons are attached. Bone is a living tissue that contains nerves and receives oxygen and nutrients from the arterial system. Therefore, when a bone breaks, a patient typically experiences severe pain and bleeding. Bone marrow, located in the center of each bone, is constantly producing red blood cells to provide oxygen and nourishment to the body and remove waste.

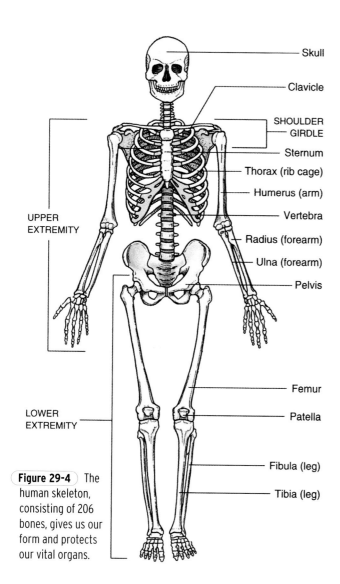

Figure 29-4 The human skeleton, consisting of 206 bones, gives us our form and protects our vital organs.

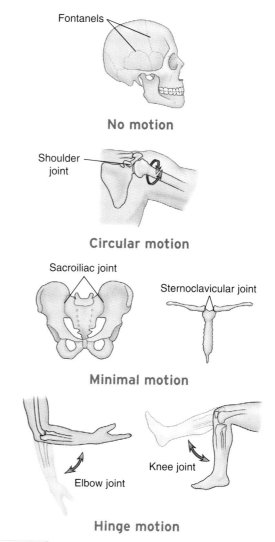

Figure 29-5 Joints have many functions. Some joints allow for motion to occur in a circular fashion; others act as hinges. Still others allow only a minimum amount of motion, or none at all.

A **joint** is formed wherever two bones come into contact. The sternoclavicular joint, for example, is where the sternum and the clavicle come together. Joints are held together in a tough fibrous structure known as a capsule, which is supported and strengthened in certain key areas by bands of fibrous tissue called **ligaments**. In moving joints, the ends of the bones are covered with a thin layer of cartilage known as **articular cartilage**. This cartilage is a pearly substance that allows the ends of the bones to glide easily. Joints are bathed and lubricated by synovial fluid.

Most joints, such as the shoulder, allow motion to occur in a circling fashion. Other joints, such as the knee and elbow, act as hinges. Still other joints, including the sacroiliac joint in the lower back and the sternoclavicular joints, allow only a minimum amount

of motion. Certain joints, such as the fontanels in the skull, fuse two bones together to create a solid, immobile, bony structure ▲ **Figure 29-5**.

Musculoskeletal Injuries

A **fracture** is a broken bone. More precisely, it is a break in the continuity of the bone, often occurring as a result of an external force ▶ **Figure 29-6**. The break can occur anywhere on the surface of the bone.

A **dislocation** is a disruption of a joint in which the bone ends are no longer in contact. The supporting ligaments are torn, usually completely, allowing the bone ends to separate completely from each other ▶ **Figure 29-7**. A fracture-dislocation is a combination injury at the joint in which the joint is dislocated and there is a fracture of the end of the bone.

Figure 29-6 A fracture can occur anywhere on the surface of a bone and may or may not break the skin.

Figure 29-7 A dislocation is a disruption of a joint in which the bone ends are no longer in contact. **A.** The clinical appearance of an elbow dislocation. **B.** X-ray appearance of the same elbow.

A **sprain** is a joint injury in which there is both some partial or temporary dislocation of the bone ends and partial stretching or tearing of the supporting ligaments. After the injury, the joint surfaces generally fall back into alignment, so the joint is not significantly

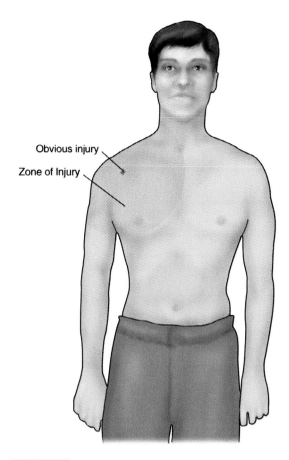

Figure 29-8 The zone of injury is the area of soft tissue, including the adjacent nerves and blood vessels, that surrounds the obvious injury of a bone or joint.

displaced. Sprains can range from mild to severe, depending on the amount of damage done to the supporting ligaments. The most severe sprains involve complete dislocation of the joint; mild sprains typically heal rather quickly.

A **strain**, or muscle pull, is a stretching or tearing of the muscle, causing pain, swelling, and bruising of the soft tissues in the area. Unlike a sprain, no ligament or joint damage occurs.

Injury to bones and joints is often associated with injury to the surrounding soft tissues, especially to the adjacent nerves and blood vessels. The entire area is known as the zone of injury ◢ **Figure 29-8** . Depending on the amount of kinetic energy the tissues absorb from forces acting on the body, the zone may extend to a distant point. For this reason, you should not focus on a patient's obvious injury without first completing an initial assessment to check for associated injuries, which may be even more serious. This is especially true in assessing damage from gunshots and falls from a height.

Mechanism of Injury

Significant force is generally required to cause fractures or dislocations. This force may be applied to the limb in any of the following ways (▼ **Figure 29-9**):

- Direct blows
- Indirect forces
- Twisting forces
- High-energy injury

A direct blow fractures the bone at the point of impact. An example is the <u>patella</u> (kneecap) that fractures when it strikes the dashboard in an automobile crash.

Indirect force may cause a fracture or dislocation at a distant point, as when a person falls and lands on an outstretched hand. The direct impact may cause a wrist fracture, but the indirect force can cause dislocation of the elbow or a fracture of the forearm, humerus, or even clavicle. Therefore, when caring for patients who have fallen, you must identify the point of contact and the mechanism of injury so that you will not overlook associated injuries.

Twisting forces are a common cause of musculoskeletal injury, especially to the anterior cruciate ligament at the knee. Skiing injuries often happen this way. A ski becomes caught, and the skier falls, applying a twisting force to the lower extremity.

High-energy injuries, such as those that occur in automobile crashes, falls from heights, gunshot wounds, and other extreme forces, produce severe damage to the skeleton, surrounding soft tissues, and vital internal organs. A patient may have multiple injuries to many body parts, including more than one fracture or dislocation in a single limb.

A significant MOI is not necessary to fracture a bone. A slight force can easily fracture a bone that is weakened by a tumor or *osteoporosis*, a generalized bone disease that is common among postmenopausal women. In elderly patients with osteoporosis, minor falls, simple twisting injuries, or even a muscle contraction can cause a fracture, most often of the wrist, spine, or hip. You should suspect the presence of a fracture in any older patient who has sustained even a mild injury.

Fractures

Fractures are classified as either closed or open. In assessing and treating patients with possible fractures or dislocations, your first priority is to determine whether the overlying skin has been damaged. If it is not, the patient has a <u>closed fracture</u>. However, making this determination is not always as easy as it sounds. With an <u>open fracture</u>, there is an external wound, caused either by the same blow that fractured the bone or by the broken bone ends lacerating the skin. The wound may vary in size from a very small puncture to a gaping tear that exposes bone and soft tissue. Regardless of the extent and severity of the damage to the skin, you should treat any injury that breaks the skin as a possible open fracture. Greater blood loss and a higher likelihood of infection, possibilities that you must try to prevent, tend to occur with open fractures.

Fractures are also described by whether the bone is moved from its normal position. A <u>nondisplaced fracture</u> (also known as a hairline fracture) is a simple crack of the bone that may be difficult to distinguish from a sprain or simple contusion. In fact, X-rays may be required for hospital personnel to diagnose a nondisplaced fracture. A <u>displaced fracture</u> produces actual

Figure 29-9 Significant force is required to cause fractures or dislocations. Among these are **A.** Direct blows, **B.** Indirect forces, **C.** Twisting forces, and **D.** High-energy injuries.

deformity, or distortion, of the limb by shortening, rotating, or angulating it. Often, the deformity is very obvious and can be associated with crepitus; however, in some cases, the deformity is minimal. Be sure to look for differences between the injured limb and the opposite uninjured limb in any patient with a fracture of an extremity ▼ **Figure 29-10** .

Medical personnel often use the following special terms to describe particular types of fractures ▶ **Figure 29-11** :

- **Greenstick fracture.** An incomplete fracture that passes only partway through the shaft of a bone but may still cause severe angulation; occurs in children.

- **Comminuted fracture.** A fracture in which the bone is broken into more than two fragments.

- **Pathologic fracture.** A fracture of weakened or diseased bone, seen in patients with osteoporosis or cancer; generally produced by minimal force.

- **Epiphyseal fracture.** A fracture that occurs in a growth section of a child's bone, which may prematurely stop growth if not properly treated.

You should suspect a fracture if one or more of the following signs is present in any patient who has a history of injury and reports pain.

DEFORMITY. The limb may appear to be shortened, rotated, or angulated at a point where there is no joint ▼ **Figure 29-12** . Always use the opposite limb as a mirror image for comparison.

TENDERNESS. <u>Point tenderness</u> on palpation in the zone of injury is the most reliable indicator of an

Figure 29-11 Special terms to describe fractures.
A. Greenstick fracture.
B. Comminuted fracture.
C. Pathologic fracture.
D. Epiphyseal fracture.

Figure 29-10 You should always compare the injured limb with the uninjured limb when checking for deformity.

Figure 29-12 Obvious deformity, shortening, rotation, or angulation suggests a fracture. Remember to compare the injured limb with the opposite, uninjured limb.

Figure 29-13 Point tenderness is the sensitive spot at the site of injury that can be located by gentle palpation along the bone with the tip of your finger.

Figure 29-14 Fractures almost always have associated bruising into the surrounding soft tissue.

Figure 29-15 Swelling that occurs in association with a fracture can often mask deformity of the limb.

Figure 29-16 Bone ends may protrude through the skin or be visible within the wound of an open fracture.

underlying fracture, although it does not tell you the type of fracture (▲ **Figure 29-13**). Be sure to wear gloves if there are any open wounds.

GUARDING. An inability to use the extremity is the patient's way of immobilizing it to minimize pain. The muscles around the fracture contract in an attempt to prevent any movement of the broken bone. Guarding does not occur with all fractures; some patients may continue to use the injured part for a period of time. Occasionally, nondisplaced fractures are not very painful, and there is minimal soft-tissue damage.

SWELLING. Rapid swelling usually indicates bleeding from a fracture site and is typically followed by severe pain. Often, if the swelling is severe enough, it may mask deformity of the limb (▲ **Figure 29-14**). Generalized swelling from fluid buildup may occur several hours after an injury.

BRUISING. Fractures are almost always associated with **ecchymosis** (discoloration) of the surrounding soft

tissues (▲ **Figure 29-15**). Bruising may be present after almost any injury; it is not specific for bone or joint injuries.

CREPITUS. A grating or grinding sensation known as **crepitus** can be felt and sometimes even heard when fractured bone ends rub together.

FALSE MOTION. Motion at a point in the limb where there is no joint is a positive indication of a fracture.

EXPOSED FRAGMENTS. In open fractures, bone ends may protrude through the skin or be visible within the wound (▲ **Figure 29-16**).

PAIN. Pain, along with tenderness and bruising, commonly occurs in association with fractures.

LOCKED JOINT. A joint that is locked into position makes any attempt to move the joint both difficult and painful.

Keep in mind that crepitus and false motion appear only when a limb is moved or manipulated and are

Figure 29-17 Joint dislocations, such as this shoulder, are characterized by deformity, swelling, pain with any movement, tenderness, locking, and impaired circulation.

Figure 29-18 Sprains most often occur in the knee or ankle and are characterized by swelling, bruising, point tenderness, pain, and joint instability.

associated with injuries that are extremely painful. Do not manipulate the limb excessively in an effort to elicit these signs.

Dislocations

A dislocated joint sometimes will spontaneously **reduce**, or return to its normal position, before your assessment. In this situation, you will be able to confirm the dislocation only by taking a patient history. Often, however, injury to the supporting ligaments and capsule is so severe that the joint surfaces remain completely separated from one another. A dislocation that does not spontaneously reduce is a serious problem. The ends of the bone can be locked in a displaced position, making any attempt at motion of the joint very difficult and very painful. The most commonly dislocated joints are the fingers, shoulder, elbow, hip, and ankle.

The signs and symptoms of a dislocated joint are similar to those of a fracture ▲ **Figure 29-17** :

- Marked deformity
- Swelling
- Pain that is aggravated by any attempt at movement
- Tenderness on palpation
- Virtually complete loss of normal joint motion (locked joint)
- Numbness or impaired circulation to the limb or digit

Sprains

A sprain occurs when a joint is twisted or stretched beyond its normal range of motion. As a result,

the supporting capsule and ligaments are stretched or torn. A sprain should be considered a partial dislocation or subluxation. The alignment generally returns to a fairly normal position, although there may be some displacement. Note that severe deformity does not typically occur with a sprain. Sprains most often occur in the knee and the ankle, but a sprain can occur in any joint. The following signs and symptoms often indicate that the patient may have a sprain ▲ **Figure 29-18** :

- Point tenderness can be elicited over the injured ligaments.
- Swelling and ecchymosis appear at the point of injury to the ligament as a result of torn blood vessels.
- Pain prevents the patient from moving or using the limb normally.
- Instability of the joint is indicated by increased motion, especially at the knee; however, this may be masked by severe swelling and guarding.

A fracture can look like a sprain, and vice versa. You will not be able to distinguish a nondisplaced fracture from a sprain, especially at the ankle. Therefore, remember to document the mechanism of injury, as certain sprains and fractures occur more consistently with certain mechanisms. This is especially true at the ankle. In general, your approach should always be to try to rule out the possibility of fracture first. The basic principles of field management for sprains, dislocations, and fractures are essentially the same.

Assessing Musculoskeletal Injuries

As an EMT-B, you are the point person in the team approach to the trauma patient. Therefore, your assessments, attempts to splint, and work to stabilize the patient are very important. Look at the big picture, evaluating the overall complexity of the situation. Always carefully assess the mechanism of injury to try to determine the amount of kinetic energy that an injured limb has absorbed.

Assessment of patients with musculoskeletal injuries must include an initial assessment of the patient; followed by a focused physical exam of the painful, swollen, deformed extremity; including evaluation of neurovascular function. Be sure to follow BSI precautions. If oxygen is indicated and you have not already applied it, be sure to do so.

For musculoskeletal trauma, use the DCAP-BTLS approach. Identify any extremity **D**eformities which likely represent significant musculoskeletal injury and stabilize appropriately. **C**ontusions and **A**brasions may overlie more subtle injuries and should prompt you to carefully evaluate the stability and neurovascular status of the limb. The presence of **P**uncture wounds or other signs of Penetrating injury should alert you to the possibility of an open fracture. Associated **B**urns must be identified and treated appropriately. Palpate for **T**enderness, which, like contusions or abrasions, may be the only significant sign of an underlying musculoskeletal injury. When **L**acerations are present on an extremity, open fracture must be considered, bleeding controlled, and dressings applied. Careful inspection for **S**welling with attention to comparison with the opposite limb may also reveal occult musculoskeletal injury.

Because patients often have multiple injuries, you must assess their overall condition, stabilize the ABCs, and control any serious bleeding before further treating the injured extremity. In a critically injured patient, you should secure the patient to a long spine board to rapidly immobilize the spine, pelvis, and extremities and provide prompt transport to a trauma center. In this situation, extensive evaluation and splinting of limb injuries in the field are a waste of valuable time.

If the patient has no life-threatening injuries, you may take extra time at the scene to stabilize the patient's overall condition and more completely evaluate the injured extremity. During the detailed physical exam, you can inspect and gently palpate the other extremities and the spine to identify areas of point tenderness that may indicate underlying fractures, dislocations, or sprains. Remember to compare

> Always assess the mechanism of injury to determine the amount of kinetic energy absorbed.

the injured limb with the opposite, uninjured limb. If possible, gently and carefully remove the patient's clothing to look for open fractures or dislocations, severe deformity, swelling, and/or ecchymosis.

Again, it is not important to distinguish among fractures, dislocations, sprains, and contusions. In most instances, your assessment will be reported as an "injury to the limb." However, you must be able to distinguish mild injuries from severe injuries, since some severe injuries may compromise neurovascular functioning.

If your assessment turns up no external signs of injury, ask the patient to move each limb carefully, stopping immediately if a movement causes pain. Skip this step in your evaluation if the patient reports neck or back pain; even the slightest motion could cause permanent damage to the spinal cord.

Be on the alert for compartment syndrome, which most commonly occurs in the fractured tibia or forearm of children and is often overlooked, especially in patients with an altered level of consciousness. The name **compartment syndrome** refers to elevated pressure in the fascial compartment, which is the fibrous tissue that surrounds and supports the muscles and neurovascular structures. Compartment syndrome occurs within 6 to 12 hours after injury, usually as a result of excessive bleeding, a severely crushed extremity, or the rapid return of blood to an ischemic limb. This syndrome is characterized by pain that is out of proportion to the injury, pallor, decreased sensation, and decreased power (ranging from decreased strength and movement of the limb to complete palsy).

If you suspect that a patient has compartment syndrome, splint the affected limb, keeping it at the level of the heart, and provide immediate transport, checking neurovascular status frequently during transport. Compartment syndrome must be managed surgically.

EMT-B Tips

Extremity injuries that impair circulation or nerve function in distal tissues are urgent situations. These patients need careful assessment, prompt transport, and frequent reassessment of distal functions. It is also crucial to report this information in your initial radio contact with the hospital, to let personnel prepare for a condition in which prompt surgery may be necessary to save the limb.

If you suspect compartment syndrome, splint the limb and transport immediately, checking neurovascular status frequently.

Assessing Pulse, Motor, and Sensory Function

Many important blood vessels and nerves lie close to the bone, especially around the major joints. Therefore, any injury or deformity of the bone may have associated vessel or nerve injury. For this reason, you must assess neurovascular function during the detailed physical exam, repeating it every 5 to 10 minutes, depending on the patient's condition, until the patient is at the hospital. Always recheck the neurovascular function before and after you splint or otherwise manipulate the limb. Manipulation can cause a bone fragment to press against or impale a nerve or vessel. Failure to restore circulation in this situation can lead to death of the limb. Always give priority to patients with impaired circulation resulting from bone fragments.

Examination of the injured limb should include assessment of four major signs that are good indicators of circulatory and nervous status distal to the injury: pulse, capillary refill, motor function, and sensory function. Follow the steps in ▶ Skill Drill 29-1:

1. **Pulse.** Palpate the pulse distal to point of injury.
   - Palpate the radial pulse in the upper extremity **(Step 1)**.
   - In the lower extremity, palpate the posterior tibial and dorsalis pedis pulses **(Step 2)**.

2. **Capillary refill.** Note and record the skin color, identifying any pallor or cyanosis. Then apply firm pressure to the tip of the fingernail or toenail, which will cause the skin to blanch (turn white). If normal color does not return within 2 seconds after you release the nail, you can assume that circulation is impaired. This test is typically recommended for use in children, although it can be used in adults as well **(Step 3)**.

3. **Sensation.** In the hand, check the feeling on the flesh near the tip of the index finger and thumb, as well as the little finger **(Step 4)**. In the foot, check the feeling on the flesh of the big toe **(Step 5)** and on the lateral side of the foot **(Step 6)**. The patient's ability to sense light touch in the fingers or toes distal to the site of a fracture is a good indication that the nerve supply is intact.

4. **Motor function.** Evaluate muscular activity when the injury is proximal to the patient's hand or foot. Ask the patient to open and close a fist for an upper extremity injury and to wiggle the toes and move the foot up and down for a lower extremity injury **(Steps 7-10)**. Sometimes, an attempt at motion will produce pain at the injury site. If this happens, do not continue this part of the examination. To avoid causing pain, do not perform this test at all if the injury involves the hand or foot itself.

Because many of the steps require patient cooperation, you will not be able to assess sensory and motor function in an unconscious patient, but you can still evaluate the limb for deformity, swelling, ecchymosis, false motion, and crepitus. If a patient is unconscious, first perform an initial assessment and then examine the extremities. Assume that an unconscious patient has a spinal fracture, and immobilize the spine.

Assessing the Severity of Injury

You must become skilled at quickly and accurately assessing the severity of injury. The Golden Hour is critical not just for life, but for limb as well. In an extremity with anything less than complete circulation, prolonged hypotension can cause significant damage. For this reason, any suspected open fracture or vascular injury is considered a medical emergency, especially in a patient with multiple trauma.

Remember that most injuries are not critical; you can identify critical injuries by using the musculoskeletal injury grading system shown in ▶ Table 29-1.

SkillDrill 29-1 Assessing Neurovascular Pulse

1 Palpate the radial pulse in the upper extremity.

2 Palpate the posterior tibial pulse in the lower extremity.

3 Assess capillary refill by blanching a fingernail or toenail.

4 Assess sensation on the flesh near the tip of the index finger.

5 On the foot, first check sensation on the flesh near the tip of the great toe.

6 Also check foot sensation on the lateral side.

7 Evaluate motor function by asking the patient to open the hand. (Perform motor tests only if the hand or foot is not injured. Stop a test if it causes pain.)

8 Also ask the patient to make a fist.

9 To evaluate motor function in the foot, ask the patient to extend the foot.

10 Also have the patient flex the foot and wiggle the toes.

TABLE 29-1 Musculoskeletal Injury Grading System

Minor Injuries	Serious Injuries	Severe, Life-Threatening Injuries (survival is probable)
• Minor sprains • Fractures or dislocations of digits	• Displaced long bone fractures • Multiple hand and foot fractures • Single open long bone fractures	• Multiple closed fractures • Limb amputations
Moderate Injuries • Open fractures of digits • Nondisplaced long bone fractures • Nondisplaced pelvic fractures • Major sprains of a major joint	• Displaced pelvic fractures • Dislocations of major joints • Multiple digit amputations • Laceration of major nerves or blood vessels	**Critical Injuries (survival is uncertain)** • Multiple open fractures of the limbs • Pelvic fractures with hemodynamic instability

Emergency Medical Care

Your first steps in providing care for any patient are the initial assessment and stabilizing the patient's ABCs. After you have done so, you can focus on specific injuries. Remember to always follow BSI precautions.

Follow the steps in (▶ **Skill Drill 29-2**) when caring for patients with musculoskeletal injuries:

1. **Completely cover open wounds** with a dry, sterile dressing, and apply local pressure to control bleeding. Once you have applied a sterile dressing, treat an open fracture in the same way as a closed fracture **(Step 1)**.

2. **Apply the appropriate splint,** and elevate the extremity. Patients with lower extremity injuries should lie supine with the limb elevated about 6″ to minimize swelling. For any patient, be sure to position the injured limb slightly above the level of the heart. Never allow the injured limb to flop about or dangle from the edge of the backboard. Always assess pulse, and motor and sensory function before and after the application of splints **(Step 2)**.

3. **If swelling is present,** apply cold packs to the area; however, avoid placing cold packs directly on the skin or other exposed tissues. Placing a cold pack on top of an air splint or other thick, insulating material will not help to reduce swelling **(Step 3)**.

4. **Prepare the patient for transport.** A patient with an isolated upper extremity will most likely be more comfortable in a semiseated position rather than lying flat; however, either position is acceptable. Ensure that the extremity is elevated above the level of the heart and secured so that it does not dangle from the edge of the backboard **(Step 4)**.

5. **Always inform hospital personnel** about all wounds that have been dressed and splinted.

Splinting

A **splint** is a flexible or rigid device that is used to protect and maintain the position of an injured extremity (▼ **Figure 29-19**). Unless the patient's life is in immediate

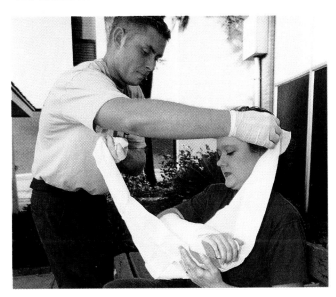

Figure 29-19 Splinting reduces pain and prevents additional damage to the injured extremity.

Skill Drill 29-2 — Caring for Musculoskeletal Injuries

1 Cover open wounds with a dry, sterile dressing, and apply pressure to control bleeding.

2 Apply a splint and elevate the extremity about 6" (slightly above the level of the heart).

3 Apply cold packs if there is swelling, but do not place them directly on the skin.

4 Position the patient for transport and secure the injured area.

danger, you should splint all fractures, dislocations, and sprains before moving the patient. By preventing movement of fracture fragments, bone ends, a dislocated joint, or damaged soft tissues, splinting reduces pain and makes it easier to transfer and transport the patient. In addition, splinting will help to prevent the following:

- Further damage to muscles, the spinal cord, peripheral nerves, and blood vessels from broken bone ends
- Laceration of the skin by broken bone ends. One of the primary indications for splinting is to prevent a closed fracture from becoming an open fracture (conversion)

- Restriction of distal blood flow resulting from pressure of the bone ends on blood vessels
- Excessive bleeding of the tissues at the injury site caused by broken bone ends
- Increased pain from movement of bone ends
- Paralysis of extremities resulting from a damaged spine

A splint is simply a device to prevent motion of the injured part. It can be made from any material on occasions when you need to improvise. However, you should have an adequate supply of standard commercial splints on hand.

GENERAL PRINCIPLES OF SPLINTING. The following principles of splinting apply to most situations:

1. **Remove clothing from the area** of any suspected fracture or dislocation so that you can inspect extremity for DCAP-BTLS.

2. **Note and record the patient's neurovascular status** distal to the site of the injury, including pulse, sensation, and movement. Continue to monitor the neurovascular status until the patient reaches the hospital.

3. **Cover all wounds with a dry, sterile dressing** before splinting. Be sure to follow BSI precautions. Do not intentionally replace protruding bones. Notify the receiving hospital of all open wounds.

4. **Do not move the patient before splinting** an extremity unless there is an immediate hazard to the patient or yourself.

5. In a suspected fracture of the shaft of any bone, be sure to **immobilize the joints** above and below the fracture.

6. With injuries in and around the joint, be sure to **immobilize the bones** above and below the injured joint.

7. **Pad all rigid splints** to prevent local pressure and discomfort to the patient.

8. While applying the splint, **maintain manual immobilization** to minimize movement of the limb and to support the injury site.

9. If fracture of a long bone shaft has resulted in severe deformity, **use constant, gentle manual traction** to align the limb so that it can be splinted. This is especially important if the distal part of the extremity is cyanotic or pulseless.

10. **If you encounter resistance** to limb alignment, splint the limb in its deformed position.

11. **Immobilize all suspected spinal injuries** in a neutral in-line position on a backboard.

12. **If the patient has signs of shock** (hypoperfusion), align the limb in the normal anatomic position and provide transport (total body immobilization).

13. **When in doubt, splint.**

GENERAL PRINCIPLES OF IN-LINE TRACTION SPLINTING. In-line <u>traction</u> is the act of exerting a pulling force on a body structure in the direction of its normal alignment. It is the most effective way to realign a fracture of the shaft of a long bone so that the limb can be splinted more effectively. Excessive traction can be very harmful to an injured limb. When applied correctly,

Documentation Tips

Straightening or splinting an injured limb can compromise distal functions, just as the initial injury can. Record the status of distal circulation and nervous function (neurovascular status) both before *and* after splinting. At a minimum, your written record should describe these functions before splinting, and confirm that they were normal immediately after splinting and upon hospital arrival. For any but the shortest transports, also indicate the results of reassessments while en route.

however, traction stabilizes the bone fragments and improves the overall alignment of the limb. You should not attempt to reduce the fracture or force all the bone fragments back into alignment. This is the physician's responsibility. In the field, the goals of in-line traction are as follows:

1. To stabilize the fracture fragments to prevent excessive movement

2. To align the limb sufficiently to allow it to be placed in a splint

3. To avoid potential neurovascular compromise

The amount of pull that is required to accomplish these objectives varies but rarely exceeds 15 lb. You should use the least amount of force necessary. Grasp the foot or hand at the end of the injured limb firmly; once you start pulling, you should not stop until the limb is fully splinted. The direction of traction pull is always along the long axis of the limb. Imagine where the normal, uninjured limb would lie, and pull gently along the line of that imaginary limb until the injured limb is in approximately that position (▼ **Figure 29-20**).

Figure 29-20   To apply traction, imagine the position where the normal uninjured limb would lie, then gently pull along that line until the injured limb is in that position. Do not release traction once you have applied it.

Skill Drill 29-3 Applying a Rigid Splint

Provide gentle support and in-line traction of the limb.

Second EMT places the splint alongside or under the limb.
Pad between the limb and the splint as needed to ensure even pressure and contact.

Secure the splint to the limb with bindings.

Assess and record distal neurovascular function.

Grasping the foot or hand and the initial pull of traction usually cause some discomfort as the bone fragments move. It helps if a second person can support the injured limb directly under the site of the fracture. This initial discomfort quickly subsides, and you can then apply further gentle traction. However, if the patient strongly resists the traction or if it causes more pain that persists, you must stop and splint the limb in the deformed position.

Remember that many different materials can be used as splints if necessary. When no splinting materials are available, the arm can be bound to the chest wall, and an injured leg can be bound to the uninjured leg to provide at least temporary stability. The three basic types of splints are rigid, formable, and traction splints.

RIGID SPLINTS. Rigid (nonformable) splints are made from firm material and are applied to the sides, front, and/or back of an injured extremity to prevent motion at the injury site. Common examples of rigid splints include padded board splints, molded plastic and metal splints, padded wire ladder splints, and folded cardboard splints. As always, be sure to follow BSI precautions. It takes two EMT-Bs to apply a rigid splint. Follow the steps in (▲ **Skill Drill 29-3**):

1. First EMT-B: **Gently support the limb** at the site of injury as others prepare and begin to position the equipment. Apply steady, in-line traction if necessary. Maintain this support until the splint is completely applied **(Step 1)**.

Skill Drill 29-4 — Applying a Zippered Air Splint

① Support the injured limb and apply gentle traction as your partner applies the open, deflated splint.

② Zip up the splint, inflate it by pump or by mouth, and test the pressure. Check and record distal neurovascular function.

2. Second EMT-B: **Place the rigid splint under or alongside the limb (Step 2)**.

3. Second EMT-B: **Place padding between the limb and the splint** to make sure there is even pressure and even contact. Look for bony prominences, and pad them.

4. Second EMT-B: **Apply bindings** to hold the splint securely to the limb **(Step 3)**.

5. Second EMT-B: **Check and record** the distal nervous and circulatory (neurovascular) function **(Step 4)**.

There are two situations in which you must splint the limb in the position of deformity: when the deformity is severe, as is the case with many dislocations, or when you encounter resistance or extreme pain when applying gentle traction to the fracture of a shaft of a long bone. In either situation, you should apply padded board splints to each side of the limb and secure them with soft roller bandages ▶ **Figure 29-21** .

FORMABLE SPLINTS. The most commonly used formable or soft splint is the precontoured, inflatable, clear plastic air splint. These are available in a variety of sizes and shapes, with or without a zipper that runs the length of the splint. Always inflate the splint after applying it. The air splint is comfortable, provides uniform contact, and has the added advantage of applying firm pressure to a bleeding wound. Air splints are used to immobilize injuries below the elbow or below the knee.

Figure 29-21 If you encounter resistance or extreme pain when applying traction to a long bone, apply padded board splints to each side of the limb, and secure them with soft roller bandages, immobilizing the limb in its deformed position.

Air splints have some drawbacks, particularly in cold weather areas. The zipper can stick, clog with dirt, or freeze. Significant changes in the weather affect the pressure of the air in the splint, decreasing as the environment grows colder and increasing as the environment grows warmer. The same thing happens when there are changes in altitude, which can be a problem with helicopter transport of patients. Therefore, you should carefully monitor the splint and let air out if the splint becomes overinflated.

The method of applying an air splint depends on whether it has a zipper. With either type, you must first cover all wounds with a dry, sterile dressing, making sure that you use BSI precautions. For a splint that has a zipper, follow the steps in ▲ **Skill Drill 29-4** :

Skill Drill 29-5 Applying an Unzipped Air Splint

Support the injured limb.
Have your partner place his or her arm
through the splint to grasp the patient's hand
or foot.

Apply gentle traction while sliding the splint
onto the injured limb.

Inflate the splint.

1. **Hold the injured limb** slightly off the ground, applying gentle traction and supporting the site of injury. Have your partner place the open, deflated splint around the limb **(Step 1)**.

2. **Zip the splint up and inflate it** by pump or by mouth. When this is done, test the pressure in the splint. With proper inflation, you should just be able to compress the walls of the splint together with a firm pinch between the thumb and index finger near the edge of the splint.

3. **Check and record pulse, motor, and sensory functions,** and monitor them periodically until the patient reaches the hospital **(Step 2)**.

If you use an unzipped or partially zippered type of air splint, have another person help you follow the steps in (▲ **Skill Drill 29-5**):

1. First EMT-B: **Support the patient's injured limb** until splinting is accomplished.

2. Second EMT-B: **Place your arm through the splint.** Extend your hand beyond the splint, and grasp the hand or foot of the injured limb **(Step 1)**.

3. Second EMT-B: **Apply gentle traction** to the hand or foot while sliding the splint onto the injured limb. The hand or foot of the injured limb should always be included in the splint **(Step 2)**.

4. First EMT-B: **Inflate the splint** by pump or by mouth **(Step 3)**.

5. Second EMT-B: **Test the pressure** in the splint. This is something that you must do with either type of air splint.

6. Second EMT-B: **Check and record pulse, motor, and sensory functions,** and monitor them en route.

Other formable splints include vacuum splints, pillow splints, SAM splints, a sling and swathe, and the pneumatic antishock garment (PASG) for pelvic fractures. Just like an air splint, a vacuum splint can be easily shaped to fit around a deformed limb. Instead of pumping air in, however, you can use a hand pump to pull the air out through a valve. Follow the steps in ▶ **Skill Drill 29-6**) to apply a vacuum splint:

1. **Support and stabilize the injured limb,** applying traction if needed, while your partner applies the splint **(Step 1)**.

2. **Gently place the injured limb onto the vacuum splint** and wrap the splint around the limb **(Step 2)**.

3. **Draw the air out of the splint** through the suction valve, and then seal the valve. Once the valve is sealed, the vacuum splint becomes rigid, conforming to the shape of the deformed limb and immobilizing it **(Step 3)**.

4. **Check distal circulation and nervous functions,** and monitor them en route.

SkillDrill 29-6 Applying a Vacuum Splint

Stabilize and support the injury.

Place the splint and wrap it around the limb.

Draw the air out of the splint and seal the valve.

TRACTION SPLINTS. Traction splints are used primarily to secure fractures of the shaft of the femur, which are characterized by pain, swelling, and deformity of the midthigh. A traction splint should not be used if the patient has a joint or lower leg injury. Several different types of lower extremity traction splints are commercially available, such as the Hare traction splint, the Sager splint, and the Kendrick splint, each with its own unique method of application with which you must be familiar. The use of the Hare and Sager splints is described in this chapter.

The Hare traction splint uses a force called counter-traction, which is applied by the upper end of the splint against the ischial tuberosity of the patient's pelvis. This splint is not suitable for use on the upper extremity because the major nerves and blood vessels in the patient's axilla cannot tolerate countertraction forces.

Do not use traction splints for any of the following conditions:

- Injuries of the upper extremity
- Injuries close to or involving the knee
- Injuries of the hip
- Injuries of the pelvis
- Partial amputations or avulsions with bone separation
- Lower leg or ankle injury

Proper application of a traction splint requires two well-trained EMT-Bs working together. Practice the steps in ▶ Skill Drill 29-7 with your partner until the sequence and necessary teamwork have become routine:

1. **Cut open the patient's pant leg,** or otherwise expose the injured lower extremity. Follow BSI precautions as needed. Be sure to assess and record the pulse, motor function, and sensation distal to the injury.

2. **Place the splint beside the patient's uninjured leg,** and adjust it to the proper length, with the ring at the ischial tuberosity and the splint extending 12″ beyond the foot. Open and adjust the four Velcro support straps, which should be positioned at the midthigh, above the knee, below the knee, and above the ankle **(Step 1)**.

3. First EMT-B: **Manually support and stabilize** the injured limb so that no motion will occur at the fracture site while the second EMT-B fastens the appropriate-sized ankle hitch about the patient's ankle and foot. Normally, the patient's shoe is removed for this procedure **(Step 2)**.

4. First EMT-B: **Support the leg at the site of the suspected injury** while the second EMT-B manually applies gentle longitudinal traction to the

Skill Drill 29-7 Applying a Hare Traction Splint

1 Expose the injured limb and check pulse, motor, and sensory function.

Place the splint beside the uninjured limb, adjust the splint to proper length, and prepare the straps.

2 Support the injured limb as your partner fastens the ankle hitch about the foot and ankle.

3 Continue to support the limb as your partner applies gentle in-line traction to the ankle hitch and foot.

4 Slide the splint into position under the injured limb.

5 Pad the groin and fasten the ischial strap.

6 Connect the loops of the ankle hitch to the end of the splint as your partner continues to maintain traction. Carefully tighten the ratchet to the point that the splint holds adequate traction.

7 Secure and check support straps.

Assess pulse, motor, and sensory functions.

8 Secure the patient and splint to the backboard in a way that will prevent movement of the splint during patient movement and transport.

ankle hitch and foot. Use only enough to force to align (reposition) the limb so that it will fit into the splint; do not attempt to align the fracture fragments anatomically **(Step 3)**.

5. First EMT-B: **Slide the splint into position** under the patient's injured limb, making certain that the ring is seated well on the ischial tuberosity **(Step 4)**.

6. **Pad the groin area**, and gently apply the ischial strap **(Step 5)**.

7. First EMT-B: While the second EMT-B continues to maintain traction, **connect the loops of the ankle hitch** to the end of the splint. Then apply gentle traction to the connecting strap between the ankle hitch and the splint, just strongly enough to maintain limb alignment. Use caution. This splint comes with a ratchet mechanism to tighten the strap, which can overstretch the limb and further injure the patient. Adequate traction has been applied when the leg is the same length as the other leg or the patient feels relief **(Step 6)**.

8. Once proper traction has been applied, **fasten the support straps** so that the limb is securely held in the splint. Check all proximal and distal support straps to make sure they are secure **(Step 7)**.

9. At this point, **reassess distal pulses,** motor function, and sensation.

10. **Place the patient securely on a long spine board** for transport to the emergency department. You may need to load the patient feet first into the ambulance so that you do not shut the door against the splint **(Step 8)**.

Because this traction splint immobilizes the limb by producing countertraction on the ischium and in the groin, use care to pad these areas well. You must avoid excessive pressure on the external genitalia. Always use commercially available padded ankle hitches rather than pieces of rope, cord, or tape. Such improvised hitches can sometimes be painful and can potentially obstruct circulation in the foot.

The Sager splint is lightweight, is easy to store, applies a measurable amount of traction, and can be used with a PASG. Best of all, you can apply it by yourself when necessary. As with any splint, in addition to knowing the precise sequence of steps to apply the splint properly, you must practice the splinting technique frequently to maintain the necessary skills. Follow the steps in to apply a Sager splint

▶ Skill Drill 29-8 :

1. **Expose the injured extremity.** Using BSI precautions as needed, assess and record the pulse, motor function, and sensation distal to the injury.

2. Before applying the splint, **adjust the thigh strap** so that it will lie anteriorly when secured in place **(Step 1)**.

3. **Estimate the proper splint length** by placing it alongside the injured limb, so that the wheel is at the level of the heel.

4. **Arrange the ankle pads** to fit the size of the patient's ankle **(Step 2)**.

5. **Place the splint along the inner aspect of the limb,** and slide the thigh strap around the upper thigh so that the perineal cushion is snug against the groin and the ischial tuberosity. Tighten the thigh strap snugly **(Step 3)**.

6. **Secure the ankle harness** tightly around the patient's ankle just above the malleoli.

7. **Pull the cable ring** snugly up against the bottom of the foot **(Step 4)**.

8. **Pull out the inner shaft** of the splint to apply traction of approximately 10% of body weight, using a maximum of 15 lb **(Step 5)**.

9. **Secure the limb** to the splint using elasticized cravats **(Step 6)**.

10. **Secure the patient** to a long spine board.

11. **Check pulse, motor, and sensory function** **(Step 7)**.

HAZARDS OF IMPROPER SPLINTING. You must be aware of the hazards associated with the improper application of splints, including the following:

- Compression of nerves, tissues, and blood vessels
- Delay in transport of a patient with a life-threatening injury
- Reduction of distal circulation
- Aggravation of the injury
- Injury to tissue, nerves, blood vessels, or muscles as a result of excessive movement of the bone or joint

SkillDrill 29-8 Applying a Sager Traction Splint

After exposing the injured area, check the patient's pulse and motor and sensory function.
Adjust the thigh strap so that it lies anteriorly when secured.

Estimate the proper length of the splint by placing it next to the injured limb.
Fit the ankle pads to the ankle.

Place the splint at the inner thigh, apply the thigh strap at the upper thigh, and secure snugly.

Tighten the ankle harness just above the malleoli.
Snug the cable ring against the bottom of the foot.

Extend the splint's inner shaft to apply traction of about 10% of body weight.

Secure the splint with elasticized cravats.

Secure the patient to a long spine board.
Check pulse, motor and sensory functions.

Transportation

Once an injured limb is adequately splinted, the patient is ready to be transferred to a backboard or stretcher and transported.

Very few, if any, musculoskeletal injuries justify the use of excessive speed during transport. The limb will be stable once a dressing and splint have been applied. However, the patient with a pulseless limb must be given a higher priority. Still, if the hospital is only a few minutes away, speeding to the emergency department will make little or no difference to the patient's eventual outcome. If the treatment facility is an hour or more away, the patient with a pulseless limb should be transported by helicopter or immediate ground transportation. If circulation in the distal limb is impaired, always notify medical control so that proper steps can be taken quickly once the patient arrives in the emergency department.

Specific Musculoskeletal Injuries

Injuries of the Clavicle and Scapula

The <u>clavicle</u>, or collarbone, is one of the most commonly fractured bones in the body. Fractures of the clavicle occur most often in children when they fall on an outstretched hand. They can also occur with crushing injuries of the chest. A patient with a fracture of the clavicle will report pain in the shoulder and will usually hold the arm across the front of his or her body. A young child often reports pain throughout the entire arm and is unwilling to use any part of that limb. These complaints may make it difficult to localize the point of injury, but, generally, swelling and point tenderness occur over the clavicle ▼ **Figure 29-22** . Because the clavicle is subcutaneous (just beneath the skin), the skin will occasionally "tent" over the fracture fragment. The clavicle lies directly over major arteries, veins, and nerves; therefore, fracture of the clavicle may lead to neurovascular compromise.

Fractures of the <u>scapula</u>, or shoulder blade, occur much less frequently because this bone is well protected by many large muscles. Fractures of the scapula are almost always the result of a forceful, direct blow to the back, directly over the scapula, which may also injure the thoracic cage, lungs, and heart. For this reason, you must carefully assess the patient for signs of breathing problems. Provide supplemental oxygen and prompt transport for patients who are having difficulty breathing. Remember, it is the associated chest injuries, not the fractured scapula, that pose the greatest threat of long-term disability.

Abrasions, contusions, and significant swelling may also occur, and the patient will often limit use of the arm because of pain at the fracture site ▼ **Figure 29-23** . The scapula also has bony projections that may be fractured with a lesser degree of force.

The joint between the outer end of the clavicle and the acromion process of the scapula is called the <u>acromioclavicular (A/C) joint</u>. This joint is frequently separated during football and hockey play when a player falls and lands on the point of the shoulder, driving the scapula away from the outer end of the clavicle. This dislocation is often called an A/C separation. The distal end of the clavicle will usually stick out, and

Figure 29-22   A clavicle injury is characterized by swelling, point tenderness, and "tenting" over the fracture fragment.

Figure 29-23   Contusions or abrasions over the scapular area may indicate a fracture.

the patient will complain of pain, including point tenderness over the A/C joint (▶ **Figure 29-24**).

Fractures of the clavicle and scapula and A/C separations can all be splinted effectively with a sling and swathe. A **sling** is any bandage or material that helps support the weight of an injured upper extremity, relieving the downward pull of gravity on the injured site. To be effective, a sling must apply gentle upward support to the olecranon process of the ulna. The knot of the sling should be tied to one side of the neck so that it does not press uncomfortably on the cervical spine (▶ **Figure 29-25A**).

To fully immobilize the shoulder region, a **swathe**, a bandage that passes completely around the chest, must be used to bind the arm to the chest wall. The swathe should be tight enough to prevent the arm from swinging freely but not so tight as to compress the chest and compromise breathing. Leave the patient's fingers exposed so that you can assess neurovascular function at regular intervals (▶ **Figure 29-25B**).

Commercially available shoulder immobilizers or slings will provide adequate splinting for injuries of the shoulder region, as will triangular bandage slings. When all else fails, place a T-shirt over the arm.

Dislocation of the Shoulder

The glenohumeral joint (shoulder joint) is where the head of the **humerus**, the supporting bone of the upper arm, meets the glenoid fossa of the scapula. The **glenoid fossa** joins with the humeral head to form the glenohumeral joint. It is the most commonly dislocated large joint in the body. Almost always, the humeral head will dislocate anteriorly, coming to lie in front of the scapula as a result of forced abduction (away from the midline) and external rotation of the arm (▶ **Figure 29-26**).

Shoulder dislocations are extremely painful. The patient will guard the shoulder and try to protect it by holding the dislocated arm in a fixed position away from the chest wall (▶ **Figure 29-27**). The shoulder joint will usually be locked, and the shoulder will appear squared off or flattened. The humeral head will protrude anteriorly underneath the pectoris major on the anterior chest wall. As a result, the axillary nerve may be compressed, causing a numb patch on the outer aspect of the shoulder. Be sure to document this finding. Some patients may also report some numbness in the hand because either the nerves or the circulation is compromised.

Immobilizing an anterior shoulder dislocation is difficult, because any attempt to bring the arm in toward

Figure 29-24 With A/C separations, the distal end of the clavicle usually sticks out.

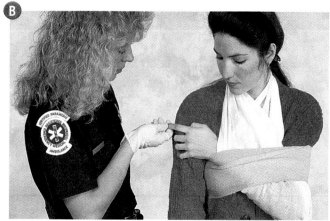

Figure 29-25 **A.** Apply the sling so that the knot is tied to one side of the neck. **B.** Bind the arm to the chest wall with a swathe so that the arm cannot swing freely. Leave the patient's fingers exposed so that you can assess distal circulation.

Figure 29-26 The shoulder almost always dislocates anteriorly. Note the absence of the normal rounded appearance of the shoulder.

Figure 29-27 A patient with a dislocated shoulder will guard the shoulder, trying to protect it by holding the arm in a fixed position away from the chest wall.

Figure 29-28 Splint the joint in a position of comfort, and place a pillow or towel between the arm and the chest wall to stabilize the arm, after which the elbow can be flexed to 90°. Apply a sling, and secure the arm to the chest with a swathe.

the chest will produce pain. You must splint the joint in whatever position is most comfortable for the patient. If necessary, place a pillow or rolled blankets or towels between the arm and chest to fill up the space between them (◄ **Figure 29-28**). Once the arm is stabilized in this way, the elbow can usually be flexed to 90° without causing further pain. At this point, you can apply a sling to the forearm and wrist to support the weight of the arm. Finally, secure the arm in the sling to the pillow and chest with a swathe. Transport the patient in a sitting or semiseated position.

Dislocation of the shoulder disrupts the supporting ligaments of the anterior aspect of the shoulder. Often, these ligaments fail to heal properly, so dislocation recurs, each time causing further neurovascular compromise and joint injury. In certain cases, surgical repair may be required. Some patients are able to reduce (set) their own dislocated shoulders. Generally, however, this maneuver must be done in a hospital setting and only after X-rays have been obtained.

A shoulder will dislocate posteriorly instead of anteriorly about once in every 20 occurrences. Football players, especially linemen, are susceptible to this injury. The arm will often be locked in an adduction (toward the midline), so it cannot be rotated. Reducing the dislocation usually requires medical supervision.

Fracture of the Humerus

Fractures of the humerus occur either proximally, in the midshaft, or distally at the elbow (► **Table 29-2**). Fractures of the proximal humerus resulting from falls are common among the elderly. Fractures of the midshaft occur more often in young patients, usually as the result of a violent injury.

With any severely angulated fracture, you should consider applying traction to realign the fracture fragments before splinting them. Check your local protocols for indications and techniques for applying traction to a severely angulated fracture. Support the site of the fracture with one hand, and with the other hand, grasp the two humeral condyles (its lateral and medial protrusions) just above the elbow. Pull gently in line with the normal axis of the limb (► **Figure 29-29**). Once you achieve gross alignment of the limb, splint the arm with a sling and swathe, supplemented by a padded board splint on the lateral aspect of the arm (► **Figure 29-30**). If the patient reports significant pain or resists gentle traction, splint the fracture in the deformed position with a padded wire ladder or a padded board splint, using pillows to support the injured limb. Note that

TABLE 29-2 Characteristics and Treatment of Fractures of the Humerus

Type	Characteristics	Treatment
Proximal Humeral Fractures	• Significant swelling, but no deformity, of the upper arm • Neurovascular compromise • Any or all of the brachial plexus affected, depending on the degree of displacement • Concurrent soft-tissue injuries • Possible rotator cuff injury (if X-rays show no fracture, a tear of the rotator cuff is possible, especially if the patient cannot move the arm toward the medial plane)	• Immobilize in a sling and swathe or a shoulder immobilizer. • Use the chest wall as a splint, and secure the injured arm to the chest wall. • Place a short, padded board splint on the lateral side of the arm under the sling and swathe for additional support.
Midshaft Fractures	• Gross angulation of the arm • Marked instability and crepitus of fracture fragments • Possible neurovascular compromise • Possible entrapment of the radial nerve (The patient cannot extend or dorsiflex the wrist or fingers and may report numbness on the dorsum of the hand; classic "wrist drop.")	• Immobilize with a sling and swathe or a shoulder immobilizer. • Use the chest wall as a splint, and secure the injured arm to the chest wall. • Place a short, padded board splint on the lateral side of the arm under the sling and swathe for additional support.
Distal Humeral Fractures	• Significant swelling at the elbow • Possible neurovascular compromise • Possible injury to the ulnar or median nerves (document nerve status before and after any attempt to reduce the fracture)	• Immobilize in a splint, in addition to a sling and swathe or a shoulder immobilizer.

Figure 29-29 To align a severe deformity associated with a humeral shaft fracture, apply gentle pressure to the humeral condyles, as shown in this uninjured arm.

Figure 29-30 Splint a humeral shaft fracture with a sling and swathe supplemented by a padded board splint on the lateral aspect of the arm.

compartment syndrome can develop in the forearm in children with these fractures.

Elbow Injuries

Fractures and dislocations often occur around the elbow, and the different types of injuries are difficult to distinguish without X-rays. However, they all produce similar limb deformities and require the same emergency care. Injuries to nerves and blood vessels are quite common in this region. Such injuries can be caused or worsened by inappropriate emergency care, particularly by excessive manipulation of the injured joint.

FRACTURE OF THE DISTAL HUMERUS. This type of fracture, also known as a supracondylar or intercondylar fracture, is common in children. Frequently, the fracture fragments rotate significantly, producing deformity and causing injuries to nearby vessels and nerves. Swelling occurs rapidly and is often severe.

DISLOCATION OF THE ELBOW. This type of injury typically occurs in athletes and does not appear in young children. The ulna and radius are most often displaced posteriorly. The **ulna**, the bone on the small finger side of the forearm, and the **radius**, the bone on the thumb side of the forearm, both join the distal humerus. The posterior displacement makes the olecranon process of the ulna much more prominent (▶ **Figure 29-31**). The joint is usually locked, with the forearm moderately flexed on the arm; this position makes any attempt at motion extremely painful. As with a fracture of the distal humerus, there is swelling and significant potential for vessel or nerve injury.

ELBOW JOINT SPRAIN. This injury is rare and is usually diagnosed by X-ray. Often, the real problem is a hard-to-detect fracture.

FRACTURE OF THE OLECRANON PROCESS OF THE ULNA. This fracture is usually the result of a direct blow and is often characterized by lacerations and abrasions. Often, the patient will be unable to extend the elbow.

FRACTURE OF THE RADIAL HEAD. Often missed during diagnosis, this fracture generally occurs as a result of a fall on an outstretched arm or a direct blow to the lateral aspect of the elbow. Attempts to rotate the elbow or wrist are very uncomfortable.

CARE OF ELBOW INJURIES. All elbow injuries are serious and require careful management. Always assess distal neurovascular functions periodically in patients with elbow injuries. If you find strong pulses and good capillary refill, then splint the elbow injury in the position in which you found it, adding a wrist sling if this seems helpful. Two padded board splints, applied to each side of the limb and secured with soft roller bandages, usu-

ally are enough to stabilize the arm (▼ **Figure 29-32A**). Make sure the board extends from the shoulder joint to the wrist joint, immobilizing the entire bone above and below the injured joint. Alternatively, you can mold a padded wire ladder splint or a SAM splint to the shape of the limb (▼ **Figure 29-32B**). If necessary, you may add further support to the limb with a pillow.

Figure 29-31 Posterior dislocation of the elbow makes the olecranon process of the ulna much more prominent.

A

B

Figure 29-32 **A.** Two padded board splints provide adequate stabilization for an injured elbow. A wrist sling provides additional support. **B.** A SAM splint can be molded to the shape of the limb so that you can splint it in the position in which it was found.

Pediatric Needs

Growth plate injuries in children are common, especially around the wrist, elbow, knee, and ankle. Injuries tend to occur through these cartilaginous growth centers because they are inherently weaker than the surrounding bone. Since longitudinal growth of the limb is dependent upon the function of the growth plate, it is extremely important to recognize the possibility of growth plate injuries, stabilize the injured limb, and transport the patient in timely fashion to an appropriate center with pediatric, pediatric orthopaedic, and pediatric surgical coverage. Proper functioning of the injured growth plate throughout the remainder of skeletal growth is dependent upon urgent anatomic reduction of the fracture and close follow-up by an orthopaedist.

Any deformity in close proximity to a joint in children younger than 16 years should be assumed to be a growth plate injury and transported and treated appropriately.

Figure 29-33 Fractures of the forearm often occur in children as a result of a fall on an outstretched hand.

A cold, pale hand or a weak or absent pulse and poor capillary refill indicate that the blood vessels have likely been injured. Further care of this patient must be dictated by a physician. Notify medical control immediately. If you are within 10 to 15 minutes of the hospital, splint the limb in the position in which you found it and provide prompt transport. Otherwise, medical control may direct you to try to realign the limb to improve circulation in the hand.

If the limb is pulseless and significantly deformed at the elbow, apply gentle manual traction in line with the long axis of the limb to decrease the deformity. This maneuver may restore the pulse. Be careful, as excessive manipulation will only worsen the vascular problem. If no pulse returns *after one attempt*, splint the limb in the most comfortable position for the patient. If the pulse is restored by gentle longitudinal traction, splint the limb in whatever position allows the strongest pulse. Provide prompt transport for all patients with impaired distal circulation.

Fractures of the Forearm

Fractures of the shaft of the radius and ulna are common in people of all age groups but are seen most often in children and the elderly. Usually, both bones break at the same time when the injury is the result of a fall on an outstretched hand (▲ **Figure 29-33**). An isolated fracture of the shaft of the ulna may occur as the result of a direct blow to it; this is known as a nightstick fracture.

Fractures of the distal radius, which are especially common in elderly patients with osteoporosis, are often known as Colles fractures. The term "silver fork deformity" is used to describe the distinctive appearance of the patient's arm (▶ **Figure 29-34**). In children, this fracture may occur through the growth plate and can have long-term consequences.

To immobilize fractures of the forearm or wrist, you can use a padded board, air, vacuum, or pillow splint. If the shaft of the bone has been fractured, be sure to include the elbow joint in the splint. Splinting of the elbow joint is not essential with fractures near the wrist; however, the patient will be more comfortable if you add a sling or pillow for more support.

Injuries of the Wrist and Hand

Injuries of the wrist, ranging from dislocations to sprains, must be confirmed by X-ray. Dislocations are usually associated with a fracture, resulting in a fracture dislocation. Another common wrist injury is the isolated, nondisplaced fracture of a carpal bone, especially the scaphoid. Any questionable wrist sprain must be splinted and evaluated in the emergency department.

There is a great variety of hand injuries, some with potentially serious consequences. Industrial, recreational, and home accidents often result in dislocations, fractures, lacerations, burns, and amputations. Because the fingers and hands are required to function in such intricate ways, any injury that is not treated properly may result in permanent disability, as well as deformity. For this reason, all injuries to the hand, including simple lacerations, must be evaluated promptly by a physician. For example, you should not attempt to "pop" a dislocated finger joint back in place (▶ **Figure 29-35**). Always bring any amputated parts to the hospital with the patient. Be sure to wrap the ampu-

Figure 29-34 **A.** Fractures of the distal radius produce a characteristic silver fork deformity. **B.** An artist's illustration of same.

tated part in a dry or moist sterile dressing depending on your local protocol and place it in a dry plastic bag. Put the bag in a cooled container; do not soak the part in water or allow it to freeze.

A bulky forearm dressing makes an effective splint for any hand or wrist injury. Follow the steps in ▶ **Skill Drill 29-9** :

1. **Follow BSI precautions.**

2. **Cover all wounds** with a dry, sterile dressing.

3. Supporting the injured limb, **form the injured hand into the <u>position of function</u>,** with the wrist slightly bent down and all finger joints moderately flexed. This is the position that is used to hold a can most comfortably.

4. **Place a soft roller bandage into the palm of the hand** (Step 1).

5. **Apply a padded board splint to the palmar side of the wrist,** leaving the fingers exposed (Step 2).

6. **Secure the entire length of the splint** with a soft roller bandage (Step 3).

7. **Apply a sling and swathe** or prop the splinted hand and wrist on a pillow or on the patient's chest during transport to the hospital.

Fractures of the Pelvis

Fracture of the pelvis is most often a result of direct compression in the form of a heavy blow that literally crushes the pelvis. The blow may be from a motor vehicle crash, a weapon used deliberately, a falling object, or a fall from a height. Injuries to the pelvis can also be caused by indirect forces. For example, when the knee strikes the dashboard in an automobile crash, the impact of the force is transmitted along the line of

Figure 29-35 Dislocation of the finger joint. Do not be tempted to try to "pop" the joint back into place.

the <u>femur</u>, the thigh bone, which is the longest and largest bone in the body. The head of the femur is driven into the pelvis, causing it to fracture. However, not all pelvic fractures result from violent trauma. Even a simple fall can produce a fracture of the pelvis, especially in elderly individuals with osteoporosis.

Fractures of the pelvis may be accompanied by life-threatening loss of blood from the laceration of blood vessels affixed to the pelvis at certain key points. Up to several liters of blood may drain into the pelvic space and the retroperitoneal space, which lies between the abdominal cavity and the posterior abdominal wall. The kidneys and pancreas are contained in the **retroperitoneal space**. The result is significant hypotension, shock, and sometimes death. For this reason, you must take immediate steps to treat shock, even if there is only minimal swelling. Often, there are no visible signs of bleeding until severe blood loss has occurred. You should be prepared to resuscitate the patient rapidly if this becomes necessary.

Because the pelvis is surrounded by heavy muscle, open fractures of the pelvis are quite uncommon.

Skill Drill 29-9 Splinting the Hand and Wrist

Move the hand into the position of function. Place a soft roller bandage in the palm.

Apply a padded board splint on the palmar side with fingers exposed.

Secure the splint with a roller bandage.

However, pelvis fracture fragments can lacerate the rectum and vagina, creating an open fracture that is often overlooked. Once the protective pelvic ring is broken, the structures it is designed to protect, including the urinary bladder, are open to injury. The bladder may be lacerated by pelvic bone fragments, but more often, it tears or ruptures as a result of tension on either the bladder or the urethra.

You should suspect a fracture of the pelvis in any patient who has sustained a high-velocity injury and complains of discomfort in the lower back or abdomen. Because the area is covered by heavy muscle and other soft tissue, deformity or swelling may be very difficult to see. The most reliable sign of fracture of the pelvis is simple tenderness on firm compression and palpation. Firm compression on the two iliac crests will produce pain at a fracture site in the pelvic ring. Assess for tenderness by taking the following steps (▶ Figure 29-36):

1. Place the palms of your hands over the lateral aspect of each iliac crest, and **apply firm but gentle inward pressure** on the pelvic ring.

2. With the patient lying supine, **place a palm over the anterior aspect of each iliac crest, and apply firm downward pressure.**

3. Use the palm of your hand to firmly but gently **palpate the pubic symphysis**, the firm cartilaginous joint between the two pubic bones. This area will be tender if there is injury to the anterior portion of the pelvic ring.

If there has been injury to the bladder or the urethra, the patient will have lower abdominal tenderness and may have evidence of **hematuria** (blood in the urine) or blood at the urethral opening.

Perform an initial assessment, and carefully monitor the general condition of any patient who you suspect has a pelvic fracture, because he or she is at high risk for hypovolemic shock. Stable patients can be secured to a long spine board or a scoop stretcher to immobilize isolated fractures of the pelvis. Place a PASG on the spine board or stretcher before transferring the patient to the backboard (▶ Figure 29-37). The PASG will be ready to apply and inflate if the patient develops signs of shock. Remember, the PASG is only a temporary stabilization device and must be removed within 24 hours. Such a critically injured patient must be transferred to the hospital immediately.

Dislocation of the Hip

The hip joint is a very stable ball-and-socket joint that dislocates only after significant injury. Almost all dislocations of the hip are posterior. The femoral head is displaced posteriorly to lie in the muscles of the buttock. Posterior dislocation of the hip most commonly occurs during automobile accidents in which the knee meets with a direct force, such as the dashboard, and the entire femur is driven posteriorly, dislocating the joint (▶ Figure 29-38). Thus, you should suspect a hip dislocation in any patient who has been in an automobile crash and has a contusion, laceration, or obvious

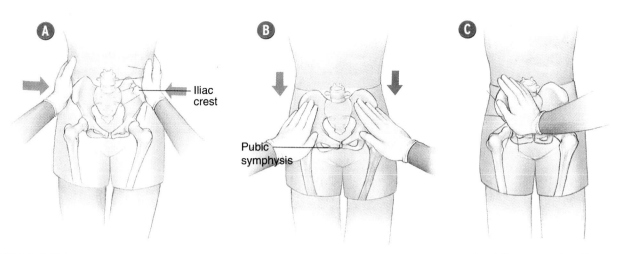

Figure 29-36 **A.** To assess for tenderness in the pelvic region, place your hands over the lateral aspect of each iliac crest, and gently compress the pelvis. **B.** With the patient in a supine position, place your palms over the anterior aspect of each iliac crest, and apply firm but gentle downward pressure. **C.** Palpate the pubic symphysis with the palm of your hand.

Figure 29-37 Place a PASG on the spine board before log-rolling a patient with a suspected pelvic fracture.

Figure 29-38 Posterior dislocation of the hip can occur as a result of the knee hitting the dashboard in an automobile crash. The impact drives the femur posteriorly (see arrow), dislocating the joint.

fracture in the knee region. Very rarely does the femoral head dislocate anteriorly; in this circumstance, the legs are suddenly and forcibly spread wide apart and locked in this position.

Posterior dislocation of the hip is frequently complicated by injury to the sciatic nerve, which is located directly behind the hip joint. The <u>sciatic nerve</u> is the most important nerve in the lower extremity; it controls the activity of muscles in the thigh and below the knee,

as well as sensation in the entire leg and foot. When the head of the femur is forced out of the hip socket, it may compress or stretch the sciatic nerve, leading to partial or complete paralysis of the nerve. The result is decreased sensation in the leg and foot and frequently weakness in the foot muscles. Generally, only the dorsi-flexors, the muscles that raise the toes or foot, are involved, causing the "foot drop" that is characteristic of damage to the peroneal portion of the sciatic nerve.

Figure 29-39 **A.** The usual position of a patient with a posterior dislocation of the hip. The hip joint is flexed, and the thigh is rotated inward and adducted across the midline of the body. **B.** Support the affected limb with pillows and blankets, particularly under the flexed knee. Secure the entire limb to a long board with long straps to prevent movement during transport.

Patients with a posterior dislocation of the hip typically lie with the hip joint flexed (the knee joint drawn up toward the chest) and the thigh rotated inward toward the midline of the body over the top of the opposite thigh (▲ **Figure 29-39A**). With the rare anterior dislocation, the limb is in the opposite position, extended straight out, rotated, and pointing away from the midline of the body.

Dislocation of the hip is associated with very distinctive signs. The patient will have severe pain in the hip and will strongly resist any attempt to move the joint. The lateral and posterior aspects of the hip region will be tender on palpation. With some thin individuals, you can palpate the femoral head deep within the muscles of the buttock. Check for a sciatic nerve injury by carefully assessing sensation and motor function in the lower extremity. Occasionally, sciatic nerve function will be normal at first and then slowly diminish.

As with any other extremity injury, you should make no attempt to reduce the dislocated hip in the field. Splint the dislocation in the position of the deformity and place the patient supine on a long spine board. Support the affected limb with pillows and rolled blankets, particularly under the flexed knee (◀ **Figure 29-39B**). Then secure the entire limb to the spine board with long straps so that the hip region will not move. Be sure to provide prompt transport.

Fractures of the Proximal Femur

Fractures of the proximal (upper) end of the femur are among the most common fractures, especially in elderly people. Although they are usually called hip fractures, they rarely involve the hip joint. Instead, the break goes through the neck of the femur, the intertrochanteric (middle) region, or across the proximal shaft of the femur (subtrochanteric fractures). Although these three fracture types occur most often in older patients, particularly patients with osteoporosis, they may also be seen as a result of high-energy injuries in young adults.

All patients with displaced fractures of the proximal femur display a very characteristic deformity. They lie with the leg externally rotated, and the injured leg is usually shorter than the opposite, uninjured limb. When the fracture is not displaced, this deformity is not present. With any kind of hip fracture, patients typically are unable to walk or move the leg because of pain in the hip region or in the groin or inner aspect of the thigh. The hip region is usually tender on palpation, and gentle rolling of the leg will cause pain but will not do further damage. On occasion, the pain is referred to the knee, and it is not uncommon for an elderly patient with a hip fracture to complain of knee pain after a fall. You should splint the lower extremity of an elderly patient who has fallen and complains of pain in either the hip or the knee, even if there is no deformity, and then transport the patient to the emergency department.

The age of the patient and the severity of the injury will dictate how you splint the fracture. With young people, fractures of the hip resulting from violent injury are best immobilized with a traction splint or the combination of a PASG and a spine board. The PASG offers an added advantage: It will help to control bleeding in the region. Apply the traction splint as you would for a femoral shaft fracture, taking special care to protect the injured region from excessive pressure from the ring of a Hare traction splint.

An elderly patient with an isolated hip fracture does not require a traction splint (▶ **Figure 29-40A**). You can

There is always significant blood loss with fractures of the femoral shaft.

Figure 29-40 **A.** A patient with a fracture of the proximal femur will typically lie still with the extremity rotated, making the injured leg appear shorter than the other leg. **B.** Splint the injured leg to the uninjured leg and secure the patient on a scoop stretcher or spine board.

effectively immobilize such a fracture by placing the patient on a long spine board or scoop stretcher, using pillows or rolled blankets to support the injured limb in the deformed position. Then secure the injured limb carefully to the stretcher with long straps

▲ **Figure 29-40B** .

All patients with hip fractures may lose significant amounts of blood. Therefore, you should treat with high-flow oxygen and monitor vital signs frequently, being alert for signs of shock.

Femoral Shaft Fractures

Fractures of the femur can occur in any part of the shaft, from the hip region to the femoral condyles just above the knee joint. Following a fracture, the large muscles of the thigh spasm in an attempt to "splint" the unstable limb. The muscle spasm often produces significant deformity of the limb, with severe angulation or external rotation at the fracture site. Usually, the limb shortens significantly as well. Fractures of the femoral

shaft are often open, and fragments of bone may protrude through the skin.

There is always a significant amount of blood loss, as much as 500 to 1,000 mL, after a fracture of the shaft of the femur. With open fractures, the amount of blood loss may be even greater. Thus, it is not unusual for hypovolemic shock to develop. Handle these patients with extreme care, because any extra movement or fracture manipulation will increase the amount of blood loss.

Because of the severe deformity that occurs with these fractures, bone fragments may penetrate or press on important nerves and vessels and produce significant damage. For this reason, you must carefully and periodically assess the distal neurovascular function in patients who have sustained a fracture of the femoral shaft. Remove the clothing from the affected limb so that you can adequately inspect the injury site for any open wounds. Remember to follow BSI precautions when any blood or body fluids are present. Monitor the patient's vital signs closely, and continue to watch for the onset of hypovolemic shock. You must provide immediate transport in this situation.

Cover any wound with a dry sterile dressing. If the foot or leg below the level of the fracture shows signs of impaired circulation (is pale, cold, or pulseless), apply gentle longitudinal traction to the deformed limb in line with the long axis of the limb. Gradually turn the leg from the deformed position to restore the limb's overall alignment. Often, this restores or improves circulation to the foot. If it does not, the patient may have sustained a serious vascular injury and is in need of prompt medical attention.

A fracture of the femoral shaft is best immobilized with a traction splint, such as a Hare traction splint or a Sager splint (see Skill Drills 29-7 and 29-8).

Injuries of Knee Ligaments

The knee is very vulnerable to injury; therefore, many different types of injuries occur in this region. Ligament injuries, for example, range from mild sprains to complete dislocation of the joint. The patella can also dislocate. In addition, all the bony elements of the knee (distal femur, upper tibia, and patella) can fracture.

The knee is especially susceptible to ligament injuries, which occur when abnormal bending or twisting forces are applied to the joint. Such injuries are often seen in both recreational and competitive athletes. The ligaments on the medial side of the knee are the ones that are most frequently injured, typically when the foot is fixed to the ground and the lateral aspect of the knee is struck by a heavy object, such as when a football player is clipped or tackled from the side.

Usually, the patient with a knee ligament injury will report pain in the joint and be unable to use the extremity normally. When you examine the patient, you will generally find swelling, occasional ecchymosis, point tenderness at the injury site, and joint effusion (excess fluid in the joint).

You must splint all suspected knee ligament injuries. The splint should extend from the hip joint to the foot, immobilizing the bone above the injured joint (the femur) and the bone below it (the tibia). A variety of splints can be used, including a padded, rigid, long leg splint or two padded board splints securely applied to the medial and lateral aspects of the limb. A long spine board, a pillow splint, or simply binding the injured limb to its uninjured mate are acceptable but less effective splinting techniques. The patient will usually be able to straighten the knee to allow you to apply the splint. However, if you encounter resistance or pain when trying to straighten the knee, splint it in the flexed position. Then continue to monitor the distal neurovascular function until the patient reaches the hospital.

Dislocation of the Knee

Complete disruption of the ligaments supporting the knee may result in dislocation of the joint. When this happens, the proximal end of the tibia completely displaces from its juncture with the lower end of the femur, usually producing a significant deformity. Although substantial ligament damage always occurs with a knee dislocation, the more urgent injury is to the popliteal artery, which is often lacerated or compressed by the displaced tibia. When gross deformity, severe pain, and an inability to move the joint cause you to suspect a dislocation of the knee, always check the distal circulation carefully before taking any other step. If the distal pulses are absent, contact medical control immediately for further stabilization instructions.

If adequate distal pulses are present, splint the knee in the position in which you found it, and transport the

patient promptly. Do not attempt to manipulate or straighten any severe knee injury if there are good distal pulses. If the limb is straight, apply standard rigid long leg splints to at least two sides of the limb to immobilize it (▼ **Figure 29-41A**). If the knee is bent and the foot has a good pulse, splint the joint in the bent position, using parallel padded board splints secured at the hip and ankle joint to provide a stable A-frame (▼ **Figure 29-41B**).

Figure 29-41 **A.** When the injured knee is straight, apply padded board splints extending from the hip to the ankle. **B.** If the knee is flexed and the foot has good pulses, apply padded board splints with the knee in the flexed position.

Secure the limb to a spine board or stretcher with pillows and straps to eliminate any motion during transport.

On rare occasions, medical control may instruct you to realign a deformed, pulseless limb to reduce compression of the popliteal artery and thus restore distal circulation. You should make only one attempt to do this. First, straighten the limb by applying gentle longitudinal traction in the axis of the limb. Once you apply manual traction, maintain it until the limb is fully splinted; otherwise, the limb will return to its deformed position. If traction significantly increases the patient's pain, do not continue. As you apply traction, monitor the posterior tibial pulse to see whether it returns. Splint the limb in the position in which you feel the strongest pulse. If you are unable to restore the distal pulse, splint the limb in the position that is most comfortable for the patient, and then provide prompt transport to the hospital. Notify medical control of the status of the distal pulse so that arrangements to treat the patient can be made in advance.

Fractures About the Knee

Fractures about the knee may occur at the distal end of the femur, at the proximal end of the tibia, or in the patella. Because of local tenderness and swelling, it is easy to confuse a nondisplaced or minimally displaced fracture about the knee with a ligament injury. Likewise, a displaced fracture about the knee may produce significant deformity that makes it look like a dislocation. Management of the two types of injuries is as follows:

- If there is an adequate distal pulse and no significant deformity, splint the limb with the knee straight.
- If there is an adequate pulse and significant deformity, splint the joint in the position of deformity.
- If the pulse is absent below the level of the injury, contact medical control immediately for further instructions.

Dislocation of the Patella

A dislocated patella most commonly occurs in teenagers and young adults who are engaged in athletic activities. Some patients have recurrent dislocations of the patella. As with recurrent dislocation of the shoulder, a minor twisting may be enough to produce the problem. Usually, the dislocated patella displaces to the lateral side, and the knee is held in a partially flexed position. The displacement of the

Figure 29-42 A dislocated patella will typically appear with the patella displaced lateral to the knee and with the knee moderately flexed.

patella produces a significant deformity in which the knee is held in a moderately flexed position and the patella is displaced to the lateral side of the knee ▲ **Figure 29-42** .

Splint the knee in the position in which you found it; most often, this is with the knee flexed to a moderate degree. To immobilize the knee, apply padded board splints to the medial and lateral aspects of the joint, extending from the hip to the ankle. Use pillows to support the limb on the stretcher.

Occasionally, as you apply the splint, the patella will return to its normal position spontaneously. When this occurs, immobilize the limb as for a knee ligament injury, in a padded long leg splint. The patient still needs to be transported to the emergency department. Report the spontaneous reduction as soon as you arrive at the hospital so that the medical staff is aware of the severity of the injury.

Injuries of the Tibia and Fibula

The **tibia** (shinbone) is the larger of the two leg bones that are responsible for supporting the major weight-bearing surface of the knee and ankle; the **fibula** is the smaller of them. Fracture of the shaft of the tibia or the fibula may occur at any place between the knee joint and the ankle joint. Usually, both bones fracture at the same time. Even a single fracture may result in severe deformity, with significant angulation or rotation. Because the

Figure 29-43 Because the tibia is so close to the skin, open fractures are quite common.

Figure 29-44 Swelling about the ankle is characteristic of both sprains and fractures.

tibia is located just beneath the skin, open fractures of this bone are quite common ▲ **Figure 29-43** .

Fractures of the tibia and fibula should be immobilized with a padded, rigid long leg splint or an air splint that extends from the foot to the upper thigh. Traction splints are not indicated for isolated tibial fractures. As with most other fractures of the shaft of long bones, you should correct severe deformity before splinting by applying gentle longitudinal traction. The goal here is to restore a position that will take a standard splint; it is not necessary to replace the fracture fragments in their anatomic position.

Fractures of the tibia and fibula are often associated with vascular injury as a result of the distorted position of the limb following injury. Realigning the limb frequently restores an adequate blood supply to the foot. If it does not, transport the patient promptly and notify medical control while you are en route.

Ankle Injuries

The ankle is the most commonly injured joint. Ankle injuries occur in individuals of all ages and range in severity from a simple sprain, which heals after a few days' rest, to severe fracture-dislocations. As with other joints, it is sometimes difficult to tell a nondisplaced ankle fracture from a simple sprain without X-rays ▲ **Figure 29-44** . Therefore, any ankle injury that produces pain, swelling, localized tenderness, or the inability to bear weight must be evaluated by a physician. The most frequent mechanism of ankle injury is twisting, which stretches or tears the supporting ligaments. A more extensive twisting force may result in

fracture of one or both malleoli. Dislocation of the ankle is usually associated with fractures of both malleoli.

You can manage the wide spectrum of injuries to the ankle in the same way, as follows:

1. Dress all open wounds.

2. Assess distal neurovascular function.

3. Correct any gross deformity by applying gentle longitudinal traction to the heel.

4. Before releasing traction, apply a splint.

You can use a padded rigid splint, an air splint, or a pillow splint. Just make sure it includes the entire foot and extends up the leg to the level of the knee joint.

Foot Injuries

Injuries to the foot can result in the fracture of one or more of the tarsals, metatarsals, or phalanges of the toes. Toe fractures are especially common.

Of the tarsal bones, the **calcaneus**, the heel bone, is the most frequently fractured. Injury usually occurs when the patient falls or jumps from a height and lands directly on the heel. The force of injury compresses the calcaneus, producing immediate swelling and ecchymosis. If the force of impact is great enough, as from a fall from a roof or tree, there may be other fractures as well.

Frequently, the force of injury is transmitted up the legs to the spine, producing a fracture of the lumbar spine ▶ **Figure 29-45** . When a patient who has jumped or fallen from a height complains of heel pain, be sure

Figure 29-45 The force of injury is transmitted up the legs to the spine, often resulting in a fracture of the lumbar spine.

Figure 29-46 A pillow splint provides excellent immobilization of the foot.

to question him or her about back pain and carefully check the spine for tenderness or deformity.

Injuries of the foot are associated with significant swelling but rarely with gross deformity. Vascular injuries are not common. As in the hand, lacerations about the ankle and foot may damage important underlying nerves and tendons. Puncture wounds of the foot are common and may cause serious infection if not treated early. All of these injuries must be evaluated and treated by a physician.

To splint the foot, apply a rigid padded board splint, an air splint, or a pillow splint, immobilizing the ankle

joint as well as the foot **▲ Figure 29-46** . Leave the toes exposed so that you can periodically assess neurovascular function.

When the patient is lying on the stretcher, elevate the foot approximately 6″ to minimize swelling. All patients with lower extremity injuries should be transported in the supine position to allow for elevation of the limb. Never allow the foot and leg to dangle off the stretcher onto the floor or ground.

If a patient has fallen from a height and complains of heel pain, use a long spine board to immobilize any possible spinal injury in addition to splinting the foot.

Prep Kit

Ready for Review

Skeletal or voluntary muscle, which attaches to bone and forms the major muscle mass of the body, is supplied with arteries, veins, and nerves. The 206 bones of the skeleton are living tissue that, when fractured, can bleed and cause severe pain. Wherever two bones come into contact, a joint is formed, strengthened in key areas by ligaments. A fracture is a broken bone; a dislocation is a disruption of a joint; a sprain is a joint injury that involves partial or temporary dislocation of bone ends and partial stretching or tearing of ligaments; and a strain is a muscle pull. Depending on the amount of kinetic energy absorbed by the tissues, the zone of injury may extend to a distant point, so you must always check for associated injuries beyond the obvious ones. Fractures are either open or closed, displaced or nondisplaced. Signs of fracture and dislocation include pain, deformity, point tenderness, guarding, swelling, crepitus, and false motion. Signs of sprain include ecchymosis and instability of the joint.

Your approach to patients with all painful, swollen, deformed extremities should include a rapid initial assessment, stabilization of vital functions and control of serious bleeding, focused physical exam of the injured body part, assessment of neurovascular function in the affected limb, an attempt to reduce fractures and dislocations, splinting to immobilize the affected part, and prompt transport to the hospital. For each limb, your neurovascular examination should include pulse, sensation, and motor function. Repeat this exam every 5 to 10 minutes.

The principles of splinting include the following: If you suspect a fracture of the shaft of any bone, make sure the splint immobilizes the joints above and below the fracture; with injuries in and around a joint, make sure the splint immobilizes the bones above and below the injured joint; where fracture of a long bone shaft has resulted in severe deformity, use constant, gentle, manual traction (pull) to align the limb so that it can be splinted, unless this is too painful. There are three types of splints: rigid splints and traction splints, which require two people to apply, and formable splints, including air splints. In addition, slings and swathes are used to help support the weight of an injured upper extremity and immobilize the shoulder region, respectively.

Provide immediate transport to any patient if you are unable to restore a pulse to a pulseless limb by applying traction. The only life-threatening musculoskeletal injuries are multiple fractures, fractures with arterial injuries, severe open fractures, limb amputations, and pelvic fractures with hemodynamic instability.

Vital Vocabulary

acromioclavicular (A/C) joint A simple joint where the bony projections of the scapula and the clavicle meet at the top of the shoulder.

articular cartilage A pearly layer of specialized cartilage covering the articular surfaces (contact surfaces on the ends) of bones in synovial joints.

calcaneus The heel bone.

clavicle The collarbone.

closed fracture A fracture in which the skin is not broken.

compartment syndrome An elevation of pressure within the fascial compartment, characterized by extreme pain, decreased pain sensation, pain on stretching of affected muscles, and decreased power; most frequently seen in fractures below the elbow or knee in children.

crepitus A grating or grinding sensation or sound caused by fractured bone ends or joints rubbing together.

dislocation Disruption of a joint in which ligaments are damaged and the bone ends are completely displaced.

displaced fracture A fracture in which bone fragments are separated from one another and not in anatomic alignment.

ecchymosis Bruising or discoloration associated with bleeding within or under the skin.

femur The thigh bone, which extends from the pelvis to the knee and is responsible for formation of the hip; the longest and largest bone in the body.

fibula The outer and smaller bone of the two bones of the lower leg.

fracture A break in the continuity of a bone.

glenoid fossa The part of the scapula that joins with the humeral head to form the glenohumeral joint.

hematuria Blood in the urine.

humerus The supporting bone of the upper arm that joins with the scapula (glenoid) to form the shoulder joint and with the ulna and radius to form the elbow joint.

joint The place where two bones come into contact.

ligament A band of fibrous tissue that connects bones to bones, and supports and strengthens a joint.

nondisplaced fracture A simple crack in the bone that has not caused the bone to move from its normal anatomic position; also called a hairline fracture.

open fracture Any break in a bone in which the overlying skin has been damaged.

patella The kneecap.

point tenderness Tenderness that is sharply localized at the site of the injury, found by gently palpating along the bone with the tip of one finger.

position of function A hand position in which the wrist is slightly dorsiflexed and all finger joints are moderately flexed.

pubic symphysis The firm cartilaginous joint between the two pubic bones.

radius The bone on the thumb side of the forearm; most important in wrist function.

reduce Return a dislocated joint or fractured bone to its normal position; set.

retroperitoneal space The space between the abdominal cavity and the posterior abdominal wall, containing the kidneys, certain large vessels, and parts of the gastrointestinal tract.

scapula Shoulder blade.

sciatic nerve The major nerve to the lower extremity; controls much of muscle function in the leg, and sensation in the entire leg and foot.

skeletal muscle Striated muscles that are attached to bones and usually cross at least one joint.

sling A bandage or material that helps to support the weight of an injured upper extremity.

splint A flexible or rigid appliance used to protect and maintain the position of an injured extremity.

sprain A joint injury involving damage to supporting ligaments, and partial or temporary dislocation of bone ends.

strain Stretching or tearing of a muscle; also called a muscle pull.

swathe A bandage that passes around the chest to secure an injured arm to the chest.

tendon A tough, ropelike cord of fibrous tissue that attaches a skeletal muscle to a bone.

tibia The larger of the two lower leg bones responsible for supporting the major weight-bearing surface of the knee and the ankle; the shinbone.

traction The act of exerting a pulling force on a structure.

ulna The bone on the small finger side of the forearm; most important for elbow function.

Assessment in Action

You are dispatched to a "fall." En route the dispatcher tells you a tree trimmer has fallen about 15 feet from a tree he was working on. On arrival you find your 35-year-old patient with his legs still tangled in the ladder, lying on the ground. He tells you he slipped off the rung and his leg slid through, causing him to fall.

He is complaining of severe pain. Injured areas include his left upper leg, hip, and shoulder. His skin is warm and moist. He is alert to person, place, and time. Vital signs include a pulse of 120 beats/min, respirations of 22 breaths/min, and a blood pressure of 136/88 mm Hg. An obvious bone end, from his midthigh, protrudes through the jeans of his left leg.

1. What is the most accurate description of the mechanism of injury?
   A. Direct force only.
   B. Twisting and direct force.
   C. Twisting force only.
   D. High-energy force.

2. Which type of splint is the best choice for the patient's upper left leg fracture?
   A. Ladder
   B. Pillow
   C. Traction
   D. Cardboard

3. Appropriate assessment for this patient's fractured limb includes:
   A. a complete set of vital signs.
   B. assessing pulses, motor, and sensory function.
   C. determining the zone of injury.
   D. palpation of the chest or abdomen.

4. When assessing an extremity, it is best to:
   A. compare your findings to your own extremities.
   B. compare the findings to the patient's other extremity.
   C. compare the lower extremities to the upper extremities.
   D. evaluate each extremity separately.

5. When you assess your patient's distal pulse, you note that it is noticeably weaker than the pulse in his other foot. Appropriate action would be to:
   A. try gentle longitudinal traction.
   B. use the ladder splint instead.
   C. use the leg portion of the PASG.
   D. secure the extremity to the long board.

6. Appropriate care of the open wound on his left thigh would be to:
   A. leave it alone.
   B. cover with a moist dressing.
   C. cover with an occlusive dressing.
   D. cover with a dry, sterile dressing.

7. His injured shoulder appears squared or flattened and he is unable to move his upper arm. He is also complaining of some numbness in his arm and hand. How would you manage this injury?
   A. Apply a traction splint to the humerus.
   B. Apply a sling and swathe.
   C. Have him straighten his arm for a ladder splint.
   D. Immobilize to the back board.

Challenging Questions

8. Of all his injuries, which presents the greatest potential for a threat to his life?

9. If you are called to the scene of a person with leg pain, and you discover a patient that had a cast application the day before for a fractured tibia/fibula, why is it very important that you assess the degree of pain and immediately transport?

10. It is very important that you handle patients with fractures very gently. Besides not wanting to cause more pain, why is this so important?

Points to Ponder

You are dispatched to an auto accident near the border of your jurisdiction. When you arrive, you find that a unit from the bordering jurisdiction is already on scene and started patient care. There are two cars and five victims, so you are happy to have the help. When you introduce yourself the other EMTs show no sign of giving you control of the scene. All five patients have injuries, but the worst is a man with multiple fractures of both legs including bilateral femur fractures, one of which is an open fracture. You have contacted your dispatch and requested an additional ambulance and have contacted your hospital to let them know what to expect. The other EMTs are employing rapid extrication and as they are headed for their ambulance you ask them if they need directions to your hospital. They tell you that they are headed to the hospital in their jurisdiction even though it is a little further away. Your partner steps in their way and insists that they transport to your hospital because the accident happened in your jurisdiction. A brief shoving match occurs between your partner and the other EMTs. Where should this patient be transported? How will you decide where to transport the patient? How will you convince the other EMTs if they disagree? How much time should be spent on this discussion?

Issues Liability, Jurisdiction, Mutual Aid Agreements, Scene Management, Transport Decisions.

Online Outlook

Because musculoskeletal injuries occur so often, you must be able to evaluate them properly. Injury to the bones and joints is often associated with injury to the surrounding soft tissue. To improve your knowledge of injuries to the skeletal system, complete Exercise 29 at <u>www.emtb.com</u>.

Head and Spine Injuries

Objectives

Cognitive

1. State the components of the nervous system (p 682).
2. List the functions of the central nervous system (p 683).
3. Define the structure of the skeletal system as it relates to the nervous system (p 683).
4. Relate mechanism of injury to potential injuries of the head and spine (p 686).
5. Describe the implications of not properly caring for potential spinal injuries (p 687).
6. State the signs and symptoms of a potential spinal injury (p 687).
7. Describe the method of determining if a responsive patient may have a spinal injury (p 687).
8. Relate the airway emergency medical care techniques to the patient with a suspected spinal injury (p 688).
9. Describe how to stabilize the cervical spine (p 688).
10. Discuss indications for sizing and using a cervical spine immobilization device (p 690).
11. Establish the relationship between airway management and the patient with head and spinal injuries (p 688).
12. Describe a method for sizing a cervical spine immobilization device (p 702).
13. Describe how to log roll a patient with a suspected spinal injury (p 690).
14. Describe how to secure a patient to a long spine board (p 690).
15. List instances when a short spine board should be used (p 692).
16. Describe how to immobilize a patient using a short spine board (p 692).
17. Describe the indications for the use of rapid extrication (p 692).
18. List the steps in performing rapid extrication (p 161).
19. State the circumstance when a helmet should be left on the patient (p 704).
20. Discuss the circumstances when a helmet should be removed (p 704).
21. Identify different types of helmets (p 704).
22. Describe the unique characteristics of sports helmets (p 704).
23. Explain the preferred methods to remove a helmet (p 704).
24. Discuss alternative methods for removal of a helmet (p 706).
25. Describe how the patient's head is stabilized to remove the helmet (p 704).
26. Differentiate how the head is stabilized with a helmet compared to without a helmet (p 701).

Affective

27. Explain the rationale for immobilization of the entire spine when a cervical spine injury is suspected (p 688).
28. Explain the rationale for utilizing immobilization methods apart from the straps on the cots (p 690).
29. Explain the rationale for utilizing a short spine immobilization device when moving a patient from the sitting to the supine position (p 692).
30. Explain the rationale for utilizing rapid extrication approaches only when they indeed will make the difference between life and death (p 692).
31. Defend the reasons for leaving a helmet in place for transport of a patient (p 704).
32. Defend the reasons for removal of a helmet prior to transport of a patient (p 704).

Psychomotor

33. Demonstrate opening the airway in a patient with a suspected spinal cord injury (p 688).
34. Demonstrate evaluating a responsive patient with a suspected spinal cord injury (p 687).
35. Demonstrate stabilization of the cervical spine (p 689).
36. Demonstrate the four-person log roll for a patient with a suspected spinal cord injury (p 690).
37. Demonstrate how to log roll a patient with a suspected spinal cord injury using two people (p 690).
38. Demonstrate securing a patient to a long spine board (p 691).
39. Demonstrate using the short board immobilization technique (p 694).
40. Demonstrate the procedure for rapid extrication (p 692).
41. Demonstrate preferred methods for stabilization of a helmet (p 704).
42. Demonstrate helmet removal techniques (p 706).
43. Demonstrate alternative methods for stabilization of a helmet (p 706).
44. Demonstrate completing a prehospital care report for patients with head and spinal injuries (p 299).

www.emtb.com

TECHNOLOGY

Online Chapter Pretest
Interactivities
Vocabulary Explorer
Anatomy Review
Web Links
Online Review Manual
Distance Learning

Chapter **FEATURES**

Skill Drills
Vital Vocabulary
Pediatric Needs
Geriatric Needs
EMT-B Safety
EMT-B Tips
Documentation Tips
Remember
Prep Kit

Your unit is on standby at the fairgrounds when you are requested to respond for a parachutist who had a partial chute failure. His chief complaint along with neck pain is that he "can't feel his legs."

Spinal cord injuries are some of the most devastating of all types of trauma for a number of reasons. This chapter will teach you the principles of good spinal care along with care for head and brain injuries. It will also help you answer the following questions:

1. Why is it important to take spinal motion restriction precautions for a trauma patient with a significant mechanism of injury but who has no neurologic deficits?

2. Describe the signs and symptoms that might make you suspect that your patient has a brain injury.

Head and Spine Injuries

The nervous system is a complex network of nerve cells that enables all parts of the body to function. It includes the brain, the spinal cord, and several billion nerve fibers that carry information to and from all parts of the body. Because the nervous system is so vital, it is well protected. The brain lies within the skull, and the spinal cord is inside the bony spinal canal. Despite this protection, serious blows can damage the nervous system.

This chapter first briefly reviews the anatomy and function of the central and peripheral nervous systems and of the skeletal system, knowledge that you will need to make an accurate assessment of injuries to these systems. It then discusses specific head and spinal injuries, including signs, symptoms, and treatment. Extrication of patients with possible spinal injuries and removal of helmets are also described.

Anatomy and Physiology of the Nervous System

The nervous system is divided into two anatomic parts: the central nervous system and the peripheral nervous system (▼ Figure 30-1). The **central nervous system (CNS)** consists of the parts of the nervous system that are covered and protected by bones: the brain and the

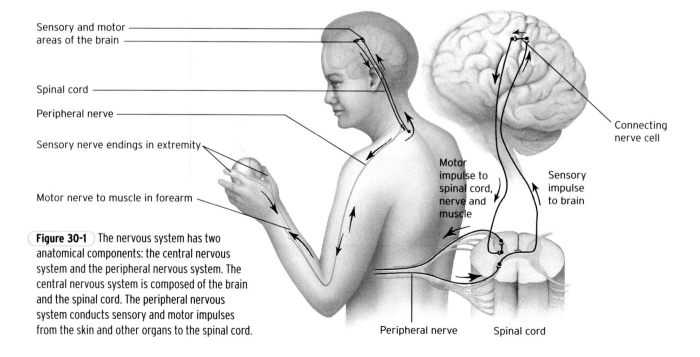

Sensory and motor areas of the brain

Spinal cord

Peripheral nerve

Sensory nerve endings in extremity

Motor nerve to muscle in forearm

Connecting nerve cell

Motor impulse to spinal cord, nerve and muscle

Sensory impulse to brain

Peripheral nerve

Spinal cord

Figure 30-1 The nervous system has two anatomical components: the central nervous system and the peripheral nervous system. The central nervous system is composed of the brain and the spinal cord. The peripheral nervous system conducts sensory and motor impulses from the skin and other organs to the spinal cord.

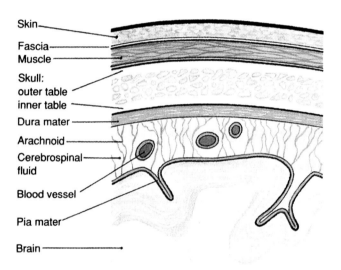

Parietal lobe
Temporal lobe
Occipital lobe
Cerebellum
Foramen magnum
Spinal cord

CEREBRUM
Frontal lobe
Brain stem

Figure 30-2 The brain is part of the central nervous system and is the organ that controls the body. It is divided into three major areas: the cerebrum, the cerebellum, and the brain stem.

spinal cord, including the nuclei and cell bodies of most nerve cells. Long fibers link these cells to the body's various organs through openings in the bony coverings. These cables of nerve fibers make up the **peripheral nervous system**.

Central Nervous System

The central nervous system (CNS) is composed of the brain and spinal cord. The brain is the organ that controls the body, the center of consciousness. It is divided into three major areas: the cerebrum, the cerebellum, and the brain stem (▲ **Figure 30-2**).

The **cerebrum**, which contains about 75% of the brain's total volume, controls a wide variety of activities. Underneath the cerebrum lies the **cerebellum**, which coordinates body movements. The most primitive part of the central nervous system, the **brain stem**, controls virtually all the functions that are necessary for life, including the cardiac and respiratory systems. Deep within the cranium, the brain stem is the best-protected part of the central nervous system.

The spinal cord, the other major portion of the central nervous system, is mostly made of fibers that extend from the brain's nerve cells. The spinal cord carries messages between the brain and the body.

Protective Coverings

The cells of the brain and spinal cord are soft and easily injured. Once damaged, they cannot be regenerated or reproduced. Therefore, the entire central nervous system is contained within a protective framework.

The thick, bony structures of the skull and spinal canal withstand injury very well. The skull is covered by a layer of muscle fascia and above that the scalp,

Skin
Fascia
Muscle
Skull:
outer table
inner table
Dura mater
Arachnoid
Cerebrospinal fluid
Blood vessel
Pia mater
Brain

Figure 30-3 The central nervous system has several layers of protective coverings: the skin, muscles and their fascia, bone, and the meninges. The three layers of the meninges include the dura mater, the arachnoid, and the pia mater.

(a thick vascular layer of skin). The spinal canal, too, is surrounded by a thick layer of skin and muscles.

The central nervous system is further protected by the **meninges**, three distinct layers of tissue that suspend the brain and the spinal cord within the skull and the spinal canal (▲ **Figure 30-3**). The outer layer, the dura mater, is a tough, fibrous layer that closely resembles leather. This layer forms a sac to contain the central nervous system, with small openings through which the peripheral nerves exit.

The inner two layers of the meninges, called the arachnoid and the pia mater, are much thinner than the dura mater. They contain the blood vessels that nourish the brain and spinal cord. Both the arachnoid and the pia mater produce CSF, which fills the spaces between them and acts as an excellent shock absorber. The brain and spinal cord essentially float in this fluid, buffered from injury.

When an injury does penetrate all these protective layers, clear, watery CSF may leak from the nose, the ears, or an open skull fracture. Therefore, if a patient with a head injury has what looks like a runny nose or has a salty taste at the back of the throat, you should assume that the fluid is CSF.

Ironically, the very layers of tissue that isolate and protect the central nervous system can lead to serious problems in closed head injuries. Severe injury may cause bleeding of the vessels under the dura mater. This, in turn, causes blood to collect in this space (a subdural hematoma), increasing the pressure inside the skull and compressing softer brain tissue. In many cases, only prompt surgery can prevent permanent brain damage.

Peripheral Nervous System

The peripheral nervous system has two anatomic parts: 31 pairs of spinal nerves and 12 pairs of cranial nerves ▶ **Figure 30-4**.

The 31 pairs of spinal nerves conduct sensory impulses from the skin and other organs to the spinal cord. They also conduct motor impulses from the spinal cord to the muscles. Because the arms and legs have so many muscles, the spinal nerves serving the extremities are arranged in complex networks. The brachial plexus controls the arms, and the lumbosacral plexus controls the legs.

Cranial nerves are the 12 pairs of nerves that pass through holes in the skull and transmit sensations directly to or from the brain. For the most part, they perform special functions in the head and face, including sight, smell, taste, hearing, and facial expressions.

There are three major types of peripheral nerves. The <u>sensory nerves</u>, with endings that can perceive only one type of information each, carry that information from the body to the brain via the spinal cord. The <u>motor nerves</u>, one for each muscle, carry information from the central nervous system to the muscles. The <u>connecting nerves</u>, found only in the brain and

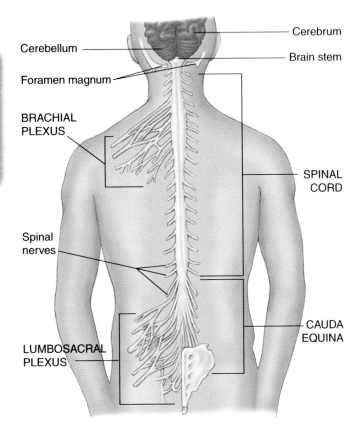

Figure 30-4 The peripheral nervous system is a complex network of motor and sensory nerves. The brachial plexus controls the arms, and the lumbosacral plexus controls the legs.

spinal cord, connect the sensory and motor nerves with short fibers, which allow the cells on either end to exchange messages.

How the Nervous System Works

The nervous system controls virtually all of our body's activities, including reflex, voluntary, and involuntary activities.

In connecting the sensory and motor nerves of the limbs, the connecting nerves in the spinal cord form a reflex arc. If a sensory nerve in this arc detects an irritating stimulus, such as heat, it will bypass the brain and send a message directly to the motor nerve ▶ **Figure 30-5**.

<u>Voluntary activities</u> are the actions that we consciously perform, in which sensory input determines the specific muscular activity—for example, reaching across the table for a salt shaker or to pass a dish. <u>Involuntary activities</u> are the actions that are not under the control of our will, such as breathing; in most instances, we inhale and exhale without consciously thinking about it. Many of our body's functions occur independently of thought, or involuntarily.

The part of the nervous system that regulates or controls our voluntary activities, including almost all coordinated muscular activities, is called the <u>somatic</u>

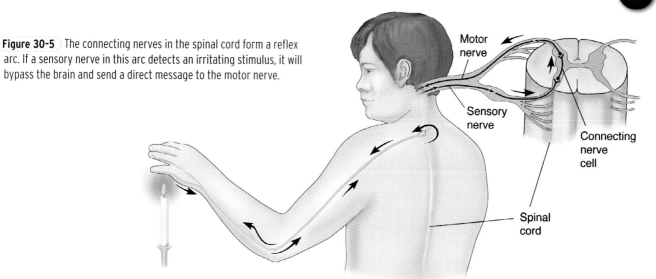

Figure 30-5 The connecting nerves in the spinal cord form a reflex arc. If a sensory nerve in this arc detects an irritating stimulus, it will bypass the brain and send a direct message to the motor nerve.

(voluntary) nervous system. The mechanism of the somatic nervous system is simple. The brain interprets the sensory information that it receives from the peripheral nerves and responds by sending signals to the voluntary muscles.

The body functions that occur without conscious effort are regulated by the much more primitive autonomic (involuntary) nervous system. The autonomic nervous system controls the functions of many of the body's vital organs, over which the brain has no voluntary control.

The autonomic nervous system, like so much in our nervous system, is composed of two parts: the sympathetic nervous system and the parasympathetic nervous system. Confronted with a threatening situation, the sympathetic nervous system reacts to the stress with the fight-or-flight response. The parasympathetic nervous

system has the opposite effect on the body, causing blood vessels to dilate, slowing the heart rate, and relaxing the muscle sphincters. These two divisions of the autonomic nervous system tend to balance each other so that basic body functions remain stable and effective.

Anatomy and Physiology of the Skeletal System

The skull has two layers of bone, the outer and inner tables, that protect the brain. It is divided into two large structures: the cranium and the face ▼ **Figure 30-6** . The mandible (lower jaw), the only movable facial bone, is connected to the cranium by the temporomandibular joint (TMJ) just in front of each ear.

Figure 30-6 The skull has two large structures: the cranium and the face.

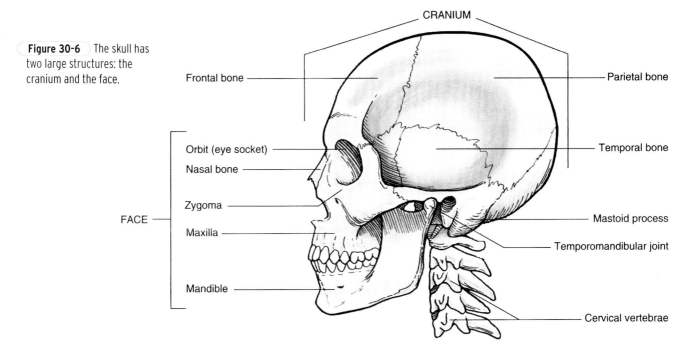

The spinal column is the body's central supporting structure. It has 33 bones, called vertebrae, and is divided into five sections: cervical, thoracic, lumbar, sacral, and coccygeal ▶ **Figure 30-7** . Injury to the vertebrae, depending on the level at which the injury occurs, can result in paralysis.

The front part of each vertebra consists of a round, solid block of bone called the "body"; the back part forms a bony arch. From one vertebra to the next, the series of arches form a tunnel running the length of the spine. This is the spinal canal, which encases and protects the spinal cord ▶ **Figure 30-8** .

The vertebrae are connected by ligaments and separated by cushions, called **intervertebral disks**. While allowing the trunk to bend forward and back, these ligaments and disks also limit motion so that the spinal cord is not injured. When the spine is injured or fractured, the spinal cord and its nerves are left unprotected. Therefore, until the spine is stabilized, you must keep it aligned as best you can to prevent further injury to the spinal cord.

The spinal column itself is almost entirely surrounded by muscles. However, you can palpate the posterior spinous process of each vertebra, which lies just under the skin in the midline of the back. The most prominent and most easily palpable spinous process is at the seventh cervical vertebra at the base of the neck.

Injuries of the Spine

The cervical, thoracic, and lumbar portions of the spine can be injured in a variety of ways. Compression injuries can occur as a result of a fall, regardless of whether the patient landed on his or her feet, coccyx, or, as in diving accidents, top of the head. Motor vehicle crashes or other types of trauma can overextend, flex, or rotate the spine. Any one of these unnatural motions, as well as excessive lateral bending, can result in fractures or neurologic deficit.

Any time the spine is **distracted**, or pulled along its length, you can expect to find serious injuries to the spine. For example, hangings typically fracture the vertebrae high up in the cervical spine.

Assessment of Spinal Injuries

You should always suspect a possible spinal injury any time you encounter one of the following mechanisms of injury:

- Motor vehicle crashes
- Pedestrian-motor vehicle collisions
- Falls
- Blunt trauma

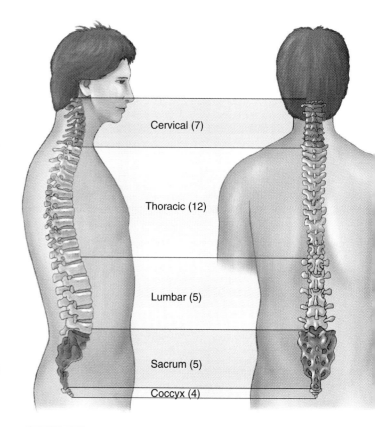

Figure 30-7 The spinal column is the body's central supporting system and consists of 33 bones divided into five sections. Injury to the vertebrae can cause paralysis.

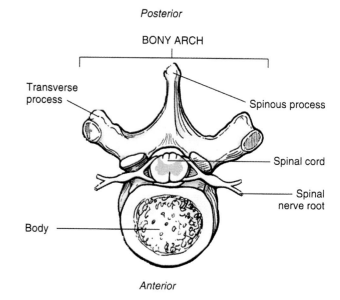

Figure 30-8 The spinal canal is formed by the vertebral body in the front (or anteriorly) and the bony arch in the back (or posteriorly).

- Penetrating trauma to the head, neck, or torso
- Motorcycle crashes
- Hangings
- Diving accidents
- Recreational accidents

> If a trauma patient is unconscious
> and you do not know the mechanism of injury,
> you should always assume that he or she has
> a spinal injury.

Documentation Tips

Proper care of a patient with a possible spinal injury requires assessment of motor and sensory functions both before and after immobilizing the patient. Likewise, careful observation of level of consciousness at different stages of your care for a head-injured patient provides crucial information. Document your detailed findings of these repeated neurologic exams to make the information available to hospital personnel and establish that your care has been thorough and appropriate.

If a trauma patient is unconscious and you do not know the mechanism of injury, you should always assume that he or she has a spinal injury. Take great care to avoid any movement that could cause further injury.

In fact, this is the safest approach to any injured patient, conscious or unconscious. The reason is that complications of spinal cord injuries are serious, often leading to death or lifelong disability. Examples include respiratory failure resulting from direct injury to the brain stem or upper spinal cord, and partial or complete paralysis below the point of injury.

When assessing a patient for possible spinal injury, you should begin with an initial assessment, focusing on the ABCs. If the patient is responsive, make sure you ask about the mechanism of injury and about his or her symptoms, starting with these five questions:

1. Does your neck or back hurt?

2. What happened?

3. Where does it hurt?

4. Can you move your hands and feet?

5. Can you feel me touching your fingers? Your toes?

As part of your focused physical exam, inspect the spinal area for DCAP-BTLS: Deformities, Contusions, Abrasions, Punctures/penetrations, Burns, Tenderness, Lacerations, and Swelling. Make sure that you do not move any body parts excessively. Determine whether the strength in each extremity is equal by asking the patient to squeeze your hands and to gently push each foot against your hands (◄ **Figure 30-9**). Finally, assess the equality of strength of the extremities by comparing the right limb to the left limb.

With unresponsive patients, you should try to identify the mechanism of injury. As part of your assessment, inspect the patient for DCAP-BTLS. First responders, family members, or bystanders may have helpful information, including when the patient lost consciousness or what his or her previous level of consciousness was.

Remember that the ability to walk, move the extremities, or feel sensation does not necessarily rule out a spinal cord injury. Nor does an absence of pain. Do not ask patients with possible spinal injuries to move as a test for pain. On the contrary, you should instruct them to be still.

However, pain or tenderness when you palpate the spinal area is certainly a warning sign that a spinal injury may exist. Patients with spinal injuries may complain of constant or intermittent pain along the spinal column or in their extremities. A spinal cord injury

Figure 30-9 **A.** Assess the equality of strength of each extremity by asking the patient to squeeze your hands. **B.** Next, ask the patient to gently push each foot against your hands.

may also produce pain independent of movement or palpation.

Other signs and symptoms of spinal injury include an obvious deformity as you palpate the spine; numbness, weakness, or tingling in the extremities; and soft-tissue injuries in the spinal region. Patients with severe spinal injury may lose sensation or experience paralysis below the suspected level of injury or be incontinent (▼ **Figure 30-10**). Obvious injury to the head and neck may indicate injury to the cervical spine. Injury to the shoulders, back, or abdomen may indicate injury to the thoracic or lumbar spine. Injuries of the lower extremities may indicate a problem with the lumbar spine or sacrum.

Emergency Medical Care

Emergency medical care of a patient with a possible spinal injury begins, as does all patient care, with your protection; therefore, you must remember to follow BSI precautions. Next, you must maintain the airway in the proper position, assess respirations, and give supplemental oxygen.

MANAGING THE AIRWAY. Knowing that improper handling of a spinal injury can leave a patient permanently paralyzed should not paralyze you in the presence of an airway obstruction. Remember, all patients without an airway will die. If a patient with a spinal injury has an airway obstruction, you should perform the jaw-thrust maneuver to open the airway (▼ **Figure 30-11**). Do not use the head tilt-chin lift maneuver, as it extends the neck and may further damage the cervical spine. If the patient is unconscious, you can lift or pull the tongue forward so that you do not have to move the neck. Once the airway is open, hold the head still, in a neutral, in-line position, until it can be fully immobilized.

After you open the airway, consider inserting an oropharyngeal airway. If you do so, be sure to monitor the airway closely and have a suctioning unit available as you will often need to clear away blood, saliva, or vomitus. Give oxygen to any patient who is having trouble breathing.

If you cannot open the airway because of the position of the head, realign the neck. Firmly grasp the patient's head with both hands, pull the head gently and firmly away from the trunk, and turn it to the front. Maintain the head in this position while you or your partner repeats the jaw-thrust maneuver.

STABILIZATION OF THE CERVICAL SPINE. Stabilizing the airway is your first priority. You must then stabilize the

Figure 30-10 With severe spinal injuries, patients may lose sensation or experience paralysis below the suspected level of injury.

Quadriplegia

Paraplegia

C5-6

L1

Figure 30-11 Jaw-thrust maneuver **A.** Stabilize the neck in a neutral, in-line position. **B.** Push the angle of the lower jaw forward.

Skill Drill 30-1   Performing Manual In-Line Stabilization

Kneel behind the patient and place your hands firmly around the base of the skull on either side.

Support the lower jaw with your index and long fingers, and the head with your palms.

Gently lift the head into a neutral, eyes-forward position, aligned with the torso. Do not move the head or neck excessively.

Continue to support the head manually while your partner places a rigid cervical collar around the neck. Maintain manual support until you have the patient secured to a backboard.

head and trunk so that bone fragments do not do further damage. Even small movements can significantly injure the spinal cord. Follow the steps in

▲ Skill Drill 30-1 :

1. **Begin manual in-line stabilization** by holding the head firmly with both hands. Whenever possible, kneel behind the patient, and place your hands around the base of the skull on either side (Step 1).

2. **Support the lower jaw** with your index and long fingers, while you are supporting the head with your palms (Step 2).

3. **Then gently lift the head** until the patient's eyes are looking straight ahead and the head and torso are in line. This neutral **eyes-forward position** makes stabilization easier. Align the nose with the navel. Never twist, flex, or extend the head or neck excessively (Step 3).

4. **Manually maintain this position** as you continue to maintain the airway. Have your partner place a rigid cervical collar around the neck to provide more stability. Do not remove your hands from the patient's head until the patient is properly secured to a backboard and the head is immobilized. The patient must remain immobilized until he or she is examined at the hospital (Step 4).

Even small movements can significantly injure the spinal cord.

Once the patient's head and neck are manually immobilized, assess the pulse, motor functions, and sensation in all extremities. Then assess the cervical spine area and neck. Keep in mind that the c-collar is used to provide increased stability to the neck. It is used in addition to, not instead of, manual c-spine immobilization. An improperly fitting collar will do more harm than good. If you do not have the proper size, place a rolled towel around the head, and tape it to the backboard as you immobilize the patient on the board. In any case, maintain manual support until the patient is fully secured to a backboard.

There are some situations in which you should not force the head into a neutral, in-line position. Do not move the head if any of the following causes the patient to complain of pain:

- Muscle spasms in the neck
- Increased pain
- Numbness, tingling, or weakness
- Compromised airway or ventilations

In these situations, immobilize the patient in the position in which you found him or her.

Preparation for Transport

Supine Patients

A patient who is supine can be effectively immobilized by securing him or her to a long backboard. The ideal procedure for moving a patient from the ground to a backboard is the **four-person log roll**. This procedure is recommended any time you suspect a spinal injury. In other cases, you may choose instead to slide the patient onto a backboard or use a scoop stretcher. The patient's condition, the scene, and the available resources will dictate the method you choose.

You should first take the necessary precautions and then direct the team from a kneeling position by the patient's head so that you can maintain manual in-line immobilization. Your job is to ensure that the head, torso, and pelvis move as a unit, with your teammates controlling the movement of the body. If necessary, you

may recruit bystanders to the team, but be sure to instruct them fully before moving the patient. To immobilize a patient on a backboard, follow the steps in
▶ **Skill Drill 30-2** :

1. **Maintain in-line stabilization** from a kneeling position at the patient's head. This EMT-B directs the log roll.

2. **Assess pulse, motor, and sensory function** in each extremity **(Step 1)**.

3. **Apply an appropriately sized cervical collar** **(Step 2)**.

4. **The other team members** should position the immobilization device (backboard) and place their hands on the far side of the patient to increase their leverage. Instruct them to use their body weight and their shoulder and back muscles to ensure a smooth, coordinated pull, concentrating their pull on the heavier portions of the patient's body **(Step 3)**.

5. **On command** from the EMT-B at the head, the rescuers roll the patient toward themselves. One rescuer quickly examines the back while the patient is rolled on the side, then slides the backboard behind and under the patient. The team rolls the patient back onto the board, avoiding rotating the head, shoulders, or pelvis **(Step 4)**.

6. **Ensure the patient is centered** on the board **(Step 5)**.

7. **Secure the upper torso** to the board once the patient is centered on the backboard **(Step 6)**.

8. **Secure the pelvis and upper legs,** using padding as needed. For the pelvis, use straps over the iliac crests, and/or groin loops **(Step 7)**.

9. **Begin to immobilize the head to the board** by positioning a commercial immobilization device, or towel rolls **(Step 8)**.

10. **Secure the head by taping** the head-immobilization device, or towels, across the forehead. To prevent airway problems and leave access to the airway, do not tape over the throat or chin **(Step 9)**.

11. **Check and readjust straps** as needed to ensure that the entire body is snugly secured and will not slide during patient movement.

12. **Reassess pulse, motor, and sensory function** in each extremity, and continue to do so periodically **(Step 10)**.

SkillDrill 30-2   Immobilizing a Patient to a Long Backboard

Apply and maintain cervical stabilization.
Assess distal functions in all extremities.

Apply a cervical collar.

Rescuers kneel on one side of the patient and place hands on the far side of the patient.

On command, rescuers roll the patient toward themselves, quickly examine the back, slide the backboard under the patient, and roll the patient onto the board.

Center the patient on the board.

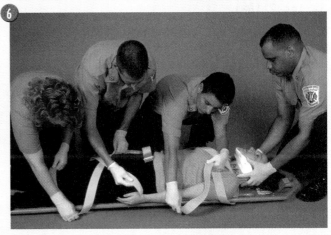

Secure the upper torso first.

Skill Drill 30-2　Immobilizing a Patient to a Long Backboard—continued.

Secure the chest, pelvis, and upper legs.

Begin to secure the patient's head using a commercial immobilization device or rolled towels.

Place tape across the patient's forehead.

Check all straps and readjust as needed.
Reassess distal functions in all extremities.

Sitting Patients

Some patients with a possible spinal injury will be in a sitting position, such as after an automobile crash. With these patients, you should use a short backboard or other short spinal extrication device to immobilize the cervical and thoracic spine. The short board is then secured to the long board.

The exceptions to this rule are situations in which you do not have time to first secure the patient to the short board, including the following situations:

- You or the patient is in danger.
- You need to gain immediate access to other patients.
- The patient's injuries justify urgent removal.

In these situations, your team should lower the patient directly onto a long backboard, using the rapid extrication technique as described in Chapter 6. Be sure that you provide manual stabilization of the cervical spine as you move the patient. Rapid extrication is indicated only in cases of life-threatening injury or loss of life or limb. In all other cases, follow the steps in ▶ **Skill Drill 30-3** to immobilize a sitting patient:

1. As with the supine patient, you must **first stabilize the head** and then maintain manual in-line stabilization until the patient is secured to the long backboard.

2. **Assess pulse, motor, and sensory function** in each extremity.

3. Apply the cervical collar (Step 1).

4. **Insert a short spine immobilization device** between the patient's upper back and the seat back (Step 2).

5. **Open the board's side flaps (if present),** and position them around the patient's torso and snug to the armpits (Step 3).

6. Once the board is properly positioned, **secure the upper torso straps first** and then the midtorso straps (Step 4).

7. **Position and fasten both groin loops** (leg straps). Check all torso straps to make sure they are secure. Make any adjustments necessary without excessive movement of the patient (Step 5).

8. **Pad any space** between the patient's head and the board as necessary.

9. **Secure the forehead strap,** and then fasten the lower head strap around the cervical collar (Step 6).

10. **Place the long backboard** next to the patient's buttocks, perpendicular to the trunk (Step 7).

11. **Turn the patient parallel** to the long board, and slowly lower him or her onto it.

12. **Lift the patient** (without rotating him or her), and slip the long board under the short board (Step 8).

13. **Secure the short and long boards** together.

14. **Reassess the pulse, motor function, and sensation** in all four extremities. Note your findings, and prepare for immediate transport (Step 9).

Standing Patients

You may arrive at a scene in which you find a patient standing or wandering around after an accident or injury. If you suspect that there may be underlying head, neck, or spinal injuries, you should immobilize the patient to a long backboard before proceeding to assess him or her. This will require three EMT-Bs. Follow the steps in ▶ **Skill Drill 30-4** :

1. **Establish manual, in-line stabilization,** apply a cervical collar, and instruct the patient to remain still.

2. **Position the board upright** directly behind the patient (Step 1).

3. **Two EMT-Bs stand on either side** of the patient and the third is directly behind the patient, maintaining immobilization.

4. **The two EMT-Bs grasp the handholds at shoulder level** or slightly above by reaching under the patient's arms while standing at either side (Step 2).

5. **Prepare to lower** the patient to the ground (Step 3).

6. **Carefully lower the patient** as a unit under the direction of the EMT-B at the head. The EMT-B at the head will have to make sure the head stays against the board and carefully rotate his hands as the patient is being lowered in order to maintain in-line stabilization (Step 4).

Head Injuries

All head injuries are potentially serious. If not properly treated, those that at first seem minor may end up being life threatening. On the other hand, severe lacerations of the scalp or fractures of the skull may occur with little or no brain injury and may produce minimal or no long-term conditions.

Scalp Lacerations

Scalp lacerations can be minor or very serious. Because both the face and the scalp have unusually rich blood supplies, even small lacerations can quickly lead to significant blood loss ▼ **Figure 30-12** . Occasionally, this blood loss may be severe enough to cause hypovolemic shock, particularly in children. In any patient with multiple injuries, bleeding from scalp or facial lacerations contributes to hypovolemia. In addition, since scalp lacerations are usually the result of direct blows to the head, they often indicate deeper, more serious injuries.

You can almost always control bleeding from a scalp laceration by applying direct pressure over the wound. Remember to follow BSI techniques. Use a dry sterile dressing, folding any torn skin flaps back down onto

Figure 30-12 The scalp has an unusually rich blood supply; therefore, even small lacerations can result in significant blood loss.

Skill Drill 30-3 Immobilizing a Patient Found in a Sitting Position

1 Stabilize the head and neck in a neutral, in-line position.

Assess pulse, motor, and sensory function in each extremity.

Apply a cervical collar.

2 Insert a short spine immobilization device between the patient's upper back and the seat.

3 Open the side flaps, and position them around the patient's torso, snug around the armpits.

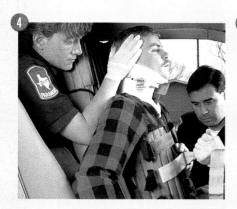

4 Secure the upper torso flaps, then the midtorso flaps.

5 Secure the groin (leg) straps. Check and adjust torso straps.

6 Pad between the head and the device as needed.

Secure the forehead strap and fasten the lower head strap around the collar.

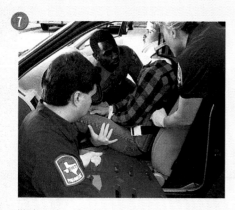

7 Wedge a long backboard next to the patient's buttocks.

8 Turn and lower the patient onto the long board.

Lift the patient, and slip the long board under the spine device.

9 Secure the immobilization devices to each other.

Reassess pulse, motor, and sensory functions in each extremity.

SkillDrill 30-4 Immobilizing a Patient Found in a Standing Position

1 After manually stabilizing the head and neck, apply a cervical collar. Position the board behind the patient.

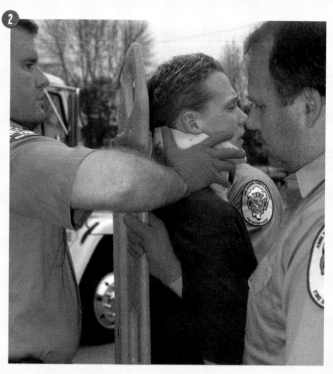

2 Position EMT-Bs at sides and behind the patient. Side EMT-Bs reach under patient's arms and grasp handholds at or slightly above shoulder level.

3 Prepare to lower the patient. EMT-Bs on the sides should be facing the EMT-B at the head and wait for his or her direction.

4 On command, lower the backboard to the ground.

the skin bed before applying pressure (▼ Figure 30-13A). In some instances, you will have to apply firm compression for several minutes to control the bleeding (▼ Figure 30-13B). If you suspect a skull fracture, do not apply excessive pressure to the open wound. Otherwise, you may increase intracranial pressure or push bone fragments into the brain.

If the dressing becomes soaked, do not remove it. Instead, place a second dressing over the first. Continue applying manual pressure until the bleeding is controlled, then secure the dressing in place with a soft, self-adhering roller bandage (▼ Figure 30-13C).

Skull Fracture

Fracture of the skull is an indication that a significant force has been applied to the head. As with any fracture,

a skull fracture may be open or closed, depending on whether there is an overlying laceration of the scalp. Injuries from bullets or other penetrating weapons frequently result in fracture of the skull. The diagnosis of a skull fracture is usually made in the hospital by X-ray examination, but you can conclude that a fracture is present if the patient's head appears deformed or if there is a visible crack in the skull within a scalp laceration. Another sign of skull fracture that you may see is ecchymosis (bruising) that develops under the eyes (**raccoon eyes**) (▼ Figure 30-14A) or behind one ear over the mastoid process (**Battle's sign**) (▼ Figure 30-14B).

Brain Injuries

CONCUSSION. A blow to the head or face may cause **concussion** of the brain. There is no universal agreement on the exact definition of a concussion, but in general, it means a temporary loss or alteration of part or all of the brain's abilities to function without actual physical damage to the brain. For example, a person who "sees stars" after being struck in the head has had

Figure 30-13 **A.** Apply pressure with a sterile dressing to fold any torn skin flaps back down onto the skin bed. **B.** Apply firm compression for several minutes to control the bleeding. **C.** Secure the compression dressing in place with a soft, self-adhering roller bandage.

Figure 30-14 Skull fracture is a possibility if a patient has ecchymosis, **A.** Under the eyes (raccoon eyes), or **B.** Behind one ear over the mastoid process (Battle's sign).

> You can almost always
> control bleeding from a scalp laceration
> by applying direct pressure
> over the wound.

a concussion that affects the occipital portion of the brain. A concussion may result in unconsciousness and even the inability to breathe for short periods of time.

A patient with a concussion may be confused or have amnesia (loss of memory). Occasionally, the patient can remember everything but the events leading up to the injury; this is called <u>retrograde amnesia</u>. Inability to remember events after the injury is called <u>anterograde (posttraumatic) amnesia</u>.

Usually, a concussion lasts only a short time. In fact, it is often over by the time you arrive. Nevertheless, you should ask about symptoms of concussion in any patient who has sustained an injury to the head; these symptoms include dizziness, weakness, or visual changes.

CONTUSION. Like any other soft tissue in the body, the brain can sustain a contusion, or bruise, when the skull is struck. A contusion is far more serious than a concussion, because it involves physical injury to the brain tissue, which may suffer long-lasting and even permanent damage. As with contusions elsewhere, there is associated bleeding and swelling from injured blood vessels. Injury of brain tissue or bleeding inside the skull will cause an increase of pressure within the skull. A patient who has had a brain contusion may exhibit any or all of the signs of brain injury described later in this chapter.

INTRACRANIAL BLEEDING. Laceration or rupture of a blood vessel inside the brain or in the meninges that cover the brain will produce intracranial bleeding (hematoma) in one of three areas ▶ **Figure 30-15** :

- Beneath the dura but outside the brain: a subdural hematoma
- Within the substance of the brain tissue itself: an intracerebral hematoma
- Outside the dura and under the skull: an epidural hematoma

A hematoma may develop rapidly, usually because of arterial injury, as in an epidural hematoma; or it may develop very slowly, as with a subdural hematoma. In any case, because the brain occupies nearly the entire space inside the skull, the result is increased pressure inside the skull, leading to compression of the brain tissue. The expanding hematoma will cause progressive loss of brain function and, if not treated properly, death.

Rapid deterioration of neurologic signs following a head injury is a sign of intracranial hematoma. You must act quickly to evaluate and treat such patients. Provide oxygen, monitor the airway, elevate the head of the stretcher, and provide immediate transport.

Other Brain Injuries

Brain injuries are not always a result of trauma. Certain medical conditions, such as blood clots or hemorrhaging, can also cause brain injuries that produce significant bleeding or swelling. Problems with the blood vessels, high blood pressure, or any number of other causes may cause spontaneous bleeding in the brain, affecting the patient's level of consciousness. This is known as altered mental status. The signs and symptoms of nontraumatic injuries are the same as those of traumatic brain injuries, except that there is no obvious mechanism of injury or any evidence of trauma.

TYPES OF INTRACRANIAL HEMATOMAS

A Subdural

B Intracerebral

C Epidural

Figure 30-15 Intracranial bleeding can occur in one of three areas. **A.** Beneath the dura but outside the brain (subdural hematoma). **B.** Within the substance of the brain tissue (intracerebral hematoma). **C.** Outside the dura and under the skull (epidural hematoma).

Complications of Head Injury

<u>Cerebral edema</u>, or swelling of the brain, is one of the most common complications of any head injury. It is also one of the most serious, because, as we have seen, swelling in the skull compresses the brain tissue, resulting in a loss of brain function.

Cerebral edema is aggravated by low oxygen levels in the blood and improved by high ones. For this reason, you must make sure that the airway is open and that adequate ventilations and high-flow oxygen are given to any patient with a head injury. This is especially true if the patient is unconscious. Do not wait for cyanosis or other obvious signs of hypoxia to develop.

It is not uncommon for the patient with a head injury to have a convulsion, or seizure. This is the result of excessive excitability of the brain, caused by direct injury or the accumulation of fluid within the brain (edema). You should be prepared to manage seizures in all patients who have had a head injury. Another effect of cerebral edema and increased intracranial pressure may be increased blood pressure, decreased pulse, and irregular respirations.

A common response to head injuries, even among children with very slight head injuries, is vomiting. This is usually the result of increased intracranial pressure. In managing such vomiting, you should pay particular attention to protecting the airway.

As was discussed earlier, the appearance of clear or pink watery CSF from the nose, the ear, or an open scalp wound indicates that the dura and the skull have both been penetrated. You should make no attempt to pack the wound, ear, or nose in this situation. Cover the scalp wound, if there is one, with sterile gauze to prevent further contamination, but do not bandage it tightly.

Assessing Head Injuries

Motor vehicle crashes, direct blows, falls from heights, assault, and sports injuries are common causes of head injury. A patient who has experienced any of these events should immediately arouse your suspicion and cause you to start looking for specific signs and symptoms of head injury. A deformed windshield or dented helmet may indicate a major blow to the head, which is likely to have caused injury ▲ **Figure 30-16** . It is especially important to evaluate and monitor the level of consciousness in patients with suspected head injuries, paying particular attention to any changes that may occur.

Figure 30-16 The classic "star" on the windshield after an automobile crash is a significant indicator of injury. Be alert for the signs and symptoms of head injury.

Types of Head Injuries

<u>Closed head injuries</u>, usually associated with trauma, are those in which the brain has been injured but the skin has not been broken and there is no obvious bleeding. In assessing a patient with a possible closed head injury, consider the mechanism of injury. Did the patient fall? Was he or she in an automobile crash or the victim of an assault? Was there deformity of the windshield or deformity of the helmet? Look for scalp lacerations, contusions, hematomas, or skull deformities. Sometimes, the skull will appear to have been pushed into the brain.

Decreased level of consciousness is the most reliable sign of this type of injury. Monitor the patient for changes in level of consciousness, including signs of confusion, disorientation, or deteriorating mental status. Is the patient unresponsive or repeating questions? Experiencing seizures? Nauseous or vomiting? Next, assess the patient for decreased movement and/or numbness and tingling in the extremities. Assess the vital signs carefully. People with head injuries may have irregular respirations, depending on which region of the brain is affected. Look for blood or CSF leaking from

Figure 30-17 Assess pupil size if you suspect a head injury. Unequal pupil size may signal a serious problem.

the ears, nose, or mouth and for bruising around the eyes and behind the ears.

You should also evaluate the patient's pupils, especially if he or she has a decreased level of consciousness. Often, unequal pupil size after a head injury signals a serious problem. Developing blood clots may be pressing on the third cranial nerve, causing one pupil to dilate ▲ **Figure 30-17**.

Scalp contusions, lacerations, hematomas, and obvious skull deformities are all signs of **open head injuries**, which are often caused by a penetrating object. There may be bleeding and exposed brain tissue. Do not probe open scalp lacerations with your gloved finger, as this may push bone fragments into the brain. Do not remove an impaled object.

Signs and Symptoms of Head Injury

Open and closed head injuries have essentially the same signs and symptoms.

Following an injury, any patient who exhibits one or more of these signs or symptoms should be evaluated promptly in the emergency department:

- Lacerations, contusions, or hematomas to the scalp
- Soft area or depression upon palpation
- Visible fractures or deformities of the skull
- Ecchymosis about the eyes or behind the ear over the mastoid process
- Clear or pink CSF leakage from a scalp wound, the nose, or the ear
- Failure of the pupils to respond to light
- Unequal pupil size
- Loss of sensation and/or motor function
- A period of unconsciousness

> Change in the level of consciousness is the single most important observation you can make in assessing the severity of brain injury.

- Amnesia
- Seizures
- Numbness or tingling in the extremities
- Irregular respirations
- Dizziness
- Visual complaints
- Combative or other abnormal behavior
- Nausea or vomiting

LEVEL OF CONSCIOUSNESS. Change in the level of consciousness is the single most important observation that you can make in assessing the severity of brain injury. Level of consciousness usually corresponds to the extent of loss of brain function. As soon as you determine that a head injury is present, you should perform a baseline assessment using the AVPU scale and record the time. Reevaluate the patient and record your observations every 15 minutes if the patient's condition is stable and at least every 5 minutes if the patient's condition is unstable, until you reach the hospital.

Frequently, the levels will fluctuate, improving, deteriorating, then improving again over time. On other occasions, there is a gradual, progressive deterioration in the patient's response to stimuli; this usually indicates serious brain damage that may need aggressive medical and/or surgical treatment. The physicians who treat the patient will need to know when loss of consciousness occurred. They will want to compare their neurologic evaluation with the one you performed in the field.

Your EMS system may choose to use the more detailed **Glasgow Coma Scale** instead of the AVPU scale to a assess a patient's level of consciousness ▶ **Figure 30-18**. In either case, you should always use simple, easily understood terms when reporting the level of consciousness, such as "does not remember events immediately preceding injury" or "confused about date and time." Terms such as "obtunded" or "dazed" have different meanings to different people and should not be used in either written or verbal reports.

GLASGOW COMA SCALE

Eye Opening

Spontaneous	4
To Voice	3
To Pain	2
None	1

Verbal Response

Oriented	5
Confused	4
Inappropriate Words	3
Incomprehensible Words	2
None	1

Motor Response

Obeys Command	6
Localizes Pain	5
Withdraws (pain)	4
Flexion (pain)	3
Extension (pain)	2
None	1

Glasgow Coma Score Total	**15**

Figure 30-18 The Glasgow Coma Scale is one method of evaluating level of consciousness. Note that the lower the score, the more severe the extent of brain injury.

CHANGES IN PUPIL SIZE. The nerves that control dilation and constriction of the pupils are very sensitive to pressure within the skull. When you beam a bright light into the eye, the pupil should constrict. Failure to do so is an early and important sign of increased intracranial pressure. Unequal pupil size may indicate increased pressure on one side of the brain.

As soon as you have assessed the patient's level of consciousness, determine the reaction of each pupil to light. Sketch the size of both pupils on the ambulance report to indicate any difference between the two eyes. Continue to monitor the pupils. Any change in their reactions over time may indicate progressive brain damage.

EMT-B Safety

Many mechanisms that cause head and spine injuries for the patient can also entail risk to emergency responders. Before you approach the patient, get the "big picture" of scene safety and take any actions necessary to ensure your own well-being. Do not rely *entirely* on assistance from fire or police personnel; maintain your own awareness of the scene.

Emergency Medical Care

Patients with head injuries often have injuries to the cervical spine as well. Therefore, when treating a patient with a head injury, you must keep in mind the need to protect and stabilize the cervical spine at all times. Avoid moving the neck unnecessarily until the spine can be appropriately splinted. An initial assessment with spinal immobilization should be done on scene with a complete, detailed physical examination en route.

Beyond this, you should treat the patient with a head injury according to three general principles, which are designed to protect and maintain the critical functions of the central nervous system:

1. **Establish an adequate airway.** If necessary, begin and maintain ventilation and always provide high-flow supplemental oxygen.

2. **Control bleeding,** and provide adequate circulation to maintain cerebral perfusion. Begin CPR, if necessary. Be sure to follow BSI precautions.

3. **Assess the patient's baseline** level of consciousness, and continuously monitor it.

As you continue to treat the patient, do not apply pressure to an open or depressed skull injury. In addition, you must assess and treat other injuries, dress and bandage open wounds as indicated in the treatment of soft-tissue injuries, splint fractures, anticipate and deal with vomiting to prevent aspiration, be prepared for convulsions and changes in the patient's condition, and transport the patient promptly and with extreme care.

MANAGING THE AIRWAY. The most important step in the treatment of patients with head injury, regardless of the severity, is to establish an adequate airway. If the patient has an airway obstruction, you should perform the jaw-thrust maneuver to open the airway. Once the airway is open, maintain the head and cervical spine in a neutral,

Figure 30-19 **A.** Maintain the head and cervical spine in a neutral in-line position. **B.** Apply a cervical collar as you finish the initial assessment.

in-line position until the person can be fully immobilized with a cervical collar ▲ **Figure 30-19** . Remove any foreign bodies, secretions, or vomitus from the airway. Make sure a suctioning unit is available, because you will often need to clear blood, saliva, or vomitus from the airway.

Once you have cleared the airway, check ventilation. If the respiratory control center of the brain has been injured, the rate and/or depth of breathing may be ineffective. Ventilation may also be limited by chest injuries or, if the spinal cord is injured, by paralysis of some or all of the muscles of respiration. Give high-flow oxygen to any patient who is having trouble breathing. This reduces hypoxia and possible cerebral edema. An injured brain is even less tolerant of hypoxia than a healthy brain, and studies have shown that supplemental oxygen can reduce brain damage. However, to be effective, it must be started as soon as possible. Do not wait until the patient becomes cyanotic. Continue to assist ventilations and administer supplemental oxygen until the patient reaches the hospital.

CIRCULATION. If the heart is not beating, providing airway maintenance, ventilation, and oxygen accomplishes nothing. You must also begin CPR if the patient is in cardiac arrest.

Active blood loss aggravates hypoxia by reducing the available number of oxygen-carrying red blood cells. Although they rarely cause shock except in infants and children, scalp lacerations often cause the loss of large volumes of blood, which must be controlled. Bleeding inside the skull may cause intracranial pressure to rise to life-threatening levels, even though the actual volume of blood lost inside the skull is relatively small.

Shock that develops in a patient with a head injury is usually due to hypovolemia caused by bleeding for other injuries. As with other trauma patients, shock in these cases indicates that the situation is critical. Such patients must be transported immediately to a trauma center. Maintain the airway while you protect the patient's cervical spine, ensure adequate ventilation, administer 100% oxygen, control obvious sites of bleeding with direct pressure, place the patient supine on a spine board, keep the patient warm, and provide immediate transport.

If the patient has a medical condition or nontraumatic injury along with the head injury, place him or her on the left side to prevent aspiration if the patient happens to vomit. *Be sure to maintain the head in the in-line neutral position, with the cervical collar in place.* You should also have a suctioning unit available.

Immobilization Devices

An injured spine is often very difficult to evaluate in a patient with a head injury. Sometimes, there is no neurologic loss. Pain in the spine may be missed because of shock or because the patient's attention is directed to more painful injuries. Evaluation is even more difficult if the patient is unconscious. Because any manipulation of the unstable cervical spine may cause permanent damage to the spinal cord, you must assume the presence of spinal injury in all patients who have sustained head injuries. Use manual in-line immobilization or a cervical collar and long backboard.

CERVICAL COLLARS. Rigid cervical immobilization devices, or cervical collars, provide preliminary, partial support. A cervical collar should be applied to every patient who has a possible spinal injury based on mechanism of injury, history, or signs and symptoms. Keep in mind, however, that cervical collars do not fully immobilize the cervical spine. Therefore, you must maintain manual support until the patient is completely secured to a spinal immobilization device, such as a long or a short backboard.

To be effective, a rigid cervical collar must be the correct size for the patient. It should rest on the shoulder girdle and provide firm support under both sides of the mandible, without obstructing the airway or ventilation efforts in any way (▶ **Figure 30-20**). Follow the steps in (▶ **Skill Drill 30-5**):

1. **One EMT-B** provides continuous manual in-line support of the head while the other prepares the collar **(Step 1)**.

2. **Measure the proper size collar** according to manufacturer's specifications. It is essential that the cervical collar fits properly. An improperly sized immobilization device has a potential for further injury. If you do not have the correct size, use a rolled towel; tape it to the backboard around the patient's head, and provide continuous manual support (▶ **Figure 30-21**) **(Step 2)**.

3. **Begin by placing the chin support** snugly underneath the chin **(Step 3)**.

4. **Maintaining head stabilization** and neutral neck alignment, wrap the collar around the neck and secure the collar to the far side of the chin support **(Step 4)**.

5. **Assure that the collar fits properly** and recheck that the patient is in a neutral, in-line position. Maintain in-line stabilization until the patient is completely secured to the board **(Step 5)**.

SHORT BACKBOARDS. There are several types of short-board immobilization devices. The most common are the vest-type device and the rigid short board (▶ **Figure 30-22**). These devices are designed to stabilize and immobilize the head, neck, and torso. They are used to immobilize noncritical patients who are found in a sitting position and have possible spinal injuries.

As was described earlier in this chapter, the first step in securing a patient to a short board or device is to provide manual, in-line support of the cervical spine. Assess the pulse, motor function, and sensation in all extremities, and then assess the cervical area. Then apply an appropriately sized cervical collar.

Position the device behind the patient, and secure it to the torso. Evaluate how well the torso and groin are secured, and make adjustments as necessary. Avoid excessive movement of the patient. Next, evaluate the position of the patient's head. Pad behind the head as needed to maintain neutral, in-line immobilization.

Now secure the patient's head to the device. Once you have done that, you may release manual support of the head. Rotate or lift the patient to the long backboard. At this point, you must reassess the pulses, motor function, and sensation in all four

Figure 30-20 Proper fit is essential in applying a cervical collar. The collar should rest on the shoulder girdle and provide firm support under both sides of the mandible without obstructing the airway or any ventilation efforts.

Figure 30-21 If you do not have an appropriately sized cervical collar, you may use a rolled towel. Tape it to the backboard around the patient's head, and provide continuous manual support.

Figure 30-22 The most common types of short-board immobilization devices are vest-type devices.

Skill Drill 30-5   Application of a Cervical Collar

Apply in-line stabilization.

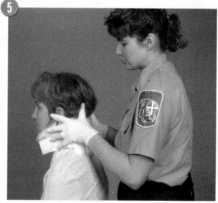

Measure the proper collar size.

Place the chin support first.

Wrap the collar around the neck and secure the collar.

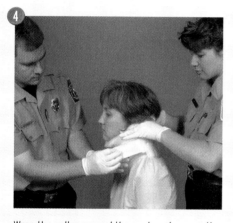

Assure proper fit and maintain neutral, in-line stabilization.

---

extremities to determine whether the change in position has affected the patient's vital signs or neurologic status. Finally you should immobilize the patient to the long backboard.

LONG BACKBOARDS. There are several types of long backboard immobilization devices that provide full body spinal immobilization ▶ **Figure 30-23** . They also provide stabilization and immobilization to the head, neck and torso, pelvis, and extremities. Long backboards are used to immobilize patients who are found in any position (standing, sitting, supine), sometimes in conjunction with short backboards.

Securing a patient to a long board was described in detail earlier in this chapter. Briefly, you should begin by providing manual, in-line support of the head. Assess pulse, motor function, and sensation in all extremities,

Figure 30-23 Long-board immobilization devices provide full body spinal immobilization, including stabilization of the head, neck and torso, pelvis, and extremities.

and assess the cervical area. Then apply an appropriately sized cervical collar, and proceed as follows:

1. **Position the device.**

2. **Log roll the patient onto the device.** You may also move the patient onto the device by suitable lift or slide or by scoop stretcher. As you maintain in-line support, your partner should kneel by the patient's head and direct the other two EMT-Bs as you roll the patient. Your partner's job is to make sure that the head, torso, and pelvis move as a unit. As the patient's back comes into view, quickly assess its condition if you did not do so during initial assessment. One EMT-B should position the device under the patient. Then, at your partner's command, roll the patient onto the board.

3. **If there are spaces** between the patient's head and torso and the board, fill them with padding. In an adult, these spaces are usually under the head and torso. In a child, place padding from the shoulders to the toes to establish a neutral position.

4. **Secure the torso to the device** by applying straps across the chest, pelvis, and legs. Adjust these straps as needed. Then secure the patient's head to the board.

5. **Reassess pulse,** motor function, and sensation in all extremities.

6. **When the patient is properly secured,** you can safely lift the board or turn it on its side, if necessary.

Helmet Removal

As you plan your care of a patient wearing a helmet, ask yourself the following questions:

- Is the patient's airway clear?
- Is the patient breathing adequately?
- Can you maintain the airway and assist ventilations if the helmet remains in place?
- How well does the helmet fit?
- Can the patient move within the helmet?
- Can the spine be immobilized in a neutral position with the helmet on?

A helmet that fits well prevents the patient's head from moving and should be left on, as long as (1) there are no impending airway or breathing problems, (2) it does not interfere with assessment and treatment of airway or ventilation problems, and (3) you can properly immobilize the spine. You should also leave the helmet on if there is any chance that removing it will further injure the patient. Remove a helmet if (1) it makes assessing or managing

airway problems difficult, (2) it prevents you from properly immobilizing the spine, or (3) it allows excessive head movement. Finally, always remove a helmet from a patient who is in cardiac arrest.

Sports helmets are typically open in the front and may or may not include an attached face mask. The mask can be removed without affecting helmet position or function by simply removing or cutting the straps that hold it to the helmet. In this way, sports helmets allow easy access to the airway ▶ **Figure 30-24** . Motorcycle helmets often have a shield covering the face. This, too, can be unbuckled to allow access to the airway ▶ **Figure 30-25** . If a shield cannot be removed, then the helmet must be removed.

Preferred Method

Removing a helmet is at least a two-person job; however, the technique for helmet removal depends on the actual type of helmet worn by the patient. One EMT-B provides constant in-line support as the other moves; you and your partner should not move at the same time. You should first consult with medical control, if possible, about your decision to remove a helmet. When you decide to do so, follow the steps in ▶ **Skill Drill 30-6** :

1. **Begin by kneeling down** at the patient's head. Your partner should kneel on one side of the patient, at the shoulder area.

2. **Open the face shield,** if there is one, and assess the patient's airway and breathing. Remove eyeglasses if the patient is wearing them **(Step 1)**.

3. **Stabilize the helmet** by placing your hands on either side of it, with your fingers on the patient's lower jaw to prevent movement of the head. Once your hands are in position, your partner can loosen the face strap **(Step 2)**.

4. **Once the strap is loosened,** your partner should place one hand on the patient's lower jaw at the angle of the jaw and the other behind the head at the occipital region. Once your partner's hands are in position, you may pull the sides of the helmet away from the patient's head **(Step 3)**.

5. **Gently slip the helmet** halfway off the patient's head, stopping when the helmet reaches the halfway point **(Step 4)**.

6. **Your partner then slides** his or her hand from the occiput to the back of the head. This will prevent the head from snapping back once the helmet is completely removed **(Step 5)**.

7. With your partner's hand in place, **remove the helmet,** and immobilize the cervical spine.

Figure 30-24 Removing the mask on a sports helmet can be done without affecting helmet position or function. **A.** Stabilize the patient's head and helmet. Then remove the facemask in one of two ways: **B.** Use a trainer's tool designed for cutting retaining clips, or, **C.** Unscrew the retaining clips for the facemask. **D.** Once the facemask is removed, the helmet can be immobilized against the backboard and a BVM can be used effectively.

Figure 30-25 Motorcycle helmets often have a shield covering the face that can be removed. **A.** Stabilize the neck in a neutral, in-line position. **B.** Unbuckle or snap off the face shield to access the airway.

Skill Drill 30-6   Removing a Helmet

Kneel down at the patient's head with your partner at one side.

Open the face shield to assess airway and breathing. Remove eyeglasses if present.

Prevent head movement by placing your hands on either side of the helmet and fingers on the lower jaw. Have your partner loosen the strap.

Have your partner place one hand at the angle of the lower jaw and the other at the occiput.

Gently slip the helmet about halfway off, then stop.

Have your partner slide the hand from the occiput to the back of the head to prevent it from snapping back.

Remove the helmet and stabilize the cervical spine.

Apply a cervical collar and secure the patient to a long backboard.

Pad as needed to prevent neck flexion or extension.

8. **Apply the cervical collar,** and then secure the patient to the backboard.

9. **With large helmets** or small patients, you may need to pad under the shoulders. This will prevent flexion of the neck. If shoulder pads or a heavy jacket is in place, you may need to pad behind the patient's head to prevent extension of the neck **(Step 6)**.

Remember, you do not need to remove a helmet if you can access the patient's airway, if the head is snug inside the helmet, and if the helmet can be secured to an immobilization device.

Alternate Method

An alternate method for removal of football helmets is possible. The advantage of this method is that it allows the helmet to be removed with less force applied, therefore reducing the possibility of motion at the neck. The disadvantage of this method is that it is slightly more time consuming. The first step involves removal of the chinstrap. This can be cut or unsnapped carefully. Be careful during removal of the chinstrap to avoid jarring the neck or head and causing excessive motion. Next, remove the face mask. The face mask is anchored to the helmet by plastic clips secured with screws. These can be removed with a screwdriver or, alternately, cut with a knife (Figure 30-24). After the face mask has been removed, the jaw pads can be popped out of place. This can be accomplished with the use of a tongue depressor ▶ **Figure 30-26A** . The fingers can be placed inside the helmet allowing greater control of the helmet during removal as the helmet is gently rocked back off the top of the head. The person at the foot of the

Figure 30-26   **A.** The jaw pads can be removed from the inside of the helmet with the aid of a tongue depressor.   **B.** Place the fingers inside the helmet and gently rock it out of place. The person at the foot controls the lower jaw with one hand and the occiput with the other. Insert padding behind the occiput to prevent neck extension.

patient controls the head by holding the jaw with one hand and the occiput with the other ▲ **Figure 30-26B** . Padding is inserted behind the occiput to prevent neck extension. If the shoulder pads are in place, appropriate padding must be applied behind the head to prevent hyperextension. Just as with the previously described method, the person over the patient's chest is responsible for making sure that the head and neck do not move during removal of the helmet.

Remember that small children may require additional padding to maintain the in-line neutral position. Children are not small adults. They have smaller airways, so padding is important to maintain the airway.

Pediatric Needs

You are likely to find infants and children who have been in automobile crashes still in their car seats. Your best course of action is to immobilize the child in the car seat if possible. Whenever you apply a cervical collar, make sure it is properly sized. If a properly fitting collar is not available, use a rolled towel and tape it to the car seat. Pad the sides of the car seat, if necessary, to prevent lateral movement ▼ **Figure 30-27** , and place additional padding in any spaces between the patient and the car seat. If the child is not in a car seat or was removed before your arrival, use an appropriately sized immobilization device. If the cervical immobilization device does not fit, use a rolled towel, and tape it to the board and manually support the head.

Figure 30-27   If you do not have an appropriately sized cervical collar for a child, you may use a rolled towel and tape it to the car seat. Pad the sides of the car seat, if needed, to prevent lateral movement.

Pad under the shoulders to the toes, as needed, to avoid excessive neck flexion ▼ **Figure 30-28** . In addition, place blanket rolls between the child and the sides of an adult-sized board to prevent the child from slipping to one side or the other ▼ **Figure 30-29** . Appropriately sized backboards are available for children.

Figure 30-28   Children have proportionately larger heads than adults, so you may need to place padding under the shoulders to avoid excessive flexion of the head.

Figure 30-29   Place blanket rolls between the child and the sides of an adult-sized board to prevent the child from slipping to one side or the other.

Prep Kit

Ready for Review

The nervous system is divided into two parts: the central nervous system and the peripheral nervous system. The central nervous system consists of the brain and the spinal cord. The cables of nerve fibers linking nerve cells in the brain and spinal cord to the body's organs make up the peripheral nervous system. In addition to the skull and spinal canal, the central nervous system is protected by the meninges, three layers of tissue called the dura mater, arachnoid, and pia mater. The peripheral nervous system consists of 31 pairs of spinal nerves, which conduct sensory impulses from the skin and other organs to the spinal cord and conduct motor impulses from the spinal cord to the muscles, and 12 pairs of cranial nerves, which transmit sensations relating to sight, smell, taste, and hearing directly to the brain. The three major types of peripheral nerves are sensory nerves, motor nerves, and connecting nerves.

The part of the nervous system that regulates our voluntary activities is called the somatic or voluntary nervous system. The much more primitive autonomic or involuntary nervous system regulates involuntary body functions. The autonomic nervous system is composed of the sympathetic and parasympathetic nervous systems, which balance each other.

The skull is divided into two large bony structures that protect the brain: the cranium and the face. The spinal column has 33 bones, called vertebrae, in five sections: cervical, thoracic or dorsal, lumbar, sacral, and coccygeal.

The cervical, thoracic, and lumbar portions of the spine can be injured through compression resulting from a fall; through unnatural motions such as overextension caused by motor vehicle crashes and other types of trauma; and through distraction (pulling) along the length of the spine, as in hanging. Start your assessment of a patient with a possible spinal injury by focusing on ABC and, if he or she is responsive, by asking five questions: Does your neck or back hurt? What happened? Where does it hurt? Can you move your hands and feet? Can you feel me touching your fingers and toes? Look for contusions, punctures, or skull deformities; test for strength in the extremities; ask about pain; and check for numbness, weakness, or tingling in the extremities. Patients with severe spinal injury may lose sensation or be paralyzed below the suspected injury.

Keep the head in a neutral, in-line position while you open and maintain the airway, assess respirations, and give supplemental oxygen. Provide manual immobilization until the patient is properly secured to a backboard. A patient who is supine can be immobilized with a long backboard, using the four-person log roll. With sitting patients, you should use a short backboard, then secure the short board to a long board. If the patient is standing, immobilize him or her to a long backboard before starting your assessment; this requires three EMT-Bs.

Common head injuries include skull wounds (scalp lacerations and skull fracture) and brain injuries (concussion, contusion, intracranial bleeding), typically caused by direct blows, car crashes, falls from heights, assault, and sports injuries. Cerebral edema, seizures, vomiting, and leakage of cerebrospinal fluid are common complications of both open and closed head injuries. Common signs and symptoms of head injuries include lacerations, visible deformities of the skull, ecchymosis about the eyes or behind the ear, unequal pupil size and failure of the pupils to respond to light, loss of sensation and/or motor function, visual complaints, and irregular respirations.

The single most important observation that you can make in assessing a brain injury is of change in the level of consciousness. Use the AVPU scale or the Glasgow Coma Scale to assess consciousness immediately and every 15 minutes for a stable patient and every 5 minutes for an unstable patient, recording scores and times as you do so. Also monitor pupil size and reactions.

Patients with head injuries often have injuries to the cervical spine as well. Therefore, when treating a patient with a head injury, you must protect and stabilize the cervical spine at all times. Three principles govern treatment of head injuries: airway, ventilation, and high-flow supplemental oxygen; bleeding and circulation; and assessing/monitoring level of consciousness.

Immobilization devices include cervical collars, which must be the correct size; short backboards, including vest-type devices and rigid short boards; and long backboards.

A helmet that fits well prevents the patient's head from moving and should be left on, as long as it does not interfere with assessment/treatment of airway or ventilation problems and you can properly immobilize the spine. Remove a helmet if it makes assessing or managing airway problems difficult, prevents you from immobilizing the spine, or allows excessive head movement. Never remove a helmet if doing so will further injure the patient. Always remove a helmet if the patient is in cardiac arrest.

Vital Vocabulary

anterograde (posttraumatic) amnesia Inability to remember events after an injury.

autonomic (involuntary) nervous system The part of the nervous system that regulates functions that are not controlled by conscious will, such as digestion and sweating.

Battle's sign Bruising behind an ear over the mastoid process that may indicate skull fracture.

brain stem The part of the central nervous system that controls virtually all functions that are necessary for life, including the cardiac and respiratory systems.

central nervous system (CNS) The brain and spinal cord.

cerebellum The part of the brain that coordinates body movements.

cerebral edema Swelling of the brain.

cerebrum The largest part of the brain, containing about 75% of the brain's total volume.

closed head injury Injury in which the brain has been injured but the skin has not been broken and there is no obvious bleeding.

concussion A temporary loss or alteration of part or all of the brain's abilities to function without actual physical damage to the brain.

connecting nerves Nerves in the brain and spinal cord that connect the motor and sensory nerves.

distracted The action of pulling the spine along its length.

eyes-forward position A head position in which the patient's eyes are looking straight ahead and the head and torso are in line.

four-person log roll The recommended procedure for moving a patient with a suspected spinal injury from the ground to a long spine board.

Glasgow Coma Scale A method of evaluating level of consciousness that uses a scoring system for neurologic responses to specific stimuli.

intervertebral disk The cushion that lies between two vertebrae.

involuntary activity The actions that we do not consciously control.

meninges Three distinct layers of tissue that surround and protect the brain and the spinal cord within the skull and the spinal canal.

motor nerves Nerves that carry information from the central nervous system to the muscles.

open head injury Injury to the head often caused by a penetrating object in which there may be bleeding and exposed brain tissue.

peripheral nervous system The 31 pairs of spinal nerves and 12 pairs of cranial nerves that link the body's other organs to the central nervous system.

raccoon eyes Bruising under the eyes that may indicate skull fracture.

retrograde amnesia The inability to remember events leading up to a head injury.

sensory nerves Nerves that transmit sensory input, such as touch, taste, heat, cold, and pain, from the body to the central nervous system.

somatic (voluntary) nervous system The part of the nervous system that regulates our voluntary activities, such as walking, talking, and writing.

voluntary activity Actions that we consciously perform, in which sensory input determines the specific muscular activity.

Assessment in Action

On the first nice weekend of April, two young men take their mountain bikes to the Elk Ridge Trails. With taunts as to who is "King of the Mountain," they race off down the trail. One of the cyclists loses control of his bike and crashes into the underbrush. He is launched over the handlebars and lands on the ground, shaken and confused.

His friend quickly rides back to the ranger station to call 9-1-1. You and your partner arrive to find a 23-year-old man still down on the trail. He is wearing shorts, sandals, and sunglasses but no helmet. The patient is confused and disoriented but responds to pain by withdrawing when you move his arms or legs. Vital signs include a pulse of 60 beats/min, respirations of 28 breaths/min and irregular, and a blood pressure of 166/98 mm Hg. Additional examination shows multiple abrasions over his entire body and an angulated fracture of his left tibia.

1. Based on the patient's presenting signs and symptoms, which presents the most likely threat to his life?
   A. Fractured tibia
   B. Multiple abrasions
   C. Possible spinal cord injury
   D. Head injury

2. Whenever possible, in what position should you immobilize a patient's head and cervical spine?
   A. Slight flexion
   B. Moderate extension
   C. Moderate flexion
   D. Neutral

3. Just as you finish securing the patient to the long spine board, he starts to retch in preparation for vomiting. You should immediately:
   A. leave him supine but prepare to suction the airway.
   B. remove all the straps and roll him over onto his stomach.
   C. keep the patient strapped to the board and turn him on his side.
   D. remove the head strap and turn the patient's head to the side.

4. En route, you notice a watery, blood-tinged fluid leaking from the patient's nose. You should:
   A. place loose sterile dressing over the area.
   B. apply direct pressure with sterile dressings.
   C. pack the nostrils and apply direct pressure.
   D. pack the nostrils with tight, sterile dressings.

5. The presence of irregular respirations in this head-injured patient indicates which part of the brain is involved?
   A. Cerebrum
   B. Cerebellum
   C. Brain stem
   D. Meninges

6. In this case, with the signs of confusion/disorientation, irregular respirations, and watery, bloody fluid from the nose, this patient is at risk for which of the following problems?
   A. Aspiration
   B. Seizures
   C. Uncontrollable speech
   D. Tachycardia and low BP

7. Which of the following is the best way to administer oxygen in this patient, provided that the patient accepted any method you chose?
   A. Mask, nonrebreathing at 12 to 15 L/min
   B. BVM at a rate of 24 to 30/min
   C. Mask, nonrebreathing at 6 to 10 L/min
   D. BVM at a rate of 12 to 16/min

Challenging Questions

8. Patients with neck injuries causing paralysis are at risk for developing breathing problems. Why?

9. If a patient is talking, alert, and oriented, the presence of unequal pupils does not mean a serious head injury is present. Why?

10. A more detailed method of assessing the level of consciousness in a patient is called the Glasgow Coma Scale. What three parameters does it measure?

Points to Ponder

You have been an EMT for just under 2 months. You respond to a construction site where an employee has fallen two stories. The patient is not breathing and you are not sure whether she has a pulse. You have sent your partner for the cervical collar and backboard. You need to roll the patient over and ask a couple firefighters to help you. A very veteran firefighter yells, "this is the street, not a classroom, save the life and worry about spinal later." He then grabs the woman and rolls her over without any spinal support. You feel embarrassed as you open her airway using jaw-thrust and check her breathing. How would you deal with this veteran firefighter? Who was right? Would you report his actions and if so, to whom? Is "street care" different from "book care?"

Issues Interagency Relationships, "Street Care," Scene Management, Triage.

Online Outlook

Bleeding from a lacerated or torn brain vessel compresses the brain tissue, resulting in a loss of brain function. Review your knowledge of intracranial hematomas by completing Exercise 30 at www.emtb.com.

Special Populations

Section

6

Pediatric Assessment

Objectives

Cognitive

1. Describe differences in anatomy and physiology of the infant, child, and adult patient (p 716).
2. Identify the developmental considerations for the following age groups: infants, toddlers, preschool, school age, and adolescent (p 718).
3. Differentiate the response of the ill or injured infant or child (age specific) from that of an adult (p 718).
4. Attend to the feelings of the family when dealing with an ill or injured infant or child (p 728).
5. Recognize the need for EMT-B debriefing following a difficult infant or child transport (p 783).

Affective

6. Explain the rationale for having knowledge and skills appropriate for dealing with the infant and child patient (p 716).
7. Attend to the feelings of the family when dealing with an ill or injured infant or child (p 718).
8. Understand the provider's own response (emotional) to caring for infants or children (p 728).

Psychomotor

9. Demonstrate an assessment of an infant, toddler and school-aged child (p 722).

www.emtb.com

TECHNOLOGY

Online Chapter Pretest
Interactivities
Vocabulary Explorer
Anatomy Review
Web Links
Online Review Manual
Distance Learning

Chapter FEATURES

Skill Drills
Vital Vocabulary
Pediatric Needs
Geriatric Needs
EMT-B Safety
EMT-B Tips
Documentation Tips
Remember
Prep Kit

A career day show-and-tell at the Longfellow Elementary School is interrupted when a teacher runs up to you and tells you that "one of her students is having an asthma attack." Across the board, pediatric calls are considered by many prehospital providers to be some of the most stressful of all calls.

This chapter will focus on pediatric patient assessment along with the most common pediatric emergencies. It will also help you answer the following questions:

1. How does the age of a child affect both your assessment and management? Give two age-specific examples.

2. Why is it poor medical practice to think of pediatric patients as being "just little adults?"

Pediatric Assessment

This chapter first describes the different developmental stages of childhood and provides some general advice on examining and coping with pain in children at each stage. The chapter then outlines the challenges of assessing children.

Children have many unique health problems. Similarly, many problems that are common in adults do not occur in children. Therefore, there is a specialized medical practice devoted to the care of the young, called **pediatrics**. Handling a sick or injured child can be extremely challenging, and it is almost always a trying experience to care for a child who is seriously ill or injured. Not everyone is comfortable caring for children. In most situations, handling an infant or child means that you must manage the parents as well. Therefore, it is vital that you remain calm and professional when you care for a child (▶ **Figure 31-1**). Hard as it is, you must keep your personal feelings in check as you work with infants, children, and their families. Despite these challenges, you have an opportunity to make a real difference in the lives of these individuals.

However, once you learn how to approach children of different ages and what to expect while caring for them, you will find that they also offer some very special rewards. Not only are their innocence and openness appealing, but they often respond to treatment much more rapidly than adults do.

Anatomy and Physiology

There is no other time in our lives that our bodies are growing and changing as fast as during childhood. Infants quickly change once outside the mother's body.

Toddlers learn to walk and talk. School-age children explore the world without thought of consequences. These changes can create difficulties with assessment of the child if the EMT-B does not expect these differences.

The airway changes greatly during the early years of life. The tongue is larger and more rounded compared with the size of the mandible, or lower jaw, in younger children. This makes the tongue a greater risk for obstruction. The mandible will grow and pull the tongue forward while it flattens with age (▶ **Figure 31-2**).

The soft tissue in the rear of the mouth can also contribute to airway problems in the youngest of children. The tonsils, adenoids, and soft palate in combination with the tongue produce a smaller opening to move air

Figure 31-1 Handling a sick or injured child can be extremely challenging. A calm, professional demeanor is of utmost importance as you care for both the child and the parents.

easily. Upper airway colds can make a child work hard just to breathe. Also, the trachea is softer and narrower. The cartilage that makes up the support matures as we grow; however, the trachea can be occluded from compression. Even during the head tilt-chin lift technique, the airway can be occluded if the maneuver is performed too aggressively.

An infant needs to breathe faster than an older child. The child's lungs will grow and develop better abilities to handle the exchange of oxygen as they age. A respiratory rate of 40 to 60 breaths/min is normal for the newborn, while the teenager is expected to have rates closer to the adult range. Breathing also requires the use of the chest muscles and diaphragm. Infants have very little use of their chest muscles to make their chests expand during inspiration. They use their diaphragm. Anything that puts pressure on the abdomen of a young child can block the movement of the diaphragm and cause respiratory compromise. Young children also experience muscle fatigue much more quickly than older ones. This can lead to respiratory failure if a child has had to breathe hard for long periods.

An infant's heart rate can become as high as 200 beats or more per minute if the body needs to compensate for injury or illness. This is the primary method for the body to compensate for decreased oxygenation. It is important to know the normal ranges when evaluating children. The ability of children to constrict their blood vessels gives them the ability to keep the vital organs well perfused. Pale skin is an early sign that the child may be compensating for decreased perfusion. Constriction of the vessels can be so profound that blood flow to the extremities can be diminished. Signs of vasoconstriction can include weak distal (eg radial) pulses in the extremities, delayed capillary refill and cool hands or feet.

Documentation Tips

The unique aspects of caring for children make it wise to carry charts and measuring tools that place detailed information at your fingertips. Many services also carry specialized pediatric protocols as part of their standing orders. Refer to these at-hand information sources during your care, and remember to make notes about your specific observations and treatment decisions. This "information-intensive" approach to pediatric care helps ensure both good care and thorough documentation.

The skeletal system contains growth plates at the ends of long bones, which enable these bones to grow during childhood. As a result of the active growth plates, children's bones are weaker and more flexible, making them prone to fracture with stress. The bones of the skull also grow, but during infancy. Infants have two soft openings within the skull called fontanels. These will usually close completely by about 18 months of age; before that time, handle an infant's head with care.

Figure 31-2 The anatomy of a child's airway differs from that of an adult's in several ways. The back of the head is larger in a child, so head positioning requires more care. The tongue is proportionally larger and more anterior in the mouth. The trachea is smaller in diameter and more flexible. The airway itself is lower and narrower.

TABLE 31-1 Helpful Tips in Caring for Infants and Children

1. **Try to remain calm and appear confident.** Children are used to having other people take charge. They are also easily frightened by noise, so speak with a soft voice whenever possible.

2. **Remember that you are caring for the whole family, not just the child.** Children are quick to pick up on their caregivers' anxiety. It may calm both parties if you can establish good rapport with the caregivers and allow them to help with the child's care. To avoid confusion, avoid using technical terms.

3. **Honesty is the best policy.** Telling a child or a caregiver that a procedure won't hurt (when you know that it will) or that it will be over quickly (when it won't) can boomerang: Once you lose their trust, any additional procedures that you attempt are more likely to meet with resistance.

4. **Tell both the caregivers and the child what is happening as often as you can.** Lack of information is very stressful for everyone; the imagination can run wild in an effort to make sense of what is going on. In children, we call this frightening fantasies; in caregivers, we call it worst-case scenarios.

5. **Keep the family together as much as possible.** This is not always possible, but children and their caregivers generally feel safer when they are together. Parents can sometimes be encouraged to help by holding the child's hand, talking to the child, or telling a story.

6. **Provide hope and reassurance to the caregivers and to the child.** Even when you are very concerned about the child's condition, be careful not to eliminate hope in the patient and family. Children especially need reassurance, rewards, and praise during painful events. Remember that no one can be absolutely certain about the outcome. Children have an amazing ability to bounce back from what looks to be death's door.

Growth and Development

Adulthood begins at age 21. On this, the medical community has agreed. But when does childhood end? Many EMS systems use 18 years of age, others use 14, and still others use 12 or 16. Even though there are specific issues that are important to different age groups, there are also some general rules that apply when you care for children of any age ◀ Table 31-1 .

Between birth and adulthood, many physical and emotional changes occur in children. While each child is unique, the thoughts and behaviors of children as a whole are often grouped into stages: infancy, the toddler years, preschool age, school age, and adolescence. Children in each stage grapple with different developmental issues.

How you examine children and how you help them to cope with the emergency depend on several practical considerations, including the child's stability and mental status, the anticipated transport time, the availability of other personnel, and the protocols in your area. However, there are a number of simple techniques that will let you calm and comfort most children during emergency treatment and transport. Here are some suggestions about approaching and caring for the different childhood age groups.

The Infant

Infancy is usually defined as the first year of life; the first month after birth is called the **neonatal** or newborn period. At first, infants respond mainly to physical stimuli such as light, warmth, cold, hunger, sound, and taste. Crying is one of their main avenues of expression during this period. After the first few months, however, they learn to coo, smile, roll over, and recognize their parents or caregivers. Infants are usually not afraid of strangers, because they become the center of attention in most families. However, by the end of their first year, they may show signs of preferring to be with their caregivers and may cry if they are separated ▶ Figure 31-3 .

Begin your assessment by observing the infant from a distance, preferably in a caregiver's arms ▶ Figure 31-4 . This initial size up can reward the EMT-B with valuable information. The work of breathing, skin color, alertness, and level of activity provide a good overall picture of the infant's condition. Older infants, from 6 months to a year, may begin to cry when touched or picked up by a stranger, so let the caregiver continue to hold the baby as you start your examination. Warm your hands and the end of the stethoscope, then begin by listening to the chest and assessing the heart rate. Next examine the abdomen, then the head, and then the rest of the body. This torso-to-head approach works well because the infant sees their world centered around their head. Near the end of their first year, an infant's world will increase in size to include their torso as well.

Provide as much sensory comfort as you can: Keep the infant warm, and offer a pacifier if the caregiver allows it. Have a caregiver hold the infant, if possible, during procedures. Plan to complete any painful procedure in an efficient manner. When splinting a suspected fracture be sure to have all of the equipment you will need in order to avoid making the procedure take longer than necessary.

The Toddler

After infancy, until about 3 years of age, a child is called a **toddler**. During this period, children begin to walk and to explore the environment. They are able to open doors, drawers, boxes, and bottles. Because they are explorers by nature and are not afraid, injuries in this age group are more frequent.

Stranger anxiety develops early in this period. Toddlers may resist separation from caregivers and be afraid to let others come near them. Because of their newly found independence, they may also be very

Between birth and adulthood, many physical and emotional changes occur in children.

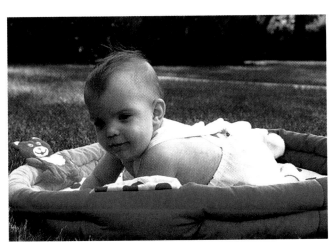

Figure 31-3 Infants are usually not afraid of strangers, but as they reach 6 months to 1 year, they may show signs that they prefer to be with their caregivers.

Figure 31-4 **A.** Begin assessing an infant from a distance, preferably in the caregiver's arms. **B.** Warm the end of the stethoscope with your hands. **C.** Listen to the chest and assess heart rate first.

Figure 31-5 Because of their newly found independence, toddlers may be unhappy about being restrained or held for procedures.

Figure 31-6 Leave a toddler on the caregiver's lap during your assessment, and use a toy to distract him or her.

unhappy about being restrained or held for procedures **▲ Figure 31-5** . Two-year-olds in particular have a well-deserved reputation for having their own ideas about almost everything, which is why these years are often called the "terrible twos." Toddlers have a hard time describing or localizing pain. Pain in the abdomen may be "My tummy hurts," and examination may reveal tenderness throughout the body. This is not because the child is trying to be difficult but because he or she cannot tell the difference.

Make as many observations as you can before touching the child: level of alertness, work of breathing, and skin color. When appropriate, examine the child on the caregiver's lap, and use toys or puppets to distract him or her **▲ Figure 31-6** .

Toddlers can be curious and adventuresome, so you may able to distract them. For example, you might allow the child to play with a tongue depressor. Restrain the child for as short a time as possible, and allow him or her to be comforted immediately after a painful procedure. Begin your assessment at the hands or feet in order to keep from upsetting the child when possible.

The Preschool-Age Child

Preschool-age children (ages 3 to 6 years) are able to use simple language quite effectively and have lively imaginations **▶ Figure 31-7** . They can understand directions, be much more specific in describing their sensations, and identify painful areas when questioned. Much of their history must still be obtained from caregivers, however. Preschool-age children have a rich fantasy life, which can make them particularly fearful about pain and change involving their bodies. At this age, they often believe that their thoughts or wishes can cause injury or harm to themselves or to

Figure 31-7 Preschool children have a vivid imagination, so much of the history must still be obtained from the caregiver.

others. They can believe that an injury was due to a bad deed they did earlier in the day.

Try to distract the child during the examination with simple conversation and questions, or use a toy, game, or puppet. Make the examination less threatening by allowing the child to handle some pieces of equipment, such as your stethoscope or a tongue blade **▶ Figure 31-8** . Do not use words that suggest invading the child's body, such as "shot," "cut," "poke," or "stick."

Tell the child what you are going to do immediately before you do it; this way, the child has no time to develop frightening fantasies. At this age, children are easily distracted with counting games, small toys, or conversation. Be sure to adjust the level of game to the

Figure 31-8 Make the exam less threatening by allowing the patient to handle some pieces of equipment.

Figure 31-9 School-age children are more like adults in that they can answer your questions and can help to take care of themselves.

developmental level of the child; health care providers often assume that preschool children understand more than they actually do. Use adhesive bandages to cover the site of an injection or other small wound, because the child might be worried about keeping his or her body together in one piece.

The School-Age Child

School-age children (ages 6 to 12 years) are beginning to act more like adults. They can think in concrete terms, respond sensibly to direct questions, and help take care of themselves. Your assessment, therefore, is more like an adult assessment; talk to the child, not just the parent, in taking the medical history
▲ **Figure 31-9**.

The school-age child is usually familiar with the process of physical examination. They have been to the doctor for childhood check-ups and immunizations. Whenever possible, give the child appropriate choices: Would you like to sit up or lie down? Would you like to take off your clothes yourself? Only ask questions that you can control the answer. If you ask "Can I take your blood pressure?" and the answer is NO! you will not be able to take it without upsetting the child. Encourage cooperation by allowing the child to listen to his or her own heartbeat through the stethoscope ▶ **Figure 31-10**.

School-age children can understand the difference between emotional and physical pain; they have concerns about the meaning of pain. Give them simple explanations about what is causing their pain and what will be done about it ▶ **Figure 31-11**). Games and conversation may distract them. Ask them to describe their favorite place, their pets, or their toys. Ask the caregiver's advice in choosing the right distraction.

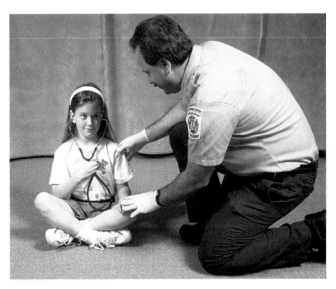

Figure 31-10 Encourage cooperation by allowing the child to listen to his or her own heartbeat through the stethoscope.

Figure 31-11 School-age children can understand simple explanations about their physical condition and the need for simple procedures.

> Even though there are specific issues that are important to different age groups, there are also some general rules that apply when you care for children of any age.

Rewarding the school-age child after a procedure can be very helpful in his or her recovery, but only reward a child for completing the procedure.

The Adolescent

Most **adolescents** (ages 12 to 18 years) are able to think abstractly and can participate in decision making. This is a period where the focus of their strength has moved from parents to peers. They are very concerned about body image and how they appear to their peers and to others. They may have very strong feelings about being observed during procedures, even—or especially—by their caregivers.

Respect the adolescent's privacy at all times. Remember that adolescents can often understand very complex concepts and treatment options; you should provide them with information when they request it (▼ Figure 31-12). You will find them more helpful and understanding of necessary procedures.

Adolescents have a clear understanding of the purpose and meaning of pain. Whenever possible, explain any necessary procedures well in advance. Assess their pain by facial and body expression as well as by asking questions; adolescents can be very stoic and may not request relief from pain even when they need

it. To distract them, find out what they are interested in, such as sports, books, movies, or friends, and get them talking about this.

Assessing Pediatric Patients
Approach to Assessment

When a child becomes sick or injured, the young body begins to compensate for the extra needs of the body. The work-of-breathing (WOB) increases. This is often seen as faster breathing, retractions along the chest wall (▼ Figure 31-13), or the way the child sits and positions himself or herself. The heart rate increases to allow more oxygenated blood to pass through the body. The skin color may turn pale or cyanotic depending on the problem. The child will become anxious as the oxygen level in the brain decreases. Assessment of the level of responsiveness will give clues to the amount of oxygen reaching the end-organs of the body. If the brain is feeling oxygen starved, other parts of the body will also.

Although each child and situation is unique, you should follow a few basic guidelines when assessing and caring for infants and children. First, you should follow the same general approach to children that you use for adults (▶ Figure 31-14).

You should take a child's vital signs in the field because you are the eyes, ears, and hands of medical control. During your assessment, you should obtain a complete set of baseline vital signs, including respirations, pulse, blood pressure (when possible), skin signs, level of activity, muscle tone, and movement. You must also decide whether to call for ALS backup or provide immediate transport. This decision is often made with the assistance of either off-line protocols or on-line medical direction. It is always a good idea to inform

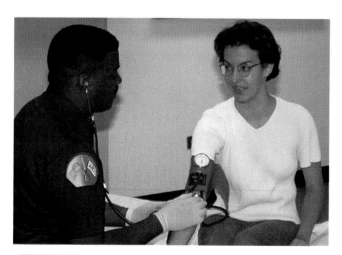

Figure 31-12 Respect the adolescent's privacy at all times; give the patient whatever information he or she requests.

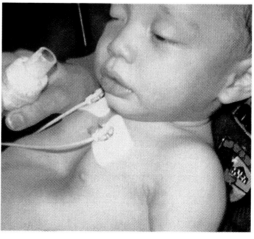

Figure 31-13 Retractions are seen along the rib cage, above the sternum, and along the clavicles.

Pediatric Patient Assessment

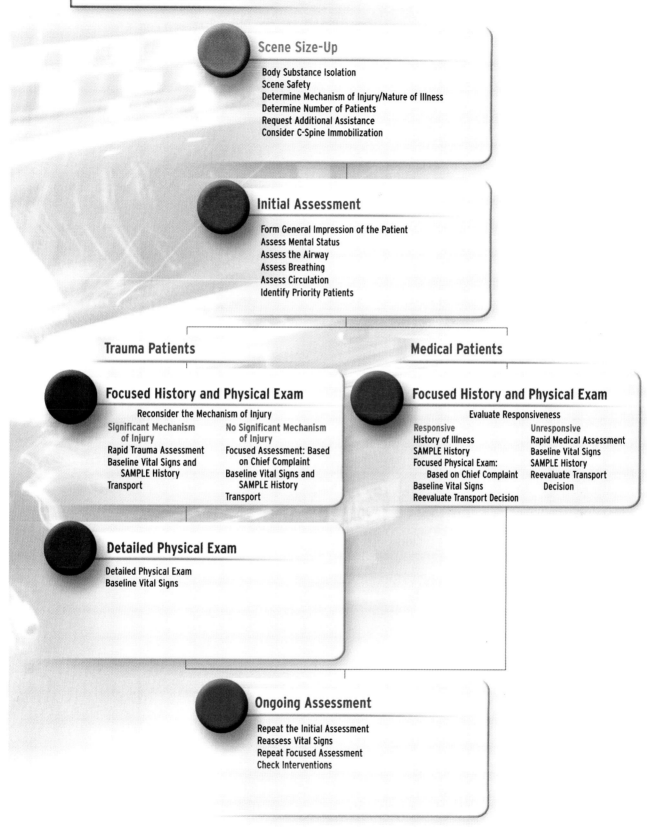

Scene Size-Up

Body Substance Isolation
Scene Safety
Determine Mechanism of Injury/Nature of Illness
Determine Number of Patients
Request Additional Assistance
Consider C-Spine Immobilization

Initial Assessment

Form General Impression of the Patient
Assess Mental Status
Assess the Airway
Assess Breathing
Assess Circulation
Identify Priority Patients

Trauma Patients

Focused History and Physical Exam

Reconsider the Mechanism of Injury

Significant Mechanism of Injury	No Significant Mechanism of Injury
Rapid Trauma Assessment	Focused Assessment: Based on Chief Complaint
Baseline Vital Signs and SAMPLE History	Baseline Vital Signs and SAMPLE History
Transport	Transport

Detailed Physical Exam

Detailed Physical Exam
Baseline Vital Signs

Medical Patients

Focused History and Physical Exam

Evaluate Responsiveness

Responsive	Unresponsive
History of Illness	Rapid Medical Assessment
SAMPLE History	Baseline Vital Signs
Focused Physical Exam: Based on Chief Complaint	SAMPLE History
Baseline Vital Signs	Reevaluate Transport Decision
Reevaluate Transport Decision	

Ongoing Assessment

Repeat the Initial Assessment
Reassess Vital Signs
Repeat Focused Assessment
Check Interventions

Figure 31-14 Base your approach to a child on the same general steps you use for adults.

> You should take
> a child's vital signs in the field because
> you are the eyes, ears, and hands
> of medical control.

the base or receiving hospital about the status of a pediatric patient so that the facility can prepare to meet the child's particular needs.

The condition of infants and children may deteriorate rapidly during transport. You should have pediatric resuscitation equipment ready to use at all times, including a pediatric resuscitation tape measure for quick determination of height and weight in small patients. This is important in selecting proper airway equipment sizes, a subject that Chapter 32 covers in more detail. Transport infants and children to facilities that are capable of providing the appropriate level of care whenever possible. Not all community hospitals offer all higher levels of care for children. You may have to bypass closer emergency care facilities to reach a pediatric center. When this is not possible, as in many rural areas, a hospital may arrange for secondary transportation after stabilizing the child's condition. Always follow your local protocols.

Vital Signs

Note that normal vital signs in pediatric patients vary with the age of the child (▼ Table 31-2). Remember that

your approach to taking vital signs also varies with the age of the child. Be gentle, talk to the child, assess respirations and pulse next, and assess blood pressure last (▼ Figure 31-15). Warm your stethoscope on your hands or a cloth before placing it on the skin. You may also want to let the child hold the equipment or stethoscope before placing it on him or her.

RESPIRATIONS. Abnormal respirations are a common sign of illness or injury in children. Respirations should be counted for at least 30 seconds. However, do not base your evaluation by counting the number of times the chest rises and falls in infants and children younger than 3 years. Rather, count the rise and fall of the

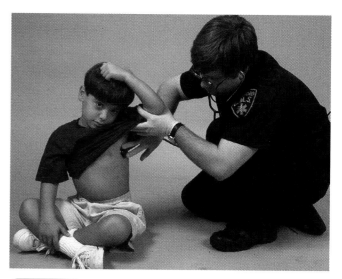

Figure 31-15 Always take vital signs in the field. Begin by talking to the child, then assess respirations and pulse.

TABLE 31-2 Vital Signs by Age			
Age	Respirations (breaths/min)	Pulse (beats/min)	Systolic Blood Pressure (mm Hg)
Newborn: 0 to 1 month	40 to 60	120 to 160	50 to 70
Infant: 1 month to 1 year	30 to 60	100 to 160	70 to 95
Toddler: 1 to 3 years	24 to 40	90 to 150	80 to 100
Preschool-Age: 3 to 6 years	22 to 34	80 to 140	80 to 100
School-Age: 6 to 12 years	18 to 30	70 to 120	80 to 110
Adolescent: 12 to 18 years	12 to 16	60 to 100	90 to 110
Over 18 years	12 to 20	60 to 100	90 to 140

Figure 31-16   **A.** Palpate over the brachial area to assess the pulse of an infant.   **B.** Palpate over the femoral area as a second choice. **C.** In older children, use the carotid artery.

Figure 31-17   When measuring a child's blood pressure, use the proper size cuff, which should cover two thirds of the patient's upper arm.

Figure 31-18   Estimate capillary refill by squeezing the end of a finger or toe for several seconds until the fingertip blanches. Normal color should return within 2 seconds after you let go.

abdomen. This is usually easier to do with the child in the caregiver's lap. Note the effort the child makes in breathing, and listen for noises during respiration.

PULSE. Pulses may be difficult to feel if they are very weak, very fast, or slow   ▲ **Figure 31-16** . In infants, feel over the brachial area or in the femoral area. In older children, use the carotid artery. Count the pulse for at

least 1 minute. Note the strength of the pulse: Is it weak or strong?

BLOOD PRESSURE. Measuring a child's blood pressure in the field can be tricky. To get an accurate reading, you must have a cuff that covers two thirds of the patient's upper arm   ▲ **Figure 31-17** . If conditions at the scene make it impossible to measure blood pressure accurately, do not waste a lot of time trying. For patients 3 years of age or younger, technical difficulties reduce the value of a blood pressure in the field.

SKIN SIGNS. Feel the skin for temperature and moisture at the same time that you measure the other vital signs. Is the skin warm and dry, or cold and clammy? Estimate capillary refill by squeezing the end of a finger or toe for several seconds and then observing the return of blood to the area   ▲ **Figure 31-18** . Color should return in less than 2 seconds after you let go.

Infants and Children with Special Needs

The approach to health care in our society continues to focus on decreasing lengths of hospitalization, and technology continues to improve. As a result of these two factors, the number of infants and children with chronic diseases who are living at home or in other environments outside of the hospital continues to grow. You should be familiar with some of the special needs created by these chronic diseases or conditions, particularly as they relate to the potential need for emergency medical care.

Some examples of infants and children with special needs include the following:

- Children who were born prematurely and have associated lung disease problems

- Small children or infants with congenital heart disease

- Children with neurologic disease (occasionally caused by hypoxemia at the time of birth, as with cerebral palsy)

- Children with chronic disease or with functions that have been altered since birth

The parent or caregiver of a special needs child will be an important part of your assessment. The EMT-B must first determine the child's normal baseline status before an assessment of the current condition can be made. It is often helpful to ask, "What is different today?" These parents/guardians often know their child's history and condition better than some skilled health care workers might.

Occasionally, these children live at home but depend on artificial ventilators or other devices to maintain life. You assess and care for these children the same as for all other patients. Your focus on the ABCs remains the priority.

Tracheostomy Tubes

Children who depend on home artificial ventilators or those who have chronic pulmonary medical conditions may breathe through a tracheostomy tube. A **tracheostomy tube** is a tube placed in the neck that passes directly into the major airways ▶ **Figure 31-19** . Because this tube bypasses the nose and

EMT-B Tips

As EMT-Bs finish initial training and begin their field response work, it is common for them to feel a strong need for additional knowledge about the special-needs patients and their equipment that this section describes. Be aggressive during training in pursuing opportunities to learn the details about these special subjects. Over time, experience will be one of your primary teachers.

mouth, the body can build up secretions in or around the tube. These tubes are prone to become obstructed by mucous plugs or foreign bodies. There may be bleeding or air leaking around the tube, which usually happens with new tracheostomies, and the tube can become loose or dislodged. Occasionally, the opening around the tube may become infected. Your care of a patient with a tracheostomy tube includes maintaining an open airway. This can include suctioning the tube if necessary to clear a mucous plug, maintaining the patient in a position of comfort, and providing transport to the hospital. Call for ALS back-up.

Figure 31-19 Some children require a tracheostomy to breathe.

Artificial Ventilators

Children who are on a ventilator at home cannot breath without help. If the ventilator malfunctions, remove the child from the ventilator and begin ventilations with a BVM device. To do this, remove the mask from a BVM device and directly attach the bag and valve to the tracheostomy tube; this will allow you to ventilate through the tracheostomy tube.

Children on home artificial ventilators will need artificial ventilation throughout transport. Artificial ventilation is provided through the tracheostomy tube. Remember that the patient's caregivers will know how the ventilator works and will be of great help to you in attaching the BVM device to the tube in preparation for transport.

Central IV Lines

Children with chronic medical conditions such as gastrointestinal disturbances that require prolonged IV feeding or those with infections that require prolonged IV antibiotics will have indwelling IV catheters placed near the heart for long-term use. These catheters can be in the chest or in the arm (▼ Figure 31-20). Problems associated with these devices may include broken lines, infections around the lines, clotted lines, and bleeding around the line or from the tubing attached to the line. If bleeding occurs, you should apply direct pressure to the tubing and provide transport to the hospital.

Gastrostomy Tubes

Gastrostomy tubes, sometimes referred to as G-tubes, are tubes placed through the wall of the abdomen directly into the stomach for feeding in children who cannot be fed by mouth (▼ Figure 31-21). Because food is pumped into the stomach, it can back up the esophagus and into the lungs. Breathing problems in these children may be complicated by aspiration of the tube contents into the lungs. You should always have suction readily available to clear any materials from the mouth and to prevent airway problems. Patients with gastrostomy tubes who have difficulty breathing should be transported either sitting or lying on the right side with the head elevated to prevent the contents of the stomach from passing into the lungs.

Figure 31-20 Children who require frequent IV medications may have a central line in place.

Figure 31-21 Gastrostomy tubes are placed through the skin into the stomach for children who cannot be fed by mouth.

> It is important to remember that when children are injured, especially those with chronic illnesses, you may have several patients to treat rather than just one

Give supplemental oxygen if the patient has any difficulty breathing. Children with diabetes who receive insulin and tube feedings may become hypoglycemic quickly if tube feedings are discontinued. Be alert for altered mental status.

Shunts

Some children with chronic neurologic conditions may have shunts in place. <u>Shunts</u> are tubes that extend from the brain to the abdomen to drain excess cerebrospinal fluid that may accumulate near the brain. These shunts keep pressures in the head from building up. If a shunt becomes clogged due to infection, changes in mental status and respiratory arrest may occur. Emergency medical care includes airway management and artificial ventilation during transport. During assessment, you will likely feel a device on the side of the head, behind the ear, beneath the skin. This device is a fluid reservoir, and the presence of this device should alert you to the possibility that the child has an underlying shunt. Should the shunt become dysfunctional, the child could be predisposed to respiratory arrest.

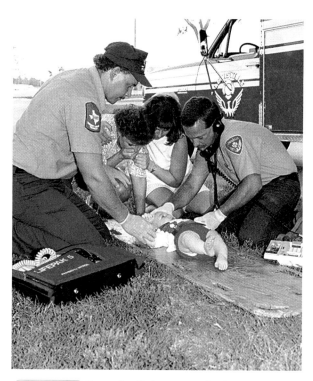

Figure 31-22 Remember that you are caring for at least two patients: the infant or child, and the parent or caregiver.

Family Matters

It is important to remember that when children are injured, especially those with chronic illnesses, you may have several patients to treat rather than just one **▲ Figure 31-22** . Family members, especially the primary caregiver, often need help or support when medical emergencies or problems develop. A calm parent usually helps to contribute to a calm child. An agitated parent usually means that the child will act the same way. Make sure that you are calm, efficient, professional, and sensitive as you deal with children and their families.

EMT-B Tips

Sick and injured children should be left with their parents unless aggressive resuscitation is needed. The stress produced by separation anxiety can make a sick child worse. If you need to separate the parent and child, try to leave them within eyesight and talking distance to minimize the stresses.

> When transporting children, do not allow the parent or EMT to hold the child during the actual transport.

Transporting Infants and Children

Before you transport a sick or injured child, you should be aware of special transport considerations for infants and children. Infants and small children are very susceptible to temperature changes. They lose body heat rapidly and must always be transported wrapped in blankets. Very young, sick children are also extremely susceptible to infection. Therefore, you should avoid breathing or coughing directly on a small or sick child. Isolate an infant or child from bacterial contamination, particularly from your own nose, mouth, and hands.

Newborns should be transported in special incubators. If an incubator is not available, wrap the newborn in blankets or silver swaddlers. Be sure to keep the newborn's face uncovered, and make sure the ambulance is warm. Many large medical centers maintain specially equipped vehicles for transporting infants and small children. You should know the location and availability of these vehicles.

When transporting children, do not allow the parent or EMT to hold the child during the actual transport. Always drive with due care. The child may not fit into the ambulance as well as an adult would, so slower speeds and cautious turning will provide extra safety for the pediatric patient. Do not allow your emotions to get control of the situation.

Prep Kit

Ready for Review

Child anatomy contributes to some special challenges in assessment and care. The tongue is large relative to other structures, so it poses a higher risk of airway obstruction than in an adult. Tonsils and other tissue more posterior can also pose this problem, as does a relatively soft and narrow trachea. Head size and shape also make airway positioning a specialized task in children. Newborns and infants have high respiratory rates, and breathe primarily with their abdomens. Vasoconstriction in the skin and increased heart rate are the major means of compensating for decreased perfusion of vital organs.

There are five development stages in childhood: infancy, the toddler years, preschool age, school age, and adolescence. Each stage requires a slightly different approach to assessment and pain management. General rules for dealing with children of all ages include appearing confident, being honest, and keeping caregivers together with the patient as much as possible.

Always take the patient's vital signs in the field and have pediatric resuscitation equipment ready. To measure respirations in children younger than 3 years, count the rise and fall of the abdomen rather than the chest. Feel for a pulse in the brachial or femoral artery in infants and small children, and in the carotid artery in older children.

The number of children living at home who have chronic diseases and special needs is increasing. These patients will test your knowledge of special equipment and care procedures, your skills in obtaining pertinent history from family and caregivers, and your ability to detect urgent problems when you may not be completely familiar with the technical details involved. Learning everything you can from each special situation will help prepare you for similar responses in the future.

When you care for a seriously ill or injured child, remember also that attending to the stress of others involved will help calm the patient. Try to keep the child with—or at least near—a parent or caregiver during transport.

Vital Vocabulary

adolescents Children between 12 to 18 years of age.

gastrostomy tube A feeding tube placed directly through the wall of the abdomen; used in patients who cannot ingest liquids or solids.

infant The first year of life.

neonatal The first month after birth.

pediatrics A specialized medical practice devoted to the care of the young.

preschool-age Children between 3 to 6 years of age.

school-age Children between 6 to 12 years of age.

shunt A tube that diverts excess cerebrospinal fluid from the brain to the abdomen.

toddler The period following infancy until 3 years of age.

tracheostomy tube A tube inserted into the trachea in children who cannot breathe on their own; passes through the neck directly into the major airways.

www.emtb.com

Assessment in Action

You and your partner are dispatched to the apartment of a child who is having "difficulty breathing." On arrival, you find a 6-year-old girl sitting at the kitchen table, hunched forward with her arms on the kitchen table, bracing herself. Her mother explains that this is the first time they have had to use the inhaler since the girl was diagnosed with asthma.

They tried the inhaler twice with minimal results and were reluctant to try it again. The family doctor did not return a page, and they called EMS. Your patient appears slightly pale. She does not pay attention to you or your partner and does not respond when you say her name. Her gaze is vacant and she appears tired. The mother also states that her daughter has had the "flu" for the past 2 days, including a low-grade fever. They state that she is allergic to animal dander and penicillin and is receiving no other medication other than her albuterol inhaler. She has no other medical problem.

1. Which of the following signs should be used to determine whether this child is sick or well during your initial assessment? Her:
   A. body position and skin color
   B. skin color and pupil size
   C. pupil size and attention to you
   D. attention to you and body position

2. In this patient, which of the following observations of respiratory distress can only be observed if her shirt is removed?
   A. Nasal flaring   B. Sternal retraction
   C. Audible wheezing   D. Grunting

3. Tripoding is significant because it suggests:
   A. severe abdominal pain.   B. accessory muscle use.
   C. abnormal circulation.   D. impending seizures.

4. As you are conducting your assessment you find that this child has sternal retractions, intercostal retractions, and nasal flaring. Vital signs include a pulse of 150 beats/min, respirations of 46 breaths/min, and a blood pressure of 96/68 mm Hg. Her skin is very warm, slightly pale, and dry. Her mother says her last temperature, taken just prior to your arrival, was 102°F (38.8°C). Lung sounds have wheezes in all lobes. Assuming that local protocols would allow, which of the following treatments is appropriate for this patient?
   A. Administering oxygen by nasal cannula and rapid transport to the hospital

   B. Sponging with tepid water to lower her fever, then transport
   C. Administering metered dose inhaler and oxygen, then transport
   D. Administering aspirin and oxygen by mask, then rapid transport

5. Given all her assessment signs, which of the following statements is accurate for this child? She is in:
   A. respiratory failure.   B. respiratory arrest.
   C. no acute distress.   D. the recovery phase.

6. Your partner states that this patient is tachypneic. What does that mean?
   A. Her heart rate is too fast.   B. Her respiratory rate is too fast.
   C. She has poor perfusion.   D. She has poor attention.

7. As your partner is administering treatment, you complete the assessment and note that her legs are mottled. You know this indicates:
   A. fever.   B. infection.
   C. poor perfusion.   D. a cold environment.

8. You complete your detailed physical assessment and note petechiae. Petechiae is/are:
   A. bruise marks.   B. cerebrospinal fluid.
   C. hematomas.   D. a fine red or maroon rash.

Challenging Questions

9. Why may blood pressure be inaccurate as an indicator of perfusion in a child?
   A. The blood pressure becomes more accurate as the child grows because of the total blood volume.
   B. The blood pressure is only accurate when compared to the pulse of a child that is awake and alert.
   C. Blood pressure cuffs do not come properly sized for the pediatric patient.
   D. A child with poor perfusion frequently has a normal blood pressure because of compensation.

10. What would the appropriate description of this child's AVPU scale be?
   A. She is alert.   B. She is unresponsive.
   C. She does not respond to   D. She responds to painful stimuli.
      her name.

Points to Ponder

You are dispatched to a non-breathing infant. When you arrive, you find a mother holding the infant and the infant appears fine. You can see that the mother has been crying and you ask what happened. The mother indicates that she checked on the baby and it did not appear to be breathing so she called 911. The dispatcher had told her what to do for the baby and as soon as she picked-up the baby it started crying. You check the baby and find nothing wrong. There is no indication that the baby was not breathing. You suspect that the first-time mother over reacted and that the baby was breathing the entire time. The mother insists that you take the baby to the hospital, but when you contact the hospital they agree with you and the physician says not to transport. The mother continues to insist that you transport,

but you are hesitant because of the cost to the mother and because it will take you out of service for an hour on a busy Friday night. Would you transport the baby? Is there a compromise?

Issues Dispatch Assisted Patient Care, Calming Excited Participants, Non-Emergent Transports, Duty to Transport, Alternative Resources, Liability.

Online Outlook

Infants and children are not simply small adults; they come in a wide variety of sizes with anatomy and physiology that are different from those of adults. To learn more about pediatric medical emergencies, complete Exercise 31 at www.emtb.com.

www.emtb.com

Pediatric Airway and Medical Emergencies

Objectives

Cognitive

1. Describe differences in anatomy and physiology of the infant, child, and adult patient as they relate to medical emergencies (p 734).
2. Identify the usual cause of cardiac arrest in infants and children versus adults (p 757).
3. Describe the steps in positioning an infant and/or child to maintain an open airway (p 735).
4. Summarize neonatal resuscitation procedures (p 755).
5. Indicate various causes of respiratory emergencies (p 742).
6. Differentiate between respiratory distress and respiratory failure (p 746).
7. List the steps in the management of foreign body airway obstruction (p 743).
8. Summarize emergency medical care strategies for respiratory distress and respiratory failure (p 747).
9. Identify the signs and symptoms of shock (hypoperfusion) in the infant and child patient (p 752).
10. Describe the methods of determining end organ perfusion in the infant and child patient (p 753).
11. List the common causes of seizures in the infant and child patient (p 747).
12. Describe the management of seizures in the infant and child patient (p 748).

Affective

13. Explain the rationale for having knowledge and skills appropriate for dealing with the infant and child patient (p 734).

Psychomotor

14. Demonstrate the techniques necessary in neonatal resuscitation (p 755).
15. Demonstrate bag-valve-mask artificial ventilations for the infant (p 740).
16. Demonstrate bag-valve-mask artificial ventilations for the child (p 740).
17. Demonstrate oxygen delivery for the infant and child (p 741).
18. Demonstrate the techniques of foreign body airway obstruction removal in the infant (p 745).
19. Demonstrate the techniques of foreign body airway obstruction removal in the child (p 744).

TECHNOLOGY

www.emtb.com

Online Chapter Pretest ◄
Interactivities
Vocabulary Explorer
Anatomy Review
Web Links
Online Review Manual
Distance Learning

"Medic 16, respond to Careland Day Care for a child with an unknown medical emergency." En route, dispatch updates you that your patient is a 3-year-old girl who has jammed several peanuts up her nose.

As children grow and experience more and more of the world, they will occasionally make some poor decisions, such as the case described above. This chapter will introduce you to the world of pediatric care, focusing specifically on airway management and resuscitation. It will also help you answer the following questions:

1. What is the most common cause of cardiac arrest in children?

2. Why is it a good idea to carry written reference material specific to pediatric patients, such as vital signs by age, airway sizes, and so on, when working in the prehospital setting?

Pediatric Airway and Medical Emergencies

There are many causes of respiratory distress and failure in children. Although you might not be able to identify the exact cause, you must be able to intervene appropriately to restore breathing in all cases. You will face some special challenges in caring for sick and injured children. Infants and children are not simply small adults. They come in a variety of sizes, and their anatomy and physiology differ from those of adults. Despite the differences between children and adults, like adults, providing adequate oxygenation and ventilation is the first step to achieving the best possible outcome for the patient, regardless of the underlying problem.

This chapter begins by identifying the signs and symptoms of respiratory distress along with management techniques. A discussion of how to open and maintain the airway in infants and children follows, including placement of airway adjuncts and the use of oxygen delivery devices, including the bag-valve-mask (BVM) device. The causes and management of airway obstruction from foreign objects are discussed next. After a description of the management of children with seizures, altered level of consciousness, poisoning, meningitis, shock, and dehydration, a brief review of neonatal resuscitation and a review of BLS precautions for infants and children are provided. Finally, an in-depth discussion of the troubling problem of sudden infant death syndrome (SIDS) and other circumstances resulting in a child's death is presented. Some simple techniques for coping with the emotional stress surrounding the death of a child are presented in this section.

EMTs who are calm when caring for adults often find themselves anxious when dealing with critically ill or injured infants or children. However, treatment of children is the same as that of adults in most emergency situations. Once you understand the differences in anatomy between children and adults and learn to recognize signs of respiratory distress in children, you will find it easier to approach even the youngest patients in a relaxed, professional manner.

Because a young child might not be able to speak, your assessment of his or her condition must be based in large part on what you can see and hear. In addition, families may be helpful in providing vital information about an accident or illness. You should think of families as part of the caregiving team and, whenever possible, include them in all decisions about care and transportation.

Understanding the Pediatric Airway

To manage the pediatric airway effectively, you must first understand the anatomic differences between adults and children. To start with, the heart is higher in a child's chest, and the lungs are smaller. The opening to the trachea is higher in the neck, and the neck itself is shorter.

The anatomy of a child's airway differs from that of an adult in five principal ways. These differences will influence the treatment decisions that you make about pediatric patients, including whether or not intervention is needed and, if so, what procedure to use. The anatomy of a child's airway and other important structures differs from that of an adult's in the following ways:

- A larger, rounder <u>occiput</u>, or back of the head, which requires more careful positioning of the airway.

- A proportionately larger tongue relative to the size of the mouth and a more anterior location in the mouth. The child's tongue is also larger relative to the small mandible and can easily block the airway.

- A floppy, U-shaped epiglottis that is larger than an adult's, relative to the size of the airway.

- Less well-developed rings of cartilage in the trachea that may easily collapse if the neck is flexed or hyperextended.

- A narrower, lower airway.

Because of the smaller diameter of the trachea in infants, which is about the same diameter as a drinking straw, their airway is easily obstructed by secretions, blood, or swelling. Also, since intercostal muscles are not well developed in children, movement of the diaphragm, their major muscle of respiration, dictates the amount of air they inspire. Gastric distention can interfere with movement of the diaphragm and lead to <u>hypoventilation</u>.

The Pediatric Airway

Positioning the Airway

Positioning the airway correctly is critical in pediatric emergency care. Always position the airway in a neutral sniffing position (▼ **Figure 32-1**). This accomplishes two goals at once: It keeps the trachea from kinking when the neck is bent back (hyperextended) or forward (flexed), and it maintains the proper alignment if you have to immobilize the spine. If the child has been involved in trauma or trauma is suspected, use the jaw-thrust maneuver to open the airway.

Follow the steps in (▶ **Skill Drill 32-1**) to position the airway in a child or infant:

1. **Place the patient on a firm surface** such as a short backboard or pediatric immobilization device **(Step 1)**.

2. **Fold a small towel to a thickness of approximately 1″, and place it under the patient's shoulders and back (Step 2)**.

3. **Place tape across the child's forehead** to limit rolling of the head during transport **(Step 3)**.

Airway Adjuncts

In children with inadequate ventilation, whatever the reason, you should use an airway adjunct to maintain an open airway. Airway adjuncts are devices that help to maintain the airway or assist in providing artificial ventilation, including oral and nasal airways, bite blocks, and BVM devices. Placing the adjuncts correctly starts with choosing the appropriately sized equipment (▶ **Table 32-1**).

OROPHARYNGEAL AIRWAY. An oropharyngeal airway is designed to keep the tongue from blocking the airway, and it makes suctioning the airway, if necessary, easier. An oropharyngeal airway should be used for pediatric patients who are unconscious and in possible respiratory failure. However, this adjunct should not be used in either conscious patients or those who have a gag reflex. Patients with a gag reflex do not tolerate an oropharyngeal airway. In addition, this adjunct should not be used in children who may have ingested a caustic or petroleum-based product, as it may induce vomiting.

(▶ **Skill Drill 32-2**) shows the steps for inserting an oropharyngeal airway in a child:

1. **Determine the appropriately sized airway,** by measuring from the corner of the patient's mouth to the earlobe, or by using the length-based resuscitation tape to measure the patient.

2. **Place the airway next to the face** with the flange at the level of the central incisors and the bite block segment parallel to the hard palate.

Figure 32-1 The airway should be placed in a neutral sniffing position to keep the trachea from kinking when the neck is flexed or hyperextended.

SkillDrill 32-1   Positioning the Airway in a Child

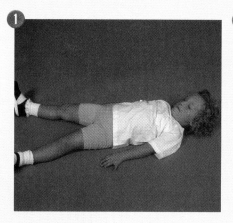

Position the child on a firm surface.

Place a folded towel about 1" thick under the shoulders and back.

Immobilize the forehead to limit movement.

TABLE 32-1 Pediatric Equipment: Getting the Size Right

The best way to identify the appropriately sized equipment for a pediatric patient is to use the length-based **pediatric resuscitation tape measure**, which can determine weight as well as height in patients weighing up to 34 kg (▼ **Figure 32-2**). The proper sequence for using the tape is the following:

Figure 32-2 Use of a pediatric resuscitation tape measure is one way to identify the correct size for airway adjuncts.

1. Place the patient supine on a flat surface.

2. Lay the tape next to the patient with the multi-colored side up.

3. Place the red end of the tape at the top of the patient's head.

4. Place one hand, side down, on top of the patient's head, covering the red box at the end of the tape.

5. Starting from the patient's head, run the side of your free hand down the tape.

6. Stretch the tape out the full length of the child, stopping at the heel. If the child is longer than the tape, stop here and use the appropriate adult technique.

7. Place your free hand, side down, at the bottom of the child's heel.

8. Note the color or letter block and weight range on the edge of the tape where your hand is. Say the color or letter out loud.

9. Select the appropriately sized equipment by matching the color or letter on the tape to the color or letter on the equipment.

SkillDrill 32-2 Inserting an Oropharyngeal Airway in a Child

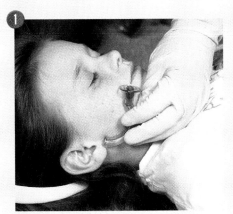

Determine the appropriately sized airway. Confirm the correct size visually, next to the patient's face.

Position the patient's airway with the appropriate method.

Open the mouth.
Insert the airway until the flange rests against the lips.
Reassess the airway.

The tip of the airway should reach the angle of the jaw **(Step 1)**.

3. **Position the patient's airway.** If the emergency is medical, use the head tilt-chin lift technique, avoiding hyperextension; you may place a towel under the patient's shoulders. If the patient has a traumatic injury, use the jaw-thrust maneuver and provide in-line spinal stabilization **(Step 2)**.

4. **Open the mouth** by applying pressure on the chin with your thumb.

5. **Insert the airway** by depressing the tongue with a tongue blade to the base of the tongue and inserting the airway directly over the tongue blade. If a tongue blade is not available, point the airway tip toward the roof of the mouth to depress the tongue. Gently rotate the airway into position as it passes through the mouth toward the curve of the tongue. Insert the airway until the flange rests against the lips.

6. **Reassess the airway** after insertion **(Step 3)**. Take care to avoid injuring the hard palate as you insert the airway. Rough insertion can cause bleeding, which may aggravate airway problems and may even cause vomiting. Note also that if the patient's airway is too small, the tongue may be pushed back into the pharynx, obstructing the airway. If the airway is too large, it may obstruct the larynx.

NASOPHARYNGEAL AIRWAY. A nasopharyngeal airway is also an airway adjunct. It is usually well tolerated and is not as likely as the oropharyngeal airway to cause vomiting. Unlike the oropharyngeal airway, the nasopharyngeal airway is used for conscious patients or for patients with altered levels of consciousness. In pediatric patients, the nasopharyngeal airway is typically used in association with possible respiratory failure. It is rarely used in infants younger than 1 year.

A nasopharyngeal airway should not be used in patients with nasal obstruction or head trauma (possible basal skull fracture) or in patients with moderate to severe head trauma, as this adjunct could increase intracranial pressure in these patients.

Follow the steps in ▶ **Skill Drill 32-3** to insert a nasopharyngeal airway in a child:

1. **Determine the appropriately sized airway.** The external diameter of the airway should not be larger than the diameter of the external openings of the nose, called **nares**, and there should be no **blanching** (turning white) of the naris after insertion.

2. **Place the airway next to the patient's face** to make sure the length is correct. The airway should extend from the tip of the nose to the tragus of the ear. The **tragus** is the small cartilaginous projection in front of the opening of the ear.

Skill Drill 32-3 Inserting a Nasopharyngeal Airway in a Child

Determine the correct airway size by comparing its diameter to the opening of the nostril (naris).

Place the airway next to the patient's face to confirm correct length.

Position the airway.

Lubricate the airway.

Insert the tip into the right naris with the bevel pointing toward the septum.

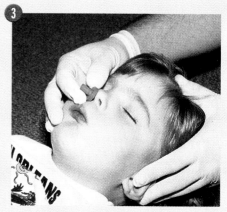

Carefully move the tip forward until the flange rests against the outside of the nostril.

Reassess the airway.

3. **Position the patient's airway,** using the techniques described above for the oropharyngeal airway **(Step 1)**.

4. **Lubricate the airway** with a water-soluble lubricant.

5. **Insert the tip into the right naris** (nostril opening) with the bevel pointing toward the **septum**, or central divider in the nose **(Step 2)**.

6. **Carefully move the tip forward following the roof of the mouth,** until the flange rests against the outside of the nostril. If you are inserting the airway on the left side, insert the tip into the left naris upside down, with the bevel pointing toward the septum. Move the airway forward slowly about 1″ until you feel a slight resistance, and then rotate the airway 180°.

7. **Reassess the airway** after insertion **(Step 3)**.

As with the oropharyngeal airway, there can be problems with the nasopharyngeal airway. An airway with a small diameter may easily become obstructed by mucus, blood, vomitus, or the soft tissues of the pharynx. If the airway is too long, it may stimulate the vagus nerve and slow the heart rate or enter the esophagus, causing gastric distention. Inserting the airway in responsive patients may cause a spasm of the larynx and result in vomiting. Nasopharyngeal airways should not be used when patients have facial trauma, as the airway may tear soft tissues and cause bleeding into the airway.

Assisting Ventilation and Oxygenation

After opening the airway, you should assess the patient's ventilation status. Look, listen, and feel for breathing. Remember to observe chest rise in older children and abdominal rise in younger children and infants. Skin condition indicates the amount of oxygen getting to the organs of the body. Patient's who are pale, mottled, or blue may have inadequate levels of oxygen in their blood. All trauma patients should receive oxygen. If the patient has sustained trauma to the face, assisting ventilations may be difficult.

Oxygen Delivery Devices

In treating infants and children who require more than the usual 21% oxygen found in room air, you have several options, as follows:

- Nonrebreathing mask at 10 to 12 L/min provides up to 90% oxygen concentration.

- Blow-by technique at 6 L/min provides more than 21% oxygen concentration.

- Nasal cannula at 2 to 6 L/min provides 24% to 44% oxygen concentration.

• BVM device (with oxygen reservoir) at 10 to 15 L/min provides L90% oxygen concentration.

Children need enough air to be delivered for adequate gas exchange in the lungs. Therefore, use of a nonrebreathing mask, a nasal cannula, or a simple face mask is indicated only for patients who have adequate respirations and/or tidal volumes. The **tidal volume** is the amount of air that is delivered to the lungs and airways in one inhalation. Children with respirations of less than 12 breaths/min or more than 60 breaths/min, an altered level of consciousness, and/or an inadequate tidal volume should receive assisted ventilations with a BVM device.

Blow-by oxygen is not an effective method for delivering oxygen. With this technique, an oxygen tube is held near the infant or child's nose and mouth. It is often used after childbirth to deliver a small amount of oxygen to the newborn. On rare occasions when other adjuncts cannot be used or the child will not tolerate any other adjunct, this technique may be necessary.

Nonrebreathing mask

A nonrebreathing mask delivers up to 90% oxygen to the patient and allows the patient to exhale all carbon dioxide without rebreathing it ⏷ **Figure 32-3** . To apply a nonrebreathing mask:

1. **Select the appropriately sized** pediatric nonrebreathing mask. The mask should extend from the bridge of the nose to the cleft of the chin.

2. **Connect the tubing** to an oxygen source set at 10 to 12 L/min.

3. **Adjust oxygen flow** as needed to match the patient's respiratory rate and depth. The reservoir bag should neither deflate completely nor fill to bulging during the respiratory cycle.

Blow-by technique

The blow-by technique does not provide a high concentration of oxygen. However, if no other adjuncts are available, the blow-by technique is better than no oxygen. To administer blow-by oxygen:

1. **Place oxygen tubing through a small hole in the bottom of a 6- to 8-oz paper or Styrofoam cup** ⏷ **Figure 32-4** . A cup is a familiar object that is less likely than an oxygen mask to frighten young children. You may be able to use an oxygen mask with an older child if you make it a game. For example, have the child pretend that the mask belongs to a popular action hero.

2. **Connect tubing to an oxygen source** set at 6 L/min.

3. **Hold the cup approximately 1″ to 2″ away from the child's nose and mouth.**

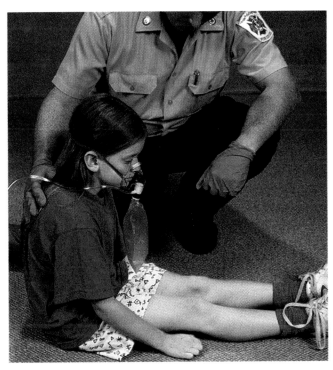

Figure 32-3 A pediatric nonrebreathing mask delivers up to 90% oxygen and allows the patient to exhale carbon dioxide without rebreathing it.

Figure 32-4 Blow-by techniques may be used, as oxygen masks frighten children. Make a small hole in a 6- to 8-oz paper or Styrofoam cup. Connect tubing to an oxygen source, and hold the cup about 2″ from the child's face.

Nasal cannula

Some patients prefer this adjunct while others find it uncomfortable. To apply a nasal cannula:

1. **Choose the appropriately sized pediatric nasal cannula** (▶ **Figure 32-5**). The prongs should not fill the nares entirely. If the nares blanch, select a smaller cannula.

2. **Connect the tubing** to an oxygen source set at 2 to 6 L/min.

BVM Device

Assisting ventilations with a BVM device is indicated for patients who have respirations that are either too slow or too fast to provide an adequate volume of inhaled oxygen, who are unresponsive, or who do not respond in a purposeful way to painful stimuli.

Assist ventilation of an infant or child using a BVM device in the following way:

1. **Ensure that you have the appropriate equipment in the right size.** The mask should be the proper size so that it extends from the bridge of the nose to the cleft of the chin, avoiding compression of the eyes (▶ **Figure 32-6**). The mask is transparent, so you can watch for cyanosis and vomiting. In addition, mask volume should be small to decrease dead space and avoid rebreathing; however, the bag should contain at least 450 mL of air. Use an infant bag, not a neonatal bag, for infants younger than 1 year and a pediatric bag for children older than age 1 year. Older children and adolescents may need an adult bag. Make sure that there is no pop-off valve on the bag, or, if there is one, make sure that you can hold it shut as necessary to achieve chest rise.

2. **Maintain a good seal** with the mask on the face.

3. **Ventilate at the appropriate rate and volume** using a slow, gentle squeeze, not a sharp, quick one. Stop squeezing and begin to release the bag as soon as the chest wall begins to rise, indicating that the lungs are filled to capacity. To keep from ventilating too rapidly, use the phrase "squeeze, release, release." Say "squeeze" as you squeeze the bag; when you see the chest start to rise, release pressure on the bag and say "release, release."

Errors in technique, including providing too much volume with each breath, squeezing the bag too force-

Figure 32-5 The prongs of a pediatric nasal cannula should not fill the nares entirely.

Figure 32-6 Proper mask size for BVM ventilation is critical. The mask should extend from the bridge of the nose to the cleft of the chin, avoiding compression of the eyes.

fully, or ventilating at too fast a rate, can result in gastric distention. An inadequate mask seal or improper head position can lead to hypoventilation or hypoxia. Even with the best technique in the world, the patient may regurgitate and aspirate the contents of his or her stomach.

ONE-RESCUER BVM VENTILATION. Perform one-rescuer BVM ventilation according to the steps in ▶ **Skill Drill 32-4** :

SkillDrill 32-4   One-Person BVM Ventilation on a Child

Open the airway and insert the appropriate airway adjunct.

Hold the mask on the patient's face with a one-handed head tilt-chin lift technique ("E-C grip").
Ensure a good mask-face seal while maintaining the airway.

Squeeze the bag 20 times/min for a child, or 30 times/min for an infant. Allow adequate time for exhalation.

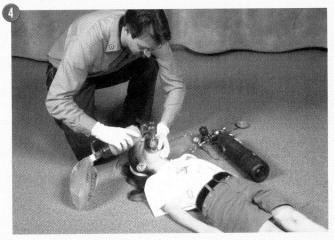

Assess effectiveness of ventilation by watching bilateral rise and fall of the chest.

1. **Open the airway,** and insert the appropriate airway adjunct **(Step 1)**.

2. **Hold the mask on the patient's face** by using the E-C grip. Form a C with the thumb and index finger along the mask while the other three fingers form an E along the mandible With infants and toddlers, support the jaw with only your third finger. Be careful not to compress the area under the chin, as you may push the tongue into the back of the mouth and block the airway. Keep fingers on the mandible.

3. **Make sure the mask forms an airtight seal** on the face. Maintain the seal while checking that the airway is open **(Step 2)**.

4. **Squeeze the bag,** using the correct ventilation rate. This is 20 breaths/min for children, and 30 breaths/min for infants.

5. **Allow 1 to 1½ seconds per ventilation,** providing adequate time for exhalation by using the phrase "squeeze, release, release" **(Step 3)**.

6. **Assess effectiveness** of ventilation by watching for adequate bilateral rise and fall of the chest. **(Step 4)**.

Figure 32-7 Any number of objects can obstruct a child's airway. Some of the more common ones include batteries, coins, toys, buttons, and candy.

TWO-RESCUER **BVM** VENTILATION. This procedure is similar to one-rescuer ventilation except that it requires two rescuers, one to hold the mask to the patient's face and maintain the patient's head position, the other to ventilate the patient. This technique is usually more effective in maintaining a tight seal.

Airway Obstruction

Children, especially those younger than 5 years, can (and do) obstruct their airway with any object that they can fit into their mouth: hot dogs, balloons, grapes, or coins (▲ **Figure 32-7**). In cases of trauma, a child's teeth may have been dislodged into the airway. Blood, vomitus, or other secretions can also cause partial or complete obstruction.

Another source of airway obstructions are infections, including pneumonia, croup, and epiglottitis (▶ **Figure 32-8**). **Croup** is an infection of the airway below the level of the vocal cords, usually caused by a virus. **Epiglottitis** is an infection of the soft tissue in the area above the vocal cords. Infection should be considered as a possible cause of airway obstruction if a child has congestion, fever, drooling, and cold symptoms. Such children must be taken immediately to the emergency department. Without special equipment and training, attempts to clear an airway that is blocked by infection can worsen the obstruction.

Signs and Symptoms

Obstruction by a foreign object may involve the upper or the lower airway. Signs and symptoms that are frequently associated with an upper airway obstruction include decreased or absent breath sounds and stridor. **Stridor** has been described as a high-pitched noise heard mainly on inspiration and is usually caused by swelling of the area surrounding the vocal cords or upper airway obstruction. In children with croup, it resembles the bark of a seal.

Figure 32-8 Epiglottitis is an infection that can cause airway obstruction in children.

Signs and symptoms of a lower airway obstruction include **wheezing**, a whistling sound caused by air traveling through narrowed air passages within the bronchioles, and/or rales. **Rales** are caused by the flow of air through liquid, present in the air pouches and smaller airways in the lungs. They produce a crackling sound like that of blowing bubbles through a straw in a glass filled with liquid. The best way to auscultate breath sounds in a child is to listen on both sides of the chest at the level of the armpit (▶ **Figure 32-9**).

Emergency Medical Care

Treatment of the child with an airway obstruction depends on whether or not the patient is unconscious and whether the obstruction is partial or complete.

If the child is conscious and you know for sure that there is a foreign body in the airway—that is, if someone actually saw the object go into the child's mouth—encourage the child to cough to clear the airway. Abdominal thrusts are also recommended to

Figure 32-9 The best way to auscultate breath sounds in children is to listen on both sides of the chest at the level of the armpit.

Figure 32-10 If a child has a partial airway obstruction, do not intervene except to give supplemental oxygen and allow the child to remain in whatever position is most comfortable.

relieve a complete airway obstruction in a child. If the material in the airway does not completely block the flow of air, the obstruction is not complete and the child may be able to breathe adequately on his or her own without any intervention. If the obstruction is only partial, do not intervene except to provide supplemental oxygen (▲ **Figure 32-10**). Allow the child to remain in whatever position is most comfortable, and monitor his or her condition.

If you see signs of complete obstruction, however, you must attempt to clear the airway at once. The signs include the following:

- Ineffective cough (no sound)
- Inability to speak or cry
- Increasing respiratory difficulty, with stridor
- Cyanosis
- Loss of consciousness

MANAGEMENT OF AIRWAY OBSTRUCTION IN A CHILD. If there is reason to believe that an unconscious child has a foreign body obstruction, check the upper airway to see whether the obstructing object is visible. The best way to do this is to grasp the tongue and jaw between your finger and thumb and lift to open the mouth; this is called the tongue-jaw lift (▶ **Figure 32-11A**). If the object is visible, try to remove it using a finger sweep motion (▶ **Figure 32-11B**). Never use finger sweeps in infants or children if you cannot see the object, as you may push it further into the airway.

Abdominal thrusts are recommended to relieve a complete airway obstruction in a child. These thrusts increase the pressure in the chest, creating an artificial

Figure 32-11 **A.** Use the tongue-jaw-lift to open the mouth in an unconscious child. **B.** If the object is visible, try to remove it by using a finger sweep.

cough that may force a foreign body from the airway.

(▶ **Skill Drill 32-5**) shows the following steps for applying abdominal thrusts to the unconscious child who you suspect has a foreign body airway obstruction:

1. **Place the child in a supine position** on a firm, flat surface **(Step 1)**.

2. **Inspect the upper airway** using the tongue-jaw lift. If you see the foreign object, try to remove it **(Step 2)**.

Skill Drill 32-5 Removing a Foreign Body Airway Obstruction in an Unconscious Child

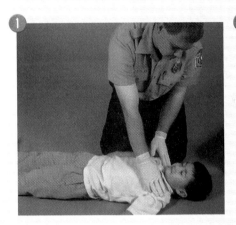

Position the child on a firm, flat surface.

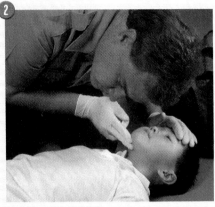

Inspect the airway. Remove any visible foreign object, if you can see it.

Attempt rescue breathing. If unsuccessful, reposition the head and try again.

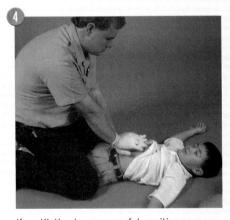

If ventilation is unsuccessful, position your hands on the abdomen above the navel and well below the chest cage.
Give five abdominal thrusts.

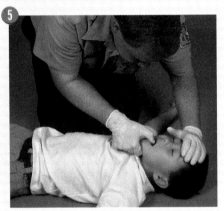

Open the airway again to try to see the object.

Only try to remove the obstruction if you can see it.
Attempt rescue breathing. If unsuccessful, reposition the head and try again.
Repeat abdominal thrusts if obstruction persists.

3. **Attempt rescue breathing.** If the first try is unsuccessful, reposition the child's head and try again **(Step 3)**.

4. **If ventilation is still unsuccessful, kneel beside or straddle the child's hips.** Place the heel of one hand on the front of the child's abdomen just above the navel and well below the rib cage and sternum. Place your other hand on top of the first hand.

5. **Press both hands into the abdomen** in an upward motion, giving five distinct thrusts. **(Step 4)**

6. **Open the airway** using the tongue-jaw lift and visualize the airway **(Step 5)**.

7. **If you see the foreign body,** remove it. Only attempt to remove objects you can actually see. Blind sweeps may push the object back into the airway.

8. **Attempt rescue breathing.** If the foreign body is not expelled on the first attempt, reposition the child's head and try again.

9. **If the airway remains obstructed,** repeat the abdominal thrusts **(Step 6)**.

The following steps are used to remove a foreign body obstruction from a conscious child who is in a standing or sitting position (▶ **Figure 32-12**):

1. **Kneel on one knee behind the child,** and circle his or her body with both arms around the patient's chest. Prepare to give abdominal thrusts by placing your fist just above the patient's navel and well below the lower tip of the sternum. Place your other hand over that fist.

2. **Give the child five rapid, distinct abdominal thrusts** in an upward direction. Be careful to avoid applying force to the lower rib cage or sternum.

3. **Repeat this standing technique** until the child expels the foreign body or fully loses consciousness.

4. **If the child becomes unconscious,** inspect the airway using the tongue-jaw lift. If you see the foreign body, try to remove it.

5. **Attempt rescue breathing.** If the first attempt fails, reposition the head and try again.

6. **If the airway remains obstructed,** repeat the abdominal thrusts.

If you manage to clear the airway obstruction in an unconscious child but he or she remains without spontaneous breathing or circulation, perform CPR.

MANAGEMENT OF AIRWAY OBSTRUCTION IN AN INFANT. Abdominal thrusts are not recommended for infants because of the risk of injury to the immature organs of the abdomen. Instead, use back blows and chest thrusts to try to clear a complete airway obstruction in an infant, as follows (▼ **Figure 32-13**):

1. **Hold the infant face down,** with the body resting on your forearm. Support the infant's jaw and face with your hand, and keep the head lower than the rest of the body.

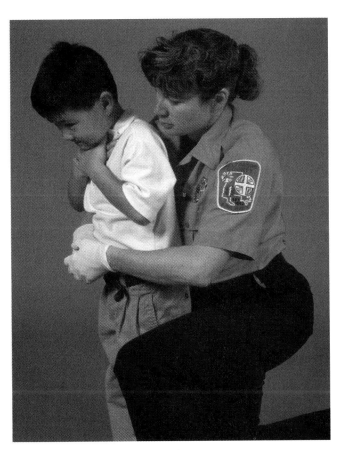

Figure 32-12 Kneel behind the child, wrap your arms around his or her body, and place your fist just above the navel and well below the lower tip of the sternum.

Figure 32-13 **A.** Hold the infant face down with the body resting on your forearm. Support the jaw and face with your hand, and keep the head lower than the rest of the body. Give the infant five back blows between the shoulder blades, using the heel of your hand. **B.** Give the infant five quick chest thrusts, using two fingers placed on the lower half of the sternum.

2. **Deliver five back blows** between the shoulder blades, using the heel of your hand.

3. **Place your free hand behind the infant's head and back,** and bring the infant upright on your thigh, sandwiching the infant's body between your two hands and arms. The infant's head should remain below the level of the body.

4. **Give five quick chest thrusts** in the same location and manner as chest compressions, using two fingers placed on the lower half of the sternum. For larger infants, or if you have small hands, you can perform this step by placing the infant in your lap and turning the infant's whole body as a unit between back blows and chest thrusts.

5. **Check the airway.** If you can see the foreign body now, remove it. If not, repeat the cycle as often as necessary.

6. **If the infant is still unconscious** after removal of the object, check for circulation and perform CPR, if necessary.

If the infant regains consciousness, keep him or her in the recovery position during transport.

Respiratory Emergencies

In the early stages of respiratory distress or failure, respirations may be too slow or too fast for the patient's age. This suggests that gases are not moving effectively into and out of the lungs. If, like most people, you find it hard to memorize normal vital sign ranges for infants and children, keep reference charts handy for this purpose. Respirations of greater than 60 breaths/min are a sign of a problem. In most cases, you should begin to assist ventilation immediately, even if the child appears to be breathing adequately. But remember, you are treating the child, not the numbers. A child breathing 60 breaths/min who is playing happily does not need assisted ventilation; a child breathing 60 breaths/min who is lying unconscious on the floor does.

Signs and Symptoms

In the early stages of respiratory distress, you may note changes in the child's behavior, such as combativeness, restlessness, and anxiety. As the body attempts to maximize the amount of air going into the lungs, the work of breathing (WOB) increases. Signs and symptoms of increased WOB include the following:

Respirations of greater than 60 breaths/min are a sign of a problem.

- Nasal flaring, as the body tries to increase the size of the airway

- Grunting respirations, as the body attempts to keep the alveoli expanded at the end of expiration

- Wheezing, stridor, or other abnormal airway sounds

- Accessory (intercostal) muscle use; remember that in young children, the diaphragm is the major muscle of ventilation

- Retractions, or movements of the child's flexible rib cage

- The **tripod position**; in older children this position will maximize their airway.

As the child progresses to possible respiratory failure, efforts to breathe decrease; the chest rises less with inspiration. A definite diagnosis of respiratory failure is made in the hospital. The body has used up its available energy stores and cannot continue to support the extra work of breathing under these conditions. At this point, cyanosis may develop (cyanosis is a late sign). Be aware that not all children become cyanotic. You should be just as concerned about a child with pale skin as one with bluish skin.

Changes in behavior will also occur until the child demonstrates an altered level of consciousness. The patient may experience periods of **apnea** (absence of breathing). As the lack of oxygen becomes more serious, the heart muscle itself becomes hypoxic and slows down. This leads to **bradycardia**, a condition in which the heart rate is less than 60 beats/min in children or less than 80 beats/min in newborns. Bradycardia is almost always related to a lack of oxygen and is an ominous sign in pediatric patients. If the heart rate is fast, you need to investigate the cause. However, if the heart rate is slow or absent, you must intervene immediately. Without aggressive airway management, bradycardia may quickly progress to cardiopulmonary arrest.

Of course, respiratory failure does not always indicate airway obstruction. It may indicate trauma, problems with the nervous system, dehydration (often caused by vomiting and diarrhea), or metabolic disturbances. For example, a child with diabetes might have a blood glucose level that is too high or too low; a child might have a pH imbalance, as can happen with some rare childhood diseases. Regardless of the cause, your first step is always to focus on ensuring adequate oxygenation and ventilation.

Never forget that a child can progress from respiratory distress to respiratory failure at any time. For this reason, you must reassess the child frequently.

Emergency Medical Care

A child or infant in respiratory distress or possible respiratory failure needs supplemental oxygen. Remember, anxiety, agitation, or crying may increase the effort or work of breathing, so use whichever method seems least upsetting to the child: mask, blow-by, or nasal cannula (▼ **Figure 32-14**). You may need to get creative by distracting the child with games, a toy, or talking.

Allow the child to remain in a comfortable position. For a small child, this may mean sitting on the caregiver's lap. Give nothing by mouth, in case the child's condition deteriorates suddenly.

If the patient has progressed to respiratory failure, you must begin assisted ventilation immediately and continue to provide supplemental oxygen.

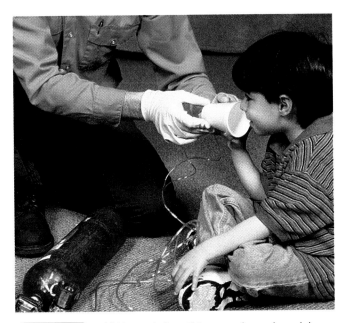

Figure 32-14 A child in respiratory distress needs supplemental oxygen; you should select whichever method seems least upsetting to the child.

Other Medical Emergencies

Seizures

A seizure is the result of disorganized electrical activity in the brain. It can be very frightening to people around the patient. Therefore, it is important to reassure the family and to approach assessment and management in a calm, step-by-step manner.

Signs and symptoms. Seizures in children may appear in several different ways, including shaking of the whole body or movement in just a single arm or leg. Seizures can also appear as lip smacking, eyes blinking, or staring off into space. In a true seizure, movements cannot be stopped on command or by holding an extremity. The duration of movement varies from patient to patient.

There are several general categories of seizures. In the course of an epileptic episode, a patient may experience one or more of these types of seizures:

- **Generalized (grand mal) seizures** appear as back-and-forth motions of both upper and lower extremities. The patient is unresponsive to verbal commands or painful stimulation.

- **Partial seizures** may appear as movement in one limb, lip smacking, or eye deviation only (eyes turned to either side or up or down).

- **Absence (petit mal) seizures** appear as an unresponsiveness with or without any movement and may last seconds to minutes.

Altered mental status and the inability of others to stop a movement or range of movements in the affected limb are common to all seizures. Some patients may feel pins and needles, hear sounds, and see hallucinations. In all but absence seizures, there is a **postictal period** of extreme fatigue or unresponsiveness after the seizure for anywhere from a few minutes to several hours. During this time, the patient may appear sleepy and/or confused and is not able to interact appropriately. A short period of seizure activity (under 30 minutes) is not in itself harmful to the patient. After 30 to 45 minutes, however, the brain may run low on energy stores, and continued activity can be harmful. **Status epilepticus** is a continuous seizure, or multiple seizures without a return to consciousness, for 30 minutes or more.

If you can identify the cause of the seizure, you will be better able to monitor the patient for any potential complications associated with the underlying problem (▶ **Table 32-2**). In particular, be alert to the presence of medications, possible poisons, and indications of abuse or neglect.

TABLE 32-2 Common Causes of Seizures

- Child abuse
- Electrolyte imbalance
- Fever
- Hypoglycemia (low blood glucose level)
- Idiopathic (no cause can be found)
- Infection
- Ingestion
- Lack of oxygen
- Medications
- Poisoning
- Previous seizure disorder
- Recreational drug use
- Trauma

FEBRILE SEIZURES. **Febrile seizures** are common in children between the ages of 6 months and 6 years. Most pediatric seizures are due to fever alone, which is why they are called febrile seizures. These seizures typically occur on the first day of a febrile illness, are characterized by generalized **tonic-clonic seizure** activity, and last less than 15 minutes with a short postictal phase or none at all. They may be a sign of a more serious problem, such as meningitis. Obtain a history from the caregivers, as these children may have had a prior febrile seizure.

If you are called to care for a child who has had a febrile seizure, you often will find that the patient is awake, alert, and fully interactive when you arrive. Keep in mind that a persistent fever can lead to another seizure. Carefully assess the ABCs, begin cooling measures with tepid water (not cold), and provide prompt transport; all children with febrile seizures need to be seen in the hospital setting ▶ Figure 32-15.

EMERGENCY MEDICAL CARE. Although medical management of seizures in the hospital setting may vary according to cause, your assessment and management of these patients remain essentially the same from patient to patient. First, ensure that the scene is safe for you and your partner and for the patient. Next, perform an initial assessment, focusing on the ABCs. If possible, obtain a brief history from the caregivers about previous serious illnesses or seizures and current medication or trauma.

Securing and protecting the airway are your priority. To avoid obstruction from the tongue falling back into the airway, place a child who is having a seizure or who is postictal in the recovery position if you can do so without having to use extreme force against the seizure activity ▶ Figure 32-16. In the case of trauma, place the head in a neutral in-line position and ensure that the cervical spine is protected with spinal precautions. Be ready to use suction to prevent aspiration of stomach contents, blood, or vomitus. Do not place your fingers in the mouth of a patient who is having a seizure.

A patient who is actively seizing or who is postictal may not be breathing adequately. Assessing the rate and depth of respirations in this situation can be difficult but is essential. Patients may have shallow, rapid breathing or may have occasional deep respirations. Signs that a patient is not breathing adequately include the following:

- Very slow respirations
- Very shallow breaths
- Bluish tint to lips or pale lips
- Snoring respirations caused by the tongue blocking the airway

Figure 32-15 Following a febrile seizure, carefully assess the child's ABCs. Then begin cooling measures, and prepare the child for transport.

Deliver oxygen by mask, blow-by, or nasal cannula. If there are no signs of improvement, begin BVM ventilation with appropriately sized equipment.

Patients who are experiencing a seizure usually maintain adequate blood pressure and pulse rate unless the seizure is caused by an underlying circulatory or neurologic problem or trauma, including bleeding, heart problems, or brain injury. Nevertheless, you must evaluate the pulse and blood pressure and re-evaluate them. Once the ABCs have been addressed, assessment and management should proceed as follows. If the patient is actively seizing, note the type of movement and position of the eyes, as this information may be very helpful for hospital staff in making a diagnosis. If there is a fever, begin cooling measures such as removing clothing and placing towels moistened with tepid water on the child. A child with febrile seizures can seize again if the temperature remains high. Do not use alcohol or cold water to cool a patient. Make sure the patient is protected from hitting the sides of the stretcher or nearby equipment. Bring any medications or possible poisons at the scene to the hospital with the patient. If patient is in status epilepticus, call for ALS backup, as medication is required to stop the seizures. In fact, you should always call for ALS backup when appropriate.

Altered Level of Consciousness

People who are aware of themselves and their surroundings are said to be conscious. Nonverbal infants may demonstrate consciousness by following a person's face or an object (tracking), by babbling and cooing, or by crying. Infants and children may exhibit an **altered level of consciousness** (also called altered mental status) in many ways, including lack of response to vocal commands and pain, combative behavior, confusion, thrashing about, drifting into and out of an alert state, or a change in the pitch and nature of their cry.

Common causes of altered level of consciousness in a pediatric patient can be found in the mnemonic AEIOU-TIPS:

* **A**lcohol
* **E**pilepsy, endocrine, or electrolyte abnormalities
* **I**nsulin or low blood glucose levels
* **O**piates or other drugs
* **U**remia
* **T**rauma or temperature
* **I**nfection
* **P**sychogenic or poison
* **S**hock, stroke, or shunt obstruction

Your first step in caring for a patient with an altered level of consciousness is to assess the ABCs and provide appropriate care as necessary. As you determine responsiveness, remember to use the AVPU scale. Then obtain a brief history from the patient's caregivers, focusing on the following points:

* Does the patient have any illnesses?
* Does the patient take any medications? When was the last dose?
* Did the patient ingest any substances (eg, poisons, drugs, or plant material)?
* Has the patient been ill?
* Has the patient had any behavior problems?

Next, observe the patient's pupils: Are they dilated or pinpoint? Do they react to a light by constricting ▼ **Figure 32-17** ? Are the eyes turned to the right, left,

Figure 32-16 A child in the postictal (confused) state following a seizure should be placed in the recovery position.

Figure 32-17 Observe a child's eyes for changes in pupillary size.

Figure 32-18 Observe a child for posturing.

Figure 32-19 A curious child will try to taste or swallow almost any substance. A common victim of accidental ingestion of dangerous compounds is the unwatched toddler.

up, or down? Is the patient staring without moving his/her eyes? Is the patient posturing ▲ **Figure 32-18** ?

Once you have completed your initial assessment, immediately secure the airway. If respirations are inadequate, provide assisted ventilation with a BVM device. If you suspect trauma, log roll the child onto a backboard, and apply a cervical collar. Give supplemental oxygen by mask or nasal cannula. If the child is actively seizing, follow the care described earlier in this chapter on seizures. Remember to call for ALS backup as necessary. No matter what the cause, you should support the patient's vital functions and provide prompt transport.

Poisoning

Poisoning is common among children. It can occur by ingesting, inhaling, injecting, or absorbing a toxic substance ▲ **Figure 32-19** . The signs and symptoms of poisoning vary widely, depending on the substance and the age and weight of the child ▶ **Table 32-3** . The child may appear normal at first, even in serious cases, or he or she may be confused, sleepy, or unconscious.

Infants may be poisoned as a result of being fed a harmful substance by a sibling or a caregiver or as a result of child abuse. Infants can be exposed to drugs and poisons left on floors and carpeting. They can also be exposed in a room or automobile in which harmful drugs, such as crack, cocaine, or PCP, are being smoked. Toddlers are curious and often ingest poisons when they find them in the home or garage. For example, some people store petroleum products in soda bottles. Toddlers may believe the substance to be soda. Adolescents are more likely to have ingested

alcohol and street drugs while "partying" or in a suicide attempt.

After you have completed your initial assessment, you should ask the caregiver the following questions:

- What is the substance(s) involved?
- Approximately how much of the substance was ingested or involved in the exposure (eg, number of pills, amount of liquid)?
- What time did the incident occur?
- Are there any changes in behavior or level of consciousness?
- Was there any choking or coughing after the exposure? (These can be signs of airway involvement.)

TABLE 32-3 Common Sources of Poisoning in Children

- Alcohol
- Aspirin and acetaminophen
- Household cleaning products such as bleach and furniture polish
- Houseplants
- Iron
- Prescription medications of family members
- Street drugs
- Vitamins

Because a child's level of consciousness may be affected by the poison, your care will be guided by how awake and alert the child appears. For a child who is responsive, your protocols may dictate that you contact medical control and your local poison control center to report the situation. Focus on the ABCs, keeping in mind that the child's condition may change over time. Assess the patient's level of consciousness, and support the vital functions as necessary, including giving supplemental oxygen. If the patient is combative and/or agitated, protect yourself from injury. Do not administer syrup of ipecac (if this is still used in your EMS system) unless directed to do so by medical control. Call for ALS backup if the patient's condition becomes unstable. As you prepare the patient for transport, try to find the container that held the suspected poison, collect any vomitus from the child and place it in a plastic bag, and take both to the emergency department.

If the child is unresponsive, make sure that you focus immediately on the ABCs, and be prepared to provide artificial ventilation if necessary. Give supplemental oxygen, and then call medical control to report the situation. Provide transport to the emergency department, keeping in mind that the child's condition could change at any time.

Fever

Fever is a common reason parents call 9-1-1. Simply defined, fever is an increase in body temperature, usually in response to an infection. Body temperatures of 100.4°F (38°C) or higher are considered to be abnormal. Fevers have many causes and are rarely life-threatening events. However, you should not underestimate the potential seriousness of fevers, such as those that occur in conjunction with a rash. You should try to determine whether the fever is a sign of serious illness, such as meningitis. Common causes of a high temperature in a child include the following:

- Infection, such as pneumonia, meningitis, or urinary tract infection

- Neoplasm (cancer)

- Drug ingestion

- Collagen vascular disease, including arthritis and systemic lupus erythematosus

- High environmental temperature

Note that there are other conditions in which the body temperature increases that are not a fever. Hyperthermia differs from fever in that it is an increase in body temperature caused by an inability of the body

> **Because untreated meningitis can lead to permanent brain damage or death, being able to recognize its possible presence is an important EMT-B skill.**

to cool itself. Hyperthermia is typically seen in warm environments, such as a closed car on a hot day.

Emergency medical care of a child with a fever begins with an initial assessment of the ABCs, caring for immediate life threats as needed. Be sure to wear personal protective equipment, especially if meningitis is a possibility. Look carefully at the child to obtain a general impression: Does the child look sick? Then report your findings to medical control. Assess the patient's level of consciousness, and obtain vital signs. Evaluate the child for signs and symptoms of shock. If the child feels very warm, remove any covering so that the skin is exposed. Begin cooling measures en route, preferably by placing wet, cool towels over the child's body and head.

Meningitis

Meningitis is an inflammation of the tissue, called the meninges, that covers the spinal cord and brain. It is caused by an infection by bacteria, viruses, fungi, or parasites. If left untreated, meningitis can lead to permanent brain damage or death. Being able to recognize a patient who may have meningitis is an important skill for the EMT-B.

Meningitis can occur in both children and adults, but some individuals are at greater risk than others, as follows:

- Males

- Newborn infants

- The elderly

- People whose immune systems have been weakened by AIDS or cancer

- People who have any past history of brain, spinal cord, or back surgery

- Children who have had head trauma

- Children with shunts, pins, or other foreign bodies within their brain or spinal cord

At especially high risk are children with a ventriculoperitoneal (VP) shunt. These special needs children have tubing that can usually be seen and felt just under the scalp.

The signs and symptoms of meningitis vary, depending on the age of the patient. Fever and altered level of consciousness are common symptoms of meningitis in patients of all ages. Changes in level of consciousness can range from a mild or severe headache to confusion, lethargy, and/or an inability to understand commands or interact appropriately. The child may also experience a seizure, which as described earlier may be a first sign of meningitis. Assess the level of consciousness using the AVPU scale. Infants younger than 2 to 3 months can have apnea, cyanosis, fever, or hypothermia.

In describing children with meningitis, physicians often use the term "meningeal irritation" or "meningeal signs" to describe pain that accompanies movement. Bending the neck forward or back increases the tension within the spinal canal and stretches the meninges, causing a great deal of pain. This results in the characteristic stiff neck of children with meningitis, who will often refuse to move their neck, lift their legs, or curl into a "C" position, even if coached to do so. One sign of meningitis in an infant is increasing irritability, especially when being handled. Another sign is a bulging fontanel.

One form of meningitis deserves special attention. **Neisseria meningitidis** is a bacterium that causes a rapid onset of meningitis symptoms, often leading to shock and death. Children with *N meningitidis* typically have small, pinpoint, cherry-red spots or a larger purple/black rash. This rash may be on part of the face or body. These children are at serious risk of sepsis, shock, and death.

All patients with possible meningitis should be considered highly contagious and infectious. Therefore, you should use BSI precautions whenever you suspect meningitis and follow up with the hospital to learn the patient's final diagnosis. If you have been exposed to saliva and respiratory secretions from a child with *N meningitidis,* you should receive antibiotics to protect yourself and others from the bacteria. This is particularly true if you managed the patient's airway. If you were not in close contact with the patient or his or her respiratory secretions, you do not need treatment.

In taking the history of a child with meningitis, pay particular attention to the following details:

- Onset of illness, including any upper respiratory symptoms such as runny nose, cough, or other cold symptoms
- Presence and duration of fever
- Level of activity
- Change in behavior in older children, irritability in younger children

EMT-B Safety

Some forms of meningitis are highly contagious. Use BSI precautions whenever you suspect meningitis, including mask and eye protection when there is coughing, sneezing, or any other possibility of contact with the patient's respiratory secretions. Local protocols may also call for putting a mask on the patient.

Emergency medical care of a patient who is believed to have meningitis should begin with an initial assessment of the ABCs and immediate care of life threats. Some patients may experience episodes of cyanosis and/or apnea. If the patient is old enough to follow commands and respond, either verbally or nonverbally, determine responsiveness by asking, " What is your name?" "How old are you?" and "Hold up two fingers." Remember that you should be wearing appropriate protective equipment before you start caring for the child.

After you have secured the airway, give supplemental oxygen by mask or nasal cannula, as tolerated. You should be prepared to manage the airway with a BVM device if necessary. Assess the patient's vital signs, keep him or her warm, and watch for signs and symptoms of shock. If the patient's vital signs are unstable, call for ALS backup.

Shock

Shock is a condition that develops when the circulatory system is unable to deliver a sufficient amount of blood to the organs of the body. This results in organ failure and eventually cardiopulmonary arrest. In children, shock is rarely due to a primary cardiac event, such as a heart attack. Shock may be due to many things; the most common causes include the following:

- Traumatic injury with blood loss (especially abdominal)
- Dehydration from diarrhea and vomiting
- Severe infection
- Neurologic injury such as severe head trauma
- A severe allergic reaction to an insect bite or allergy (anaphylaxis)
- Diseases of the heart
- A collapsed lung (pneumothorax)
- Blood or fluid around the heart (cardiac tamponade or pericarditis)

TABLE 32-4 Vital Signs by Age

Age	Respirations (breaths/min)	Pulse (beats/min)	Systolic Blood Pressure (mm Hg)
Newborn: 0 to 1 month	40 to 60	120 to 160	50 to 70
Infant: 1 month to 1 year	30 to 60	100 to 160	70 to 95
Toddler: 1 to 3 years	24 to 40	90 to 150	80 to 100
Preschool-Age: 3 to 6 years	22 to 34	80 to 140	80 to 100
School-Age: 6 to 12 years	18 to 30	70 to 120	80 to 110
Adolescent: 12 to 18 years	12 to 16	60 to 100	90 to 110
Over 18 years	12 to 20	60 to 100	90 to 140

Infants and children have less blood circulating in their bodies than adults do, so the loss of even a small volume of fluid or blood may lead to shock. Pediatric patients also respond differently than adults to fluid loss. They may respond by increasing their heart rate, increasing their respirations and showing signs of pale or blue skin. You must be able to recognize the signs of shock in infants and children.

Begin by assessing the ABCs, intervening immediately as required; do not wait until you have completed a detailed assessment to take action. Children in shock often have increased respirations but do not demonstrate a fall in blood pressure until shock is severe.

In assessing circulation, you should pay particular attention to the following:

- **Pulse.** Assess both the rate and the quality of the pulse. A weak, "thready" pulse is a sign that there is a problem. The appropriate rate depends on the age; anything over 160 beats/min suggests shock (▲ Table 32-4).

- **Skin signs.** Assess the temperature and moisture on the hands and feet. How does this compare with the temperature of the skin on the trunk of the body? Is the skin dry and warm, or cold and clammy?

- **Capillary refill.** Squeeze a finger or toe for several seconds until the skin blanches, then release it. The time it takes for the blood to return to the area is the capillary refill time. Does the fingertip return to its normal color within 2 seconds, or is it delayed?

- **Color.** Assess the patient's skin color. Is it pink, pale, ashen, or blue?

Changes in pulse rate, color, skin signs, and capillary refill are all important clues suggesting shock.

Blood pressure is the most difficult vital sign to take in pediatric patients. The cuff must be the proper size: two-thirds the length of the upper arm. The value for normal blood pressure is also age-specific. Remember that blood pressure may be normal; this is called compensated shock. If the blood pressure is low, this is a sign of decompensated shock, a serious condition that requires care an ALS team can provide.

Part of your assessment should also include talking with the caregivers to determine when the signs and symptoms first appeared and whether any of the following has occurred:

- Decrease in urine output (with infants, are there fewer than 6 to 10 wet diapers?)

- Absence of tears, even when the child is crying

- Changes in level of consciousness and behavior

Shock is a serious condition; limit your care to the steps in (▶ Skill Drill 32-6):

1. **Ensure that the airway is open.**

2. **Be prepared to provide artificial ventilation** if necessary.

3. **Control bleeding** if present **(Step 1)**.

4. **Give supplemental oxygen** by mask or nasal cannula as tolerated. Continue to monitor airway and breathing **(Step 2)**.

5. **Position the patient** with the head lower than the feet by elevating the feet with blankets **(Step 3)**.

6. **Keep the patient warm** with blankets and by turning up the heat in the patient compartment.

SkillDrill 32-6   Caring for a Child in Shock

Open the airway.
Be prepared to ventilate.
Control any bleeding.

Begin supplemental oxygen.

Position the patient with the head lower than the feet.

Keep the patient warm with blankets.
Transport immediately.
Continue to monitor vital signs.
Consider ALS backup.
Allow a caregiver to accompany the child if possible.

7. **Provide immediate transport** to the nearest appropriate facility.

8. **Continue monitoring vital signs** en route to the hospital.

9. **Contact ALS** backup as needed.

10. **Allow a caregiver** to accompany the child whenever possible **(Step 4)**.

Limit your management to these simple interventions. Time should not be wasted in field procedures. Immediate transport is of utmost importance.

Dehydration

Dehydration occurs when fluid losses are greater than fluid intake. The most common cause of dehydration in children is vomiting and diarrhea. If left untreated, dehydration can lead to shock and eventually death. Infants and children are at greater risk than adults for dehydration because their fluid reserves are smaller than those in adults. Life-threatening dehydration can overcome an infant in a matter of hours. Again, your ability to recognize a child with this condition is a critical part of your job.

TABLE 32-5 Vital Signs and Symptoms of Dehydration

	Mild Dehydration	Moderate Dehydration	Severe Dehydration
Pulse	Normal	Increased	Increased; 160+ is sign of impending shock.
Level of Activity	Normal or slowed	Slowed	Variable, weak to unresponsive
Urine Output	Decreased	Decreased	No output
Skin	Normal	Cool, mottled; poor turgor	Cool, clammy; poor turgor; delayed capillary refill time
Mouth	Saliva may have drooling, bubbles	Dry mucous membranes	Dry mucous membranes
Eyes	Normal	Tears	Sunken eyes
Anterior Fontanel	Normal to sunken	Sunken	Very sunken
Level of Consciousness	Normal	Altered	Altered; lethargic
Blood Pressure	Normal	Normal	Normal to low when shock sets in

Dehydration can be described as mild, moderate, or severe. The severity of the dehydration can be gauged by looking at several clues ▲ Table 32-5 . For example, an infant with mild dehydration may have dry lips and gums, decreased saliva, and fewer wet diapers throughout the day ▶ Figure 32-20 . As the dehydration grows more severe, the lips and gums may become very dry, the eyes may look sunken, and the infant may be sleepy and/or irritable, refusing bottles. The skin may be loose and have no elasticity (tenting); this is called poor skin turgor. Also, infants may have sunken fontanels.

Young children can compensate for fluid losses by decreasing blood flow to the extremities and directing it to vital organs such as the brain and heart. Children who are moderately to severely dehydrated may have mottled, cool, clammy skin and delayed capillary refill. Respirations will usually be increased. Be aware that blood pressure may remain normal until the child is in shock.

Emergency medical care should include careful attention assessing the ABCs and obtaining baseline vital signs. However, if the dehydration is severe, ALS backup may be necessary so that IV access can be obtained and rehydration can begin. All children with signs and symptoms of moderate to severe

Figure 32-20 An infant with mild dehydration may exhibit "tenting" or poor skin turgor.

dehydration should be transported to the emergency department.

Neonatal Resuscitation

At birth, most infants require only the resuscitation measures shown at the top of the American Heart Association's inverse pyramid, which are designed to stimulate the newborn to breathe air and begin circulation of blood through the lungs (▶ Figure 32-21). These measures include positioning of the airway, drying, warming, suctioning, and tactile stimulation. Here are some tips to help you maximize the effects of the measures:

- Position the infant on his or her back with the head down and the neck slightly extended. Place a towel or blanket under the infant's shoulder to help maintain this position.

- Suction the mouth and then nose using a bulb syringe or suction device with an 8- or 10-French catheter. Suction both sides of the back of the mouth, where secretions tend to collect, but avoid deep suctioning of the mouth and throat; this can cause the heart to slow down. It is always good practice to aim blow-by oxygen at the infant's mouth and nose during resuscitation.

- In addition to drying the infant's head, back, and body vigorously with dry towels, you may rub the infant's back and slap the soles of his or her feet.

In instances when a newborn is in distress, you should be properly equipped for resuscitation measures. All ambulances should have the following equipment and supplies for newborn resuscitation (▶ Figure 32-22):

- A bulb syringe
- Clean dry towels
- An infant blanket
- A BVM device with a 450-mL reservoir
- Clear masks in both infant and premature infant sizes
- 2 umbilical clamps
- Sterile 4 × 4 gauze
- A stocking cap
- An oxygen source with tubing

Additional Resuscitation Efforts

Observe the infant for spontaneous respirations, skin color, and movement of the extremities. If the respiratory effort appears appropriate, evaluate the heart rate by palpating the pulse at the base of the umbilical cord or at the brachial artery. The heart rate is the most important measure in determining the need for further resuscitation (▶ Table 32-6).

If chest compressions are required, give them at a rate of 120 beats/min using either the hand-encircling

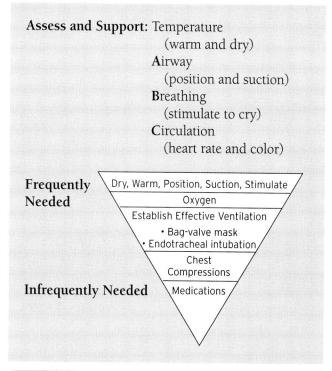

Assess and Support: Temperature
(warm and dry)
Airway
(position and suction)
Breathing
(stimulate to cry)
Circulation
(heart rate and color)

Frequently Needed

Dry, Warm, Position, Suction, Stimulate
Oxygen
Establish Effective Ventilation
• Bag-valve mask
• Endotracheal intubation
Chest Compressions

Infrequently Needed — Medications

Figure 32-21 The American Heart Association's resuscitation process for the newborn is designed to stimulate the newborn to breathe air and begin circulation of the blood through the lungs.

Figure 32-22 The proper equipment for neonatal resuscitation includes a bulb syringe, towels, an infant blanket, a BVM device, clear masks in two sizes, two umbilical clamps, sterile gauze, a stocking cap, and an oxygen source with tubing.

technique or the two-finger technique (▶ Figure 32-23). Coordinate chest compressions with ventilations at a ratio of 3:1.

Any newborn who requires more than routine resuscitation requires transport, when possible, to a center with a level III neonatal intensive care unit. This type of unit is especially for newborns who require specialized care, including mechanical ventilation.

TABLE 32-6 Additional Neonatal Resuscitation Efforts

If the Heart Rate Is . . .	More Than 100 Beats/Min	60 to 100 Beats/Min	Fewer Than 60 Beats/Min
Do this:	Keep the infant warm.	Begin assisted ventilation with a BVM device and 100% oxygen.	Begin assisted ventilation with a BVM device and 100% oxygen.
	Transport the infant.	Reassess the infant every 15 to 30 seconds until heart rate and respirations are normal.	Reassess the infant every 15 to 30 seconds until heart rate and respirations are normal.
	Assess the infant continuously.	Continue to reassess the infant. Call for ALS backup.	Begin chest compressions. Call for ALS backup.
		Keep the infant warm.	If the heart rate does not increase, medication and ALS will be necessary.

About 12% of deliveries are complicated by the presence of **meconium**, a dark green material in the amniotic fluid. Meconium can be thick or thin. If the newborn aspirates thick meconium, serious lung disease and sometimes death can occur. Therefore, if you see meconium in the amniotic fluid or meconium staining, you should continue vigorous suctioning of the infant after delivery.

Basic Life Support Review

The reasons for cardiopulmonary arrest differ in children and adults. In adults, cardiac arrest is usually the result of an abnormal cardiac rhythm, which is itself caused by underlying cardiac disease. Because most children have healthy hearts, sudden cardiac arrest is rare. More commonly, children have cardiopulmonary arrest because of respiratory or circulatory failure from illness or injury. For this reason, the airway and breathing are the focus of pediatric basic life support (BLS) ▶ **Table 32-7** .

Respiratory problems leading to cardiopulmonary arrest in children can have a number of different causes, including the following:

- Injury, both blunt and penetrating
- Infections of the respiratory tract or another organ system
- A foreign body in the airway
- Near drowning
- Electrocution
- Poisoning or drug overdose
- Sudden infant death syndrome (SIDS)

Figure 32-23 **A.** Chest compressions should be given with the hands encircling the infant and thumbs side by side. **B.** In very small infants, you may need to overlap the thumbs. **C.** In larger infants, you may use the two-finger technique, using the middle and ring fingers.

TABLE 32-7 Review of Pediatric BLS

Action	Infants Younger Than 1 Year	Children Between Ages 1 and 8 Years
Airway	Head tilt-chin lift; jaw-thrust if spine injury is suspected	Head tilt-chin lift; jaw-thrust if spine injury is suspected
Breathing		
Initial	2 breaths at a rate of 1 to 1½ seconds/breath (Use a BVM with oxygen connected if available.)	2 breaths at a rate of 1 to 1½ seconds/breath (Use a BVM with oxygen connected if available.)
Subsequent	20 breaths/min	20 breaths/min
Circulation		
Pulse check	Brachial/femoral arteries	Carotid artery
Compression area	Lower half of sternum	Lower half of sternum
Compression width	2 or 3 fingers or 2 thumb encircled hands	Heel of hand
Compression depth	½" to 1"	1" to 1½"
Compression rate	At least 100/min	100/min
Ratio of Compressions to Ventilations	5:1 (pause for ventilation)	5:1 (pause for ventilation)
Foreign Body Obstruction	Back blows and chest thrusts	Abdominal thrusts

For purposes of pediatric BLS, infancy ends at 1 year of age, and childhood extends to 8 years. Although children older than 8 years are still considered pediatric patients, they are treated with adult BLS methods. The goal, of course, is the same for all patients: To restore breathing and circulation of the blood.

Pediatric BLS can be divided into four steps, as follows:

1. Determining responsiveness

2. Airway

3. Breathing

4. Circulation

Determining Responsiveness

Never shake a child to determine whether he or she is responsive, especially if there is a possible neck or back injury. Instead, gently tap the child on the shoulder, and speak loudly (▶ **Figure 32-24**). If a child is responsive but struggling to breathe, allow him or her to remain in whatever position is most comfortable.

If you find an unresponsive child while you are alone and not on duty, provide BLS for approximately 1 minute, and then stop to call the EMS system. Why not call right away, as you would with an adult? Because unlike an adult, an unconscious child may respond quickly to ventilation and oxygenation. Indeed, these

Figure 32-24 Never shake a child to determine responsiveness. Rather, gently tap the child on the shoulder, and speak loudly.

actions may prevent the child from progressing to full cardiopulmonary arrest.

Airway

Because children often put toys and other objects, as well as food, in their mouths, foreign body obstruction of the upper airway is common. The steps for removing a foreign object are reviewed earlier in this chapter. You must make sure that the upper airway is open when dealing with pediatric respiratory emergencies or cardiopulmonary arrest. If the child is unconscious and lying in a supine position, the airway may become obstructed when the tongue and throat muscles relax and the tongue falls backward ▶ **Figure 32-25** .

If the child is unconscious but breathing, place him or her on one side or the other in the recovery position, in which the upper leg is flexed and bent forward for stabilization and the head is positioned to allow drainage of saliva or vomitus ▶ **Figure 32-26** . Do not use this position if you suspect a spinal injury unless you can secure the child to a backboard that can be tilted to the side. Do not attempt to open the airway at all if the child is conscious and breathing, but in a labored fashion. Instead, provide immediate transport to the nearest hospital.

There are two common techniques for manually opening the airway in a child who is neither conscious nor breathing: the head tilt-chin lift technique and the jaw-thrust maneuver ▼ **Figure 32-27** . The latter is safer if there is a possibility of a neck injury.

HEAD TILT–CHIN LIFT TECHNIQUE. Perform this technique in a child in the following way:

1. **Place one hand on the child's forehead,** and tilt the head back gently, with the neck slightly extended.

2. **Place the fingers (not the thumb) of your other hand under the child's chin,** and lift the jaw upward and outward. Do not close the mouth or push under the chin; either move may obstruct rather than open the airway.

3. **Remove any visible foreign body or vomitus.**

Figure 32-25 The airway may be obstructed when the tongue and throat muscles relax and the tongue falls back into the throat.

Figure 32-26 A child who is unconscious but breathing should be placed in the recovery position to allow saliva or vomitus to drain from the mouth.

Figure 32-27 **A.** Use the head tilt-chin lift technique to open the airway in a child who has not sustained a traumatic injury. Do not overextend the neck. **B.** Use the jaw-thrust maneuver to open the airway if there is a possibility that a traumatic injury has occurred.

JAW-THRUST MANEUVER. Perform this maneuver in a child in the following way:

1. **Place two or three fingers** under each side of the angle of the lower jaw; lift the jaw upward and outward.

2. **If the jaw thrust alone** does not open the airway and cervical spine injury is not a consideration, tilt the head slightly. If cervical spine injury is suspected, use a second rescuer to immobilize the cervical spine.

Remember that the head of an infant or young child is disproportionately large in comparison to the chest and shoulders. As a result, when a child is lying flat on his or her back, especially on a backboard, the head will bend forward onto the upper chest. This can partially or completely obstruct the upper airway. To avoid this possibility, place a wedge of padding under the upper chest and shoulders.

Breathing

Once the airway is open, determine if the child is breathing spontaneously, using the look, listen, and feel technique (▼ **Figure 32-28**):

- **Look** for rise and fall of the chest or abdomen.
- **Listen** for exhalation of breath.
- **Feel** for exhaled air flow at the mouth.

If an infant or small child is breathing, provide immediate transport. Again, a child who is in respiratory distress should be allowed to stay in whatever position is most comfortable. Larger children who are unconscious and breathing with difficulty should be kept in the recovery position if possible.

If an infant or child is not breathing, provide rescue breathing while keeping the airway open. If you are using mouth-to-mouth resuscitation with an infant, place your mouth over the infant's mouth and nose to create a seal. If you are using a bag-valve-mask device to assist ventilations in an infant, use the proper sized mask and the technique described earlier.

When two rescuers are available, use your thumb and index finger to apply pressure over the area just below the Adam's apple (the Sellick maneuver) (▼ **Figure 32-29**). This will decrease the risk of gastric distention and aspiration of vomitus by pushing the larynx back to compress and close off the esophagus.

In a child with tracheostomy (breathing) tubes in the neck, remove the mask from the bag-valve device and connect it directly to the tracheostomy tube to ventilate the child. If a bag-valve-mask device is unavailable, a mask, barrier device, or your mouth over the tracheotomy site can be used. Place your hand firmly over the child's mouth and nose to prevent the artificial breaths from leaking out of the upper airway.

Circulation

Once you have opened the airway and provided two rescue breaths, you must determine the state of the child's circulation. Check for pulses in the carotid artery in older children and the brachial or femoral artery in young children and infants. During your pulse check also evaluate the child for other signs of circulation that may include; breathing, coughing, or movement. Locate the carotid artery by placing one or two fingers over the groove between the Adam's apple and the neck muscles. Locate the brachial artery by placing two or three fingers on the inside of an infant's upper

Figure 32-28 After you have opened the airway, use the look, listen, and feel technique to determine if the child is breathing spontaneously.

Figure 32-29 Perform the Sellick maneuver to decrease the risk of gastric distention and aspiration of vomitus

Skill Drill 32-7 Performing Infant Chest Compressions

1

Position the infant on a firm surface while maintaining the airway.
Place two fingers in the middle of the sternum just below a line between the nipples.

2

Use two fingers to compress the chest about ½" to 1" at a rate of 100 times/min.
Allow the sternum to return briefly to its normal position between compressions.

3

Coordinate rapid compressions and ventilations in a 5:1 ratio.
Check for return of breathing and pulse after 1 minute, then every few minutes.

arm, between the elbow and the shoulder. The femoral artery can be felt in the crease between the upper leg and the groin. However, palpating the pulse in an infant or child is difficult; therefore, do not spend more than 10 seconds trying. If an infant or child is not breathing, you can assume that there is no pulse.

For chest compressions to be effective, the patient should be placed on a firm, flat surface with the head at the same level as the body. If you need to carry an infant while providing CPR, your forearm and hand can serve as the flat surface. Follow these steps in (▲ **Skill Drill 32-7**) to perform infant chest compressions:

1. **Place the infant on a firm surface,** using one hand to keep the head in an open airway position. You can also use a pad or wedge under the shoulders and upper body to keep the head from tilting forward.

2. Imagine a line drawn between the nipples. **Place two fingers in the middle of the sternum,** about ½" below the level of the imaginary line (one fingerwidth) **(Step 1)**.

3. **Using two fingers, compress the sternum** about one third to one half the depth of the chest; this is usually about ½" to 1". Compress the chest at a rate of 100 compressions/min. With pauses for ventilation, you will actually compress the chest about 80 compressions/min.

4. **After each compression, allow the sternum to return briefly to its normal position.** Allow equal time for compression and relaxation of the chest. Do not remove your fingers from the sternum, and avoid jerky movements **(Step 2)**.

5. **Coordinate rapid compressions and ventilations** in a 5:1 ratio, making sure the infant's chest rises with each ventilation. You will find this easier to do if you use your free hand to keep the head in the open airway position. If the chest does not rise, or rises only a little, use a chin lift to open the airway.

6. **Reassess the infant for signs of spontaneous breathing or pulses** after 1 minute and again after every few minutes **(Step 3)**.

(▶ **Skill Drill 32-8**) shows the steps for performing CPR in children between ages 1 and 8 years:

1. **Place the child on a firm surface,** and use one hand to maintain the head in a tilted-back position **(Step 1)**.

2. **Using two fingers of the other hand, locate the bottom of the sternum** by tracing the lower margin of the rib cage to the notch where the ribs and sternum meet. Place the heel of your hand over the lower half of the sternum; this is the area between the meeting place of the ribs and

Skill Drill 32-8 Performing CPR on a Child

Place the child on a firm surface and maintain the airway with one hand.

Place the heel of your other hand over the lower half of the sternum, avoiding the xiphoid.

Compress the chest about 1" to 1½" at a rate of 100/min (about 80/min with pauses for ventilations).
Coordinate compressions with ventilations in a 5:1 ratio, pausing for ventilations.

Reassess for breathing and pulse after about 1 minute, and then every few minutes.
If the child resumes effective breathing, place him or her in the recovery position.

sternum and an imaginary line drawn between the nipples. Avoid compression over the lower tip of the sternum, which is called the **xiphoid process (Step 2)**.

3. **Compress the chest** about one third to one half its total depth; this is usually 1" to 1½". Compress the chest at a rate of 100 compressions/min. With pauses for ventilation, the actual number of compressions will be about 80/min. Compression and relaxation should be about the same duration. Use smooth movements. Hold your fingers off the child's ribs, and keep the heel of your hand on the sternum.

4. **Coordinate rapid compressions and ventilations** in a 5:1 ratio, making sure the chest rises with each ventilation. At the end of every fifth compression, pause for 1 to 1½ seconds for artificial ventilation **(Step 3)**.

5. **Reassess the child for signs of spontaneous breathing and pulses** after about a minute and again every few minutes.

6. **If the child resumes effective breathing,** place him or her in the recovery position **(Step 4)**.

Remember, if the child is older than 8 years or is equivalent to an adult in size, use the adult CPR sequence, including the use of the AED.

Sudden Infant Death Syndrome

The death of an infant or a young child is called **sudden infant death syndrome (SIDS)** when, after a complete autopsy, the cause of death remains unexplained. SIDS is the leading cause of death in infants younger than 1 year; most cases occur in infants younger than age 6 months.

Although it is impossible to predict SIDS, there are several known risk factors:

- Mother younger than 20 years old
- Mother smoked during pregnancy
- Low birth weight

Deaths due to SIDS can occur at any time of the day; however, these children are often discovered in the morning when the parents go in to check on the infant. If you are the first provider at the scene of suspected SIDS, you will face three tasks: assessment and management of the patient, communication and support of the family, and assessment of the scene.

Assessment and Management

SIDS is a diagnosis of exclusion. All other potential causes must first be ruled out, a process that may take physicians quite a while. An infant who has been a victim of SIDS will be pale or blue, not breathing, and unresponsive. Other causes for such a condition include the following:

- Overwhelming infection
- Child abuse
- Airway obstruction from a foreign object or as a result of infection
- Meningitis
- Accidental or intentional poisoning
- Hypoglycemia (low blood glucose level)
- Congenital metabolic defects

Regardless of the cause, assessment and management of the infant remain the same. Remember that what you find in assessing the infant and the scene may provide important diagnostic information.

Begin with an assessment of the ABCs, and provide interventions as necessary. Depending on how much time has passed since the child was discovered, he or she may show signs of postmortem changes. These include stiffening of the body, called **rigor mortis**, and **dependent lividity**, which is the pooling of blood in the lower parts of body or those that are in contact with the floor or bed.

If the child shows such signs, call medical control. In some EMS systems, a victim of SIDS may be declared dead on the scene. Deciding whether to start CPR on a child who shows clear signs of rigor mortis or dependent lividity can be very difficult. Family members may consider anything less as withholding critical care. In this situation, the best course of action may be to initiate CPR and transport the patient and the family to the nearest emergency department, where the family can receive more extensive support (follow local protocols). If there is no evidence of postmortem changes, begin CPR immediately.

As you assess the infant, pay special attention to any marks or bruises on the child before performing any procedures, including CPR. Also note any intervention such as CPR that was done by the parents before you arrived.

Communication and Support of the Family

The death of a child is a very stressful event for a family; it also tends to evoke strong emotional responses among health care providers, including EMS personnel. Part of your job at this point is to allow the family to express their grief in ways that may differ from your own cultural, religious, and personal practices. Provide support in whatever ways you can.

Many times family members will ask specific questions about the event: Why did this happen? How did this happen? Let them know that their concerns will be addressed but that answers are not immediately available. Always use the infant's name in speaking to family members. If possible, allow the family to spend time with the infant and to ride in the ambulance to the hospital.

Scene Assessment

Carefully inspect the environment, following local protocols, noting the condition of the scene where the caregivers found the infant. Your assessment of the scene should concentrate on the following:

- Signs of illness, including medications, humidifiers, thermometers, etc.
- The general condition of the house (Note any signs of poor hygiene.)
- Family interaction. Do not allow yourself to be judgmental about family interactions at this time. Do note and report any behavior that is clearly not within the acceptable range, such as physical and verbal abuse.
- The site where the infant was discovered. Note all items in the infant's crib or bed, including pillows, stuffed animals, toys, and small objects.

The death of a child is difficult for everyone involved: parents, relatives, friends, and health care professionals. You should arrange for a proper debriefing after your involvement with the case comes to a close. This can

EMT-B Tips

Most parents of children who die suddenly will experience extremely strong emotional responses for a long time after the death. Counseling and support services begin with your care, including immediate referral to longer-term services. You can usually make this referral through social services personnel in a hospital you work with, something you should know about in advance. Many communities also support groups for families who lose children, including SIDS deaths. Make sure the parents are aware of available services, offer to put them in touch while you are there, and leave the contact information in written form for their later reference even if you have helped them make the contact.

be a session with a trained counselor or a group discussion with your colleagues or the entire health care team.

Apparent Life-Threatening Event

Infants who are not breathing and are cyanotic and unresponsive when found by their families sometimes resume breathing and color with stimulation. These children have had what is called an **apparent life-threatening event (ALTE)**, sometimes called "near-miss SIDS" in the past. In addition to cyanosis and apnea, a classic ALTE is characterized by a distinct change in muscle tone (limpness) and choking or gagging. After the event, a child may appear healthy and show no signs of illness or distress. Nevertheless, you must complete a careful assessment and provide immediate transport to the emergency department.

Pay strict attention to management of the airway. Assess the infant's history and, if possible, the environment. Allow caregivers to ride in the ambulance. If asked, explain that you cannot say what caused the event, and that this is something that doctors will have to determine at the hospital.

Death of a Child

As with SIDS, the death of a child from any cause poses special challenges for EMS personnel. In addition to any medical treatment the child may require, you must be prepared to offer the family a high level of support and understanding as they begin the grieving process ▶ Table 32-8 . First, the family may want you to initiate resuscitation efforts, which may or may not conflict with your EMS protocols. If the child is clearly deceased and, under protocol, can be declared dead in the field, but the family is so distraught that they insist that resuscitation efforts be made, initiate CPR and transport the child.

The extent of your interaction with the family will depend, to some degree, on the number of providers

available at the scene. Always introduce yourself to the child's caregivers, and ask about the child's date of birth and medical history. If and when the decision is made to start or stop resuscitation efforts, inform the family immediately. Find a place for family members from which they can watch resuscitation without being in the way. Do not, in any case, speculate on the cause of the child's death. The family will want to see the child and should be asked whether they want to hold the child and say good-bye. Parents may be experiencing strong feelings of denial.

The following interventions are helpful in caring for the family at this time:

- Learn and use the child's name rather than the impersonal "your child."
- Speak to family members at eye level, maintaining good eye contact with them.
- Use the word "dead" or "died" when informing the family of the child's death; euphemisms such as "passed away" or "gone" are not effective.
- Acknowledge the family's feelings ("I know this is devastating for you"), but never say "I know how you feel," even if you have experienced a similar event; the statement will anger many people.
- Offer to call other family members or clergy if the family wishes.
- Keep any instructions short, simple, and basic. Emotional distress may limit their ability to process information.
- Ask each adult family member individually whether he or she wants to hold the child.
- Wrap the dead child in a blanket, as you would if he or she were alive, and stay with the family while they hold the child. Ask them not to remove tubes or other equipment that was used in an attempted resuscitation.

Remember that each individual and each culture expresses grief in a different way, some more visibly than others. Some will require intervention; others will not. Most caregivers feel directly or indirectly responsible for the death of a child and may express this immediately; this does not mean that they actually are responsible. Sometimes, it is helpful to address the issue of guilt by saying, "Many caregivers feel responsible for their child's death. Are you feeling that?" Parents often have questions that you should be prepared to answer ▶ Table 32-9 . Although you should keep the possibility of abuse or neglect in mind, your role is not that of investigator. Any further inquiry is the responsibility of law enforcement.

Some EMS systems arrange for home visits after the death of a child so that EMS providers and family members can come to some sort of closure together. This also

TABLE 32-8 How You Can Help the Family of a Deceased Child

When Arriving on Site:

- Introduce yourself quickly.
- Obtain a brief history.
- When possible, one provider should stay with the family.

If Resuscitation is Attempted:

- Give brief, frequent updates and explanations.
- Allow family members to stay within viewing distance if they wish.
- Allow family members to accompany child to hospital when possible.

If No Resuscitation is Performed:

- Sit down with the family.
- Inform the family immediately.
- Explain why no resuscitation will be attempted.
- Offer to arrange for religious support, including baptism or last rites.

Beginning the Grieving Process:

- Learn and use the child's name.
- Allow family to express emotions; be nonjudgmental.
- Give brief explanations and answers.
- Explain to the family that the cause of death is still unknown.
- Allow time for questions.

DO:

- Tell the family how sorry you are.
- Tell the family whom they can call if they have questions later.
- Give written instructions and referrals.

DON'T:

- Say, "I know how you feel."
- Say, "You have other children" or "You can have other children."
- Attempt to answer the question "Why did this happen?"
- Try to tell family that they will be feeling better in time.

TABLE 32-9 Common Questions Following Death of a Child

Q Was there pain?

A This often can be answered by a simple "No." If you are uncertain, you may give an indirect answer such as "We really don't know what patients feel in these circumstances."

Q What did he/she die of?

A Do not answer this question; you would probably be guessing at this point.

Q Why did this happen?

A Do not attempt to answer this question either, as the answer depends on one's own individual philosophy, or religion. "I wish I had an answer for you" is usually the most appropriate response.

Q What happens now?

A This question usually concerns the next few minutes or the next hour. If you know, you should give the family a general idea of what will happen. For example, if there is no history of illness, you can say that "the coroner (or medical examiner) will be examining [the child's name], and then he (or she) will be taken to the mortuary."

gives the family an opportunity to ask any remaining questions about the event. However, you need special training for such visits.

Again, coping with the death of a child can be very stressful for health care professionals. You may find yourself with unexpected feelings of pain and loss. It is helpful to take some time before going back on the job to work through your feelings and to talk about the event with your EMS colleagues. Be alert for signs of posttraumatic stress in yourself and others: nightmares, restlessness, difficulty sleeping, lack of appetite, a constant need for food, and the like. Consider the need for professional help if these signs or symptoms continue. All EMS programs should have critical incident stress management protocols and debriefing teams available for traumatic incidents.

Although you may experience the death of a child as a failure, your skill at coping with this kind of emotional event can be a great comfort to the family, helping them to accept their loss and begin the long process of grieving.

Prep Kit

Ready for Review

The airway in a child has a smaller diameter than the airway in an adult and is therefore more easily obstructed. Because the diaphragm is the principal muscle of respiration in children and infants, gastric distention can create breathing difficulties. The three fundamentals of pediatric emergency care are to provide basic life support as needed, prevent disability by stabilizing the spine, and consult with an ALS unit when appropriate.

You will need to carry special sizes of airway equipment for pediatric patients. Use a pediatric resuscitation tape measure to determine the appropriately sized equipment for children.

In treating possible respiratory failure in a child, always position the airway in a neutral position. Use an airway adjunct to maintain an open airway: an oropharyngeal airway in an unconscious patient (unless he or she has ingested a caustic or petroleum-based product), and a nasopharyngeal airway in a conscious patient (unless he or she is younger than 1 year and/or has sustained head trauma). Appropriate oxygen delivery devices include the blow-by technique at 6 L/min, a nasal cannula at 4 to 6 L/min, a simple face mask at 6 to 10 L/min, a nonrebreathing mask at 10 to 12 L/min, and a BVM device at 10 to 15 L/min.

Use a BVM device with a child whose breathing and tidal volume are inadequate and who has an altered level of consciousness. There are three keys to successful use of the BVM device in a child: (1) Have the appropriate equipment in the right size, (2) maintain a good face to mask seal, and (3) ventilate at the appropriate rate and volume: 20 breaths/min for an infant or child, 30 for a neonate, 1 to 1 1/2 seconds per ventilation. Squeeze gently, and stop squeezing as the chest wall begins to rise; use the phrase "squeeze, release, release" to maintain a proper rhythm.

Children younger than 5 years often obstruct their upper and lower airway with a variety of foreign objects. If the child is conscious, encourage him or her to cough to clear the airway. If the child is unconscious, you should first use the tongue-jaw lift and finger sweeps to try to remove an object that you can see. In treating an unconscious child with complete airway obstruction, use abdominal thrusts (in a series of five), alternating with attempts at artificial breathing; in infants, substitute back blows and chest thrusts. In a conscious child who is sitting or standing, apply abdominal thrusts from behind.

A child who is in early respiratory distress may be breathing too slowly or too fast. Rates greater than 60 breaths/min are a sign of a problem requiring assisted ventilation in most cases. Look for signs of extra effort to breathe, including nasal flaring and grunting respirations; these may give way to cyanosis. You must intervene immediately if bradycardia develops in a child in respiratory distress. Use the least upsetting method to administer supplemental oxygen, adding assisted ventilations if these become necessary; use a BVM device without an artificial airway.

Seizures in children may appear as a shaking of the whole body (generalized), a movement in a single arm or leg or eye (partial), or a momentary unresponsiveness (absence seizure). Complications of seizures are due to injury from seizure motion, airway obstruction, or poor breathing effort. Do not put anything into the mouth of a seizing child. Do position the child so that the tongue is not an obstruction, and be prepared to suction secretions or vomitus. Febrile seizures, occurring on the first day of a fever, may be a sign of a more serious problem such as meningitis. Begin cooling measures, and transport the patient to the hospital.

Other childhood conditions that require immediate transport include altered level of consciousness, which you may assess using the AVPU scale; severe dehydration; and poisoning. The best way to cool a child with a fever is with wet towels that are at room temperature, not cold. Children with meningitis will have a fever, altered level of consciousness, and irritability, along with neck pain. All patients with possible meningitis should be considered highly contagious and infectious. *Neisseria meningitides* infection, characterized by tiny red spots or a large purple rash, is a fast-moving, dangerous form of meningitis. If you have been exposed to respiratory secretions from a child with this form of the disease, you should take antibiotics.

Infants and children can go into shock after the loss of even a small volume of fluid or blood, which may be caused by an injury, dehydration, severe infection or allergic reaction, heart disease, or a collapsed lung. Children who are in shock often have increased respirations but normal blood pressure until the condition is severe. Changes in skin color and capillary refill are important signs of shock.

The most common cause of dehydration in children is vomiting and diarrhea. Life-threatening diarrhea can develop in an infant in hours. You can determine whether a child's dehydration is mild, moderate, or severe by assessing the child's urine output, level of activity, mental status, skin tone, and pulse. For severe dehydration, ALS backup is necessary so that IV fluids can be given.

The heart rate is the most important measure in determining the need for extra resuscitation efforts in a normal newborn. If the heart rate is 80 to 100 beats/min, you should give blow-by oxygen and continue to reassess the infant. If the rate does not rise to more than 100 beats/min, begin assisted ventilations with a BVM device and 100% oxygen, and reassess the infant every 15 to 30 seconds. If the rate remains low, begin chest compressions, continue assisted ventilations, and call for ALS backup.

BLS for infants and children consists of determining responsiveness and assessing airway, breathing, and circulation. If the child is unconscious but breathing, place him or her in the recovery position unless you suspect a spinal injury. Use the head tilt-chin lift or jaw-thrust maneuver to open the airway in a child who is unconscious and not breathing. If a child is not breathing, provide rescue breathing while keeping the airway open. Breathe for an infant at a rate of 1 to $1\frac{1}{2}$ breaths/second at first, then 20 breaths/min. Breathe for a child between ages 1 and 8 years at a rate of 2 breaths/second at first, then 20 breaths/min. Do not spend more than a few seconds trying to feel a pulse in an infant or child; if he or she is not breathing, you can assume there is no pulse.

To provide CPR in an infant, compress the chest 100 compressions/min, pausing after every five compressions for ventilation; use two or three fingers, and compress the lower half of the sternum to a depth $\frac{1}{2}$" to 1". In children, use the same rate and compressions to a depth of 1" to $1\frac{1}{2}$" and the same 5:1 ratio of compressions to ventilations, but use the heel of your hand to compress the chest; avoid compressing the xiphoid process.

A victim of sudden infant death syndrome (SIDS) will be pale or blue, not breathing, and unresponsive. He or she may show signs of postmortem changes, including rigor mortis and dependent lividity; if so, call medical control to report the situation. If family members insist or protocols mandate, you should initiate CPR and transport infant and family to the emergency department, where the family can receive more extensive support. If the child does not have any evidence of postmortem changes, begin CPR immediately. Carefully inspect the environment where a SIDS victim was found, looking for signs of illness, abusive family interactions, and objects in the child's crib. Provide support for the family in whatever way you can, but do not make judgmental statements. Allow them to spend time with the child and ride in the ambulance to the hospital.

Any death of a child is stressful for family members and for health care providers. In dealing with the family, acknowledge their feelings, keep any instructions short and simple, use the child's name, and maintain eye contact. Be prepared to respond to philosophical as well as medical questions, in most cases by indicating concern and understanding; do not be specific about the cause of death. Be alert for signs of posttraumatic stress in yourself and others after dealing with the death of a child. It can help to talk about the event and your feelings with your EMS colleagues.

Prep Kit

Vital Vocabulary

altered level of consciousnes A mental state in which infants and children may be unresponsive, combative, or confused, may thrash about, or may drift into and out of an alert state; also called altered mental status.

apnea Absence of breathing.

apparent life-threatening event (ALTE) An event that causes unresponsiveness, cyanosis, and apnea in an infant, who then resumes breathing with stimulation.

blanching Turning white.

bradycardia A heart rate of less than 60 beats/min in children or less than 80 beats/min in infants.

croup Infection of the airway below the level of the vocal cords, usually caused by a virus.

dehydration A state in which fluid losses are greater than fluid intake into the body, leading to shock and death if untreated.

dependent lividity Pooling of the blood in the lower parts of the body after death.

epiglottitis An infection of the soft tissue in the area above the vocal cords.

febrile seizure Seizure relating to a fever.

hypoventilation Reduced minute volume, either from reduced rate and/or depth of breathing.

meconium A dark green material in the amniotic fluid that can cause lung disease in the newborn.

meningitis Inflammation of the meninges that cover the spinal cord and the brain.

nares The external openings of the nostrils.

Neisseria meningitides A form of bacterial meningitis characterized by rapid onset of symptoms, often leading to shock and death.

occiput The back of the head.

pediatric resuscitation tape measure A tape that estimates an infant or child's weight on the basis of length and lists appropriate drug doses and equipment sizes on the tape.

postictal period The period immediately following a seizure, characterized by extreme tiredness or listlessness.

rales A crackling breath sound caused by the flow of air through liquid in the lungs; a sign of lower airway obstruction.

rigor mortis Stiffening of the body after death.

shock A condition that develops when the circulatory system is not able to deliver sufficient blood to body organs, resulting in organ failure and eventual death if untreated.

septum The central divider in the nose.

status epilepticus The term used to describe a continuous seizure, or multiple seizures without a return to consciousness, for 30 minutes or more.

stridor A high-pitched breath sound heard mainly on inspiration that is a sign of upper airway obstruction.

sudden infant death syndrome (SIDS) Death of an infant or young child that remains unexplained after a complete autopsy.

tidal volume The amount of air that is delivered to the lungs and airways in one inhalation.

tonic-clonic seizure A seizure that features rhythmic back-and-forth motion of an extremity and body stiffness.

tragus The small cartilaginous projection in front of the opening of the ear.

tripod position An abnormal position to keep the airway open; it involves leaning forward onto two arms stretched forward.

wheezing A whistling breath sound caused by air traveling through narrowed air passages within the bronchioles; a sign of lower airway obstruction.

xiphoid process The lower tip of the sternum.

Assessment in Action

You are dispatched to an unconscious 2-year-old child. On arrival, a woman rushes out of the house with a baby in her arms. She is screaming "Help me, help me, my baby isn't breathing!" She thrusts a limp child with a gray-blue face in your arms. The child's eyes are half open with a vacant stare.

1. Your priority of assessment is to:
   A. check mental status.   B. check airway patency.
   C. check pulse.   D. check for responsiveness.

2. You check for airway patency, it seems clear, and you check for breathing. The child is breathing at 6 breaths/min. An apical pulse is 20 beats/min. Which of the following is appropriate?
   A. Check for capillary return
   B. Start ventilating and giving chest compressions
   C. Ventilate with a BVM device and reassess
   D. Check pupil size and reaction

3. The most appropriate way to assess for adequate tidal volume in this patient is to:
   A. check the pulse for increased rate.
   B. check for good rise and fall of the chest.
   C. check the pulse oximetry value.
   D. check for responsiveness.

4. After a few minutes of CPR, the child's heart rate increases to 150 beats/min, he has a weak cry, and his color begins to slowly improve. Appropriate oxygen administration at this point would include:
   A. blow-by.   B. nasal cannula.
   C. nonrebreathing mask. D. continuing to use the BVM device.

5. Appropriate positioning of this patient at this time would be:
   A. picking him up and cuddling him.
   B. sitting him up to help his breathing.
   C. keeping him lying flat.
   D. tipping the cot so his hips are higher than his chest.

6. Your partner is trying to get a blood pressure reading. You know that an appropriately sized blood pressure cuff is:
   A. One third the length of the upper arm.
   B. Two thirds the length of the upper arm.
   C. One half the length of the upper arm.
   D. One fourth the length of the upper arm.

7. Part of necessary treatment for this child includes:
   A. administering an inhaler if the child has one.
   B. keeping the child warm.
   C. administering glucose gel.
   D. administering activated charcoal.

8. Information that is extremely important for the hospital to know is the suspected substance that the child overdosed on and:
   A. time of suspected ingestion. B. known allergies.
   C. previous illnesses.   D. behavior change in the child.

9. On the way to the emergency department your 2-year-old patient has a seizure. Appropriate treatment includes:
   A. immediate suctioning.
   B. restraining the child.
   C. using the BVM to force ventilation.
   D. turning the child on his side.

10. After a minute of seizure-like activity, your 2-year-old patient stops skeletal muscle movement and appears to be sleeping. Appropriate actions include:
    A. assessing the airway and breathing.
    B. immediately suctioning the airway.
    C. checking the child's heart rate.
    D. starting ventilations with a BVM device.

Points to Ponder

You are dispatched to an "unconscious child." When you arrive at the address you find a house that looks like no one is living in it. The yard has junked cars in it and the grass has not been mowed in months. As you walk up on the wooden porch it sags and you are concerned you will fall through. There are three young children playing in the yard, two are wearing only diapers and the third is naked. When you enter the house the smell of old food, feces and animals is overwhelming. The mother leads you to a child lying on a cot in a bedroom. In the bedroom you find three filthy mattresses on the floor and the cot against the wall. A 2-year-old boy is on the cot and he is wearing only underwear and he is laying in vomit and feces. The mother tells you that he has "had the flu" for 5 days and she could not wake him up for lunch. The child has a high fever and is very lethargic. The mother explains that her husband left her 2 years ago and that she cannot work and take care of the children. It is not their home, it was empty and they just moved in one day and no one has kicked them out. The mother says that she cannot go with you because she has to stay with the other four children. You transport the child to the hospital. What are your feelings about this mother and family? Is this a reportable problem and if so, to whom? How would your feelings impact the care you would provide in this situation?

Issues Low-Income Patients, Personal Biases, Reportable Conditions, Realities of Life.

Online Outlook

There are many causes of respiratory distress and failure in children. Although you might not be able to identify the exact cause in every patient, you must be able to intervene appropriately to restore breathing in all of them. To learn more about upper airway problems in children, complete Exercise 32 at www.emtb.com.

Pediatric Trauma

TECHNOLOGY

www.emtb.com

Online Chapter Pretest

Interactivities

Vocabulary Explorer

Anatomy Review

Web Links

Online Review Manual

Distance Learning

"Rescue 23, you are needed at the Bay Street Entertainment Center for a child injured in a go-cart crash."

As with the other aspects of prehospital pediatric care, pediatric trauma has its own unique characteristics. This chapter concludes the pediatric-specific material and will also help you answer the following questions:

1. What signs, symptoms, or other clues might lead you to suspect that a child has been the victim of physical abuse?

2. Are there certain physical characteristics that make children more at risk when they are injured? What are they?

Pediatric Trauma

Trauma is the number one killer of children in the United States. More children die of trauma-related injuries in 1 year than of all other causes combined. As an EMT-B, you will frequently treat injured children; therefore, you must have a thorough understanding of how trauma affects them. The quality of care in the first few minutes after a child has been injured can have an enormous impact on that child's chances for complete recovery.

Treatment of traumatic injuries in children starts with understanding these injuries as completely as possible. The types of injuries differ, depending on the age of the child. Infants and toddlers are most commonly hurt as a result of falls or abuse. Older children and adolescents are usually injured as a result of mishaps involving automobiles. According to information collected by the National Pediatric Trauma Registry (NPTR) over the last 10 years, the automobile is the most significant threat to the well-being of the child. Approximately 41% of all injuries that the NPTR recorded in this time period were related to vehicular mishaps, including those involving bicycles and pedestrians. Other common causes of traumatic injury and death include falls, gunshot wounds, blunt injuries, and sports activities. Another extremely serious and troublesome cause of injury is child abuse.

Anatomic Differences

By now, you know that children are not simply small adults; they differ in many ways other than size. Children have less circulating blood than adults do. Children also lose body heat more easily than adults do because children have a larger body surface area in relation to body mass. A child's bones have not finished growing; they are more flexible and elastic than those in an adult's skeleton. Fat is distributed in a child in a somewhat different way than in an adult, so vital organs in the abdomen and the chest of a child are less well insulated. Therefore, a child may experience significant injuries to internal organs but have little or no evidence of external trauma. This is especially true of chest injuries. Because a child's ribs are softer and more flexible than those of an adult, they may compress the underlying lungs and heart, causing life-threatening conditions without obvious external damage ▼ Figure 33-1 .

Given these anatomic differences, you must be able to recognize severe injuries in children, as well as to identify potentially life-threatening injuries so that you

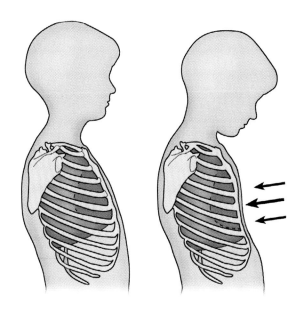

Figure 33-1 A child's ribs are softer and more flexible than an adult's. As a result, they may compress the lungs and heart, causing serious injury with no obvious external damage.

can provide prompt emergency medical care. This begins with your scene size-up. Look for the child's level of activity, work of breathing, and skin color. This information is quickly gained and is the beginning of your ABCs. Complete the initial assessment by:

- Evaluating the child's responsiveness
- Ensuring that the child has an open airway and is breathing
- Assisting ventilation and giving supplemental oxygen to the child, if necessary
- Assessing the child's circulation by obtaining a pulse (brachial, carotid, femoral) and blood pressure, evaluating for external bleeding, and assessing skin color, temperature, and capillary refill

Injury Patterns

Although you are not responsible for diagnosing injuries in children, your ability to recognize and report serious injuries will provide critical information to hospital staff. For this reason, it is important for you to understand the special physical and psychological characteristics of children and what makes them more likely to have certain kinds of injuries. Situations that are unique to children also make them more susceptible to injury, such as their need to ride in child safety seats, their involvement in specific mishaps with motor vehicles, and their participation in organized sports.

Physical Differences

Children are smaller than adults; therefore, when they are hurt in the same type of accident as an adult, the location of their injuries may differ from those in an adult. For example, the bumper of a car will strike an adult in the lower leg, whereas that same bumper will strike a child in the pelvis. In a crash involving sudden deceleration, an adult might injure a ligament in the knee; in that same accident, a child might injure the bones in the leg.

Children's bones and soft tissues are less well developed than those of adults; therefore, the force of an injury affects these structures somewhat differently than it does in an adult. Because a child's head is proportionately larger than an adult's, it exerts greater stress on the neck structures during a deceleration injury. Because of these anatomic differences, you should always carefully assess for head and neck injuries in children.

Psychological Differences

Children are also less mature psychologically than adults; therefore, they are often injured because of their undeveloped judgment and their lack of experience. For example, children are more likely than adults to cross the street without looking for oncoming traffic. As a result, children are more likely than adults to be struck by cars. Children and adolescents are also more likely to sustain injuries from diving into shallow water because they forget to check the depth of the water before they dive. In such situations, you should always assume that the child has serious head and neck injuries. Other common injuries include wrist injuries from in-line roller skating and ankle fractures from bicycle crashes. Note that these examples do not apply to all children or all adults. In fact, some children have more common sense than some adults. However, you should be aware of these injury patterns when you are called to respond to pediatric emergencies.

Child Safety Seats

Children are often injured or killed in motor vehicle crashes. Those who are not restrained in child safety seats are at greater risk for head, neck, and spinal injuries. Although child safety seats are effective in decreasing the severity of injuries, children may still sustain abdominal and lower spinal injuries as the result of trauma caused by improperly used passenger restraints. Infants are especially prone to injuries of the head and neck due to weaker neck muscles and their larger head and should be in a rear-facing seat until 1 year of age. Although head, neck, and spinal injuries are less common in restrained passengers, they are certainly possible. Therefore, you should always immobilize the patient's cervical spine ▼ **Figure 33-2** .

Young children, especially those who have been restrained in a child safety seat, may be critically injured

Figure 33-2 Even though head, neck, and spinal injuries are less common in children who are restrained, they are still possible. Therefore, you should always immobilize the patient's cervical spine.

Figure 33-3 Children riding in a child safety seat in the front passenger seat of a car may be injured or killed by the force of a deploying airbag.

or killed by airbags if they are riding in the front passenger seat of a car (▲ **Figure 33-3**). This occurs because the child safety seat positions the child too close to the airbag. When the airbag deploys, the child may sustain a devastating spinal or head injury. For this reason, child safety seats should never be placed in the front seat of a vehicle that is equipped with passenger airbags.

Automobile Collisions

Children playing or riding a bicycle can dart out in front of motor vehicles without looking. In such a situation, the driver may have very little time to slow down or stop to prevent hitting the child. The area of greatest injury varies, depending on the size of the child and the height of the bumper at the time of impact (▼ **Figure 33-4**). When vehicles slow down at the moment of impact, the bumper dips slightly, causing the point of impact with the child to be lowered. The exact area that is struck depends on the child's height and the final position of the bumper at the time of impact. Children who are injured in these situations

often sustain high-energy injuries to the head, spine, abdomen, pelvis, or legs.

Sports Activities

Children, especially those who are older or adolescents, are often injured in organized sports activities. Head and neck injuries can occur after high-speed collisions in contact sports such as football, wrestling, ice hockey, field hockey, soccer, or lacrosse. Remember to immobilize the cervical spine when caring for children with sports-related injuries. You should also be familiar with your local protocols related to helmet removal, and/or follow the guidelines presented in Chapter 30.

Injuries to Specific Body Systems

Head Injuries

Head injuries are common in children. This is due, in part, to the fact that the size of a child's head, in relation to the body, is larger than that of an adult. The signs and symptoms of head injury in a child are similar to those in an adult, but there are some important differences. Nausea and vomiting are common signs and symptoms of head injury in children; however, it is easy to mistake these for an abdominal injury or illness. You should suspect a serious head injury in any child who experiences nausea and vomiting after a traumatic event.

Your single most important step in caring for a child with a head injury is to ensure that the airway is open. Whenever you suspect trauma, you should immobilize the cervical spine and use the jaw-thrust maneuver to open the airway, as the child's tongue may have relaxed back into the throat, blocking the airway. As you immobilize the child onto a backboard, avoid using sandbags

Thorax

Femur

Ground

Head

Figure 33-4 The exact area that is struck depends on the child's height relative to the position of the bumper at the time of impact.

to immobilize the head (▼ **Figure 33-5**). If the child begins to vomit and the board has to be turned to the side, the weight of the bags on the head could cause additional injury. <u>Hyperventilation</u> (rapid ventilation) of the child with a head injury should not be attempted until normal ventilations have been established with a bag-valve-mask device for several minutes.

Respiratory arrest can also occur as a result of head injuries in children. You should be prepared to assist ventilations or provide rescue breaths in any child who has evidence of severe head injury.

Chest Injuries

Chest injuries in children are usually the result of blunt trauma rather than penetrating objects. Remember that children have very soft, flexible ribs that can be compressed a great deal without breaking. Keep this in mind as you assess a child who has sustained high-energy blunt trauma to the chest. Even though there may be no external sign of injury, such as broken ribs, contusions, or bleeding, there may be significant injuries within the chest.

Abdominal Injuries

Abdominal injuries are very common in children. Remember, though, that children can compensate for significant blood loss better than adults without signs or symptoms of shock developing. They can also have a serious injury without early external evidence of a problem. All children with abdominal injuries should be monitored for signs and symptoms of shock, including a weak, rapid pulse; cold, clammy skin; decreased capillary refill (an early sign); confusion, and decreased systolic blood pressure (a late sign). Even in the absence of signs and symptoms of shock, or with only very few signs and symptoms, you should remain cautious about the possibility of internal injuries.

Children can lose a greater proportion of their blood volume than adults can before signs or symptoms of

Figure 33-5 Use a proper pediatric immobilization device rather than sandbags to immobilize the head of a child. If you need to turn the board to the side if the child vomits, sandbags could shift and cause further injury.

shock develop. What makes this situation dangerous is that infants and children have less blood circulating in their bodies than adults do, so the loss of even a small volume of fluid or blood may lead to shock (▶ **Figure 33-6**).

Greater than 25% blood volume loss significantly increases the risk of shock.

Signs of Shock in Children

- Tachycardia
- Poor capillary refill
- Mental status changes

Signs of Shock in Adults

- Tachycardia
- Hypotension
- Mental status changes

Greater than 30%–40% blood volume loss significantly increases risk of shock.

You should always suspect hidden internal injuries in children after a high-energy trauma. One of the problems associated with abdominal injuries in children is the presence of air in the stomach. Children, especially those who have had a traumatic injury, tend to swallow air. Air in the stomach can cause distention and interfere with your assessment. Air can also accumulate in the stomach with artificial ventilation, making it less effective. This is one of the reasons to use the jaw-thrust maneuver to position the airway, as it decreases the amount of air accumulating in the stomach.

Injuries of the Extremities

Children have immature bones with active growth centers. Growth of long bones occurs from the ends at specialized growth plates. These growth plates are potential weak spots in the bone and are often injured as a result of trauma. In general, children's bones bend more easily than adults' bones. As a result, incomplete or greenstick fractures can occur.

Greater than 25% blood volume
loss significantly increases risk
of shock

Signs of Shock in Children
• Tachycardia
• Poor capillary refill
• Mental status changes

Developing shock

Blood
volume

25% 50% 75% 100%

Signs of Shock in Adults
• Tachycardia
• Hypotension
• Mental status changes

Greater than 30-40% blood
volume loss significantly
increases risk of shock

Developing shock

Blood
volume

25% 50% 75% 100%

Figure 33-6 Children can lose a greater proportion of their blood volume than adults can before signs or symptoms of shock develop.

Extremity injuries in children are generally managed in the same manner as those in adults. Painful deformed limbs with evidence of broken bones should be splinted. Specialized splinting equipment, such as a traction splint for fractures of the femur, should be used only if it fits the child. You should not attempt to use adult immobilization devices on a child unless the child is large enough to properly fit in the device.

Other Considerations

Pneumatic Antishock Garments

A **pneumatic antishock garment** (PASG) is rarely used in treating children. One situation in which you would use a PASG is when the child has obvious lower extremity trauma, particularly to both legs; pelvic instability; and clear signs and symptoms of decompensated shock. However, one problem with the use of this device for children is that it rarely fits. The PASG

should be used on children only if it fits properly. Techniques such as placing the child in one leg of the garment are absolutely contraindicated and should never be used. The abdominal compartment of the garment should never be inflated on children because excessive pressure on the abdomen will cause pressure on the diaphragm and compromise breathing.

Burns

Children can be burned in a variety of ways. The most common involve exposure to hot substances such as scalding water in a bathtub, hot items on a stove, or exposure to caustic substances such as cleaning solvents or paint thinners ▶ **Figure 33-7** . You should suspect possible internal injuries from chemical ingestion when you see a child who has burns, particularly around the face and mouth.

One common problem following burn injuries in children is infection. Burned skin cannot resist infection as effectively as normal skin can. For this reason, sterile techniques should be used in handling the skin of children with burn wounds.

As when you are caring for adults, you should first remove all clothing from the burned skin as part of a complete exposure of the patient. Leaving charred clothing in place prevents you from clearly assessing the patient. In addition, the clothing may still be hot and continue to burn the underlying skin if it is not removed. After chemical burns, it is particularly important to remove the clothing rapidly, since chemical materials that are retained within the clothing may also cause damage to the underlying skin. After the skin has been exposed, you should place dry sterile dressings on the skin as soon as possible to decrease the risk of infection.

You must learn your local protocols regarding the immediate referral of children to burn centers.

▶ **Table 33-1** provides some general guidelines to follow in assessing a child who has been burned. These guidelines may help you to determine which children should be treated primarily at specialized burn centers. Also note that you should consider the possibility of child abuse in any burn situation. Make sure you report any information about your suspicions to hospital staff.

Submersion Injury

Submersion injuries include near drowning and drowning. In submersion situations, you must always take steps to ensure your own safety when retrieving the patient from the water.

Drowning is the second most common cause of unintentional death among children in the United States; children under age 5 years are at particular risk. At this age, children often fall into swimming pools and lakes,

TABLE 33-1 Severity of Burns in Children	
Severity of Burn	**Body Area Involved**
Minor	Partial-thickness burns involving less than 10% of the body surface
Moderate	Partial-thickness burns involving 10% to 20% of the body surface
Critical	Any full-thickness burn
	Any partial-thickness burn involving more than 20% of the body surface
	Any burn involving the hands, feet, face, airway, or genitalia

but many drown in bathtubs and even buckets. Older adolescents, who account for the most drownings after toddlers, drown when swimming or boating; alcohol is frequently a factor.

The principal injury from submersion is lack of oxygen. Even a few minutes (or less) without oxygen affect the heart, lungs, and brain, causing life-threatening problems such as cardiac arrest, respiratory difficulty, and coma. Submersion in icy water can rob the body of heat, causing hypothermia. While a very few, very cold victims of submersion hypothermia have survived long periods in cardiac arrest in icy water, most people in this situation die. Diving into the water, of course, increases the risk of neck and spinal cord injuries.

Assessment and reassessment of the ABCs are critical in submersion injuries. First assess breathing and pulse, because the patient may be in cardiac or respiratory arrest. Immediately check breathing effort, skin color, and capillary refill in addition to vital signs. Always immobilize the cervical spine of patients who were diving. Lung injuries may progress, causing breathing difficulty over time, so be sure to reassess the patient frequently during transport.

If you cannot effectively ventilate the patient, consider the possibility of a foreign body airway obstruction; water alone does not obstruct the airway. If you can see the object, be sure to use removal techniques that are appropriate to the patient's age.

If it is within your scope of practice, consider using a nasogastric tube to protect the airway in unresponsive

Figure 33-7 The most common burns in children involve exposure to hot surfaces. This child's buttocks were placed against a hot heating grate.

In submersion situations, you must always take steps to ensure your own safety when retrieving the patient from the water.

patients, as they will usually vomit. Always have a suction device ready in case of vomiting or water in the airway. Call for an ALS team if transport times are long and in your protocol.

Remove wet clothing so that the patient does not get colder. Keep the patient warm and monitor vital functions during transport.

A child may appear completely normal after being submersed and then develop problems minutes or hours later. This is called secondary drowning and happens when the lungs are filled with fluid from within the lung (pulmonary edema).

Emergency Medical Care

Emergency medical care of a child who has experienced a traumatic injury immediately focuses on the ABCs, as with all patients.

Airway

You should be alert for airway problems in all children who have sustained traumatic injuries. Children who are awake, alert, and talking generally have open airways; however, unconscious children, even those who are initially breathing on their own with signs of an open airway, are at risk for airway obstruction. Look and listen for signs indicating abnormal airflow

Figure 33-8 Turn the backboard to the side and suction the mouth when an immobilized child vomits.

through the upper airway. If stridor—an abnormal airway sound made by turbulent airflow—is present, use the jaw-thrust maneuver to keep the airway open. One advantage of this maneuver is that it minimizes the risk of damage to the cervical spine because it keeps the head in a neutral position.

Because nausea and vomiting are common in children with traumatic head injuries, you must be prepared for it. Keep suctioning equipment readily available so that you can suction the mouth and oropharynx as necessary to keep the airway open. Be prepared to turn a backboard to one side if the child vomits ▼ **Figure 33-8** . Remember that you should not use sandbags to stabilize the cervical spine in children. If you must turn the backboard to allow for vomiting, the weight of the sandbags may cause additional head injury when the backboard and patient are turned.

Breathing

You should give supplemental oxygen to all children with possible head, chest, or abdominal injuries or any evidence of shock, to correct for any hypoxia. Children who are breathing on their own should be given high-concentration oxygen via a nonrebreathing mask. Care should be taken to ensure that the mask fits the child properly; adult masks used on children typically leak, making oxygen administration less effective ▶ **Figure 33-9** .

You should be prepared to assist with ventilation in children who are in respiratory distress. For children who have had traumatic injuries, use a child-sized BVM device at a rate of 20 breaths/min, or one breath every 3 seconds. A faster rate of ventilation, hyperventilation, is indicated in children with head trauma only when signs of brain swelling are present. Signs include one dilated, nonreactive pupil, decorticate (pull in) or decerebrate (push away) posturing, or altered breathing patterns. To hyperventilate your patient, increase the rate to 5 breaths/min above the normal rate until the symptoms resolve (eg, the dilated pupil decreases, posturing stops, or ventilation patterns normalize), then return to normal rate of ventilations; follow your local protocols.

Immobilization

Immobilization is necessary for all children who have possible head or spinal injuries after a traumatic event. Follow the steps in ▶ **Skill Drill 33-1** :

1. **Maintain the child's head in a neutral position** by placing a towel under the child's shoulders **(Step 1)**.

2. **Place an appropriately sized cervical collar on the patient (Step 2)**.

Figure 33-9 **A.** Use a properly fitting nonrebreathing mask to deliver supplemental oxygen. **B.** Area covered on a child's face with a properly fitting mask.

3. **Carefully log roll the child** onto the immobilization device **(Step 3)**.

4. **Secure the patient's torso** to the immobilization device first **(Step 4)**.

5. **Secure the child's head** to the immobilization device **(Step 5)**.

6. **Complete immobilization** by ensuring that the child is strapped in properly **(Step 6)**.

Immobilization can be difficult to perform due to the child's body proportions. Young children require padding under the torso to maintain a neutral position. At around 8 to 10 years of age, children no longer require padding underneath the torso in order to form a neutral position. Instead, they can simply lie supine on the board. However, another complication may occur if a child is put onto an adult-sized long board. Because a child's body is narrower than an adult's, it will require padding along the sides in order to be properly secured on an adult-sized long board

EMT-B Tips

An injured child with serious airway or breathing problems is likely to need full-time attention from two EMT-Bs. The need for a driver, and often for added help with patient care, makes it important to start arranging early for backup from another unit—possibly even before you arrive at the scene.

Follow the steps in ▶ **Skill Drill 33-2** to immobilize an infant:

1. **Carefully stabilize the infant's head in a neutral position** and lay the seat down into a reclined position on a hard surface **(Step 1)**.

2. **Position a pediatric board or other similar device** between the patient and the surface on which the infant is resting **(Step 2)**.

3. **Carefully slide the infant into position** on the board **(Step 3)**.

4. **Make sure the infant's head is in a neutral position** by placing a towel under the infant's shoulders **(Step 4)**.

5. **Secure the torso first** and place any padding to fill any voids **(Step 5)**.

6. **Secure the infant's head** to the board **(Step 6)**.

As with all patients who have unstable or potentially unstable injuries, immediate transport is indicated. The identification of the nearest appropriate facility depends on local protocols and the capabilities of local hospitals. In some areas of the country, you may be directed to take the patient directly to a pediatric trauma center or to arrange for air transport to a pediatric trauma center. In other areas of the country, children are evaluated primarily at local hospitals and are then transferred to a pediatric trauma center. You should be familiar with the local guidelines and protocols regarding transport issues.

Child Abuse

The term **child abuse** means any improper or excessive action that injures or otherwise harms a child or infant; it includes physical abuse, sexual abuse, neglect, and emotional abuse. The intentional injury of a child, whether physical or emotional, is not rare in our society. More than 2 million cases of child abuse are reported to child protection agencies annually. Many of these children suffer life-threatening injuries, and some die. If suspected child abuse is not reported, the child is likely

SkillDrill 33-1 Immobilizing a Child

Use a towel under the shoulders to maintain the head in neutral position.

Apply an appropriately sized cervical collar.

Log roll the child onto the immobilization device.

Secure the torso first.

Secure the head.

Ensure that the child is strapped in properly.

Skill Drill 33-2 Immobilization of an Infant

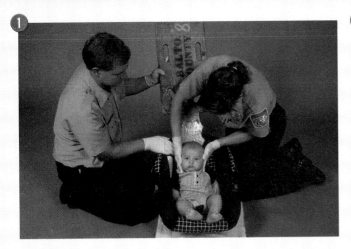

Stabilize the head in neutral position.

Place an immobilization device between the patient and the surface he or she is resting on.

Slide the infant onto the board.

Place a towel under the shoulders to ensure neutral head position.

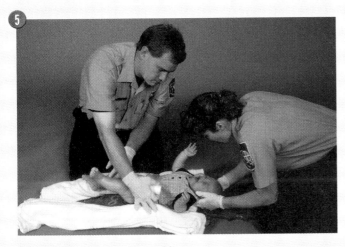

Secure the torso first; pad any voids.

Secure the head.

to be abused again and again, perhaps suffering permanent injuries or even dying. Therefore, you must be aware of the signs of child abuse and neglect, and of your responsibility to report suspected abuse to law enforcement or child protection agencies.

Signs of Abuse

As an EMT-B, you will be called to homes because of a reported injury to a child. If you suspect that physical or sexual abuse is involved, you should ask yourself the following questions:

- Is the injury typical for the developmental level of the child?
- Is the method of injury reported by the parent or caregiver consistent with the child's injuries?
- Is the caregiver behaving appropriately (concerned about the child's well-being)?
- Is there evidence of drinking or drug use at the scene?
- Was there a delay in seeking care for the child?
- Is there a good relationship between the child and the caregiver?
- Does the child have multiple injuries at different stages of healing?
- Does the child have any unusual marks or bruises that may have been caused by cigarettes, grids, or branding injuries?
- Does the child have several types of injuries, such as burns, fractures, and bruises?
- Does the child have any burns on the hands or feet that involve a glove distribution (marks that encircle a hand or foot in a pattern that looks like a glove)?
- Is there an unexplained decreased level of consciousness?
- Is the child clean and an appropriate weight for his or her age?
- Is there any rectal or vaginal bleeding?
- What does the home look like? Clean or dirty? Is it warm or cold? Is there food?

Your assessment in the field will allow a better assessment by the medical staff later. An easy way to remember these is the mnemonic CHILD ABUSE shown in (▲ **Table 33-2**).

As you assess the child, look for and pay particular attention to the following signs (▶ **Figure 33-10**).

BRUISES. Observe the color and location of any bruises. New bruises are pink or red. Over time, bruises turn blue, then green, then yellow-brown and faded. Note the location. Bruises to the back, buttocks, or face are suspicious and are usually inflicted by a person.

Table 33-2 CHILD ABUSE Mnemonic for Assessing Possible Child Abuse
Consistency of the injury with the child's developmental age
History inconsistent with injury
Inappropriate parental concerns
Lack of supervision
Delay in seeking care
Affect
Bruises of varying ages
Unusual injury patterns
Suspicious circumstances
Environmental clues

Figure 33-10 Signs of child abuse. **A.** Scald. **B.** Multiple injuries at different stages of healing.

BURNS. Burns to the penis, testicles, vagina, or buttocks are usually inflicted by someone else, as are burns that encircle a hand or foot to look like a glove. You should suspect abuse if the child has cigarette burns or grid pattern burns.

FRACTURES. Fractures of the humerus or femur do not normally occur without major trauma, such as a fall from a high place or a motor vehicle crash. Falls from bed are not usually associated with fractures.

SHAKEN BABY SYNDROME. Infants may sustain life-threatening head trauma by being shaken or struck on the head, a life-threatening condition called **shaken**

baby syndrome. With this condition, there is bleeding within the head and damage to the cervical spine as a result of intentional, forceful shaking. The infant will be found unconscious, often without evidence of external trauma. The call for help may be for an infant who has stopped breathing or is unresponsive. The infant may appear to be in cardiopulmonary arrest, but what has likely occurred is that the shaking tore blood vessels in the brain, resulting in bleeding around the brain. The pressure from the blood results in a coma.

NEGLECT. Children who are neglected are often dirty or too thin or appear developmentally delayed because of lack of stimulation. You may observe such children when you are making calls for unrelated problems. Report all cases of suspicious neglect.

Symptoms and Other Indicators of Abuse

An abused child may appear withdrawn, fearful, or hostile. You should be particularly concerned if the child refuses to discuss how an injury occurred. Occasionally, the parent or caregiver will reveal a history of several "accidents." Be alert for conflicting stories or a marked lack of concern from the parents or caregiver. Remember, the abuser may be a parent, caregiver, relative, or friend of the family. Sometimes the abuser is an acquaintance of a single parent.

Emergency Medical Care

Your priority is to care for ABCs, as in all other instances. Care for all wounds, splint fractures, and keep the infant or child warm and comfortable. Provide transport in all instances in which you suspect abuse has occurred. You are not there to solve the problem or to accuse a parent or caregiver. In fact, you need their cooperation, as you cannot transport a child without consent from the parent or guardian. Sometimes, you can persuade a parent to allow transport if you say that the child may need special X-rays or tests. If the parent still refuses and you are concerned about the child's well-being, consult law enforcement.

EMT-Bs in all states must report all cases of suspected abuse, even if the emergency department fails to do so. Most states have special forms for reporting. Supervisors are generally forbidden to interfere with the reporting of suspected abuse, even if they disagree with the assessment. You do not have to prove that there has been abuse. Law enforcement and child protection agencies are mandated to investigate all reported cases.

Sexual Abuse

Children of any age and either gender can be victims of sexual abuse. Most victims of rape are older than age 10 years, although younger children may be victims as well. This type of sexual abuse is often the result of longstanding abuse by relatives.

Your assessment of a child who has been sexually abused should be limited to determining the type of dressing any injuries require. Sometimes, a sexually abused child is also beaten. Therefore, you should treat any bruises or fractures as well. Do not examine the genitalia of a young child unless there is evidence of bleeding, or there is an injury that must be treated.

In addition, if you suspect that a child is a victim of sexual abuse, do not allow the child to wash, urinate, or defecate before a physician completes an exam. Although this step is difficult, it is important to preserve evidence. If the molested child is a girl, ensure that a female EMT or police officer remains with the child unless locating one will delay transport.

You must maintain professional composure the entire time you are assessing and caring for a sexually abused child. Assume a concerned, caring approach, and shield the child from onlookers and curious bystanders. Obtain as much information as possible from the child and any witnesses. The child may be hysterical or unwilling to say anything at all, especially if the abuser is a relative or family friend. You are in the best position to obtain the most accurate firsthand information about the incident. Therefore, you should record any information carefully and completely on the patient care report.

Transport all children who are victims of sexual assault. Sexual abuse of a child is a crime. Cooperate with law enforcement officials in their investigations.

EMS Response to Pediatric Emergencies

After care and transport of a sick or injured child, you may experience a wide range of powerful emotions. These emotions result from the call itself or from your previous experience (or inexperience) in caring for infants and children. You may feel anxious if you have not had much experience in dealing with infants and children. You may also think of your own children or the children of a loved one.

As a result, you must be prepared to care for children. Practice with children and pediatric equipment is necessary. As you know, children are not simply small adults. However, many of the skills and principles you use to care for adults can be applied to children. You must simply remember there are differences in anatomy and emotions.

After difficult incidents involving children, debriefing is helpful in working through the stress and trauma. It is also a means to help you in the future if you are faced with similar situations. The ability to seek help after difficult episodes is a sign of maturity and confidence.

Prep Kit

Ready for Review

For several reasons, you face special challenges when you are called on to care for children who have traumatic injuries. Children are not only smaller than adults and more vulnerable; they are also anatomically, physiologically, and psychologically different from adults in some important ways. You must understand these differences to provide the best possible care for children who have been injured.

You should remember that children's bones are more flexible and bend more with injury and that the ends of the long bones, where growth occurs, are weaker and may be injured more easily. Children's heads are proportionately larger and are more likely to be injured in automobile mishaps. Children's internal organs are not as insulated by fat and may be injured more severely, and children have less circulating blood, so that, although children exhibit the signs of shock more slowly, they go into shock faster. Children are not always as cautious as adults and tend to have more accidental poisoning, diving, and bicycle injuries.

If you cannot effectively ventilate a victim of submersion, consider the possibility of a foreign body airway obstruction, as water alone does not obstruct the airway. If permitted, use a nasogastric tube to protect the airway in unresponsive patients who have been submersed.

You should also remember that infants and small children cannot communicate the source or cause of their injuries, and children of any age and background are at risk for child abuse and neglect.

There is rarely anything more satisfying than helping or saving the life of an injured child, but injured children who are unconscious or in pain can be difficult. Therefore, you must always be prepared emotionally to care for children who have been injured and seek counseling or debriefing if necessary after caring for a traumatically injured child.

Vital Vocabulary

child abuse Any improper or excessive action that injures or otherwise harms a child or infant; includes neglect and physical, sexual, and emotional abuse.

hyperventilation Rapid or deep breathing that lowers blood carbon dioxide levels below normal.

pneumatic antishock garment (PASG) An inflatable device that covers the legs and abdomen; used to splint the lower extremities or pelvis, or to control bleeding in lower extremities, pelvis, or abdominal cavity.

shaken baby syndrome Bleeding within the head and damage to the cervical spine of an infant who has been intentionally and forcibly shaken; a form of child abuse.

Assessment in Action

You are called to the scene of a motor vehicle crash involving a 5-year-old who was unrestrained. The child was ejected from the vehicle and flew approximately 20 ft and landed in the median. She is pale but awake and lying still. She does not respond to voice and withdraws her arms to a pinch. Her skin is pale, cool, and dry. Her vital signs include a pulse of 160 beats/min and respirations of 40 breaths/min. She has abrasions the length of the right side of her face and down her right arm and right leg. Her pants are torn on the right side as is her shirt. There are intercostal and supraclavicular retractions noted.

1. Your first priority for treatment is to:
   A. oxygenate and ensure adequate ventilations.
   B. take a blood pressure.
   C. immobilize her on a long backboard.
   D. place a c-collar.

2. Which of the following statements regarding her mental status would be appropriate to suspect?
   A. She is scared and frightened.
   B. She may have a head injury.
   C. She is shy and normally quiet.
   D. She may be pouting.

3. Your partner takes her blood pressure and states that he thinks she just has some bad scrapes because her pressure is 86/42 mm Hg. Which of the following statements is most accurate concerning her blood pressure?
   A. Children have more efficient body systems so blood pressure is a sensitive indicator of blood volume.
   B. Because children have a lower blood volume, even small changes are quickly noticed by falling blood pressure.
   C. Because children have more total body water, blood pressure is maintained longer.
   D. Children can lose a greater proportion of their blood volume before hypotension develops.

4. During your initial assessment you noted the intercostal and supraclavicular retractions and you observed equal chest rise and fall. Her lung sounds were equal and clear. Those retractions suggest what type of problem?
   A. A cardiac injury
   B. Broken ribs
   C. Flail chest
   D. Lung injury

5. The best way to manage this child's airway is to:
   A. find out if she has a prescribed inhaler.
   B. apply a nasal cannula at 4 to 6 L/min.
   C. apply a nonrebreathing mask.
   D. sit her up to ease her breathing.

6. Because she has abrasions down the entire right side of her body, it would be appropriate to suspect that internal bleeding would most likely involve organs on that side. Which of the following organs are located on that side?
   A. Spleen
   B. Liver
   C. Pancreas
   D. Thymus

7. You are palpating the pelvis and legs of your patient and suspect a pelvic fracture. Appropriate treatment includes:
   A. applying the PASG, inflating all three compartments.
   B. placing her in one leg of the PASG and inflating.
   C. keeping her immobilized on the backboard.
   D. using the pediatric traction splint.

8. Your detailed physical exam includes pupil size and reaction. In this case, her pupil size and reaction will help indicate if:
   A. shock is present.
   B. a head injury is present.
   C. she is alert and oriented.
   D. she has a skull fracture.

Challenging Questions

9. During your detailed exam of her head, you note clear fluid coming from her right ear. This indicates:
   A. water was spilled.
   B. this is a non-trauma problem.
   C. a basilar skull fracture.
   D. she ruptured the globe of her eye.

10. When trying to assess perfusion in this patient, when should capillary refill be assessed?
    A. As soon as possible at the scene
    B. As soon as possible inside the rescue squad
    C. When she starts responding
    D. When she is warm

Points to Ponder

You arrive at the scene of an auto-pedestrian accident involving a 5-year-old girl. Your assessment finds her to be unresponsive, with multiple small wounds and contusions. She has a large contusion on her left hip and you suspect spinal injury. When you go for the pediatric spinal immobilization equipment you find it missing. You want to wait for another ambulance to bring the proper equipment but you partner wants to load and go. What are the risks of using equipment that is too large? What are the risks of waiting for the proper equipment? How would you decide which to do? What if you and your partner cannot agree on what to do?

Issues Decision-Making Skills, Partner-to-Partner Communication, Problems Without Clear Answers, Pre-shift Equipment Check.

Online Outlook

The treatment priorities in children who sustain serious trauma are similar to those in adults—the stabilization of the child and management of life-threatening injuries. To learn more about the diagnosis and treatment of pediatric trauma, complete Exercise 33 at www.emtb.com.

www.emtb.com

Geriatric Assessment

TECHNOLOGY

www.emtb.com

- Online Chapter Pretest
- Interactivities
- Vocabulary Explorer
- Anatomy Review
- Web Links
- Online Review Manual
- Distance Learning

Chapter FEATURES

- Skill Drills
- Vital Vocabulary
- Pediatric Needs
- Geriatric Needs
- EMT-B Safety
- EMT-B Tips
- Documentation Tips
- Remember
- Prep Kit

"Squad 11, see the woman in apartment 2D at the Soundview Apartments. Her husband has fallen in the shower and she can't get him up."

Falls involving the elderly are very common, and unfortunately are often a pivotal event that signals a decline in their health and wellness. With the aging and graying of America comes a proportionate increase in this group's use of the EMS system.

This chapter will help you understand the unique aspects of assessing the elderly as well as when you transfer/transport them. It will also help you answer the following questions:

1. Can you name at least three areas that differentiate elderly care from that of routine adult care?

2. What are some of the common challenges encountered when transferring the elderly to or from an extended care facility?

Geriatric Assessment

Geriatric or elderly patients are individuals who are older than 65 years. It stands to reason that we do not age overnight. A decline in our body systems starts in our late 20s and progresses slowly throughout our lifespan. We use the age of 65 in order to be consistent with other medical groups and governmental agencies. No one relishes the thought of growing old, but the reality is that we all will, and the elderly will continue to grow into a larger percentage of the population in the new century. According to US Census Data, almost 35 million individuals are older than 65 years. It is projected that by the year 2030, the elderly population will be greater than 70 million. This is a very significant evolutionary trend for the EMT-B because the elderly are major users of the EMS and health care systems in general. These calls may be confusing to the EMT-B because the "classic" presentation of medical conditions common in younger patients may not be presented. An acute MI may present as jaw or neck pain, and some older patients may not experience chest pain at all. Their aging body can mask serious medical conditions. Elderly patients frequently have chronic medical problems and may be taking numerous medications for their illnesses. Providing effective treatment for this growing number of patients will require that all EMT-Bs understand the issues related to aging and that they modify some of their assessment and treatment approaches.

While many EMT-Bs may relish the action of high-profile calls, the reality is that a large percentage of your patient contacts will involve the elderly. Lifesaving interventions for geriatric patients may include reviewing the home environment to assure safe and liveable conditions exist, providing information on preventing falls, and making referrals to appropriate social services agencies when needed. EMT-Bs who respond to the homes of elderly patients are in an ideal position not only to provide immediate help, but also to provide key information to others in the health care and social services systems. Often, simple preventive measures can help the elderly to avoid further injury, costly medical treatment, and death. The EMT-B is on the front line in helping to prevent and care for geriatric emergencies.

Leading Causes of Death

The leading causes of death in the elderly include heart disease, cancer, stroke, diabetes, and trauma. The aging physiology of the elderly makes them more vulnerable to the affects of disease and injury than a younger individual. In addition, acute illness and trauma are more likely to involve organ systems beyond those initially involved. For example, an elderly patient who has fallen and fractured a hip may develop pneumonia during his recovery.

▶ **Table 34-1** shows the risk factors that affect mortality in elderly patients.

Physiologic Changes That Accompany Age

As we get older, our physiology changes. In general, a 65-year-old person cannot expect to have the same degree of physical performance as when he or she was 30 years old. By the time a person reaches age 65 years, the amount of total body water and the number of total body cells have decreased by as much as 30%. Generally, after age 30 years, organ systems

Table 34-1 Risk Factors Affecting Mortality in Elderly Patients

- Age greater than 75 years
- Living alone
- Recent death of a significant other
- Recent hospitalization
- Incontinence (inability to hold urine or feces)
- Immobility
- Unsound mind

begin to deteriorate at roughly 1% per year. However, the aging process does not necessarily mean disease.

Common stereotypes about the elderly include the presence of mental confusion, illness, a sedentary lifestyle, and immobility. Although these perceptions are common, they are usually very far from the norm. The elderly can continue to stay fit and active even though they will not be able to perform at the same level as they did in their youth ▶ Figure 34-1 . Most elderly individuals lead very active lives, participating in sports and in the community, and they are generally healthy in spite of the aging process. What happens when we age?

Skin

Collagen, a protein that is the chief component of connective tissue and bones, is lost as we age, making the skin wrinkled, thinner, and more susceptible to injury. Because the elasticity of the skin has declined, bruising becomes more common because the skin cannot constrict and stop the bleeding as quickly. This causes a greater number of bruises and more that are larger from minimal trauma. There are also fewer sweat glands, and older skin feels dry. Less fat rests under the skin, making pressure sores more common in the elderly bed bound patient. These sores are made by the patient lying in the same position for a long period of time, allowing the body to cut off the blood flow to an area of skin, which in turn lets the skin die and a sore to develop.

Senses

The pupils of the eyes begin to lose the ability to handle changes in light and require more time to adjust, which can make driving and walking more hazardous. Light changes can cause problems of visual acuity and depth perception. Cataracts, clouding of the lenses or their surrounding membranes, interfere with vision and make it difficult to distinguish colors and see clearly, increasing the likelihood of falls and accidents, and account for some mistakes in taking various medications. Changes in the inner ear make hearing high-frequency sounds difficult; these changes can also cause problems with balance and make falls more likely. Changes in appetite may occur because of a decrease in the number of taste buds. The sense of touch lessens from loss of the end nerve fibers. This loss, in conjunction with the slowing of the peripheral nervous system, can create situations where an elderly person can have a delayed reaction when touching something hot, resulting in a burn.

Respiratory System

Although the alveoli become enlarged, their elasticity decreases, making it harder to expel the used air in an elderly person's lung tissue. This lack of elasticity results in a decreased ability to exchange oxygen and carbon dioxide. The body's receptors that monitor the changes in oxygen and carbon dioxide slow with age, which causes lower pulse oximetry readings even in healthy individuals. A decrease in the number of cilia that line the bronchial tree lessens the ability to cough and therefore increases the chances of infection. A patient who is having trouble breathing may get less

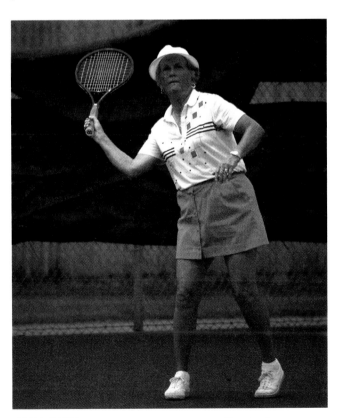

Figure 34-1 The elderly can continue to stay fit and active.

help from muscles in the chest wall because of the decrease in muscle mass that accompanies aging.

Cardiovascular System

Cardiac output is a measure of the workload of the heart. We normally compensate for an increased demand on the cardiovascular system by increasing our heart rate, increasing the contraction of the heart, and constricting the blood vessels to nonvital organs. Aging decreases a person's ability to speed up contractions, to increase contraction strength, and to constrict, or narrow, blood vessels (called **vasoconstriction**) because of stiffer vessels. Many elderly patients are at risk for **atherosclerosis**, an accumulation of fatty material in the arteries. Major complications of atherosclerosis include myocardial infarction and stroke. The presence of **arteriosclerosis**, a disease that causes the arteries to thicken, harden, and calcify, makes stroke, heart disease, hypertension, and bowel infarction more likely. The elderly are also at an increased risk for **aneurysm**, an abnormal, blood-filled dilation of the wall of a blood vessel. Severe blood loss occurs when an aneurysm bursts.

Renal System

Kidney function in the elderly declines because of a 30% to 40% decrease in nephron function, the working part of the kidney. The kidneys are important in eliminating certain medications from a person's system. With a decrease in renal function, levels of medications may rise, creating the impression of an overdose. Electrolyte disturbances are also more likely to occur with the lowered filtering of the blood.

Nervous System

The number of brain cells in some areas may decrease by as much as 45%. By age 85, a 10% reduction in brain weight can result in increased risk of head trauma. Short-term memory impairment, a decrease in the ability to perform psychomotor skills, and slower reflex times are all normal in the aging process. This decline may make assessment of the older patient challenging. It is important to compare the older patients' current status with their normal abilities.

Musculoskeletal System

The disks between the vertebrae begin to narrow, and a decrease in height of between 2″ and 3″ may occur through the lifespan. A decrease in the amount of muscle mass often results in less strength, and fractures are more likely to occur because of a decrease in bone density also known as osteoporosis. Posture also changes as flexion at the neck and a forward curling of

> Generally, after age 30 years, organ systems begin to deteriorate at roughly 1% per year.

the shoulders produce a condition called *kyphosis* (also called *humpback, hunchback,* or *Pott's curvature*), making immobilization of the elderly more challenging.

Gastrointestinal System

A decrease in the volume of saliva and gastric juices causes a dry mouth, making it harder to chew and begin to digest foods. A slowing of the intestinal tract may cause constipation or bowel impaction. Decreased liver function makes it harder to detoxify the blood and eliminate substances such as medications and alcohol. This can make it difficult for patients and their physician to find the appropriate dosage when taking new medications.

Patient Assessment

Any time you assess a patient, you use the same basic approach: scene size-up, initial assessment, and a focused history and physical exam. Assessing an elderly patient is really no different. However, there are some issues that may indicate that you should modify your approach to the initial assessment or become more aware of some conditions that may affect the elderly patient.

Scene Size-Up

As you approach any scene, you must be keenly aware of the environment and the reason you were called. Activities of daily living such as the ability to move around, talk on the telephone, prepare and eat meals, perform basic cleaning skills, and attend to personal hygiene are essential for continued health in all individuals. For the elderly, normal aging or a disease process may make activities of daily living difficult and cause a cascade of problems. For example, suppose that a 70-year-old woman who trips on a loose carpet, falls, and breaks her hip. She lives alone and has no one to help her with cooking and other daily activities. Her hip is treated, but in the following months of therapy, she fears the thought of falling again and does as little as she can. She becomes weaker and begins to have some difficulty walking, lifting even small objects, shopping, and making meals. She loses some weight and becomes

Figure 34-2 Interview family members, friends, and caregivers as part of your assessment of an elderly patient.

weaker and is eventually forced to move to an adult care facility because of her need for constant help. All this was the result of a simple fall.

When you first arrive at a patient's residence, you should look for important clues to determine not only your safety, but also that of the occupant. The environment will provide a great deal of important information if you know what to look for.

The general condition of the home will give you some important clues. Are there hazards, such as steep stairs, missing handrails, or other things that could cause a fall? Is it evident that the person may be having difficulty keeping the house clean? Is there evidence of adequate food, water, heat, lights, and ventilation? Are there many pill bottles around, indicating treatment for some type of disease process? Does someone else live there who can help to answer questions? These are very important scene clues that can provide much information before you even contact the patient.

Initial Assessment

The sequence of the initial assessment is the same for pediatric, adult, and geriatric patients. However, you should not make any assumptions about an elderly patient's level of consciousness. Never assume that an altered mental status is normal. Altered mental status indicates some level of brain dysfunction and is a serious problem. The best rule of thumb is to always compare the patient's current level of consciousness or ability to function with the level or ability before the problem began. Do not assume that confusion or unresponsiveness is normal behavior for anyone. In many cases, you will have to rely on a family member or caregiver to help establish what the patient's baseline level

of consciousness was before the complaint began.
◄ Figure 34-2.

During the initial assessment, you will assess the patient's chief complaint and ABCs. If a life-threatening condition exists, you will have to perform emergency treatment before continuing your assessment. The initial assessment sets the tone and helps you to decide whether the patient requires a rapid resuscitative approach or a slower, contemplative one. In most cases, the slower, contemplative approach is all that is needed.

Focused History and Physical Exam

It is often said that 80% of a medical diagnosis is based on the patient's history. The history is usually the key in helping to assess a patient's problem. In addition to clearing the airway and managing the ABCs, obtaining a thorough history is one of the most important things you can do. An inaccurate or inadequate history can cause you to make incorrect presumptions and pursue a flawed treatment plan.

To obtain an accurate history, patience and good communication skills are essential. An elderly patient's diminished sight, hearing, and speaking ability may hamper communications ▼ Figure 34-3. If possible, take a few moments to have the patient put in his

Figure 34-3 As you assess an elderly patient, make eye contact, and grasp the patient's hand to feel for temperature, grip, and skin condition.

dentures, glasses, or hearing aid. All of these items can help the patient to communicate with you more effectively.

A poor history-gathering technique can hamper communications. You must be able to gain a patient's confidence, which is best accomplished by treating the patient with respect, taking a slow deliberate approach, and explaining what you are doing. First, ask the patient what his or her name is, and then address the patient using courtesy titles, such as "Mr.," "Mrs.," or "Ms.," and his or her last name. Avoid being overly familiar with the patient, and do not use first names or nicknames unless the patient asks you to.

When there are multiple responders everyone asks questions, sometimes several at a time. This is a poor technique that results in a haphazard history regardless of the patient's age. For elderly patients who may have communication or perceptual problems, it makes obtaining a thorough or SAMPLE history almost impossible. In addition, many individuals are reluctant to discuss their problems in front of a crowd. Be sure to have one EMT-B obtain the patient's history, one question at a time, providing as much privacy as possible
▼ Figure 34-4 .

When speaking to an elderly patient, bend down so that you are eye to eye with the patient. Be sure that the patient can see your face. A patient that has difficulty hearing will often look for clues in the speaker's face to assist in understanding the subject matter. Turn on a light if you are in a dimly lit room. Turn off any TVs or radios that are on. Use a normal tone of voice, especially if the patient is wearing a hearing aid. A loud tone may

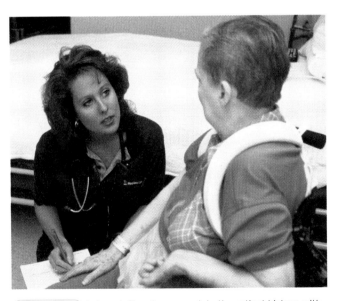

Figure 34-4 A slow, deliberate approach to the patient history, with one EMT-B asking the questions, is generally the best strategy in assessing an elderly patient.

actually cause sound distortion in the hearing aid and make communication worse. Ask as many open-ended questions as possible, and use closed-ended questions to clarify points. It is better to ask "please tell me about the pain you are feeling" rather than "is the pain sharp or dull?" While taking the history, write down any key points on a notepad so that you do not ask the same question repeatedly because you forgot the answer. After interviewing the patient, ask family members or caregivers to clarify what you just learned from the patient. Be careful not to offend the patient. Taking a few minutes to obtain an accurate history saves time in the long run by providing information on which accurate decisions can be based.

Past medical conditions can provide information about the patient's current problem. Elderly patients often suffer from more than one disease process at a time, and the symptoms of one disease may make the assessment of another more difficult.

Elderly patients are often prescribed multiple medications. A condition known as polypharmacy is common in the elderly. Elderly patients often seek medical care from multiple doctors and may feel embarassed to tell one what another has prescribed. This can lead to the patient taking the same drug twice. This can be even more difficult when the bottles are marked with different names for the same medication. Obtain a list of medications and dosages. Information about which medications are currently being taken is vital. In addition, find out whether the patient has recently started or stopped taking any of the medications, is taking any over the counter medications or has taken any "home remedies." Medication interactions and noncompliance with instructions for taking prescribed drugs are common and may contribute to the patient's symptoms or problem.

Be aware that the sensation of pain may be diminished in an elderly patient, leading you to underestimate the severity of a condition. This is associated with the aging nervous system. For example, 20% to 30% of elderly patients have "silent" heart attacks, without the typical symptom of chest pain. In addition, fear of hospitalization often causes the patient to either understate or minimize symptoms.

During the focused physical examination, be aware that elderly people are more prone to hypothermia than younger people are. Be sure to keep the patient warm and maintain the body temperature. Inspection and palpation can be hampered by multiple layers of clothing. Remove only the clothing that is necessary for examining the patient, and cover the patient back up when you are finished.

Response to Nursing and Skilled Care Facilities

Responding to a nursing home or skilled care facility is a common patient contact for EMT-Bs. Before you provide transport for the patient, you should find out the following critical information from the nursing staff:

- What is the patient's chief complaint today?
- What initial problem caused the patient to be admitted to the facility?

To determine the nature of the problem, you will usually have to compare the patient's present condition with his or her condition before onset of the symptoms. Ask the staff about the patient's mobility, activities of daily living, and ability to speak. This will help to paint a picture of the patient's baseline condition and indicate whether today's behavior differs from it.

Many facilities that are transferring patients will include a transfer record that contains the patient's history, medication lists and dosages, previous diagnosis, vital signs, allergies, and more ▼ Figure 34-5 . These records provide members of the medical team with essential information and save time, especially when

the patient cannot speak for himself or herself. Be sure to obtain this essential record before leaving for the hospital, and relay it to the hospital staff when giving your report.

Trauma
Mechanism of Injury

Falls are the leading cause of trauma, death, and disability in the elderly. Most patients survive; however, a significant number require hospitalization. Motor vehicle trauma is the second leading cause of trauma death in the geriatric population. An elderly patient is five times more likely than a younger patient to be fatally injured in a car crash, even though excessive speed is rarely a causative factor in the older age group. Pedestrian accidents and burns are also common mechanisms of injury in elderly patients, resulting in death, serious injury, or disability.

Systemic Impact of Aging and Trauma

You must consider the body's decreasing ability to isolate simple trauma when you are assessing and caring for an elderly patient. An isolated hip fracture in a

Figure 34-5 A transfer record from a long-term care facility contains vital information for members of the medical team.

A cleaning service and a social worker sent by the city find an 80-year-old man, John, frozen to death in his second-floor apartment. For months, John's neighbors tried to help him because he did not seem to be able to care for himself. Neighbors gave him money for food and ran an extension cord to his apartment when his electricity was turned off. When John was found dead, the radiator in his apartment was working, but most of the heat was being lost through a broken window. The apartment was so cold that a half-empty can of beer near the window was frozen. Filthy clothing and sheets, soiled mattresses, and paint chips littered the apartment.

Jane is a 75-year-old woman with Alzheimer's disease who is confined to her apartment, where she lives with her husband, son, and daughter-in-law, Gail. Gail works full time as a waitress and provides most of Jane's support. Jane's 77-year-old husband, Bob, is retired and is a chronic alcohol abuser with a history of violence directed at his family. One morning, a neighbor sees a chair crash through the kitchen window and calls the police. The police find Gail unconscious on the kitchen floor and Jane bound and gagged on a mattress in the bedroom. Feces and urine are all over Jane's body. EMTs arriving at the scene find that the bed springs have broken Jane's skin. She also appears extremely malnourished and dehydrated.

Do you think John or Jane have been victims of elder abuse? Why or why not?

healthy 25-year-old adult is rarely associated with systemic decline. However, the same injury in an 85-year-old patient can produce a systemic impact that results in deterioration, shock, and life-threatening **hypoxia**, a dangerous condition in which the body tissues and cells do not have enough oxygen. Although an injury may be considered isolated and not alarming in most adults, an elderly patient's overall physical condition may lessen the body's ability to compensate for the effects of even simple injuries. Younger patients have the ability to increase their heart rate, constrict their blood vessels, and breathe faster and deeper to compensate for injuries. The aging body has a heart that can no longer beat faster, vessels that cannot constrict due to atherosclerosis, and lungs that do not exchange oxygen as well.

Your assessment of the patient's condition and stability must include past medical conditions, even if they are not currently acute or symptomatic. For example, suppose you respond to a call about a patient with a history of unstable angina who sustains a simple isolated fracture of the ankle. You must consider this

patient to be unstable and provide prompt transport before the stress and simple trauma worsen the angina and patient instability occurs.

Falls and Trauma

A medical condition such as fainting, a cardiac rhythm disturbance, or a medication interaction may lead to a fall that causes injury to the patient. Whenever you assess an elderly patient who has fallen, it is important to find out why the fall occurred. Was the patient dizzy before the fall? Do they remember the fall? Did a fainting episode cause the fall and injury, or did the patient trip on something or lose his or her balance? Sometimes, a recent history of starting or stopping blood pressure medication is enough to cause a patient to become dizzy and fall. Consider that the fall may have been caused by a medical condition, and look carefully for clues from the patient, bystanders, and the environment. Although the trauma that the patient sustains from the fall can be serious, you should also consider that if a medical condition caused the fall it may continue to be life threatening.

When you respond to a motor vehicle crash, be alert to the possibility that a medical emergency may have caused the accident, especially in single vehicle collisions with no apparent cause.

Because brain tissue shrinks with age, the elderly are more likely to sustain closed head injuries, such as subdural hematomas. These hematomas can go unnoticed because the blood has a void to fill before it can produce pressure in the skull showing the familiar signs of head trauma.

As a result of bone loss from **osteoporosis**, a generalized bone disease that is commonly associated with postmenopausal women, elderly patients of both sexes are prone to fractures, especially in areas such as the hip. With age, the spine stiffens as a result of shrinkage of disk spaces, and vertebrae become brittle. Compression fractures of the spine are more likely to occur.

Because of the amount of flexion that occurs in the spinal column, hip, or knee of elderly patients, use of conventional splints and backboards to immobilize the patient may be difficult or impossible unless a lot of padding is used. What is considered a normal anatomic position for children and adults is often very abnormal for some elderly trauma patients. You should try to determine the patient's baseline condition and what was normal for the patient before the accident. Trying to force a patient with pronounced joint flexion into "normal" anatomic position can be very painful for the

Figure 34-6 Vacuum mattresses that conform to body contours are a good choice for immobilizing the elderly.

patient and frustrating for you. Some devices, such as traction splints, simply do not work on patients with flexed hips and knees. Splinting devices, such as vacuum mattresses that conform to body contours, may be a better choice for immobilization than a conventional backboard ▲ **Figure 34-6** .

Remember that when you treat an elderly trauma patient, you must assess the injuries and carefully look for the cause of the fall or crash.

Cardiovascular Emergencies

Syncope

You should always assume that **syncope**, or fainting, in the elderly is a life-threatening problem until proven otherwise. Syncope is often caused by an interruption of blood flow to the brain. Syncope has many causes; some are serious and others are not. Regardless, an elderly person who has a period of unconsciousness should be examined to determine the cause of the syncope. ▶ **Table 34-2** shows some of the causes of syncope in an elderly patient.

Heart Attack

The classic symptoms of a heart attack are often not present in the elderly. As many as one third of elderly patients have "silent" heart attacks in which the usual chest pain is not present. ▶ **Table 34-3** shows signs and symptoms that are commonly noted in elderly patients who are experiencing a heart attack.

The Acute Abdomen

Because of an aging nervous system, abdominal complaints in the elderly are extremely difficult to assess. A number of life-threatening abdominal problems are common in elderly patients. In the field the one real threat from abdominal complaints is blood loss, which can lead to shock and death. Abdominal aortic aneurysm (AAA) is one of the most rapidly fatal conditions. AAA tends to develop in individuals who have a history of hypertension and atherosclerosis. The walls of the aorta weaken, and blood begins to leak into the layers of the vessel, causing the aorta to bulge like a bubble on a tire. If enough blood is lost into the vessel wall itself, shock occurs. If the wall bursts, it rapidly leads to fatal blood loss. When the problem is caught early, there is a chance to repair the vessel before rupture and fatal blood loss occur.

A patient with an abdominal aortic aneurysm most commonly reports abdominal pain radiating through to the back with occasional flank pain. If the AAA becomes large enough, it can be felt as a pulsating mass just above and slightly to the left of the navel during your physical examination. Occasionally, the AAA causes a decrease in blood flow to one of the legs, and the patient complains of some discomfort in the affected extremity. Assessment may also reveal diminished or absent pulses in the extremity. **Compensated shock** (early shock) and **decompensated shock** (late shock) as a result of blood loss are common occurrences. Because of a decrease in blood volume and decreased blood flow to the brain, the patient may experience syncope. You should treat the patient for shock and provide prompt transport to the hospital.

Another cause of abdominal pain and shock is gastrointestinal bleeding, which can occur for a variety of reasons and is usually heralded by the vomiting of blood or material that looks like coffee grounds. Bleeding that travels through the lower digestive tract is usually manifested by black or tarry stools, while frank red blood usually means a local source of bleeding such as hemorrhoids. A patient with gastrointestinal bleeding may experience weakness, dizziness, or syncope. Bleeding into the gastrointestinal system can be life threatening because of the potential for blood loss and shock.

Bowel obstructions occur frequently in the elderly population. The gastrointestinal tract slows with aging and the patient can experience problems having bowel movements. When these patients go into the bathroom and are straining to have a bowel movement, they can stimulate the vagus nerve and produce a syndrome called vaso-vagal, where the heart rate drops dramati-

Table 34-2 Possible Causes of Syncope in an Elderly Patient

Cardiac Dysrhythmias/ Dysrhythmias/ Heart Attack	The heart is beating too fast or too slowly, the cardiac output drops, and blood flow to the brain is interrupted. A heart attack can also cause syncope.
Vascular and Volume	Medication interactions can cause venous pooling, and **vasodilation**, widening of a blood vessel, results in a drop in blood pressure and inadequate blood flow to the brain. Another cause of syncope can be a drop in blood volume because of hidden bleeding from a condition such as an aneurysm.
Neurologic	A transient ischemic attack or a "brain attack" can sometimes mimic syncope.

Table 34-3 Common Signs and Symptoms of Heart Attack in an Elderly Patient

Dyspnea	**Dyspnea**, the feeling of shortness of breath or difficulty in breathing, is a common complaint in the elderly and is most often associated with heart attack. It is often combined with other symptoms, such as nausea, weakness, and sweating. Chest pain associated with angina typically has an onset during periods of stress or exertion. In the elderly, chest pain is often not present, but exertional dyspnea is. As the disease progresses, dyspnea may have an onset without exertion. Dyspnea in the elderly is often the equivalent of chest pain in younger patients who are having angina or a heart attack. In addition, congestive heart failure and acute pulmonary edema may result from the "silent" heart attack.
A Weak Feeling	Weakness can be caused by many things. However, you should suspect a heart attack in a patient with a sudden onset of weakness. Weakness is often associated with sweating.
Syncope/Confusion/ Altered Mental Status	Syncope can have many causes, and in the elderly, none of these causes should be presumed to be minor. Major life-threatening causes of syncope are often cardiac in origin. Altered mental status is usually a signal of poor blood supply to the brain, often from cardiac dysrhythmia and heart attack.

cally and the patient becomes dizzy or passes out. This patient will usually be stable upon your arrival, but requires transport to rule out other conditions.

Altered Mental Status

Because of our stereotypical perceptions about the elderly, we may expect them to forget names or not be able to remember events or learn new things. However, these types of changes in mental status are not part of the normal aging process. They may be part of a slow deterioration of a condition or a disease of rapid onset, neither of which is normal. To determine the onset of this change in mental status, you must compare the patient's ability to function with that of the recent past. This will help to establish a baseline and give some per-

spective on the onset of the change. The two terms that are often used to describe a change in mental status are "delirium" and "dementia."

Delirium is a change in mental status that is marked by the inability to focus, think logically, and maintain attention. Acute anxiety may be present in addition to the other symptoms. Usually, memory remains mostly intact. Delirium is commonly marked by an acute or recent onset and is a "red flag" for some type of new health problem. Delirium may be caused by tumors, fever, or drug or alcohol intoxication or withdrawal. Delirium can be present from metabolic causes as well. Any time a patient has an acute onset of delirious behavior, you should rapidly assess the patient for the following three conditions:

> Comparing the patient's mental status with that of the recent past will help establish a baseline and give some perspective on the onset of the change.

- Hypoxia
- Hypovolemia
- Hypoglycemia

Any of these three conditions, if left unrecognized or untreated, may be rapidly fatal. Delerium is short in its onset and usually cureable if identified early.

<u>Dementia</u> is the slow onset of progressive disorientation, shortened attention span, and loss of cognitive function. Dementia develops slowly over a period of years rather than a few days. Alzheimer's disease, CVAs, or genetic factors may cause dementia. Dementia is usually considered irreversible and is an expected course of the pathophysiologic neurologic disease process. The patient's history and determination of function in the recent past are key factors in determining the baseline. A demented patient may be experiencing a delerious event. Delirium is caused by emergent problems; dementia is not.

Advance Directives

Many individuals today are making use of <u>advance directives</u>, specific legal papers that direct relatives and caregivers about what kind of medical treatment may be given to patients who cannot speak for themselves. An advance directive is also commonly called a living will. Mentally competent adults and emancipated minors have the right to consent to or decline treatment, provided that they are competent to do so. The definition of competence is often hotly debated, but a person who is older than 18 years of age, alert, and not intoxicated and who understands the consequences of his or her decision is generally deemed competent. Unfortunately, patients who are unconscious or in a medical crisis are not able to inform medical personnel about their wishes to consent to or decline treatment. It is dangerous to take someone else's word for what the patient's wishes are; this is the reason that written advance directives have been developed.

Advance directives may also take the form of "Do Not Resuscitate" (DNR) orders. DNR orders give you permission not to attempt resuscitation for a patient in cardiac arrest. However, for a DNR order to be valid, in general, the patient's medical problems must be clearly stated, and the form must be signed by the patient or legal guardian and by one or more physicians. In most states, the form must be dated within the preceding 12 months. Even in the presence of a DNR order, you are still obligated to provide supportive measures that may include oxygen delivery, pain relief, and comfort when you can. Learn and become familiar with your state laws regarding this issue.

A health care power of attorney is an advance directive that is exercised by an individual who has been authorized by the patient to make medical decisions for the patient. Be sure to follow your service's protocol when faced with any advance directive.

Dealing with advance directives has become more common for EMS providers as more individuals are electing to use hospice services and spend their final days at home. Although advance directives may be in place, family members or caregivers who are faced with the final moments of life or when the patient's condition worsens often become alarmed and call 9-1-1. Family members and caregivers may then become upset when you take resuscitative action and begin transportation to the hospital.

Another common situation is the transportation of patients from nursing facilities. Specific guidelines vary from state to state; however, you should consider the following general guidelines:

- Patients have the right to refuse treatment, including resuscitative efforts, provided that they are able to communicate their wishes.
- A DNR order is valid in a health care facility only if it is in the form of a written order by a physician.
- You should periodically review state and local protocols and legislation regarding advance directives.
- When you are in doubt or when there are no written orders, you should try to resuscitate the patient.

It is absolutely essential that every EMT-B becomes familiar with his or her state regulations regarding advance directives. Every service should also provide additional training on the actions you should take when presented with advance directives. When in doubt, your best course of action is to take resuscitative action that is appropriate to the situation and to practice sound medical treatment.

Elder Abuse

Reports and complaints of abuse, neglect, and other related problems among the nation's elderly are on the rise. **Elder abuse** is defined as any action on the part of an elderly individual's family member, caregiver, or other associated person that takes advantage of the elderly individual's person, property, or emotional state; it is also called granny beating or parent battering.

The exact extent of elder abuse is not known for several reasons, including the following:

- Elder abuse is a problem that has been largely hidden from society.

- The definitions of abuse and neglect among the elderly vary.

- Victims of elder abuse are often hesitant to report the problem to law enforcement agencies or human and social welfare personnel.

A parent who feels ashamed or guilty because he or she raised the abuser is a typical victim of elder abuse. The abused individual may also feel traumatized by the situation or be afraid that the abuser will try to get back at him or her. In some areas of the country, there is a lack of formal reporting mechanisms, and some states lack statutory provisions that require that elder abuse be reported.

The physical and emotional signs of abuse, such as rape, spouse beating, or nutritional deprivation, are often overlooked or not accurately identified. Older women in particular are not likely to report incidents of sexual assault to law enforcement agencies. Patients with sensory deficits, senility, and other forms of altered mental status, such as drug-induced depression, may not be able to report abuse.

Elder abuse occurs most often in women older than 75 years of age. The abused person is often frail with multiple chronic medical conditions, has dementia, and may suffer from an impaired sleep cycle, sleepwalking, and periods of shouting at others. The individual may be incontinent and in general is dependent on others for activities of daily living.

Abusers of the elderly are often products of child abuse themselves, and the abuse that is inflicted upon the elderly may be a retaliatory matter. Most of these abusers are not trained in the particular care that the elderly require and have little relief time from the constant care demands of their own family, children, and spouse. Their lives are now complicated by the often less-than-flexible elderly individual they have to care for.

The abuser may also suffer from marked fatigue, be unemployed with financial difficulties, and be a substance abuser. With a careful eye, the EMT-B can recognize the clues to these stressful situations and help guide the family toward programs in their community that are geared to helping the whole family. Programs such as adult daycare, meals on wheels, or many local individualized programs help to decrease the stress put on the family and lower the chances of abuse.

Abuse is not restricted to the home; environments such as nursing, convalescent, and continuing care centers are also sites where the elderly sustain physical, psychological, or pharmacologic harm. Often, care providers in these environments consider the elderly to represent management problems or categorize them as obstinate and undesirable patients.

Assessment of Elder Abuse

While assessing the patient, you should try to obtain an explanation of what happened. You should suspect abuse when answers to questions about what caused the injury are concealed or avoided.

You must also suspect abuse when you are given unbelievable answers from anyone other than the patient, the possible abuser, or significant witnesses. You should be suspicious if you think "Does this make sense?" or "Do I really believe this story?" while reviewing the patient's history. If you see burns, especially cigarette burns or physical marks that indicate that certain parts of the patient's body have been scalded systematically, you must also suspect abuse. As an EMT-B, you may be the first health care provider to observe the signs of possible abuse. Information that may be important in assessing possible abuse includes the following:

- Repeated visits to the emergency department or clinic

- A history of being "accident prone"

- Soft-tissue injuries

- Unbelievable or vague explanations of injuries

- Psychosomatic complaints

- Chronic pain

- Self-destructive behavior

- Eating and sleep disorders

- Depression or a lack of energy

- Substance and/or sexual abuse

Table 34-4 Categories of Elder Abuse

Physical	• Assault • Neglect • Dietary • Poor maintenance of home • Poor personal care
Psychological	• Benign neglect • Verbal • Being treated as an infant • Deprivation of sensory stimulation
Financial	• Theft of valuables • Embezzlement

Documentation Tips

As with other legally complex and emotionally charged issues, the possibility of elder abuse demands particularly careful documentation. Be thorough, objective, and factual, avoiding unsupported opinions and personal judgments. You may be called on to explain your report in a legal proceeding.

You should remember that many patients who are being abused are so afraid of retribution that they make false statements. An elderly patient who is being abused by family members may lie about the origin of abuse for fear of being thrown out of the home. In other cases of elder abuse, sensory deprivation or dementia may hinder adequate explanation.

In addition to the lifesaving care that you can provide the patient, your examination of the patient can help to reduce further trauma from abuse through its very identification. Repeated abuse can lead to a high risk of death. A preventive measure in reducing additional maltreatment of the patient is identification of the abuse by emergency medical providers. This may allow for referral and protective services of human, social, and public safety agencies ▲ Table 34-4 .

Signs of Physical Abuse

Signs of abuse may be quite obvious or subtle. Inflicted bruises are usually found on the buttocks and lower back, genitals and inner thighs, cheeks or earlobes, upper lip and inside the mouth, and neck. Pressure bruises caused by the human hand may be identified by oval grab marks, pinch marks, or hand prints. Human bites are typically inflicted on the upper extremities and can cause lacerations, and infection. You should inspect the patient's ears for indications of twisting, pulling, or pinching or evidence of frequent blows to the outer ears.

You should also investigate multiple bruises in various states of healing by questioning the patient and reviewing the patient's activities of daily living.

Burns are a common form of abuse. Typical abuse from burns are caused by contact with cigarettes, matches, heated metal, forced immersion in hot liquids, chemicals, and electrical power sources.

It may be difficult to see a failure to thrive in an elderly patient who has been abused. You should observe the patient's weight and try to determine whether the patient appears undernourished or has been unable to gain weight in the current environment. Does the patient have a ravenous appetite? Has medication been withheld? Is money being withheld, so the patient cannot buy food or medicine? You should also check for signs of neglect, such as evidence of a lack of hygiene, poor dental hygiene, poor temperature regulation, or lack of reasonable amenities in the home.

You must regard injuries to the genitals or rectum with no reported trauma as evidence of sexual abuse in any patient. Elderly patients with altered mental status may never be able to report sexual abuse. In addition, many women do not report cases of sexual abuse because of shame and the pressure to forget.

Prep Kit

Ready for Review

Management of elderly patients can present you with many challenges that are not encountered with younger patients and confront you with a host of different problems that may be quite difficult and frustrating to solve. The health problems of the elderly are multifaceted, and frequent barriers to communication can be expected. In managing the elderly patient, things may not always be what they seem.

Although assessment of the elderly patient involves the same basic approach as with any other patient, you must take a more wary approach to the elderly patient. To obtain an adequate history and physical exam will require patience on the part of the EMT-B but it will be time well spent. The injury or medical condition may be worse than is indicated by the existing signs and symptoms, and the injuries and conditions that are found will have a more profound effect than they would in a younger patient. In addition to the critical needs that an underlying medical problem may cause, the elderly patient is more unstable than a younger patient and has an increased possibility for sudden rapid deterioration.

The exact extent of elder abuse is not known because many patients do not report it. Abusers are often family members who must care for the elderly person in addition to caring for their own spouses and children. Elder abuse also occurs in nursing, convalescent, and continuing care centers. Elder abuse can be gruesome, vulgar, and barbaric; however, your responsibility is to provide lifesaving care to the patient and try to reduce additional abuse through identification of the problem.

Whether because of better medical care, genetics, or some other factor, the elderly patient you are caring for has survived. Growing old is not easy, and neither is the emergency medical care of the elderly patient. You must be careful to obtain an accurate history of the patient, be compassionate, and communicate your findings effectively. The duty that we owe to our elders should be no less than we would expect in our golden years.

Vital Vocabulary

advance directives Written documentation that specifies medical treatment for a competent patient should he or she become unable to make decisions.

aneurysm An abnormal, blood-filled dilation of a blood vessel.

atherosclerosis The most common form of arteriosclerosis in which fatty material is deposited and accumulates in the innermost layer of medium- and large-sized arteries.

arteriosclerosis A disease that is characterized by hardening, thickening, and calcification of the arterial walls.

cataract Clouding of the lens of the eye or its surrounding transparent membrane.

collagen A protein that is the chief component of connective tissue and bones.

compensated shock Early shock.

decompensated shock Late shock.

delirium A change in mental status marked by the inability to focus, think logically, and maintain attention.

dementia The slow onset of progressive disorientation, shortened attention span, and loss of cognitive function.

dyspnea Shortness of breath or difficulty breathing.

elder abuse Any action on the part of an elderly individual's family member, caregiver, or other associated person that takes advantage of the elderly individual's person, property, or emotional state; also called granny beating or parent battering.

hypoxia A dangerous condition in which the body does not have enough oxygen.

osteoporosis A generalized bone disease, commonly associated with postmenopausal women, in which there is a reduction in the amount of bone mass leading to fractures after minimal trauma in either sex.

syncope Fainting, often caused by an interruption of blood flow to the brain.

vasodilation Widening of a blood vessel.

vasoconstriction Narrowing of a blood vessel.

Online Outlook

In order to provide effective treatment to the growing number of elderly patients, all EMTs must have an increased understanding of geriatric care issues. Learn more about the health of geriatric Americans by completing Exercise 34 at www.emtb.com.

www.emtb.com

Assessment in Action

You and your partner are called to a private residence for a woman who had fallen. Upon arrival, you are met at the door by the patient, an 83-year-old woman. She states that she does not think she needs an ambulance but her neighbor, who was visiting at the time she fell, insisted on calling EMS. You find out that the woman actually fell about an hour ago. She landed squarely on her buttocks.

You note that the patient is limping markedly, but your assessment reveals only minimal swelling and no obvious deformity, but you note a large bruise forming on her right hip and upper leg. She also has some bleeding of an area on her right forearm where she has a bandage. The patient is alert and seems oriented but appears very pale. She states she has "soreness" in her hip and dizziness. Her vital signs include a pulse of 68 beats/min, respirations of 26 breaths/min, and a blood pressure of 88/56 mm Hg. She has a history of high blood pressure and a "sugar problem." She takes medication for both. She has no allergies.

1. An appropriate way to address this patient is by making eye contact and:
   A. raising your voice so she can hear you.
   B. using familiar terms such as "grandma."
   C. asking the neighbor to tell you the patient's name.
   D. using her last name and "Mr." or "Mrs."

2. Which of this patient's vital signs are within normal limits for her age group?
   A. Pulse
   B. Blood pressure
   C. Respirations
   D. Skin color

3. Given her mental status, mechanism of injury, and her vital signs, how serious is this patient's problem?
   A. Not serious; she is alert and oriented.
   B. Serious; she is alert and oriented but probably fractured her hip.
   C. Not serious; her pulse is stable and she is able to move on her own.
   D. Very serious; her blood pressure, skin color, and dizziness indicate a serious condition.

4. An acceptable method to evaluate for a hip injury is to:
   A. ask how well the patient can walk.
   B. watch the patient as he or she walks.
   C. palpate the entire extremity.
   D. ask how the fall occurred.

5. As part of the history taking, which question may indicate the presence of another immediate problem?
   A. When did you eat last?
   B. Why did you fall?
   C. Where are your medications?
   D. Are you allergic to anything?

6. To assess patient complaints adequately in an elderly patient, questions should be phrased as:
   A. simple yes-no questions.
   B. all open-ended questions.
   C. specific questions with choices.
   D. words to see what the patient agrees with.

7. You look under her bandage and note what appears to be a skin tear on her arm. This tear has occurred because:
   A. loss of collagen causes skin to tear as opposed to lacerate.
   B. she did not fall against anything sharp or pointed.
   C. pre-existing diseases that have affected the skin.
   D. lowered metabolism contributes to fragile skin.

Challenging Questions

8. You attempt to secure a bandage around the skin tear. Because of her fragile skin, you will:
   A. secure only one edge of the tape to her skin.
   B. tape dressing to dressing, not dressing to skin.
   C. use paper tape instead of adhesive tape.
   D. leave the skin tear uncovered.

9. Because of her history she needs to be immobilized. Her posture is stooped and she has a history of arthritis in her knees. What is the best method to immobilize her?
   A. Use a backboard.
   B. Use a scoop stretcher.
   C. Try a vacuum mattress.
   D. Try multiple rigid splints.

10. What more could you do to treat this elderly patient that is in shock?

Points to Ponder

You arrive at a home and are met at the door by a middle-aged man who immediately tells you not to listen to his mother. As you gather a little more information, you find that the son called for you to take his father to the hospital, but the mother insists that the "Do Not Resuscitate" (DNR) orders be followed. You find the man in bed, and it appears that he has been there for several days. He is unresponsive, and his breathing rate is 8 breaths/min and shallow. His pulse is 130 beats/min and is weak and irregular. His wife explains that he is in end stages of cancer and that he

lost consciousness several hours ago. He has not eaten in 3 days and stopped taking water yesterday. The wife produces all of the DNR documents and they appear to be in order. The son is insisting that you take him to the hospital and says that if you don't, he will. Whose wishes do you follow? How can you help negotiate between the family members? What are your feelings about DNR orders? If his heart suddenly stopped, could you stand by and watch the man die without trying to help him?

Issues Working with Families, DNR Orders, Emotional Well-being of EMTs.

Operations

7

Section

Ambulance Operations

Objectives

Cognitive

1. Discuss the medical and nonmedical equipment needed to respond to a call (p 808).
2. List the phases of an ambulance call (p 807).
3. Describe the general provisions of state laws relating to the operation of the ambulance and privileges in any or all of the following categories (p 820):
   - speed
   - warning lights
   - sirens
   - right-of-way
   - parking
   - turning
4. List contributing factors to unsafe driving conditions (p 819).
5. Describe the considerations that should be given to (p 821):
   - request for escorts
   - following an escort vehicle
   - intersections
6. Discuss "Due Regard for Safety of All Others" while operating an emergency vehicle (p 816).
7. State what information is essential in order to respond to a call (p 816).
8. Discuss various situations that may affect response to a call (p 819).
9. Differentiate between the various methods of moving a patient to the unit based upon injury or illness (p 813).
10. Apply the components of the essential patient information in a written report (p 824).
11. Discuss the elements that dictate the use of lights and siren to the scene and to the hospital (p 821).*
12. Summarize the importance of preparing the unit for the next response (p 808).
13. Identify what is essential for completion of a call (p 824).
14. Distinguish among the terms cleaning, disinfection, high-level disinfection, and sterilization (p 825).
15. Describe how to clean or disinfect items following patient care (p 825).

Affective

16. Explain the rationale for appropriate reporting of patient information (p 824).
17. Explain the rationale for having the unit prepared to respond (p 808).

Psychomotor

None

* These are noncurriculum objectives.

35

www.emtb.com

Online Chapter Pretest
Interactivities
Vocabulary Explorer
Anatomy Review
Web Links
Online Review Manual
Distance Learning

Skill Drills
Vital Vocabulary
Pediatric Needs
Geriatric Needs
EMT-B Safety
EMT-B Tips
Documentation Tips
Remember
Prep Kit

You are the EMT

Every day, thousands of Americans will dial 9-1-1 for some emergency. Within minutes, an ambulance is en route to the scene bringing specially trained and equipped prehospital providers to their side.

This chapter will begin to acquaint you with the emergency response vehicle along with its contents that are your "tools of the trade." It will also help you answer the following questions:

1. What are the nine phases of an ambulance call?

2. Why is having "due regard for the safety of others" essential when responding to a call?

Ambulance Operations

Many patients have said that one of the most frightening parts of being suddenly ill or injured is the ambulance ride to the hospital. Already anxious, a patient may be made more so by a fast, bumpy ride with a siren blaring. Sometimes, such a ride is truly lifesaving. However, in most cases, excessive speed is unnecessary and dangerous. What is necessary is that the patient be safely transported to an appropriate medical care facility in the shortest practical time. This takes common sense and defensive driving techniques. Speed is no substitute for these qualities.

This chapter focuses on the techniques and judgment that you will need to learn to drive an ambulance or ambulance service vehicle. It begins with a look at ambulance design, then discusses emergency vehicle control and operation, both important factors in safe driving. The chapter also discusses how to equip and maintain an ambulance, parking considerations, the effects of weather on driving, and common hazards that are encountered in driving an ambulance. Finally, it describes how to work safely with air ambulances.

Emergency Vehicle Design

An **ambulance** is a vehicle that is used for treating and transporting patients who need emergency medical care to a hospital. The first motor-powered ambulance was introduced in 1906. For many decades after that, a hearse was the vehicle that was most often used as an ambulance, because it was the only vehicle with room enough for a person to lie down. Few supplies were carried on board, and there was little space for attendants.

The hearse-ambulance has gone the way of its horse-drawn predecessor. Ambulances today are designed according to strict government regulations based on

national standards. The standards themselves are based in large part on suggestions from the ambulance industry, including EMS personnel. One of the most significant developments in ambulance design has been the enlargement of the patient compartment. Another development is the use of **first-responder vehicles**, which respond initially to the scene with personnel and equipment to treat the sick and injured until an ambulance can arrive.

As defined by the National Academy of Sciences-National Research Council, the modern ambulance is a vehicle for emergency medical care that has the following features:

- A driver's compartment

- A patient compartment that can accommodate two EMTs and two patients on stretchers, positioned so that at least one of the patients can receive CPR during transit

- Equipment and supplies to provide emergency medical care at the scene and during transport, to safeguard personnel and patients from hazardous conditions, and to carry out light extrication procedures

- Two-way radio communication so that ambulance personnel can speak with the dispatcher, the hospital, public safety authorities, and medical control

- Design and construction that ensure maximum safety and comfort

Each state establishes its own standards for licensing or certifying ambulances; however, most use the federal specifications (KKK-A-1822C, 1990) that cover the following three types of basic ambulance designs ▶ Figure 35-1 and ▶ Table 35-1 .

Figure 35-1 **A.** The conventional, truck cab-chassis has a modular ambulance body that can be transferred to a newer chassis (Type I). **B.** The standard van ambulance has a forward-control integral cab body (Type II). **C.** The specialty van ambulance has a forward-control integral cab body (Type III).

The six-pointed **Star of Life®** emblem (▶ **Figure 35-2**) identifies vehicles that meet federal specifications as licensed or certified ambulances. It should be affixed to the sides, rear, and roof of the ambulance. Local regulatory authorities determine what emblems may be displayed on the side of a prehospital care ambulance.
(▶ **Figure 35-3**) illustrates some of the required features of a licensed or certified ambulance.

Figure 35-2
The Star of Life®.

Phases of an Ambulance Call

An ambulance call has nine phases: preparation, dispatch, en route, arrival at scene, transfer of patient to ambulance, en route to receiving facility (transport), at receiving facility (delivery), en route to station, and postrun, as shown in (▼ **Table 35-2**). These nine phases address the vehicle and its crew, and their roles in a response to a medical emergency. The details of patient care are not included in these nine phases.

The Preparation Phase

Making sure that equipment and supplies are in their proper place and ready for use is an important part of

Figure 35-3 Warning lights and public address systems are necessary on licensed or certified ambulances.

TABLE 35-1 Basic Ambulance Designs	
Type I	Conventional, truck cab-chassis with a modular ambulance body that can be transferred to a newer chassis as needed
Type II	Standard van, forward-control integral cab-body ambulance
Type III	Specialty van, forward-control integral cab-body ambulance

TABLE 35-2 Phases of an Ambulance Call
• Preparation for the call
• Dispatch
• En route
• Arrival at scene
• Transfer of the patient to the ambulance
• En route to the receiving facility (transport)
• At the receiving facility (delivery)
• En route to the station
• Postrun

preparing for the call. Items that are missing or that do not work are of no use to you or the patient. As a general rule of thumb, the more complex a piece of equipment is, and the harder it is to learn to use, the more likely it is to malfunction during an emergency. Many EMS items have never been rigorously tested under field conditions and could turn out to be expensive mistakes. For this reason, new equipment should only be placed on an ambulance after consulting with the medical director.

Equipment and supplies should be durable and, to the extent possible, standardized. This makes it easy to quickly exchange equipment with other ambulances or with the emergency department, thus saving time during patient transfer.

Store equipment and supplies in the ambulance according to how urgently and how often they are used ▶ **Figure 35-4** . Give priority to items that are needed to care for life-threatening conditions. These include equipment for airway management, artificial ventilation, and oxygen delivery. Place these items within easy reach, at the head of the primary stretcher. Place items for cardiac care, control of external bleeding, and monitoring blood pressure at the side of the stretcher.

Storage cabinets and kits should open easily. They should also close securely so that they do not fly open while the ambulance is in motion. Cabinet and drawer fronts should be transparent so that you can quickly identify their contents; if they are not, be sure to label each container ▶ **Figure 35-5** .

MEDICAL EQUIPMENT. As an EMT-B, you have access to a large variety of medical equipment and supplies, far more than can be described here. Certain items must be available on the ambulance at all times.

Basic supplies. ▶ **Table 35-3** lists the common supplies carried on ambulances.

Airway management. Airway management equipment that should be carried on ambulances includes the following:

- Oropharyngeal airways for adults, children, and infants
- Nasopharyngeal airways for adults and children
- Two sets of equipment for advanced airway procedures if your service is authorized by state regulation and the medical director to perform these: one in the ambulance and one in the jump kit that you carry to the patient

Ventilation devices. It is important that two portable artificial ventilation devices that operate independently

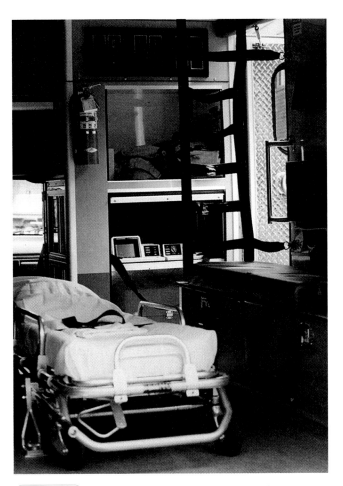

Figure 35-4 Store equipment and supplies in the ambulance according to how urgently and how often they are used.

Figure 35-5 Containers should be placed in cabinets and drawers with transparent fronts for quick identification.

of an oxygen supply are carried on the ambulance: one for use in the ambulance and one for use outside the ambulance or as a spare. These devices include pocket masks and bag-valve-mask (BVM) devices. In addition, BVM devices capable of oxygen enrichment that, when

TABLE 35-3 Common Supplies

- Pillows and pillowcases
- Sterile sheets
- Blankets
- Towels
- Disposable emesis bags or basins
- Boxes of disposable tissue
- Bedpan (optional)
- Urinals (one male, one female; optional)
- Thermometers (one oral, one rectal, one hypothermia)
- Blood pressure cuffs (pediatric, adult, large adult)
- Stethoscope
- Pair of trauma shears
- Package of disposable drinking cups
- Unbreakable container of water
- Package of wet wipes
- Chemical cold packs
- Sterile irrigation fluid
- Restraining devices
- Package of plastic bags for waste or severed parts
- Latex, vinyl, or other disposable gloves (various sizes)
- Sharps container (minimum)
- Set of hearing protectors
- Infection control kits (goggles, masks, waterproof gowns)

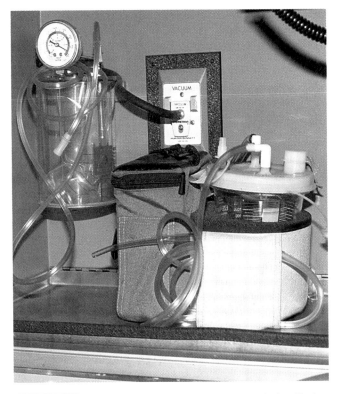

Figure 35-6 The ambulance should carry both a mounted suctioning unit and a portable unit.

Masks for these devices come in a variety of sizes, from infant to adult, and are necessary materials to carry on the ambulance. The masks should be transparent so that you can monitor the patient's respirations, notice any color changes in the patient, and detect vomiting. Adult- and pediatric-size BVMs should be used with the appropriately sized mask to deliver the proper volume of oxygen-enriched air to the patient. In some regions, barrier devices for ventilation may be carried on the ambulance, depending on the preference of the medical director. Oxygen-powered devices are also available to provide ventilation to a patient. The EMT-B should follow local guidelines in identifying the specific ventilation equipment carried on the ambulance.

Suctioning unit. The ambulance should carry both portable and mounted suctioning units ▲ **Figure 35-6** . These units must be powerful enough to provide an airflow of 30 L/min at the end of the tube and a vacuum of 300 mm Hg when the tube is clamped. The suctioning force must be adjustable for use on infants and children. The units should include large-bore, nonkinking suction tubing with a semirigid pharyngeal tip, with additional semirigid tips available.

The installed unit should include a suction yoke, an unbreakable collection bottle, water for rinsing the

attached to an oxygen supply with the oxygen reservoir in place, are able to supply almost 100% oxygen, should also be carried on the ambulance. The nonrebreathing valve on the mask must allow patients to inhale oxygen during both artificial ventilation and spontaneous respirations. Devices should be either disposable or easy to clean and **decontaminate**, which means to remove radiation, chemical, or other hazardous materials.

suction tips, and suction tubing, all easily accessible when you are sitting at the head of the stretcher. The tubing must reach the patient's airway, regardless of the patient's position. All components of the suctioning unit must be disposable or made of material that is easily cleaned and decontaminated.

Oxygen delivery. The ambulance should carry at least two oxygen supply units: one portable and one installed. The portable unit should be located near a door or in the jump kit, for easy use outside the ambulance. It should have a capacity of minimum 300 L of oxygen and be equipped with a yoke, pressure gauge, flowmeter, oxygen supply tubing, nonrebreathing mask, and nasal cannula. This unit must be able to deliver oxygen at a variable rate between 2 and 15–25 L/min. At least one extra portable 300-L cylinder should be kept on the ambulance. Many services equip the backup cylinder with its own yoke, gauge, regulator, and tubing so that it can be used for a second patient.

The mounted oxygen unit should have a capacity of 3,000 L of oxygen (▼ **Figure 35-7**). It should also be equipped with visible flowmeters that are capable of

delivering 2 to 25 L/min that are accessible when you are at the head of the stretcher. Oxygen masks, with and without nonbreathing bags, should be transparent, and disposable, in sizes for adults, children, and infants.

Ambulance services that often transport patients on runs lasting longer than 1 hour should consider using a disposable, single-use humidifier for the mounted oxygen system. On runs of less than 1 hour, humidification may increase a patient's risk of infection unless the equipment is rigorously maintained.

CPR equipment. A **CPR board** provides a firm surface under the patient's torso so that you can give effective chest compressions (▼ **Figure 35-8A**). It also establishes an appropriate degree of head tilt (▼ **Figure 35-8B**). If you do not have a special CPR board, you can place a long or short backboard under the patient on the stretcher. Use a tightly rolled sheet or towel to raise the patient's shoulders 3" to 4"; this will also keep the patient's head in a position of maximum backward tilt and keep the shoulders and chest in a straight position. Caution: Do not use this roll to hyperextend the neck if you suspect a spinal injury.

Figure 35-7 An oxygen unit with a capacity of 3,000 L of oxygen should be mounted on the ambulance.

Figure 35-8 **A.** A CPR board should be carried on the ambulance. **B.** A patient on a CPR board has the appropriate degree of head tilt for effective artificial ventilation.

TABLE 35-4 Basic Wound Care Supplies

- Sterile sheets
- Large safety pins
- Adhesive tape in several widths
- Self-adhering, soft roller bandages, 4" × 5 yd
- Self-adhering, soft roller bandages, 2" × 5 yd
- Sterile dressings, gauze, 4" × 4"
- Sterile dressings, ABD or laparotomy pads, usually 6" × 9" or 8" × 10"
- Sterile universal trauma dressings, usually 10" × 36", folded into 9" × 10" packages
- Sterile, occlusive, nonadherent dressings (aluminum foil sterilized in original package)
- An assortment of band-aids

TABLE 35-5 Splinting Supplies

- Adult-size traction splint
- Child-size traction splint
- A variety of arm and leg splints, such as inflatable, vacuum, cardboard, plastic, foam wire-ladder, or padded board. The number and type of splints should be determined by state regulations and your medical director.
- A variety of triangular bandages and roller bandages
- A short backboard device
- A long backboard
- Cervical collars in an adjustable size or a variety of sizes
- Adult-size pneumatic antishock garment (PASG), previously called MAST trousers

Mechanical devices that operate on compressed gas and deliver chest compressions and ventilations are also available.

Basic wound care supplies. (▲ **Table 35-4**) lists the basic supplies for dressing open wounds that should be included on the ambulance.

Splinting supplies. Examples of supplies for splinting fractures and dislocations that may be carried on ambulances (▼ **Figure 35-9**) are listed in (▲ **Table 35-5**).

Childbirth supplies. You must carry a sterile emergency obstetric (OB) kit (▼ **Figure 35-10**) that includes the supplies listed in (▶ **Table 35-6**).

Medications. It is important that the ambulance carry the items listed in (▶ **Table 35-7**). Be certain that you have the telephone number and radio frequency of medical control or the local poison control center with you on the ambulance. The back of your clipboard is a good place to keep this information.

Figure 35-9 Supplies for splinting fractures and dislocations should be carried on the ambulance.

Figure 35-10 A sterile emergency obstetric kit must be carried on the ambulance.

TABLE 35-6 Emergency OB Kit

- Pair of surgical scissors
- Hemostats or special cord clamps
- Umbilical tape or sterilized cord
- Small rubber bulb syringe
- Towels
- Gauze sponges
- Pairs of sterile gloves
- Sanitary napkins
- A plastic bag
- Baby blanket

Figure 35-11 Every ambulance should carry an automated external defibrillator.

TABLE 35-7 Medications and Other Supplies Carried on the Ambulance

- Activated charcoal
- Drinkable water and cups
- Oral glucose
- Oxygen
- Supplies for irrigating the skin and eyes
- A snake bite kit or other regional equipment, depending on the area and local protocol

Figure 35-12 A portable jump kit contains anything you may need during the first 5 minutes with the patient except for the semiautomated external defibrillator and possibly the oxygen cylinder and portable suctioning unit.

Automated external defibrillator. Semiautomated defibrillation equipment, as permitted by regulation and the local medical director, should always be carried on the ambulance ▲ **Figure 35-11** .

The jump kit. The ambulance must be equipped with a portable, durable, and waterproof **jump kit** that you can carry to the patient ▲ **Figure 35-12** . Think of the jump kit as the "5-minute kit," containing anything you might need in the first 5 minutes with the patient except for the semiautomated external defibrillator, possibly the oxygen cylinder, and portable suctioning unit. The jump kit must be easy to open and secure. ▶ **Table 35-8** lists the items that are typically contained in a jump kit.

Patient transfer equipment. Each ambulance should carry the following patient transfer equipment:

- A primary wheeled ambulance stretcher
- A folding stretcher
- A collapsible chair device or stair chair for use in narrow spaces
- A roll up backboard (Reeve's stretcher)

The collapsible and folding stretchers may be combined into one unit. Stretchers must be easy to move, store, clean, and disinfect. The folding stretcher should keep the patient elevated above the floor when in the flat, extended position ▶ **Figure 35-13** . The wheeled stretcher should be adjustable in height ▶ **Figure 35-14** . When it is secured in the lowest position, the top should be 11″ to 15″ above the floor of the ambulance. You should be able to tilt the head of the stretcher upward to at least a 60° semisitting position and tilt the

TABLE 35-8 Items Carried in a Jump Kit

- Latex, vinyl, or other gloves
- Triangular bandages
- Trauma shears
- Adhesive tape in various widths
- Universal trauma dressings
- Self-adhering soft roller bandages, 4″ × 5 yd and 2″ × 5 yd
- Oropharyngeal airways in adult, child, and infant sizes*
- BVM device with masks for adults, children, and infants*
- Blood pressure cuff
- Stethoscope
- Penlight
- Sterile gauze dressings, 4″ × 4″
- Sterile dressings (ABD or laparotomy pads), 6″ × 9″ or 8″ × 10″
- Thermometer
- Adhesive strips
- Oral glucose
- Activated charcoal

* These might be carried in a separate airway kit, along with the portable oxygen cylinder.

Figure 35-13 A folding stretcher is one type of patient transfer equipment that may be carried on the ambulance.

Figure 35-14 The wheeled ambulance stretcher is adjustable in height.

entire stretcher into 10° to 15° of Trendelenburg's position (head down) for airway care and treatment of shock. Stretchers must be at least 76″ long and 23″ wide and must be provided with fasteners to secure them firmly to the floor or side of the ambulance during transport. Stretcher restraints should be capable of holding the stretcher in place in case the vehicle rolls over. Make sure there are at least two restraining devices for the patient, such as deceleration or stopping straps over the shoulders, to prevent the patient from continuing to move forward in case the ambulance suddenly slows or stops.

Moving the patient to the ambulance can be done in different ways, depending on the injury or illness. Some patients can walk easily to the ambulance, which is sometimes easier and safer than trying to use a stretcher. For patients with spinal injuries, using a backboard or

other immobilizing device, such as a Kendrick Extrication Device (KED), is usually best. For some patients with medical problems, especially patients with respiratory problems, transport with the patient sitting upright may allow the patient the most comfort and safety.

SAFETY AND OPERATIONS EQUIPMENT. In addition to medical equipment, a properly stocked ambulance carries several kinds of equipment for responder safety, rescue operations, and locating emergency scenes. To do the job effectively, the EMT team will need the following equipment:

- Personal protective equipment
- Equipment for work areas
- Preplanning/navigation guides
- Extrication equipment

Personal safety equipment. You should always carry personal protective equipment that allows you to work safely in a limited variety of hazardous or contaminated situations. These situations include the edges of a structural fire or explosion, vehicle extrication, and in crowds. The equipment should protect you from exposure to blood and other potentially infectious body fluids. Note that you will not be equipped to face all HazMat and other exposure situations that you may encounter; this is the job of specially trained HazMat technicians and response teams. Your equipment might include the following:

- Face shields
- Gowns, shoe covers, caps
- Turnout gear
- Helmets with face shields or safety goggles
- Safety shoes or boots

Equipment for work areas. A weatherproof compartment that you can reach from outside the patient compartment should hold equipment for safeguarding patients and EMTs, controlling traffic and bystanders, and illuminating work areas ▼ **Figure 35-15** . The following items are recommended:

- Warning devices that flash intermittently or have reflectors (road flares are not acceptable because they can pose an additional hazard, such as ignition of flammable liquids or gases)
- Two high-intensity halogen 20,000 candle flashlights of the recharging battery-powered, stand-up type

Figure 35-15 The ambulance should have a weatherproof compartment that can be reached from outside the patient compartment. It should hold equipment for safeguarding patients and EMTs, controlling traffic, and illuminating work areas.

- Fire extinguisher, type BC, dry powder, size 5 lb minimum
- Hard hats or helmets with face shields or safety goggles
- Portable floodlights

Preplanning and navigation. Make sure you have detailed street and area maps in the driver's compartment of the ambulance, along with directions to key locations, such as local hospitals. Become familiar with the roads and traffic patterns in your town or city so that you can plan alternative routes to common destinations. Pay particular attention to ways around frequently opened bridges, congested traffic, or blocked railroad crossings. Often, switching to an alternative route will save more time than driving faster. Also become familiar with special facilities and locations within your regional operating area, such as other medical facilities, airports, arenas and stadiums, and chemical or research facilities that might pose unusual problems (staging areas may be pre-defined for emergency operations).

Extrication equipment. A weatherproof compartment outside the patient compartment should contain equipment that is needed for simple, light extrication, even if an extrication and rescue unit is readily available. ▶ **Table 35-9** lists the items that should be included in the compartment.

If rescue and extrication services are not readily available, additional equipment may be needed.

PERSONNEL. Every ambulance must be staffed with at least one EMT-B in the patient compartment whenever a patient is being transported; two EMTs are strongly recommended. Some services may operate with a non-EMT driver and a single EMT-B in the patient compartment.

DAILY INSPECTIONS. Being fully prepared means that you and your team must inspect both the ambulance and equipment daily to ensure that everything is in proper working order. The ambulance inspection should include the following:

- Fuel levels
- Oil levels
- Transmission fluid levels
- Engine cooling system and fluid levels
- Batteries
- Brake fluid
- Engine belts
- Wheels and tires, including the spare, if there is one. Check inflation pressure and look for signs of unusual or uneven wear.

TABLE 35-9 Extrication Equipment

- 12" wrench, adjustable, open-end
- 12" screwdriver, standard square bar
- 8" screwdriver, Phillips head #2
- Hacksaw with 12" carbide wire blades
- Vise-grip pliers, 10"
- 5-lb hammer with 15" handle
- Fire ax, butt, 24" handle
- Wrecking bar with 24" handle. This may be in a combination tool with a hammer and ax.
- 51" crowbar, pinch point
- Bolt cutter with 1" to 1¼" jaw opening
- Folding shovel, pointed blade
- Tin snips, double action, 8" minimum
- Gauntlets, reinforced, leather covering past midforearm; one pair per crew member
- Rescue blanket
- Ropes, 5,400-lb tensile strength in 50' lengths in protective bags
- Mastic knife (able to cut seat belt webbing)
- Spring-load center punch
- Pruning saw
- Heavy duty 2" × 4" and 4" × 4" shoring (cribbing) blocks, various lengths

---

- All interior and exterior lights
- Windshield wipers and fluid
- Horn
- Siren
- Air conditioners and heaters
- Ventilating system
- Doors. Make sure they open, close, latch, and lock properly.
- Communication systems, vehicle and portable
- All windows and mirrors. Check for cleanliness and position.

Check all medical equipment and supplies at least daily, including all the oxygen supplies, the jump kit,

Documentation Tips

Because mechanical aspects of emergency work such as driving and moving patients strongly impact your safety and that of others, your service should have specific procedures for daily inspections. Following them protects you physically, and documenting your compliance is an important legal protection. Procedures should call for dating and either signing or initialing the checksheets, and for storing them where they can be found later if needed.

splints, dressings and bandages, backboards and other immobilization equipment, and emergency OB kit. Is the equipment functioning properly? Are the supplies clean? Are there enough of them? All battery-operated equipment, including the defibrillator, should be operated and checked each day. Rotate the batteries according to an established schedule.

SAFETY PRECAUTIONS. A final part of the preparation phase is reviewing safety precautions. These precautions, which include standard traffic safety rules and regulations, should be followed on every call. Check to make sure that safety devices, such as seat belts, are in proper working order.

The Dispatch Phase

Dispatch must be easy to access and in service 24 hours a day (▼ **Figure 35-16**). It may be operated by the local EMS or by a shared service that also covers law enforcement and the fire department. The dispatch center might serve only one jurisdiction, such as a single city or town, or it might be an area or regional center serving several communities or an entire county. In either case,

Figure 35-16 The dispatcher is the key communications link throughout all phases of the ambulance run.

it should be staffed by trained personnel who are familiar with the agencies they are dispatching and the geography of the service area. For every emergency request, the dispatcher should gather and record the following minimum information:

- The nature of the call
- The name, present location, and call-back telephone number of the caller
- The location of the patient(s)
- The number of patients and some idea of the severity of their conditions
- Any other special problems or pertinent information about hazards or weather conditions

Many areas implement emergency medical dispatching, which provides the caller with instructions for patient care before the ambulance arrives.

En Route to the Scene

As you and your partner prepare to respond to the scene, make sure you fasten your seat belts and shoulder harnesses before you move the ambulance. At this point, you should inform dispatch that your unit is responding and confirm the nature and location of the call. This is also an excellent time to ask for any other available information about the location. For example, you might learn that the patient is on the third floor or that the best door to use is around the side of the house.

While en route, the team should prepare to assess and care for the patient. Review dispatch information about the nature of the call and the location of the patient. Assign specific initial duties and scene management tasks to each team member, and decide what type of equipment to take initially. Depending on your operation procedures, you may also decide which stretcher to bring to the patient.

DRIVER CHARACTERISTICS. In many ways, the en route or response phase of the call is the most dangerous for you. Collisions between automobiles and emergency vehicles cause many serious injuries among EMS personnel (▶ **Figure 35-17**). Therefore, drivers should be screened carefully. Not everyone who drives an automobile is qualified to drive an emergency vehicle. In some states, you must successfully complete an approved emergency vehicle operations course before you are allowed to drive the ambulance on emergency calls. In any state, diligence and caution are important characteristics, as are a positive attitude about your ability and tolerance of other drivers.

> The proper attitude is very important for an ambulance driver. The good judgment needed to drive an ambulance requires practice —even for the best drivers.

One basic requirement is physical fitness. Many crashes occur as a result of physical impairment of the driver. You should not be driving if you are taking medications that may cause drowsiness or slow your reaction times. These include cold remedies, analgesics, or tranquilizers. And, of course, you should never drive or provide medical care after drinking alcohol.

Another requirement is emotional fitness. Emotions should not be taken lightly. Personality often changes once an individual gets behind a steering wheel. Emotional stability is closely related to the ability to operate under stress. In addition to knowing exactly what to do, you must be able to do it under trying conditions.

The proper attitude is very important for an ambulance driver. Being able to drive to your destination without interruption and to move into the opposite lane are valuable, time-saving skills that must be practiced consistently. Do not ever get behind the wheel thinking that you can do whatever you like.

In addition to training and experience, the good judgment and knowledge that you need to drive an ambulance requires practice. Remember, even the best drivers can benefit from practice.

SAFE DRIVING PRACTICES. Safe driving is a very important part of the emergency care of sick and injured patients.

Figure 35-17 The en route or response phase may be the most dangerous part of the call.

The first rule of safe driving in an emergency vehicle is that speed does not save lives; good care does. The second rule is that the driver and all passengers must wear seat belts and shoulder restraints at all times. These are the most important items of safety equipment on every ambulance. Other EMTs should wear restraints en route to the scene and whenever they are not performing direct patient care. Patients should also be properly restrained.

Learn how your vehicle accelerates, corners, sways, and stops. For example, disc booster brakes make braking more efficient but increase sway. You must know exactly how your particular vehicle will respond to steering, braking, and accelerating under various conditions.

Getting a feel for the proper brake pressure comes with experience and practice. Each vehicle has a different braking action. For example, the brakes on types I and III vehicles have a heavier feel than the brakes on a type II vehicle. Braking on a diesel-powered unit will be different from braking on an identically equipped gasoline-powered unit. Certain heavy vehicles use air brakes, which have yet another feel. Get to know each vehicle you drive, and be sure you understand its braking characteristics and the best downshifting techniques.

The EMT driver often assumes that motorists and pedestrians will do the right thing when an emergency vehicle is in the vicinity. This is a mistake. Motorists may indeed pull over to the nearest curb and stop or drive as close to the curb as possible, but you cannot take this behavior for granted. At any time, a motorist might stop suddenly in front of the ambulance or pull to the left. Both of these motorist responses may result in a crash. Always assume the driver has not heard your siren or seen you until proven otherwise by his or her actions.

When you are driving an ambulance on a multi-lane highway, you should usually stay in the extreme left-hand (fast) lane. This allows other motorists to move over to the right when they see or hear you approach.

Most important, you must always drive defensively. Never rely on what another motorist will do unless you get a clear visual signal. Even then, you must be prepared to take defensive action in the case of a misunderstanding, panic, or careless driving on the part of the other driver.

The problem of excessive speed. Only in extreme life-and-death emergencies is speed an important factor. In most instances, if you properly assess and stabilize the patient at the scene, speed during transport is unnecessary and undesirable. No matter what the situation, you should never travel at a speed that is unsafe for the given road conditions.

EMT-B Safety

Ambulance crashes that kill EMTs, patients, or occupants of other vehicles are disturbingly common. Most of them could be prevented by the driver of the ambulance. Attending thoroughly to your own driving skills, driving according to established standards, and dealing with any obvious deficiencies in your partner's driving skills are all crucial to your safety on the job.

Studies have shown conclusively that excessive speeds are unnecessary and, in most cases, do not add to patient survivability. More often, using excessive speed while driving to and from the scene has resulted in crashes in which the EMT, patient, and occupants of other vehicles are killed.

Consider these factors:

1. **Expertise** on the part of the dispatcher, resulting in calls being given a high priority only when this is truly indicated. Dispatching requires a trained, experienced EMT or emergency medical dispatcher. Only someone with training and a working knowledge of emergency calls can determine the urgency of a call, especially when the caller is excited and distraught.

2. **Adequate equipment in the ambulance.** If you have the equipment and supplies that are necessary to stabilize the patient, you will be able to properly care for the patient en route without the need for speeding to the hospital.

3. **Adequate training of the EMT.** With adequate training and confidence in your ability to care for the patient, your role extends beyond simply acting as a chauffeur.

4. **Adequate driving ability.** This is the most important factor. If you understand the added risks that go with high-speed driving and the principles of safe ambulance operation, you will tend to choose safety over speed.

5. **Recognition of siren syndrome.** The siren may have a psychological effect on drivers. Recognizing this will help you become aware of your or other drivers' tendencies to drive faster and faster in the presence of sirens. Although a siren signifies a request for drivers to yield right of way, drivers do not always yield right of way.

Emergency vehicle control. As the driver of an ambulance, you have only two ways to control the vehicle: by changing its direction or changing its speed. Either maneuver requires a continuous rolling contact between the surface of the tires and the surface of the road. Two factors are involved in this contact. The first is the <u>coefficient of friction</u>, which is a measure of the tire's grip on the road; <u>friction</u> is resistance to the motion of one body against another. The second factor is the <u>footprint</u> of the tire, which is the area of contact between the tire and surface of the road. On the typical ambulance, the footprint is about 8″ long and as wide as the tire.

The coefficient of friction may vary widely on different parts of the same road, depending on the condition of the surface, the age of the road, and the weather. It also varies according to the tire's tread design and wear. As a driver, you must constantly evaluate the road surface: At a given speed, how much frictional force can the tires apply before the ambulance becomes unstable? This is especially important in cornering, in which additional centrifugal force is acting on the vehicle.

Steering techniques. Steering technique includes the way you hold the steering wheel, the way it moves, and the timing of the movements. Hold the wheel with your hands at the ten-o'clock and two-o'clock positions ▶ **Figure 35-18A** . This allows you to turn the wheel without removing either hand; one hand pulls while the other slides so that they remain parallel ▶ **Figure 35-18B** . Your hands should not pass the twelve-o'clock or six-o'clock positions, because they will cross and become tangled; instead, let the hand that was pulling start to slide, and use the opposite hand to pull.

Timing of steering wheel movements relates to the speed of the vehicle. All vehicles lag somewhat when responding to steering input. The faster the speed, the greater the lag.

Chassis set. The <u>chassis</u> is the vehicle frame of the ambulance. <u>Chassis set</u> is the transfer of weight (center of mass) to different points on the chassis. Basically, the weight of a vehicle is concentrated over one of three points on the chassis: the front wheels, the rear wheels, or the center between the front and rear wheels. The transfer of weight from one point to another is caused by <u>acceleration</u>, or increasing speed, or <u>deceleration</u>, or slowing down. When a vehicle accelerates, the weight is transferred to the rear; the front wheels lose some traction, which means that you lose some ability to steer. The ambulance will have a tendency to travel in a straight line. With

braking, the opposite weight shift occurs; this is why the rear end of the vehicle tends to slide to the outside of a curve when cornering.

Vehicle size and distance judgment. Vehicle length and width are critical factors in maneuvering, driving, and parking an emergency vehicle. They are especially important with types I and III vehicles, which are wider than they look from behind the steering wheel. To brake and pass effectively, you must know the width and length of your vehicle. Crashes often occur when the vehicle is backing up. Always use someone outside the ambulance as a ground guide when you are backing up, to avoid any surprises. Vehicle size and weight will greatly influence braking and stopping distances. Good peripheral vision and depth perception will help you to judge distances, but they are no substitute for intensive training, experience, and frequent evaluation of the vehicle.

Road positioning and cornering. Road position means the position of the vehicle on the roadway

(**Figure 35-18**) **A.** Hold the steering wheel with your hands at the ten-o'clock and two-o'clock positions so that you can turn the wheel without removing either hand. **B.** Turn the wheel by pulling with one hand and sliding the other. Make sure that both hands remain parallel.

relative to the inside or outside edge of the paved surface. To corner efficiently, you must know the vehicle's present position and its projected path. The aim is to take the corner at the speed that will put you in the proper road position as you exit the curve

▼ **Figure 35-19** . The process works in the following way: The apex of the turn through a curve is the point at which the vehicle is closest to the inside edge of the curve. If you reach the apex early in the curve, the vehicle will be forced toward the outside of the roadway as it exits the curve. If you reach the apex late in the curve, the vehicle will tend to stay on the inside of the roadway; this helps you to keep the vehicle in the proper lane.

Controlled acceleration. Controlled acceleration is the use of acceleration to control the vehicle; it is done by applying foot pressure on the accelerator pedal. Acceleration is most efficient when the vehicle is traveling in a straight line, because the force of linear acceleration is equally distributed to the rear wheels. If you accelerate in a curve or during a turn, however, you force the vehicle to the outside of the curve. If acceleration in this direction becomes excessive, the vehicle may drift out of control and become unstable.

Controlled braking. Controlled braking is the use of the brakes to control the vehicle. Brakes not only control the movement of the vehicle, causing it to slow or stop; they also help to control its direction. Braking

> Brakes help control the vehicle's direction. Braking when traveling in a straight line is safest. Braking in a turn is inefficient and may cause a skid or spin.

while the vehicle is traveling in a straight line is the safest, most efficient method. Braking in a turn causes a loss of efficiency. You might not notice this at low speed, but it becomes more apparent at higher speeds. Applying the brakes while cornering is not an effective way to slow the vehicle and may actually cause a skid or spin. Instead, maintain your speed by simultaneously easing off brake pressure and increasing accelerator pressure. Getting the feel for the proper brake pressure comes with experience and practice driving your assigned vehicle.

WEATHER AND ROAD CONDITIONS. You should be constantly alert to changing weather, road, and driving conditions ▼ **Figure 35-20** . Whether going to or coming from an emergency, you must modify your speed according to road conditions. Take warnings of ice or hazardous conditions seriously, and be prepared to take an alternative route, if necessary. During a major disaster, all public safety and emergency services should be coordinated. If you run into unexpected traffic congestion, notify the dispatcher so that other emergency vehicles can select alternative routes.

Figure 35-19 To keep the ambulance in the proper lane on a curve, you must know the vehicle's present position and projected path and take the corner at the correct speed.

Figure 35-20 Modify your speed according to changing weather, road, and driving conditions.

Even the most careful drivers will occasionally run into unexpected situations that may require special driving skills. However, if you drive at a speed that is appropriate for the weather and road conditions, you will minimize these situations. For example, it is safer if you decrease speed in weather situations involving fog, rain, snow, or ice.

Hydroplaning. On a wet road, a tire usually displaces the water on the road surface and stays in direct contact with the road. However, at speeds greater than 30 mph, the tire may be lifted off the road as water "piles up" under it; the vehicle feels as if it were floating. This is known as **hydroplaning**. At higher speeds on wet roadways, the front wheels may actually be riding on a sheet of water, robbing the driver of control of the vehicle. If hydroplaning occurs, you should gradually slow down without jamming on the brakes. Shimmying the steering wheel may also help to cut through the water and allow the tires to regain road surface, but this technique requires a great deal of practice.

Water on the roadway. Wet brakes will slow the vehicle and pull it to one side or the other. If at all possible, avoid driving through large pools of standing water; often, you cannot tell how deep they are. If you must drive through standing water, make sure to slow down and turn on the windshield wipers. After driving out of the pool, lightly tap the brakes several times until they are dry. If the vehicle is equipped with anti-lock brakes, apply a steady, light pressure to dry the brakes. Driving through moving water should be avoided at all times.

Decreased visibility. In areas where there is fog, smog, snow, or heavy rain, common sense tells you to slow down after warning cars behind you. At night, use only low headlight beams for maximum visibility without reflection. You should always use headlights during the day to increase your visibility to other drivers. Also, watch carefully for stopped or slow-moving cars.

Ice and slippery surfaces. A light mist on an oily, dusty road can be just as slippery as a patch of ice. Good all-weather tires and an appropriate speed will reduce traction problems significantly. If you are in an area that often has snowy or icy conditions, consider using studded snow tires, if they are permitted by law. You should be especially careful on bridges and overpasses when temperatures are close to freezing. These road surfaces will freeze much faster than surrounding road surfaces because they lack the warming effect of the ground underneath.

EMT-B Tips

Although preventing skids and sliding is ideal, you are likely to skid or slide at least occasionally, especially if you live in climates with ice and snow. Your training should include the technique for correcting slides during turns. If you are likely to drive on ice and snow, you should practice until it becomes automatic—at low speeds in an area where there is no danger of collisions. Remember that four-wheel-drive and front-wheel-drive vehicles behave differently in slides than their rear-wheel-drive counterparts.

LAWS AND REGULATIONS. Regulations regarding vehicle operations vary from state to state and from city to city, but some things are the same everywhere. Drivers of emergency vehicles have certain limited privileges in every state. However, these privileges do not lessen their liability in a crash. In fact, in most cases, the driver is presumed to be guilty if a collision occurs while the ambulance is operating with warning lights and siren. Motor vehicle crashes are the single largest source of lawsuits against EMS personnel and services.

While on a valid emergency call, emergency vehicles typically are exempt from usual vehicle operations. If you are on an emergency call and are using your warning lights and siren, you may be allowed to do the following:

- Park or stand in an otherwise illegal location
- Proceed through a red traffic light or stop sign
- Drive faster than the posted speed limit
- Drive against the flow of traffic on a one-way street, or make a turn that is normally illegal
- Travel left of center to make an otherwise illegal pass

Remember that these exemptions vary by state and local jurisdiction. Therefore, you should check your local statutes for regulations in your area.

An emergency vehicle is almost never allowed to pass a school bus that has stopped to load or unload children and is displaying its flashing red lights or extended "stop arm." If you approach a school bus that has its lights flashing, you should stop before reaching the bus and wait for the driver to make sure the children are safe, close the bus door, and turn off the warning lights. Only then may you carefully proceed past the stopped school bus.

Use of warning lights and siren. Three basic principles govern the use of warning lights and siren on an ambulance:

1. The unit must be on a true emergency call to the best of your knowledge.

2. Both audible and visual warning devices must be used simultaneously.

3. The unit must be operated with due regard for the safety of all others, on and off the roadway.

The siren is probably the most overused piece of equipment on an ambulance. In general, the siren does not help you as you drive, nor does it really help other motorists. Motorists who are driving at the speed limit with the windows up, the radio on, and the air conditioner or heater set on high cannot hear the siren until the ambulance is very close. If the radio is particularly loud, they may not hear the siren at all.

If you do have to use the siren, be sure to warn the patient before you turn it on. Be especially mindful not to increase the speed of the ambulance just because the siren is in use. Always travel at a speed that will allow you to stop safely at all times, especially so that you are prepared for drivers who do not give you the right-of-way. Never assume that warning lights and sirens will allow you to drive through a congested area without stopping or slowing down. Slow down to ensure that all drivers are stopping as you approach an intersection, then proceed with due caution.

Some ambulance headlights are equipped with a high-beam flasher unit. These are the most visible, effective warning devices for clearing traffic in front of the vehicle.

Right-of-way privileges. A right-of-way privilege is just that: a privilege. State motor vehicle statutes or codes often grant an emergency vehicle, such as an ambulance, the right to disregard the rules of the road when responding to an emergency. However, in doing so, the operator of an emergency vehicle must not endanger people or property under any circumstances.

Consider this case: An ambulance is approaching an intersection that is controlled by a four-way stop sign. The ambulance, with lights and audible warning device functioning, proceeds through the intersection without slowing or stopping and crashes into a car coming from its right. Did the operator of the ambulance act appropriately by going through the intersection in this manner?

Right-of-way privileges for ambulances vary from state to state. Some states allow you to proceed through a red light or stop sign after you stop and make sure it is safe to go on. Other states allow you to proceed through a controlled intersection "with due regard," using flashing lights and siren. This means that you may proceed only if you consider the safety of all people who are using the highway. If you fail to use due regard, your service might be sued. If you are found to be at fault, you may personally have to pay punitive damages or face both civil and criminal sanctions.

Get to know your local right-of-way privileges. Exercise them only when it is absolutely necessary for the patient's well-being. The use of lights and audible warning devices is a matter of state and local practice and protocol.

Use of escorts. Using a police escort is an extremely dangerous practice. When other motorists hear a siren and see a police car passing, they might assume that the police car is the only emergency vehicle and not see the ambulance. The only time an escort is justified is when you are in unfamiliar territory and truly need a guide more than an escort. In such cases, neither vehicle should use any warning lights or sirens. If you are being guided by a police car, make sure that you follow at a safe distance.

Intersection hazards. Intersection crashes are the most common and usually the most serious type of collision in which ambulances are involved. Always be alert and careful when approaching an intersection. If you are on an urgent call and cannot wait for traffic lights to change, you should still come to a momentary stop at the light; look around for other motorists and pedestrians before proceeding into the intersection.

Motorists who "time the traffic lights" present a serious hazard. You may arrive at an intersection while the light is green. At the same time, a motorist who is timing the lights on the cross street arrives at the intersection. The motorist has a red light but knows that it is about to turn green and is expecting to go through. The stage is now set for a serious crash.

Another common intersection hazard occurs when the driver of one emergency vehicle follows another emergency vehicle through an intersection without assessing the situation carefully. A motorist who has yielded the right-of-way to the first vehicle may proceed into the intersection without expecting a second vehicle. You should exercise extreme caution in these situations. To signal motorists that a second unit is approaching, use a siren tone that is different from that of the first vehicle.

TABLE 35-10 Guidelines for Safe Ambulance Driving

Keep in mind the following guidelines whenever you are en route to a call:

1. Select the shortest and least congested route to the scene at the time of the dispatch.

2. Avoid routes with heavy traffic congestion; know alternative routes to each hospital during rush hours.

3. Avoid one-way streets; they may become clogged. Do not go against the flow of traffic on a one-way street, unless absolutely necessary.

4. Watch carefully for bystanders as you approach the scene. Curiosity seekers rarely move out of the way.

5. Park the ambulance in a safe place once you arrive at the scene. If you park facing into traffic, turn off your headlights so that they do not blind oncoming cars unless they are needed to illuminate the scene. If the vehicle is blocking part of the road, keep your warning lights on to alert oncoming motorists; otherwise, turn them off.

6. Drive within the speed limit while transporting patients, except in the rare extreme emergency.

7. Go with the flow of the traffic.

8. Use the siren as little as possible en route.

9. Always drive defensively.

10. Always maintain a safe following distance. Use the "4-second rule": Stay at least 4 seconds behind another vehicle in the same lane.

11. Try to maintain an open space or cushion in the lane next to you as an escape route in case the vehicle in front of you stops suddenly.

12. Use your siren if you turn on the emergency lights, except when you are on a freeway.

13. Always assume that other drivers will not hear the siren or see your emergency lights.

GUIDELINES FOR SAFE AMBULANCE DRIVING. ◄ Table 35-10 lists the guidelines to follow when you are en route to a call.

Arrival at the Scene

Once you reach the scene, you should inform dispatch that you have arrived and give a brief report of what you see. Also report any unexpected situations, such as the need for backup units, a heavy rescue unit, or a HazMat team ► Figure 35-21 . Do not enter the scene if there are any hazards to you. If there are dangerous hazards at the scene, the patient should be moved before you begin care. The patient may have to be moved by others if you are not appropriately equipped.

Immediately size up the scene by using the following guidelines:

• Look for safety hazards.

• Evaluate the need for additional units or other assistance.

• Determine the mechanism of injury in trauma patients or the nature of the illness on medical calls.

• Evaluate the need to stabilize the spine.

• Make sure that you follow BSI precautions. The type of care that you expect to give will dictate what personal protective equipment you should wear.

If you are the first EMT-B at the scene of a mass casualty incident, quickly estimate the number of patients ► Figure 35-22 . Inform dispatch that backup units are needed at the scene. Mass casualty incidents involve complex organization of personnel under the incident command system (see Chapter 37). In this system, individual EMT-Bs may be assigned roles to do such things as begin the triage process, assist in treating patients, and loading patients for transportation to a hospital.

SAFE PARKING. In assessing the situation, you must decide where to park the ambulance. Pick a position that will allow for efficient traffic control and flow around a crash scene. Do not park alongside the scene, as you may block the movement of other emergency vehicles. Instead, park about 100′ past the scene on the same side of the road. It is best to park uphill and/or upwind of the scene if smoke or hazardous materials are present ► Figure 35-23 . If you must park on the back side of a hill or curve, leave your warning lights or devices on. Do the same when parking at night. Always park so as to provide a cushion of space between your vehicle and operations at the scene.

Figure 35-21 Once you arrive at the scene, you should report to dispatch and ask for backup, rescue, or HazMat units as needed.

Figure 35-22 At a mass casualty incident, follow instructions from the incident commander assigning your roles. These could include assisting with triage, treating patients, or loading patients for transportation to the hospital.

Figure 35-23 Park the ambulance about 100' past the scene on the same side of the road. Park uphill or upwind of the scene if hazardous materials are present.

Assume that someone will collide with your vehicle and strike personnel on the scene.

Stay away from any fires, explosive hazards, downed wires, or structures that might collapse. Be sure to set the parking brake. If your vehicle is blocking part of the roadway, leave the emergency warning lights on. If your vehicle has them, leave only the flashing yellow lights on. Other drivers tend to drive toward emergency vehicles with flashing red or red and white lights. Within these safety guidelines, you should try to park your ambulance as close to the scene as possible to facilitate emergency medical care. If necessary, you can temporarily block traffic to unload equipment and to load patients quickly and safely. If you must do this, try to do it quickly so that traffic is not blocked any longer than is absolutely necessary. Also, park in a location that will not hamper your leaving the scene.

TRAFFIC CONTROL. After ensuring your own safety, your first responsibility at a crash scene is to care for the patients. Only when all the patients have been treated and the emergency situation is under control should you be concerned with restoring the flow of traffic. If the police are slow to arrive at the scene, you might then need to take action.

The purpose of traffic control is to ensure an orderly traffic flow and to prevent another crash. Under ordinary circumstances, traffic control is difficult. A crash or disaster scene presents serious additional problems. Passing motorists often "rubberneck," paying little attention to the roadway in front of them. Some curiosity seekers may park down the road and return on foot, creating still other hazards. As soon as possible, place appropriate warning devices, such as reflectors, on both sides of the crash. Remember, the main objectives in directing traffic are to warn other drivers, to prevent additional crashes, and to keep vehicles moving in an orderly fashion so that care of the injured is not interrupted.

The Transfer Phase

In almost every case, you will provide lifesaving care right where you find the patient, before moving the patient to the ambulance. You may then begin less critical measures, such as bandaging and splinting. Next, you must package the patient for transport, securing him or her to a device such as a backboard, a scoop stretcher, or the wheeled ambulance stretcher. Then move to the ambulance, and properly lift the patient into the patient compartment.

No matter how careful the driver may be, riding to the hospital while lying on one's back on a stretcher can be uncomfortable and even dangerous. So be sure to secure the patient with at least three straps across the body ▶ **Figure 35-24** . Use deceleration or stopping straps over the shoulders to prevent the patient from continuing to move forward in case the ambulance suddenly slows or stops.

The Transport Phase

Inform dispatch when you are ready to leave with the patient. Report the number of patients you have and the name of the receiving hospital. Even though you have already assessed and treated the patient, you should continue to monitor him or her en route. These ongoing assessments may uncover changes in the patient's vital signs and overall condition. Be sure to recheck the patient's vital signs en route. The frequency of checking vital signs depends on the situation, but checking them every 15 minutes for a stable patient and every 5 minutes for an unstable patient is a practice that many services use. In addition, it is important that you continually reassess the patient's clinical situation, and record and address new problems and the patient's responses to earlier treatment.

At this time, you should also contact the receiving hospital. Inform medical control about your patient(s) and the nature of the problem(s). Depending on the number of EMT-Bs on your team and how much care the patient needs, you might also want to begin working on your written report while en route.

Finally, and most importantly, do not abandon the patient emotionally. Do not become so involved in paperwork and ongoing assessments that you ignore the patient's fears. You are there to help the patient as a person, so use this time to reassure him or her. Some patients, such as the very young or elderly, may benefit from added attention during transport. Be aware of the differing levels of need of different patients.

The Delivery Phase

Inform dispatch as soon as you arrive at the hospital. Then follow these steps to transfer the patient to the receiving hospital:

1. Report your arrival to the triage nurse or other arrival personnel.

2. Physically transfer the patient from the stretcher to the bed directed for your patient.

3. Present a complete verbal report at the bedside to the nurse or physician who is taking over the patient's care.

4. Complete a detailed written report, and leave a copy with an appropriate staff member.

Figure 35-24 Be sure to secure the patient appropriately for protection during transport.

Figure 35-25 After transferring the patient and relating patient information to the hospital staff, you should restock any items that were used during the run.

The written report should include a summary of the history of the patient's current illness or injury with pertinent positives and negatives, mechanism of injury, and findings on your arrival. In addition, you should list vital signs and briefly mention relevant past medical or surgical history, as well as information regarding medication and allergies. Also, be sure to include any treatment and its effect that occurred in the prehospital setting.

While at the hospital, you may be able to restock any items that were used during the run, such as oxygen masks or dressings and bandages ▲ **Figure 35-25** . Remember, though, that your priority is transfer of the patient and patient information to the hospital staff. Restocking the ambulance comes second.

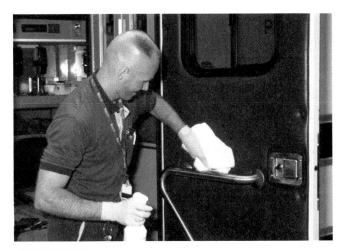

Figure 35-26 Be sure to clean and disinfect the ambulance and equipment at the station if you did not do so at the hospital.

En Route to the Station

Once you leave the hospital, inform dispatch whether or not you are in service and where you are going. As soon as you are back at the station, you should do the following:

- Clean and disinfect the ambulance and any equipment that was used, if you did not do so before leaving the hospital ▲ **Figure 35-26** .

- Restock any supplies you did not get at the hospital.

The Postrun Phase

During the postrun phase, you should complete and file any additional written reports and again inform dispatch of your status, location, and availability.

You are also responsible for maintaining the ambulance so that it is safe and available on a moment's notice. This means routine inspections. Use a written checklist to document needed repairs or replacement of equipment and supplies. In addition, you must ensure that the following steps are taken after each trip:

- Scrub blood, vomitus, and other substances from the floors, walls, and ceilings with soap and water.

- Clean and decontaminate the inside of the ambulance, according to state and local regulations. (You can use a 10% solution of bleach in water to clean the ambulance after any contamination.)

- Dispose of any contaminated waste in the manner prescribed by your agency.

- Clean the outside of the ambulance as needed.

- Replace or repair broken or damaged equipment without delay.

- Replace any other equipment or supplies that were used.

- Refuel the vehicle if the fuel tank is below required reserves. The oil level should be checked each time the vehicle is refueled.

It is important that you know the meanings of the terms "cleaning," "disinfection," "high-level disinfection," and "sterilization," as follows:

- **Cleaning**. The process of removing dirt, dust, blood, or other visible contaminants from a surface.

- **Disinfection**. The killing of pathogenic agents by directly applying a chemical made for that purpose to a surface.

- **High-level disinfection**. The killing of pathogenic agents by the use of potent means of disinfection.

- **Sterilization**. A process, such as the use of heat, that removes all microbial contamination.

Dispose of any contaminated materials that are not disinfected by placing them in the appropriate containers used for biohazard disposal.

Prescheduled preventive maintenance checks. The ambulance chassis and engine components are subjected to significantly greater stresses than the typical automobile or truck. For this reason, the manufacturer's recommendations for periodic maintenance must be strictly followed, especially regarding lubrication, oil and filter changes, transmission and differential service, brakes, wheel alignment, wheel bearings, and steering components. Many services now use a Hobbs or engineer hour meter, which assesses hours of engine use, in addition to the odometer to help determine periodic maintenance requirements.

As is the case with emergency medical care report forms, local and individual differences will affect inspection routines. Your ambulance service should develop its own inspection forms for all three kinds of inspections so that nothing is overlooked. These forms should be filed for inspection and legal documentation and should be kept for at least 3 years.

Air Medical Operations

<u>Air ambulances</u> are used to evacuate medical patients. They land at or near the scene, and transport patients to trauma facilities every day in many areas.

There are two basic types of air medical units: fixed-wing and rotary-wing, otherwise known as helicopters ▶ **Figure 35-27** . Fixed-wing aircraft generally are used for interhospital patient transfers over distances greater than 100 to 150 miles. For shorter distances, ground transport or rotary-wing aircraft are more efficient.

Specially trained medical flight crews accompany all air ambulance flights. Your role in fixed-wing aircraft transfers probably will be limited to providing ground transport for the patient and medical flight crew between the hospital and the airport.

Rotary-wing aircraft have become an important tool in providing emergency medical care. Trauma patient survival is directly related to the time that elapses between injury and definitive treatment. Most helicopters that are used for emergency medical operations fly well in excess of 100 mph in a straight line, without road or traffic hazards. The crew may include EMTs, paramedics, flight nurses, or physicians.

You should be familiar with the capabilities, protocols, and methods for accessing helicopters in your area. Helicopter services provide training for EMT-Bs in ground operations and safety. The following discussion is an introduction to safe operations, and is not intended to be substituted for the more extensive courses available locally.

Safety Precautions Around Helicopters

Helicopter safety is nothing more than good common sense, along with a constant awareness of the need for personal safety. The types of helicopters that are used for medical operations vary, but the dangers are the same. If you are familiar with the way helicopters work and follow the pilot's instructions, you will minimize these dangers. You should be sure to do nothing near the helicopter and go only where the pilot or crew directs you.

The most important rule is to keep a safe distance from the aircraft whenever it is on the ground and "hot," which means when the tail rotor is spinning. This means that every EMT-B should stay outside the landing zone perimeter unless directed by the pilot or a member of the flight crew that they are to come to the aircraft. Usually, the flight crew will come to the EMT-Bs carrying their own equipment and not require any assistance inside the landing zone. If you are asked to enter the landing zone, stay away from the tail rotor; the tips of its blades move so rapidly that they are invisible. In fact, never approach the helicopter from the rear, even if it is not hot. If you must move from one side of the helicopter to another, go around the front. Never duck under the body, the tail boom, or the rear section of the helicopter; the pilot

Figure 35-27 **A.** Fixed-wing aircraft are generally used to transfer patients from one hospital to another over distances greater than 100 to 150 miles. **B.** A rotary-wing aircraft, or helicopter, is used to help provide emergency medical care to patients who need to be transported quickly over shorter distances.

cannot see in these areas. The proper approach area is between the nine-o'clock and three-o'clock positions as the pilot faces forward ▶ **Figure 35-28** .

Another area of concern is the height of the main rotor blade. On many aircraft, it is flexible and may dip as low as 4′ off the ground ▶ **Figure 35-29** . When you approach the aircraft, walk in a crouched position. Wind gusts can alter the blade height without warning, so be sure to protect equipment as you carry it under the blades. Air turbulence created by the rotor blades can blow off hats and loose equipment. These, in turn, can become a danger to the aircraft and personnel in the area.

When accompanying a flight crew member, you must follow directions exactly. Never try to open any aircraft door or move equipment unless a crew member tells you to. When told to approach the aircraft, use extreme caution and pay constant attention to hazards.

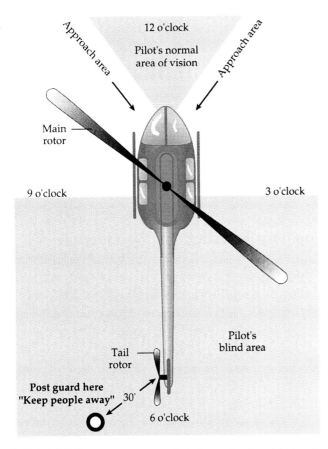

Figure 35-28 Approach a helicopter between the nine-o'clock and three-o'clock positions as the pilot faces forward.

Figure 35-29 The main rotor blade of the helicopter is flexible and may dip as low as 4' off the ground.

Landing Sites

Although a helicopter can fly straight up and down, this is the most dangerous mode of operation. The safest and most effective way to land and take off is similar to that used by fixed-wing aircraft. Landing at a slight angle allows for safer operations. Takeoff combines a gradual lift and forward motion to travel up and out on a slight angle.

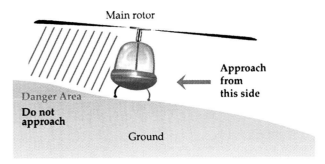

Figure 35-30 Approach a helicopter on a grade from the downhill side only.

Clearing a landing site is another important role you can play. Look for loose debris, electric or telephone wires, poles, or any other hazards that might interfere with the safe operation of the helicopter. If you note any hazards, inform the pilot by radio or other signal. The pilot will usually "overfly," or survey the site, before final approach and landing to ensure that all potential dangers are identified. Depending on the time, temperature, winds, and the aircraft's weight, you might need to mark the proposed site with flags, lights, or other signaling devices. A clear landing zone that is at least 100' by 100' is recommended.

If the helicopter must land on a grade, extra caution is advised. The main rotor blade will be closer to the ground on the uphill side. In this situation, approach the aircraft from the downhill side only ▲ Figure 35-30 . Do not move the patient to the helicopter until the crew has signaled that they are ready to receive you. A flight crew member will direct and assist you in loading the patient.

Nighttime operations are considerably more hazardous than daytime operations because of the darkness. The pilot may fly over the area with the helicopter's lights on to spot obstacles and the shadows of overhead wires, which can be hard to see. Do not shine spotlights, flashlights, or any other lights in the air to help the pilot; they may temporarily blind the pilot. Instead, direct light beams toward the ground at the landing site. Even after the helicopter has landed, you should not aim lights anywhere near it. Of course, smoking, open lights or flames, and flares are prohibited within 50' of the aircraft at all times.

For further information on air ambulances, see the following publications:

- DOT publication HS805-703, Air Ambulance Guidelines, February 1981

- DOT publication HS806-841, Proceedings: National MEDEVAC Helicopter Conference

Prep Kit

Ready for Review

An ambulance is an emergency medical vehicle that contains a driver's compartment, a patient compartment, equipment and supplies to provide care at the scene and during transport, and two-way radio communication. It must be designed and constructed to ensure maximum safety and comfort. Ambulances should be white on the outside with an orange stripe, and should have blue lettering and reflectorized emblems. The Star of Life, a six-pointed emblem that identifies ambulances that meet federal specifications, may be displayed on the sides, rear, and roof of the ambulance.

The ambulance should be climate-controlled, insulated, and easy to clean. The patient compartment should be large enough to accommodate two stretcher patients, two EMTs, and all the necessary equipment and supplies to take care of patients.

The nine phases of an ambulance call are preparation for the call, dispatch, en route to the scene, arrival at the scene, transferring the patient to the ambulance, en route to the receiving facility, at the receiving facility, en route to the station, and postrun.

Specific patient care supplies should be carried on the ambulance, including basic medical equipment, airway management equipment and ventilation devices, suctioning equipment, oxygen delivery equipment, CPR equipment, and basic wound care supplies. In addition, you must ensure that splinting supplies, childbirth supplies, and appropriate medications are on board. An automated external defibrillator, as permitted by medical control, should always be carried on the ambulance. A jump kit, patient transfer equipment, nonmedical supplies, and initial extrication and rescue equipment are also needed.

The driver must be qualified to drive the ambulance; he or she must be physically and emotionally fit, and have the proper attitude. The driver must know and follow safe driving practices.

In addition to ground ambulances, air ambulances in the form of fixed-wing aircraft or helicopters are used to evacuate patients, land at a crash scene, and transport patients to trauma facilities.

Vital Vocabulary

acceleration The process of increasing speed.

air ambulances Fixed-wing aircraft and helicopters that have been modified for medical care; used to evacuate and transport patients with life-threatening injuries to treatment facilities.

ambulance A specialized vehicle for treating and transporting sick and injured patients.

chassis The vehicle frame.

chassis set Transfer of the weight (center of mass) of the ambulance to different points on the chassis.

cleaning The process of removing dirt, dust, blood, or other visible contaminants from a surface.

coefficient of friction A measure of the grip of the tire on the road surface.

CPR board A device that provides a firm surface under the patient's torso.

deceleration The process of slowing down.

decontaminate To remove or neutralize radiation, chemical, or other hazardous material from clothing, equipment, vehicles, and personnel.

disinfection The killing of pathogenic agents by direct application of chemicals.

first-responder vehicle A specialized vehicle used to transport EMS equipment and personnel to the scenes of medical emergencies.

footprint The area of contact between the ambulance tire and the road surface.

friction Resistance to the motion of one body against another.

high-level disinfection The killing of pathogenic agents by using potent means of disinfection.

hydroplaning A condition in which the tires of a vehicle may be lifted off the road surface as water "piles up" under them, making the vehicle feel as though it is floating.

jump kit A portable kit containing items that are used in the initial care of the patient.

Star of Life The six-pointed star that identifies vehicles that meet federal specifications as licensed or certified ambulances.

sterilization A process, such as heating, that removes microbial contamination.

Assessment in Action

All of your hard work has paid off. You have completed the EMT-B course, passed the state test, and have been certified. In addition, you have a new job as an EMT-B with a local private ambulance service. You put on your uniform and report to headquarters where you are introduced to your new partner. You shake hands, say your hellos, and head out to the bay to check out your rig and start your orientation.

1. Of the following, which issue with the ambulance is **LEAST** important to tell your supervisor about?
   A. Strange-sounding brakes
   B. Oil dripping under the engine
   C. A full tank of gas
   D. A screw stuck in the front tire

2. As you are checking the patient compartment, you find a small, dried puddle of blood under the stretcher. What should you do next?
   A. Wipe up the blood with a wet paper towel.
   B. Wait until the end of your shift to clean up the blood.
   C. Clean up the blood using appropriate BSI precautions.
   D. Leave the problem for the crew that left the ambulance dirty.

3. You notice that there are no cervical collars in the trauma bag. If you respond to a call without the required equipment on the ambulance, you could legally be charged with:
   A. slander.
   B. negligence.
   C. abandonment.
   D. malfeasance.

4. As you wait for your first call, you begin to review ambulance operations. According to state laws that govern ambulance operations, you are NOT allowed to:
   A. park in a no parking zone.
   B. endanger people's lives and property.
   C. go the wrong way down a one-way street.
   D. drive faster than the posted speed limit.

5. Which of the following statements about transporting a patient is **FALSE**?
   A. A patient who is in stable condition can ride alone in the patient compartment.
   B. Safety precautions should be observed for patients and providers alike whenever possible.
   C. All equipment that is not currently being used for patient care should be stowed.
   D. A patient on the cot should be strapped securely into place and the cot secured in place as well.

6. As a general rule of thumb, the more complex a piece of equipment is:
   A. the less often one needs to train on it.
   B. the more often it needs to be checked to see if it is working.
   C. the less often it needs medical control before it can be used.
   D. the more often it will need to be cleaned.

7. The ambulance should carry both:
   A. a fixed or mounted suction unit and a portable one.
   B. a rigid and a folding stretcher or cot.
   C. a fixed or mounted CPR board and a portable one.
   D. a rigid and a folding long backboard.

Challenging Questions

8. Which of the following supplies for splinting fractures and dislocations should be carried on the ambulance?
   A. Rolled up magazines and gauze bandaging
   B. Cravats and trauma dressings
   C. An ambulance stretcher with linen and blankets
   D. A long backboard and extrication device

9. Which of the following equipment is designed to be used during the first 5 minutes of an emergency situation?
   A. Sterile dressings and roller bandages
   B. A traction splint
   C. A semiautomated external defibrillator
   D. An extrication device

10. When you are working around or near an EMS helicopter or air medical unit:
    A. only go when and where the pilot or flight crew direct.
    B. take equipment from the aircraft but only when you see that something may be needed.
    C. move freely about the area when the aircraft is "cold" (when its engines are turned off and the rotors are not turning).
    D. do not enter the landing zone unless given permission by the fire personnel at the scene.

Points to Ponder

You have responded to a patient whose chief complaint is difficulty of breathing. He does not have an address locally and appears to have been living in the streets for a few days. He has a history of hypertension and asthma and is experiencing some difficulty breathing and has a moderate wound above his eye from a fall 2 days ago. You load him into your ambulance and head toward the nearest hospital. When you contact the hospital for a pre-arrival report, they "divert" you to another hospital. There has been no divert announced and they did not tell you until after you described your patient. You believe that they are "dumping" this patient in violation of EMTALA. What should you do?

Issues Patient "Dumping," Divert Declarations, EMTALA, Working with Hospital Personnel, Relationships with Hospitals, Outcome of Reporting the Hospital.

Online Outlook

Ambulance vehicles are classified as Type I, II, or III. To learn more about ambulance vehicle classifications, complete Exercise 35 at www.emtb.com.

www.emtb.com

Gaining Access

Objectives

Cognitive

1. Describe the purpose of extrication (p 832).
2. Discuss the role of the EMT-B in extrication (p 833).
3. Identify what equipment for personal safety is required for the EMT-B (p 834).
4. Define the fundamental components of extrication (p 832).
5. State the steps that should be taken to protect the patient during extrication (p 834).
6. Evaluate various methods of gaining access to the patient (p 835).
7. Distinguish between simple and complex access (p 836).

Affective

None

Psychomotor

None

3

www.emtb.com

Online Chapter Pretest
Interactivities
Vocabulary Explorer
Anatomy Review
Web Links
Online Review Manual
Distance Learning

Skill Drills
Vital Vocabulary
Pediatric Needs
Geriatric Needs
EMT-B Safety
EMT-B Tips
Documentation Tips
Remember
Prep Kit

"Unit 2, respond to a motor vehicle crash with two critically injured patients pinned inside the wreckage. The fire department is on scene." On arrival, you report to the fire captain in charge and he asks for your assistance with patient care inside the vehicle while rescue personnel proceed with extrication.

This chapter will help you understand what is going on around you, how to act safely when asked to be with the patient, and the importance of coordinating with those in charge before entering the area or wreckage. It will also help you answer the following questions:

1. What protective gear should you wear if you are asked to enter a crashed vehicle to assess a patient?

2. If you are treating a trapped patient in a car wreck, when do you need to communicate with rescue personnel? What can you ask them to do to allow you to do your job better?

Gaining Access

As an EMT-B, you will usually not be responsible for rescue and extrication. Rescue involves many different processes and environments. It also requires training beyond the level of the EMT-B. In this chapter, you will learn basic concepts of extrication.

The chapter begins with a discussion of personal safety and patient safety. Gaining access is the next phase of extrication discussed. This includes how to gain access to patients and how to keep patients and bystanders safe in the process. Your main concern is reaching the patient so that you can begin providing care. In most instances, once you have reached the patient, extrication will occur around you and the patient. Communication between the EMT-B caring for the patient and fire personnel performing the extrication is vital. Removal is the final phase of extrication, and this usually results in the patient being placed on the ambulance stretcher.

Fundamentals of Extrication

During all phases of rescue, your primary concern is safety, and your primary role is to provide emergency medical care and prevent further injury to the patient. You will provide care as extrication goes on around you unless this proves to be too dangerous for you or the patient. **Extrication** is the removal from entrapment or from a dangerous situation or position. **Entrapment** means to be caught within a closed area with no way out, or to have a limb or other body part trapped. In the context of this chapter, extrication means removal of a patient from a wrecked automo-

bile. However, the same principles and concepts apply to other situations.

You will need to coordinate your efforts with those of the rescue team. If you respect their job, they will respect yours. You should communicate with members of the rescue team throughout the extrication process. Start talking to the rescue team leader as soon as you arrive at the scene. Under the incident command system (described in Chapter 37), the rescue operations are integrated as a separate group. The EMT-B becomes a member of this group, and will enter the vehicle and provide care for the patient(s) when approved by the extrication leader.

At any accident scene, four different basic functions must be addressed ▶ **Figure 36-1** . When possible, responders work in well-defined separate teams to ensure clear lines of responsibility and organization. Each team focuses on and is responsible for a different function:

- Firefighters are responsible for extinguishing any fire, preventing additional ignition, ensuring that the scene is safe, and washing down any spilled fuel.

- Law enforcement is responsible for traffic control and direction, maintaining order at the scene, investigating the crash or crime scene, and establishing and maintaining lines so that bystanders are kept at a safe distance and out of the way of rescuers.

- The rescue team is responsible for properly securing and stabilizing the vehicle, providing safe entrance and **access** to patients (the ability to reach the patient), extricating any patients, ensuring that patients are properly protected during extrication or other rescue activities, and providing adequate room so that patients can be removed properly.

- EMS personnel are responsible for assessing and providing immediate medical care, triage and assigning priority to patients, packaging the patient, providing additional assessment and care as needed once the patient has been removed, and providing transport to the emergency department.

Good communication among team members and clear leadership are essential to safe, efficient provision of proper emergency care. Although your input at the scene is important, one member of your team must be clearly in charge. The team leader's assessment of the patient and the situation will dictate the way in which medical care, packaging, and transport will proceed. Customarily, the crew chief, who typically is clearly

indicated on the shift schedule, is responsible for this role. If not, a team leader must be identified and agreed to before you arrive at the scene.

In some areas, there might not be enough personnel for two or multiple separate units. In these areas, you and your team may have two roles. However, one person must still be in charge of the overall rescue operation. If there is no identifiable leadership at the scene, the rescue effort and patient care will suffer. Leaders should be identified as part of a larger incident command system. They should be medically trained and qualified to judge the priorities of patient care, and they must also be experienced in extrication.

Scene Size-Up

You must always be prepared, mentally and physically, for any incident that requires rescue or extrication. The most important part of this preparation is thinking about your safety and the safety of your team. Safety begins with the proper mind-set and the proper protective equipment.

When you arrive, you should position the unit in a safe location that does not add a hazard to the scene. Before proceeding, make sure that the scene is properly marked and that either the road is closed or traffic flow is controlled safely around the scene ▼ Figure 36-2 . One of the important responsibilities of scene size-up is to determine what, if any, additional resources will be needed. These resources may include additional EMS units and personnel. If you are first on the scene, you may need to initiate a rescue response or call for law enforcement or specialized crews, such as HazMat or utility departments.

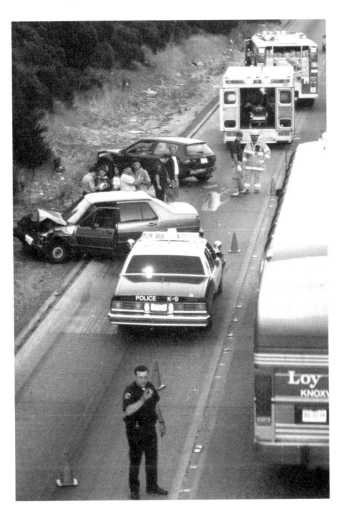

Figure 36-1 Every crash requires cooperation, as each responder has a specific role at the scene. Firefighters, law enforcement, the rescue team, and EMS personnel all have individual roles.

Figure 36-2 The scene of a crash should be marked properly, and traffic should be diverted so that responders have enough room to work.

Figure 36-3 Proper protective equipment varies depending on the situation.

Figure 36-4 Always explain to the patient why you are there and what you are doing.

The equipment that you use and the gear that you wear will depend on the situation (▲ **Figure 36-3**). However, the importance of wearing blood- and fluid-impermeable gloves at all times during patient contact cannot be emphasized enough. If you will be involved with extrication, you should wear a pair of leather gloves over your disposable gloves to protect you from injury in handling ropes, tools, broken glass, hot or cold objects, or sharp metal.

Remember, you should not attempt to gain access to the patient or enter the vehicle until you are sure that the vehicle is stable and that any hazards have been identified and either properly controlled or eliminated. When there is a rescue leader present, you will only be authorized to enter when these considerations have been met.

Patient and Bystander Safety

While you are gaining access to the patient and during extrication, you must make sure that the patient remains safe. Always talk to the patient and describe what you are going to do before you do it and as you are doing it, even if you think the patient is unconscious (▲ **Figure 36-4**). In many instances, you or your partner may be providing cervical spine immobilization or other care during extrication. EMS personnel should wear proper protective gear while in the working area. The patient and the EMS personnel should be covered with a heavy, nonflammable blanket to protect them against flying glass or other objects. A backboard may also be used as a protective shield (▲ **Figure 36-5**). Try to keep heat, noise, and force to a minimum. Use only what is necessary to extricate the patient safely.

Bystanders and family members can be hazards themselves. If they are allowed to get too close,

Figure 36-5 Use a spine board or blanket to protect the patient and any rescuers who are providing care.

they are at risk of injury and may also interfere with the overall management of the incident. For these reasons, the rescue group will set up a danger zone that is off-limits to bystanders (▶ **Figure 36-6**). A **danger zone** (hot zone) is an area where individuals can be exposed to sharp metal edges, broken glass, toxic substances, lethal rays, or ignition or explosion of hazardous materials. You should help to set up and enforce this zone. If you arrive before the rescue group, you should coordinate crowd control with law enforcement officials.

Occasionally, a bystander may prove difficult to manage. This situation is especially challenging when the bystander claims to have medical credentials. Your EMS service should have a protocol for dealing with this situation. Many states provide physicians with wallet-sized copies of their medical license to use as identification (▶ **Figure 36-7**). However, not all physicians have training

Figure 36-6 A danger zone should be established to prevent bystanders from entering the area around an incident.

Figure 36-8 The exact way to gain access depends on many factors, including the terrain, the way in which the vehicle is situated, and the weather.

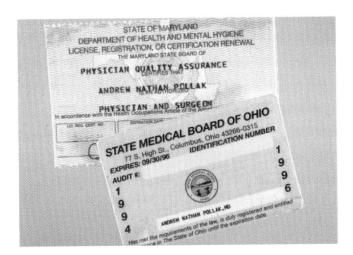

Figure 36-7 Many physicians carry a wallet-sized copy of their medical license.

in emergency medical care. If this situation occurs, inform medical control immediately. Communication between medical control and the physician at the scene may eliminate some of the problems. You may also assign such individuals duties that will allow them to become involved in a small way. This will reduce the risk of a possible confrontation.

Gaining Access to the Patient

The exact way you gain access to or reach the patient(s) depends on the situation. It is up to you to identify the safest, most efficient way to gain access. Darkness, uneven terrain, tall grass, shrubbery, or wreckage may make patients hard to find **▲ Figure 36-8** . Multiple vehicles with multiple patients may be involved. If this is the case, you should locate and rapidly triage each patient to determine who needs urgent care. This step

is important before you proceed with any treatment and patient packaging. Be sure to take these factors into account in your scene size-up. Remember that scene size-up is a continuing process, because the situation often changes. As a result, you may need to change your plans for gaining access and providing treatment.

To determine the exact location and position of the patient, you and your team should consider the following questions:

- Is the patient in a vehicle or in some other structure?
- Is the vehicle or structure severely damaged?
- What hazards exist that pose risk to the patient and rescuers?
- In what position is the vehicle? On what type of surface? Is the vehicle stable or is it apt to roll or tip?

You must also take into account the patient's injuries and their severity. You may have to change your course of action as you learn more about the patient's condition. Do not try to access the patient until you are sure that the vehicle is stable and that hazards have been identified and rendered safe. Hazards might include electrical or gas lines.

What should you do if you have to remove a patient quickly because the environment is threatening or you need to perform CPR? CPR is not effective when the patient is in a sitting position or lying on the soft seat of a vehicle. In these instances, you and your team may have to use the rapid extrication technique to move a patient from a sitting position inside a vehicle to a supine position on a long backboard. A team of

Figure 36-9 Get to the patient as quickly and simply as possible by opening the door without using tools or breaking any glass.

EMT-Bs who are experienced in using this technique should be able to rapidly remove a patient who is not entrapped keeping in mind the patient's condition and the group's safety. Use the rapid extrication technique only as a last resort.

SIMPLE ACCESS. Your first step is **simple access**, trying to get to the patient as quickly and simply as possible without using any tools or breaking any glass. Automobiles are built for easy entry and exit; however, it may be necessary to use tools or other forcible entry methods. Whenever possible, you should first try to unlock the doors (or ask the patient to unlock them) or roll down the windows. Try to open every door using the door handles to gain access before breaking any windows or using other methods of forced entry ▲ Figure 36-9 . Enter through the doors when there is no danger to the patient. The rescue group should provide the entrance you need to gain access to the patient.

COMPLEX ACCESS. **Complex access** requires the use of special tools and special training and includes breaking windows or other forcible entry. Most of these skills are too advanced for the 110-hour EMT-B course and are not covered in this text.

Patient Care During Entrapment and Extrication

Providing medical care to a patient who is trapped in a vehicle is principally the same as that for any other patient. Unless there is an immediate threat of fire, explosion, or other danger, once entrance and access to the patient have been provided, you should perform an initial assessment and provide care before further extrication begins, as follows:

1. Provide manual stabilization to protect the cervical spine, as needed.

2. Open the airway.

3. Provide high-flow oxygen.

4. Assist or provide for adequate ventilation.

5. Control any significant external bleeding.

6. Treat all critical injuries.

Preparation for Removal

As a part of your assessment, you should participate in the preparation for removal. Determine how urgently the patient must be extricated, where you should be positioned to best protect the patient during extrication, and, once the patient has been freed, how you will best move the patient from within the vehicle onto the long backboard and onto the stretcher. Carefully examine the exposed area of the limb or other part of the patient that is trapped to determine the extent of injury and whether there is a possibility of hidden bleeding. If possible, you should also evaluate sensation in the trapped area so that you will know whether increased pain indicates that an object is pressing on or impaled in the patient during extrication.

During this time, the rescue group is assessing exactly how the patient is trapped and determining the safest, easiest way to extricate him or her. Your input is essential so that the patient's injuries are considered as the rescue group plans a move that protects the patient from further harm. Once the plan has been devised and everyone understands what will be done, you should determine how best to protect the patient. Often, you or another EMT-B will be placed in the vehicle alongside the patient to monitor his or her condition and well-being as the vehicle is being forcibly cut, bent, or disassembled. Be sure to wear proper protective clothing.

Naturally, your safety and that of the patient are paramount during this process. Both you and the patient should be covered by a thick, fire-resistant canvas or blanket for protection from broken glass, flying particles, tools, or other hazards during any cutting or forceful extrication maneuvers. Extrication is often extremely noisy. You must be sure that you can communicate effectively with both the patient and the rescue group so that you can instantly let the rescuers know if it is necessary that they stop.

Once the patient has been freed, rapidly assess any previously unaccessible patient, and reassess the patient. Make sure that the spine is manually immobilized, and apply a cervical collar if this was not previously done.

Reevaluate whether the patient needs to be immediately removed by using manual immobilization and the rapid extrication technique, or whether the patient's condition and the scene allow for immobilization using an extrication vest or short backboard before he or she is moved further. In most cases, it is impractical and difficult to properly apply extremity splints within the vehicle. Extremity injuries can generally be rapidly supported and immobilized while the patient is being removed by securing an injured arm to the body and, if a leg is injured, securing one leg to the other. This will be adequate until the patient is secured to the backboard or time allows for more detailed assessment and splinting of each injury.

Removal

Moving the patient in one fast, continuous step increases the risk of harm and confusion. To ensure that each EMT-B can be positioned so that he or she can lift and carry properly at all times, move the patient in a series of smooth, slow, controlled steps, with stops designed between them to allow for the repositioning and adjustments that are needed. Plan the exact steps and pathway that you will follow in moving the patient from sitting in the vehicle to lying supine on the backboard and prepared ambulance cot. Choose a path that requires the least manipulation of the patient or equipment. Make sure that sufficient personnel are available. Once you are sure that everyone understands the steps and is ready, you can move the patient safely. Make sure that you move the patient as a unit, resisting the temptation to move the immobilization device instead. While moving the patient, continue to protect him or her from any hazards.

Once the patient has been placed on the stretcher, continue with any additional assessment and treatment that was deferred. If it is extremely cold or hot, raining or snowing, you will want to load the stretcher and patient into the climate-controlled ambulance before continuing assessment and treatment. If the patient's condition requires that transport be initiated without further delay, you should provide only the additional care that is essential or necessary to package the patient. Leave the remaining steps to be performed while you are en route to the hospital.

Specialized Rescue Situations

On most calls, you can drive the ambulance to within a short distance of the patient's location and, with either simple or complex access, you can reach and treat the patient. However, in some situations, the patient can be

EMT-B Safety

A vehicle crash scene can present many of the hazards to rescuer and patient safety that you will encounter in emergency responses: fuel spills that pose fire and explosion risks, downed electrical lines, broken glass and torn metal, and exposure to potentially infectious body fluids. Your safety at every type of emergency scene begins with, and depends on, an initial scene size-up that leads to decisions about what kind of personal protective equipment to use and whether to call for additional or specialized assistance.

reached only by teams that are trained in making special technical rescues. Specialized skills of these teams include the following:

- Technical rope rescue (low- and high-angle rescue)
- Mountain, rock, and ice-climbing rescue
- Cross-field and trail rescue (park rangers)
- Water and small craft rescue
- White-water rescue
- Dive rescue (SCUBA)
- Cave rescue
- Mine rescue
- Confined space rescue
- Ski slope and cross-country or trail snow rescue (ski patrol)
- Lost person search and rescue (SAR)
- Tactical response and rescue (SWAT)

THE EMT AND TECHNICAL RESCUE SITUATIONS. **Technical rescue situations** may contain hidden dangers, and special technical skills are needed for personnel to safely enter and move around. It is not safe to include any personnel who do not have the necessary special training and experience in such a rescue. A **technical rescue group** is made up of individuals from one or more departments in a region who are trained and on call for certain types of technical rescue. Many members of a technical rescue group are also trained as first responders or EMT-Bs so that they can provide the necessary immediate care when only they can safely reach the patient. Even when the technical rescue group includes a paramedic or physician, generally nothing but essential simple care is provided until the rescuers can bring the patient to the nearest point where a safe, stable setting exists.

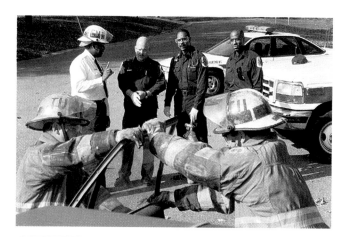

Figure 36-10 The incident commander is the individual who has overall command of the scene.

If a technical rescue group is necessary but is not present when you arrive, you should immediately check with the incident commander to make sure that the group has been summoned and is en route to your location. The **incident commander** is the individual who has overall command of the scene in the field ▲ **Figure 36-10** . If no incident commander is present, follow local guidelines. (Chapter 37 discusses Incident Command in more detail.)

When you arrive at a scene where a technical rescue is already in progress, you will usually be met by a member of the rescue group and directed or led to the actual rescue site. If the rescue scene is at some distance from the road, you may need to leave the ambulance on the road. The use of the ambulance stretcher is impractical in these situations; you should instead bring a long backboard and/or basket stretcher or similar rescue stretcher to carry the patient back to the waiting ambulance. Be sure that you take all of the carry-in kits and other equipment you may need to treat and immobilize the patient at the actual rescue operation site.

When you arrive at the rescue operation site, identify the stable location to which the rescue group will bring the patient, and set up your equipment there. As soon as the rescue group has brought the patient to this staging area, you should perform a rapid assessment and, after providing the treatment indicated, package the patient without delay. Although you and the other EMTs who responded with the ambulance will assume the primary responsibility for the patient's care at this point, it usually requires a cooperative effort by both the rescue group and EMS teams to carry the patient to the waiting ambulance. Consider using an air medical unit if the patient will need to be carried and/or transported an extensive distance.

LOST PERSONS SEARCH AND RESCUE. When someone is lost in the outdoors and a search effort is initiated, an ambulance is usually summoned to the search base. Each search team will be organized to include a member who is trained to either the first responder or EMT-B level, carrying the essential equipment to provide simple immediate care. Your role, and that of the other EMT-Bs who arrived with the ambulance, is to stand by at the search base until the lost person or people have been found.

As soon as you arrive at the scene and have been briefed on the situation, you should isolate and prepare the equipment you will need to carry in to the patient's location so that no time is lost once the patient has been found or a member of the search team becomes injured. The prepared carry-in equipment, including a long backboard and other equipment you will need to immobilize the patient, should be left in the back of the ambulance so that it is protected from the weather. In addition, if the ambulance should need to be relocated, the equipment will not need to be reloaded or possibly be left behind. You will usually be given a portable radio that is tuned to the search frequency so that you can monitor the progress of the search and communicate with and be contacted by those in charge of the search operation.

Sometimes, you may be asked to stay with relatives of the lost individual who are at the scene. Find out from relatives whether the lost person has any medical history that may need to be addressed, and pass this information on to those who are in charge of the search. Unless you have been instructed otherwise, only incident command should communicate any news or progress of the search to the family. For this reason, you must be sure that your radio is set at a discreet volume.

Once the lost person has been found, you will be guided by search personnel to that location or a prearranged intersecting point where the patient will be carried to decrease the amount of time you need to reach the patient and begin treatment. You should be sure that the carry-in equipment is evenly distributed among personnel and that the pace is such that all can stay together easily. Sometimes, the time and effort that are needed to reach and carry out the patient can be decreased by relocating the ambulance or, if available, by using a four-wheel drive or all-terrain vehicle. As with other technical rescues, although the ambulance crew will assume the responsibility for patient care once they are at the patient's side, a cooperative effort of both EMS and the search team is necessary to safely carry the patient to the base and waiting ambulance.

TACTICAL SITUATIONS. If you are called to a scene where a **tactical situation** is taking place, such as an armed hostage situation, presence of a sniper, or exchange of shots, and the threat of violence remains, you should turn off the lights and sirens as you come close to the scene. In such situations, you should request direction from the incident commander or another appropriate authority in control of the scene. When you arrive at the outer perimeter barrier line that the police have established, you should ask a police officer to notify the incident commander of your arrival and for an officer to guide you to the shielded, safe staging area that has been selected for the ambulance and for care of the wounded and injured.

For your safety, you should exit the ambulance, stay low, and remain near the side of the vehicle unless you are directed to another place of safety. Do not turn on the vehicle's outside speakers, and turn down the volume of any radios that you are carrying. No matter how tempting it is to look, be sure that you do not look around the corner of any building or around the sides or over the top of any structure that may be serving to shield you. If it is dark outside, turn off the headlights and all clearance lights, and do not display any other light that might be reflected and serve to highlight your general location.

As in other technical rescue situations, your role, and that of the other EMT-Bs, is to stand by at the staging area and treat and package injured patients after the SWAT team or other law enforcement officers have evacuated them to your shielded, safe location. When you are ready to transport a patient, you should ask a law enforcement officer to notify the incident commander. You should leave only after the incident commander has verified that it is safe for the ambulance to move. Be sure that you follow the specific route that is indicated by the incident commander or a law enforcement officer assigned to guide you. You should proceed slowly for a good distance from the incident perimeter before using your emergency lights and siren.

STRUCTURE FIRES. In most areas, an ambulance is dispatched with the fire department apparatus to any structure fire, whether or not any injuries are reported. A fire in a house, apartment building, office, school, plant, warehouse, or other building is considered a **structure fire**. When responding to a major fire scene, you should determine whether, because of the fire, any special route will be necessary. Once you arrive at the scene, you should ask the incident commander where the ambulance should be parked. It is essential that the ambulance be parked far enough away from the fire to be safe from the fire itself or a collapsing building.

EMT-B Safety

Physical dangers such as fire, infectious disease, and electricity are not the only risks to your safety on emergency responses. Some calls involve the possibility of deliberate violence against rescuers. Formal tactical situations are the obvious examples, but "simple" calls involving assaults, possible alcohol or drug use, and domestic disputes can be just as dangerous. Your training, your attitude when responding to calls, and your routine daily procedures should all take these risks into account.

You must also ensure that the ambulance will not block or hinder other arriving equipment or become locked in by other equipment or hose lines. However, you must also make sure that the ambulance will be close enough to be visible and that patients can be brought to it easily. The fire officer who is the incident commander will decide where this location should be.

Your next step is to determine whether there are any injured patients at the scene or whether you have been called to stand by. A number of ambulances may be dispatched to a major fire to ensure that one or more units will always remain immediately available at the scene if others leave to transport the injured.

As with other technical rescue situations, search and rescue in a burning building requires special training and equipment. Search and rescue is performed by teams of firefighters wearing full turnout gear and self-contained breathing apparatus (SCBA), and carrying tools and fully charged hose lines. These teams will bring patients out of the burning building to the area where the ambulance is standing by. Therefore, unless otherwise ordered, you should always stay with the ambulance. Do not wander off even after the fire is basically out, in case a firefighter becomes injured during salvage and overhaul. The ambulance should leave the scene only if transporting a patient or if the incident commander has released it.

Sometimes, the scene at a crash or fire is further complicated by the presence of hazardous materials. A **hazardous material** is any substance that is toxic, poisonous, radioactive, flammable, or explosive and can cause injury or death with exposure. In addition to posing a threat to you and others at the immediate scene, hazardous materials may pose a threat to a much larger area and population. Whenever there is a possibility that a hazardous material is involved, you will have to follow a number of additional special procedures. (Chapter 37 covers the specifics of hazardous material procedures.)

Prep Kit

Ready for Review

During all phases of rescue, your primary concern is safety, and your primary role is to provide emergency medical care and prevent further injury to the patient. When there are not enough personnel for both an EMS team and a rescue team, you and your team may have to act as rescuers as well. Safety during rescue or extrication begins with the proper mind-set and the proper protective equipment. During size-up, you should identify the safest, most efficient way to access the patient. Try to get to the patient as simply and quickly as possible without using any tools or breaking any glass. Make sure that you and the patient are protected with a fireproof blanket. Unless there is immediate danger, perform an initial assessment of a patient while he or she is still in the vehicle. Immobilize the cervical spine before moving the patient from the vehicle. If you see that a special rescue team is needed, inform the dispatcher.

When a scene calls for a search or for specialized rescue, you may have to call for a technical rescue group, or you may find one already at work when you arrive. Your interaction and cooperation with this group, and with an incident commander when one has been designated, are important to a smooth rescue. You will be involved to some degree in the logistics of vehicle staging and patient movement, as well as patient care.

Tactical situations are best directly handled by teams with specialized training. Your role will often largely consist of remaining out of danger, cooperating with the incident commander, or with police or other specialized personnel if incident command is not in effect, and remaining ready to care for any patients that are brought to you.

Vital Vocabulary

access The ability to gain entry to an enclosed area and reach a patient.

complex access Complicated entry that requires special tools and training and includes breaking windows or using other force.

danger zone (hot zone) An area where individuals can be exposed to sharp metal edges, broken glass, toxic substances, lethal rays, or ignition or explosion of hazardous materials.

entrapment To be caught (trapped) within a vehicle, room, or container with no way out, or to have a limb or other body part trapped.

extrication Removal of a patient from entrapment or a dangerous situation or position, such as removal from a wrecked vehicle, industrial accident, or building collapse.

hazardous material Any substance that is toxic, poisonous, radioactive, flammable, or explosive and causes injury or death with exposure.

incident commander The individual who has overall command of the scene in the field.

simple access Access that is easily achieved without the use of tools or force.

structure fire A fire in a house, apartment building, office, school, plant, warehouse, or other building.

tactical situation A hostage, robbery, or other situation in which armed conflict is threatened or shots have been fired and the threat of violence remains.

technical rescue situation A rescue that requires special technical skills and equipment in one of many specialized rescue areas, such as technical rope rescue, cave rescue, and dive rescue.

technical rescue group A team of individuals from one or more departments in a region that is trained and on call for certain types of technical rescue.

Points to Ponder

You respond to a rollover on the freeway involving a van. When you arrive, you find the van upside down with the side door partially open, but stuck in that position and the driver's door jammed closed. A highway patrol officer has his shotgun in hand and is standing back from the van. When you look into the van you notice that the driver is wearing a uniform and the passengers are all wearing orange jumpsuits. There are seven people in the van with a variety of obvious injuries. The highway patrol officer tells you that it was a prisoner transfer between the county jail and the state prison and that he has called for assistance and others should arrive soon. He says that he will stand in the side door and protect you. The van rocks if you push on it, but does not look like it would roll over very easily. It will be necessary to climb into the van to provide adequate treatment for the patients. Would you enter the van to provide treatment? The driver does not appear to be too seriously injured and may be able to help protect you. Would you take the time to clear him or treat more seriously injured inmates? How much of a risk would you be taking treating the inmates? If the two of the inmates have life threatening injuries, are you willing to allow them to die while you wait for extrication equipment to stabilize the van and police officers to ensure your safety?

Issues Scene Safety, Determining Risk, Duty to Treat, Personal Biases, Delaying Patient Care.

Assessment in Action

Today is the beginning of the second month you have been going out on calls. This call is the first one involving a motor vehicle crash. Your partner is an experienced EMT-B and he goes over a few important facts with you as you respond. You remember your training in the classroom.

1. When you arrive, after parking the ambulance safely, the next thing you should do is:
   A. gain access to the patient as quickly as possible to correct any life-threatening conditions.
   B. go to the nearest rescue truck to help bring rescue tools over to the crashed vehicle.
   C. report to the fire officer in charge and take direction from that individual.
   D. wait in your ambulance until someone comes over or calls you by radio asking you to come to the wreck.

2. What are the phases of extrication?
   A. Safety, gaining access, life-saving care, preparation for removal, and removal
   B. Safety, gaining access, life-saving care, and transportation to a hospital
   C. Safety, preparation for removal, removal, and communication to the hospital
   D. Safety, removal, transportation to a hospital, and communication before you arrive

3. Under the incident command system,
   A. rescue and medical operations are combined into one group.
   B. the rescue operation is coordinated as a separate group with the EMT-B joining it.
   C. the EMT-B is part of the medical operations and works outside the rescue group.
   D. there are no separate teams, but each person works independently on assigned tasks.

4. During an extrication, which of the following can you expect to be asked to wear when entering a wrecked vehicle to treat a patient who is trapped inside?
   A. Full turnout gear including fire-retardant coat and pants, boots, and a fire helmet
   B. A jump suit with good protection for your arms and legs
   C. Your normal duty uniform
   D. Leather gloves over your disposable gloves

5. When gaining access, the EMT-B should always:
   A. enter a vehicle from the driver's side.
   B. make certain the vehicle is stable before entering.
   C. wait until the fire department has removed the roof.
   D. before entering, place into the vehicle all the equipment needed for the care that will be given.

6. If you are standing by at a fire, you should always:
   A. report to the command post to take direction if needed elsewhere.
   B. park your vehicle in the staging area and walk over to the fire ground to be closer if needed.
   C. stay near your vehicle so people can find you if they need you.
   D. leave as soon as it is obvious the fire has been extinguished.

7. The incident commander at a rescue scene:
   A. has overall responsibility for managing the incident.
   B. will direct EMT-B personnel on what patient care equipment to use and how to care for patients.
   C. is responsible for doing all the tasks required to manage the incident.
   D. will only allow the EMT-B access to the patient once the patient has been brought to the ambulance.

Challenging Questions

8. You are at the scene of a motor vehicle crash and there are four patients. Which one of these patients would you or your partner go to first if each was the same distance away?
   A. Sucking chest wound with patient breathing but unresponsive
   B. Fractured femur with the patient conscious and experiencing great pain
   C. Unresponsive patient with all the characteristics of cardiopulmonary arrest, even when viewed at a distance
   D. A severe laceration to the upper arm with arterial bleeding, with the patient conscious and sitting leaning against a tree

9. During vehicle extrication, the EMT-B often:
   A. uses a blanket to help drag the patient out of the wreckage.
   B. holds the tools for the firefighters cutting open the wreckage.
   C. places a spine board or blanket over the patient or other rescuers to protect them from glass and metal fragments.
   D. directs the fire personnel to delay removal until all splints, dressings, and bandaging have been completed in the wrecked car.

10. At a crash scene, different groups have different responsibilities. Which of the following is true?
    A. Fire rescue personnel are responsible for safety, extrication, and directing traffic.
    B. EMS is responsible for safety, patient care, and extrication.
    C. Police are responsible for safety, maintaining order, and the investigation of the cause of the crash.
    D. Fire fighters are responsible for safety, fire suppression, and patient care.

Online Outlook

Learn more about urban search and rescue by completing Exercise 36 at www.emtb.com.

www.emtb.com

Special Operations

Objectives

Cognitive

1. Explain the EMT-B's role during a call involving hazardous materials (p 849).
2. Describe what the EMT-B should do if there is reason to believe that there is a hazard at the scene (p 846).
3. Describe the actions that an EMT-B should take to ensure bystander safety (p 849).
4. State the role the EMT-B should perform until appropriately trained personnel arrive at the scene of a hazardous materials situation (p 848).
5. Break down the steps to approaching a hazardous situation (p 848).
6. Discuss the various environmental hazards that affect EMS (p 846).
7. Describe the criteria for a multiple-casualty situation (p 853).
8. Evaluate the role of the EMT-B in the multiple-casualty situation (p 854).
9. Summarize the components of basic triage (p 853).
10. Define the role of the EMT-B in a disaster operation (p 858).
11. Describe basic concepts of incident management (p 845).
12. Explain the methods for preventing contamination of self, equipment, and facilities (p 849).
13. Review the local mass-casualty incident plan (p 855).

Affective

14. Discuss the psychological impact of wanting to act but recognizing that a scene is not safe to enter (p 847).*

Psychomotor

15. Given a scenario of a mass-casualty incident, perform triage (p 854).

    * These are noncurriculum objectives.

www.emtb.com

Online Chapter Pretest
Interactivities
Vocabulary Explorer
Anatomy Review
Web Links
Online Review Manual
Distance Learning

Skill Drills
Vital Vocabulary
Pediatric Needs
Geriatric Needs
EMT-B Safety
EMT-B Tips
Documentation Tips
Remember
Prep Kit

You are the EMT

You are sent to a condominium for an unexplained illness. When you arrive, you are told that the fire department has removed 15 people. Each person has been overcome by carbon monoxide poisoning. As many as 10 more people inside have been found and rescue is under way. There are only 5 other ambulances on your dispatcher's back up list. These have all been called. Additional ambulances may be more than 30 minutes away.

The prehospital environment is an unpredictable and often uncontrolled place to work. Some types of responses will require much more from you than patient care. Managing scenes that you find in disarray, avoiding risks at those scenes and helping others avoid them, and calling for and coordinating the arrival of additional resources-all of these can be your responsibility. You will also be called on to assist with complex scenes already being managed by other agencies. This chapter introduces several subjects related to complex and dangerous scenes. It will help you answer the following questions:

1. Describe the general procedures for initial responses to a mass-casualty incident in your area.

2. How is triage done at a mass-casualty incident?

3. What is the role of the EMT-B at a hazardous materials spill?

4. Define the different roles an EMT-B may be asked to serve within a local incident command system.

Special Operations

The first section of this chapter will introduce you to incident command systems. The purpose of this section is to give you an idea of what happens during complex incidents. The role of the EMT-B within the system is explained.

The next section describes your responsibilities at a hazardous materials incident. When you are responding to this type of incident, you cannot rush in to provide patient care. Rather, you must cooperate with the incident command system, taking time to accurately assess the scene by identifying the size of the hazard area, finding a safe location to which patients can be removed, and taking self-protective measures. Safety is your primary consideration. If a hazardous materials incident is not carefully handled, many people, including rescue personnel, can become patients or casualties.

The final section describes the several roles of the EMT-B at mass-casualty incidents. Again under the incident command system, EMS personnel will have one of several roles identified to manage a large number of patients at a single event. The usual EMS response of triaging three or four patients will be difficult when there are 25 or more casualties. To ensure that every patient receives appropriate care and transportation to a hospital consistent with the severity of his or her condition, a more organized operation is required with three major responsibilities assigned: triage, treatment, and transportation.

Incident Command Systems

In recent years, a number of leadership and command systems have been developed to improve the on-scene management of emergency situations. The fire service has taken the lead in developing these programs to help control, direct, and coordinate emergency responders and resources. These programs are called incident command systems. They have been adapted and used by many EMS organizations to better organize their own operations. The **incident command system** is designed for use in daily operations. However, it is most effective when used to organize large numbers of personnel at complex incidents such as hazardous materials spills and mass-casualty incidents.

Components and Structure of an Incident Command System

At a large fire, a hazardous materials incident, or a mass-casualty incident, fire, rescue, HazMat, police, and EMS units from many different areas usually will become involved in some way. To ensure clear lines of responsibility and authority, a preestablished system is needed to identify who is in charge of different activities and who reports to whom. Even on a call with only one patient and no need for any other services, the implementation of an incident command system is helpful to identify the roles and responsibilities of each crew member, particularly if the event begins to escalate.

The incident command system is structured such that there is a single authority with overall responsibility to manage the incident. This person is identified as the **incident commander**. The incident commander usually remains at a **command post**, the designated field command center. A field command center is typically a vehicle or building at the scene where the incident commander establishes an "office." From here, the commander oversees and coordinates the activities of the various groups and leaders.

Functions normally centered at the command post include information, safety, and liaison with other agencies and groups who are responding. In a typical incident command system operation, all information to the public and the news media originates at the command post. The incident commander will usually appoint a safety officer who will circulate among responding personnel. It is essential that every EMT-B understand that any order or directive issued by a safety officer has the full authority of the incident commander and must be immediately followed. Many times EMT-Bs cannot see a hazard or problem they are walking into, and the safety officer is responsible for protecting all personnel and any victims of the incident. Finally, an officer may be named by the incident commander to coordinate incoming fire, police, and EMS units.

In the initial response, the incident commander may assume direct control over the groups and task forces being set up. In this circumstance, a medical group supervisor may be named to coordinate all EMS activity, or a rescue group supervisor may be appointed to deal with people entrapped in the wreckage. In extended operations that may go on for hours, days, or longer, the typical incident command structure may have multiple sectors including operations, planning, logistics, finance. (▼ Figure 37-1) shows a sample incident command system organization chart that includes these sectors. Each of these sections will have a single officer acting as the person in charge, the **sector commander**. Not all positions are used at every incident. The incident commander will select the individual positions and teams, and will choose which to use depending on the nature of the incident.

Major incidents often require another level of management, known as unified command. With unified command, the incident commander is joined at the command post by one officer who is in charge of all fire operations, one who is in charge of all rescue or HazMat operations, one who is in charge of all EMS operations, and one who is in charge of all law enforcement. This group, under the direction of the incident commander, directs the overall operations at the scene. Because the different public safety officers are stationed at the command post, they can be easily found and can collectively advise the incident commander of changes and problems that are communicated to them. The incident commander can also involve them in making the necessary decisions and in rapidly conveying orders to those

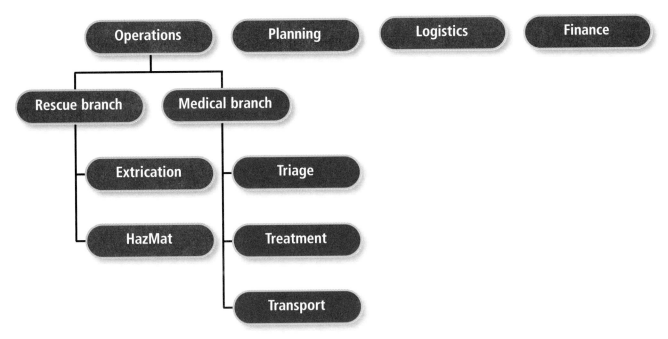

Figure 37-1 Incident command structure. Not all positions will be filled in every incident. However, the incident commander is responsible for all activity until subordinates are appointed to assist in managing the incident.

(c) National Wildlife Coordinating Group

under their command. In addition to unified command, this system ensures that the actions of each different type of responder are properly coordinated.

How these systems work together depends on the nature of the event. For example, with a major airplane crash, the leading agency is typically the fire department. In this situation, EMS is usually one aspect of the overall fire incident command system. Within their own system, EMS personnel establish and carry out their tasks. However, ultimate control of the incident will rest with the fire commander. Other situations, such as widespread injuries at a rock concert, are primarily civil events. Law enforcement would take the lead, establishing an incident command plan. Fire and EMS would follow the law enforcement commander's decision. EMS is seldom the lead agency.

At one time or another, your unit will probably be the first to respond to an incident that will involve more than one EMS unit or one or more non-EMS agencies. An example might be 10 or 20 teenagers suffering from adverse reactions to pepper spray one student brought to school, or another event where there is a limited role for immediate fire or police intervention. In this situation, the senior EMT-B should establish command and inform the dispatcher by saying, for example, "Dispatch, this is Squad 71, establishing Route 43 command." From that point on, all communications from the dispatcher to the scene will be directed to "Route 43 Command." If you arrive after command has already been established, advise the dispatcher that you are on scene and "reporting to command." Then find the command post, and report for assignment.

These systems will vary from place to place, and different terms may be used. You should become familiar with the specific terms and chain of command that are used in your area.

Introduction to Hazardous Materials

Your training has taught you that rapid response to the scene of a crash can save lives. You and your team can make quick decisions and act on them. Even so, you may sometimes be criticized for taking too much time at the crash scene. Such critics fail to appreciate a very important rule: When you arrive at the scene of a possible **hazardous materials incident**, you must first step back and assess the situation. This can be very stressful for you, particularly if you can see a patient. However, rushing into such events can have catastrophic results. Because of the unique aspects of responding to and working at a HazMat incident, OSHA has set specific additional training requirements in publication "29 CFR 1910.120—Hazardous Waste

Operations and Emergency Response Standard," which all individuals, including EMT-Bs, must meet before becoming involved in these situations. Because this text does not include the information to meet these requirements, you need to check with your agency for information about additional specific training.

Hazardous materials may be involved in any of the following situations ▼ Figure 37-2 :

- A truck or train crash in which a substance is leaking from a tank truck or railroad tank car
- A leak, fire, or other emergency at an industrial plant, refinery, or other complex where chemicals or explosives are produced, used, or stored
- A leak or rupture of an underground natural gas pipe
- Deterioration of underground fuel tanks and seepage of oil or gasoline into the surrounding ground
- Buildup of methane or other by-products of waste decomposition in sewers or sewage-processing plants
- A motor vehicle crash in which a gas tank has ruptured

Figure 37-2 Two examples of hazardous materials incidents.

Figure 37-3 **A.** Warning placards are found on railroad cars that carry hazardous materials. **B.** Labels are also affixed to boxes that contain hazardous materials.

Often, the presence of hazardous materials is easily recognized from warning signs, placards, or labels found in the following locations **▲ Figure 37-3** :

- On buildings or areas where hazardous materials are produced, used, or stored
- On trucks and railroad cars that carry any amount of hazardous material
- On barrels or boxes that contain hazardous material

Unfortunately, identifying materials still can be difficult. Little consistency is used on labels and placards. The laws and regulations that cover labeling of packages and transport vehicles can also be misleading. In most cases, the package or tank must contain a certain amount of a hazardous material before a placard is required. For example, because of the small quantities of hazardous materials that are involved, a truck carrying 99 lb of HazMat #1 and 99 lb of both HazMat #2 and HazMat #3 may not be required by law to display any labels or placards. The truck may show only a "Please Drive Carefully" placard. This placard implies that the truck carries no hazardous materials. An experienced HazMat technician knows that this is the most dangerous placard. However, other motorists are not aware that the truck is carrying a combination of hazardous materials. A crash involving this truck is a serious situation, but you would not know this if you relied on labels and placards.

Some substances are not hazardous; however, when mixed with another substance, they may become toxic or volatile. There may be no regulations against carrying such substances together on one truck or railroad car (or adjacent tank cars). No warnings are required.

The driver of a commercial truck and the conductor of a train, however, must carry papers that identify what is being transported in their care. These papers may be your first clue that there is a possible HazMat problem; although, depending on the nature of the incident, the papers may not be available to you.

In the event of a leak or spill, a hazardous materials incident is often indicated by presence of the following:

- A visible cloud or strange-looking smoke resulting from the escaping substance
- A leak or spill from a tank, container, truck, or railroad car with or without hazardous material placards or labels
- An unusual, strong, noxious, acrid odor in the area

To indicate the presence of normally odorless toxic gases or fluids during a leak or spill, manufacturers may add a substance that produces a strong noxious odor. However, a large number of hazardous gases and fluids are essentially odorless (or do not have a distinctive unpleasant smell) even when a substantial leak or spill has occurred. In some incidents, a large number of people are exposed and may be injured or killed before the presence of a hazardous material incident is identified. If you approach a scene where more than one person has collapsed or is unconscious or in respiratory distress, you should assume that there has been a hazardous material leak or spill and that it is unsafe to enter the area.

It is important for you to understand the potential danger of hazardous materials and know how to operate safely at a hazardous materials incident. If you do not follow the proper safety measures, you and many others could end up needlessly injured or dead. Safety—of you and your team, the other responders, and the public—must be your most important concern.

EMT-B Safety

Safety considerations at hazardous materials scenes differ considerably from those involved in emergency response in general. Hazardous materials require an even higher degree of alertness than usual to avoid entering a dangerous environment, and to help others avoid it. There is also a need to prevent the spread of contamination to yourself or your ambulance. Understanding these two concepts is a good start toward safe operations in the presence of hazardous materials.

There will be times when the ambulance is the first to arrive at the scene. If, as you approach, any signs suggest that a hazardous material incident has occurred, you should stop at a safe distance; after rapidly sizing up the scene, call for a HazMat team. If you do not recognize the danger until you are too close, immediately leave the **danger zone**. Once you have reached a safe place, try to rapidly assess the situation and provide as much information as possible when calling for the HazMat team, including your specific location, the size and shape of the containers of the hazardous material, and what you have observed and been told has occurred. Do not reenter the scene. Do not leave the area until you have been cleared by the HazMat team, or you may contribute to the situation by spreading hazardous material.

Identifying Hazardous Materials

Until the HazMat team arrives to determine the hazard zone, you should be aware of the safety perimeters that are necessary for hazardous materials that are toxic

(poisons) and those in which there is danger of fire or explosion. When toxic gas, fumes, or airborne droplets or particles are involved, the safe area is upwind and at least 100′ from the site of any visible cloud or other discharge; in a hilly area, you should be uphill as well as upwind. Remember, wind direction can change quickly. A piece of narrow roller bandage, approximately 2′ long, tied to the top of your antenna will serve as a wind direction guide. Be sure to check the wind direction periodically, and relocate if a change in wind direction dictates.

If you can see and read the placard or other warning sign, note its color, wording, any symbols that it contains, and, if included, the four-digit number that appears on it or on any orange panel near it
▼ **Figure 37-4**). This number, which may be preceded by the letters UN or NA, identifies the specific hazardous material. The name of the material may also be displayed along with the number. The same number and name can also be found on the shipping papers and packaging of the material. If you are unable to read the placard or labels, do not move closer and risk exposure.

Figure 37-4 The four-digit number that appears on the warning placard identifies the specific hazardous material.

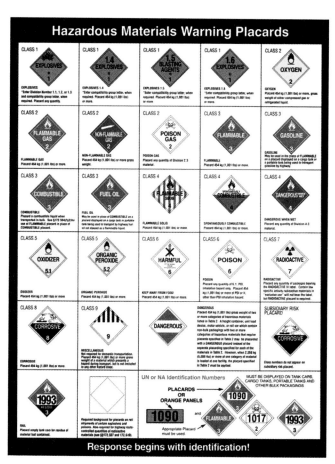

Figure 37-5 Hazardous materials warning placards.

The HazMat team will have binoculars that allow team members to read the placards or labels from a safe distance. If you are able to read the placard with the naked eye, you may be too close and should consider moving farther away. ◄ **Figure 37-5** shows a chart illustrating the hazardous materials warning placards, and ▼ **Figure 37-6** shows a chart illustrating the warning labels. You should study and be familiar with these warning materials.

You must also be sure to keep bystanders away. Often, well-meaning individuals try to help. However, unless they are trained for these types of incidents, you should move them from the area.

Once you have called for the HazMat Team, you should focus your efforts on activities that will ensure the safety and survival of the greatest number of people. Use the ambulance's public address system to alert individuals who are near the scene and direct them to move to a location where they will be sufficiently far from and out of the line of danger. With the aid of others on your team, try to set up a perimeter to stop traffic and individuals from entering the danger zone.

The HazMat team is equipped to identify the specific substance that is involved and, using a number of complex factors, determine the size, direction or shape, and perimeter of the danger zone. Knowing the type, toxicity or concentration, and quantity of the hazardous material that is involved will help the team to determine the location of and safe distance from the danger zone. Determination of the danger zone will also be affected by the amount of wind and other weather factors.

When a material is hazardous because of its flammability or potential for explosion rather than its toxicity, you will need to be at an even greater distance and behind a windowless wall or other strong barrier that will shield you and others from heat, the blast force, and flying debris.

Once firefighters and the HazMat team have arrived at a small incident, they will determine which specific hazardous material is involved and will mark the perimeter of the danger or hazard zone with warning tape. At a large incident, they may broadcast the zone's limits. Only individuals who are trained in HazMat and wearing the proper level of protective gear should enter the hazard zone. As an EMT-B, you do not have this role. Your job is to stand by at a designated **treatment area** outside of the hazard zone and provide treatment when HazMat team members bring patients to you.

Patients' skin and clothing may contain hazardous material, so a **decontamination area** should be set up between the hazard zone and the treatment area. The decontamination area is the designated area where contaminants are removed before an individual can go to another area. **Decontamination** is the process of removing or neutralizing and properly disposing of hazardous materials from equipment, patients, and rescue personnel. The decontamination area must include special containers for contaminated clothing and special bags to isolate each patient's personal effects safely until they can be decontaminated at a later time. The area will also contain a number of special facilities to thoroughly wash and rinse patients and backboards. The water that is used must be captured and delivered into special sealable containers.

Anyone who leaves the hazard zone must pass through the decontamination area. Firefighters' and HazMat team members' outer protective gear is rinsed and washed in the decontamination area before it is removed ▶ **Figure 37-7**. To prevent needless contact and communication of splash or residues, different personnel are used in the decontamination and treatment

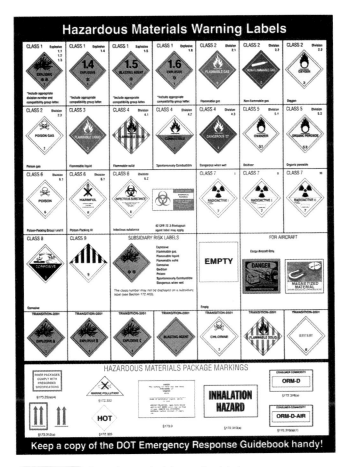

Figure 37-6 Hazardous materials warning labels.

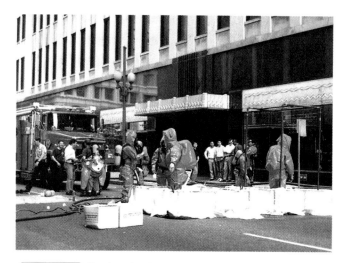

Figure 37-7 The decontamination zone is where fire fighters and HazMat team members' outer protective gear is rinsed and washed before removal.

areas. You should not move into the decontamination area unless you are properly trained and equipped. You should wait for the patients to be brought to you.

Caring for Patients at a Hazardous Materials Incident

Most HazMat team members are trained to the first responder or EMT-B level. Because of the dangers, time constraints, and inhibiting bulky protective gear, it is practical only to provide the simplest assessment and essential care in both the hazard zone and the decontamination area. In addition, to avoid entrapment and communication of contaminants, no bandages or splints are applied, except pressure dressings that are needed to control bleeding, until the "clean" patient has been moved to the treatment area. Therefore, the EMT-Bs providing care in the treatment area should

Classification of Hazardous Materials

The NFPA 704 Hazardous Materials Clasification standard classifies hazardous materials according to health hazard or toxicity levels, fire hazard, and reactive hazard. Toxicity protection levels are also classified according to the level of protection provided. Even chemicals that are in the same category, on the basis of their chemical makeup, form, and concentration, will have different hazard levels. The degree of health, fire, reactive hazard, and type of protection needed to operate safely near these substances must be known.

Toxicity Level. **Toxicity levels** are measures of the risk that a substance poses to someone who comes into contact with it. There are five toxicity levels: 0, 1, 2, 3, and 4 ▼ **Table 37-1** . The higher the number, the greater the toxicity, as follows:

- **Level 0** includes materials that would cause little, if any, health hazard if you came into contact with them.
- **Level 1** includes materials that would cause irritation on contact but only mild residual injury, even without treatment.
- **Level 2** includes materials that could cause temporary damage or residual injury unless prompt medical treatment is provided. Both Levels 1 and 2 are considered to be slightly hazardous but require use of SCBA if you are going to come into contact with them.
- **Level 3** includes materials that are extremely hazardous to health. Contact with these materials requires full protective gear so that none of your skin surface is exposed.
- **Level 4** includes materials that are so hazardous that minimal contact will cause death. For Level 4 substances, you need specialized gear that is designed for protection against that particular hazard.

TABLE 37-1 Toxicity Levels of Hazardous Materials

Level	Health Hazard	Protection Needed
0	Little to no hazard	None
1	Slightly hazardous	Self-contained breathing apparatus (level C suit) only
2	Slightly hazardous	Self-contained breathing apparatus (level C suit) only
3	Extremely hazardous	Full protection, with no exposed skin (level A or B suit)
4	Minimal exposure causes death	Special HazMat gear (level A suit)

assess and treat the patient in the same way as they would a patient who has not been previously assessed or treated.

Your care of patients at a HazMat incident must address the following two issues:

- Any trauma that has resulted from other related mechanisms, such as vehicle collision, fire, or explosion

- The injury and harm that have resulted from exposure to the toxic hazardous substance

You should treat the patient's injuries in the same way that you would treat any injury. There are very few specific antidotes or treatments for exposure to most hazardous materials. Different people may respond differently to contact with the same hazardous material. Therefore, your treatment for the patient's exposure to

the toxic substance should focus mainly on supportive care and initiating transport to the hospital with a minimum of additional delay.

Most serious injuries and deaths from hazardous materials result from airway and breathing problems. Therefore, you should be sure to maintain the airway and, if the patient appears to be in distress, give oxygen at 10 to 15 L/min with a nonrebreathing mask. Monitor the patient's breathing at all times. If you see signs that would indicate that respiratory distress is increasing, you may need to provide assisted ventilation with a BVM device and high-flow oxygen.

If special antidotes or other special treatments need to be initiated in the field, they will be ordered by the medical control and relayed to the officer who is in charge of EMS operations at the scene. If special treatment includes medications, IVs, or other advanced care,

Protection Level. **Protection levels** indicate the amount and type of protective gear that you need to prevent injury from a particular substance. The four recognized protection levels, A, B, C, and D, are as follows (▼ **Figure 37-8**):

- **Level A,** the most hazardous, requires fully encapsulated, chemical-resistant protective clothing that provides full body protection, as well as SCBA and special, sealed equipment.

- **Level B** requires nonencapsulated protective clothing, or clothing that is designed to protect against a particular hazard. Usually, this clothing is made of material that will let only limited amounts of moisture and vapor pass through (nonpermeable). Level B also requires breathing devices that contain their own air supply, such as SCBA, and eye protection.

- **Level C,** like Level B, requires the use of nonpermeable clothing and eye protection. In addition, face masks that filter all inhaled outside air must be used.

- **Level D** requires a work uniform, such as coveralls, that affords minimal protection.

All levels of protection require the use of gloves. Two pairs of rubber gloves are needed for protection in case one pair must be removed because of heavy contamination.

Figure 37-8 Four levels of protection. **A.** Level A protection. **B.** Level B protection. **C.** Level C protection. **D.** Level D protection.

paramedics or other advanced personnel will be sent to work with you at the treatment area.

SPECIAL CARE. In some cases, before the decontamination area has been completely set up, the HazMat Team will find one or two patients who need immediate treatment and transport without further delay if they are to survive. Even after the decontamination area is set up and functioning, some patients may have such respiratory distress or another urgent critical condition that the time necessary for full decontamination may prove fatal. If additional delay for proper decontamination appears to be life threatening in nontoxic exposure situations, it may be necessary to simply cut away all of the patient's clothing and do a rapid rinse to remove the majority of the contaminating matter before transport.

If you are treating and transporting a patient who has not been fully and properly decontaminated, you will need to increase the amount of protective clothing you wear, including the use of SCBA. At the least, this should include two pairs of gloves, goggles or a face shield, a protective coat, respiratory protection, and a disposable fluid-impervious apron or similar outfit. Many HazMat teams carry easy-to-use disposable fluid-impervious light protective suits for such a purpose. Remember, however, that transporting a contaminated patient merely increases the size of the event. The decision to transport even a patient with critical injuries rests with the incident commander, who bases his or her decision on recommendations made by the HazMat team.

To make decontaminating the ambulance afterwards easier, tape the cabinet doors shut. Any equipment kits, monitors, and other items that will not be used en route should be removed from the patient compartment and placed in the front of the ambulance or in outside compartments. Before loading the patient, you should turn on the power vent ceiling fan and patient compartment air-conditioning unit fan. Unless the weather is too severe, the windows in the driver's area and sliding side windows in the patient compartment should also be partially opened to prevent creating a "closed box" in the patient compartment and to ensure that the ambulance is properly ventilated for the patient's and EMTs' safety.

When you leave the scene, inform the hospital that you are transporting a critically injured patient who has not been fully decontaminated at the scene. This will allow the hospital to prepare to receive the patient. Many emergency departments have a room with a separate outside entrance and decontamination facilities for such an event. You may be diverted to a facility with these capabilities if the receiving hospital is not so

> Most serious injuries and deaths from hazardous materials result from airway and breathing problems.

equipped. Be sure that one EMT-B enters the emergency department and, after giving hospital staff the report and advising them again of the incomplete decontamination, obtains directions before the patient is unloaded and brought in. If there are enough ambulances at a hazardous materials scene, one may be isolated and used only to transport such patients. Remember, the ambulance needs to be decontaminated before transporting another patient.

Resources

Every ambulance, as well as the dispatch center, should have a copy of *2000 Emergency Response Guidebook*, prepared by Transport Canada, the US Department of Transportation, and the Secretariat of Communications and Transportation of Mexico ▼ **Figure 37-9** . This publication lists most hazardous materials. For each one, it describes the proper initial emergency action to control the scene and provide emergency medical care. Some state and local government agencies may also have information about hazardous materials that are commonly found in their areas. Be sure to keep these publications up to date and close at hand on the unit.

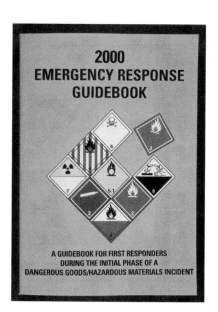

Figure 37-9 The *2000 Emergency Response Guidebook.*

Another valuable resource is the **Chemical Transportation Emergency Center (CHEMTREC)**, located in Washington, DC. CHEMTREC was established by the Chemical Manufacturers Association to assist emergency personnel in identifying and handling hazardous materials transport incidents. The center operates 24 hours a day, 7 days a week. Its toll-free number is 1-800-424-9300 from anywhere within the United States or Canada.

CHEMTREC provides information, warnings, and guidance for proper emergency management and treatment. However, it cannot identify an unknown substance. You must provide CHEMTREC with the correct DOT identification number, the chemical name, or the product name of the material.

If you are interested in learning more about hazardous materials incidents and rescue requirements, you can look to the following:

- National Fire Protection Association (NFPA) standard #479
- OSHA standard #1910.120
- Federal Emergency Management Agency (FEMA) guidelines for coping with hazardous materials incidents
- EPA protective clothing

Mass-Casualty Incidents

In this text, a **mass-casualty incident** refers to any call that involves more than one patient, as well as any situation that places such a great demand on available equipment or personnel that the system is stretched to its limit or beyond. Airplane, bus, or railroad crashes, and earthquakes are obvious examples of mass-casualty incidents. However, other causes of these incidents are far more common than such disasters and are usually much smaller in scope.

Ask yourself the following questions:

- How many seriously injured patients can you care for effectively and transport in your ambulance? One? Two?
- What happens when you have three patients to deal with?
- What do you do when two cars crash head-on, resulting in eight critically injured patients, and you only have three ambulances available?

Obviously, you and your team cannot treat and transport all injured patients at the same time. At a mass-casualty incident, you will often experience a demand for equipment and personnel. For example, you may

---

EMT-B Tips

The terminology used to describe an incident with multiple patients varies in different communities. Many communities use the term *multiple-casualty situation* to describe an emergency that involves more than one patient, but use the term *mass-casualty incident* to describe larger scale events, such as those with more than 20 patients. In this text, the term *mass-casualty incident* is used to describe any call that involves more than one patient.

---

realize that there may be 15 or more minutes to wait before the next ambulance will arrive. Should you stay at the scene, placing the patients who are ready to go at some risk? Or should you leave with the patients who are loaded, leaving those at the scene without sufficient resources to manage all their needs?

If there are more patients at the scene than you can transport in your ambulance, call for back up ambulances and other mutual aid resources to assist (**▼ Figure 37-10**). While this may cause some delay in initiating treatment to all patients, this will not adversely affect the patient care if the EMS resources on scene begin to work with the most severely injured first. Always follow local protocol.

Triage

Triage is essential at all mass-casualty incidents. Triage is the sorting of two or more patients based on the

Figure 37-10 Mass-casualty incidents require additional ambulances and EMS providers from the immediate region.

severity of their conditions to establish priorities for care based on available resources (▶ Figure 37-11).

In a smaller scale mass-casualty incident, the first provider on scene with the highest level of training usually begins the triage process. When back up ambulances and crews are readily available, patients are ranked in order of severity. The patient with the most severe injuries is given priority attention. After counting the number of patients and notifying the dispatcher of additional help that is needed, initial assessment of all patients begins. As personnel arrive, the EMT-B should assign crews and equipment to priority patients first.

Triage at a large-scale mass-casualty incident should be done in several steps. The following triage steps are accepted by the majority of larger scale mass-casualty operations:

- Life-saving care rapidly administered to those in need

- Color coding to indicate priority for treatment and transportation at the scene (▼ Table 37-2). Red-tagged patients are the first priority,

Figure 37-11 Triage is an essential component of operations at a mass-casualty incident.

Table 37-2 Triage Priorities	
Triage Category	**Typical Injuries**
First Priority (Red) Patients who need immediate care and transport. Treat these patients first, and transport as soon as possible.	• Airway and breathing difficulties • Uncontrolled or severe bleeding • Decreased level of consciousness • Severe medical problems • Shock (hypoperfusion) • Severe burns
Second Priority (Yellow) Patients whose treatment and transportation can be temporarily delayed	• Burns without airway problems • Major or multiple bone or joint injuries • Back injuries with or without spinal cord damage
Third Priority (Green) Patients whose treatment and transportation can be delayed until last	• Minor fractures • Minor soft-tissue injuries
Fourth Priority (Black) Patients who are already dead or have little chance for survival. If resources are limited, treat salvageable patients before these patients.	• Obvious death • Obviously nonsurvivable injury, such as major open brain trauma • Full cardiac arrest

EMT-B Tips

Definitions of mass-casualty incidents vary from one place to another, and training on such specialized topics may not be frequent. As a new EMT-B, you may have to do some research and studying on your own to be sure that you understand and can apply local policy and procedure for large-scale incidents.

yellow-tagged patients are the second priority, and those tagged green or black are the lowest priority.

- Rapid removal of red-tagged patients for field treatment and transportation as ambulances are available.

- Use of a separate treatment area to care for red-tagged patients if transport is not immediately available. Yellow-tagged patients can also be monitored and cared for in the treatment area while waiting for transportation.

What would you do?

You are at the scene of a car crash in which three individuals have been injured. One patient is an alert 19-year-old woman with a profusely bleeding open fracture of the femur. The second patient is a conscious and distressed 68-year-old man with a sucking wound of the chest. The third patient is a 30-year-old man who is unconscious with massive head and chest injuries. His breathing is rapid, shallow, and irregular.

You can treat only one patient at a time. If you start treatment by resuscitating the 30-year-old patient, you will be treating him for a long time. Probably, he will die anyway. In addition, one or both of the other two patients will die. However, if you first occlude the sucking chest wound in the 68-year-old patient and then stop the bleeding in the 19-year-old patient with a pressure dressing, both, or at least one, of these patients will survive. If you treat the 30-year-old patient last, he will probably die, but you will have done the greatest good for the greatest number. The principle of triage is to treat the patient with survivable injuries first.

Special triage situations

Patients who have been contaminated by radiation or other hazardous materials are placed in a separate category of triage. This is the highest and most urgent category of all. Contaminated patients must be moved away from all other patients. They must not be allowed to contaminate other patients, EMS personnel, ambulances, or hospitals.

Certain large urban areas that offer regionalized care use another concept of triage. Single patients with specific medical problems, such as burns, trauma, cardiac, or neonatal, are triaged to specialized regional centers for treatment. Making the decision to transport a patient to a special treatment center is difficult. The decision is based on many factors, including (but not limited to) the following:

- The specific illness or injury

- The severity of the illness or injury

- The availability of local resources at the time of the event

- Local rules and protocols

These decisions are often made only after online communication with medical control.

If there are special treatment centers in your area, you must know the specific triage protocols that apply. Also note that in the event of a mass-casualty incident, these protocols might not be used. For example, a school bus crash in which all 30 or 40 patients are children can overwhelm a pediatric hospital. Similarly, 10 burn patients from a petroleum plant fire could immobilize a burn center. In these cases, good triage and communication with medical control are essential in providing each patient with the best available treatment.

Most urban areas have regional trauma care centers. Severe, life-threatening injuries should be treated in facilities that are prepared to deal immediately and completely with the problem. Ideally, severely injured patients should be identified in the field and sent to a designated level one trauma center.

It is not enough to know the triage techniques that your EMS system uses to identify patients for transport to specialized treatment facilities. As with the other skills you are learning, you must practice these techniques as well. Your EMS system should conduct disaster drills yearly, preferably with the participation of local hospitals and other public safety and rescue units. Disaster plans must be developed and practiced in advance of need. The mass confusion of a disaster site is no time to experiment with organization.

- When there are more patients waiting for transport than there are ambulances, the Transportation Sector Officer decides which patient is the next to be loaded.

- Specialized transportation resources (air ambulance, paramedic ambulances, etc) require separate decisions when these resources are available but limited.

TRIAGE PRIORITIES. Patients should be color coded early to visually identify the severity of the condition and to eliminate the need for individual patient assessments to be performed by each EMT-B who comes along later.

Patients who are tagged red should later be reassessed in the treatment area to determine who should receive limited resources such as paramedic assessment and care. The sorting of multiple red-tagged patients in the treatment area who need to be seen immediately by paramedics will depend on the number of paramedics available at that time. The order in which the patients will be transported is determined after the initial triage and treatment is completed.

If patients are entrapped, extrication is required. If circumstances such as heavy smoke or a potential haz-ardous materials exposure exist, triage will be difficult if not impossible. The immediate concern will be the removal of the patients to a safe area for triage to be done later. The triage area is the name usually given to such a collecting area for patients to be initially triaged and color coded. For patients located in nonhazardous areas, this initial triage can begin right away.

INCIDENT COMMAND. To be effective, the various decision points for triage must be linked into the incident command system. The command structure must be established early and expanded as needed and as resources become available over time. Incident command systems may vary in different communities. When an EMT-B responds to another community as back up for a mass-casualty incident, he or she must follow the directions and orders given.

Table 37-3 shows the important components of an incident command system in a mass-casualty incident. As an example of how responsibilities may be assigned at a major EMS incident, consider the following typical assignments (◄ **Table 37-3**):

- **Command center.** This is typically a vehicle or building at the scene where the EMS commander establishes an "office." From here, the commander oversees and coordinates the activities of the various groups and leaders.

- **Staging area.** This is a holding area for arriving ambulances and crews until they can be assigned a particular task.

- **Extrication area.** This is where patients are disentangled and removed from a hazardous environment, allowing them to be moved to the triage area.

- **Triage area.** The **triage area** is a sorting point, run by a **triage officer**, where each patient is assessed and tagged, using color-coded tags or tape (► **Figure 37-12**), according to their injuries. These triaged patients are then directed to specific locations in the treatment area(s), according to their assigned priority.

- **Treatment area.** This is where a more thorough assessment is made and on-scene treatment is begun while transport is being arranged. The treatment area is organized and managed under the authority of the **treatment officer**. Patients are given care under the standards of the EMS system in the treatment area before being transported. This means that all fractures should be

---

Table 37-3	Key Components at a Mass-Casualty Incident

- Incident commander, command post, and incident command system

- On-site communications system

- Adequate supply of long backboards, straps, or ties

- Extrication/retrieval team

- Triage officer and designated triage area

- Staffed patient collection area

- Staffed patient treatment area

- Supply location adjacent to the treatment area

- Transportation officer and transport area

- Staging area to hold resources until they are needed

- Fire and law enforcement personnel

- A secure perimeter

splinted, and all care normally rendered under a focused assessment should be accomplished before the patient is released for transportation.

- **Supply area.** This is an area in which to assemble extra equipment and supplies, such as blankets, oxygen cylinders, bandages, and backboards, for dispersal to other areas as needed.

- <u>Transportation area.</u> This is where ambulances and crews are organized to transport patients from the treatment sector to area hospitals. The transportation area is managed by the <u>transportation officer</u>, who will assign patients to waiting ambulances.

- <u>Rehabilitation area.</u> This area provides protection and treatment to firefighters and other personnel working at the emergency scene. As workers enter and leave the scene, they are medically monitored and provided any needed care. This helps to ensure the safety and health of emergency workers who could become injured or ill while on the job.

When you respond to a mass-casualty incident, you will be assigned to a specified area and its designated officer. Report at once to this officer for your assignment. When you have finished your assigned task, report back to that same officer for another assignment. If your duties are complete, you may be reassigned.

Figure 37-12 Triage tag. **A.** Front. **B.** Back.

TRIAGE PROCEDURES. If medical control is not willing or able to determine the appropriate destination hospital for each patient, a rotation system can be used to distribute patients properly to each hospital on the basis of hospital capacity and capabilities. Of course, any designated trauma centers should be used to receive the most critical patients, following locol protocols. The transport officer is responsible for sending the ambulance to the appropriate hospital or the next hospital in turn. This rotation must occasionally be altered to allow specific patients to be taken to the most appropriate facility, such as a pediatric center, or to another hospital because a hospital has notified the field that it needs to be skipped for one rotation.

Normally, no more than two patients are placed in the same ambulance. However, with severe weather, a patient who has been tagged green may be seated in an ambulance next to the driver to move the patient to a comfortable, safe indoor holding area at the hospital.

As the patients are loaded into the ambulance, the transport officer logs each patient's mass-casualty tag number, each patient's overall condition, and the hospital to which they will be taken. As the ambulance leaves the scene, the transport officer radios the receiving hospital and briefly describes the patients, the unit transporting them, and the time they left the scene. To minimize radio traffic during such incidents, personnel on individual ambulances do not usually use their radios except to obtain advice from medical control or to notify the transport officer that they are leaving the hospital and returning to the field.

After giving a verbal report to hospital staff and transferring the patients, the ambulance returns to the staging area without further delay, helping to keep a continuous flow of ambulances moving between the mass-casualty incident site and the hospital. Equipment that is collected at the hospital or additional supplies that are needed in the field are brought to the staging area.

If additional ambulances are needed, the transport officer radios the command center, which then directs the resources from the staging area. If none are available at the staging area, the EMS chief notifies the dispatcher to obtain them elsewhere. To prevent a lack of ambulances, request extra ambulances as early as possible in a triage situation.

After all the first-priority (red-tagged) patients have been transported, the second-priority (yellow-tagged) patients are transported, followed by the third-priority (green-tagged) patients. After all patients have been transported, several units usually stay at the incident site to protect the other responders who will remain in case of injury. Often, ambulances will still be needed to transfer patients from the facility to which they were initially brought for stabilization to another, more appropriate facility.

Treatment and triage continue until all patients have been treated and transported. After the mass-casualty incident has ended, all personnel who were involved should be debriefed and evaluated to determine whether they need counseling. Mass-casualty incidents require regional preplanning and periodic simulation drills in which the fire, rescue, EMS, and police units are all involved. These drills usually include a large number of mock victims who are triaged and treated from the onset of the incident to delivery and re-triage at the hospital.

The success of any incident command system depends on all personnel performing their assigned tasks and working within the system. An EMT-B who is assigned to perform triage and decides instead to transport patients from the scene, bypasses the triage, treatment, and transport areas. As a result, those patients who were not yet triaged would not receive the care they need. Always remember that the cost of "doing your own thing" may include the loss of lives.

Disaster Management

A **disaster** is a widespread event that disrupts functions and resources of a community and threatens lives and property. Many disasters may not involve personal injuries. Droughts causing widespread crop damage are an example. On the other hand, many disasters such as floods, fires, and hurricanes also result in widespread injuries.

> The success of any incident command system depends on all personnel performing their assigned tasks and working within the system.

The role of the EMT-B in a disaster is to respond when requested and to report to the incident command system for assigned roles. One such role might be to record baseline vital signs and assessment of other response personnel before they enter the area. Later, the EMT-B may provide medical care and support to those who become exhausted or injured and return to the rehabilitation area.

In a disaster with an overwhelming number of casualties, area hospitals may decide that they cannot treat all patients at their facility. In this case, they may mobilize medical and nursing teams with equipment. Using a facility such as a warehouse near the disaster scene, they will set up a casualty collection area. The EMT-B would then be requested to transport patients to this alternative facility instead of to the local emergency department. Once at the **casualty collection area**, triage can be performed, medical care provided, and patients transported to the hospital on a priority basis.

If a casualty collection area is established, it will be coordinated through the incident command system in the same way as all other branches and areas of the operation. This is usually done only in a major disaster such as an earthquake when transportation to a hospital facility is impossible or has prolonged delays. It may take several hours to establish a casualty collection area. This delay can limit the number of events where such an area is an effective method for handling the incident.

Weapons of Mass Destruction

The intent of terrorism is to create chaos. To be prepared for a terrorist event, community leaders, including fire, police, and EMS officials, need to take appropriate actions to reduce the risks created by terrorism.

Six principles outline the role of the EMT-B at an incident involving a weapon of mass destruction:

1. **Carry out frequently used procedures and techniques in an emergency.** Appropriate responses to an incident involving a weapon of mass destruction must be familiar and uncomplicated.

2. **Indentify an incident involving a weapon of mass destruction in one of two ways: sudden onset or delayed onset.** An incident of sudden onset can be identified almost immediately, such as a bomb blast. An incident with delayed onset can take hours or even days to appear, such as bizarre medical symptoms after exposure to some biological and chemical agents.

3. **Treat an event that is potentially or actually caused by a weapon of mass destruction as a HazMat situation.** EMS personnel should not enter the area until properly trained and equipped personnel identify the agent involved. EMS personnel should decide whether the known number of patients will require a mass-casualty response. If so, a command structure can be established immediately.

4. **Control the convergence of people.** Although public safety personnel, including EMT-Bs, will tend to want to rush into the incident to help, all incidents involving a suspected weapon of mass destruction must be carefully assessed by specially trained and equipped personnel before others can enter. EMS and all safety personnel should keep all others from converging into the area where patients are located.

5. **Treat the event as a crime scene once the incident has been identified as being caused by a weapon of mass destruction.** This approach will preserve evidence and assist in later prosecution. Local and state police and the Federal Bureau of Investigation should be notified.

6. **Turn victims into patients.** People who plan and execute acts of terrorism want to create victims. Appropriate responses by EMS personnel and others can enable the treatment of these patients through local resources.

When all of these steps have been taken, the risk to public safety personnel and others is greatly reduced, which, in turn, helps those in the community return to a normal state in a shorter time.

Read the complete article at www.emtb.com.

Prep Kit

Ready for Review

At a hazardous materials incident, safety—of you and your team, the patient, and the public—is your most important concern. If you arrive first, assess the situation, taking care to protect yourself, and then call for a trained HazMat team. The most important step in such an incident is to identify the substances involved. Do not enter the hazard zone; your job is to provide supportive care once the patient can be safely moved out of the area. Hazardous materials are classified according to five toxicity levels. Four protection levels are indicated for the amount and type of protective gear you need. Levels indicate the amount and type of protective gear that you need to prevent injury from a particular substance. Most serious injuries and deaths from hazardous materials incidents result from airway and breathing problems. Patients' injuries should be treated in the same way that you would treat any injury. Resources for HazMat incidents include the *2000 Emergency Response Guidebook* and The Chemical Transportation Emergency Center (CHEMTREC). CHEMTREC is open 24 hours a day to help you identify and handle hazardous materials transport incidents.

Incident command systems allow for coordination of police, fire, and EMS activities in an emergency situation. In major incidents, there is usually a unified command, with a single command post where decisions are made by agency leaders. If your unit arrives first at an incident that will involve more than one unit or agency, command should be established. Otherwise, you should report to the command post for assignment. You may be assigned to one of the following sectors: staging, extrication, triage, treatment, supply, transportation, or rehabilitation.

In a mass-casualty incident, the most highly trained medical person on the scene directs triage. This means assigning treatment and transport priorities according to the severity and survivability of patients' injuries. There are four triage levels, each with a separate treatment area. Highest priority is given to patients whose injuries are critical but probably survivable with prompt treatment. The cardinal rule of triage is to do the greatest good for the greatest number. Treatment and triage continue until all patients have been transported. In urban areas with special treatment centers, special protocols are used to triage patients with specific injuries to the appropriate centers. Communication with medical control is essential for good triage.

Disasters are widespread events that can threaten lives and property, and sometimes can cause personal injuries. The incident command system is used for disasters just as for other types of mass-casualty incidents. However, if the number of patients overwhelms the area's hospitals, an alternate facility and casualty collection area can be set up for triage and treatment.

Vital Vocabulary

casualty collection area An area set up by physicians, nurses, and other hospital staff near a major disaster scene, where patients can receive further triage and medical care.

Chemical Transportation Emergency Center (CHEMTREC) An agency that assists emergency personnel in identifying and handling hazardous materials transport incidents.

command post The designated field command center where the incident commander and support personnel are located.

danger zone An area where individuals can be exposed to toxic substances, lethal rays, or ignition or explosion of hazardous materials.

decontamination The process of removing or neutralizing and properly disposing of hazardous materials from equipment, patients, and rescue personnel.

decontamination area The designated area in a hazardous materials incident where all patients and rescuers must be decontaminated before going to another area.

disaster A widespread event that disrupts community resources and functions, in turn threatening public safety, citizens' lives, and property.

hazardous material Any substance that is toxic, poisonous, radioactive, flammable, or explosive and causes injury or death with exposure.

hazardous materials incident An incident in which a hazardous material is no longer properly contained and isolated.

incident commander The individual who has overall command of the scene in the field.

incident command system An organizational system to help control, direct, and coordinate emergency responders and resources; known more generally as an incident management system (IMS).

mass-casualty incident An emergency situation involving more than one patient, and which can place such great demand on equipment or personnel that the system is stretched to its limit or beyond.

protection level A measure of the amount and type of protective equipment that an individual needs to avoid injury during contact with a hazardous material.

rehabilitation area This area provides protection and treatment to firefighters and other personnel working at an emergency. Here, workers are medically monitored and receive any needed care as they enter and leave the scene.

sector commander The individual delegated to oversee and coordinate activity in an incident command sector; works under the incident commander.

toxicity level A measure of the risk that a hazardous material poses to the health of an individual who comes into contact with it.

transportation area The area in a mass-casualty incident where ambulances and crews are organized to transport patients from the treatment area to receiving hospitals.

transportation officer The individual in charge of the transportation sector in a mass-casualty incident, who assigns patients from the treatment area to awaiting ambulances in the transportation area.

treatment area Location in a mass-casualty incident where patients are brought after being triaged and assigned a priority, where they are reassessed, treated, and monitored until transport to the hospital.

treatment officer The individual, usually a physician, who is in charge of and directs EMS personnel at the treatment area in a mass-casualty incident.

triage The process of sorting patients based on the severity of injury and medical need, to establish treatment and transportation priorities.

triage area Designated area in a mass-casualty incident where the triage officer is located and patients are initially triaged before being taken to the treatment center.

triage officer The individual in charge of the incident command triage sector, who directs the sorting of patients into triage categories in a mass-casualty incident.

Assessment in Action

You have been responding to ambulance calls for some time now. You have seen all types of medical and trauma situations. Your confidence has been growing and you feel good about your new role. There are a few things you have not yet encountered, however. You have just returned from a routine call, and you are restocking the ambulance. You and your partner review some of the things you have not yet seen.

1. You arrive at the scene of a tractor trailer truck leaking liquid contents of several barrels onto the highway. The driver has walked away from the cab into this liquid, and has now fallen. What should you do?
   A. Stay back even if you can see the driver is injured. Wait for the fire department to arrive and declare the area safe to enter.
   B. Rush in quickly to pull the driver out of the liquid. This way, care can be given safely.
   C. Ask the driver to come out on his own if he can. Once he is away from the truck you can start to treat him.
   D. Only one of you should go in to treat the patient. You can switch places later, reducing the time each of you will have to be in the hazardous area.

2. One of the roles of the EMT-B at the scene of a hazardous materials spill is to assist:
   A. in keeping bystanders back.
   B. in decontamination.
   C. in stopping any chemical spills from containers.
   D. the firefighters in moving rescue equipment nearer the scene.

3. The word "triage" means deciding which:
   A. crews will transport patients, allowing the others to stay and work at the scene to render care to those remaining.
   B. patient will be treated first, depending on the severity of his or her condition.
   C. equipment is appropriate for each patient being treated.
   D. of two or more patients will receive priority care.

4. The incident command system should be used at every event. For large operations such as a mass-casualty incident, which of the following best describes how the incident command system will function?
   A. Not all of the positions will necessarily be filled.
   B. All of the positions will usually be filled.
   C. Only the medical branch or group positions will be filled.
   D. Only the logistics section positions will be filled.

5. Triage at a mass-casualty incident includes applying colored tags to patients to identify their priority need for care and transportation. Which color indicates first-priority patients to be transported first?

A. Black-tagged patients B. Green-tagged patients
C. Yellow-tagged patients D. Red-tagged patients

6. Placards often identify what types of hazardous materials are being carried on trucks. When a truck carrying a placard "Please Drive Safely" has been in a crash, you should assume that:
   A. there are no hazardous materials on board.
   B. there may be several different types of hazardous materials on board.
   C. personnel responding to the crash do not need to worry about becoming contaminated.
   D. no one should go in until authorized by a trained fire fighter.

7. The three main functions of a mass-casualty operation include:
   A. triage, transportation, and communications.
   B. triage, tagging, and transportation.
   C. triage, treatment, and transportation.
   D. tagging, communications, and transfer of patients to hospital staff.

Challenging Questions

8. If you approach a scene where several people have collapsed but there is no vehicle crash or other logical explanation, you should suspect:
   A. a HazMat incident. B. an infectious disease.
   C. trauma from a hit-and-run driver. D. a shooting incident.

9. EMT-Bs may serve a role of "rehabilitation" at the scene of any large event. This term refers to:
   A. providing assistance to those with minor injuries to allow them to return to duty.
   B. offering exercises for those who have become stiff and sore from exertion during the operation.
   C. establishing baseline vital signs for all rescue and fire fighting personnel, and later using this information to assist those who become exhausted or injured in the line of duty.
   D. supervising physical therapists who may be called in to provide treatments to those with minor injuries.

Points to Ponder

You are dispatched to a "heart attack" at an auto body repair shop. When you arrive, the receptionist in the front office tells you it is back in the paint area. When you get back in the shop area someone tells you "they are in the spray booth." You and your partner enter the spray booth to find a person performing CPR on someone in a "tyvek suit." You start setting up and the person performing CPR collapses. You take him and your partner starts attaching the AED on the original patient. You realize that you are feeling light-headed about the time your partner collapses. You crawl toward your partner and the exit. Would you try to drag your partner out or would you go out alone? What about the two patients, would you try to drag them out also? Would you

feel responsible for your partner's death if you got out and she did not? What are some clues that this is a HAZMAT problem that you should have recognized prior to your partner's collapse?

Issues Scene Safety, HAZMAT, Backing Up Your Partner, Risks of Being an EMT, Critical Incident Stress Debriefing (CISD).

Online Outlook

Incident command systems allow for coordination of police, fire, and EMS activities in an emergency situation. In major incidents, there is usually a unified command, with a single command post where decisions are made by agency leaders. To learn more about major incident command systems, complete Exercise 37 at www.emtb.com.

www.emtb.com

Enrichment

Section **8**

Advanced Airway Management

Objectives

Cognitive

1. Identify and describe the airway anatomy in the adult (p 867).
2. Explain the pathophysiology of airway compromise (p 867).
3. Describe the proper use of airway adjuncts (p 868).
4. Review the use of oxygen therapy in airway management (p 866).
5. Describe the indications, contraindications, and technique for insertion of nasogastric tubes (p 868).
6. Describe how to perform the Sellick maneuver (cricoid pressure) (p 869).
7. Describe the indications for advanced airway management (p 868).
8. List the equipment required for orotracheal intubation (p 871).
9. Describe the proper use of the curved blade for orotracheal intubation (p 872).
10. Describe the proper use of the straight blade for orotracheal intubation (p 872).
11. State the reasons for and proper use of the stylet in orotracheal intubation (p 872).
12. Describe the methods of choosing the appropriate size endotracheal tube in an adult patient (p 873).
13. State the formula for sizing an infant or child endotracheal tube (p 874).
14. List complications associated with advanced airway management (p 881).
15. Describe the skill of orotracheal intubation in the adult patient (p 876).
16. Describe the skill of orotracheal intubation in the infant and child patient (p 874).
17. Describe the skill of confirming endotracheal tube placement in the adult, infant, and child patient (p 879).
18. State the consequences of and the need to recognize unintentional esophageal intubation (p 881).
19. Describe the skill of securing the endotracheal tube in the adult, infant, and child patient (p 875).

Affective

20. Recognize and respect the feelings of the patient and family during advanced airway procedures (p 867).
21. Explain the value of performing advanced airway procedures (p 866).
22. Defend the need for the EMT-B to perform advanced airway procedures (p 868).
23. Explain the rationale for the use of a stylet (p 874).
24. Explain the rationale for having a suction unit immediately available during intubation attempts (p 876).
25. Explain the rationale for confirming breath sounds (p 879).
26. Explain the rationale for securing the endotracheal tube (p 875).

Psychomotor

27. Demonstrate how to perform the Sellick maneuver (cricoid pressure) (p 870).
28. Demonstrate the skill of orotracheal intubation in the adult patient (p 876).
29. Demonstrate the skill of orotracheal intubation in the infant and child patient (p 874).
30. Demonstrate the skill of confirming endotracheal tube placement in the adult patient (p 879).
31. Demonstrate the skill of confirming endotracheal tube placement in the infant and child patient (p 874).
32. Demonstrate the skill of securing the endotracheal tube in the adult patient (p 879).

TECHNOLOGY

www.emtb.com

Online Chapter Pretest
Interactivities
Vocabulary Explorer
Anatomy Review
Web Links
Online Review Manual
Distance Learning

Chapter FEATURES

Skill Drills
Vital Vocabulary
Pediatric Needs
Geriatric Needs
EMT-B Safety
EMT-B Tips
Documentation Tips
Remember
Prep Kit

"Medic 12, respond to the Franklin High School football field for a 'player down.'"
As you approach the patient, you see an athletic trainer providing rescue breathing.
The player still has a pulse.

This chilling scenario addresses a true medical quandary, as you must juggle spinal care and airway management as you provide care. This chapter will present both the knowledge and skills needed to manage calls like this, and will also help you answer the following questions:

1. Are there procedural variations that occur when intubating a trauma patient? What are they?

2. For the trauma patient, does airway management take precedence over spinal care?

Advanced Airway Management

T he single most important manipulative skill you will use as an EMT-B is establishing and maintaining a patient's airway. While the obviously broken leg or amputated finger may be eye-catching, the blocked airway must be cleared immediately, or the patient will die. As long as the gag reflex is present, most patients can clear their own airways. Therefore, in managing the conscious patient, you may need only to provide oxygen and monitor the patient closely for any changes. Patients whose consciousness is altered may require an oropharyngeal or nasopharyngeal airway and suctioning. However, patients who are unresponsive and not breathing on their own will fare better with advanced airway techniques. The purpose of advanced airway management is to protect and

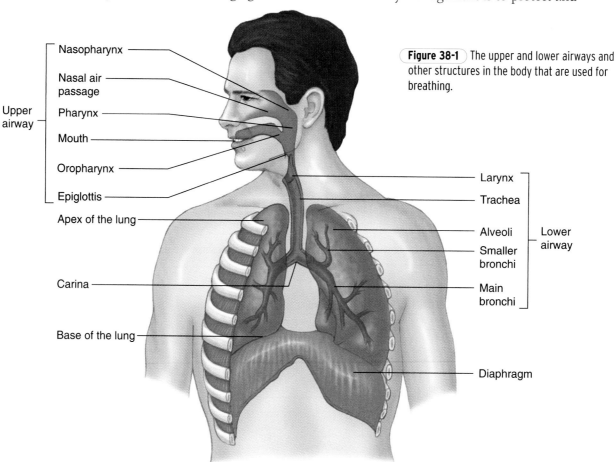

Figure 38-1 The upper and lower airways and other structures in the body that are used for breathing.

Nasopharynx

Nasal air passage

Upper airway

Pharynx

Mouth

Oropharynx

Epiglottis

Apex of the lung

Carina

Base of the lung

Larynx

Trachea

Alveoli

Smaller bronchi

Lower airway

Main bronchi

Diaphragm

improve ventilation in such patients by using a tube to create a direct channel to the trachea. Endotracheal intubation, or simply intubation, is a difficult skill to master and requires additional training for the EMT-B. Blind intubation using a lighted stylet is another technique for establishing endotracheal tube placement. Additional options include using a multi-lumen airway or a laryngeal mask airway. All these techniques require additional training, appropriate approval for their use, and medical oversight. During advanced procedures, as with basic procedures, the EMT-B needs to recognize and respect the feelings of the patient and family.

The chapter begins with a brief review of the anatomy and physiology of the respiratory system, followed by a discussion of gastric tube endotracheal intubation. The chapter concludes with a section on the use of a lighted stylet, multi-lumen airway adjuncts, and laryngeal mask airways.

Anatomy and Physiology of the Airway

As you learned earlier, the respiratory system consists of all the structures in the body that are used for breathing ◀ **Figure 38-1** . The upper airway begins with the nose, mouth, and throat (pharynx). The lower airway includes the larynx (vocal cords), trachea, bronchi, and lungs. The epiglottis is a leaf-shaped structure located at the glottic opening (or top of the trachea) that prevents food and liquid from entering the lower airway during swallowing. The bronchi and other air passages branch off from the trachea, extending into each lung, subdividing into bronchioles (smaller passages) down to the alveoli, where the exchange of gases occurs.

The mechanical process of breathing occurs through the use of the diaphragm and intercostal muscles. The diaphragm is a thin, dome-shaped muscle that separates the thoracic cavity from the abdominal cavity. The diaphragm and intercostal muscles contract during the active phase of breathing (inhalation), increasing the size of the chest cavity. Contraction of the diaphragm pulls the chest cavity down; contraction of the intercostal muscles pulls the rib cage up and out. The increased size of the chest cavity allows air to flow into the lungs. During the passive phase of breathing (exhalation), air flows out of the lungs. The diaphragm and intercostal muscles relax, and the size of the chest cavity decreases. The diaphragm moves up, and the ribs move down.

The respiratory system delivers oxygen to the body and removes carbon dioxide, a process that takes place on two levels: the alveolar/capillary exchange and the capillary/cellular exchange ▶ **Figure 38-2** .

The alveolar/capillary exchange works in the following way:

1. **Air breathed in during inspiration** travels through the airways to the alveoli.

2. **As this oxygen-containing air** enters the alveoli, oxygen-poor blood is circulated through the capillaries around each alveoli.

3. **Oxygen in the alveoli** crosses over into the bloodstream. Carbon dioxide in the blood from the capillaries crosses over into the alveoli, creating a shift of oxygen and carbon dioxide.

Capillary to tissue cells

O_2 and nutrients

CO_2 and waste

Pulmonary arteriole

CO_2

O_2

Lung alveoli capillaries

Pulmonary venule

CO_2

O_2
Lung alveolus

Figure 38-2 The exchange of oxygen and carbon dioxide occurs at the cellular level, where cells give up carbon dioxide into the capillaries and the capillaries give up oxygen to the cells.

> After 4 to 6
> minutes without oxygen,
> cells in the brain and nervous system
> may die.

The capillary/cellular exchange occurs throughout the body's cells. Cells give up carbon dioxide into the capillaries, and capillaries give up oxygen to the cells.

Each living cell in the body requires a regular supply of oxygen; some cells, such as those in the heart, brain, and nervous system, need a constant supply of oxygen to survive. Cells in the heart will be damaged if the oxygen supply is interrupted for more than a few minutes. After 4 to 6 minutes without oxygen, cells in the brain and nervous system may die. Dead brain cells can never be replaced. Brain damage and other permanent changes in the body result from damage caused by a lack of oxygen.

Other cells in the body that are not as dependent on a constant oxygen supply can tolerate short periods without oxygen and still survive.

Basic Airway Management

You should always assess the airway first in an injured or ill patient. This rule applies to both the basic and advanced levels of airway management. Advanced airway techniques are begun only after proper basic airway management has been completed.

As you have already learned, the first step in airway management is opening a patient's airway. You should use the head tilt-chin lift maneuver in the patient with no spinal injury and the jaw-thrust maneuver in a patient you suspect has a spinal injury. After you have opened the airway, you should assess the airway and evaluate the need for suctioning to remove foreign bodies, liquid, or blood from the patient's mouth.

After the airway has been cleared, you need to determine whether the patient needs an airway adjunct. The basic airway adjuncts that are already available to you are oropharyngeal and nasopharyngeal airways. The more advanced airway adjuncts that may be available to you, with approval of your medical director, will be discussed in this chapter.

Gastric Tubes

Patients who have gastric distention or are vomiting are especially challenging to manage. You must use basic suctioning techniques to prevent aspiration in a patient who is vomiting. Patients with gastric distention are prone to vomiting; therefore, you should consider using a gastric tube in these patients.

A **gastric tube** is an advanced airway adjunct that provides a channel directly into a patient's stomach, allowing you to remove gas, blood, and toxins or to insert medications and nutrition. In the field, you will use a gastric tube primarily to decompress the stomach of a patient with gastric distention, a problem that is most common in children but is also seen in adults.

There are two types of gastric tubes: nasogastric tubes, which are inserted through the nose, and orogastric tubes, which are inserted through the mouth. A nasogastric tube is contraindicated in a patient with major facial, head, or spinal trauma. In these patients, an orogastric tube is safer. A nasogastric tube can cause nasal trauma with bleeding, or it can accidentally be passed into the trachea, interfering with the airway and ventilation. In a patient with a basal skull fracture, a nasogastric tube can accidentally be passed into the brain.

Inserting a gastric tube can activate a patient's gag reflex, causing vomiting and aspiration. Clearly, inserting a gastric tube is a delicate task that must be done strictly according to local EMS protocol and medical direction. Special care is called for if the patient has head, spinal, or major facial trauma. Be sure to follow local protocol.

You will need the following equipment for gastric intubation ▶ **Figure 38-3** :

- Proper-sized tubes
  —newborn/infant, 8 French
  —toddler/preschool, 10 French
  —school-age child, 12 French
  —adolescent, 14 to 16 French

- Catheter-tipped 20-mL syringe

- Water-soluble lubricant

- Emesis container

- Tape

- Stethoscope

- Suctioning unit and catheters

Once you have prepared and assembled the proper equipment, use the following procedure to insert a nasogastric tube:

1. **Measure the tube** from the tip of the nose, around the ear, to the epigastric area below the xiphoid process. (If you are using an orogastric tube, measure from the teeth to the angle of the jaw and down to the epigastric area.) Mark the

▶ **Skill Drill 38-1**

Figure 38-3 Equipment for gastric intubation includes gastric tubes, a catheter-tipped 20-mL syringe, water-soluble lubricant, an emesis container, tape, a stethoscope, and a suctioning unit.

measured length on the tube with a piece of tape, or note the number on the tube.

2. **Lubricate the distal end** of the tube with a water-soluble lubricant.

3. **Place the patient** in the proper position. If you do not suspect a spinal injury, place the patient supine, with the head turned to the left side.

4. **Pass the tube** along the nasal floor (or, for an orogastric tube, over the tongue to the back of the throat) until you reach the tape marker.

5. **Confirm proper tube placement** by aspirating stomach contents with the syringe or injecting 20 mL of air into the tube and listening for gurgling over the stomach with the stethoscope.

6. **Aspirate air and stomach contents** with the syringe, once placement is confirmed, to decompress the stomach, or attach to on-board suction. Follow local protocols concerning the type of suction to use (intermittent or continuous).

7. **Secure the tube** in place with tape.

The Sellick Maneuver

Intubating an unresponsive patient who has no cough and/or gag reflex may cause vomiting and aspiration, which can ultimately damage tissues and block the lower airway passages. A procedure called the <u>Sellick maneuver</u>, which was originally developed for intubating patients during surgery, can be helpful in avoiding these complications in the field.

The <u>cricoid cartilage</u>, located just below the thyroid cartilage (Adam's apple), is a rigid, ring-shaped structure that completely encircles the larynx at the top of the trachea. It can be hard to locate in infants, children, and small adults. The depression between the thyroid cartilage and the cricoid cartilage is called the cricothyroid membrane. (In certain cases, ALS providers will insert an emergency airway though this membrane.) The esophagus is much softer than the trachea and does not have rings of cartilage to hold it open. It is normally closed, opening only as we eat or drink. By applying pressure on the cricoid cartilage, you can squeeze the esophagus shut and thus prevent solids and fluids from leaving the esophagus and eventually being aspirated into the larynx and trachea.

To perform this maneuver, follow the steps in
▶ **Skill Drill 38-1** :

1. **With the patient's neck slightly extended** (only if there is no suspicion of spinal injury), **visualize the cricoid cartilage**, just inferior to the thyroid cartilage (Adam's apple) **(Step 1)**.

2. **Confirm location of the cricoid cartilage** by palpating with the tip of your index finger **(Step 2)**.

3. **Place a thumb and index finger on either side of the midline of the cricoid cartilage.** Apply firm—but not excessive—posterior pressure on the cricoid cartilage to compress and shut off the esophagus behind it. Too much pressure could collapse the larynx. Maintain this pressure until the patient is intubated **(Step 3)**.

The Sellick maneuver should be performed by a third EMT-B and might not be possible if you and your partner are alone. When performing this maneuver, be sure to correctly identify anatomic landmarks to avoid damaging other structures.

Endotracheal Intubation

<u>Endotracheal intubation</u> is the insertion of a tube into the trachea to maintain the airway. This can be done through the mouth (called <u>orotracheal intubation</u>) or through the nose (called <u>nasotracheal intubation</u>). In either case, the tube passes directly through the larynx between the vocal cords and then into the trachea.

Endotracheal intubation on patients who are conscious or drifting into and out of consciousness is extremely difficult. As an EMT-B, you will be intubating only patients who are unresponsive with no gag reflex, or in cardiac arrest. However, you should not immediately intubate a patient who is unresponsive or in cardiac arrest. First, you must try to open the airway with the appropriate BLS maneuver, clear the airway, and

Skill Drill 38-1 Performing the Sellick Maneuver

Visualize the cricoid cartilage.

Palpate to confirm its location.

Apply firm pressure on the cricoid ring with your thumb and index finger on either side of midline. Maintain pressure until intubated.

ventilate the patient with a BVM. When BLS maneuvers fail to open the airway, you should then consider endotracheal intubation based on your local medical protocols.

The remainder of this section will focus on orotracheal, rather than nasotracheal, intubation.

Orotracheal Intubation

Orotracheal intubation is the most effective way to control a patient's airway and has many advantages over other airway management techniques (▶ **Table 38-1**). It is indicated for patients who cannot protect their own airways as a result of unconsciousness or cardiac arrest (▼ **Figure 38-4**). It is also used for patients who need prolonged artificial ventilation, are unresponsive to

Figure 38-4 Endotracheal intubation is indicated for patients who are unconscious and cannot protect their own airways.

TABLE 38-1 Advantages of Orotracheal Intubation

- Completely controls and protects the airway

- Delivers better minute volume without the difficulty of maintaining an adequate mask seal, as is needed with a BVM device. (The minute volume is the volume of air cycled through the alveoli in 1 minute.)

- If prolonged ventilation is required, it may be left in place for a long time.

- Prevents gastric distention, which means less regurgitation of stomach contents and greater opportunity for good tidal volume

- Minimizes the risk of aspiration of stomach contents into the respiratory system because a balloon seals off the trachea

- Allows for direct access to the trachea for suctioning

- Allows for the delivery of high volumes of oxygen at higher than normal pressures

- Provides a route for administration of certain medications painful stimuli, or have no gag reflex or ability to cough. Remember that defibrillation is the priority for patients in cardiac arrest from ventricular fibrillation. Intubation is performed only after defibrillation and during the 1-minute time lapse for CPR.

Equipment

Endotracheal intubation requires all your attention. You should not be searching for forgotten or misplaced equipment as you work. Therefore, you should assemble all the equipment that you will need before starting the procedure, while the patient is being hyperventilated (▼ **Figure 38-5**). As in all patient care situations, be sure to follow BSI precautions. You will be working in close proximity to the patient's airway, so the minimum BSI includes gloves, eye protection, and a mask.

There are two methods for placing an endotracheal tube. Both use endotracheal tubes with slight differences in equipment. The visualized technique uses a laryngoscope. The layrngoscope enables the provider to observe the vocal cords visually to manually place the endotracheal tube between the vocal cords into the trachea. The blind technique uses a **lighted stylet**. The light at the end of the stylet is extremely bright. The light can be visualized on the outside of the body when placed in the trachea. The light cannot be seen if it is placed in the esophagus (there is too much tissue for the light to penetrate to the outside). Because the vocal cords are normally located in the midline of the neck, a light seen in the sternal notch is below the vocal cords and in the trachea. An endotracheal tube, slipped over the stylet, will then lie in the trachea. Because the vocal cords are not actually visualized, the technique is termed "blind."

The equipment for both visualized and blind endotracheal intubation is basically the same with the exception of the insertion device. The following is a list of equipment needed:

- BSI equipment
- Proper-sized endotracheal tube (ETT)
- Laryngoscope handle and blade (visualized technique)
- Stylet (visualized technique) or lighted stylet (blind technique)
- 10-mL syringe
- Oxygen, with BVM device for ventilation before and after intubation
- A suctioning unit with rigid and soft-tip catheters
- Magill forceps
- Towels for raising the patient's head and/or shoulders
- A stethoscope
- Water-soluble lubricant for tubes and scopes
- A commercial securing device or tape

You must check your equipment daily to ensure that it is all available and to be certain that it is properly assembled and working, especially before you try to intubate a patient.

LARYNGOSCOPE. The purpose of a **laryngoscope** is to sweep the tongue out of the way and align the airway so that you can see the vocal cords and pass the ETT through them (▼ **Figure 38-6**). The handle of the laryngoscope contains two C or D cell batteries to provide power to the light and has a locking bar to connect the handle to the blade; the blade is detachable from

Figure 38-5 Assemble all necessary equipment before you begin intubation.

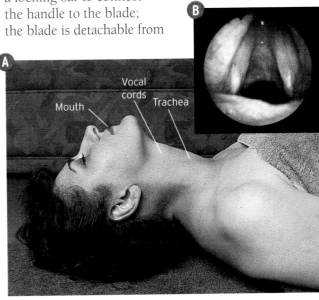

Figure 38-6 **A.** You must see the vocal cords to pass an ETT through them. The vocal cords are located in the upper airway at the entrance to the larynx. **B.** A view of the vocal cords.

Figure 38-7 Laryngoscope blades are curved or straight and come in different sizes.

A

Tongue
Trachea
Vallecula
Epiglottis
Esophagus

B

Tongue
Trachea
Vallecula
Epiglottis
Esophagus

Figure 38-8 **A.** Insert a curved blade just in front of the epiglottis into the vallecula. **B.** Insert a straight blade past the epiglottis.

the handle. Blades are either curved or straight and range in size from 0 to 4 (◄ **Figure 38-7**). The two blade designs function differently to align the structures so that you can visualize the vocal cords. The curved blade is inserted just in front of the epiglottis, into the **vallecula** (the space between the base of the tongue and the epiglottis), allowing you to see the glottic opening and vocal cords (◄ **Figure 38-8A**). The straight blade is inserted past the epiglottis (◄ **Figure 38-8B**). Because its broader base and flange provide better displacement of the tongue, a curved blade is preferred for use in older children. A straight blade, which actually lifts the epiglottis out of the way to allow for visualization of the glottic opening and vocal cords, is preferred for use in infants. You should practice intubation with both curved and straight blades so that you will feel comfortable using both techniques in a real patient situation.

A notch on the blade locks onto the locking bar of the handle. Because adequate lighting is essential for you to visualize the epiglottis and vocal cords, the light source is near the tip of the blade. You can activate the light by lifting the blade away from the handle until it locks at a right angle (▼ **Figure 38-9**). The light should be bright white. However, the bulb will not come on if the blade is not attached properly, the bulb is burned out or loose, or the batteries in the handle are dead. Always carry extra batteries for the handle and extra light bulbs in assorted sizes for each blade.

LIGHTED STYLET. The lighted stylet comes in one size that fits all adult and many pediatric endotracheal tubes. The lighted stylet consists of a malleable metal wand with a light source at one end and a handle with an energy source at the other. The wand is designed to provide stiffness and shaping to the tube. Once an endotracheal tube is threaded onto the wand, the handle will have a locking device to secure the proximal end of the

Figure 38-9 Once the blade is locked in place at a 90° angle, the light will turn on.

endotracheal tube. This prevents the endotracheal tube from moving prior to insertion, and the stylet from protruding beyond the end of the endotracheal tube.

ENDOTRACHEAL TUBES. Endotracheal tubes come in many sizes; the size is specified by the measurement of the inside diameter of the tube. Sizes range from 2.5 mm to 9 mm. The length of the ETT is marked on the outside of the tube in centimeters. The usual length of a tube for an adult is 33 cm. The following are general guidelines to use when you are intubating an average-sized adult patient (▼ Figure 38-10):

- The centimeter markings on the outside of the tube will usually indicate that it is 15 cm to the vocal cords, 20 to 21 cm to the sternal notch, and 25 cm to the carina.

- You can mark the length placement of the ETT by looking at where the tube lines up with the

teeth on an intubated patient. This tube-to-teeth mark is usually at around 22 cm.

The proper-sized tube for adult male patients ranges from 7.5 to 8.5 mm; for adult female patients, it ranges from 6.5 to 8.0 mm (▼ Figure 38-11). For most efficient use of the tube, use the largest-diameter ETT you can. A good rule of thumb is to always have a 7.5-mm ETT on hand; this size tube will fit most male or female adult patients. However, you should carry a complete selection of tube sizes in the unit to ensure that no matter what size you choose, you have one tube smaller and one tube larger, in case you need it.

Tube components include a standard 15-mm adapter, which attaches to the BVM device (▼ Figure 38-12). Make sure that the adapter is securely pushed into the tube so that it does not pull off when you ventilate the patient. The tube has a pilot balloon attached to it to indicate

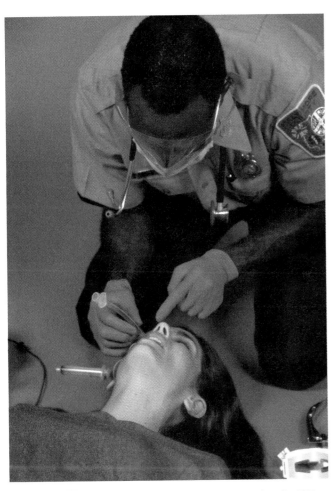

Figure 38-10 Prior to securing the tube, note the mark on the ETT. The ETT typically lines up with the teeth on an intubated patient around the 22-cm mark.

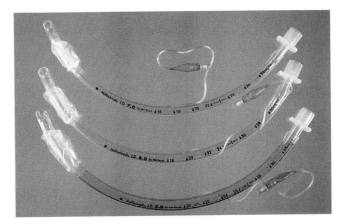

Figure 38-11 Endotracheal tubes that are used on adults generally range in size from 6.5 to 8.5 mm. Note the centimeter markings.

Figure 38-12 The components of the adult endotracheal tube include a 15-mm adapter that attaches to a ventilating device, a pilot balloon, the tube, a balloon cuff (shown inflated), and the Murphy eye. The pediatric tube shown at the bottom includes an adapter and a Murphy eye at the uncuffed distal end of the tube.

how well the balloon cuff at the end of the ETT is inflated. The cuff at the end of the tube holds about 10 mL of air. The small hole at the distal end of the tube across from the bevel end, called a Murphy eye, helps to prevent tube obstruction.

For children, it is best to have a chart or tape device to help you with sizing the ETT (▼ **Figure 38-13**). Generally, for newborns and small infants, the proper tube size ranges from 3.0 to 3.5 mm; for infants up to 1 year, it is 4.0 mm. You may also follow a formula for sizing tubes in children. You can calculate tube size in children by adding 16 to the child's age and then dividing by 4. Another method is to select a tube that roughly equals the size of the diameter of the patient's little finger across the nailbed (▼ **Figure 38-14**). No matter what size you decide to use, you should also have one tube larger and one tube smaller available, in case you need it.

With children older than age 8 years and with adults, you will use cuffed tubes. However, in younger children, the circular narrowing of the trachea at the level of the cricoid cartilage functions as a cuff. Therefore, uncuffed tubes are used in children younger than 8 years. Always watch the tube pass through the vocal cords in a child (as well as in an adult) to make sure that the tip of the ETT is in the proper position.

STYLET. A plastic-coated wire called a **stylet** may be inserted into the ETT to add rigidity and shape to the tube (▼ **Figure 38-15**). You should bend the tip of the stylet to form a gentle curve in adults. Because an infant's or child's airway is more angular and less aligned than an adult's, you should bend the tip of the stylet into a hockey stick shape for use in an infant or child (▼ **Figure 38-16**). You should also apply a little

Figure 38-13 A chart or tape device is best for estimating the size of an ETT for children.

Figure 38-15 A wire stylet, which adds rigidity and shape to the tube, must be removed after tube placement.

Figure 38-14 Another method of sizing endotracheal tubes in children is to select a tube that roughly equals the size of the diameter of the patient's little finger across the nailbed.

Figure 38-16 Bend the tip of the stylet into a hockey stick shape for a pediatric patient, as shown at the top. Bend the stylet to form a gentle curve for an adult patient, as shown at the bottom.

water-soluble lubricant to the tube to make it easier to insert and to the end of the stylet to make it easier to remove once the tube is in place. Do not insert the stylet past the Murphy eye, as it could puncture or lacerate delicate airway tissues (▶ **Figure 38-17**). A good rule of thumb is to keep the stylet ¼" from the cuff, or proximal end in adults and 1" from the end of the tube in infants and children. Before you attempt intubation, you should always confirm that the stylet is not sticking out past the end of the ETT.

These principles are also followed for the lighted stylet. The lighted stylet may or may not be disposable, depending on the manufacturer. Because the light source is in the handle, make sure you have replacement handles or batteries, whichever is appropriate for your device.

SYRINGE. You will use the 10-mL syringe to test for air leaks in the ETT before intubation (▶ **Figure 38-18**). You will use it again after the ETT is in place to inflate the cuff and provide a seal inside the trachea to prevent aspiration and help to secure the ETT. Note that this step is done only in ETTs with cuffs; therefore, you will not perform this step with the uncuffed tubes that are used on infants and children.

Take the following steps to use the syringe properly:

1. **As you are assembling** and checking your equipment before intubation, pull back on the plunger of the syringe to the 10-mL mark to fill the syringe with the amount of air that is needed to inflate the cuff.

2. **Attach the syringe** to the pilot balloon, and test the cuff by inflating it with 5 to 10 mL of air.

3. **Deflate the cuff** after you have confirmed that there are no air leaks.

4. **With the syringe still attached,** remove the air from the cuff by pulling back on the plunger to the 10-mL mark. Be sure that the syringe remains attached to the pilot balloon with the plunger pulled back to the 10-mL mark.

After the ETT has been properly inserted in the patient, you will inflate the cuff with 5 to 10 mL of air and then remove the syringe from the pilot balloon to prevent air from leaking out back into the syringe (▶ **Figure 38-19**).

OTHER EQUIPMENT. You must also have a device available to secure the ETT in place. The use of a commercial securing device is recommended over using tape. There are many manufacturers of securing devices;

Figure 38-17 Do not insert the stylet past the Murphy eye, as it could damage airway tissues. Keep the stylet 1/4" from the cuff in the adult tube and 1" from the end of the pediatric tube.

Figure 38-18 Inflate the cuff with 5 to 10 mL of air to check for air leaks.

Figure 38-19 Inflate the cuff with 5 to 10 mL of air, and then remove the syringe from the pilot balloon to prevent air from leaking out back into the syringe.

you should become familiar with the device used in your system. There are some EMS systems that use tape to secure the ETT (▶ **Figure 38-20**). Tape can also be used as a back-up system to a commercial device. Medical control may also advise you to use an oral airway or similar device as a bite block in the intubated patient.

Figure 38-20 You must secure the ETT in place with either tape or a commercial device. Note that the cervical collar alone does not ensure spinal immobilization.

Figure 38-21 Magill forceps can be used to help guide the tube.

In addition, you will need the following equipment:

- Oxygen
- A suctioning unit
- A BVM device
- Magill forceps (can be used to help guide the tube in the visualized technique) ▲ **Figure 38-21**
- Towels for raising the patient's head or shoulders if necessary
- Secondary confirmation device
- C-collar backboard

You will use the BVM device to ventilate the patient before you first try to intubate and then to ventilate the intubated patient. The suctioning unit should be readily available to clear any fluid or particles from the mouth ▶ **Figure 38-22**. Use a rigid, large-bore suction catheter to clear the mouth before intubation. Once the patient is intubated, you might need to use a French catheter to suction any fluids from inside the ETT.

The Intubation Procedure

VISUALIZED (ORAL) INTUBATION. You may intubate only if authorized to do so by off-line or online medical control, according to your local medical protocols. Once you and medical control have made the decision to intubate, you must act quickly, carefully, and efficiently. If environmental light is too bright and you are using a lighted stylet, move the patient to your ambulance or another place where ambient light can be controlled. Be sure to follow BSI precautions, including gloves, eye protection, and a mask. You should not use more than 30 seconds in an attempt to properly position the ETT. The 30-second time limit begins when you stop ventilation and insert either the laryngoscope blade or the lighted stylet into

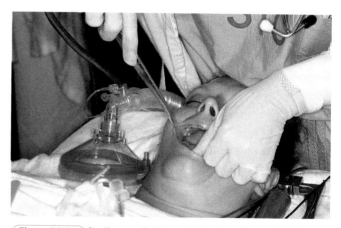

Figure 38-22 Suction any fluid or particles from the mouth before any attempt to intubate.

the patient's mouth; it ends when the ETT has been properly placed. If you are not successful in placing the ETT, stop, withdraw the tube, hyperventilate the patient, and try again according to your local protocols.

Intubation is a multiple-person task, especially in a situation involving cardiac arrest and use of an AED. The following tasks should be divided among the EMT-Bs who are present:

- First EMT-B applies and uses the AED.
- Second EMT-B ventilates the patient with a BVM device with 100% oxygen at a rate of one ventilation every 5 seconds.
- Third EMT-B provides CPR.
- Fourth EMT-B prepares and intubates the patient.

You should note that defibrillation with an AED remains the highest priority. Intubating a patient who is in cardiac arrest should occur only after the necessary defibrillations and CPR have been performed for

1 minute. Consult with medical control regarding protocol on the sequence of these events.

Follow the steps in ▶ **Skill Drill 38-2** to perform visualized orotracheal intubation:

1. **Open the patient's airway** with a BLS maneuver, and clear the airway of any foreign material.

2. **Insert an oropharyngeal airway** and ventilate the patient with a BVM device at the appropriate rate, which will vary depending on the age of the patient. You should hyperventilate the patient at a rate of at least 24 breaths/min before attempting intubation **(Step 1)**.

3. **As your partner ventilates the patient,** you should quickly assemble and test your equipment. Verify that the bulb on the laryngoscope or lighted stylet is working, make sure the ETT cuff has no leaks, and select the proper-sized tube. If you are using a non-lighted stylet, insert it in the ETT. Lubricate the tube and stylet as needed **(Step 2)**.

4. **Confirm that the patient has been properly hyperventilated.** Remove the oral airway if it is in place.

5. **If another EMT-B is available,** have him or her perform the Sellick maneuver to improve visualization of the vocal cords or positioning of the lighted stylet. This maneuver will also prevent vomiting and aspiration. Maintain pressure on the cricoid cartilage until the ETT cuff is inflated.

6. **Position the patient's head and neck** to allow for the best visualization of the vocal cords. In a patient with no spinal cord injury, use the head tilt-chin lift maneuver to align the structures. When you are using the laryngoscope, place towels under the patient's shoulders, if necessary, to raise the head for a better view of the vocal cords. When you are using the lighted stylet, grasping the tongue and jaw and pulling upward will aid in insertion **(Step 3)**.

7. **To intubate a patient** who you suspect has a spinal cord injury, you should make sure that your partner maintains manual in-line stabilization of the head and neck in the neutral position with a cervical collar in place while you attempt the intubation. If using the laryngoscope, you might need to lie on your stomach or straddle the patient's head while leaning back to visualize the vocal cords adequately **(Step 4)**.

8. **Grasp the laryngoscope** handle in your left hand. Make sure the blade is locked into place and the bulb is illuminated. Open the patient's mouth with the gloved fingers of your right hand. Gently place the blade in the right side of the patient's mouth, then move it toward the center of the mouth, gently pushing the tongue to the left. The tongue must be displaced for you to visualize the vocal cords. Visualize the epiglottis. Advance a curved blade along the base of the tongue until its tip rests at the vallecula; advance a straight blade along the base of the tongue until you see it catch the epiglottis. Lift the laryngoscope away from the posterior pharynx so that you can see the vocal cords. The lifting force is directed straight up, parallel to the long axis of the laryngoscope handle, not back toward the patient's head. It should feel as if you are picking up the patient's head by the jaw. To avoid breaking the patient's teeth or lacerating the lips, never use the blade as a lever or fulcrum against the upper teeth. Do not lose sight of the vocal cords at any time after you have visualized them. Proper placement of the ETT depends on your visualization of the ETT as it is placed through the vocal cords.

   With the lighted stylet, grasp the tongue and jaw, and pull upward, turn the stylet on and advance the tube until resistance is felt. Check to see if light is seen midline, then advance the tube further through the vocal chords. Light should be visible at the anterior wall of the trachea. If ambient light is too bright, cover the working area with a blanket.

9. **Insert the ETT** with your right hand, keeping the vocal cords and the tip of the tube in sight at all times. Do not advance the ETT down the center of the laryngoscope blade, or your view of the vocal cords will be obstructed.

   Advance the tube from the right side of the patient's mouth. Watch the uninflated cuff on the tube as it passes through the vocal cords, then advance the ETT until the cuff is just past the vocal cords. Note and document the centimeter markings on the outside of the ETT at the level of the teeth.

   Once the tube has been inserted through the vocal cords into the trachea, gently remove the laryngoscope and stylet, if a stylet was used. *Do not let go of the ETT until it is secured.*

Skill Drill 38-2 Performing Orotracheal Intubation

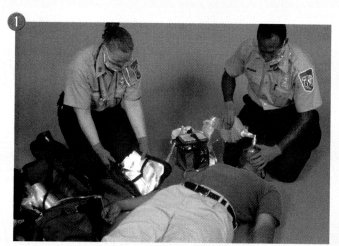

Open and clear the airway.
Place an oropharyngeal airway and hyperventilate with a BVM.

Assemble and test intubation equipment as your partner continues to ventilate.

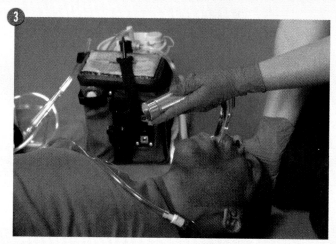

Confirm adequate hyperventilation and remove the oral airway.

If available, have another rescuer perform the Sellick manuever to improve visualization of the cords.

Use the head tilt-chin lift maneuver to position the nontrauma patient for insertion of the laryngoscope.

In a trauma patient, maintain the cervical spine in-line and neutral as your partner lies down or straddles the patient's head to visualize the vocal cords.

With the lighted stylet, you will release the jaw and retract the stylet approximately 10 cm. Advance the stylet until the glow illuminates the sternal notch. Hold the tube against the patient's lips, release the locking lever and pull the stylet out of the tube. *Do not let go of the ETT until it is secured* **(Step 5)**.

10. **Inflate the soft balloon cuff** on the end of the tube with 5 to 10 mL of air. This will seal the trachea and anchor the tube so that air can be blown directly into the lungs. Gently squeeze the pilot balloon cuff to verify the amount of air you should use. The pilot balloon should be full but easily compressed between your fingers. Detach

Insert the laryngoscope from the right side of mouth and move the tongue to the left. Lift the laryngoscope away from the posterior pharynx to visualize the vocal cords.

9. Insert the ETT from the right side. Remove laryngoscope and stylet. Hold the tube carefully until secured.

Inflate the balloon cuff and remove the syringe as your partner prepares to ventilate.

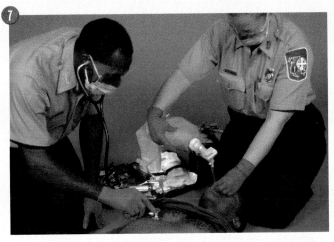

Begin ventilating and confirm placement of the ETT by listening over both lungs and the stomach. Also confirm placement with an end tidal carbon dioxide detector, if available.

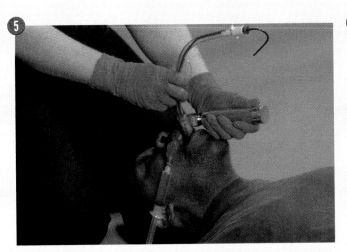

Secure the tube and continue to ventilate.

Note and record depth of insertion, and reconfirm position after each time you move the patient.

the syringe so that the air in the cuff will not empty back into it **(Step 6)**.

11. **You or your partner** (whoever is not holding the ETT in place) **should begin ventilating** the patient with a BVM device. Confirm placement of the ETT. Listen with a stethoscope over both lungs and the stomach as you ventilate the patient through the tube. You should be able to hear equal breath sounds over both right and left lung fields. Also listen at the sternal notch in children. You should see both sides of the chest rise and fall with each ventilation. This is especially important in children, as breath sounds in

children may be misleading. You may hear them even if the tube is in the esophagus. You should not be able to hear breath sounds in the stomach.

Proper confirmation of ETT placement is essential for care of the patient. If you do not actually visualize the ETT passing through the vocal cords, or see the light at the midline, you may place the ETT in the esophagus rather than in the trachea, which can prove fatal for the patient. The actual visualization of the ETT as it passes through the vocal cords is the best way to confirm proper placement.

It is recommended that you use a secondary method of confirming proper tube placement. There are several devices available—esophageal detector devices, **end-tidal carbon dioxide detectors** (including colorimetric detectors) and portable capnography monitors.

Esophageal detector devices (EDD) are designed to connect directly to the ET tube adapter end (where the BVM is attached) once the patient has been intubated. Two common devices use a syringe with plunger or a bulb syringe design. The device works by attempting to withdraw air from the ETT. If the tube is properly placed, air will freely withdraw through the syringe or will inflate the bulb, as the trachea will not collapse around the end of the ETT. However, if the ETT is in the esophagus, the soft tissues of the esophagus will collapse around the end of the ETT and there will be noticeable resistance to the withdrawing of air through the syringe/plunger or to the inflation of the bulb.

End-tidal CO_2 detectors and capnography monitors sense the amount of carbon dioxide during ventilation. Patients in respiratory and/or cardiac arrest will not be producing any carbon dioxide. Therefore, you cannot get a reading until you are providing ventilations to the patient.

One example of an end-tidal CO_2 detector is a disposable plastic indicator with chemically treated paper that changes from purple to yellow in the presence of carbon dioxide (usually takes several ventilations to obtain a reading). The device connects between the ET tube and the BVM. Secondary confirmation is made by verifying the appropriate color change. If carbon dioxide is present, it will change the color of the indicator to yellow. If the ETT is in the esophagus, ventilations

EMT-B Tips

The EMT-B who is ventilating the patient is responsible for monitoring tube placement and preventing it from being dislodged. This EMT, who should not be physically involved in lifting or moving the patient, has a good viewpoint from which to plan and coordinate team movements.

will not produce any carbon dioxide and there will be no color change on the indicator (may change to tan, but generally will stay purple).

Capnography monitors can also be used for secondary confirmation of ET tube placement. These devices monitor for the presence of carbon dioxide through an adapter that connects between the ETT and the BVM device. During ventilations, the amount of carbon dioxide present is either displayed as a number or as a positive waveform on the monitor. Positive waveforms and/or carbon dioxide readings provide secondary confirmation of proper placement. If the ETT is in the esophagus, waveforms and readings will not be present.

Remember that these are all devices used as secondary confirmation of ET tube placement. All of the devices are not guaranteed 100% that your tube is in the correct location. Your primary confirmation is direct visualization of the tube passing through the vocal cords, ausculating good bilateral breath sounds (no epigastric sounds) and seeing the patien's chest rise and fall with each ventilation **(Step 7)**.

12. **Once you have verified** that the tube is properly placed, secure the ETT in place with the device and technique that have been approved by your medical director.

13. **Keep in mind that,** even when placed properly, the ETT will move if it is not secured. For this reason, you must never let go of the ETT until it is secured. Even then, you must continuously check the tube to make sure it is secure and in the correct place. It is recommended that immobilization of the head and c-collars be placed on patients that are intubated (even if there is no trauma) to avoid unnecessary movement of the head during transport. Excessive head movement is thought to contribute to dislodgment of initially properly

TABLE 38-2   Benefits and Complications of Endotracheal Intubation

Benefits	Complications
Provides complete protection of airway	Intubating the right mainstem bronchus
Can be left in for long periods of time	Intubating the esophagus
Delivers better oxygen concentration than a BVM device	Aggravating a spinal injury
Prevents gastric distention and aspiration	Vomiting and/or removing the tube
Allows for deep suctioning of the trachea	Causing soft-tissue trauma
Allows for administration of certain medications	Mechanical failure
	Patient intolerance

placed ET tubes. Continue to artificially ventilate the patient at an age-appropriate rate. Also, again, remember to note the distance the tube has been inserted. Be sure to reassess breath sounds each time you move the patient **(Step 8)**.

BLIND (NASAL) INTUBATION. Many of the procedural steps for blind intubation are the same as the ones for visualized intubation.

1. Use BSI precautions.

2. Ensure adequate artificial ventilation by bag-valve-mask (BVM) device and oxygen.

3. Hyperventilate the patient at a rate of 20 to 24 breaths/min prior to any advanced airway placement. Oxygenate the patient for 1 to 2 minutes.

4. Assemble and test all equipment, including preparation for securing the device.

5. Check for a gag reflex.

6. Check for and remove, if possible, any sharp debris in the patient's mouth.

7. Position the patient's head in a neutral position and move the tongue forward.

8. Grasp the tongue and jaw, and pull upward.

9. Turn the light on.

10. Advance the tube until resistance is felt.

11. Check to see if light is midline, then advance further through the vocal cords. Light should be visible at the anterior wall of the trachea.

12. Release the jaw and hold the tube against the lips.

13. Retract the stylet approximately 10 cm.

14. Lift the tongue and jaw again and advance the stylet until the glow illuminates the sternal notch. If the ambient light is too strong, cover the working area with a blanket.

15. Holding the tube against the lips, release the locking lever and pull the stylet out of the tube.

16. Secure the tube.

17. Attach BVM and ventilate the patient.

Complications

Endotracheal intubation is a difficult skill to master. If intubation takes longer than 30 seconds, the resulting delay in oxygenation may lead to brain damage. Obviously, you will need a great deal of expert instruction and practice to master this skill. Among the possible complications of endotracheal intubation are the following, as summarized in ▲ **Table 38-2**.

INTUBATING THE RIGHT MAINSTEM BRONCHUS. This is the most common error that is made during intubation. If you push or accidentally slip the tube in too far, the ETT will pass into the right mainstem bronchus. In this position, it will ventilate the right lung only. Therefore, you will hear breath sounds on the right side only. The best way to correct this problem is to deflate the cuff and pull the ETT back about 1". Listen again for bilateral breath sounds. Make sure you do not completely remove the ETT.

INTUBATING THE ESOPHAGUS. This often occurs when you insert the ETT without first seeing the vocal cords, or without seeing the light in the midline. As a result, the ETT is inserted into the esophagus rather than the trachea. The result is rapid inflation of the patient's stomach rather than ventilation of the lungs; if the situation is not corrected, the patient will die. To avoid this, carefully watch the ETT as it passes through the vocal cords or monitor the midline position of the light. Next, check breath sounds over the left and right apices and bases of the lungs. Watch for the rise and fall of the chest. If there is any doubt, pull out the ETT, hyperventilate the patient for 2 to 3 minutes, and then try to intubate the patient again. Some EMS systems allow a maximum of two attempts at intubation. Be sure that you follow the protocol established by your medical director. If you are still unsuccessful after two attempts at intubation, consider using different advanced airway adjunct (LMA, Combitube, or PtL) or insert an oral airway and ventilate with a BVM.

AGGRAVATING A SPINAL INJURY. Whenever there is concern about a spinal injury, you must intubate without moving the patient's neck from the neutral, in-line position. This makes it difficult to lift the lower jaw and tongue enough to see the vocal cords; indeed, this can be done only by two EMT-Bs working together.

TAKING TOO LONG TO INTUBATE. Do not take any longer than 30 seconds trying to intubate, or the patient will become more hypoxic. Your partner or another member of the team should actually time the intubation. If you cannot complete the procedure within 30 seconds, you should ventilate the patient again with a BVM device at 100% oxygen for 2 to 3 minutes before trying again. Ask a third EMT-B to perform the Sellick maneuver so that you can see the vocal cords better. If after two tries the tube cannot be passed, try another airway technique, or ask another qualified rescuer to try. If the patient is difficult to intubate, you should not waste time in the field. Use another airway adjunct, and provide immediate transport, assisting ventilations as needed.

PATIENT VOMITING. A patient who is not totally unresponsive may begin to gag or try to remove the tube. Gagging may cause the patient to vomit and aspirate stomach contents. To avoid this, always check for a gag reflex before intubation, using a tongue blade, the laryngoscope blade, or an oral airway. Patients who tolerate an oral airway do not have an intact gag reflex and may need intubation. Be aware that checking for a gag reflex can make the patient vomit. You should always have a suctioning unit ready. Trying to insert an ETT through the vocal cords can also cause the cords to spasm. This is called **laryngospasm**. If this occurs, stop intubating, and ventilate the patient with a BVM device.

SOFT-TISSUE TRAUMA. The laryngoscope and the tip of the ETT can injure the lips, teeth, tongue, gums, and other airway structures. Used as a lever, the laryngo-

> You may intubate only if authorized to do so by off-line or online medical direction, according to your local medical protocols.

scope blade can easily break teeth, while a tube pushed blindly through the vocal cords can lacerate the oropharynx. Careful attention to your technique will minimize the risk of these complications.

MECHANICAL FAILURE. You may hear or feel air coming from the oropharynx when ventilating the patient. In an adult, this means that the cuff does not have enough air in it or that it has been torn and is leaking. If this occurs, you must get more air into the cuff (check the pilot balloon), or you must replace the tube. In a child, an air leak means that the uncuffed tube is too small or the child is large enough to need a cuffed tube.

PATIENT INTOLERANT OF ETT. Because of the reversal of hypoxia from direct oxygenation, a patient may regain a gag reflex or regain consciousness and try to remove the ETT. Before extubating the patient in these circumstances, you should determine that the patient can obey commands. If he or she can, ensure that the suctioning unit is nearby and turned on. Then deflate the cuff, and carefully withdraw the ETT as the patient inhales. Sometimes, you may have to ask the patient to cough. Provide immediate suctioning if the patient vomits, then reassess the airway and administer supplemental oxygen. Always consult medical control before removing the ETT.

DECREASE IN HEART RATE. Be sure to monitor the patient's vital signs carefully and continuously, particularly the heart rate. In children, it is important to check heart rate and skin color. With endotracheal intubation, the heart rate may decrease when the airway has been stimulated. Also be sure to evaluate the lung sounds and chest wall motion any time you move the patient. It is easy to dislodge the ETT while moving the patient. Always re-confirm placement after the patient has been moved in any way.

Multi-Lumen Airways

In addition to endotracheal intubation, other advanced airway devices are available to the EMT-B. These devices are called **multi-lumen airways**, and depending on local protocol and your medical director,

TABLE 38-3 Benefits and Complications of Multi-Lumen Airways	
Benefits	**Complications**
Ease of proper placement	Loses effectiveness (cuff malfunction)
No mask seal necessary	Requires deeply comatose patient
Requires minimal skill and practice to maintain	Requires constant balloon observation
Easily used in spinal injury patients	Cannot be used on patients shorter than 5′ tall
May be inserted blindly	Requires great care in listening for breath sounds
Protects the airway from upper airway secretions	Large balloon is easily broken and tends to push the PtL out of the mouth when inflated
Stays in place well (ETC)	
Sturdy balloon (ETC)	

you may be trained in the use of these airways. The benefits and complications associated with use of the multi-lumen airway are shown in ▲ Table 38-3.

The multi-lumen airways, which are inserted without direct visualization of the vocal cords, have been designed to provide lung ventilation when placed in either the trachea or the esophagus, making them much easier to insert than an ETT. Two of these adjuncts are described here: the Esophageal Tracheal Combitube (ETC), and the Pharyngeotracheal Lumen Airway (PtL). Remember that you must be trained and authorized to use these devices.

Esophageal Tracheal Combitube

The **ETC** consists of a double-lumen tube and two balloon cuffs ▼ Figure 38-23. The blue lumen (No. 1) is

Figure 38-23 The ETC consists of a double-lumen tube and two balloon cuffs. The blue lumen is the primary ventilation port, and the clear lumen is the ventilation port if the tube is placed in the trachea.

the primary ventilation port when the tube is inserted in the esophagus. The clear lumen (No. 2) is the ventilation port if the tube is placed in the trachea. The clear cuff at the tip of the tube (distal cuff) seals off the esophagus or the trachea; the larger, flesh-colored cuff near the midway point seals off the oropharynx and nasopharynx. A blue pilot balloon and a white pilot balloon correspond to the flesh-colored and distal cuffs. Two syringes are also included in the kit. The ETC is a single-use item and must be discarded after use. It should not be cleaned and reused.

The ETC is inserted blindly ► Figure 38-24. If the tube happens to go into the trachea, ventilations are provided directly into the trachea. If the tube goes into the esophagus, as occurs most often, ventilations can still be provided to the patient. You do not need to maintain a constant face mask seal with either placement. Instead, the ETC forms an inflated cuff seal in the oropharynx, so you can ventilate the trachea via a tube, rather than a mask. This ease of ventilation is an advantage of the ETC.

CONTRAINDICATIONS. You should not attempt to insert an ETC in the following individuals:

- Conscious or semiconscious patients with a gag reflex
- Children younger than 16 years
- Adults shorter than 5′ tall
- Patients who have ingested a caustic substance
- Patients who have a known esophageal disease

INSERTING THE ETC. As with endotracheal intubation, you must act quickly and carefully once you have received permission from medical control to use the

Figure 38-24 **A.** If the ETC is inserted into the trachea, it functions as an ETT with ventilations provided directly into the trachea. **B.** If the ETC is inserted into the esophagus, ventilations can still be provided to the patient.

ETC. Remember to follow BSI precautions, including the use of gloves, eye protection, and a mask, any time you may be exposed to blood or other body fluids.

The steps for insertion of the ETC are as follows:

1. **Assemble and check** the proper equipment, including the following:
   —BSI equipment
   —ETC kit with syringes
   —Water-soluble lubricant
   —Suctioning unit with suction catheters
   —BVM device and oxygen

2. **Apply a water-soluble lubricant** to the ETC.

3. **Position the patient.** Open the patient's mouth and clear it of any foreign objects, including vomitus, dentures, and blood clots. Remove the oral airway if one has been inserted. Open the airway of a patient who has no possible spinal injury by hyperextending the patient's head and neck. Note that with an unconscious patient who may have a spinal injury, you must maintain the neck in a neutral, in-line position during insertion of the ETC.

4. **Hyperventilate the patient** with 100% oxygen using a BVM device.

5. **Lift the lower jaw and tongue** away from the posterior pharynx by inserting your thumb deep into the patient's mouth and grasping the tongue and lower jaw between your thumb and index finger.

6. **Gently guide the ETC** along the base of the tongue and into the airway. Hold the ETC so that it curves in the same direction as the natural curva-

ture of the pharynx. Insert the tip into the mouth, and advance it carefully along the tongue. Do not use force. If you meet resistance, pull back and redirect the ETC. When the ETC is at the proper depth, the teeth will be between the heavy black lines.

7. **Inflate the blue pilot balloon** (and flesh-colored cuff) with the predrawn 100-mL blue-tipped syringe. Once the cuff is inflated and the pilot balloon is tense, immediately inflate the white pilot balloon (and the distal cuff) with the smaller, predrawn 15-mL syringe. The ETC may move forward a bit, but this is normal.

8. **Ventilate the patient** through the blue (No. 1) tube with a BVM device.

9. **Confirm the placement** of the tube. If the chest rises and falls and you hear breath sounds, the ETC is in the esophagus. When this is the case, continue to ventilate through the blue (No. 1) tube. If the chest does not rise and fall, and you do not hear breath sounds, the ETC is in the trachea. In this case, apply the BVM device to the shorter, clear tube, and ventilate the patient through it. Again, listen for breath sounds in all lung fields and in both axillae. Also listen over the stomach to verify that proper placement has occurred.

10. **Continuously monitor the patient.** Watch for balloon cuff leaks by carefully squeezing the pilot balloon. Use the syringes to keep the balloon cuffs properly inflated. Balloon cuffs may be torn by broken teeth, dentures, and bones. Therefore, you must use special care with this device, especially in the event of facial trauma.

Documentation Tips

After placement of any advanced airway device—ET tube, ETC, PtL, or LMA—document the intubation and exactly how you confirmed correct tube position. Also record your reconfirmation of tube position after each patient move. Note tube size where this is applicable, and the position of any measurement marks on the tube relative to the patient's teeth.

REMOVING THE ETC. Removal of the ETC airway is fairly simple. If the patient will no longer tolerate the ETC, you should remove it. Remember that the patient will likely vomit when the ETC is removed, so you must have a suctioning unit readily available. Be sure to turn the patient on his or her side to keep the airway clear of vomitus. When you are ready, simply deflate both balloon cuffs, and gently remove the tube.

Pharyngeotracheal Lumen Airway

The **Pharyngeotracheal Lumen Airway (PtL)** consists of two tubes, two balloon cuffs, a bite block, and a neck-retaining strap (▲ **Figure 38-25**). The long, clear (No. 3) tube contains a stylet and a low-pressure balloon cuff near its tip. The stylet is left in as a plug if the tube is placed in the esophagus but is removed if the tube ends up in the trachea. In either case, the balloon cuff prevents gastric contents from entering the lungs when the cuff is inflated.

The No. 3 tube passes through the larger-diameter green (No. 2) tube. The No. 2 tube has a large balloon cuff designed to seal the oropharynx. This allows ventilation gas to pass through it into the trachea (if the No. 3 tube is placed in the esophagus) but also prevents blood and debris from entering the airway from above. The balloon cuff in the No. 2 tube functions as the mask seal. The No. 1 tube is connected to these balloon cuffs to assist with inflation of these important airway seals.

As with the ETC, this device is designed to be inserted blindly into the oropharynx and esophagus, but you must be trained and authorized to use it (▶ **Figure 38-26**). If the tube happens to go into the trachea when blindly inserted, it acts like an endotracheal tube. If the long tube goes into the esophagus, you can still provide adequate ventilations to the patient. However, with the PtL, you need not maintain a constant face mask seal. The PtL forms an inflated cuff seal in the oropharynx, and the trachea may be ventilated via a tube rather than a mask.

Figure 38-25 The PtL consists of two tubes, two balloon cuffs, a bite block, and a neck-retaining strap.

Figure 38-26 The PtL is inserted blindly into the oropharynx. **A.** If the PtL is inserted into the trachea, it functions as an ETT with ventilations provided directly into the trachea. **B.** If the PtL is inserted into the esophagus, ventilations can still be provided to the patient.

EMT-B Safety

Placement of advanced airway adjuncts involves placing your own mucous membrane surfaces—eyes, nose, mouth—very near the mouths of patients likely to cough or vomit during the procedure. Without proper use of personal protective equipment, this would involve direct exposure to potentially infectious fluids such as blood, vomitus, and mucus. Follow BSI precautions faithfully: Use a mask, eye protection, and gloves.

CONTRAINDICATIONS. You should not attempt to use the PtL in the following individuals:

- Conscious or semiconscious patients with a gag reflex
- Children younger than 14 years
- Adults shorter than 5′ tall
- Patients who have ingested a caustic substance
- Patients who have a known esophageal disease

INSERTING THE PtL. Once you have confirmed with medical control your decision to insert a PtL, you must act quickly and carefully. Remember to follow BSI precautions, including gloves, eye protection, and a mask, any time you may be exposed to blood or other body fluids. Take the following steps to insert the PtL:

1. **Assemble and check** the proper equipment, including the following:
   —BSI equipment
   —PtL
   —Water-soluble lubricant
   —Suctioning unit with suction catheters
   —BVM device and oxygen

2. **Lubricate the tube** on the PtL with a water-soluble lubricant.

3. **Position the patient.** Open the patient's mouth and clear it of any foreign objects, such as vomitus, dentures, and blood clots. Remove the oral airway if one has been inserted. If the patient has no spinal injury, open the airway by hyperextending the head and neck. With a trauma patient, maintain the neck in a neutral in-line position during insertion of the PtL.

4. **Hyperventilate the patient** with 100% oxygen with the BVM device.

5. **Lift the lower jaw and tongue** away from the posterior pharynx by inserting your thumb deep into the patient's mouth and grasping the tongue and lower jaw between your thumb and index finger.

6. **Hold the PtL** so that it curves in the same direction as the natural curvature of the pharynx. Gently guide the PtL along the base of the tongue and into the airway until the teeth are against the teeth strap. If resistance is met, pull back and redirect the PtL. When the PtL is at the proper depth, place the neck strap over the patient's head and tighten.

7. **Inflate the balloon cuffs** with the No. 1 tube. Be sure to close the white cap.

8. **Ventilate the patient** through the short, green No. 2 tube, and then check the patient's chest for equal breath sounds.

9. **If you see the chest rise** and hear equal breath sounds, the No. 3 tube is in the esophagus, and you should ventilate the patient with the No. 2 tube. If the chest does not rise and fall and you do not hear equal breath sounds, the No. 3 tube is likely in the trachea. In this case, you should remove the stylet from the No. 3 tube and ventilate the patient using the No. 3 tube.

10. **Verify that the patient** is receiving adequate ventilation by listening to the lungs on both sides of the chest anteriorly, in both axillae, and over the stomach as you ventilate the patient with a BVM.

11. **Continuously monitor the patient.** Watch for balloon cuff leaks, and use inlet tube No. 1 to keep the balloon cuffs properly inflated. Jagged, broken teeth, dentures, and bones can easily tear balloon cuffs, so you must use special care if the patient has facial trauma.

REMOVING THE PtL. Removing the PtL is a simple procedure. You should remove the PtL if the patient will no longer tolerate it. The patient will likely vomit when the PtL is removed, so you must keep a suctioning unit readily available. Turn the patient to one side to help keep the airway clear of vomitus. When you are ready to remove the PtL, simply deflate the balloon cuffs and gently remove the tube.

Laryngeal Mask Airway

The **laryngeal mask airway (LMA)** was originally developed for use in anesthesia. However, since its inception, its use has been expanded to the field, especially as an alternative for BLS providers.

The LMA consists of two parts: the tube and the mask or cuff. The device is made of silicone and is designed to be reused after proper sterilization. After blind insertion, the device then molds and seals itself around the laryngeal opening by inflation of the mask. The epiglottis is contained within the mask or cuff. The device comes in seven sizes and can be used in children as well as adults ▶ **Table 38-4** .

Use of the device requires training with a manikin. Proponents advocate additional training in an operating room with anesthetized patients to become familiar with the anatomical variations that cannot be duplicated by a manikin. This type of training helps avoid malpositioning. Malpositioning may occur when the device is located somewhere other than over the laryngeal opening or when the device is "folded over" and caught on top of the epiglottis. Malpositions can sometimes be managed by repositioning the patient's head, readjusting the LMA position, or adjusting the air in the cuff. When in doubt, remove the device and start over.

CONTRAINDICATIONS. There are potential contraindications for use of the device. When positive pressure ventilation with high airway pressures occur (as in an asthma or COPD patient), the mask may leak; active vomiting may dislodge the device; esophageal diseases.

INSERTING THE LMA. After confirming your decision to insert a PtL with medical control, remember to follow BSI precautions, including the use of gloves, eye protection, and a mask. Ensure that the patient has no gag reflex, then follow the steps in ▶ **Skill Drill 38-3** to insert the LMA:

1. **Assemble and check** the proper equipment:
   —BSI equipment
   —LMA (check the cuff and valve)
   —Water-soluble lubricant
   —Suctioning unit with suctioning catheters
   —BVM device and oxygen

2. **Open the patient's airway** and clear it of any foreign material. Insert an oropharyngeal airway **(Step 1)**.

3. **Hyperventilate the patient** with a BVM device at the appropriate rate, depending on the age of the patient (24 breaths/min is typical for adults).

4. **Select the appropriate LMA size** as your partner ventilates the patient, and verify the mask has no leaks. Fully deflate the mask and lubricate it **(Step 2)**.

5. **Position the LMA** for insertion with the mask down, holding it like a pen **(Step 3)**.

6. **Remove the oropharyngeal device** and, keeping the patient's neck flexed and with your partner

Table 38-4 LMA Sizes

Size	Weight	Maximum Air in Mask
1	under 5 kg (11 lb)	4 mL
1.5	5–10 kg (11–22 lb)	7 mL
2	10–20 kg (22–44 lb)	10 mL
2.5	20–30 kg (44–66 lb)	14 mL
3	30 kg (66 lb) to a small adult	20 mL
4	Adult	30 mL
5	Large adult	40 mL

holding the mouth open, begin to insert the mask **(Step 4)**.

7. **When the widest part of the mask** is past the teeth, use the index finger to maintain a continuous forward pressure sliding the LMA over the hard palate and soft palate into the hypopharynx until definite resistance is felt **(Step 5)**.

8. **While removing your index finger,** gently press down on the tube with the other hand to prevent the LMA from being pulled out of place **(Step 6)**.

9. **After assuring** that the black line on the LMA is facing the upper lip, inflate the mask without holding the tube. Short outward movement is normal **(Step 7)**.

10. **Confirm placement of the LMA** by listening with a stethoscope over the lungs and stomach. You should hear equal breath sounds and see equal chest rise and fall. Further confirmation with a secondary confirmation device such as an end tidal carbon dioxide detector may be directed by medical control. If a previously unconscious, unresponsive patient becomes combative, this indicates that ventilations are successful and the patient has received oxygen. Once this happens, the LMA must be removed immediately to avoid stimulating vomiting.

11. **Once you have verified tube placement,** insert a bite block, such as an oropharyngeal airway, and secure the tube in place with tape or a commercial device. As with other devices, if this device is not properly secured, it will dislodge, preventing oxygen from entering the lungs **(Step 8)**.

Skill Drill 38-3   Using an LMA

Assemble and check equipment.
Open and clear the airway, and insert an oral airway.

Hyperventilate the patient.
Choose the tube size, check the mask for leaks, and deflate and lubricate it.

Grasp the tube and position it for insertion, mask down.

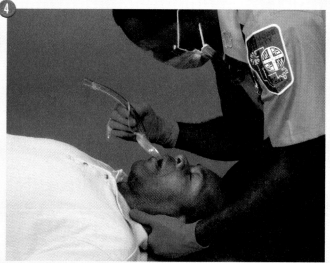

Remove the oral airway and begin to insert the mask.

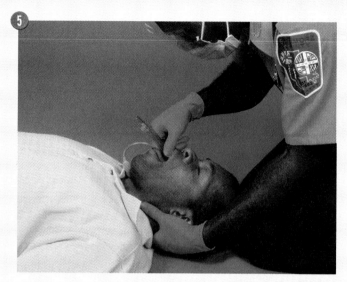

Using your index finger, push the mask up onto the hard palate and advance it until you feel resistance.

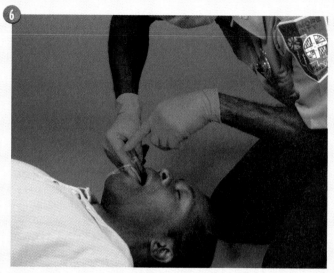

Use the other hand to stabilize the tube as you remove your index finger.

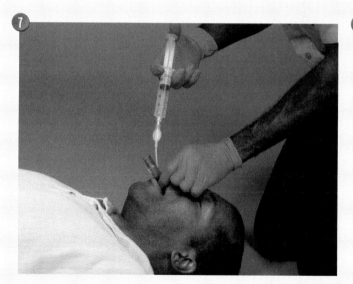

Check that the black line on the tube faces the upper lip, then inflate the tube without holding it.

Confirm tube placement by listening, and with a secondary confirmation device.

Insert a bite block and secure the LMA.

Prep Kit

Ready for Review

Gastric tubes provide a channel directly into a patient's stomach, allowing you to remove gas, blood, and toxins or to administer medications and nutrition. In the field, gastric tubes are mostly used to decompress the stomach of a patient with gastric distention.

There are two types of gastric tubes: nasogastric tubes and orogastric tubes. An orogastric tube, which is inserted through the mouth, is safer and easier to use. A nasogastric tube, which is inserted through the nose, can cause nasal trauma with bleeding and, in patients with a basal skull fracture, can be accidentally passed into the brain. Either type of tube can be accidentally passed into the trachea. Insertion of a gastric tube is a delicate task that must be done strictly according to local EMS protocol, with special care being taken for a patient who has head, spinal, or major facial trauma.

Endotracheal intubation, the insertion of a tube into the trachea to maintain a patient's airway, can be done through the mouth (orotracheal intubation) or through the nose (nasotracheal intubation). You will intubate only patients who are unconscious, unresponsive, or in cardiac arrest.

Orotracheal intubation controls and protects the airway and may be employed long-term if necessary. It also allows for direct access to the trachea for suctioning and the delivery of high volumes of oxygen at higher than normal pressures. There are two techniques for insertion of an endotracheal tube, using a laryngoscope or using a lighted stylet.

Some of the equipment that is needed for endotracheal intubation includes the correctly sized endotracheal tube; a laryngoscope or lighted stylet, stylet, and syringe; oxygen with a BVM device; a suctioning unit; and Magill forceps (if a laryngoscope is used).

Complications of endotracheal intubation include intubating the mainstem bronchus, intubating the esophagus, aggravating a spinal injury, taking too long to intubate, causing soft-tissue trauma, and mechanical failure. The patient may also vomit and/or try to remove the tube.

A patient who has been intubated must be monitored continuously to evaluate the heart rate and lung sounds. In addition, movement of the patient can cause the endotracheal tube to become dislodged.

Multi-lumen airways, such as the Esophageal Tracheal Combitube and the Pharyngeotracheal Lumen Airway, and the Laryngeal Mask Airway are inserted blindly and are easier to insert than an ETT. However, you must be trained and authorized to use these devices.

Vital Vocabulary

cricoid cartilage A rigid, ring-shaped structure that completely encircles the larynx at the top of the trachea.

cricoid pressure A technique that is used with intubation in which pressure is applied on either side of the cricoid cartilage to prevent gastric distention and allow better visualization of vocal cords; also called the Sellick maneuver.

End tidal carbon dioxide detector A plastic, disposable indicator that signals by color change when an endotracheal tube is in the proper place.

endotracheal intubation Insertion of an endotracheal tube (ETT) directly through the larynx between the vocal cords, and into the trachea, to open and maintain an airway.

Esophageal Tracheal Combitube (ETC) A multi-lumen airway that consists of a single, dual-lumen tube with two cuffs.

gastric tube An advanced airway adjunct that provides a channel directly into a patient's stomach, allowing you to remove gas, blood, and toxins, or to insert medications and nutrition.

laryngeal mask airway (LMA) Advanced airway device that is blindly inserted into the mouth to isolate the larynx for direct ventilation; consists of a tube and a mask/cuff that inflates to seal around the laryngeal opening.

laryngoscope An instrument used to give a direct view of the patient's vocal cords during endotracheal intubation.

laryngospasm Vocal cord spasm.

lighted stylet An instrument used to aid in blind insertion of an endotracheal tube.

multi-lumen airway Advanced airway devices, such as the Esophageal Tracheal Combitube and the Pharyngeotracheal Lumen Airway, that have multiple tubes to aid in ventilation and will work whether placed in the trachea or esophagus.

nasotracheal intubation Endotracheal intubation through the nose.

orotracheal intubation Endotracheal intubation through the mouth.

Pharyngeotracheal Lumen Airway (PtL) A multi-lumen airway that consists of two tubes, two masks, and a bite block.

Sellick maneuver A technique used with intubation, in which pressure is applied on either side of the cricoid cartilage to prevent gastric distention and allow better visualization of vocal cords; also called cricoid pressure.

stylet A plastic-coated wire that gives added rigidity and shape to the endotracheal tube.

vallecula The space between the base of the tongue and the epiglottis; receives the tip of a curved laryngoscope blade during endotracheal intubation.

Assessment in Action

It's Friday night. You and your partner have already been on 6 calls, and you are not even halfway through the shift. "Rescue 9, PD requests your presence at the Parkside Motor Inn for a possible overdose."

The 3-minute run across town goes without incident, and you arrive at a seedy motel. The trail of police officers points to the patient, and as you walk into the room, one of the officers states, "I think he just quit breathing." You kneel to assess the patient, and one of the man's friends asks, "He ain't doin' that breathing thing is he, man?" You confirm to your partner that the patient is in respiratory arrest, but still has a weak but regular pulse.

1. Your initial priority is:
   A. to take care of the patient's friend.
   B. establish an airway and begin ventilations.
   C. check for any bleeding.
   D. determine pupil reaction.

2. Your initial method to establish an airway and begin ventilations should be:
   A. endotracheal intubation.
   B. multi-lumen airway.
   C. oral airway and BVM device.
   D. laryngeal mask airway.

3. You have checked your patient and have found that he has no gag reflex. Of all the advanced devices, which would give the best overall control of the airway in this patient?
   A. Endotracheal intubation
   B. Multi-lumen airway
   C. Pharyngeotracheal lumen airway
   D. Laryngeal mask airway

4. Whenever possible, why is it important to hyperventilate a patient before you attempt inserting the endotracheal tube?
   A. It is required by federal law.
   B. It prevents accidental intubation of the esophagus.
   C. It provides additional oxygen for the brain and heart.
   D. It makes passing the tube through the glottic opening much easier.

5. Your first attempt took about 20 seconds, and you were still unable to visualize the vocal cords. Your most appropriate step at this time would be to:
   A. immediately attempt to revisualize the vocal cords for up to another 45 seconds.
   B. withdraw the laryngoscope and ventilate the patient before re-attempting intubation.
   C. log roll the patient onto his side and deliver five back blows.
   D. deliver five quick abdominal thrusts and then recheck the airway.

6. You realize that the patient's trachea is extremely anterior, and you are concerned about the increasing possibility of vomiting. What procedure helps prevent vomiting while at the same time improving visualization?
   A. Heimlich maneuver
   B. Gallop procedure
   C. Sellick maneuver
   D. Marriott procedure

7. Once you have inserted the ETT, you need to confirm placement by listening with the stethoscope over:
   A. either the right or left lung.
   B. one lung and then the stomach.
   C. both lungs only.
   D. both lungs and the epigastrium.

Challenging Questions

8. You note that once the patient is intubated and ventilated his heart rate becomes stronger. Why did this happen?

9. After ventilating for several minutes, the patient starts becoming combative. What happened?

10. How should you handle the patient that is reaching for the ETT and moving around on the cot?

Points to Ponder

You respond to a possible rape victim who was found between two downtown buildings. You are very nearby and are first on scene. Paramedics have also been dispatched but the closest ones were out so they are about 10 minutes behind you. You find that the patient's throat has been cut and she is bleeding moderately, but experiencing difficulty breathing and speaking. There is a trauma center about 7 minutes away. Your partner wants to wait for the paramedics who can perform advanced airway management, but you want to load and go. Local protocols are not specific but would lean toward waiting for ACLS. Her airway seems to be worsening. What would you do? How would you make the decision to transport or wait?

Issues Decision Making, Disagreements Between Partners, Dealing With Times When Protocols Are Not Clear.

www.emtb.com

BLS Review

Cognitive

1. Identify the need for basic life support, including the urgency surrounding its rapid application (p 894).
2. List the EMT-B's responsibilities in beginning and terminating CPR (p 897).
3. Describe the proper way to position an adult patient to receive basic life support (p 898).
4. Describe the proper way to position an infant and child to receive basic life support (p 904).
5. Describe the three techniques for opening the airway in infants, children, and adults (p 898).
6. List the steps in providing artificial ventilation in infants, children, and adults (p 902).
7. Describe how gastric distention occurs (p 902).
8. Define the recovery position (p 903).
9. Describe infectious disease issues related to rescue breathing (p 917).
10. List the steps in providing chest compressions in an adult (p 906).
11. List the steps in providing chest compressions in an infant and child (p 911).
12. List the steps in providing one-rescuer CPR in an infant, child, and adult (p 907).
13. List the steps in providing two-rescuer CPR in an infant, child, and adult (p 907).
14. Distinguish foreign body airway obstruction from other conditions that cause respiratory failure (p 912).
15. Distinguish a complete airway obstruction from a partial airway obstruction (p 915).
16. Describe the steps in removing a foreign body obstruction in an infant, child, and adult (p 913).

Affective

17. Recognize and respect the feelings of the patient and family during basic life support (p 897).
18. Explain the urgency surrounding the rapid initiation of basic life support measures (p 895).
19. Explain the EMT-B's responsibilities in starting and terminating CPR (p 897).
20. Explain the rationale for removing a foreign body obstruction (p 912).

Psychomotor

21. Demonstrate how to position the patient to open the airway (p 898).
22. Demonstrate how to perform the head tilt-chin lift maneuver in infants, children, and adults (p 900).
23. Demonstrate how to perform the jaw-thrust and modified jaw-thrust maneuvers in infants, children, and adults (p 901).
24. Demonstrate how to place a patient in the recovery position (p 903).
25. Demonstrate how to perform chest compressions in an adult (p 906).
26. Demonstrate how to perform chest compressions in an infant and child (p 911).
27. Demonstrate how to perform one-rescuer CPR in an infant, child, and adult (p 907).
28. Demonstrate how to perform two-rescuer CPR in an infant, child, and adult (p 907).
29. Demonstrate how to remove a foreign body obstruction in an infant, child, and adult (p 913).

* All of the objectives in this chapter are noncurriculum objectives.

www.emtb.com

TECHNOLOGY

Online Chapter Pretest
Interactivities
Vocabulary Explorer
Anatomy Review
Web Links
Online Review Manual
Distance Learning

Chapter

"Unit 9, respond to City Hall for CPR in progress in the Licensing department."
This is reported as a witnessed cardiac arrest.

In spite of years of prevention efforts, sudden cardiac death strikes down countless Americans. When you are called to scenes such as the one above, you are faced with the ultimate challenge: to revive the patient and return him or her to a normal, functional life.

This chapter will review the key concepts and the principles of basic life support and will also help you answer the following questions:

1. What are the links in the chain of survival and which, if any is the most important?

2. What are the EMT-B's responsibilities in starting and terminating CPR?

BLS Review

The principles of basic life support were first introduced in 1960. Since this time, the specific techniques have been reviewed and revised every 5 to 6 years. The updated guidelines are published in the *Journal of the American Medical Association*. The most recent revision occurred as a result of the 2000 Conference on Cardiopulmonary Resuscitation and Emergency Cardiac Care. The guidelines in this appendix follow those proposed at the 2000 conference. Note that the 1994 EMT-Basic National Standard Curriculum requires basic life support (BLS) as a prerequisite to the EMT-Basic course; it is presented here as a review.

This chapter begins with a definition and general discussion of BLS. The next sections describe methods for opening and maintaining an airway, providing artificial ventilation to a person who is not breathing, providing artificial circulation to a person with no pulse, and removing a foreign body airway obstruction. Each of these sections is followed by a review of the changes in technique that are necessary to treat infants and children. The chapter concludes with a discussion of the methods of preventing the transmission of infectious diseases during cardiopulmonary resuscitation (CPR).

Elements of Basic Life Support

<u>Basic life support</u> is noninvasive emergency lifesaving care that is used to treat airway obstruction, respiratory arrest, or cardiac arrest. This care focuses on what is often termed the ABCs: airway (obstruction), breathing (respiratory arrest), and circulation (cardiac arrest or severe bleeding) ▼ **Figure 39-1**. BLS follows a specific sequence for adults and for infants and children

Airway   Breathing   Circulation

Figure 39-1 The ABCs of basic life support are airway, breathing, and circulation.

▼**Table 39-1** . Ideally, only seconds should pass between the time you recognize that a patient needs BLS and the start of treatment. Remember, brain cells die every second that oxygen does not reach the brain. Permanent brain damage may occur if the brain is without oxygen for 4 to 6 minutes. After 6 minutes without oxygen, some brain damage is almost certain ▶**Figure 39-2** .

If a patient is not breathing well or at all, you may simply need to open the airway. Very often, this will help the patient to breathe normally again. However, if the patient has no pulse, you must combine artificial ventilation with artificial circulation. If breathing stops before the heart stops, the patient will have enough oxygen in the lungs to stay alive for several minutes. But when a patient goes into cardiac arrest first, the heart and brain stop receiving oxygen right away.

<u>Cardiopulmonary resuscitation (CPR)</u> is used to establish artificial ventilation and circulation in a patient who is not breathing and has no pulse. The steps for CPR include:

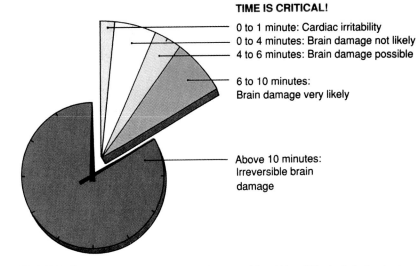

TIME IS CRITICAL!

0 to 1 minute: Cardiac irritability
0 to 4 minutes: Brain damage not likely
4 to 6 minutes: Brain damage possible
6 to 10 minutes:
Brain damage very likely

Above 10 minutes:
Irreversible brain
damage

Figure 39-2 Time is critical for patients who are not breathing. If the brain is deprived of oxygen for 4 to 6 minutes, brain damage is likely to occur.

1. Opening the airway

2. Restoring breathing by means of rescue breathing (mouth-to-mouth ventilation, mouth-to-nose ventilation, or through the use of mechanical devices)

3. Restoring circulation by means of chest compressions to circulate blood through the body

TABLE 39-1 Review of Pediatric BLS Procedures

Procedure	Infants (younger than age 1 year)	Children (age 1 to 8 years)
Airway	Head tilt-chin lift; jaw thrust if spinal injury is suspected	Head tilt-chin lift; jaw thrust if spinal injury is suspected
Breathing Initial breaths	2 breaths with duration of 1 to 1½ seconds each	2 breaths with duration of 1 to 1½ seconds each
Subsequent breaths	1 breath every 3 seconds; 20 breaths/min	1 breath every 3 seconds; 20 breaths/min
Circulation Pulse check	Brachial/femoral arteries	Carotid artery
Compression area	Lower half of sternum	Lower half of sternum
Compression width	2 or 3 fingers	Heel of hand
Compression depth	½" to 1"	1" to 1½"
Compression rate	At least 100/min	100/min
Ratio of Compressions to Ventilations	5:1 (pause for ventilation)	5:1 (pause for ventilation)
Foreign Body Obstruction	Back blows and chest thrusts	Abdominal thrusts

For CPR to be effective, you must be able to easily identify a patient who is in respiratory and/or cardiac arrest and begin treatment with BLS measures immediately (▼ Figure 39-3).

BLS can be given by one or two EMT-Bs, by first responders, or by alert bystanders. It does not require any equipment; however, you should use a barrier device to perform rescue breathing. Rescue breathing delivers exhaled gas from you to the patient. This gas contains 16% oxygen, which is more than enough to maintain the patient's life. Once you determine that the patient needs BLS, you should begin rescue breathing immediately, along with efforts to support the circulation and correct cardiac problems.

BLS differs from **advanced life support (ALS)**, which involves advanced lifesaving procedures, such as cardiac monitoring, administration of IV fluids and medications, and use of advanced airway adjuncts. However, when done correctly, BLS can maintain life for a short time until ALS measures can be started. In some instances, such as choking, near drowning, or lightning injuries, early BLS measures may be all that a patient needs to be resuscitated. Of course, these patients also require transport to the hospital for evaluation.

BLS measures are only as effective as the person who is performing them. Your skills will be very good immediately after training. However, as time goes on, your skills will deteriorate unless you practice them regularly.

Assessing the Need for BLS

Because of the urgent need to start CPR in a pulseless, nonbreathing patient, you must complete an initial assessment as soon as possible, evaluating the patient's ABCs. The first step is determining unresponsiveness (▼ Figure 39-4). A patient who is alert and oriented does not need CPR; a person who is unresponsive may need CPR, based on further assessment.

You may also suspect the presence of a cervical spine injury. If so, you must protect the spinal cord from further injury as you perform CPR. If there is even a remote possibility of this type of injury, you should begin taking appropriate precautions during the initial assessment.

The basic principles of BLS are the same for infants, children, and adults. For the purposes of BLS, anyone younger than 1 year is considered an infant. A child is between ages 1 and 8 years. For children older than 8 years, you can usually use the same techniques that you

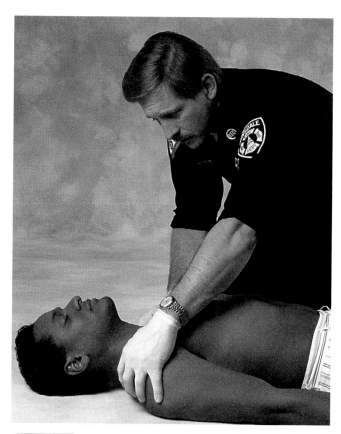

Figure 39-3 You must quickly identify patients in distress so that BLS measures can begin immediately.

Figure 39-4 Assess airway, breathing, and circulation in an unconscious patient by first attempting to rouse the patient.

The most important element for successful CPR is immediate opening of the airway.

Documentation Tips

Correct handling of situations when you choose not to start CPR on a patient in cardiac arrest begins with compliance with protocols and ends with detailed documentation. In particular, record physical exam signs that led to your choice, and make reference to the protocol that states these signs as a reason not to start. If extenuating circumstances such as entrapment physically prevent resuscitation attempts, record the conditions thoroughly. These decisions occasionally give rise to questions that can often be put to rest immediately by reference to a well-written chart.

use for adults. However, these are guidelines, not rules. Children vary in size. Some small children may best be treated as infants, some larger children as adults. There are two basic differences in providing CPR for infants, children, and adults. The first is that the emergencies in which infants and children require CPR have different underlying causes. The second is that there are anatomic differences between adults, children, and infants. These differences include smaller airways in infants and children than those of adults.

Although cardiac arrest in adults usually occurs before respiratory arrest, the reverse is true in infants and children. In most cases, cardiac arrest in children younger than 9 years results from respiratory arrest. If untreated, respiratory arrest will quickly lead to cardiac arrest and death. Respiratory arrest in infants and children has a variety of causes, including aspiration of foreign bodies into the airway, such as parts of hot dogs, peanuts, candy, or small toys; airway infections, such as croup and epiglottitis; near-drowning incidents or electrocution; and sudden infant death syndrome (SIDS).

When to Start and Stop BLS

As an EMT-B, it is your responsibility to start CPR in virtually all patients who are in cardiac arrest. There are only two general exceptions to the rule.

First, you should not start CPR if the patient has obvious signs of irreversible or biological death. These are called "dead on arrival" (DOA) criteria. Signs of irreversible or biological death include clinical death, absence of a pulse, and absence of breathing, along with any one of the following:

- Rigor mortis, or stiffening of the body after death
- Dependent lividity (livor mortis), a discoloration of the skin due to pooling of blood ▼ Figure 39-5
- Putrefaction or decomposition of the body
- Evidence of nonsurvivable injury, such as decapitation.

Rigor mortis and dependent lividity develop after a patient has been dead for a long period of time.

Second, you should not start CPR if the patient and his or her physician have previously agreed upon DNR (do not resuscitate) or no-CPR orders ▼ Figure 39-6. This may apply only to situations in which the patient is

Figure 39-5 Dependent lividity is an obvious sign of death, caused by blood settling to the lower parts of the body. The lividity in this figure is seen as purple discoloration of the back, except in areas that are in firm contact with the ground (scapula and buttock).

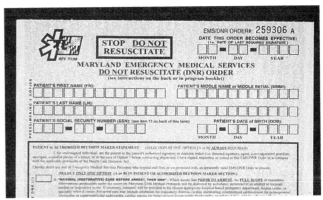

Figure 39-6 You should not start CPR if the patient and his or her physician have previously agreed upon DNR or no-CPR orders. Learn your local protocols for treating terminally ill patients.

known to be in the terminal stage of an incurable disease. In this situation, CPR serves only to prolong the patient's dying. However, this can be a complicated issue. Advance directives, such as living wills, may express the patient's wishes, but these documents are not binding for all health care providers, especially outside of a hospital or nursing home. The safest course is to assume that an emergency exists and begin CPR under the rule of implied consent. Learn your local protocols and the standards in your system for treating terminally ill patients. Some EMS systems have computer notes on patients who are preregistered with the system. These notes usually specify the amount and extent of treatment that are desired.

In all other instances, you should begin CPR on anyone who is in cardiac arrest. It is usually impossible to know how long the patient has been without oxygen to the brain and vital organs. Factors such as air temperature and the basic health of the patient's tissues and organs can affect the ability to survive. Therefore, most legal advisers recommend that, when in doubt, you should always give too much care rather than too little. You should always start CPR if any doubt exists.

You are not responsible for making the decision to stop CPR. Once you begin CPR in the field, you must continue until one of the following events occurs:

- **S** The patient **starts** breathing and has a pulse.
- **T** The patient is **transferred** to another person who is trained in BLS, ALS-trained personnel, or another emergency medical responder.
- **O** You are **out** of strength or too tired to continue.
- **P** A **physician** who is present assumes responsibility for the patient.

"Out of strength" does not mean merely weary; rather, it means no longer physically able to perform CPR. In short, CPR should always be continued until the patient's care is transferred to a physician or higher medical authority in the field. In some cases, your medical director or a designated medical control physician may order you to stop CPR on the basis of the patient's condition.

Every EMS system should have clear standing orders or protocols that provide guidelines for starting and stopping CPR. Your medical director and your system's legal adviser should agree on these protocols, which should be closely administered and reviewed by your medical director.

Pediatric Needs

Opening the airway in an infant or child is done by using the same techniques as are used for an adult. However, because a child's neck is so flexible, the head tilt-chin lift maneuver should be modified so that as you tilt the head back, you are moving it only into the neutral position or a slightly extended position (▼ **Figure 39-7**). You may also use the jaw-thrust maneuver without a head tilt. In fact, this is the best method to use if you suspect a spinal injury in a child. If a second rescuer is present, he or she should immobilize the child's cervical spine.

Figure 39-7 The head tilt-chin lift maneuver on a child is slightly modified in that as you tilt the head back, you move it only into the neutral position or a slightly extended position.

Positioning the Patient

The next step in providing CPR is to position the patient to ensure that the airway is open. For CPR to be effective, the patient must be lying supine on a firm surface, with enough clear space around the patient for two rescuers to perform CPR. If the patient is crumpled up or lying face down, you will need to reposition him or her. The few seconds that you spend to position the patient properly will greatly improve the delivery and effectiveness of CPR.

Follow the steps in (▶ **Skill Drill 39-1**) to reposition an unconscious adult patient for airway management:

1. **Kneel beside the patient.** You and your partner must be far enough away so that the patient, when rolled toward you, does not come to rest in your lap **(Step 1)**.

2. First EMT-B: **Place your hands** behind the patient's back, head, and neck to protect the cervical spine if you suspect spinal injury. Second EMT-B: Place your hands on the distant shoulder and the hip **(Step 2)**.

Skill Drill 39-1   Positioning the Patient

Kneel beside the patient, leaving room to roll the patient toward you.

Grasp the patient, stabilizing the cervical spine if needed.

Move the head and neck as a unit with the torso as your partner pulls on the distant shoulder and hip.

Move the patient to a supine position with legs straight and arms at the sides.

3. Second EMT-B: **Turn the patient toward you** by pulling on the distant shoulder and the hip. First EMT-B: Control the head and neck so that they move as a unit with the rest of the torso. This single motion will allow the head, neck, and back to stay in the same vertical plane and will minimize aggravation of any spinal injury **(Step 3)**.

4. First EMT-B: **Place the patient in a supine position,** with the legs straight and both arms at the sides **(Step 4)**.

If possible, log roll the patient onto a long backboard as you are positioning him or her for CPR.

This device will provide support during transport and emergency department care. Once the patient is properly positioned, you can easily assess airway, breathing, circulation, and disability and start CPR if necessary.

Opening the Airway in Adults

Without an open airway, rescue breathing will not be effective. There are three techniques for opening the airway in adults: the head tilt-chin lift maneuver, the jaw-thrust maneuver with head tilt, and the jaw-thrust maneuver without head tilt.

Head Tilt-Chin Lift Maneuver

Opening the airway to relieve an obstruction caused by relaxation of the tongue can often be accomplished quickly and easily with the <u>head tilt-chin lift maneuver</u> (▼ **Figure 39-8**). In patients who have not sustained trauma, this simple maneuver is sometimes all that is required for the patient to resume breathing. If the patient has any foreign material or vomitus in the mouth, you should quickly remove it. Wipe out any liquid materials from the mouth with a piece of cloth held by your index and middle fingers; use your hooked index finger to remove any solid material. You should perform the head tilt-chin lift maneuver in an adult in the following way (▼ **Figure 39-9**):

1. **Make sure the patient is supine.** Kneel close beside the patient.

2. **Place one hand on the patient's forehead,** and apply firm backward pressure with your palm to tilt the patient's head back. This extension of the neck will move the tongue forward, away from the back of the throat, and will clear the airway if the tongue is blocking it.

3. **Place the tips of the fingers** of your other hand under the lower jaw near the bony part of the chin. Do not compress the soft tissue under the chin, as this would block the airway.

4. **Lift the chin forward,** bringing the entire lower jaw with it, helping to tilt the head back. Do not use your thumb to lift the chin. Lift so that the teeth are nearly brought together, but avoid closing the mouth completely.

The chin lift has the added advantage of holding loose dentures in place, making obstruction by the lips less likely. Performing ventilation is much easier when dentures are in place. However, dentures that do not stay in place should be removed. Partial dentures (plates) may come loose as a result of an accident or as you are providing care, so check these periodically.

A

Tongue blocking air passage

Air passage

B

Air passage opened

Tongue forward

Figure 39-8 **A.** Relaxation of the tongue back into the throat causes airway obstruction. **B.** The head tilt-chin lift maneuver combines two movements to open the airway.

Figure 39-9 To perform the head tilt-chin lift maneuver, place one hand on the patient's forehead, and apply firm backward pressure with your palm to tilt the head back. Next, place the tips of the fingers of your other hand under the lower jaw near the bony part of the chin. Lift the chin forward, bringing the entire lower jaw with it, helping to tilt the head back.

Jaw-Thrust Maneuver
With and Without Head Tilt

The head tilt-chin lift maneuver is effective for opening the airway in most patients. The <u>jaw-thrust maneuver</u> is another technique for opening the airway. It can be performed with or without a head tilt. To perform a jaw-thrust maneuver, place your fingers behind the angles of the patient's lower jaw and then move the jaw forward. When no spinal injury is suspected, you may tilt the head back to open the airway further without significantly extending the cervical spine. If the patient's mouth remains closed, you can use your thumbs to pull the patient's lower lip down, to allow breathing. You can also easily apply a face mask with both hands while performing the jaw thrust with or without a head tilt.

You should perform the jaw-thrust maneuver, with a head tilt, in the following way ▶ **Figure 39-10** :

1. **Kneel above the patient's head.** Place your index or middle finger behind the angle of the patient's lower jaw on both sides, and forcefully move the jaw forward. Tilt the head backward if you do not suspect spinal injury.

2. **Use your thumbs to open the mouth** to allow breathing.

3. **The nose can be sealed with your cheek** when providing rescue breathing using the jaw-thrust maneuver.

In cases of suspected spinal injury, you want to minimize movement of the patient's neck. In this case, perform a jaw-thrust maneuver without a head tilt. Keep the head in a neutral position as you move the jaw forward and open the mouth ▶ **Figure 39-11** .

Rescue Breathing in Adults

Once you open the airway, check for breathing by placing your ear about 1″ above the patient's nose and mouth; listen carefully for sounds of breathing. Turn your head so that you can watch for movement of the patient's chest and abdomen ▶ **Figure 39-12** . This is called the look, listen, and feel technique. You know that the patient is breathing if you see the chest and abdomen rise and fall, and, more important, if you feel and hear air move during exhalation. With airway obstruction, there may be no movement of air, even though the chest and abdomen rise and fall as the patient tries to breathe. You may also have difficulty seeing movement of the chest and abdomen if the patient is fully clothed. Finally, you may see very little

Figure 39-10 To perform the jaw-thrust maneuver with a head tilt, place your index or middle finger behind the angle of the lower jaw on both sides. Move the jaw forward, and tilt the head back.

Figure 39-11 To perform the jaw-thrust maneuver without a head tilt, maintain the head in neutral alignment and use your index and long fingers to thrust the jaw forward.

Figure 39-12 Look, listen, and feel for signs of breathing.

or no chest movement at all in some patients, particularly those with chronic lung disease. Therefore, if you do not feel any air movement as you look, listen, and feel, you must begin artificial ventilation. This evaluation should take no more than 5 seconds.

A lack of oxygen, combined with too much carbon dioxide in the blood, is lethal. To correct this condition, you must provide slow, deliberate inhalations that last 2 seconds. This gentle, slow method of ventilating the patient prevents air being forced into the stomach.

Ventilation

Ventilations are now done routinely with barrier devices, such as masks. These devices feature a plastic barrier that covers the patient's mouth and nose and a one-way valve to prevent backflow of secretions and gases ▶ Figure 39-13). Such devices provide good infection control as well. Providing ventilations without a barrier device is appropriate only in extreme conditions.

You should perform rescue breathing with a simple barrier device in an adult in the following way ▶ Figure 39-14):

1. **Open the airway** with the head tilt-chin lift maneuver (nontrauma patient).

2. **Press on the forehead** to maintain the backward tilt of the head. Pinch the patient's nostrils together with your thumb and index finger.

3. **Depress the lower lip** with the thumb of the hand that is lifting the chin. This will help to keep the patient's mouth open.

4. **Open the patient's mouth widely,** and place the barrier device over the patient's mouth and nose.

5. **Take a deep breath,** then make a tight seal with your mouth around the barrier device. Give two slow rescue breaths, each lasting 2 seconds, followed by 10 to 12 breaths/min.

6. Remove your mouth, and allow the patient to exhale passively. Turn your head slightly to watch for movement of the patient's chest.

If you use the jaw-thrust maneuver to open the airway, you must move to the patient's side to provide ventilations. Keep the patient's mouth open with both thumbs, and seal the nose by placing your cheek against the patient's nostrils ▶ Figure 39-15). Note that this maneuver is very difficult; practice with a manikin will help you gain familiarity with this technique.

Figure 39-13 A barrier device is used in performing ventilation, as it prevents backflow of saliva, blood, and vomitus.

Figure 39-14 To perform ventilations, ensure that you make a tight seal with your mouth around the barrier device, and then give two slow gentle breaths, each lasting 2 seconds.

Stoma Ventilations

Patients who have undergone surgical removal of the larynx often have a permanent tracheal stoma at the midline in the neck or at the front base of the neck. A stoma is an opening that connects the trachea directly to the skin ▶ Figure 39-16). Because it is at the midline, the stoma is the only opening that will move air into the patient's lungs; you should ignore any other openings. Patients with a stoma should be ventilated with a BVM device, as described in Chapter 7.

Gastric Distention

Artificial ventilation often results in the stomach becoming filled with air, a condition called gastric distention. Although it most commonly happens in children, it also happens in adults. Gastric distention is most likely to occur if you blow too hard as you ventilate, if you give breaths too rapidly, or if the patient's

Figure 39-15 **A.** If you use the jaw-thrust maneuver to open the airway, keep the patient's mouth open with both thumbs as you move from above the patient's head to the side. **B.** Seal the nose by placing your cheek against the patient's nostrils.

Figure 39-16 **A.** A stoma is an opening that connects the trachea directly to the skin. **B.** Use a BVM device to ventilate a patient with a stoma.

airway is obstructed. Therefore, it is important for you to give slow, gentle breaths. Such breaths are also more effective in ventilating the lungs. Serious inflation of the stomach is dangerous, as it can cause the patient to vomit during CPR. It can also reduce lung volume by elevating the diaphragm.

If massive gastric distention interferes with adequate ventilation, you should contact medical control. Check the airway again and reposition the patient, watch for rise and fall of the chest, and avoid giving forceful breaths. You should continue to provide slow rescue breaths without trying to expel the stomach contents. Any attempt to do so with manual pressure over the upper part of the abdomen is likely to result in vomiting.

Recovery Position

The <u>recovery position</u> helps to maintain a clear airway in a patient with a decreased level of consciousness who has not had traumatic injuries and is breathing on his or her own ▶ **Figure 39-17** . It also allows vomitus to

Figure 39-17 The recovery position is used to maintain an open airway in a patient with a decreased level of consciousness who has not had traumatic injuries. It allows vomitus, blood, and any other secretions to drain from the mouth.

drain from the mouth. Roll the patient onto his or her side so that the head, shoulders, and torso move as a unit, without twisting. Then place the patient's hands under his or her cheek. Never place a patient who has a suspected head or spinal injury in the recovery position because maintainence of spinal alignment in this position is difficult and spinal cord injury could result.

Pediatric Needs

Children who are in respiratory distress are usually struggling to breathe. As a result, they usually position themselves in a way that keeps the airway open enough for air to move. Let them stay in that position as long as their partially obstructed airway does not become a complete airway obstruction. If you and your partner arrive at the scene and find that an infant or child is not breathing or has cyanosis, one of you should provide care while the other calls for additional help.

For infants, the preferred technique of rescue breathing is mouth-to-nose-and-mouth ventilation. With this technique, a seal must be made over the mouth and the nose. Various masks or other barrier devices are recommended for this technique. If the patient is a large child (age 1 to 8 years) for whom a tight seal cannot be made over both mouth and nose, you should provide mouth-to-mouth ventilation as you would for an adult.

Once you have made an airtight seal over the mouth, give two gentle breaths lasting 1 to 1½ seconds. These initial breaths will help you to assess for airway obstruction as well as expand the lungs. Because the lungs of infants and children are much smaller than those of adults, you do not need to blow in a great amount of air. Limit the amount of air to that needed to cause the chest to rise.

Remember, too, that a child's airway is smaller than that of an adult. Therefore, there is greater resistance to airflow. As a result, you will need to use a bit more ventilatory pressure to inflate the lungs. You know you are giving the correct amount of air volume as soon as you see the chest rise. Infants and children should be ventilated once every 3 seconds or 20 times per minute.

If air enters freely with your initial breaths and the chest rises, the airway is clear. You should then check the pulse. If air does not enter freely, you should check the airway for obstruction. Reposition the patient to open the airway, and give another two breaths. If air still does not enter freely, you must then clear the airway.

Adult CPR

Once you have arrived at the scene and determined that the patient is unresponsive and not breathing, you must position the patient and begin rescue breathing. After you begin rescue breathing, you must assess the patient's circulation.

Cardiac arrest is determined by the absence of a palpable pulse in the carotid artery. Feel for the carotid artery by locating the larynx at the front of the neck and then sliding two fingers toward one side. The pulse is

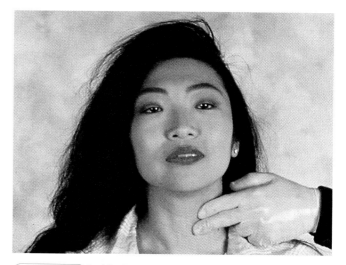

Figure 39-18 Feel for the carotid artery by locating the larynx, then sliding two fingers toward one side. You can feel the pulse in the groove between the larynx and the sternocleidomastoid muscle.

felt in the groove between the larynx and the sternocleidomastoid muscle, with the pulp of the index and long fingers held side by side (▲ **Figure 39-18**). Light pressure is sufficient to palpate the pulse. Excessive pressure must not be applied because it can obstruct the carotid circulation, dislodge blood clots, or produce marked reflex slowing of heart rate.

External Chest Compression

You can provide CPR by applying rhythmic pressure and relaxation to the lower half of the sternum. The heart is located slightly to the left of the middle of the chest between the sternum and the spine (▶ **Figure 39-19**). The blood that circulates through the lungs by chest compressions is likely to receive adequate oxygen to maintain life when accompanied by artificial ventilation. However, keep in mind that, at its best, external chest compression provides only one third of the blood that is normally pumped by the heart, so it is very important to do it properly.

The patient must be placed on a firm, flat surface, in a supine position. The head should not be elevated at a level above the heart, as this will further reduce blood flow to the brain. The surface can be the ground, the floor, or a backboard on a stretcher. You cannot perform chest compressions adequately on a bed; therefore, a patient who is in bed should be moved to the floor or have a board placed under the back. Remember, too, that external chest compressions must always be accompanied by artificial ventilation.

PROPER HAND POSITION. Correct hand position is established by sliding the index and middle fingers of the

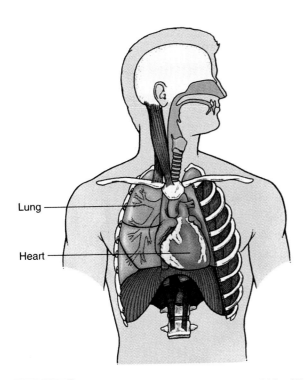

Figure 39-19 The heart lies slightly to the left of the middle of the chest between the sternum and the spine.

hand near the patient's feet along the edge of the rib cage until they reach the xiphoid notch in the center of the chest. Follow the steps in ▶ **Skill Drill 39-2** :

1. **Slide your index and middle fingers** of the hand near the patient's feet along the center of the patient's rib cage to the notch in the center of the chest **(Step 1)**.

2. **Push your middle finger** as high as possible into the notch, and then lay your index finger on the lower portion of the sternum with the two fingers touching **(Step 2)**.

3. **Place the heel of your other hand** on the lower half of the sternum so that it touches the index finger of the first hand **(Step 3)**.

4. **Remove your first hand** from the notch in the center of the rib cage, and place it over the hand that is resting on the patient's lower sternum **(Step 4)**.

5. **With your arms straight**, lock your elbows, and position your shoulders directly over your hands. Depress the sternum $1\frac{1}{2}''$ to $2''$, using a rocking motion and rising gently upward. Only the heel of one hand should be in contact with the lower half of the sternum. Take great care not to place your hand either on the xiphoid process, which

extends down over the upper abdomen and liver, or beside the sternum onto the ribs or costal cartilage. Your technique may be improved or made more comfortable if you interlock the fingers of your lower hand with the fingers of your upper hand; either way, your fingers should be kept off the patient's chest **(Step 5)**.

PROPER COMPRESSION TECHNIQUE. Complications from chest compressions are rare, but can include fractured ribs, a lacerated liver, or a fractured sternum. Although these injuries cannot be entirely avoided, you can minimize the chance that they will occur if you use good, smooth technique and proper hand placement.

Proper compressions begin by locking your elbows, with your arms straight, and positioning your shoulders directly over your hand so that the thrust of each compression is straight down on the sternum. Depress the sternum $1\frac{1}{2}''$ to $2''$ in an adult, using a rocking motion and rising gently upward. This motion allows pressure to be delivered vertically down from your shoulders. Vertical downward pressure produces a compression that must be followed immediately by an equal period of relaxation. The ratio of time devoted to compression versus relaxation should be 1:1.

Skill Drill 39-2 Performing Chest Compressions

1

Slide your index and middle fingers along the rib cage to the notch in the center of the chest.

2

Push the middle finger high into the notch, and lay the index finger on the lower portion of the sternum.

3

Place the heel of the second hand on the lower half of the sternum, touching the index finger of your first hand.

4

Remove your first hand from the notch, and place it over the hand on the sternum.

5

With your arms straight, lock your elbows, and position your shoulders directly over your hands. Depress the sternum 1¹/₂" to 2", using a rhythmic motion.

The actual motions must be smooth, rhythmic, and uninterrupted (▼ **Figure 39-20A**). Short, jabbing compressions are not effective in producing artificial blood flow. Do not remove the heel of your hand from the patient's chest during relaxation, but make sure that you completely release pressure on the sternum so that it can return to its normal resting position between compressions (▼ **Figure 39-20B**).

One-Rescuer Adult CPR

When you are doing CPR alone, you must give both artificial ventilations and chest compressions in a ratio of compressions to ventilations of 15:2. Follow the steps in (▶ **Skill Drill 39-3**):

1. **Perform the initial assessment** to determine the need for CPR (responsiveness), and then call for additional help **(Step 1)**.

2. Position the patient properly to **open the airway (Step 2)**.

3. **Determine breathlessness** by using the look, listen, and feel technique. If the patient is unconscious but breathing, place him or her in the recovery position, and maintain the open airway **(Step 3)**.

4. **If not breathing, begin rescue breathing** by delivering two breaths, for 2 seconds each **(Step 4)**.

5. **Determine pulselessness** by checking the carotid pulse **(Step 5)**.

6. **If pulseless, begin compressions.** Place your hands in the proper position for delivering external chest compressions, as described above.

7. **Give 15 compressions** at a rate of about 100/min for an adult. Each set of 15 compressions should take about 10 seconds. Using a rhythmic motion, apply pressure vertically from your shoulders down through both arms to depress the sternum 1½" to 2" in the adult, then rise up gently. Count the compressions aloud.

8. **Open the airway** and then give two ventilations, each lasting 2 seconds.

9. Locate the proper position, and **begin another cycle** of chest compressions. Perform four cycles of compressions and ventilations.

10. **After four cycles** of compressions and ventilations, stop CPR and check for the return of a carotid pulse. If there is no change, resume CPR. If the patient has a pulse, check for breathing. If the patient is not breathing, provide rescue breathing. If the patient has a pulse, is breathing, but remains unresponsive, place the patient in the recovery position and closely monitor the patient **(Step 6)**.

Two-Rescuer Adult CPR

You and your team should be able to perform both one-rescuer and two-rescuer CPR with ease. Two-rescuer CPR is always the first choice, since it is both less tiring for rescuers and more effective. Once one-rescuer CPR is in progress, a second rescuer can be added very easily. He or she should enter the procedure after a cycle of 15 compressions and two ventilations. You should use airway adjuncts, such as mouth-to-

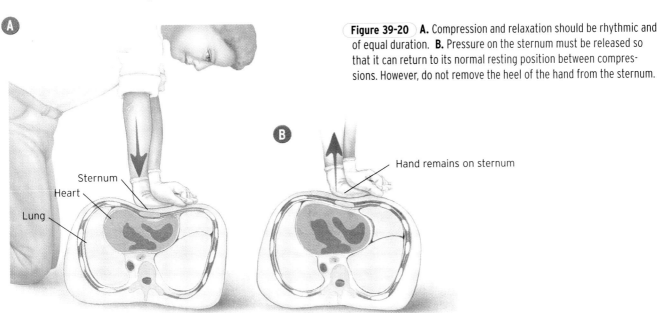

Figure 39-20 **A.** Compression and relaxation should be rhythmic and of equal duration. **B.** Pressure on the sternum must be released so that it can return to its normal resting position between compressions. However, do not remove the heel of the hand from the sternum.

Sternum

Heart

Lung

Hand remains on sternum

SkillDrill 39-3 Performing One-Rescuer Adult CPR

Establish unresponsiveness and call for help.

Open the airway.

Look, listen, and feel for breathing. If breathing, place in the recovery position and monitor.

If not breathing, give two breaths of 2 seconds each.

Check for carotid pulse.

If no pulse is found, place your hands in the proper position for chest compressions.

Give 15 compressions at about 100/min.

Open the airway and give two ventilations of 2 seconds each.

Perform four cycles of compressions.

Stop CPR and check for return of the carotid pulse. Depending on patient condition, continue CPR, continue rescue breathing only, or place in the recovery position and monitor.

mask ventilations, whenever possible. Follow the steps in ▶ **Skill Drill 39-4** :

1. Moving to the head, **establish the need for CPR** by determining responsiveness as your partner moves to the patient's side to be ready to deliver chest compressions **(Step 1)**.

2. Position the patient to **open the airway (Step 2)**.

3. **Check for breathing** by using the look, listen, and feel technique. If the patient is unconscious but breathing, place him or her in the recovery position, and maintain the open airway **(Step 3)**.

4. **If the patient is not breathing, begin rescue breathing** by delivering two breaths, for 2 seconds each **(Step 4)**.

5. **Determine pulselessness** by checking the carotid pulse **(Step 5)**.

6. **Begin chest compressions,** as described above, at a compression to ventilation ratio of 15:2. Once the airway is secured (intubated) the ratio of chest compressions to breaths can change to 5:1. As in one-rescuer CPR, compressions should be given at a rate of about 100/min.

7. **After 1 minute of CPR,** the rescuer at the head checks the patient's pulse to determine whether the carotid pulse has returned. Because chest compressions produce a pulse, you must check for the pulse after a ventilation. Continue to check for a pulse every few minutes.

8. **If there is no change, resume CPR.** If the patient has a pulse, check for breathing. If the patient is not breathing, provide rescue breathing. If the patient has a pulse, is breathing, but remains unresponsive, place the patient in the recovery position and closely monitor the patient **(Step 6)**.

Switching Positions

The best time to switch positions is during the pulse checks. However, you can switch positions any time one of you needs to change by following the same sequence of steps: The EMT-B who has been performing chest compressions checks for a carotid pulse following the final ventilation by the other EMT-B, who then moves to the chest and establishes his or her hand position on the sternum. Compressions start with the command, "No pulse. Continue CPR." You and your partner should be on opposite sides of the patient so

Pediatric Needs

In most instances, cardiac arrest in infants and children follows respiratory arrest, triggered by hypoxia and ischemia of the heart. Children consume oxygen two to three times as rapidly as adults. Therefore, you must first focus on opening the airway and providing artificial ventilation. Often, this will be enough to get the patient breathing again.

that you can easily switch positions when necessary, as follows:

1. **First EMT-B:** Move into position to begin chest compressions after giving a breath.

2. **Second EMT-B:** Give the 15th compression, then move to the patient's head.

3. **Second EMT-B:** Check the carotid pulse for 5 to 10 seconds. If the patient has no pulse, say "No pulse. Continue CPR."

Once the airway is open and you have delivered two breaths, you need to assess circulation. As with an adult, you should first check for a palpable pulse in a large central artery. Absence of a palpable pulse in a major artery means that you must begin external chest compressions. You can usually palpate the carotid pulse in children older than 1 year, but it is difficult in infants, who have short and often fat necks. Therefore, in infants, palpate the brachial artery, which is located on the inner side of the arm, midway between the elbow and shoulder. Place your thumb on the outer surface of the arm between the elbow and shoulder. Then place the tips of your index and long fingers on the medial side of the biceps, and press lightly toward the bone ▼ **Figure 39-21** .

Figure 39-21 To assess circulation in an infant, palpate the brachial artery on the inner side of the arm, midway between the elbow and shoulder.

Skill Drill 39-4   Performing Two-Rescuer Adult CPR

Establish unresponsiveness and take positions.

Open the airway.

Look, listen, and feel for breathing. If breathing, place in the recovery position and monitor.

If not breathing, give two breaths of 2 seconds each.

Check for carotid pulse.

If no pulse, begin chest compressions at about 100/min (15 compressions to two ventilations).

After 1 minute, check for a carotid pulse. Check every few minutes thereafter.

Depending on patient condition, continue CPR, continue rescue breathing only, or place in the recovery position and monitor.

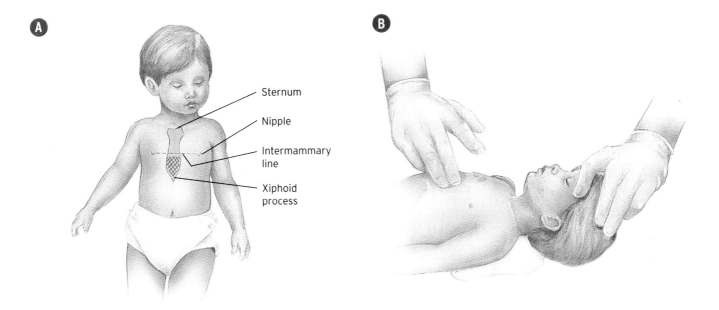

Figure 39-22 **A.** The proper location for chest compressions in an infant is in the midline, one fingerwidth below an imaginary line drawn between the nipples at the sternum. **B.** With your middle and ring fingers, compress the sternum ¹/₂" to 1" at a rate of 100/min.

EXTERNAL CHEST COMPRESSION. Most BLS techniques are the same for infants, small children, larger children, and adults. As with an adult, an infant or child must be lying on a hard surface for the best results. For an infant, the hard surface can be your hand or forearm, with your palm supporting the infant's back. In this way, the infant's shoulders are elevated, and the head is slightly tilted back in a position that will keep the airway open. However, you must ensure that the infant's head is not higher than the rest of the body. The technique for chest compressions in infants and children differs because of a number of anatomic differences, including the position of the heart, the size of the chest, and the fragile organs of a child. The liver is relatively large, immediately under the right side of the diaphragm, and very fragile, especially in infants. The spleen, on the left, is much smaller and much more fragile in children than in adults. These organs are easily injured if you are not careful in performing chest compressions, so be sure that your hand position is correct before you begin.

PROPER HAND POSITION. As the chest grows, the proportion of space occupied by the heart decreases, but the heart in the infant or child is located at about the same level as that in adults. Imagine a line drawn between the nipples, over the sternum ▲ **Figure 39-22A**. The proper area for compression is one finger width below this line on the sternum. If you place your index finger just below this line, your adjacent middle and ring fingers will be at the proper point for compression ▲ **Figure 39-22B**. Finger position is important, as you must take care to avoid compressing the xiphoid process.

PROPER COMPRESSION TECHNIQUE. The chest of an infant or child is both smaller and more pliable than that of an adult. Therefore, you should not use both hands to compress the chest. In an infant, two or three fingers are enough. With your fingers on the lower sternum, compress the sternum ¹/₂" to 1" at a rate of at least 100/min. After each compression, release pressure from the sternum without removing your fingers from the patient's chest. Use smooth, rhythmic motions to deliver compressions, as with adult CPR.

For a child older than 1 year, the way in which you deliver chest compressions differs somewhat. You might need to use more force with a child than with an infant, compressing the sternum 1" to 1¹/₂" at a rate of about 100/min with the heel of one hand. Your other hand should be used to maintain the child's head position so that you can provide rescue breathing without repositioning the head ▶ **Figure 39-23**. Compressions should be delivered in a smooth, rhythmic manner in which the chest returns to its resting position after each compression, leaving your hand on the patient's chest. Note that large children or those older than 8 years should be given chest compressions as an adult.

As with an adult, external chest compressions on a child or infant must be coordinated with ventilations.

Figure 39-23 When performing chest compressions on a child, use the heel of one hand to compress the sternum 1" to 1½" at a rate of about 100/min. The other hand should remain on the child's head to maintain the open airway.

The rate of compression to ventilation for infants and children is 5:1 for both one-rescuer and two-rescuer CPR. This means that you should open the airway and ventilate the patient once after each set of five compressions. One ventilation should take 1 to 1½ seconds.

Make sure that the hand closest to the head remains on the infant's forehead during chest compressions. Your other hand may remain on the chest as you give rescue breathing. If the chest does not rise, remove the hand that is on the patient's chest, and reposition the airway using the head tilt-chin lift maneuver. Then return the compression hand to the chest. In this instance, you do not need to physically relocate the exact position on the sternum. You can find the correct position visually to save time.

Interrupting CPR

CPR is an important holding action that provides minimal circulation and ventilation until the patient can receive definitive care in the form of defibrillation or further care at the hospital. No matter how well it is performed, however, CPR is rarely enough to save a patient's life. If ALS is not available at the scene, you must provide immediate transport, continuing two-rescuer CPR on the way.

Try not to interrupt CPR for more than a few seconds, except when it is absolutely necessary. For example, if you have to move a patient up or down stairs, you should continue CPR until you arrive at the head or foot of the stairs, interrupt CPR at an agreed-

upon signal, and move quickly to the next level where you can resume CPR. Do not move the patient until all transport arrangements are made so that your interruptions of CPR can be kept to a minimum.

Foreign Body Airway Obstruction in Adults

Airway obstruction may be caused by many things, including relaxation of the throat muscles in an unconscious patient, vomited or regurgitated stomach contents, a blood clot, bone fragments or damaged tissue after an injury, dentures, or foreign bodies in the airway.

Loose dentures, large pieces of vomited food, mucus, or blood clots in the mouth should be swept forward and out with your gloved index finger. Use suctioning to maintain a clear airway. Occasionally, a large foreign body will be aspirated and block the upper airway.

Recognizing Foreign Body Obstruction

Sudden airway obstruction by a foreign body in an adult usually occurs during a meal. In a child, it usually occurs during mealtime or at play. Children commonly choke on peanuts, large bits of hot dog, or small toys. If the foreign body is not removed quickly, the lungs will use up their oxygen supply; unconsciousness and death will follow. Your treatment will be based on the cause of the obstruction. Therefore, you must learn to tell the difference between obstructions caused by a foreign body and those due to respiratory failure or arrest, such as fainting, stroke, or heart problems.

CONSCIOUS PATIENTS. Sudden airway obstruction is usually easy to recognize in someone who is eating or has just finished eating. The person is suddenly unable to speak or cough, grasps his or her throat, turns cyanotic, and makes exaggerated efforts to breathe. Either air is not moving into and out of the airway or the air movement is so slight that it is not detectable. At first, the patient will be conscious and able to clearly indicate the nature of the problem. Ask the patient, "Are you choking?" The patient will usually answer by nodding yes. Alternatively, he or she may use the universal sign to indicate airway blockage **▶ Figure 39-24**.

UNCONSCIOUS PATIENTS. When you discover an unconscious patient, your first step is to determine whether he or she is breathing and has a pulse. The unconsciousness may be due to airway obstruction, cardiac arrest, or a number of other problems. Only after ruling out cardiac arrest can you concentrate on possible airway obstructions.

Figure 39-24 Hands at the throat are the universal sign to indicate choking.

You should suspect an airway obstruction if the standard maneuvers to open the airway and ventilate the lungs are not effective. If you feel resistance to blowing into the patient's lungs or pressure builds up in your mouth, the patient probably has some type of obstruction.

Removing a Foreign Body Obstruction

Two manual maneuvers are recommended for removing a foreign body airway obstruction: the abdominal-thrust maneuver (the Heimlich maneuver) and finger sweeps and manual removal of the object.

ABDOMINAL-THRUST MANEUVER. The <u>abdominal-thrust maneuver</u>, also called the Heimlich maneuver, is the preferred way to dislodge and force food or other material from the throat of a choking victim. Residual air, which is always present in the lungs, is compressed upward and used to expel the object. You should give abdominal thrusts in sets of five until the foreign body is dislodged.

With the patient sitting or standing, follow these steps (▲ **Figure 39-25**):

1. **Stand behind the patient,** and wrap your arms around his or her waist.

2. **Make a fist with one hand;** grasp the fist with the other hand. Place the thumb side of the fist against the patient's abdomen, just above the umbilicus and well below the xiphoid.

3. **Press your fist into the patient's abdomen** with a quick inward and upward thrust.

Figure 39-25 The abdominal-thrust maneuver. Stand behind the patient, and wrap your arms around his or her waist. Press your fists into the patient's abdomen in a series of five quick inward and upward thrusts.

4. **Repeat the thrusts in sets of five** until the object is expelled from the airway or the patient becomes unconscious.

For the patient who is crumpled up or lying flat, modify the technique as follows (▶ **Figure 39-26**):

1. **Place the patient in a supine position.**

2. **Straddle the patient's hips or legs.**

3. **Place the heel of one hand against the patient's abdomen** above the umbilicus and well below the xiphoid process. Then place your other hand on top of the first.

4. **Press the hand into the patient's abdomen** with quick inward and upward thrusts, and repeat five times.

CHEST THRUSTS. You can perform the abdominal-thrust maneuver safely on all adults and children. However, you should use chest thrusts for women in advanced stages of pregnancy, patients who are very obese, and children younger than 1 year.

Figure 39-26 The abdominal-thrust maneuver in a supine patient. Straddle the hips or legs. Place the heel of one hand against the patient's abdomen and the other hand on top of the first. Press your hands into the patient's abdomen in a series of five quick inward and upward thrusts.

To perform chest thrusts when the patient is standing or sitting, use the following technique ▶ **Figure 39-27** :

1. **Stand behind the patient** with your arms directly under the patient's armpits, and wrap your arms around the patient's chest.

2. **Make a fist with one hand**; grasp the fist with the other hand. Place the thumb side of the fist against the patient's sternum, avoiding the xiphoid process and the edges of the rib cage.

3. **Press your fist into the patient's chest** with backward thrusts until the object is expelled or the patient becomes unconscious.

If the patient is lying down, modify the technique as follows ▶ **Figure 39-28** :

1. **Place the patient in a supine position.**

2. **Kneel next to the patient.**

3. **Use the same hand position** as that for chest compressions.

4. **Deliver slow, deliberate chest thrusts** to expel the object.

Manual Removal of Foreign Objects

Use of finger sweeps should be limited to unconscious patients. If you can see a foreign object in the patient's mouth, you should remove it carefully with your gloved fingers. This may be necessary if the abdominal-

Figure 39-27 Removal of foreign body obstruction using chest thrusts. Stand behind the patient and wrap your arms around the chest. Place the thumb side of one fist against the chest while holding your fist with the other hand. Press your fists into the patient's chest with backwards thrusts.

thrust maneuver dislodges but does not expel the foreign body.

Use the following technique to remove the foreign material manually ▶ **Figure 39-29** :

1. **Place the patient in a supine position.**

2. **Open the patient's mouth** by grasping the tongue and the lower jaw between your thumb and fingers and lifting them forward (tongue-jaw lift). This pulls the tongue away from the back of the throat and from the foreign body that may be lodged there.

3. **Use the index finger of your opposite hand as a hook to sweep down inside the patient's cheek** to the base of the tongue.

4. **Dislodge any impacted foreign body** up into the mouth.

5. **When the foreign body comes up within reach, grasp and carefully remove it.**

Make sure that you do not push the dislodged foreign body farther back into the airway. Since this is very easy to do in infants and small children, blind finger sweeps are not recommended for these patients. Instead, look first, and then reach for the object with your index finger and thumb only after you see it. If you don't see anything, don't reach.

Figure 39-28 Chest thrusts with the patient in a supine position. Kneel next to the patient. Place your hands as you would to deliver chest compressions. Deliver slow chest thrusts until the object is expelled.

Partial Airway Obstruction

Some patients may have only a partial airway obstruction. They are able to exchange some air but still have signs of respiratory distress. Breathing is noisy, and the patient may be coughing. Your main concern is to prevent a partial airway obstruction from becoming a complete airway obstruction. The abdominal-thrust maneuver is generally not effective in these situations. Manual removal is dangerous because you could force the object farther down the airway, causing a complete obstruction.

Therefore, for a patient with a partial airway obstruction, you should first encourage the patient to cough. Do not interfere with the patient's attempts to expel the foreign body; rather, simply stay with and monitor the patient. Give 100% oxygen to the patient using a nonrebreathing mask, and provide prompt transport. A partial airway obstruction with poor exchange (ie, ineffective cough, high-pitched inspiratory sound, increased respiratory difficulty, and cyanosis) should be treated as a complete airway obstruction.

Foreign Body Obstruction in Infants and Children

Airway obstruction is a common problem in infants and children, usually caused by a foreign body or an infection, such as croup or epiglottitis, resulting in swelling and narrowing of the airway. You should try to identify the cause of the obstruction as soon as possible. In patients who have signs and symptoms of an

Figure 39-29 **A.** To manually remove a foreign object in an unconscious patient, use the tongue-jaw lift to open the mouth and to help see the object. **B.** Hook the index finger of your opposite hand to sweep down inside the cheek to the base of the tongue.

airway infection, you should not waste time trying to dislodge a foreign body. The child needs immediate transport to the emergency department.

A previously healthy child who is eating, playing with small toys, or crawling about the house and who suddenly has difficulty breathing has probably aspirated a foreign body. As in adults, foreign bodies may cause a partial or complete airway obstruction. With a partial airway obstruction, air exchange can be either good or poor.

With good air exchange, the patient can cough forcefully, although there may be wheezing between coughs. As long as the patient can breathe, cough, or talk, you should not interfere with his or her own attempts to expel the foreign body. In fact, you should encourage the child to continue coughing and breathing. You should attempt to remove the obstruction only if the cough becomes ineffective; if the patient has stridor, increased respiratory difficulty, or cyanosis; or if the patient loses consciousness.

Give patients with partial airway obstruction oxygen. If the oxygen does not convert poor air exchange into good air exchange, you must treat the patient as if he or she had a complete airway obstruction.

Removing a Foreign Body Airway Obstruction

For a child who is sitting or standing, use the following technique (▶ **Figure 39-30**):

1. **Stand behind the patient.** Place your arms under the patient's armpits, and wrap your arms around the patient's chest.

2. **Make a fist with one hand;** grasp the fist with the other hand. Place the thumb side of your fist against the patient's abdomen, just above the umbilicus and well below the xiphoid process.

3. **Press your fist into the patient's abdomen** with a set of five quick upward thrusts.

4. **Repeat the thrusts in sets of five** until the object is expelled or the patient loses consciousness.

For a child who is lying down or unconscious, modify the technique, as follows (▶ **Figure 39-31**):

1. **Place the patient in a supine position.**

2. **Kneel beside the patient,** or straddle the patient's hips.

3. **Place the heel of one hand against the patient's abdomen** above the umbilicus and well below the xiphoid process. Then place your other hand on top of the first.

4. **Press the hand into the patient's abdomen** with quick inward and upward thrusts, and repeat five times.

5. **Open the airway,** and attempt rescue breathing. If the obstruction is not cleared, repeat abdominal thrusts.

If the foreign body is not expelled, open the child's mouth. If you see the foreign body, perform the tongue-jaw lift, and then use a finger sweep to remove it. Do not use blind finger sweeps on infants and children, as you may force foreign objects farther into the airway. In rare instances, when you cannot remove the foreign body, perform mouth-to-mask ventilation en route to the hospital.

The abdominal-thrust maneuver might injure the liver or other abdominal organs in an infant. Therefore, use the following technique to remove a foreign body in an infant (▶ **Figure 39-32**):

Figure 39-30 Stand behind the patient, place your arms under the armpits, and wrap your arms around the patient's chest. Press your fists into the patient's abdomen in a series of five quick, upward thrusts.

Figure 39-31 Place the patient in a supine position, and kneel beside the patient or straddle the patient's hips. Place the heel of one hand against the patient's abdomen, with the other hand on top of the first. Press your hands into the patient's abdomen in a series of five quick upward thrusts.

1. **Place one hand on the infant's back and neck** and the other on his or her chest, jaws, and face, holding the jaw firmly to support the head at a level lower than the trunk. This sandwiches the infant between your hands and arms. Your forearm should rest on your thigh to support the infant.

Figure 39-32 **A.** Deliver five quick back blows between the shoulder blades, using the heel of your hand. **B.** Give five quick chest thrusts on the sternum at a slightly slower rate than you would give for CPR.

2. **Deliver five quick back blows** between the shoulder blades, using the heel of your hand.

3. **Next, turn the infant face up,** making sure that you support the head and neck. Hold the infant in a supine position on your thigh, with the head slightly lower than the trunk.

EMT-B Safety

While your chances of contracting a disease during CPR training or actual CPR on a patient are very low, common sense and OSHA guidelines both demand that you take reasonable precautions to prevent unnecessary exposure to infectious disease. Using standard precautions makes the risk *extremely* low; you then don't have to be anxious about practicing and performing the skill.

4. **Give five quick chest thrusts on the sternum** in the same fashion as for CPR, except at a slightly slower rate. If the infant is large or your hands are small, you might need to place the infant on your lap to deliver the chest thrusts.

5. **If the infant is unconscious,** you should perform the tongue-jaw lift to open the mouth. Remove the object manually if you can see it.

If the infant does not start breathing after these maneuvers, try to open the airway again, and give artificial ventilation. If the chest does not rise, reposition the head, and attempt ventilation again. If the chest still does not rise, continue giving back blows followed by chest thrusts until the obstruction is cleared or you reach the hospital.

Infectious Disease and the EMT-B

Transmission of infectious disease such as HBV, AIDS, or herpes simplex can occur while performing CPR. There is also a risk of aerosol transmission of airborne diseases, such as tuberculosis and meningitis.

The probability that you will become infected with HIV or HBV while administering CPR is minimal. In theory, at least, the risk is greater for transmission of herpes simplex or *Neisseria* meningitis. The use of plastic nose covers with filtered openings, or masks with one-way valves offer some degree of protection.

The emergence of multi-drug-resistant tuberculosis also poses a threat to the EMT-B, although transmission of tuberculosis usually involves close physical contact over long periods of time. If you know that you have been exposed to tuberculosis, you should be evaluated by a physician using the standard tests for this disease.

Prep Kit

Ready for Review

Basic life support (BLS) is a series of emergency lifesaving procedures that are carried out in order to treat respiratory arrest, cardiac arrest, or both. Commonly known as cardiopulmonary resuscitation (CPR), it is a method of providing artificial ventilation and circulation. The effectiveness of CPR depends on prompt recognition of respiratory and/or cardiac arrest and the immediate start of treatment. You are expected to be able to recognize cardiac or respiratory arrest without difficulty and quickly to institute proper BLS measures.

BLS can be given by one or two EMT-Bs, by first responders, or by alert and well-trained bystanders. It does not require any equipment; however, a barrier device should be used to perform rescue breathing.

The basic principles of BLS are the same for infants, children, and adults. For the purposes of BLS, anyone younger than 1 year is considered an infant. A child is between ages 1 and 8 years. For children older than 8 years, you should use the same techniques as you use for adults.

Several methods exist for opening the airway and providing rescue breathing. Each has specific applications for conscious or unconscious patients, with or without head or spinal injury. The head tilt-chin lift maneuver is effective for opening the airway of most patients. However, for patients who have suspected spinal injury, the jaw-thrust maneuver without a head tilt is indicated. Rescue breathing is done routinely with a barrier device, such as a mask, in order to provide infection control. Sometimes, rescue breathing results in too much air forced into the stomach. The resulting condition is called gastric distention. A patient with gastric distention may vomit during CPR. If this condition develops, you should continue to provide slow rescue breaths without trying to expel the stomach contents.

If a patient begins breathing following rescue breathing, you should place the patient in the recovery position. This position helps to maintain a clear airway in a patient with a decreased level of consciousness who has not had traumatic injuries and is breathing on his or her own.

After you begin rescue breathing, you must assess the patient's circulation. If the patient has no pulse, you must provide artificial circulation by applying rhythmic pressure and relaxation to the lower half of the sternum. Remember that the patient must be on a firm, flat surface for chest compressions to be effective. Proper hand position and proper compression technique are necessary for artificial circulation to be effective.

CPR can be done with one or two rescuers. Two-rescuer CPR is always the first choice. When a rescuer is doing adult CPR alone or with another rescuer, the ratio of compressions to ventilations is 15:2. In infants and children, the ratio of compressions to ventilations is 5:1 for both one-rescuer and two-rescuer CPR. Remember that you should try not to interrupt CPR for more than a few seconds, except when it is absolutely necessary.

Similarly, specific techniques must be used for removing foreign bodies that obstruct the airway. Obstruction may be caused by many things, including relaxation of the throat muscles in an unconscious patient, vomited or regurgitated stomach contents, a blood clot, bone fragments or damaged tissue after an injury, dentures, or foreign bodies in the airway. Recognition of the obstruction and prompt initiation of interventions are critical.

Two manual maneuvers are recommended for removing a foreign body airway obstruction: the abdominal-thrust maneuver (Heimlich maneuver) and finger sweeps and manual removal of the object. In infants and children, the cause of airway obstruction may be infectious. Therefore, you should try to identify the cause of an obstruction as soon as possible. Infants and children with these infections need immediate transport to the hospital.

Vital Vocabulary

abdominal-thrust maneuver The preferred method to dislodge and force food or other material from the throat of a choking victim; also called the Heimlich maneuver.

advanced life support (ALS) Advanced lifesaving procedures, such as cardiac monitoring, administration of IV fluids and medications, and use of advanced airway adjuncts.

basic life support (BLS) Noninvasive emergency lifesaving care that is used to treat airway obstruction, respiratory arrest, or cardiac arrest.

cardiopulmonary resuscitation (CPR) The combination of rescue breathing and chest compressions used to establish adequate ventilation and circulation in a patient who is not breathing and has no pulse.

gastric distention A condition in which air fills the stomach as a result of high volume and pressure during artificial ventilation.

head tilt-chin lift maneuver A technique to open the airway that combines tilting back the forehead and lifting the chin.

jaw-thrust maneuver A technique to open the airway by placing the fingers behind the angles of the patient's lower jaw and forcefully moving the jaw forward; can be performed without head tilt.

recovery position A position that helps to maintain a clear airway in a patient with a decreased level of consciousness who has not had traumatic injuries and is breathing on his or her own.

Assessment in Action

You and your partner are dispatched to a local restaurant for a person down. On arrival, you are escorted to the restroom where you find a middle-aged man lying on his side on the floor. Bystanders tell you they found the man down when another patron entered the restroom. No one immediately available can tell you anything about this man. He is unresponsive to voice; his facial color is cyanotic. He has no chest rise and fall and a rapid check shows no carotid pulse.

1. You should now:
   A. assess his response to painful stimuli.
   B. open his airway.
   C. turn him on his back.
   D. remove his shirt.

2. Which method of opening his airway should you perform?
   A. Head tilt-chin lift
   B. Jaw thrust
   C. Inserting an oral airway
   D. Chin lift

3. You see nothing in his airway and determine that this man is not breathing. You start rescue breathing with a barrier device. The best tidal volume will be provided by using:
   A. a bag-valve-mask device with two breaths, lasting 1 second each.
   B. your own lung capacity and two breaths, lasting 1 1/2 seconds each.
   C. a bag-valve-mask device with three breaths, lasting 1 second each.
   D. your own lung capacity and three breaths, lasting 1 1/2 seconds each.

4. Successful attempts at rescue breathing can best be initially assessed by having your partner:
   A. observe for rise and fall of the chest.
   B. observe for rise and fall of the stomach.
   C. observe for facial color change.
   D. check for the return of a pulse.

5. Your partner tells you that the patient's stomach is continually distending while you are attempting to ventilate. You now know that you must:
   A. gently press on his stomach to expel the air.
   B. roll him on his side and prepare for vomiting.
   C. reposition his airway and try again.
   D. attempt ventilations with more force.

6. While you are attempting to correct this problem, the manager tells you that a lady approached him regarding her husband. Shortly after they began eating, he suddenly got a "panicky look," got up from the table, and ran to the restroom. What important information do you need to find out?
   A. Is he allergic to anything?
   B. Is he on any medication?
   C. Did he speak?
   D. What was he eating?

7. After obtaining that information from his wife, you now will:
   A. perform chest compressions.
   B. place him in the recovery position.
   C. perform abdominal thrusts.
   D. perform a sweep of his oral airway.

8. You recheck his airway and discover several large chunks of food. You clear the airway. Your next action is to:
   A. resume rescue breathing.
   B. check for the carotid pulse.
   C. place him in the recovery position.
   D. check for return of respirations.

9. You continue treatment of this patient and shortly afterward determine that there is the return of a faint carotid pulse, but no return of respirations. Your next action is to:
   A. continue rescue breathing.
   B. place him in the recovery position.
   C. continue chest compressions.
   D. place a nonrebreathing mask.

Challenging Question

10. The manager tells you that the man's wife is waiting in the foyer. The manager told her that there was an unconscious man that the EMTs were working on but didn't tell her anything else. What should you do?

Points to Ponder

You respond to a house to find a man performing CPR on his wife. She is on the bed and while the bed is moving, it is unlikely any blood is. The man tells you that he found her about 25 minutes ago and started CPR. He stopped CPR for several minutes when he called 9-1-1 and his children to let them know what happened. When you check the woman's pulse, she is very cold and beginning to stiffen. You tell the husband that she is dead and that it is

unlikely that you can revive her. The husband wants you to start CPR and try to save her. Would you start CPR? How would you comfort the husband? What if your medical control said to stop resuscitation efforts, but the man wanted them continued?

Issues When Not to Resuscitate, Helping Grieving Family, Signs of Irreversible Death, Communicating With Medical Control.

www.emtb.com

Appendix A

National Registry Skill Sheets

Patient Assessment/Management - Medical

Start Time: _____
Stop Time: _____   Date: _____
Candidate's Name: _____
Evaluator's Name: _____

	Points Possible	Points Awarded
Takes, or verbalizes, body substance isolation precautions	1	
SCENE SIZE-UP		
Determines the scene is safe	1	
Determines the mechanism of injury/nature of illness	1	
Determines the number of patients	1	
Requests additional help if necessary	1	
Considers stabilization of spine	1	
INITIAL ASSESSMENT		
Verbalizes general impression of the patient	1	
Determines responsiveness/level of consciousness	1	
Determines chief complaint/apparent life threats	1	
Assesses airway and breathing — Assessment / Initiates appropriate oxygen therapy / Assures adequate ventilation	1 / 1 / 1	
Assesses circulation — Assesses/controls major bleeding / Assesses pulse / Assesses skin (color, temperature and condition)	1 / 1 / 1	
Identifies priority patients/makes transport decision	1	

FOCUSED HISTORY AND PHYSICAL EXAMINATION/RAPID ASSESSMENT

Signs and symptoms *(Assess history of present illness)*

Respiratory	Cardiac	Altered Mental Status	Allergic Reaction	Poisoning/ Overdose	Environmental Emergency	Obstetrics	Behavioral	Points Possible	Points Awarded
•Onset?	•Onset?	•Description of the episode.	•History of allergies?	•Substance?	•Source?	•Are you pregnant?	•How do you feel?		
•Provokes?	•Provokes?	•Onset?	•What were you exposed to?	•When did you ingest/become exposed?	•Environment?	•How long have you been pregnant?	•Determine suicidal tendencies.		
•Quality?	•Quality?	•Duration?	•How were you exposed?	•How much did you ingest?	•Duration?	•Pain or contractions?	•Is the patient a threat to self or others?		
•Radiates?	•Radiates?	•Associated Symptoms?	•Effects?	•Over what time period?	•Loss of consciousness?	•Bleeding or discharge?	•Is there a medical problem?		
•Severity?	•Severity?	•Evidence of Trauma?	•Progression?	•Interventions?	•Effects – general or local?	•Do you feel the need to push?	•Interventions?		
•Time?	•Time?	•Interventions?	•Interventions?	•Estimated weight?		•Last menstrual period?			
•Interventions?	•Interventions?	•Seizures?							
		•Fever?						1	

	Points Possible	Points Awarded
Allergies	1	
Medications	1	
Past pertinent history	1	
Last oral intake	1	
Event leading to present illness (rule out trauma)	1	
Performs focused physical examination *(assesses affected body part/system or, if indicated, completes rapid assessment)*	1	
Vitals *(obtains baseline vital signs)*	1	
Interventions *(obtains medical direction or verbalizes standing order for medication interventions and verbalizes proper additional intervention/treatment)*	1	
Transport *(re-evaluates the transport decision)*	1	
ONGOING ASSESSMENT *(verbalized)*		
Repeats initial assessment	1	
Repeats vital signs	1	
Repeats focused assessment regarding patient complaint or injuries	1	
	Total: 30	

Critical Criteria

___ Did not take, or verbalize, body substance isolation precautions when necessary
___ Did not determine scene safety
___ Did not obtain medical direction or verbalize standing orders for medical interventions
___ Did not provide high concentration of oxygen
___ Did not find or manage problems associated with airway, breathing, hemorrhage or shock (hypoperfusion)
___ Did not differentiate patient's need for transportation versus continued assessment at the scene
___ Did detailed or focused history/physical examination before assessing the airway, breathing and circulation
___ Did not ask questions about the present illness
___ Administered a dangerous or inappropriate intervention

Patient Assessment/Management - Trauma

Start Time: _____
Stop Time: _____   Date: _____
Candidate's Name: _____
Evaluator's Name: _____

	Points Possible	Points Awarded
Takes, or verbalizes, body substance isolation precautions	1	
SCENE SIZE-UP		
Determines the scene is safe	1	
Determines the mechanism of injury	1	
Determines the number of patients	1	
Requests additional help if necessary	1	
Considers stabilization of spine	1	
INITIAL ASSESSMENT		
Verbalizes general impression of the patient	1	
Determines responsiveness/level of consciousness	1	
Determines chief complaint/apparent life threats	1	
Assesses airway and breathing — Assessment / Initiates appropriate oxygen therapy / Assures adequate ventilation / Injury management	1 / 1 / 1	
Assesses circulation — Assesses/controls major bleeding / Assesses pulse / Assesses skin (color, temperature and condition)	1 / 1 / 1	
Identifies priority patients/makes transport decision	1	
FOCUSED HISTORY AND PHYSICAL EXAMINATION/RAPID TRAUMA ASSESSMENT		
Selects appropriate assessment *(focused or rapid assessment)*	1	
Obtains, or directs assistance to obtain, baseline vital signs	1	
Obtains S.A.M.P.L.E. history	1	
DETAILED PHYSICAL EXAMINATION		
Assesses the head — Inspects and palpates the scalp and ears / Assesses the eyes / Assesses the facial areas including oral and nasal areas	1 / 1 / 1	
Assesses the neck — Inspects and palpates the neck / Assesses for JVD / Assesses for tracheal deviation	1 / 1 / 1	
Assesses the chest — Inspects / Palpates / Auscultates	1 / 1 / 1	
Assesses the abdomen/pelvis — Assesses the abdomen / Assesses the pelvis / Verbalizes assessment of genitalia/perineum as needed	1 / 1 / 1	
Assesses the extremities — 1 point for each extremity includes inspection, palpation, and assessment of motor, sensory and circulatory function	4	
Assesses the posterior — Assesses thorax / Assesses lumbar	1 / 1	
Manages secondary injuries and wounds appropriately — 1 point for appropriate management of the secondary injury/wound	1	
Verbalizes re-assessment of the vital signs	1	
	Total: 40	

Critical Criteria

___ Did not take, or verbalize, body substance isolation precautions
___ Did not determine scene safety
___ Did not assess for spinal protection
___ Did not provide for spinal protection when indicated
___ Did not provide high concentration of oxygen
___ Did not find, or manage, problems associated with airway, breathing, hemorrhage or shock (hypoperfusion)
___ Did not differentiate patient's need for transportation versus continued assessment at the scene
___ Did other detailed physical examination before assessing the airway, breathing and circulation
___ Did not transport patient within (10) minute time limit

Appendix A

BAG-VALVE-MASK APNEIC PATIENT

Start Time: _____
Stop Time: _____ Date: _____
Candidate's Name: _____
Evaluator's Name: _____

	Points Possible	Points Awarded
Takes, or verbalizes, body substance isolation precautions	1	
Voices opening the airway	1	
Voices inserting an airway adjunct	1	
Selects appropriately sized mask	1	
Creates a proper mask-to-face seal	1	
Ventilates patient at no less than 800 ml volume *(The examiner must witness for at least 30 seconds)*	1	
Connects reservoir and oxygen	1	
Adjusts liter flow to 15 liters/minute or greater	1	
The examiner indicates arrival of a second EMT. The second EMT is instructed to ventilate the patient while the candidate controls the mask and the airway		
Voices re-opening the airway	1	
Creates a proper mask-to-face seal	1	
Instructs assistant to resume ventilation at proper volume per breath *(The examiner must witness for at least 30 seconds)*	1	
Total:	**11**	

Critical Criteria

____ Did not take, or verbalize, body substance isolation precautions

____ Did not immediately ventilate the patient

____ Interrupted ventilations for more than 20 seconds

____ Did not provide high concentration of oxygen

____ Did not provide, or direct assistant to provide, proper volume/breath
(more than two (2) ventilations per minute are below 800 ml)

____ Did not allow adequate exhalation

Appendix A

Cardiac Arrest Management/AED

Start Time: _____
Stop Time: _____ Date: _____
Candidate's Name: _____
Evaluator's Name: _____

	Points Possible	Points Awarded
ASSESSMENT		
Takes, or verbalizes, body substance isolation precautions	1	
Briefly questions the rescuer about arrest events	1	
Directs rescuer to stop CPR	1	
Verifies absence of spontaneous pulse (skill station examiner states "no pulse")	1	
Directs resumption of CPR	1	
Turns on defibrillator power	1	
Attaches automated defibrillator to the patient	1	
Directs rescuer to stop CPR and ensures all individuals are clear of the patient	1	
Initiates analysis of the rhythm	1	
Delivers shock (up to three successive shocks)	1	
Verifies absence of spontaneous pulse (skill station examiner states "no pulse")	1	
TRANSITION		
Directs resumption of CPR	1	
Gathers additional information about arrest event	1	
Confirms effectiveness of CPR (ventilation and compressions)	1	
INTEGRATION		
Verbalizes or directs insertion of a simple airway adjunct (oral/nasal airway)	1	
Ventilates, or directs ventilation of, the patient	1	
Assures high concentration of oxygen is delivered to the patient	1	
Assures CPR continues without unnecessary/prolonged interruption	1	
Re-evaluates patient/CPR in approximately one minute	1	
Repeats defibrillator sequence	1	
TRANSPORTATION		
Verbalizes transportation of patient	1	
Total:	**21**	

Critical Criteria

____ Did not take, or verbalize, body substance isolation precautions

____ Did not evaluate the need for immediate use of the AED

____ Did not direct initiation/resumption of ventilation/compressions at appropriate times.

____ Did not assure all individuals were clear of patient before delivering each shock

____ Did not operate the AED properly (inability to deliver shock)

____ Prevented the defibrillator from delivering indicated stacked shocks

SPINAL IMMOBILIZATION
SUPINE PATIENT

Start Time: _____

Stop Time: _____   Date: _____

Candidate's Name: _____

Evaluator's Name: _____

	Points Possible	Points Awarded
Takes, or verbalizes, body substance isolation precautions	1	
Directs assistant to place/maintain head in the neutral in-line position	1	
Directs assistant to maintain manual immobilization of the head	1	
Reassesses motor, sensory and circulatory function in each extremity	1	
Applies appropriately sized extrication collar	1	
Positions the immobilization device appropriately	1	
Directs movement of the patient onto the device without compromising the integrity of the spine	1	
Applies padding to voids between the torso and the board as necessary	1	
Immobilizes the patient's torso to the device	1	
Evaluates and pads behind the patient's head as necessary	1	
Immobilizes the patient's head to the device	1	
Secures the patient's legs to the device	1	
Secures the patient's arms to the device	1	
Reassesses motor, sensory and circulatory function in each extremity	1	
Total:	**14**	

Critical Criteria

_____ Did not immediately direct, or take, manual immobilization of the head

_____ Released, or ordered release of, manual immobilization before it was maintained mechanicall

_____ Patient manipulated, or moved excessively, causing potential spinal compromise

_____ Patient moves excessively up, down, left or right on the patient's torso

_____ Head immobilization allows for excessive movement

_____ Upon completion of immobilization, head is not in the neutral position

_____ Did not assess motor, sensory and circulatory function in each extremity after immobilization to the device

_____ Immobilized head to the board before securing the torso

---

SPINAL IMMOBILIZATION
SEATED PATIENT

Start Time: _____

Stop Time: _____   Date: _____

Candidate's Name: _____

Evaluator's Name: _____

	Points Possible	Points Awarded
Takes, or verbalizes, body substance isolation precautions	1	
Directs assistant to place/maintain head in the neutral in-line position	1	
Directs assistant to maintain manual immobilization of the head	1	
Reassesses motor, sensory and circulatory function in each extremity	1	
Applies appropriately sized extrication collar	1	
Positions the immobilization device behind the patient	1	
Secures the device to the patient's torso	1	
Evaluates torso fixation and adjusts as necessary	1	
Evaluates and pads behind the patient's head as necessary	1	
Secures the patient's head to the device	1	
Verbalizes moving the patient to a long board	1	
Reassesses motor, sensory and circulatory function in each extremity	1	
Total:	**12**	

Critical Criteria

_____ Did not immediately direct, or take, manual immobilization of the head

_____ Released, or ordered release of, manual immobilization before it was maintained mechanicall

_____ Patient manipulated, or moved excessively, causing potential spinal compromise

_____ Device moved excessively up, down, left or right on the patient's torso

_____ Head immobilization allows for excessive movement

_____ Torso fixation inhibits chest rise, resulting in respiratory compromise

_____ Upon completion of immobilization, head is not in the neutral position

_____ Did not assess motor, sensory and circulatory function in each extremity after voicing immobilization to the long board

_____ Immobilized head to the board before securing the torso

Appendix A

IMMOBILIZATION SKILLS
TRACTION SPLINTING

Start Time: _____
Stop Time: _____   Date: _____
Candidate's Name: _____

Evaluator's Name:	Points Possible	Points Awarded
Takes, or verbalizes, body substance isolation precautions	1	
Directs application of manual stabilization of the injured leg	1	
Directs the application of manual traction	1	
Assesses motor, sensory and circulatory function in the injured extremity	1	
Note: The examiner acknowledges "motor, sensory and circulatory function are present and normal"		
Prepares/adjusts splint to the proper length	1	
Positions the splint next to the injured leg	1	
Applies the proximal securing device (e.g... ischial strap)	1	
Applies the distal securing device (e.g...ankle hitch)	1	
Applies mechanical traction	1	
Positions/secures the support straps	1	
Re-evaluates the proximal/distal securing devices	1	
Reassesses motor, sensory and circulatory function in the injured extremity	1	
Note: The examiner acknowledges "motor, sensory and circulatory function are present and normal"		
Note: The examiner must ask the candidate how he/she would prepare the patient for transportation		
Verbalizes securing the torso to the long board to immobilize the hip	1	
Verbalizes securing the splint to the long board to prevent movement of the splint	1	
Total:	**14**	

Critical Criteria

_____ Loss of traction at any point after it was applied
_____ Did not reassess motor, sensory and circulatory function in the injured extremity before and after splinting
_____ The foot was excessively rotated or extended after splint was applied
_____ Did not secure the ischial strap before taking traction
_____ Final Immobilization failed to support the femur or prevent rotation of the injured leg
_____ Secured the leg to the splint before applying mechanical traction

Note: If the Sagar splint or the Kendricks Traction Device is used without elevating the patient's leg, application of manual traction is not necessary. The candidate should be awarded one (1) point as if manual traction were applied.

Note: If the leg is elevated at all, manual traction must be applied before elevating the leg. The ankle hitch may be applied before elevating the leg and used to provide manual traction.

IMMOBILIZATION SKILLS
LONG BONE INJURY

Start Time: _____
Stop Time: _____   Date: _____
Candidate's Name: _____

Evaluator's Name:	Points Possible	Points Awarded
Takes, or verbalizes, body substance isolation precautions	1	
Directs application of manual stabilization of the injury	1	
Assesses motor, sensory and circulatory function in the injured extremity	1	
Note: The examiner acknowledges "motor, sensory and circulatory function are present and normal"		
Measures the splint	1	
Applies the splint	1	
Immobilizes the joint above the injury site	1	
Immobilizes the joint below the injury site	1	
Secures the entire injured extremity	1	
Immobilizes the hand/foot in the position of function	1	
Reassesses motor, sensory and circulatory function in the injured extremity	1	
Note: The examiner acknowledges "motor, sensory and circulatory function are present and normal"		
Total:	**10**	

Critical Criteria

_____ Grossly moves the injured extremity
_____ Did not immobilize the joint above and the joint below the injury site
_____ Did not reassess motor, sensory and circulatory function in the injured extremity before and after splinting

BLEEDING CONTROL/SHOCK MANAGEMENT

Start Time: _____   Date: _____

Stop Time: _____

Candidate's Name: _____

Evaluator's Name: _____

	Points Possible	Points Awarded
Takes, or verbalizes, body substance isolation precautions	1	
Applies direct pressure to the wound	1	
Elevates the extremity	1	
Note: The examiner must now inform the candidate that the wound continues to bleed.		
Applies an additional dressing to the wound	1	
Note: The examiner must now inform the candidate that the wound still continues to bleed. The second dressing does not control the bleeding.		
Locates and applies pressure to appropriate arterial pressure point	1	
Note: The examiner must now inform the candidate that the bleeding is controlled		
Bandages the wound	1	
Note: The examiner must now inform the candidate the patient is now showing signs and symptoms indicative of hypoperfusion		
Properly positions the patient	1	
Applies high concentration oxygen	1	
Initiates steps to prevent heat loss from the patient	1	
Indicates the need for immediate transportation	1	
Total:	**10**	

Critical Criteria

_____ Did not take, or verbalize, body substance isolation precautions

_____ Did not apply high concentration of oxygen

_____ Applied a tourniquet before attempting other methods of bleeding control

_____ Did not control hemorrhage in a timely manner

_____ Did not indicate a need for immediate transportation

IMMOBILIZATION SKILLS
JOINT INJURY

Start Time: _____   Date: _____

Stop Time: _____

Candidate's Name: _____

Evaluator's Name: _____

	Points Possible	Points Awarded
Takes, or verbalizes, body substance isolation precautions	1	
Directs application of manual stabilization of the shoulder injury	1	
Assesses motor, sensory and circulatory function in the injured extremity	1	
Note: The examiner acknowledges "motor, sensory and circulatory function are present and normal."		
Selects the proper splinting material	1	
Immobilizes the site of the injury	1	
Immobilizes the bone above the injured joint	1	
Immobilizes the bone below the injured joint	1	
Reassesses motor, sensory and circulatory function in the injured extremity	1	
Note: The examiner acknowledges "motor, sensory and circulatory function are present and normal."		
Total:	**8**	

Critical Criteria

_____ Did not support the joint so that the joint did not bear distal weight

_____ Did not immobilize the bone above and below the injured site

_____ Did not reassess motor, sensory and circulatory function in the injured extremity before and after splinting

Appendix A

AIRWAY, OXYGEN AND VENTILATION SKILLS
UPPER AIRWAY ADJUNCTS AND SUCTION

Start Time: _____ Date: _____

Stop Time: _____

Candidate's Name: _____

Evaluator's Name: _____

OROPHARYNGEAL AIRWAY

	Points Possible	Points Awarded
Takes, or verbalizes, body substance isolation precautions	1	
Selects appropriately sized airway	1	
Measures airway	1	
Inserts airway without pushing the tongue posteriorly	1	
Note: The examiner must advise the candidate that the patient is gagging and becoming conscious		
Removes the oropharyngeal airway	1	

SUCTION

Note: The examiner must advise the candidate to suction the patient's airway		
Turns on/prepares suction device	1	
Assures presence of mechanical suction	1	
Inserts the suction tip without suction	1	
Applies suction to the oropharynx/nasopharynx	1	

NASOPHARYNGEAL AIRWAY

Note: The examiner must advise the candidate to insert a nasopharyngeal airway		
Selects appropriately sized airway	1	
Measures airway	1	
Verbalizes lubrication of the nasal airway	1	
Fully inserts the airway with the bevel facing toward the septum	1	
Total:	**13**	

Critical Criteria

_____ Did not take, or verbalize, body substance isolation precautions

_____ Did not obtain a patent airway with the oropharyngeal airway

_____ Did not obtain a patent airway with the nasopharyngeal airway

_____ Did not demonstrate an acceptable suction technique

_____ Inserted any adjunct in a manner dangerous to the patient

---

OXYGEN ADMINISTRATION

Start Time: _____ Date: _____

Stop Time: _____

Candidate's Name: _____

Evaluator's Name: _____

	Points Possible	Points Awarded
Takes, or verbalizes, body substance isolation precautions	1	
Assembles the regulator to the tank	1	
Opens the tank	1	
Checks for leaks	1	
Checks tank pressure	1	
Attaches non-rebreather mask to oxygen	1	
Prefills reservoir	1	
Adjusts liter flow to 12 liters per minute or greater	1	
Applies and adjusts the mask to the patient's face	1	
Note: The examiner must advise the candidate that the patient is not tolerating the non-rebreather mask. The medical director has ordered you to apply a nasal cannula to the patient.		
Attaches nasal cannula to oxygen	1	
Adjusts liter flow to six (6) liters per minute or less	1	
Applies nasal cannula to the patient	1	
Note: The examiner must advise the candidate to discontinue oxygen therapy		
Removes the nasal cannula from the patient	1	
Shuts off the regulator	1	
Relieves the pressure within the regulator	1	
Total:	**15**	

Critical Criteria

_____ Did not take, or verbalize, body substance isolation precautions

_____ Did not assemble the tank and regulator without leaks

_____ Did not prefill the reservoir bag

_____ Did not adjust the device to the correct liter flow for the non-rebreather mask *(12 liters per minute or greater)*

_____ Did not adjust the device to the correct liter flow for the nasal cannula *(6 liters per minute or less)*

MOUTH TO MASK WITH SUPPLEMENTAL OXYGEN

Start Time: _____   Date: _____

Stop Time: _____

Candidate's Name: _____

Evaluator's Name: _____

	Points Possible	Points Awarded
Takes, or verbalizes, body substance isolation precautions	1	
Connects one-way valve to mask	1	
Opens patient's airway or confirms patient's airway is open (manually or with adjunct)	1	
Establishes and maintains a proper mask to face seal	1	
Ventilates the patient at the proper volume and rate (800=1200 ml per breath/10-20 breaths per minute)	1	
Connects the mask to high concentration of oxygen	1	
Adjusts flow rate to at least 15 liters per minute	1	
Continues ventilation of the patient at the proper volume and rate (800=1200 ml per breath/10-20 breaths per minute)	1	
Note: The examiner must witness ventilations for at least 30 seconds		
Total:	**8**	

Critical Criteria

_____ Did not take, or verbalize, body substance isolation precautions

_____ Did not adjust liter flow to at least 15 liters per minute

_____ Did not provide proper volume per breath (more than 2 ventilations per minute were below 800 ml)

_____ Did not ventilate the patient at a rate a 10-20 breaths per minute

_____ Did not allow for complete exhalation

VENTILATORY MANAGEMENT
ENDOTRACHEAL INTUBATION

Start Time: _____

Stop Time: _____

Candidate's Name: _____   Date: _____

Evaluator's Name: _____

Note: If a candidate elects to initially ventilate the patient with a BVM attached to a reservoir and oxygen, full credit must be awarded for steps denoted by *** provided the first ventilation is delivered within the initial 30 seconds

	Points Possible	Points Awarded
Takes of verbalizes body substance isolation precautions	1	
Opens the airway manually	1	
Elevates the patient's tongue and inserts a simple airway adjunct (oropharyngeal/nasopharyngeal airway)	1	
Note: The examiner must now inform the candidate "no gag reflex is present and the patient accepts the airway adjunct."		
*** Ventilates the patient immediately using a BVM device unattached to oxygen	1	
*** Hyperventilates the patient with room air	1	
Note: The examiner must now inform the candidate that ventilation is being properly performed without difficulty		
Attaches the oxygen reservoir to the BVM	1	
Attaches the BVM to high flow oxygen (15 liter per minute)	1	
Ventilates the patient at the proper volume and rate (800-1200 ml/breath and 10-20 breaths/minute)	1	
Note: After 30 seconds, the examiner must auscultate the patient's chest and inform the candidate that breath sounds are present and equal bilaterally and medical direction has ordered endotracheal intubation. The examiner must now take over ventilation of the patient.		
Directs assistant to hyper-oxygenate the patient	1	
Identifies/selects the proper equipment for endotracheal intubation	1	
Checks equipment Checks for cuff leaks	1	
Checks laryngoscope operation and bulb tightness		
Note: The examiner must remove the OPA and move out of the way when the candidate is prepared to intubate the patient.		
Positions the patient's head properly	1	
Inserts the laryngoscope blade into the patient's mouth while displacing the patient's tongue laterally	1	
Elevates the patient's mandible with the laryngoscope	1	
Introduces the endotracheal tube and advances the tube to the proper depth	1	
Inflates the cuff to the proper pressure	1	
Disconnects the syringe from the cuff inlet port	1	
Directs assistant to ventilate the patient	1	
Confirms proper placement of the endotracheal tube by auscultation bilaterally and over the epigastrium	1	
Note: The examiner must ask, "If you had proper placement, what would you expect to hear?"		
Secures the endotracheal tube (may be verbalized)	1	
Total:	**21**	

Critical Criteria

_____ Did not take or verbalize body substance isolation precautions when necessary

_____ Did not initiate ventilation within 30 seconds after applying gloves or interrupts ventilations for greater than 30 seconds at any time

_____ Did not voice or provide high oxygen concentrations (15 liter/minute or greater)

_____ Did not ventilate the patient at a rate of at least 10 breaths per minute

_____ Did not provide adequate volume per breath (maximum of 2 errors per minute permissible)

_____ Did not hyper-oxygenate the patient prior to intubation

_____ Did not successfully intubate the patient within 3 attempts

_____ Used the patient's teeth as a fulcrum

_____ Did not assure proper tube placement by auscultation bilaterally over each lung and over the epigastrium

_____ The stylette (if used) extended beyond the end of the endotracheal tube

_____ Inserted any adjunct in a manner that was dangerous to the patient

_____ Did not immediately disconnect the syringe from the inlet port after inflating the cuff

Appendix A

VENTILATORY MANAGEMENT
DUAL LUMEN DEVICE INSERTION FOLLOWING
AN UNSUCCESSFUL ENDOTRACHEAL INTUBATION ATTEMPT

Start Time: _____

Stop Time: _____

Candidate's Name: _____ Date: _____

Evaluator's Name: _____

	Points Possible	Points Awarded
Continues body substance isolation precautions	1	
Confirms the patient is being properly ventilated with high percentage oxygen	1	
Directs the assistant to hyper-oxygenate the patient	1	
Checks/prepares the airway device	1	
Lubricates the distal tip of the device *(may be verbalized)*	1	
Note: The examiner should remove the OPA and move out of the way when the candidate is prepared to insert the device		
Positions the patient's head properly	1	
Performs a tongue-jaw lift	1	

USES ☐ COMBITUBE	☐ USES THE PTL		
Inserts device in the mid-line and to the depth so that the printed ring is at the level of the teeth	Inserts the device in the mid-line until the bite block flange is at the level of the teeth	1	
Inflates the pharyngeal cuff with the proper volume and removes the syringe	Secures the strap	1	
Inflates the distal cuff with the proper volume and removes the syringe	Blows into tube #1 to adequately inflate both cuffs	1	
Attaches/directs attachment of BVM to the first (esophageal placement) lumen and ventilates		1	
Confirms placement and ventilation through the correct lumen by observing chest rise, auscultation over the epigastrium and bilaterally over each lung		1	
Note: The examiner states, "You do not see rise and fall of the chest and hear sounds only over the epigastrium."			
Attaches/directs attachment of BVM to the second (endotracheal placement) lumen and ventilates		1	
Confirms placement and ventilation through the correct lumen by observing chest rise, auscultation over the epigastrium and bilaterally over each lung		1	
Note: The examiner states, "You see rise and fall of the chest, there are no sounds over the epigastrium and breath sounds are equal over each lung."			
Secures device or confirms that the device remains properly secured		1	
	Total:	**15**	

Critical Criteria

____ Did not take or verbalize body substance isolation precautions
____ Did not initiate ventilations within 30 seconds
____ Interrupted ventilations for more than 30 seconds at any time
____ Did not hyper-oxygenate the patient prior to placement of the dual lumen airway device
____ Did not provide adequate volume per breath (maximum 2 errors/minute permissible)
____ Did not ventilate the patient at a rate of at least 10 breaths per minute
____ Did not insert the dual lumen airway device at a proper depth or at the proper place within 3 attempts
____ Did not inflate both cuffs properly
____ **Combitube** - Did not remove the syringe immediately following the inflation of each cuff
____ **PTL** - Did not secure the strap prior to cuff inflation
____ Did not confirm, by observing chest rise and auscultation over the epigastrium and bilaterally over each lung, that the proper lumen of the device was being used to ventilate the patient
____ Inserted any adjunct in a manner that was dangerous to the patient

---

VENTILATORY MANAGEMENT
ESOPHAGEAL OBTURATOR AIRWAY INSERTION FOLLOWING
AN UNSUCCESSFUL ENDOTRACHEAL INTUBATION ATTEMPT

Start Time: _____

Stop Time: _____ Date: _____

Candidate's Name: _____

Evaluator's Name: _____

	Points Possible	Points Awarded
Continues body substance isolation precautions	1	
Confirms the patient is being ventilated high percentage oxygen	1	
Directs the assistant to hyper-oxygenate the patient	1	
Identifies/selects the proper equipment for insertion of EOA	1	
Assembles the EOA	1	
Tests the cuff for leaks	1	
Inflates the mask	1	
Lubricates the tube *(may be verbalized)*	1	
Note: The examiner should remove the OPA and move out of the way when the candidate is prepared to insert the device		
Positions the head properly with the neck in the neutral or slightly flexed position	1	
Grasps and elevates the patient's tongue and mandible	1	
Inserts the tube in the same direction as the curvature of the pharynx	1	
Advances the tube until the mask is sealed against the patient's face	1	
Ventilates the patient while maintaining a tight mask-to-face seal	1	
Directs confirmation of placement of EOA by observing for chest rise and auscultation over the epigastrium and bilaterally over each lung	1	
Note: The examiner must acknowledge adequate chest rise, bilateral breath sounds and absent sounds over the epigastrium		
Inflates the cuff to the proper pressure	1	
Disconnects the syringe from the inlet port	1	
Continues ventilation of the patient	1	
	Total:	**17**

Critical Criteria

____ Did not take or verbalize body substance isolation precautions
____ Did not initiate ventilations within 30 seconds
____ Interrupted ventilations for more than 30 seconds at any time
____ Did not direct hyper-oxygenation of the patient prior to placement of the EOA
____ Did not successfully place the EOA within 3 attempts
____ Did not ventilate at a rate of at least 10 breaths per minute
____ Did not provide adequate volume per breath (maximum 2 errors/minute permissible)
____ Did not assure proper tube placement by auscultation bilaterally and over the epigastrium
____ Did not remove the syringe after inflating the cuff
____ Did not successfully ventilate the patient
____ Did not provide high flow oxygen (15 liters per minute or greater)
____ Inserted any adjunct in a manner that was dangerous to the patient

Appendix B

Registry Review

These review questions are designed to help you assess your knowledge of the principles of emergency medical care, as discussed in *Emergency Care and Transportation of the Sick and Injured*, Eighth Edition. The questions are not endorsed by the National Registry of Emergency Medical Technicians.

1. Which of the following statements about a child's respiratory system is true?
   A. Children depend less heavily on the diaphragm for breathing.
   B. Infants younger than 1 month are able to breathe through the mouth.
   C. The larynx and cricoid cartilage are smaller and softer than that of an adult.
   D. The tongue takes up less space in a child's mouth than in an adult's mouth.

2. As an EMT-B, your first responsibility at the scene of a sudden illness or injury is:
   A. sorting patients based on the degree of illness or injury.
   B. maintaining the airway of an unconscious patient.
   C. your safety and the safety of others.
   D. removing trapped patients.

3. When trying to manage a disruptive patient, you should:
   A. turn your back on the patient to show that you are not a threat.
   B. attempt to disarm the patient yourself if the patient has a gun or knife.
   C. leave the patient alone for a few minutes to think about the situation.
   D. keep your eyes on the patient at all times and be alert for aggressive behavior.

4. The normal pulse rate for a child is approximately how many beats per minute?
   A. 60 to 100
   B. 80 to 100
   C. 100 to 120
   D. 70 to 140

5. You are called to a restaurant where a woman who is at least 8 months pregnant is choking on a piece of meat. She is grasping her throat and coughing as she tries to breathe. What information about the patient is most important in determining whether she has a complete airway obstruction or a partial airway obstruction?
   A. She is grasping her throat.
   B. Audible coughing is noted.
   C. The foreign body is meat.
   D. The pregnancy is almost full term.

6. Orders communicated to the EMT-B in the standing orders or protocols are known as:
   A. online medical direction.
   B. off-line medical direction.
   C. general medical orders.
   D. specific medical orders.

7. A conscious and alert woman who has severe abdominal pain refuses to go to the hospital. Her husband asks you to transport the patient regardless of her wishes. The most appropriate course of action would be to:
   A. respect the patient's wishes.
   B. transport the patient because her husband requests it.
   C. transport the patient because her condition warrants it.
   D. explain to the husband that transport is not needed because the patient's condition is not life threatening.

8. When assessing a patient's knee, you would NOT expect to find:
   A. swelling.
   B. bruising.
   C. paradoxical motion.
   D. loss of motor function.

9. To protect yourself from exposure to blood or other body fluids while in the field, you must wear:
   A. an oxygen mask.
   B. gloves and eye protection.
   C. full turnout gear and an SCBA.
   D. three protective layers of clothing.

10. The Critical Incident Stress Debriefing (CISD) program is designed to help:
    A. families deal with the sudden death of a loved one.
    B. law enforcement officials interview victims of a crime.
    C. law enforcement officials interview witnesses to a crime.
    D. emergency medical personnel cope with personal and group anxieties and stress.

11. Chest compressions on a 3-year-old patient should be performed at a depth and rate of:
    A. $1/2$" to 1", at a rate of 140/min.
    B. 1" to $1 1/2$", at a rate of 100/min.
    C. 1" to 2", at a rate of 60 to 80/min.
    D. $3/4$" to 2", at a rate of 100 to 120/min.

12. A local celebrity has severe injuries as a result of an automobile-truck crash. The highway is closed by law enforcement officials, but the media is allowed to cover the story. A reporter approaches you and asks the condition of the patient. You should:
    A. ignore the reporter.
    B. answer the reporter's questions as best you can.
    C. tell the reporter the patient will be fine to protect his privacy.
    D. explain that you cannot comment and that the reporter should contact the hospital.

13. Gastric distention during artificial ventilation is considered dangerous because it can:
    A. stimulate hyperventilation.
    B. result in bacterial pneumonia.
    C. cause the patient to vomit during CPR.
    D. increase lung volume by elevating the diaphragm.

14. The best way to estimate a patient's skin temperature is to use the:
    A. back of your hand.
    B. tips of your fingers.
    C. palm of your hand.
    D. index and middle fingers.

15. The state of the pupils is a rapid reflection of:
    A. circulation.
    B. blood pressure.
    C. retinal pressure.
    D. central nervous system injury or disease.

16. Which of the following is NOT an acceptable reason for you to stop CPR once you have started?
    A. The patient starts breathing and you feel a pulse.
    B. You are too fatigued and exhausted to continue any longer.
    C. A bystander tells you that the patient may have a living will.
    D. A physician at the scene assumes responsibility and tells you to stop.

17. In most instances, cardiac arrest in infants and children results from:
    A. electrocution.
    B. respiratory arrest.
    C. severe head trauma.
    D. severe hypothermia.

18. In which of the following situations has expressed consent been given?
    A. A 5-year-old child who says, "Make me better"
    B. An unconscious 26-year-old woman who has a bleeding head wound
    C. A 35-year-old man who has a slight concussion but holds his bleeding arm out for bandaging
    D. An 86-year-old man who stares blankly at his bleeding leg and says, "What happened to me?"

19. Which of the following signs is seen in respiratory depression?
    A. Rapid, shallow respirations
    B. Deep, labored, noisy respirations
    C. Strong airflow at the nose and mouth
    D. Little or no movement of the chest and abdomen

20. If an injured patient needs to be moved, but is not in immediate danger from fire or building collapse, you should first:
    A. determine the number of people you will need to help move the patient.
    B. remove the patient with the rapid extrication technique.
    C. check the patient's airway, breathing, and circulation.
    D. order the equipment you will need for extrication.

21. When you are dealing with an emotionally disturbed patient, the best legal situation is to:
    A. always transport the patient with restraints.
    B. try to obtain the patient's consent to medical treatment.
    C. have law enforcement restrain the patient with police-type handcuffs.
    D. allow the patient to refuse treatment when the patient presents a threat to self or others.

22. A woman in labor appears to have a part of the umbilical cord protruding from the vagina. You should first place the woman in Trendelenburg's position, and then carefully:
    A. push the cord back into the vagina and provide prompt transport.
    B. push the baby's head back into the vagina and provide prompt transport.
    C. moisten the cord with sterile saline solution and provide prompt transport.
    D. insert your gloved finger into the vagina and gently push the baby's head away from the umbilical cord.

23. The usual dosage of activated charcoal for a child is how many grams per kilogram of body weight?
    A. 1
    B. 2
    C. 3
    D. 5

24. An 8-year-old boy has a deep cut on his arm with severe bright red bleeding. You have tried to contact the parents, but they cannot be reached. Your next step would be to:
    A. phone the emergency department physician and ask for permission to proceed with treatment.
    B. take the boy to the emergency department but give no treatment.
    C. ask the police for permission to proceed with treatment.
    D. assume the parents would give consent for treatment.

25. A patient who is lying on the ground with his left leg bent out to the side appears to have a deformed knee. He is in extreme pain and states that he cannot move the leg. On assessment, you find that the patient has strong distal pulses. You should prepare the patient for transport by:
    A. wrapping the leg with a pillow.
    B. splinting the leg in the position in which it is found.
    C. straightening the leg and applying and inflating an air splint.
    D. straightening the leg and applying two standard rigid leg splints.

26. Normal systolic blood pressure in an adult male patient is approximately:
    A. 90 mm Hg plus the patient's age, up to 150 mm Hg.
    B. 95 mm Hg plus the patient's age, up to 150 mm Hg.
    C. 100 mm Hg plus the patient's age, up to 150 mm Hg.
    D. 105 mm Hg plus the patient's age, up to 150 mm Hg.

27. When evaluating respirations, you should observe and record the:
    A. rate, quality, and rhythm.
    B. rate and amount of oxygen exhaled.
    C. rate and amount of carbon dioxide exhaled.
    D. number of breaths in a 60-second period and multiply by 2.

28. What is the single most important measure, outside of wearing PPE, for controlling risk of exposure to communicable disease?
    A. Handwashing
    B. Taking antibiotics
    C. Disinfecting with alcohol
    D. Ensuring immunizations are up to date

29. Signs that an adult, conscious patient has adequate respirations include:
    A. pale or cyanotic skin.
    B. retractions on inspiration.
    C. respiratory rate of 12 to 20/min.
    D. respiratory rate of 8 to 24/min.

30. You are on the first ambulance to reach a multiple-casualty scene. As the most experienced EMT-B on the team, you serve as triage officer. You identify one critical patient and other less severely injured patients. When the next ambulance reaches the scene, you should:
    A. assign the critical patient to the second ambulance and accompany him or her on the transport.
    B. immediately transport the critical patient and transfer triage duties to the officer on the second ambulance.
    C. assign the critical patient to the second ambulance; once the critical patient is removed, you can eliminate the role of triage officer.
    D. assign the critical patient to the second ambulance, keep any extra personnel at the scene to help, and continue as triage officer.

31. What happens to the pressure inside the chest at the onset of inhalation?
    A. It increases.
    B. It decreases.
    C. It remains the same.
    D. It is always equal to atmospheric pressure.

32. A man is found sitting behind the steering wheel after a crash. He has a painful, deformed lower right leg and an open wound to his right forearm. Your care of him should include:
    A. giving him oxygen, then moving him to the ambulance and providing transport.
    B. moving him to the ambulance, then bandaging the wound and splinting the leg.
    C. applying a traction splint to the leg injury before moving him to the ambulance.
    D. performing an initial assessment and stabilizing his vital functions before extrication begins.

33. The normal respiratory rate for an infant is approximately how many breaths per minute?
    A. 6 to 12
    B. 12 to 20
    C. 15 to 30
    D. 25 to 50

34. Which of the following terms is described as an audible high-pitched breath sound that usually results from a blockage of the smaller air passages?
    A. Stridor
    B. Wheezing
    C. Exhalation
    D. Rales

35. Which of the following statements about using a bag-valve-mask (BVM) device is true?
    A. One-person BVM is more effective than two-person BVM.
    B. Two-person BVM is more effective than one-person BVM.
    C. You should try to deflate the bag simultaneously with the patient's expiratory effort.
    D. When using the BVM device with chest compressions, you should ventilate twice after every fifth compression.

36. A properly sized oropharyngeal airway should:
    A. be the same size as the little finger.
    B. reach from the nose to the forehead.
    C. reach from the lips to the epiglottis.
    D. reach from the earlobe to the corner of the mouth.

37. A man is found unconscious and slumped over the steering wheel after an automobile crash. He regains consciousness and is not able to feel pain in his legs and feet. This finding suggests that the:
    A. patient has a hematoma.
    B. spinal cord has been injured.
    C. cervical spine has been displaced.
    D. back has not been seriously injured.

38. Your patient is a 4-month-old infant who is awake but appears to be listless and has dry, tented skin. His mother states that he has had a 3-day history of diarrhea. Your treatment should include:
    A. giving two baby bottles of water.
    B. providing prompt transport.
    C. giving oxygen with a nonrebreathing face mask at 4 L/min.
    D. helping the mother give the infant 2 tablespoons of an antidiarrheal medication.

39. How many seconds should each ventilation last when you are using a BVM to ventilate an adult patient?
    A. 1
    B. 2
    C. 3
    D. 4

40. Artificial ventilation for a patient involved in a near-drowning accident should begin as soon as the patient is:
    A. positioned face up.
    B. moved into the ambulance.
    C. pulled from the water and placed on a firm surface.
    D. pulled from the water and placed on a spine board.

41. You are assisting at an emergency home delivery, and the baby's head is delivered still covered by the membranes of the unruptured amniotic sac. What should you do next?
    A. Wait for the sac to break on its own, then clear the baby's nose and mouth.
    B. Leave the sac intact, monitor the baby's vital signs, and provide immediate transport.
    C. Immediately, but carefully, puncture the sac with your gloved fingers, a sterile clamp, or scissors, and clear the baby's nose and mouth.
    D. Wait until the delivery is complete, carefully puncture the sac with your gloved fingers, a sterile clamp, or scissors, and clear the baby's nose and mouth.

42. You are called to the home of a woman who has frostbite. Upon arrival, you find that she is in her warm house, but there is a snowstorm outside. The nearest hospital is one hour away. In this situation, treatment should consist of:
    A. rubbing the affected area with snow.
    B. rubbing the affected area with your warm hands.
    C. attempting active, rapid rewarming.
    D. immersing the affected area in a cold water bath.

43. An unconscious patient with possible spinal injuries seems to have trouble breathing. The patient's chest wall is moving only slightly, but the diaphragm is moving in and out with each breath. These findings suggest that the patient:
    A. needs CPR immediately.
    B. needs ventilations assisted with a BVM and high-flow oxygen.
    C. should be placed in Trendelenburg's position to increase blood flow to the heart.
    D. is breathing normally following trauma, but requires immediate transport.

44. Respiratory distress in a child is suggested by all of the following EXCEPT:
    A. screaming.
    B. nasal flaring.
    C. active exhalation.
    D. seesaw respirations.

45. Assessment of a patient with a low blood glucose level is most likely to reveal which of the following findings?
    A. Salivation, sweating, and diarrhea
    B. Nausea, vomiting, and abdominal pain
    C. Decreased mental status and convulsions
    D. Agitation, mood swings, and cardiac abnormalities

46. A suspected fractured elbow should be immobilized in the position in which it is found because movement may result in:
    A. further injury to the bone.
    B. damage to nerves and blood vessels.
    C. unnecessary increase in pain to the patient.
    D. a separation or dislocation of the elbow joint.

47. You are called to a construction site and find a construction worker buried to midchest in mud from a trench cave-in. Other workers are trying to dig him out. The patient is cyanotic, has a pulse of 128/min, and shallow respirations of 30/min. Given the patient's vital signs, which of the following supplemental oxygen devices would be most appropriate at this time?
    A. Nasal cannula
    B. Simple face mask
    C. Nonrebreathing mask
    D. Bag-valve-mask device

48. You are called to the home of a child who has been injured in a bicycle accident. Upon arrival, you find the child sitting on the porch of his house, about 25' from the accident site. He tells you he skidded on some sand and then fell off the bicycle. He remembers everything that happened and says that he only hurt his knee. You note an abrasion on the knee with a small amount of bleeding. Given the circumstances in this situation, your first concern when assessing the patient is to:
    A. splint the knee injury.
    B. check the capillary refill in the injured extremity.
    C. find and treat all injuries in the order you find them.
    D. focus on finding and treating the most life-threatening injuries.

49. A man is conscious and alert after an automobile crash in which he was the driver. He states that his fingers are tingling and that his shoulders hurt. Your assessment should include:
    A. gently feeling along the spine for any point tenderness.
    B. gently moving the patient's arms, legs, and shoulders to determine the severity of his pain.
    C. asking the patient to move his head from side to side to determine if he has neck pain.
    D. asking the patient to roll and shrug his shoulders in an attempt to determine the severity of his pain.

50. Which of the following is the method of choice for providing artificial ventilation?
    A. Mouth-to-mask ventilation
    B. One-person bag-valve-mask
    C. Two-person bag-valve-mask
    D. Oxygen-powered manually triggered breathing device

51. A teenage boy is successfully resuscitated at the scene after a near-drowning accident. Your next step in caring for the patient is to:
    A. take the patient home.
    B. provide transport to the hospital.
    C. provide transport to the patient's doctor.
    D. advise him to visit his own doctor as soon as possible.

52. When evaluating a patient who complains of a painful left leg, your focused history and physical exam should include assessing:
    A. skin color, temperature, and moisture.
    B. distal pulse rate, sensation, and motor function.
    C. skin color, distal pulse rate, and skin temperature.
    D. deformity, proximal pulse rate, and ability to move.

53. Which of the following is considered a significant mechanism of injury for a child?
    A. A bicycle collision
    B. A fall from higher than 5′
    C. A slow-speed vehicle collision
    D. An abrasion injury of the abdomen

54. The chance to save a patient experiencing cardiac arrest from VF is greater if:
    A. CPR is initiated within 10 minutes.
    B. oxygen and rapid transport are provided.
    C. rapid transport to the hospital is provided.
    D. defibrillation or CPR is initiated within 4 minutes.

55. Your primary responsibility in the initial management of a disruptive patient is to:
    A. make a specific diagnosis.
    B. lecture the patient about the dangers of substance abuse.
    C. take charge of the situation, but protect yourself if necessary.
    D. play along with the patient if he or she sees or hears things that are not real.

56. A man is found unconscious in his car with the window open. His face is severely swollen and he is barely breathing. A law enforcement officer at the scene tells you that he saw the man's car slow down and then park at the side of the road. You should first:
    A. search for an epinephrine kit in the car.
    B. give oxygen and perform an initial assessment.
    C. place cool compresses on his face and provide immediate transport.
    D. check the patient for an embedded insect stinger and then pull it out before providing transport.

57. The primary purpose of the scene size-up is to:
    A. verify if news media have arrived.
    B. ensure the well-being of the EMT-B.
    C. get names and addresses of witnesses.
    D. determine the patient's respiratory rate.

58. Any order from medical control should be:
    A. automatically questioned.
    B. followed immediately as stated.
    C. repeated back word for word and confirmed.
    D. discussed with your partner to ascertain its accuracy.

59. Which of the following statements about the prehospital care report is true?
    A. It is only valuable as a legal document.
    B. It cannot be used for patient billing information.
    C. It helps ensure efficient continuity of patient care.
    D. It is only for the prehospital care provider's information.

60. What is the most important first step when dealing with a patient having a heart attack?
    A. Starting an IV
    B. Initiating CPR
    C. Performing defibrillation
    D. Showing support and a caring attitude

61. Which of the following parts of the body deteriorates the fastest without constant perfusion?
    A. Heart
    B. Liver
    C. Kidneys
    D. Skeletal muscle

62. A patient has severe bleeding from a chest wound, and no dressing or bandage is available. The most appropriate action in this case would be to:
    A. use a pressure point.
    B. use your gloved hand to apply direct pressure.
    C. quickly try to find a bandage, clean cloth, or sanitary napkin.
    D. wash your bare hand with soap and then apply direct pressure.

63. Altered mental status that often accompanies diabetic emergencies is often mistaken for:
    A. a migraine.
    B. alcohol intoxication.
    C. a severed spinal cord.
    D. a swollen or deformed lower extremity.

64. A 5-year-old child requires full spinal immobilization after falling from a tree. As the child is log rolled onto the backboard, you should:
    A. place blanket rolls under the child's knees to prevent the legs from moving.
    B. place a small pillow under the child's head to prevent hyperextension of the neck.
    C. place a rolled towel under the child's neck to prevent hyperextension of the neck.
    D. place padding between the shoulders and the backboard to prevent hyperflexion of the neck.

65. When ventilating a patient with a bag-valve-mask device, you should squeeze the bag until:
    A. it is empty.
    B. the patient's chest rises.
    C. 100% oxygen is delivered.
    D. the patient has spontaneous respirations.

66. A mass-casualty plan should be activated when:
    A. there is more than one patient.
    B. there are as many patients as EMT-Bs.
    C. an incident occurs on a weekend or holiday.
    D. patient needs are greater than the available resources.

67. If use of an AED is indicated and the patient has a pacemaker, you should:
    A. not defibrillate the patient.
    B. place both pads near the pacemaker.
    C. avoid placing the pads over the pacemaker.
    D. place one pad over the pacemaker and the other on the left side of the back.

68. Treatment of a patient who is hyperventilating should include:
    A. reassuring the patient and providing prompt transport.
    B. having the patient breathe into a bag without providing transport.
    C. giving oxygen, having the patient breathe into a bag, and providing transport.
    D. having the patient breathe into a bag, giving reassurance, and providing transport.

69. Chest compressions on a 9-month-old patient should be performed at a depth and rate of:
    A. $\frac{1}{4}$" to $\frac{1}{2}$", at a rate of 140/min.
    B. $\frac{1}{2}$" to 1", at a rate of 100/min.
    C. 1" to 1$\frac{1}{2}$", at a rate of 80 to 100/min.
    D. 1$\frac{1}{2}$" to 2", at a rate of 100 to 120/min.

70. You are called to care for a patient in respiratory distress. He is breathing noisily and coughing. You should consider that the patient is experiencing:
    A. gastric distention.
    B. a cyanotic episode.
    C. a partial airway obstruction.
    D. a complete airway obstruction.

71. The size of the nasopharyngeal airway is determined by measuring from the:
    A. lips to the angle of the jaw.
    B. chin to the angle of the jaw.
    C. tip of the nose to the earlobe.
    D. incisors to the base of the tongue.

72. For the purpose of administering CPR, patients classified as children are between the ages of:
    A. 1 and 3 years.
    B. 1 and 8 years.
    C. 2 and 12 years.
    D. 3 and 6 years.

73. The first question to ask yourself at the scene of a train or bus crash is:
    A. "How severe are the patients' injuries?"
    B. "How many patients are there?"
    C. "What caused the crash?"
    D. "Who will do the triage?"

74. You have been called to the scene of an automobile crash. You should park the ambulance:
    A. alongside the crash site.
    B. 25' from the crash site on the same side of the street.
    C. 50' from the crash site on the opposite side of the street.
    D. 100' from the crash site on the same side of the street.

75. A man is found slumped over the steering wheel, unconscious and making "snoring" sounds, after an automobile crash. The patient's head is turned to the side, and his neck is flexed. The first steps in caring for this patient would be to secure the airway and then:
    A. rotate the head to correct the deformity.
    B. splint the head in the position you found it.
    C. hyperextend the neck to correct the deformity.
    D. attempt manual stabilization and move the head to a neutral, in-line position.

76. During the first stage of labor, you should usually:
    A. prepare for an emergency delivery at home.
    B. have time to transport the woman to the hospital.
    C. help the woman walk around between contractions.
    D. hold the woman's legs together to slow down delivery.

77. The best way to gain the confidence of and effectively communicate with a frightened patient is to:
    A. shout at the patient.
    B. use medical terminology.
    C. let the patient have some time alone.
    D. make and keep eye contact with the patient.

78. If a life-threatening condition, such as an airway obstruction, is found during your initial assessment, you should:
    A. immediately assess the patient's circulation.
    B. note the condition and continue assessment.
    C. give priority to emergency care of the ABCs.
    D. immediately stop your assessment and provide rapid transport.

79. Pale skin generally suggests which of the following underlying problems?
    A. Heat cramps
    B. Poor oxygenation
    C. Liver abnormalities
    D. Inadequate circulation

80. The treatment of partial-thickness burns on the legs of a child should include:
    A. giving oxygen with a nasal cannula at 2 L/min.
    B. covering the burn with dry bandages and clean sheets.
    C. putting the child in ice water to stop the burning process.
    D. asking the caregiver for butter to cover the burn.

81. What are the two main purposes of the oropharyngeal airway?
    A. Prevents airway obstruction and eases suctioning
    B. Prevents airway injury and eases suctioning
    C. Prevents airway obstruction and tachycardia
    D. Prevents aspiration and airway obstruction

82. Which of the following is NOT considered a link in the Chain of Survival?
    A. Bystander CPR
    B. Advanced Cardiac Life Support
    C. Rapid Transport
    D. Early Defibrillation

83. A splint is applied to a patient with a fractured elbow. Five minutes later, the radial pulse in the injured arm is very weak, and the patient states that he has no feeling in the arm. Because the nearest hospital is 30 minutes away, the appropriate course of action would be to:
    A. transport the patient immediately.
    B. position the splinted arm lower than the patient's body.
    C. position the splinted arm higher than the patient's body.
    D. contact medical control for a decision on realigning the limb.

84. Cardiac arrest in children is usually preceded by respiratory arrest, because children:
    A. have large, overdeveloped lungs.
    B. often have long-term, chronic diseases.
    C. consume oxygen two to three times faster than adults.
    D. do not consume much oxygen due to their slower heart rate.

85. Assessment of the patient's airway begins with:
    A. assisting ventilations.
    B. checking capillary perfusion.
    C. noting skin color and temperature.
    D. noting how well the patient responds to the question, "Are you okay?"

86. The use of oxygen in treatment of shock is considered to be:
    A. a routine part of treatment.
    B. of no particular benefit to the patient.
    C. a last resort measure if all other treatment fails.
    D. useful only if the patient has difficulty breathing.

Appendix B

87. As you open the airway of an elderly man who is not breathing, you do not feel, hear, or see any air exchange. You deliver two quick breaths, mouth-to-mask. The patient's chest does not rise, and your breaths meet no resistance, but the patient's stomach inflates with each breath. Your attempts at rescue breathing have not been effective most likely because the:
    A. patient has had a laryngectomy, and the breaths are exiting via the stoma.
    B. patient has an open pneumothorax, and the breaths are exiting via the wound.
    C. seal around the mask is inadequate, and the air is leaking out around the patient's cheeks.
    D. rescue breaths are too fast or too strong, and the air is being forced into the patient's stomach.

88. A 53-year-old man leaps from a third floor apartment window to escape a fire. The man tumbles in midair, but manages to land on his feet. The most appropriate course of action is to first:
    A. assess the patient thoroughly for third-degree burns.
    B. assess and treat the patient for possible lower extremity and spinal fractures.
    C. treat any serious cuts and burns, then transport the patient to the hospital.
    D. ask the patient to come over to the ambulance immediately so he can be examined.

89. You are treating an adult patient in cardiac arrest. The AED advises "no shock." You verify that the patient is still pulseless. Your next step is to:
    A. restart CPR.
    B. shock anyway.
    C. provide immediate transport.
    D. Provide transport and deliver three stacked shocks en route.

90. The first step in caring for a patient who has an airway obstruction without spinal injury is to:
    A. apply a cervical collar.
    B. activate the EMS system.
    C. perform CPR and give supplemental oxygen.
    D. open the mouth using the head-tilt/chin-lift maneuver.

91. A woman has frostbite in both feet after walking several miles in a frozen field. Her feet are white, hard, and cold to touch. Treatment at the scene should include:
    A. rubbing her feet gently with your own warm hands.
    B. trying to restore circulation by helping her walk around.
    C. removing her wet clothing and rubbing her feet briskly with a warm, wet cloth.
    D. removing her wet clothing and covering her feet with dry, sterile dressings.

92. A general impression of a patient is formed to determine:
    A. scene safety.
    B. treatment priority.
    C. transport speed.
    D. response speed.

93. You and your partner are called to the scene of a possible crime. Upon arrival, you find one dead patient and one seriously injured patient. Law enforcement is present. Your initial responsibilities include:
    A. protecting the scene and securing potential evidence.
    B. witnessing bystander statements and assisting law enforcement.
    C. protecting yourself and your partner and providing emergency medical care.
    D. assisting law enforcement with crowd control and providing emergency medical care.

94. You are called to the scene of a crash in which a car with a lone driver has hit a utility pole. Witnesses say that the incident just happened. The driver is not breathing, has no carotid pulse, and has widely dilated pupils. The driver is also being held in an upright position by the steering wheel. An extrication team has been called. To stabilize the patient's vital functions before extrication begins, your first step should be to:
    A. give high-flow oxygen.
    B. gently shake the patient to awaken him.
    C. establish and maintain an open airway.
    D. apply direct pressure to control bleeding.

95. A man trips and falls down a flight of stairs. Upon your arrival, he does not respond to your greeting or questions. The most appropriate initial course of action would be to treat the patient as if he has had a:
    A. spinal injury.
    B. diabetic emergency.
    C. fractured extremity.
    D. reaction to medication.

96. You suspect that a 17-year-old boy has dislocated his shoulder in a game of touch football. The patient is in extreme pain and shouts for you to "do something." Your first step in caring for the patient should be to:
    A. give him pain medication.
    B. give him supplemental oxygen.
    C. immobilize the shoulder in the position you found it.
    D. attempt to reduce the shoulder or "put it back in place."

97. When communicating with an elderly patient, you should:
    A. approach the patient slowly and calmly.
    B. avoid the patient and speak only to family members.
    C. step back to avoid making the patient uncomfortable.
    D. raise your voice to ensure that the patient can hear you.

98. Which of the following conditions can occur if an unconscious patient is given oral glucose?
    A. Shock
    B. Aspiration
    C. Hypotension
    D. Hyperglycemia

99. A man has an open, bleeding gash on his forehead after an automobile crash. To control the bleeding, you should apply:
    A. pressure to the carotid artery.
    B. pressure to the subclavian artery.
    C. a sterile dressing with a snug bandage.
    D. a sterile dressing with a loose bandage.

100. The first step in the management of a patient exhibiting disruptive behavior is to:
    A. call the police.
    B. assess the situation.
    C. give supplemental oxygen.
    D. notify the emergency department.

101. Which pulse should you palpate in an infant to assess the quality of the pulse?
    A. Radial
    B. Carotid
    C. Brachial
    D. Popliteal

102. A teenage girl states that she was stung on the arm and that she knows she is allergic to bee stings. You see a raised, white area on the arm at the site of the sting. To slow the spread of the toxin, you should place which of the following directly over the site?
    A. A cold pack
    B. A warm compress
    C. A constricting band
    D. A saline-moistened dressing

103. The primary rhythm that the AED will advise to shock is:
    A. asystole
    B. supraventricular tachycardia
    C. ventricular tachycardia
    D. ventricular fibrillation

104. The treatment of hypothermia in the field should include:
    A. preventing blood loss.
    B. massaging the patient's extremities.
    C. giving the patient hot coffee to drink.
    D. stabilizing the vital signs and preventing further heat loss.

105. You are at the scene of a hazardous materials incident and are outside of the hazard zone you have established. The HazMat team has not yet arrived. An unconscious patient is lying in the danger area, and the wind is blowing from behind you toward the scene and beyond. You should:
    A. stay upwind of the materials, but remain on site.
    B. evacuate the area and await the arrival of the HazMat team.
    C. enter the zone rapidly with the wind at your back, and quickly remove the patient.
    D. approach the patient and provide only life-saving care until the HazMat team can arrive and decontaminate you both.

106. What is the most serious underlying problem that must be addressed during the initial assessment of a patient with a severe facial injury?
    A. Fracture of facial bones
    B. Injury to the lumbar spine
    C. Possible hypovolemic shock
    D. Partial or complete upper airway obstruction

107. Nitroglycerin helps a patient with chest pain by:
    A. causing coronary vasoconstriction.
    B. increasing the blood pressure.
    C. dilating the coronary arteries.
    D. relieving anxiety.

108. A 3-year-old child is found at the bottom of an ice-covered pond after being submerged for about 15 minutes. The patient is not breathing and has no palpable pulse. The most appropriate course of action would be to:
    A. pronounce the child dead.
    B. begin full resuscitation efforts.
    C. wrap the child in blankets and give back blows.
    D. give supplemental oxygen and begin rewarming.

109. How does the heart get more blood when it is working hard?
    A. The aorta constricts.
    B. The heart beats faster.
    C. The coronary arteries dilate.
    D. The pulmonary vascular resistance increases.

110. The first step in treating a patient with a head injury is to:
    A. control bleeding.
    B. immobilize the patient's head.
    C. establish and maintain an airway.
    D. check for and stabilize any cervical spine injuries.

111. You are ventilating a patient with a stoma and air is escaping from the mouth and nose. To prevent this, you should:
    A. use less pressure.
    B. suction the stoma.
    C. suction the breathing tube.
    D. seal the mouth and pinch the nostrils.

112. You are treating a 55-year-old unconscious male who was found outside of his home in a snow bank. It is unknown how long he has been down. You suspect he is suffering from severe hypothermia. Based on this information, you would expect his pulse to be:
    A. Tachycardic
    B. Bradycardic
    C. Bounding
    D. Over 140/90

113. Which of the following conditions is considered the most serious?
    A. Asystole
    B. Atrial fibrillation
    C. Ventricular fibrillation
    D. Ventricular tachycardia

114. Use of a police escort may be a dangerous practice in an intersection because:
    A. bystanders could gather to watch and cause traffic problems.
    B. too many emergency vehicles with sirens and lights could cause motorists to panic.
    C. trying to move two emergency vehicles through congested traffic is more difficult than one and may take much time.
    D. a motorist seeing the police car pass might assume it is the only emergency vehicle and could proceed, hitting the ambulance.

115. Your care of a premature baby should include:
    A. keeping the baby cool.
    B. removing the clamp on the umbilical cord.
    C. keeping the mouth and nose clear of mucus.
    D. directing a stream of oxygen directly into the baby's mouth.

116. A young boy with a severe soft-tissue injury to the leg has rather extensive bleeding, which has frightened him. The best way to control the bleeding in this situation is to apply:
    A. a conventional tourniquet.
    B. pressure to the femoral artery.
    C. direct pressure with a dry, sterile dressing.
    D. a blood pressure cuff to act as a tourniquet.

117. The proper method to perform chest compressions on an infant is the thumb-encircling technique or with:
   A. Two fingers placed on the xiphoid process.
   B. Two fingers placed on the lower half of the sternum.
   C. The heel of one hand placed at midsternum.
   D. The heel of one hand placed on the lower sternum.

118. A woman who is having her third baby tells you she must move her bowels. The most appropriate step would be to:
   A. provide prompt transport because there is still plenty of time before the delivery.
   B. ask her if she is about to deliver, and if she says no, provide prompt transport.
   C. provide immediate transport because it is always safer to deliver at the hospital.
   D. prepare to deliver the baby at the scene, because delivery is about to occur.

119. When obtaining a history from a diabetic patient, you should ask which of the following questions in addition to the SAMPLE history?
   A. "Are you allergic to insulin?"
   B. "What kind of insulin do you take?"
   C. "Have you taken your insulin today?"
   D. "How long have you been a diabetic?"

120. You are called to a scene of a one-vehicle car crash in which a car has crashed into a utility pole. Your scene size-up reveals that you have one patient. The patient is lying partially out of the car with one leg on the ground. You also note two power lines have fallen and have landed on the car. The fire department removes the patient from the vehicle. Your initial assessment reveals that the patient is pulseless, apneic, and unresponsive. You should immediately:
   A. perform CPR for one minute and reassess the patient.
   B. apply the AED and defibrillate the patient if a shock is advised.
   C. apply high-flow oxygen with a non-rebreathing mask (with c-spine precautions).
   D. apply a splint to the injured leg and perform a focused history and physical exam.

121. If you discover an error as you are writing the patient report, you should:
   A. erase the error and rewrite the correct information.
   B. draw the error to the attention of your supervisor, but do not change the form.
   C. draw a line through the error, initial it, and write the correct information next to the error.
   D. cover the incorrect information with correction fluid, initial it, and write the correct information in the corrected area.

122. What is the proper ratio of compressions to ventilations for two-rescuer adult CPR prior to an advanced airway (endrotracheal intubation, multi-lumen airway, etc) being established?
   A. 5:1
   B. 1:5
   C. 15:2
   D. Once every 5 seconds.

123. When evaluating a patient who complains of chest pain, you should find out when the pain began, what caused it, what it feels like, if it is radiating and to where, how severe it is, and whether the:
   A. pain causes nausea.
   B. pain is constant or intermittent.
   C. patient is under the influence of alcohol.
   D. patient was able to call for the ambulance.

124. Which of the following patients would be the highest priority in a triage situation?
   A. A 24-year-old man with a deformed lumbar spine and paralyzed legs
   B. A 26-year-old woman with multiple lacerations, no pulse, and no respirations
   C. A 32-year-old woman with bilateral deformed femurs and no signs of shock
   D. A 35-year-old man who is unconscious and has a significant head laceration

125. What is the most common cause of airway obstruction in an unconscious 27-year-old patient?
   A. Vomit in the mouth
   B. The tongue
   C. Blood clots
   D. The food found in the mouth

126. You have responded to the scene of a crash where a bystander who claims to have medical credentials becomes difficult to manage. You should:
    A. inform medical control immediately.
    B. inform law enforcement immediately.
    C. flatly tell the bystander to leave or he may be arrested.
    D. let the bystander take over patient care as he has higher medical credentials.

127. You should NOT assist with nitroglycerin if the patient:
    A. is older than 80 years.
    B. took a pill 5 minutes earlier.
    C. has a heart rate over 100 beats per minute.
    D. has a systolic blood pressure of less than 100 mm Hg.

128. A traffic light turns red as the ambulance on an emergency call is approaching an intersection. There are no vehicles in front of the ambulance. You should:
    A. sound the siren, maintain speed, and proceed.
    B. bypass the traffic light by turning into a side street.
    C. stop, sound the siren if necessary, and proceed when safe.
    D. turn off the lights and siren and wait for the light to change.

129. A patient who has just had a severe asthma attack is now very sleepy. This may indicate that the patient:
    A. may stop breathing.
    B. does not need transport.
    C. has recovered from the attack.
    D. is probably having a drug reaction.

130. The principal goal in treatment of heat-related emergencies is to:
    A. provide rapid transport.
    B. make the patient comfortable.
    C. replace lost fluids with salt water.
    D. reduce the patient's body temperature.

131. You are called to a scene where a 5-year-old child has ingested a poison. The child is awake and responsive. You should first:
    A. consult medical control.
    B. give the child syrup of ipecac.
    C. give the child activated charcoal.
    D. give the child an injection of epinephrine.

132. You should assist with delivery of the baby's head by:
    A. placing one hand at the top of the head and the other in back.
    B. maintaining finger pressure against the center of the baby's skull.
    C. placing the palm of your hand firmly against the back of the baby's skull.
    D. placing the flats of your fingers on the bony part of the skull and exerting very gentle pressure on it.

133. Shivering in the presence of hypothermia indicates that the:
    A. muscular system is damaged.
    B. nerve endings are damaged, causing loss of muscle control.
    C. body is trying to generate more heat through muscular activity.
    D. circulatory system is impaired, and the body cannot maintain its temperature.

134. The driver in a one-car crash has no apparent injuries, but is acting unruly. A half-full whiskey bottle is lying on the passenger seat. The appropriate course of action would be to:
    A. assume that the driver is drunk.
    B. ask bystanders to help you restrain the driver.
    C. let law enforcement officials handle the matter.
    D. assess the situation to determine why the driver is acting unruly.

135. You are called to an apartment where two men have been fighting and one has been stabbed. You should:
    A. put on body armor before entering the apartment.
    B. enter the apartment and attempt to grab the knife from the man.
    C. enter the apartment and begin treating the patient who was stabbed.
    D. remain outside, evaluate the potential for violence, and call for help from law enforcement.

136. What is the proper ratio of compressions to ventilations for one-rescuer adult CPR?
    A. 1:5
    B. 2:15
    C. 5:1
    D. 15:2

Appendix B

137. A woman who is having her first child is having contractions 2 minutes apart. You should:
    A. prepare to deliver the baby at the scene.
    B. examine for crowning before deciding whether to transport.
    C. provide slow transport while monitoring the woman's vital signs.
    D. place the woman in Trendelenburg's position and provide immediate transport.

138. Which of the following conditions may develop as a result of severe hypothermia?
    A. Jaundice
    B. Cardiac arrhythmia
    C. Congestive heart failure
    D. Cerebrovascular accident

139. Which of the following signs strongly suggests early stages of shock in a child?
    A. Delayed capillary refill time
    B. Systolic blood pressure of less than 50 mm Hg
    C. Diastolic blood pressure of less than 50 mm Hg
    D. A combined blood pressure of less than 100 mm Hg

140. Which of the following is NOT an important consideration when caring for a patient believed to have ingested or been exposed to a poison?
    A. Type of substance
    B. Time of ingestion/exposure
    C. Amount of substance ingested
    D. What kind of food was eaten last

141. A man is cut above the ankle by a lawn mower blade. If the bleeding cannot be controlled with direct pressure, you should apply pressure on which of the following arteries?
    A. Dorsalis pedis
    B. Subclavian
    C. Temporal
    D. Femoral

142. When caring for a patient with a suspected extremity fracture, you should:
    A. move the limb across the body to provide support.
    B. move the limb to determine the severity of the fracture.
    C. splint the part first, then control bleeding in open fractures.
    D. splint the part in the position you find it, whenever possible.

143. A newborn is not breathing on its own shortly after delivery. The one-minute APGAR is 4. The next action to care for this newborn would be to:
    A. begin CPR.
    B. suction the mouth and nose.
    C. stimulate the newborn with gentle shaking.
    D. assist ventilations with a BVM at a rate of 60/minute.

144. Signs of internal bleeding include:
    A. increased pulse rate and warm skin.
    B. increased pulse rate and clammy skin.
    C. reduced pulse rate and dilated pupils.
    D. reduced pulse rate and a soft abdomen.

145. To help a patient in shock maintain adequate blood flow and oxygen supply to the heart and brain, you should:
    A. tilt the entire body up at the head.
    B. elevate the lower extremities 6″ to 12″.
    C. elevate the upper part of the body 6″ to 12″.
    D. elevate the lower extremities and trunk of the body.

146. After applying both a dressing and a bandage to a laceration below the elbow, you should check for signs of impaired circulation in the patient's:
    A. neck.
    B. elbow.
    C. fingers.
    D. shoulder.

147. A 17-year-old boy is found unconscious, floating facedown in a swimming pool. You and your partner should first:
    A. roll him over as a unit and then place him on a backboard.
    B. roll him over as a unit, extend his neck to open the airway, and then prepare to float a backboard under him.
    C. place him on a backboard in a facedown position, then remove him from the pool.
    D. stabilize his neck and back with your hands while you and your partner roll him over as a unit and then establish an open airway.

148. What is the absolute minimum information that you should obtain from the dispatcher while you are en route to the scene of an emergency?
    A. Whether or not the scene is safe
    B. The number of patients and their locations
    C. The nature of the call and the number of patients
    D. The nature and location of the call

Answers

1. **C.** A child's nose and mouth are much smaller than that of an adult. The larynx, cricoid cartilage, and trachea are smaller and softer as well. This makes the mechanics of breathing much more delicate.

2. **C.** Your first responsibility at the scene is your own safety and the safety of others.

3. **D.** When trying to manage a disruptive patient, you should keep your eyes on the patient at all times and be alert for aggressive behavior.

4. **B.** The normal pulse rate for a child is 80 to 100 beats per minute.

5. **B.** In this case, audible coughing is a good sign. With a partial obstruction, the patient is able to exchange some air, but breathing is noisy and the patient may be coughing. Your main concern is to prevent a partial airway obstruction from becoming a complete airway obstruction.

6. **B.** Off-line medical direction is delivered to the EMT-B by protocols or standing orders. Online medical direction occurs when the EMT-B talks to directly to medical control via radio or telephone from the scene.

7. **A.** A competent patient has the right to refuse treatment. The EMT-B should explain to the patient why transportation to the hospital for treatment is advisable. However, the EMT-B in this case must respect the patient's wishes if she refuses treatment. In any case of patient refusal, the EMT-B should follow local protocols.

8. **C.** You would not expect to find paradoxical motion with an extremity injury. Paradoxical motion is chest movement in the opposite direction of the normal rise and fall of breathing.

9. **B.** Gloves and eye protection are the minimum standard for all patient care if there is any possibility for exposure to blood or body fluids. These are part of the body substance isolation techniques you should follow whenever exposure to blood or other body fluids is possible.

10. **D.** The purpose of Critical Incident Stress Debriefing (CISD) is to help emergency medical personnel relieve personal and group anxieties and stress. These debriefings should not be dismissed as trivial or nonessential.

11. **B.** For child CPR, the chest should be compressed 1" to 1½", at a rate of at least 100/min.

12. **D.** Confidential information cannot be disclosed without permission from the patient or a court order. The EMT-B should not comment on the condition of any patient, except to report to the hospital or to turn the patient over to equally or better trained health care professionals.

13. **C.** Serious gastric distension is dangerous, as it causes the patient to vomit during CPR. It can also reduce lung volume by elevating the diaphragm.

14. **A.** The best way to estimate skin temperature is to place the back of your hand on the patient's skin.

15. **D.** The state of the pupils, especially any progressive change, is a rapid reflection of central nervous system injury or disease.

16. **C.** If you begin CPR in the field, you must continue unless one of the following occurs: the patient starts breathing and has a pulse; the patient is transferred to a higher medical authority; you are out of strength or too fatigued to continue; or a physician present assumes responsibility for the patient.

17. **B.** With infants and children, full cardiac arrest results from respiratory arrest. If uncorrected, respiratory arrest will lead to cardiac arrest and death.

18. **C.** Expressed consent occurs when the patient expressly authorizes you to provide care or transport to the hospital. Expressed consent may take the form of words, a nod of agreement, or other expressions of approval.

19. **D.** With respiratory depression or arrest, there is little or no movement of the chest and abdomen. There is also little or no airflow felt or heard at the nose and mouth.

20. **C.** The only time your attention should be directed away from initial assessment of the patient is when the patient's life or your life is in immediate danger.

21. **B.** When dealing with emotionally disturbed patients, the best legal situation is to try to obtain the patient's consent to medical treatment. This may be difficult, since these patients often resist treatment or try to threaten you. If the patient presents a threat to self or others, you can legally care for, and even restrain, the patient against his or her will.

Appendix B

22. **D.** When presented with a prolapsed umbilical cord, you should place the woman in Trendelenburg's position, carefully insert your gloved finger into the vagina, and then gently push the baby's head away from the umbilical cord.

23. **A.** The usual dosage for a child is 1 g of activated charcoal per kilogram of body weight, to a maximum of 12.5 to 25 g.

24. **D.** You should assume that the parents would give consent for treatment.

25. **B.** A patient with a dislocated knee will be in extreme pain. If the patient has strong distal pulses in the injured leg, splint the knee in the position in which you found it.

26. **C.** Normal systolic blood pressure in an adult male patient is 100 mm Hg plus the patient's age, up to 150 mm Hg.

27. **A.** Rate, quality, and rhythm should all be assessed when evaluating respirations.

28. **A.** Most infectious diseases are spread by surface contact; therefore, handwashing remains a most effective way to prevent the spread of disease.

29. **C.** Normal respiratory rate for the adult patient is 12 to 20 times a minute. Adequate breathing includes a normal rate, normal skin vitals (pink, warm, dry), and occurs without accessory muscle use.

30. **D.** As triage officer, you must remain at the scene to coordinate prioritized patient care. The triage officer should not become involved in patient care. An incident commander, transport officer, and others will be identified, as needed, depending on the scope of the problem. Leaving the scene, even with a critical patient, defeats the concept of continuity of care and breaks down the command process.

31. **B.** Air pressure within the thorax decreases at the onset of inhalation. Air then moves from the outside into the trachea and fills the lungs.

32. **D.** Except in cases where an emergency rapid extrication is warranted by the patient's condition or safety concerns at the scene, appropriate patient care should be provided before removing the patient from the vehicle. In this case, performing the initial assessment and stabilizing the vital functions should be done before extrication.

33. **D.** The normal respiratory rate for an infant is approximately 25 to 50 breaths per minute.

34. **B.** Wheezing is described as an audible, high-pitched breath sound usually resulting from a blockage of the smaller air passages.

35. **B.** Two-person BVM is more effective than one-person BVM. It is very difficult for one EMT-B to maintain a proper seal between the mask and face with one hand while getting adequate air into the patient with the other hand.

36. **D.** The proper sized oropharyngeal airway is determined by measuring from the corner of the mouth to the earlobe.

37. **B.** In this situation, it is likely that the patient has sustained spinal injuries because the patient does not feel pain in the extremities.

38. **B.** Dehydration may cause shock in infants and children. Therefore, prompt transport is necessary.

39. **B.** When ventilating an adult patient with a BVM, the ventilation should be delivered over 2 seconds, this assures adequate tidal volume and will decrease the amount of gastric distention.

40. **A.** Artificial ventilation for a patient involved in a near-drowning accident should begin as soon as possible, even before you remove the patient from the water.

41. **C.** If the baby's head is still covered by the membranes of the amniotic sac after delivery, you must break the membranes immediately to prevent suffocation. You should then clear the baby's nose and mouth and complete the delivery.

42. **C.** For the situation where prompt hospital care is not available, you should attempt active, rapid rewarming.

43. **B.** An unconscious patient who is seen breathing with the diaphragm rather than with the chest muscles has likely sustained a severe spinal injury. When the diaphragm is unable to substitute for the chest muscles, the patient is likely to have respiratory difficulty. Therefore, you should assist ventilations with a BVM and high-flow oxygen.

44. **A.** A child in respiratory distress will show all the signs listed except screaming. In order to scream, a child must be breathing well and have a respiratory reserve.

45. **C.** Decreased level of consciousness is the most common sign of low blood glucose levels. Seizures or convulsions may also occur at a later time.

46. **B.** A fractured elbow should be immobilized in the position in which it is found because movement may result in damage to nerves and blood vessels.

47. **C.** A nonrebreathing mask would be the most beneficial to this patient. Patients breathing fewer than 12 breaths/min or more than 24 breaths/min are not breathing adequately. Fast, shallow breathing does not allow for adequate exchange of air and carbon dioxide in the alveoli. The nonrebreathing mask is capable of providing up to 95% inspired oxygen.

48. **D.** Even though the patient's injuries appear only minor, your primary concern is to find and/or rule out any obvious or hidden life-threatening injuries. Only after you have completed this step can you direct your attention to less serious problems.

49. **A.** A patient who is conscious and complaining of shoulder pain and tingling in the extremities should be treated for possible spinal injuries. Your assessment should include gently feeling along the spine for any point tenderness. To prevent further injury, you should not ask the patient to move the head, neck, or extremities.

50. **A.** The four methods for providing artificial ventilation by an EMT-B, in order of preference, are mouth-to-mask ventilation, two-person bag-valve-mask, oxygen-powered manually triggered breathing device, and one-person bag-valve-mask.

51. **B.** You must provide transport of all patients involved in near-drowning accidents. Even if initial resuscitation in the field appears completely successful, the patient can still aspirate fluids. This may result in complications lasting days or weeks.

52. **B.** During the focused physical exam, assess for DCAP-BTLS on both legs and check for PMS (pulse, motor, and sensory function). Compare the results of your exam on both legs.

53. **A.** Falls greater than 10′ for children, as well as bicycle collisions and medium-speed vehicle collisions, are considered significant mechanisms of injury.

54. **D.** The best results in resuscitating patients who have sudden cardiac death include rapid BLS (within 4 minutes) and ready availability of defibrillation.

55. **C.** Your primary responsibility in the initial management of a disruptive patient is to take charge of the situation and to be mindful of your personal safety.

56. **B.** If a patient seems to be having an allergic reaction, you should give oxygen as you complete the initial assessment. Next, obtain baseline vital signs and, if the patient is conscious, a SAMPLE history.

57. **B.** In addition to beginning the process of gathering important patient information, the scene size-up is also your first real opportunity to evaluate whether the environment is safe so that you can begin caring for the patient. If the scene is unsafe, this is the time to make it safe before entering.

58. **C.** Once you receive an order from medical control, you must repeat the order back word for word and then receive confirmation.

59. **C.** Prehospital care reports help to ensure efficient continuity of patient care. This report describes the nature of the patient's injuries or illness at the scene and the initial treatment you provide.

60. **D.** Providing support and reassurance to the patient will help reduce anxiety. This will also physically help the patient because fear can stimulate the heart and make matters worse.

61. **A.** The heart needs constant perfusion in order to function properly. Without adequate perfusion, it will deteriorate much more quickly than the liver, kidneys, or skeletal muscle. No part of the body can tolerate inadequate perfusion indefinitely.

62. **B.** Use your gloved hand to apply direct pressure. Do not waste valuable time washing or looking for a dressing of any kind.

63. **B.** Altered mental status associated with diabetes has often been mistaken for alcohol or drug intoxication.

64. **D.** As you log roll a child onto an immobilization device, make sure you place padding under the child's shoulders to prevent hyperflexion of the neck.

65. **B.** After positioning the BVM device on the patient, you should hold the mask in place while your partner squeezes the bag with two hands until the patient's chest rises.

66. **D.** A mass-casualty or multiple-casualty plan should be invoked whenever patient needs are greater than available resources. Depending on the severity of the injuries, this may involve as few as two or three patients, or as many as nine or ten.

67. **C.** Defibrillator pads should not be placed over or near a pacemaker.

68. **A.** Reassurance remains the best way to treat hyperventilation. Breathing into a bag may be dangerous. Because there usually is a cause for the hyperventilation, the patient should be transported to the hospital for evaluation.

69. **B.** For infant CPR, the chest should be compressed ½″ to 1″, at a rate of at least 100/min.

70. **C.** A patient with a partial airway obstruction will have some degree of respiratory distress, but will probably be able to cough and breathe noisily.

71. **C.** The proper sized nasopharyngeal airway is determined by measuring from the tip of the nose to the earlobe.

72. **B.** For the purposes of BLS, patients classified as children are between the ages of 1 and 8 years.

73. **B.** The first question to be answered at the scene of a multiple-casualty incident is, "How many patients are there?" Once that is determined, additional resources can be summoned immediately. Triage should be started by the most experienced EMT on the scene, and assessing the severity of injuries will be a function of the triage and treatment process. Determinations of what caused the crash are left to the proper investigating agencies.

74. **D.** When responding to an accident, the ambulance should be parked about 100′ from the accident on the same side of the street.

75. **D.** The patient's "snoring" sounds indicate an airway problem. Therefore, you should secure the airway and then hold the head still, in a neutral, in-line position, until it can be fully immobilized.

76. **B.** If the woman is in the first stage of labor, you usually have enough time to transport her to the hospital.

77. **D.** The best way to communicate with a frightened patient is to make and keep eye contact in order to help the patient keep calm.

78. **C.** Priority is always given to the emergency care of the ABCs. When a life-threatening condition is found, such as an airway obstruction, you should provide emergency care immediately—clear the obstruction and maintain the airway before moving on to assessing breathing.

79. **D.** Pale skin indicates inadequate circulation. Poor oxygenation will usually cause cyanosis, liver problems produce a jaundiced skin color, and a flushed skin color is often seen with heat cramps.

80. **B.** A burn destroys the patient's protective skin layer, and covering the skin with dry bandages and clean sheets helps minimize the risk of infection.

81. **A.** The oropharyngeal airway prevents obstruction of the airway, primarily from the tongue. It also makes it easier to suction the airway.

82. **C.** The links in the Chain of Survival include early access to EMS, early (bystander) CPR, early defibrillation, and early ACLS.

83. **D.** The appropriate course of action in this situation would be to contact medical control for a decision on realigning the limb.

84. **C.** Since children consume oxygen two to three times faster than adults, cardiac arrest is usually secondary to hypoxia and ischemia of the heart.

85. **D.** Assessment of the patient's airway begins with the evaluation of the patient's level of consciousness. Level of consciousness is assessed by the patient's response to the question, "Are you okay?"

86. **A.** Oxygen should be given to all patients in shock.

87. **D.** Blowing too fast or too vigorously can cause air to enter the esophagus and stomach rather than the trachea. This will cause inflation of the stomach (gastric distention) rather than the lungs.

88. **B.** In this situation, you should suspect impacted fractures of the lower extremities and possible fractures of the spine.

89. **A.** CPR should be performed on all pulseless patients. CPR (for one minute) is indicated whenever the AED analyzes and gives a "no shock advised" and the patient is assessed to be pulseless.

90. **D.** The first step in determining why an airway is obstructed is to open the patient's mouth using the head tilt-chin lift maneuver. You should always take care to protect the neck in a trauma situation, but remember that the priority is always the airway.

91. **D.** When treating a patient with frostbite, you should remove any wet clothing and cover the injured area with a dry cloth or dry, sterile dressings. Do not break any blisters, and do not apply heat or try to rewarm the area.

92. **B.** The general impression formed by the EMT-B determines the priority in treating the patient.

93. **C.** Your primary responsibility is always to protect yourself and to provide emergency medical care. When a crime is involved, it is important to make every effort to preserve the crime scene and protect any evidence while still providing appropriate prehospital care.

94. **C.** In this situation, although the patient appears to be dead, you must establish an open airway and attempt to ventilate so that you can begin effective CPR as soon as possible.

95. **A.** You should assume a spinal injury with any patient who is unresponsive. After checking the head and cervical spine for deformities, the cervical spine should then be immobilized.

96. **C.** A patient with a dislocated shoulder will be in extreme pain; therefore, immobilization is difficult. You should immobilize the shoulder in the position that is most comfortable for the patient. Never attempt to reduce or "put back in place" the shoulder.

97. **A.** Approach an elderly patient slowly and calmly. Allow plenty of time for the patient to respond to your questions.

98. **B.** When oral glucose is properly given, placing it between the cheek and gum of a conscious patient who is able to swallow and protect the airway, there are no side effects. However, if given to a patient who is unconscious or unable to swallow, aspiration can occur.

99. **C.** Bleeding from a wound should be treated with direct pressure from your gloved hand or with a pressure dressing. Once the bleeding has been controlled, you should firmly wrap a sterile roller bandage around the wound to maintain the pressure.

100. **B.** The first step in the management of a patient exhibiting disruptive behavior is to assess the situation.

101. **C.** The brachial pulse is the easiest to access and evaluate in an infant.

102. **A.** To slow the spread of the toxin from a bee sting, you should apply ice or cold packs to the injected site, but not directly on the skin.

103. **D.** Ventricular fibrillation (chaotic electrical activity) is the primary rhythm that the AED is designed to analyze for and to advise to shock (defibrillate). Most AED units will advise to shock a ventricular tachycardia rhythm that is faster than 180 beats per minute. The AED will not advise to shock the rhythm asystole or supraventricular tachycardia.

104. **D.** Management of hypothermia in the field focuses on stabilizing the vital signs, preventing further heat loss, and providing prompt transport.

105. **A.** Stay upwind (and uphill, when applicable) of the hazardous material, but remain on site to protect others from entering the area. Await the arrival of properly trained and equipped HazMat technicians, and NEVER knowingly enter a hazard zone without the proper protection and training.

106. **D.** The most serious underlying problem associated with a facial injury is partial or complete upper airway obstruction.

107. **C.** Nitroglycerin causes dilation of the blood vessels in the heart and elsewhere. You should watch the blood pressure closely after giving nitroglycerin.

108. **B.** Never give up on resuscitating a drowning victim. Submersion in very cold water will produce hypothermia and lower the metabolic rate, which protects the vital organs from lack of oxygen. Once the child has been removed from the water, you should begin full resuscitation efforts.

109. **C.** When the heart is working hard, the coronary arteries dilate. Oxygen-rich blood from the aorta can then nourish the heart.

110. **C.** Establishing and maintaining an airway is the first step in treating a patient with a head injury.

111. **D.** A stoma is a permanent opening in the neck that connects the trachea directly to the skin. When ventilating a patient with a stoma, the air will leak out. To prevent this, you must seal the mouth and pinch the nostrils and then ventilate through the stoma. Release the patient's mouth and nostrils for exhalation.

112. **B.** Patients suffering from severe hypothermia will present with an altered mental status, decreased respirations and a decreased pulse (bradycardia).

113. **A.** Atrial fibrillation, ventricular tachycardia, and ventricular fibrillation all involve some activity of the heart muscle. Asystole does not. A heart that has no activity will probably not recover, despite BLS and ALS.

114. **D.** Use of a police escort may be dangerous in an intersection because a motorist hearing a siren and seeing the police car pass may assume that only one emergency vehicle is passing. The motorist may then proceed into the intersection and possibly hit the ambulance.

115. **C.** Your care of a premature baby should include keeping the mouth and nose clear of mucus.

116. **C.** The best way to control bleeding in an extremity injury to a child is to apply direct pressure with a dry, sterile dressing.

117. **B.** To perform chest compressions on an infant, place both of your thumbs on the lower half of the sternum when you are using the thumb-encircling technique. When using two fingers to provide compressions, proper location is still over the lower half of the sternum (approximately one fingerbreadth below the nipple line).

118. **D.** If a woman who has had a child tells you she feels as if she must move her bowels, you should prepare to deliver the baby at the scene. The baby's head is pressing on her rectum and delivery is about to occur.

119. **C.** When called to the scene of a diabetic emergency, you should ask the patient or his or her family if insulin had been taken that day, whether a meal had been missed, if the patient had vomited after a meal, and whether the patient had done any strenuous exercise.

120 **B.** The longer a patient remains in ventricular fibrillation, the less likely that he or she can be resuscitated successfully or without serious long-term neurologic problems. Since this patient is already in ventricular fibrillation, she has most likely been fibrillating for some time and will need to be shocked as soon as possible.

121. **C.** If you discover errors as you are writing a report, draw a single horizontal line through the error, initial it, and write the correct information next to it.

122. **C.** The proper ratio of compressions to ventilations for two-rescuer adult CPR is 5:1.

123. **B.** Pertinent information to gather when evaluating a patient experiencing pain follows the OPQRST mnemonic: Onset, Provoke, Quality, Radiation, Severity, and Time. Whether the pain is constant or intermittent falls into the time category.

124. **D.** Unconsciousness qualifies as a first priority condition, while back injuries and bone or joint injuries are second priority. The pulseless patient is dead, which is considered the lowest priority.

125. **B.** In an unconscious patient, the tongue and throat tissues relax causing the airway to be obstructed.

126. **A.** Each EMS service should have a protocol for dealing with bystanders who are physicians. Not all physicians are trained in emergency medical care. Medical control may be able to communicate with the physician and help eliminate some problems.

127. **D.** Do not give nitroglycerin to a patient with a systolic blood pressure of less than 100 mm Hg. Nitroglycerin may further lower the pressure.

128. **C.** When the ambulance approaches a red light at an intersection and there is no traffic in front of it, the driver should stop at the light, sound the siren, and proceed when certain that the intersection is clear.

129. **A.** A patient having a severe asthma episode could become exhausted. This may mean that the patient may soon stop breathing.

130. **D.** The principal goal in treatment of heat exposure is to reduce the patient's body temperature.

131. **A.** Consult medical control first when caring for an alert child who has ingested a poison. You should discuss with medical control the possibility of giving activated charcoal.

132. **D.** Assist with delivery of the baby's head by placing the flats of your fingers on the bony part of the skull as it emerges and then exert very gentle pressure. Avoid pressing your fingers into the baby's fontanels.

133. **C.** Shivering in the presence of hypothermia indicates that the body is trying to generate more heat through muscular activity.

134. **D.** The appropriate course of action in this situation would be to assess the scene to determine why the driver is being disruptive. Do not "write off" the unruly or abusive patient as "just another drunk."

135. **D.** Whenever you are in doubt about your safety, do not put yourself at risk. Never enter an unstable environment. As part of your scene size-up, evaluate the potential for violence. If it is a possibility, call for additional help. Rely on the advice of law enforcement.

136. **D.** The proper ratio of compressions to ventilations for one-rescuer adult CPR is 15:2.

137. **B.** You should examine for crowning before deciding whether there is time to transport when a woman expecting her first child is having contractions 2 minutes apart.

138. **B.** One result of severe hypothermia, a core temperature of 80°F (27°C), is the possibility of cardiac arrhythmia.

139. **A.** Delayed capillary refill time in a peripheral extremity strongly suggests early stages of shock in a child.

140. **D.** When caring for a patient believed to have ingested or been exposed to a poison, determining what kind of food was eaten last is not an important consideration. Factors to consider are the type of substance, the time of ingestion/exposure, the amount of substance ingested, the amount of time exposed, and the weight of the patient.

141. **D.** Since the bleeding is above the ankle, you should use the femoral pressure point, which is proximal to the wound.

142. **D.** You should splint a suspected extremity fracture in the position in which you found it, whenever possible.

143. **B.** The first step in caring for a newborn who is not breathing spontaneously is to suction the mouth and nose.

144. **B.** An increased pulse rate and clammy skin suggest possible internal bleeding.

145. **B.** Elevation of the lower extremities increases the amount of blood available to the chest and head.

146. **C.** Once the dressing and bandage are applied, check for signs of impaired circulation or loss of sensation in the patient's fingers.

147. **D.** The first step in caring for a patient who is found unconscious, floating facedown in a pool, is for you and your partner to stabilize the patient's neck and back with your hands. You should then roll him over as a unit and establish an airway while you are still in the water.

148. **D.** The minimum information that should be obtained from the dispatcher is the location of the scene and the general nature of the situation. The dispatcher cannot reliably advise you of the scene's safety until you arrive and can survey the area yourself.

Glossary

abandonment   Unilateral termination of care by the EMT-B without the patient's consent and without making provisions for transferring care to another medical professional with skills at the same level or higher.

abdomen   The body cavity that contains the major organs of digestion and excretion.

abdominal-thrust maneuver   The preferred method to dislodge and force food or other material from the throat of a choking victim; also called the Heimlich maneuver.

abduction   Motion of a limb away from the midline.

abortion   Delivery of the fetus and placenta before 20 weeks; miscarriage.

abrasion   Loss or damage of the superficial layer of skin as a result of a body part rubbing or scraping across a rough or hard surface.

absence seizure   Seizure that may be characterized by a brief lapse of attention in which the patient may stare and does not respond. Also known as petit mal seizure.

absorption   The process by which medications travel through body tissues until they reach the bloodstream.

acceleration   The process of increasing speed.

access   The ability to gain entry to an enclosed area and reach a patient.

accessory muscles   The secondary muscles of respiration.

acetabulum   The depression on the lateral pelvis where its three component bones join, in which the femoral head fits snugly.

acidosis   A pathologic condition resulting from the accumulation of acids in the body.

acromioclavicular (A/C) joint   A simple joint where the bony projections of the scapula and the clavicle meet at the top of the shoulder.

action   The therapeutic effect of a medication on the body.

activated charcoal   An oral medication that binds and adsorbs ingested toxins in the gastrointestinal tract, for treatment of some poisonings and medication overdoses. Charcoal ground into a very fine powder that provides the greatest possible surface area for binding medications that have been taken by mouth; it is carried on the EMS unit.

activities of daily living (ADL)   The basic activities a person usually accomplishes during a normal day, such as eating, dressing, and washing.

acute abdomen   A condition of sudden onset of pain within the abdomen, usually indicating peritonitis; demands immediate medical or surgical treatment.

acute myocardial infarction (AMI)   Heart attack; death of heart muscle following obstruction of blood flow to it. Acute in this context means "new" or "happening right now."

Adam's apple   The firm prominence in the upper part of the larynx formed by the thyroid cartilage. It is more prominent in men than in women.

addiction   A state of overwhelming obsession or physical need to continue the use of a drug or agent.

adduction   Motion of a limb toward the midline.

adolescents   Children between 12 and 18 years of age.

adsorption   To bind or stick to a surface.

advance directive   Written documentation that specifies medical treatment for a competent patient should the patient become unable to make decisions; also called a living will.

advanced life support (ALS)   Advanced lifesaving procedures, such as cardiac monitoring, administration of IV fluids and medications, and use of advanced airway adjuncts.

agonal respirations   Slow, gasping respiration, sometimes seen in dying patients.

air ambulances   Fixed-wing aircraft and helicopters that have been modified for medical care; used to evacuate and transport patients with life-threatening injuries to treatment facilities.

air embolism   The presence of air in the veins, which can lead to cardiac arrest if it enters the heart.

airway   The upper airway tract or the passage above the larynx, which includes the nose, mouth, and throat.

allergen   A substance that causes an allergic reaction.

allergic reaction   The body's exaggerated immune response to an internal or surface agent.

altered level of consciousness   A mental state in which infants and children may be unresponsive, combative, or confused, may thrash about, or may drift into and out of an alert state; also called altered mental status.

altered mental status   A change in the way a person thinks and behaves that may signal disease in the central nervous system.

alveoli   The air sacs of the lungs in which the exchange of oxygen and carbon dioxide takes place.

ambient temperature   The temperature of the surrounding environment.

ambulance   A specialized vehicle for treating and transporting sick and injured patients.

Americans with Disabilities Act (ADA)   Comprehensive legislation that is designed to protect individuals with disabilities against discrimination.

American Standard System   A safety system for size D or larger oxygen cylinders, designed to prevent the accidental attachment of a regulator to a cylinder containing the wrong type of gas.

amniotic sac   The fluid-filled, baglike membrane in which the fetus develops.

anaphylactic shock   Severe shock caused by allergic reactions.

anaphylaxis   An extreme, possibly life-threatening systemic allergic reaction that may include shock and respiratory failure.

anatomic position   The position of reference in which the patient stands facing you, arms at the side, with the palms of the hands forward.

aneurysm   A swelling or enlargement of a part of an artery, resulting from weakening of the arterial wall.

angina pectoris   Transient (short-lived) chest discomfort caused by partial or temporary blockage of blood flow to the heart muscle.

angle of Louis   A ridge on the sternum that lies at the level where the second rib is attached to the sternum; provides a constant and reliable bony landmark on the anterior chest wall.

anorexia   Lack of appetite for food.

anterior   The front surface of the body; the side facing you in the standard anatomic position.

anterior superior iliac spines   The bony prominences of the pelvis (ilium) at the front on each side of the lower abdomen just below the plane of the umbilicus.

anterograde (posttraumatic) amnesia   Inability to remember events after an injury.

antidote   A substance that is used to neutralize or counteract a poison.

antivenin   A serum that counteracts the effect of venom from an animal or insect.

aorta   The principal artery leaving the left side of the heart and carrying freshly oxygenated blood to the body.

aortic valve   The one-way valve that lies between the left ventricle and the aorta. It keeps blood from flowing back into the left ventricle after the left ventricle ejects its blood into the aorta. One of four heart valves.

apex (plural: apices)   The tip or the topmost portion of a structure.

apgar score   A scoring system for assessing the status of a newborn that assigns a number value to each of five areas of assessment.

aphasia   The inability to understand or produce speech.

apnea   Absence of breathing.

apparent life-threatening event (ALTE) An event that causes unresponsiveness, cyanosis, and apnea in an infant, who then resumes breathing with stimulation.

appendicitis Inflammation of the appendix.

appendix A small tubular structure that is attached to the lower border of the cecum in the lower right quadrant of the abdomen.

arrhythmia An irregular or abnormal heart rhythm.

arterial rupture Rupture of a cerebral artery that may contribute to interruption of cerebral blood flow.

arteriole The smallest branch of an artery leading to the vast network of capillaries.

arteriosclerosis A disease that is characterized by hardening, thickening, and calcification of the arterial walls.

artery A blood vessel, consisting of three layers of tissue and smooth muscle that carries blood away from the heart.

articular cartilage A pearly layer of specialized cartilage covering the articular surfaces (contact surfaces on the ends) of bones in synovial joints.

aspiration The introduction of vomit or other foreign material into the lungs.

assault Unlawfully placing a patient in fear of bodily harm.

asthma A disease of the lungs in which muscle spasm in the small air passageways and the production of large amounts of mucus result in airway obstruction.

asystole Complete absence of heart electrical activity.

atherosclerosis A disorder in which cholesterol and calcium build up inside the walls of blood vessels, forming plaque, which eventually leads to partial or complete blockage of blood flow. An atherosclerotic plaque can also become a site where blood clots can form, break off, and embolize elsewhere in the circulation.

atrium One of two (right and left) upper chambers of the heart. The right atrium receives blood from the vena cava and delivers it to the right ventricle. The left atrium receives blood from pulmonary veins and delivers it to the left ventricle.

auscultation A method of listening to sounds within an organ with a stethoscope.

autonomic nervous system The part of the nervous system that regulates functions, such as digestion and sweating, that are not controlled voluntarily.

AVPU A method of assessing a patient's level of consciousness by determining whether a patient is Awake and alert, responsive to Verbal stimulus or Pain, or Unresponsive; used principally in the initial assessment.

avulse To pull or tear away.

avulsion An injury in which soft tissue either is torn completely loose or is hanging as a flap.

backboard A device that is used to provide support to a patient who is suspected of having a hip, pelvic, spinal, or lower extremity injury. Also called a spine board, trauma board, or longboard.

bag-valve-mask (BVM) device A device with face mask attached to a ventilation bag containing a reservoir and connected to oxygen; delivers more than 90% supplemental oxygen.

ball-and-socket joint A joint that allows internal and external rotation as well as bending.

barrier device A protective item, such as a pocket mask with a valve, that limits exposure to a patient's body fluids.

base station Any radio hardware containing a transmitter and receiver that is located in a fixed place.

basic life support (BLS) Noninvasive emergency lifesaving care that is used to treat airway obstruction, respiratory arrest, or cardiac arrest.

basket stretcher A rigid stretcher commonly used in technical and water rescues that surrounds and supports the patient yet allows water to drain through holes in the bottom. Also called a Stokes litter.

battery Touching a patient or providing emergency care without consent.

Battle's sign Bruising behind an ear over the mastoid process that may indicate skull fracture.

behavior How a person functions or acts in response to his or her environment.

behavioral crisis The point at which a person's reactions to events interfere with activities of daily living; a behavioral crisis becomes a psychiatric emergency when it causes a major life interruption, such as attempted suicide.

bends Common name for decompression sickness.

biceps The large muscle that covers the front of the humerus.

bilateral A body part or condition that appears on both sides of the midline.

bile ducts Ducts that convey bile between the liver and the intestine.

birth canal The vagina and cervix.

blanching Turning white.

blood pressure (BP) The pressure that the blood exerts against the walls of the arteries as it passes through them.

bloody show A plug of pink-tinged mucus that is discharged when the cervix begins to dilate.

blowout fracture Fracture of the orbit or of the bones that support the floor of the orbit.

blunt trauma A mechanism of injury in which force occurs over a broad area and the skin is not usually broken.

body substance isolation (BSI) An infection control concept and practice that assumes that all body fluids are potentially infectious.

brachial artery The major vessel in the upper extremity that supplies blood to the arm.

bradycardia A heart rate of less than 60 beats/min in children or less than 80 beats/min in infants.

brain The controlling organ of the body and center of consciousness; functions include perception, control of reactions to the environment, emotional responses, and judgment.

brain stem The area of the brain between the spinal cord and cerebrum, surrounded by the cerebellum; controls functions that are necessary for life, such as respirations.

breath-holding syncope Loss of consciousness caused by a decreased breathing stimulus.

breath sounds An indication of air movement in the lungs, usually assessed with a stethoscope.

breech presentation Delivery in which the buttocks come out first.

burnout A condition of chronic fatigue and frustration that results from mounting stress over time.

burns An injury in which the soft tissue receives more energy than it can absorb without injury, from thermal heat, frictional heat, toxic chemicals, electricity, or nuclear radiation.

calcaneus The heel bone.

capillary Any one of the small blood vessels that connect arteriole and venule and through whose walls various substances pass into and out of the interstitial tissues and then on to the cells.

capillary refill A test that evaluates distal circulatory system function by squeezing (blanching) blood from an area such as a nail bed and watching the speed of its return after releasing the pressure.

capillary vessels The fine end-divisions of the arterial system that allow contact between cells of the body tissues and the plasma and red blood cells.

carbon dioxide retention A condition characterized by a chronically high blood level of carbon dioxide in which the respiratory center no longer responds to high blood levels of carbon dioxide.

cardiac arrest A state in which the heart fails to generate an effective and detectable blood flow; pulses are not palpable in cardiac arrest, even if muscular and electrical activity continues in the heart.

cardiogenic shock A state in which not enough oxygen is delivered to the tissues of the body, caused by low output of blood from the heart. It can be a severe complication of a large acute myocardial infarction, as well as other conditions.

cardiopulmonary resuscitation (CPR) The combination of rescue breathing and chest compressions used to establish adequate ventilation and circulation in a patient who is not breathing and has no pulse.

carotid artery The major artery that supplies blood to the head and brain.

carpometacarpal joint The joint between the wrist and the metacarpal bones; the thumb joint.

carrier An animal or person who may transmit an infectious disease but may not display any symptoms of it.

casualty collection area An area set up by physicians, nurses, and other hospital staff near a major disaster scene, where patients can receive further triage and medical care.

cataract Clouding of the lens of the eye or its surrounding transparent membrane.

catheter A hollow, cylindrical structure that drains or delivers fluids.

cavitation A phenomenon in which speed causes a bullet to generate pressure waves, which cause damage distant from the bullet's path.

cecum The first part of the large intestine, into which the ileum opens.

cellular telephone A low-power portable radio that communicates through an interconnected series of repeater stations called "cells."

central nervous system (CNS) The brain and spinal cord.

cerebellum One of the three major subdivisions of the brain, sometimes called the "little brain"; coordinates the various activities of the brain, particularly body movements.

cerebral edema Swelling of the brain.

cerebral embolism Obstruction of a cerebral artery caused by a clot that was formed elsewhere in the body and traveled to the brain.

cerebrovascular accident (CVA) An interruption of blood flow to the brain that results in the loss of brain function.

cerebrum The largest part of the three subdivisions of the brain, sometimes called the "gray matter"; made up of several lobes that control movement, hearing, balance, speech, visual perception, emotions, and personality.

certification A process in which a person, an institution, or a program is evaluated and recognized as meeting certain predetermined standards to provide safe and ethical care.

cervical spine The portion of the spinal column consisting of the first seven vertebrae that lie in the neck.

cervix The lower one-third, or neck, of the uterus.

channel An assigned frequency or frequencies that are used to carry voice and/or data communications.

chassis The vehicle frame.

chassis set Transfer of the weight (center of mass) of the ambulance to different points on the chassis.

Chemical Transportation Emergency Center (CHEMTREC) An agency that assists emergency personnel in identifying and handling hazardous materials transport incidents.

chief complaint The reason a patient called for help; also, the patient's response to general questions such as "What's wrong?" or "What happened?"

child abuse Any improper or excessive action that injures or otherwise harms a child or infant; includes neglect and physical, sexual, and emotional abuse.

cholecystitis Inflammation of the gallbladder.

chronic bronchitis Irritation of the major lung passageways, from either infectious disease or irritants such as smoke.

chronic obstructive pulmonary disease (COPD) A slow process of dilation and disruption of the airways and alveoli, caused by chronic bronchial obstruction.

circulatory system The complex arrangement of connected tubes, including the arteries, arterioles, capillaries, venules, and veins, that moves blood, oxygen, nutrients, carbon dioxide, and cellular waste throughout the body.

clavicle The collarbone; it is lateral to the sternum and medial to the scapula.

cleaning The process of removing dirt, dust, blood, or other visible contaminants from a surface.

closed abdominal injury Any injury of the abdomen caused by a nonpenetrating instrument or force, in which the skin remains intact; also called blunt abdominal injury.

closed chest injury Injury to the chest in which the skin is not broken, usually due to blunt trauma.

closed fracture A fracture in which the skin is not broken.

closed head injury Injury in which the brain has been injured but the skin has not been broken and there is no obvious bleeding.

closed injury Injury in which damage occurs beneath the skin or mucous membrane but the surface remains intact.

coagulate To form a clot to plug an opening in an injured blood vessels and stop blood flow.

coagulation Formation of clots to plug openings in injured blood vessels and stop blood flow.

coccyx The last three or four vertebrae of the spine; the tailbone.

coefficient of friction A measure of the grip of the tire on the road surface.

colic Acute, intermittent cramping abdominal pain.

collagen A protein that is the chief component of connective tissue and bones.

command post The designated field command center where the incident commander and support personnel are located.

common cold A viral infection usually associated with swollen nasal mucous membranes and the production of fluid from the sinuses and nose.

communicable disease Any disease that can be spread from person to person, or from animal to person.

compartment syndrome An elevation of pressure within the fascial compartment, characterized by extreme pain, decreased pain sensation, pain on stretching of affected muscles, and decreased power; most frequently seen in fractures below the elbow or knee in children.

compensated shock The early stage of shock, in which the body can still compensate for blood loss.

competent Able to make rational decisions about personal well-being.

complete airway obstruction Occurs when a foreign body completely obstructs the patient's airway. Patients cannot breathe, talk, or cough.

complex access Complicated entry that requires special tools and training and includes breaking windows or using other force.

concussion A temporary loss or alteration of part or all of the brain's abilities to function without actual physical damage to the brain.

conduction The loss of heat by direct contact (eg, when a body part comes into contact with a colder object).

congestive heart failure (CHF) A disorder in which the heart loses part of its ability to effectively pump blood, usually as a result of damage to the heart muscle and usually resulting in a backup of fluid into the lungs.

conjunctiva The delicate membrane lining the eyelids and covering the exposed surface of the eye.

conjunctivitis Inflammation of the conjunctiva.

connecting nerves Nerves in the brain and spinal cord that connect the motor and sensory nerves.

consent Permission to render care.

contagious An infectious disease that is capable of being transmitted from one person to another.

contamination The presence of infectious organisms on or in objects such as dressings, water, food, needles, wounds, or a patient's body.

continuous quality improvement (CQI) A system of internal and external reviews and audits of all aspects of an EMS system.

contraindication Situations in which a medication should not be given because it would not help or may actually harm a patient.

contusion Bruising, or ecchymosis.

convection The loss of body heat caused by air movement (eg, breeze blowing across the body).

core temperature The temperature of the central part of the body (eg, the heart, lungs, and vital organs).

cornea The transparent tissue layer in front of the pupil and iris of the eye.

coronary artery A blood vessel that carries blood and nutrients to the heart muscle.

costal arch A bridge of cartilage that connects the ends of the sixth through tenth ribs with the lower portion of the sternum.

costovertebral angle An angle that is formed by the junction of the spine and the tenth rib.

cover The tactical use of an impenetrable barrier to conceal EMS personnel and protect them from projectiles (eg, bullets, bottles, rocks).

CPR board A device that provides a firm surface under the patient's torso.

cranium The area of the head above the ears and eyes; the skull. The cranium contains the brain.

crepitus A grating or grinding sensation caused by fractured bone ends or joints rubbing together; also air bubbles under the skin that produce a crackling sound or crinkly feeling.

cricoid cartilage A rigid, ring-shaped structure that completely encircles the larynx at the top of the trachea.

cricoid pressure A technique that is used with intubation in which pressure is applied on either side of the cricoid cartilage to prevent gastric distention and allow better visualization of vocal cords; also called the Sellick maneuver.

cricothyroid membrane A thin sheet of fascia that connects the thyroid and cricoid cartilages that make up the larynx.

critical incident stress debriefing (CISD) A confidential group discussion of a severely stressful incident that usually occurs within 24 to 72 hours of the incident.

critical incident stress management (CISM) A process that confronts the responses to critical incidents and defuses them, directing the emergency services personnel toward physical and emotional equilibrium.

croup An infectious disease of the upper respiratory system that may cause partial airway obstruction and is characterized by a barking cough; usually seen in children.

crowning The appearance of the infant's head at the vaginal opening during labor.

cyanosis Bluish-gray skin color that is caused by reduced oxygen levels in the blood.

cystitis Inflammation of the bladder.

danger zone (hot zone) An area where individuals can be exposed to sharp metal edges, broken glass, toxic substances, lethal rays, or ignition or explosion of hazardous materials.

DCAP-BTLS A mnemonic for assessment in which each area of the body is evaluated for Deformities, Contusions, Abrasions, Punctures/Penetrations, Burns, Tenderness, Lacerations, and Swelling.

deceleration The process of slowing down.

decompensated shock The late stage of shock, when blood pressure is falling.

decompression sickness A painful condition seen in divers who ascend too quickly, in which gas, especially nitrogen, forms bubbles in blood vessels and other tissues; also called "the bends."

decontaminate To remove or neutralize radiation, chemical, or other hazardous material from clothing, equipment, vehicles, and personnel.

decontamination The process of removing or neutralizing and properly disposing of hazardous materials from equipment, patients, and rescue personnel.

decontamination area The designated area in a hazardous materials incident where all patients and rescuers must be decontaminated before going to another area.

dedicated line A special telephone line that is used for specific point-to-point communications; also known as a "hot line."

deep Further inside the body and away from the skin.

defibrillate To shock a fibrillating (chaotically beating) heart with specialized electrical current in an attempt to restore a normal rhythmic beat.

dehydration A state in which fluid losses are greater than fluid intake into the body, leading to shock and death if untreated.

delirium A change in mental status marked by the inability to focus, think logically, and maintain attention.

delirium tremens (DTs) A severe withdrawal syndrome seen in alcoholics who are deprived of ethyl alcohol; characterized by restlessness, fever, sweating, disorientation, agitation, and convulsions; can be fatal if untreated.

dementia The slow onset of progressive disorientation, shortened attention span, and loss of cognitive function.

dependent lividity Blood settling to the lowest point of the body, causing discoloration of the skin.

depression A persistent mood of sadness, despair, and discouragement; depression may be a symptom of many different mental and physical disorders, or it may be a disorder on its own.

dermis The inner layer of the skin, containing hair follicles, sweat glands, nerve endings, and blood vessels.

designated officer The individual in the department who is charged with the responsibility of managing exposures and infection control issues.

detailed physical exam The part of the assessment process in which a detailed area-by-area exam is performed on patients whose problems cannot be readily identified or when more specific information is needed about problems identified in the focused history and physical exam.

diabetes mellitus A metabolic disorder in which the ability to metabolize carbohydrates (sugars) is impaired, usually because of a lack of insulin.

diabetic coma Unconsciousness caused by dehydration, very high blood glucose, and acidosis in diabetes.

diabetic ketoacidosis (DKA) A form of acidosis in uncontrolled diabetes in which certain acids accumulate when insulin is not available.

diamond carry A carrying technique in which one EMT-B is located at the head end, one at the foot end, and one at each side of the patient; each of the two EMT-Bs at the sides uses one hand to support the stretcher so that all are able to face forward as they walk.

diaphoretic Characterized by profuse sweating.

diaphragm A muscular dome that forms the undersurface of the thorax, separating the chest from the abdominal cavity. Contraction of the diaphragm (and the chest wall muscles) brings air into the lungs. Relaxation allows air to be expelled from the lungs.

diastole The relaxation, or period of relaxation, of the heart, especially of the ventricles.

diastolic pressure The pressure that remains in the arteries during the relaxing phase of the heart's cycle (diastole) when the left ventricle is at rest.

diffuse pain Pain that is not identified as being specific to a single location.

diffusion A process in which molecules move from an area of higher concentration of molecules to an area of lower concentration.

digestion The processing of food that nourishes the individual cells of the body.

dilation Widening of a tubular structure such as a coronary artery.

diphtheria An infectious disease in which a membrane lining the pharynx is formed that can severely obstruct passage of air into the larynx.

Glossary

direct contact Exposure or transmission of a communicable disease from one person to another by physical touching.

direct ground lift A lifting technique that is used for patients who are found lying supine on the ground with no suspected spinal injury.

disaster A widespread event that disrupts community resources and functions, in turn threatening public safety, citizens' lives, and property.

disinfection The killing of pathogenic agents by direct application of chemicals.

dislocation Disruption of a joint in which ligaments are damaged and the bone ends are completely displaced.

displaced fracture A fracture in which bone fragments are separated from one another and not in anatomic alignment.

distal Structures that are farther from the trunk or nearer to the free end of the extremity.

distracted The action of pulling the spine along its length.

diverticulitis Bulging out of intestinal rings in small pockets at weak areas in the muscle walls, creating abdominal discomfort.

diving reflex Slowing of the heart rate caused by submersion in cold water.

DNR (Do Not Resuscitate) orders Written documentation giving permission to medical personnel not to attempt resuscitation in the event of cardiac arrest.

dorsal The posterior surface of the body, including the back of the hand.

dorsalis pedis artery The artery on the anterior surface of the foot between the first and second metatarsals.

dose The amount of medication given on the basis of the patient's size and age.

drowning Death from suffocation by submersion in water.

duplex The ability to transmit and receive simultaneously.

duty to act A medicolegal term relating to certain personnel who either by statute or by function have a responsibility to provide care.

dysarthria The inability to pronounce speech clearly, often due to loss of the nerves or brain cells that control the small muscles in the larynx.

dyspnea Shortness of breath or difficulty breathing.

ecchymosis Bruising or discoloration associated with bleeding within or under the skin.

eclampsia Convulsions (seizures) resulting from severe hypertension in the pregnant woman.

ectopic pregnancy A pregnancy that develops outside the uterus, typically in a fallopian tube.

edema The presence of abnormally large amounts of fluid between cells in body tissues, causing swelling of the affected area.

elder abuse Any action on the part of an elderly individual's family member, caregiver, or other associated person that takes advantage of the elderly individual's person, property, or emotional state; also called granny beating or parent battering.

electrolytes Certain salts and other chemicals that are dissolved in body fluids and cells.

embolus A blood clot or other substance in the circulatory system that travels to a blood vessel where it causes blockage.

emergency A serious situation, such as injury or illness, that threatens the life or welfare of a person or group of people and requires immediate intervention.

emergency medical care Immediate care or treatment.

emergency medical services (EMS) A multidisciplinary system that represents the combined efforts of several professionals and agencies to provide prehospital emergency care to the sick and injured.

emergency medical technician (EMT) An EMS professional who is trained and licensed by the state to provide emergency medical care in the field.

emergency move A move in which the patient is dragged or pulled from a dangerous scene before initial assessment and care are provided.

emesis Vomiting.

emphysema A disease of the lungs in which there is extreme dilation and eventual destruction of pulmonary alveoli with poor exchange of oxygen and carbon dioxide; it is one form of chronic obstructive pulmonary disease (COPD).

EMT-Basic An EMT who has training in basic emergency care skills, including automated external defibrillation, use of a definitive airway adjunct, and assisting patients with certain medications.

EMT-Intermediate An EMT who has training in specific aspects of advanced life support, such as IV (intravenous) therapy, interpretation of cardiac rhythms and defibrillation, and orotracheal intubation.

EMT-Paramedic An EMT who has extensive training in advanced life support, including IV (intravenous) therapy, pharmacology, cardiac monitoring, and other advanced assessment and treatment skills.

End tidal carbon dioxide detector A plastic, disposable indicator that signals by color change when an endotracheal tube is in the proper place.

endocrine system The complex message and control system that integrates many body functions, including the release of hormones.

endotracheal intubation Insertion of an endotracheal tube (ETT) directly through the larynx between the vocal cords, and into the trachea, to open and maintain an airway.

entrance wound The area of the body where a penetrating trauma occurs. In knife or gunshot wounds, this would be the area where the bullet or blade entered. Also seen in serious electrical injuries.

entrapment To be caught (trapped) within a vehicle, room, or container with no way out, or to have a limb or other body part trapped.

envenomation The act of injecting venom.

epidermis The outer layer of skin, which is made up of cells that are sealed together to form a watertight protective covering for the body.

epiglottis A thin, leaf-shaped valve that allows air to pass into the trachea but prevents food or liquid from entering.

epiglottitis An infection of the soft tissue in the area above the vocal cords.

epinephrine A substance produced by the body (commonly called adrenaline), and a drug produced by pharmaceutical companies that increases pulse rate and blood pressure; the drug of choice for an anaphylactic reaction.

epistaxis Nosebleed.

Esophageal Tracheal Combitube (ETC) A multi-lumen airway that consists of a single, dual-lumen tube with two cuffs.

esophagus A collapsible tube that extends from the pharynx to the stomach; contractions of the muscle in the wall of the esophagus propel food and liquids through it to the stomach.

eustachian tube The internal auditory canal that connects the middle ear to the nasal cavity.

evaporation Conversion of water or another fluid from a liquid to a gas.

evisceration The displacement of organs outside of the body.

exit wound The area of the body where a penetrating trauma exited. In gunshot wounds, this would be the area where the bullet exited.

exhalation The part of the breathing process in which the diaphragm and the intercostal muscles relax, forcing air out of the lungs.

exposure A situation in which a person has had contact with blood, body fluids, tissues, or airborne particles in a manner that suggests that disease transmission may occur.

exposure control plan A comprehensive plan that helps employees to reduce their risk of exposure to or acquisition of communicable diseases.

expressed consent A type of consent in which a patient gives express authorization for provision of care or transport.

extend To straighten.

external auditory canal The ear canal; leads to the tympanic membrane.

extremity lift A lifting technique that is used for patients who are supine or in a sitting position with no suspected extremity or spinal injuries.

extrication Removal of a patient from entrapment or a dangerous situation or position, such as removal from a wrecked vehicle, industrial accident, or building collapse.

eyes-forward position A head position in which the patient's eyes are looking straight ahead and the head and torso are in line.

fallopian tube Long, slender tube that extends from the uterus to the region of the ovary on the same side, and through which the ovum passes from ovary to uterus.

fascia A sheet or band of tough fibrous connective tissue; lies deep under the skin and forms an outer layer for the muscles.

febrile seizures Convulsions that result from sudden high fevers, particularly in children.

Federal Communications Commission (FCC) The federal agency that has jurisdiction over interstate and international telephone and telegraph services and satellite communications, all of which may involve EMS activity.

femoral artery The principal artery of the thigh, a continuation of the external iliac artery. It supplies blood to the lower abdominal wall, external genitalia, and legs. It can be palpated in the groin area.

femoral head The proximal end of the femur, articulating with the acetabulum to form the hip joint.

femur The thigh bone, which extends from the pelvis to the knee and is responsible for formation of the hip; the longest and largest bone in the body.

fetal alcohol syndrome A condition of infants who are born to alcoholic mothers; characterized by physical and mental retardation and a variety of congenital abnormalities.

fetus The developing, unborn infant inside the uterus.

fibrillation Completely disorganized, ineffective twitching of the heart muscle.

fibula The outer and smaller bone of the two bones of the lower leg.

first responder The first trained individual, such as a police officer, fire fighter, or other rescuer, to arrive at the scene of an emergency to provide initial medical assistance.

first responder vehicle A specialized vehicle used to transport EMS equipment and personnel to the scenes of medical emergencies.

flail chest A condition in which three or more ribs are fractured in two or more places, or in association with a fracture of the sternum, so that a segment of chest wall is effectively detached from the rest of the thoracic cage.

flex To bend.

flexible stretcher A stretcher that is a rigid carrying device when secured around a patient but can be folded or rolled when not in use.

floating ribs The eleventh and twelfth ribs, which do not attach to the sternum through the costal arch.

flutter valve A one-way valve that allows air to leave the chest cavity but not return. Formed by taping three sides of an occlusive dressing to the chest wall, leaving the fourth open as the valve.

focal pain Pain that is easily identified as being specific to a single location.

focused history and physical exam The part of the assessment process in which the patient's major complaints or any problems that are immediately evident are further and more specifically evaluated.

footprint The area of contact between the ambulance tire and the road surface.

foramen magnum A large opening at the base of the skull through which the brain connects to the spinal cord.

forcible restraint The act of physically preventing an individual from treating any physical action.

four-person log roll The recommended procedure for moving a patient with a suspected spinal injury from the ground to a long spine board.

Fowler's position The position in which the patient is sitting up with the knees bent.

fracture A break in the continuity of a bone.

friction Resistance to the motion of one body against another.

frostbite Damage to tissues as the result of exposure to cold; frozen or partially frozen body parts.

full-thickness burn A burn that affects all skin layers and may affect the subcutaneous layers, muscle, bone, and internal organs, leaving the area dry, leathery, and white, dark brown, or charred; traditionally called a third-degree burn.

functional disorder A disorder in which there is no known physiologic reason for the abnormal functioning of an organ or organ system.

gag reflex A normal reflex mechanism that causes retching; activated by touching the soft palate or the back of the throat.

gallbladder A sac on the undersurface of the liver that collects bile from the liver and discharges it into the duodenum through the common bile duct.

gastric distention A condition in which air fills the stomach as a result of high volume and pressure during artificial ventilation.

gastric tube An advanced airway adjunct that provides a channel directly into a patient's stomach, allowing you to remove gas, blood, and toxins, or to insert medications and nutrition.

gel A semi-liquid substance that is administered orally through capsules or plastic tubes.

general adaptation syndrome The body's three-stage response to stress. First, stress causes the body to trigger an alarm response, followed by a stage of reaction and resistance, and then recovery, or if the stress is prolonged, exhaustion.

general impression The overall initial impression that determines the priority for patient care; based on the patient's surroundings, the mechanism of injury, signs and symptoms, and the chief complaint.

generalized seizure Seizure characterized by severe twitching of all the body's muscles that may last several minutes or more; also known as a grand mal seizure.

generic name The original chemical name of a medication (in contrast to one of its "trade names"); not capitalized.

genital system The male and female reproductive systems.

Glasgow Coma Scale A method of evaluating level of consciousness that uses a scoring system for neurologic responses to specific stimuli.

glenoid fossa The part of the scapula that joins with the humeral head to form the glenohumeral joint.

globe The eyeball.

glucose One of the basic sugars; it is the primary fuel, along with oxygen, for cellular metabolism.

Golden Hour The time from injury to definitive care, during which treatment of shock or traumatic injuries should occur because survival potential is the best.

good air exchange A term used to distinguish the degree of distress in a patient with a partial airway obstruction. With good air exchange, the patient is still conscious and able to cough forcefully, although wheezing may be heard.

Good Samaritan laws Statutory provisions enacted by many states to protect citizens from liability for errors and omissions in giving good faith emergency medical care, unless there is wanton, gross, or willful negligence.

greater trochanter A bony prominence on the proximal lateral side of the thigh, just below the hip joint.

guarding Involuntary muscle contractions (spasm) of the abdominal wall, an effort to protect the inflamed abdomen; a sign of peritonitis.

hair follicles The small organs in the skin that produce hair.

hallucinogen An agent that produces false perceptions in any one of the five senses.

hazardous material Any substance that is toxic, poisonous, radioactive, flammable, or explosive and causes injury or death with exposure.

hazardous materials incident An incident in which a hazardous material is no longer properly contained and isolated.

head tilt–chin lift maneuver A combination of two movements to open the airway by tilting the forehead back and lifting the chin; used for nontrauma patients.

heart A hollow muscular organ that receives blood from the veins and propels it into the arteries.

heart rate (pulse) The wave of pressure that is created by the heart's contracting and forcing blood out the left ventricle and into the major arteries.

heat cramps Painful muscle spasms usually associated with vigorous activity in a hot environment.

heat exhaustion A form of heat injury in which the body loses significant amounts of fluid and electrolytes because of heavy sweating; also called heat prostration or heat collapse.

heatstroke A life-threatening condition of severe hyperthermia caused by exposure to excessive natural or artificial heat, marked by warm, dry skin; severely altered mental status; and often irreversible coma.

hematemesis Vomiting blood.

hematoma The collection of blood in a space, tissue, or organ due to a break in the wall of a blood vessel.

hematuria The presence of blood in the urine.

hemiparesis Weakness on one side of the body.

hemophilia A congenital condition in which the patient lacks one or more of the blood's normal clotting factors.

hemoptysis The spitting or coughing up of blood.

hemorrhage Bleeding.

hemorrhagic stroke One of the two main types of stroke; occurs as a result of bleeding inside the brain.

hemothorax A collection of blood in the pleural cavity.

hepatitis An infection of the liver, usually caused by a virus, that causes fever, loss of appetite, jaundice, fatigue, and altered liver function.

hernia The protrusion of a loop of an organ or tissue through an abnormal body opening.

high-level disinfection The killing of pathogenic agents by using potent means of disinfection.

hinge joints Joints that can bend and straighten but cannot rotate; they restrict motion to one plane.

histamine A substance released by the immune system in allergic reactions that is responsible for many of the symptoms of anaphylaxis.

HIV infection Infection with the human immunodeficiency virus (HIV) that can progress to acquired immunodeficiency syndrome (AIDS).

hollow organs Structures through which materials pass, such as the stomach, small intestines, large intestines, ureters, and bladder.

hormone A chemical substance that regulates the activity of body organs and tissues; produced by a gland.

host The organism or individual that is attacked by the infecting agent.

humerus The supporting bone of the upper arm that joins with the scapula (glenoid) to form the shoulder joint and with the ulna and radius to form the elbow joint.

hydroplaning A condition in which the tires of a vehicle may be lifted off the road surface as water "piles up" under them, making the vehicle feel as though it is floating.

hyperbaric chamber A chamber, usually a small room, pressurized to more than atmospheric pressure.

hyperglycemia Abnormally high glucose level in the blood.

hypertension Blood pressure that is higher than the normal range.

hyperthermia A condition in which core temperature rises to 101°F (38.3°C) or more.

hyperventilation Rapid or deep breathing that lowers blood carbon dioxide levels below normal.

hyphema Bleeding into the anterior chamber of the eye, obscuring the iris.

hypnotic A sleep-inducing effect or agent.

hypoglycemia Abnormally low glucose level in the blood.

hypotension Blood pressure that is lower than the normal range.

hypothermia A condition in which the internal body temperature falls below 95°F (35°C), usually as a result of prolonged exposure to cool or freezing temperatures.

hypoventilation Reduced minute volume, either from reduced rate and/or depth of breathing.

hypovolemic shock A condition in which low blood volume, due to either massive internal or external bleeding or extensive loss of body water, results in inadequate perfusion.

hypoxia A condition in which the body's cells and tissues do not have enough oxygen.

hypoxic drive Backup system to control respirations when oxygen levels fall.

ileus Paralysis of the bowel, arising from any one of several causes; stops contractions that move material through the intestine.

iliac crest The rim, or wing, of the pelvic bone.

ilium One of three bones that fuse to form the pelvic ring.

implied consent Type of consent in which a patient who is unable to give consent is given treatment under the legal assumption that he or she would want treatment.

incident commander The individual who has overall command of the scene in the field.

incident command system An organizational system to help control, direct, and coordinate emergency responders and resources; known more generally as an incident management system (IMS).

incontinent Loss of bowel and bladder control due to a generalized seizure.

indication A therapeutic use for a specific medication.

indirect contact Exposure or transmission of disease from one person to another by contact with a contaminated object.

infant The first year of life.

infarcted cells Cells in the brain that die as a result of loss of blood flow to the brain.

infarction Death of a body tissue, usually caused by interruption of its blood supply.

infection The abnormal invasion of a host or host tissues by organisms such as bacteria, viruses, or parasites, with or without signs or symptoms of disease.

infection control Procedures to reduce transmission of infection among patients and health care personnel.

infectious disease A disease that is caused by infection, in contrast to one caused by faulty genes, metabolic or hormonal disturbances, emotional trauma, or another cause.

inferior The part of the body, or any body part, nearer to the feet.

inferior vena cava One of the two largest veins in the body; carries blood from the lower extremities and the pelvic and the abdominal organs into the heart.

informed consent Permission for treatment given by a competent patient after the potential risks, benefits, and alternatives to treatment have been explained.

ingestion Swallowing; taking a substance by mouth.

inguinal ligament The tough, fibrous ligament that stretches between the lateral edge of the pubic symphysis and the anterior superior iliac spine.

inhalation The active, muscular part of breathing that draws air into the airway and lungs.

initial assessment The part of the assessment process that helps you to identify any immediately or potentially life-threatening conditions so that you can initiate lifesaving care.

insulin A hormone produced by the pancreas that enables sugar in the blood to enter the cells of the body; used in synthetic form to treat and control diabetes mellitus.

insulin shock Unconsciousness or altered mental status in a patient with diabetes caused by significant hypoglycemia; usually the result of excessive exercise and activity or failure to eat after a routine dose of insulin.

intervertebral disk The cushion that lies between two vertebrae.

intramuscular (IM) injection Injection into a muscle; a medication delivery route.

intraosseous (IO) Into the bone; a medication delivery route.

intravenous (IV) injection Injection directly into a vein; a medication delivery route.

involuntary activity The actions that we do not consciously control.

involuntary muscle Muscle that continues to contract, rhythmically, regardless of the conscious will of the individual.

iris The muscle and surrounding tissue behind the cornea that dilate and constrict the pupil, regulating the amount of light that enters the eye; pigment in this tissue gives the eye its color.

irreversible shock The final stage of shock, resulting in death.

ischemia A lack of oxygen that deprives tissues of necessary nutrients, resulting from partial or complete blockage of blood flow; potentially reversible since permanent injury has not yet occurred.

ischemic cells Cells in the brain that receive enough blood after a cerebrovascular accident to stay alive but not to function properly.

ischemic stroke One of the two main types of stroke; occurs when blood flow to a particular part of the brain is cut off by a blockage (eg, a clot) inside a blood vessel.

ischium One of three bones that fuse to form the pelvic ring.

jaundice A yellow skin or sclera color that is caused by liver disease or dysfunction.

jaw-thrust maneuver Technique to open the airway by placing the fingers behind the angle of the jaw and bringing the jaw forward; used when a patient may have a cervical spine injury.

joint (articulation) The place where two bones come into contact.

joint capsule The fibrous sac with synovial lining that encloses a joint.

jump kit A portable kit containing items that are used in the initial care of the patient.

kidneys Two retroperitoneal organs that excrete the end products of metabolism as urine and regulate the body's salt and water content.

kinetic energy The energy of a moving object.

Kussmaul respirations Deep, rapid breathing; usually the result of an accumulation of certain acids when insulin is not available in the body.

labored breathing Breathing that requires visibly increased effort; characterized by grunting, stridor, and use of accessory muscles.

laceration A smooth or jagged open wound.

lacrimal glands The glands that produce fluids to keep the eye moist; also called tear glands.

large intestine The portion of the digestive tube that encircles the abdomen around the small bowel, consisting of the cecum, the colon, and the rectum.

laryngeal mask airway (LMA) Advanced airway device that is blindly inserted into the mouth to isolate the larynx for direct ventilation; consists of a tube and a mask/cuff that inflates to seal around the laryngeal opening.

laryngoscope An instrument used to give a direct view of the patient's vocal cords during endotracheal intubation.

laryngospasm A severe constriction of the larynx and vocal cords.

lateral Parts of the body that lie farther from the midline. Also called outer structures.

lens The transparent part of the eye through which images are focused on the retina.

leukotrienes Chemical substances that contribute to anaphylaxis; released by the immune system in allergic reactions.

ligament A band of the fibrous tissue that connects bones to bones. It supports and strengthens a joint.

lighted stylet An instrument used to aid in blind insertion of an endotracheal tube.

limb presentation A delivery in which the presenting part is a single arm, leg, or foot.

liver A large solid organ that lies in the right upper quadrant immediately below the diaphragm; it produces bile, stores sugar for immediate use by the body, and produces many substances that help regulate immune responses.

lumbar spine The lower part of the back, formed by the lowest five nonfused vertebrae; also called the dorsal spine.

lumbar vertebrae Vertebrae of the lumbar spine.

lumen The inside diameter of an artery or other hollow structure.

lung compliance The ability of the alveoli to fully expand when air is drawn in on inhalation.

mandible The bone of the lower jaw.

manubrium The upper quarter of the sternum.

mass-casualty incident An emergency situation involving more than one patient, and which can place such great demand on equipment or personnel that the system is stretched to its limit or beyond.

mastoid process A prominent bony mass at the base of the skull behind the ear.

maxillae The upper jawbones that assist in the formation of the orbit, the nasal cavity, and the palate, and lodge the upper teeth.

mechanism of injury The way in which traumatic injuries occur; the forces that act on the body to cause damage.

meconium A dark green material in the amniotic fluid that can cause lung disease in the newborn.

MED channels VHF and UHF channels that the FCC has designated exclusively for EMS use.

medial Parts of the body that lie closer to the midline; also called inner structures.

medical control Physician instructions that are given directly by radio (online/direct) or indirectly by protocol/guidelines (off-line/indirect), as authorized by the medical director of the service program.

medical director The physician who authorizes or delegates to the EMT the authority to perform medical care in the field.

medicolegal A term relating to medical jurisprudence (law) or forensic medicine.

meninges Three distinct layers of tissue that surround and protect the brain and the spinal cord within the skull and the spinal canal.

meningitis An inflammation of the meningeal coverings of the brain; it is usually caused by a virus or a bacterium.

mental disorder An illness with psychological or behavioral symptoms and/or impairment in functioning, caused by a social, psychological, genetic, physical, chemical, or biologic disturbance.

metabolism The sum of all the physical and chemical processes of living organisms; the process by which energy is made available for the uses of the organism.

metered-dose inhaler (MDI) A miniature spray canister through which droplets or particles of medication may be inhaled.

midaxillary line An imaginary vertical line drawn through the middle of the axilla (armpit), parallel to the midline.

midclavicular line An imaginary vertical line drawn through the middle portion of the clavicle and parallel to the midline.

midline An imaginary vertical line drawn from the middle of the forehead through the nose and the umbilicus (navel) to the floor.

motor nerves Nerves that carry information from the central nervous system to the muscles of the body.

mucous membranes The lining of body cavities and passages that communicate directly or indirectly with the environment outside the body.

mucus The opaque, sticky secretion of the mucous membranes that lubricates the body openings.

multigravida A woman who has had previous pregnancies.

multipara A woman who has had more than one live birth.

multi-lumen airway Advanced airway devices, such as the Esophageal Tracheal Combitube and the Pharyngeotracheal Lumen Airway, that have multiple tubes to aid in ventilation and will work whether placed in the trachea or esophagus.

musculoskeletal system The bones and voluntary muscles of the body.

myocardial contusion A bruise of the heart muscle.

myocardium The heart muscle.

nares The external openings of the nostrils.

nasal cannula An oxygen delivery device in which oxygen flows through two small, tubelike prongs that fit into the patient's nostrils.

nasal flaring Flaring out of the nostrils, indicating that there is an airway obstruction.

nasopharyngeal (nasal or trumpet) airway Airway adjunct inserted into the nostril of a conscious patient who is not able to maintain a natural airway.

nasopharynx The part of the pharynx that lies above the level of the roof of the mouth, or soft palate.

nasotracheal intubation Endotracheal intubation through the nose.

nature of illness Effort to determine the general type of illness.

near drowning Survival, at least temporarily, after suffocation in water.

negligence Failure to provide the same care that a person with similar training would provide.

Neisseria meningitides A form of bacterial meningitis characterized by rapid onset of symptoms, often leading to shock and death.

neonatal The first month after birth.

nervous system The system that controls virtually all activities of the body, both voluntary and involuntary.

neurogenic shock Circulatory failure caused by paralysis of the nerves that control the size of the blood vessels, leading to widespread dilation; seen in spinal cord injuries.

nitroglycerin Medication that increases cardiac perfusion by blood flow by causing arteries to dilate; the EMT-B may be allowed to help the patient self-administer the medication.

nondisplaced fracture A simple crack in the bone that has not caused the bone to move from its normal anatomic position; also called a hairline fracture.

nonrebreathing mask A combination mask and reservoir bag system that is the preferred way to give oxygen in the prehospital setting; delivers up to 90% inspired oxygen.

nuchal cord An umbilical cord that is wrapped around the infant's neck.

occiput The most posterior portion of the cranium.

occlusion Blockage, usually of a tubular structure such as a blood vessel.

occlusive dressing Dressing made of Vaseline gauze, aluminum foil, or plastic that prevents air and liquids from entering or exiting a wound.

Occupational Safety and Health Administration (OSHA) The federal regulatory compliance agency that develops, publishes, and enforces guidelines concerning safety in the workplace.

ongoing assessment The part of the assessment process in which problems are reevaluated and responses to treatment are assessed.

open abdominal injury An injury of the abdomen caused by a penetrating or piercing instrument or force, in which the skin is lacerated or perforated and the cavity is opened to the atmosphere; also called penetrating injury.

open chest injury Injury to the chest in which the chest wall itself is penetrated by a fractured rib or some external object.

open fracture Any break in a bone in which the overlying skin has been damaged.

open head injury Injury to the head often caused by a penetrating object in which there may be bleeding and exposed brain tissue.

open injury An injury in which there is a break in the surface of the skin or the mucous membrane, exposing deeper tissue to potential contamination.

opioids Any drug or agent with actions similar to morphine.

OPQRST The six pain questions: Onset, Provoking factors, Quality, Radiation, Severity, Time.

optic nerve A cranial nerve that transmits visual information to the brain.

oral By mouth; a medication delivery route.

oral glucose A simple sugar that is readily absorbed by the bloodstream; it is carried on the EMS unit.

orbit The eye socket, made up of the maxilla and zygoma.

organic brain syndrome Temporary or permanent dysfunction of the brain, caused by a disturbance in the physical or physiologic functioning of brain tissue.

orientation The mental status of a patient as measured by memory of person (name), place (current location), time (current year, month, and approximate date), and event (what happened).

oropharyngeal (oral) airway Airway adjunct inserted into the mouth to keep the tongue from blocking the upper airway and to make suctioning the airway easier.

oropharynx A tubular structure that extends vertically from the back of the mouth to the esophagus and trachea.

orotracheal intubation Endotracheal intubation through the mouth.

osteoporosis A generalized bone disease, commonly associated with postmenopausal women, in which there is a reduction in the amount of bone mass leading to fractures after minimal trauma in either sex.

over-the-counter (OTC) medications Medications that may be purchased directly by a patient without a prescription.

ovary A female gland that produces sex hormones and ova (eggs).

oxygen A gas that all cells need in order to metabolize; the heart and brain, especially, cannot function without oxygen.

paging The use of a radio signal and a voice or digital message that is transmitted to pagers ("beepers") or desktop monitor radios.

palmar The front region of the hand.

palpate Examine by touch.

pancreas A flat, solid organ that lies below the liver and the stomach; it is a major source of digestive enzymes and produces the hormone insulin.

pancreatitis Inflammation of the pancreas.

paradoxical motion The motion of the portion of the chest wall that is detached in a flail chest; the motion—in during inhalation, out during exhalation—is exactly the opposite of normal chest wall motion during breathing.

parietal regions The areas between the temporal and occiput regions of the cranium.

partial airway obstruction Condition in which an obstruction leaves the patient able to exchange some air, but also causes some degree of respiratory distress.

partial-thickness burn A burn affecting the epidermis and some portion of the dermis but not the subcutaneous tissue, characterized by blisters and skin that is white to red, moist, and mottled; traditionally called a second-degree burn.

patella The kneecap; a specialized bone that lies within the tendon of the quadriceps muscle.

pathogen A microorganism that is capable of causing disease in a susceptible host.

pedal edema Swelling of the feet and ankles caused by collection of fluid in the tissues; a possible sign of congestive heart failure (CHF).

pediatrics A specialized medical practice devoted to the care of the young.

pediatric resuscitation tape measure A tape that estimates an infant or child's weight on the basis of length and lists appropriate drug doses and equipment sizes on the tape.

penetrating trauma A mechanism of injury in which force occurs in a small point of contact between the skin and the object. The skin is broken and the potential for infection is high.

penetrating wound An injury resulting from a sharp, pointed object.

perfusion The circulation of blood within an organ or tissue in adequate amounts to meet the cells' current needs.

pericardial tamponade Compression of the heart due to a buildup of blood or other fluid in the pericardial sac.

pericardium The fibrous sac that surrounds the heart.

perineum The area of skin between the vagina and the anus.

peripheral nervous system The part of the nervous system that consists of 31 pairs of spinal nerves and 12 pairs of cranial nerves. These peripheral nerves may be sensory nerves, motor nerves, or connecting nerves.

peristalsis The wave-like contraction of smooth muscle by which the ureters or other tubular organs propel their contents.

peritoneal cavity The abdominal cavity.

peritoneum The membrane lining the abdominal cavity (parietal peritoneum) and covering the abdominal organs (visceral peritoneum).

peritonitis Inflammation of the peritoneum.

personal protective equipment (PPE) Protective equipment that OSHA requires to be made available to the EMT. In the case of infection risk, PPE blocks entry of an organism into the body.

per os (PO) Through the mouth; a medication delivery route; same as oral.

per rectum (PR) Through the rectum; a medication delivery route.

pharmacology The study of the properties and effects of medications.

Pharyngeotracheal Lumen Airway (PtL) A multi-lumen airway that consists of two tubes, two masks, and a bite block.

pin-indexing system A system established for portable cylinders to ensure that a regulator is not connected to a cylinder containing the wrong type of gas.

pinna The external, visible part of the ear.

placenta Tissue attached to the uterine wall that nourishes the fetus through the umbilical cord.

placenta abruptio Premature separation of the placenta from the wall of the uterus.

placenta previa A condition in which the placenta develops over and covers the cervix.

plantar The bottom of the foot.

plasma A sticky, yellow fluid that carries the blood cells and nutrients and transports cellular waste material to the organs of excretion.

platelets Tiny, disk-shaped elements that are much smaller than the cells; they are essential in the initial formation of a blood clot, the mechanism that stops bleeding.

pleura The serous membrane covering the lungs and lining the thoracic cavity, completely enclosing a potential space known as the pleural space.

pleural effusion A collection of fluid between the lung and chest wall that may compress the lung.

pleural space The potential space between the parietal pleura and the visceral pleura. It is described as "potential" because under normal conditions, the lungs fill this space.

pleuritic chest pain Sharp, stabbing pain in the chest that is worsened by a deep breath or other chest wall movement; often caused by inflammation or irritation of the pleura.

pneumonia An infectious disease of the lung that damages lung tissue.

pneumatic antishock garment (PASG) An inflatable device that covers the legs and abdomen; used to splint the lower extremities or pelvis, or to control bleeding in the lower extremities, pelvis, or abdominal cavity.

pneumothorax A partial or complete accumulation of air in the pleural space.

point tenderness Tenderness that is sharply localized at the site of the injury, found by gently palpating along the bone with the tip of one finger.

poison A substance whose chemical action could damage structures or impair function when introduced into the body.

polydipsia Excessive thirst persisting for long periods of time despite reasonable fluid intake; often the result of excessive urination.

polyphagia Excessive eating; in diabetes, the inability to use glucose properly can cause a sense of hunger.

polyuria The passage of an unusually large volume of urine in a given period; in diabetes, this can result from wasting of glucose in the urine.

poor air exchange A term used to distinguish the degree of distress in a patient with a partial airway obstruction. With poor air exchange, the patient has a weak, ineffective cough, increased difficulty breathing, possible cyanosis, and may produce a high-pitched noise on inhalation (stridor).

portable stretcher A stretcher with a strong rectangular tubular metal frame and rigid fabric stretched across it.

position of function A hand position in which the wrist is slightly dorsiflexed and all finger joints are moderately flexed.

posterior The back surface of the body; the side away from you in the standard anatomical position.

posterior tibial artery The artery just posterior to the medial malleolus; supplies blood to the foot.

postictal period The period immediately following a seizure, characterized by extreme tiredness or listlessness.

postictal state Period following a seizure that lasts between 5 and 30 minutes, characterized by labored respirations and some degree of altered mental status.

posttraumatic stress disorder (PTSD) A delayed stress reaction to a prior incident. This delayed reaction is the result of one or more unresolved issues concerning the incident that might have been alleviated with the use of critical incident stress management.

potential energy The product of mass, gravity, and height, which is converted into kinetic energy and results in injury, such as from a fall.

power grip A technique in which the cot or backboard is gripped by inserting each hand under the handle with the palm facing up and the thumb extended, fully supporting the underside of the handle on the curved palm with the fingers and thumb.

power lift A lifting technique in which the EMT-B's back is held upright, with legs bent, and the patient is lifted when the EMT-B straightens the legs to raise the upper body and arms.

Glossary

pregnancy-induced hypertension A condition of late pregnancy that also involves headache, visual changes, and swelling of the hands and feet; also called pre-eclampsia.

preschool-age Children between 3 and 6 years of age.

prescription medications Medications that are distributed to patients only by pharmacists according to a physician's order.

presentation The position in which an infant is born; the part of the infant that appears first.

pressure point A point where a blood vessel lies near a bone; useful when direct pressure and elevation do not control bleeding.

priapism A continuous and painful erection of the penis caused by certain spinal injuries and some diseases.

primary service area (PSA) The designated area in which the EMS service is responsible for the provision of prehospital emergency care and transportation to the hospital.

primigravida A woman who is experiencing her first pregnancy.

primipara A woman who has had one live birth.

prolapse of the umbilical cord A situation in which the umbilical cord comes out of the vagina before the infant.

prone position The position in which the body is lying face down.

prostate gland A small gland that surrounds the male urethra where it emerges from the urinary bladder; it secretes a fluid that is part of the ejaculatory fluid.

protection level A measure of the amount and type of protective equipment that an individual needs to avoid injury during contact with a hazardous material.

proximal Structures that are closer to the trunk.

psychogenic A symptom or illness that is caused by mental factors as opposed to physical ones.

psychogenic shock Shock caused by a sudden, temporary reduction in blood supply to the brain that causes fainting (syncope).

pubic symphysis A hard bony prominence that is found in the midline in the lowermost portion of the abdomen.

pubis One of three bones that fuse to form the pelvic ring.

pulmonary artery The major artery leading from the right ventricle of the heart to the lungs; it carries oxygen-poor blood.

pulmonary contusion A bruise of the lung.

pulmonary edema A buildup of fluid in the lungs, usually as a result of congestive heart failure.

pulmonary embolism A blood clot that breaks off from a large vein and travels to the blood vessels of the lung, causing obstruction of blood flow.

pulmonary veins The four veins that return oxygenated blood from the lungs to the left atrium of the heart.

pulse The wave of pressure created as the heart contracts and forces blood out the left ventricle and into the major arteries.

pulse oximetry An assessment method that measures oxygen saturation of hemoglobin in the capillary beds.

pupil The circular opening in the middle of the iris that admits light to the back of the eye.

putrefaction Decomposition of body tissues.

quadrants The way to describe the sections of the abdominal cavity. Imagine two lines intersecting at the umbilicus dividing the abdomen into four equal areas.

quality control The responsibility of the medical director to ensure that the appropriate medical care standards are met by EMT-Bs on each call.

rabid Describes an animal that is infected with rabies.

raccoon eyes Bruising under the eyes that may indicate skull fracture.

radial artery The major artery in the forearm; it is palpable at the wrist on the thumb side.

radiation The direct loss of body heat to colder objects in the environment, or heat gain from warmer objects such as the sun.

radiation A continuation of an area of pain or discomfort distal to the site of the origin of the pain; gives the sensation that the pain is moving (radiating) away from the origin.

radius The bone on the thumb side of the forearm; most important in wrist function.

rales Cracking, rattling breath sound that signals fluid in the air spaces of the lungs; also called crackles.

rapid extrication technique A technique to move a patient from a sitting position inside a vehicle to supine on a backboard in less than 1 minute when conditions do not allow for standard immobilization.

rapport A trusting relationship that you build with your patient.

recovery position A position that helps to maintain a clear airway in a patient with a decreased level of consciousness who has not had traumatic injuries and is breathing on his or her own.

rectum The lowermost end of the colon.

red blood cells Cells that carry oxygen to the body's tissues; also called erythrocytes.

reduce Return a dislocated joint or fractured bone to its normal position; set.

referred pain Pain felt in an area of the body other than the area where the cause of pain is located.

rehabilitation area This area provides protection and treatment to firefighters and other personnel working at an emergency. Here, workers are medically monitored and receive any needed care as they enter and leave the scene.

renal pelvis A cone-shaped collecting area that connects the ureter and the kidney.

repeater A special base station radio that receives messages and signals on one frequency and then automatically retransmits them on a second frequency.

respiration The loss of body heat as warm air in the lungs is exhaled into the atmosphere and cooler air is inhaled.

respiratory system All the structures of the body that contribute to the process of breathing, consisting of the upper and lower airways and their component parts.

responsiveness The way in which a patient responds to external stimuli, including verbal stimuli (sound), tactile stimuli (touch), and painful stimuli.

retina The light-sensitive area of the eye where images are projected; a layer of cells at the back of the eye that changes the light image into electrical impulses, which are carried by the optic nerve to the brain.

retinal detachment Separation of the retina from its attachments at the back of the eye.

retrograde amnesia The inability to remember events leading up to a head injury.

retroperitoneal Behind the abdominal cavity.

retroperitoneal space The space between the abdominal cavity and the posterior abdominal wall, containing the kidneys, certain large vessels, and parts of the gastrointestinal tract.

retractions Movements in which the skin pulls in around the ribs during inspiration.

rhonchi Coarse, low-pitched breath sounds heard in patients with chronic mucus in the airways.

rigor mortis Stiffening of the body, is a definitive sign of death.

Rule of Nines A system that assigns percentages to sections of the body, allowing calculation of the amount of skin surface involved in the burn area.

sacrum One of three bones (sacrum and two pelvic bones) that make up the pelvic ring; consists of five fused sacral vertebrae.

salivary glands The glands that produce saliva to keep the mouth and pharynx moist.

SAMPLE history A key brief history of a patient's condition to determine Signs/Symptoms, Allergies, Medications, Pertinent past history, Last oral intake, and Events leading to the illness/injury.

scalp The thick skin covering the cranium, which usually bears hair.

scanner A radio receiver that searches or "scans" across several frequencies until the message is completed; the process is then repeated.

scapula The shoulder blade.

scene size-up A quick assessment of the scene and the surroundings made to provide information about its safety and the mechanism of injury or nature of illness, before you enter and begin patient care.

school-age Children between 6 and 12 years of age.

sciatic nerve The major nerve to the lower extremity; controls much of muscle function in the leg, and sensation in the entire leg and foot.

sclera The tough, fibrous white portion of the eye that protects the more delicate inner structures.

scoop stretcher A stretcher that is designed to be split into two or four sections that can be fitted around a patient who is lying on the ground or other relatively flat surface; also called a split litter.

scuba A system that delivers air to the mouth and lungs at various atmospheric pressures, increasing with the depth of the dive; stands for **self-contained underwater breathing apparatus**.

sebaceous glands Glands that produce an oily substance called sebum, which discharges along the shafts of the hairs.

sector commander The individual delegated to oversee and coordinate activity in an incident command sector; works under the incident commander.

sedative A substance that decreases activity and excitement.

seizure Generalized, uncoordinated muscular activity associated with loss of consciousness; a convulsion.

Sellick maneuver A technique used with intubation, in which pressure is applied on either side of the cricoid cartilage to prevent gastric distention and allow better visualization of vocal cords; also called cricoid pressure.

semen Seminal fluid ejaculated from the penis and containing sperm.

seminal vesicles Storage sacs for sperm and seminal fluid, which empty into the urethra at the prostate.

sensitization Developing a sensitivity to a substance that initially caused no allergic reaction.

sensory nerves The nerves that carry sensations of touch, taste, heat, cold, pain, or other modalities from the body to the central nervous system.

septic shock Shock caused by severe bacterial infection.

septum The central divider in the nose.

shaken baby syndrome Bleeding within the head and damage to the cervical spine of an infant who has been intentionally and forcibly shaken; a form of child abuse.

shock position The position that has the head and torso (trunk) supine and the lower extremities elevated 6" to 12". This helps to increase blood flow to the brain; also referred to as the *modified Trendelenburg's* position.

shock A condition that develops when the circulatory system is not able to deliver sufficient blood to body organs, resulting in organ failure and eventual death if untreated.

shoulder girdle The proximal portion of the upper extremity, made up of the clavicle, the scapula, and the humerus.

shunt A tube that diverts excess cerebrospinal fluid from the brain to the abdomen.

side effects Any effects of a medication other than the desired ones.

sign An objective finding that can be seen, heard, felt, smelled, or measured.

simple access Access that is easily achieved without the use of tools or force.

simplex Single-frequency radio; transmissions can occur in either direction but not simultaneously in both; when one party transmits, the other can only receive, and the party that is transmitting is unable to receive.

skeletal muscle Muscle that is attached to bones and usually crosses at least one joint; striated, or voluntary, muscle.

skeleton The framework that gives us our recognizable form; also designed to allow motion of the body and protection of vital organs.

sling A bandage or material that helps to support the weight of an injured upper extremity.

small intestine The portion of the digestive tube between the stomach and the cecum, consisting of the duodenum, jejunum, and ileum.

smooth muscle Nonstriated, involuntary muscle; it constitutes the bulk of the gastrointestinal tract and is present in nearly every organ to regulate automatic activity.

sniffing position An unusually upright position in which the patient's head and chin are thrust slightly forward.

solid organs Solid masses of tissue where much of the chemical work of the body takes place (eg, the liver, spleen, pancreas, and kidneys).

solution A liquid mixture that cannot be separated by filtering or allowing the mixture to stand.

somatic nervous system The part of the nervous system that regulates our voluntary activities, such as walking, talking, and writing.

sphincters Circular muscles that encircle and, by contracting, constrict a duct, tube, or opening.

spinal cord An extension of the brain, composed of virtually all the nerves carrying messages between the brain and the rest of the body. It lies inside of, and is protected by, the spinal canal.

splint A flexible or rigid appliance used to protect and maintain the position of an injured extremity.

spontaneous pneumothorax Pneumothorax that occurs when a weak area on the lung ruptures in the absence of major injury, allowing air to leak into the pleural space.

spontaneous respirations Breathing in a patient that occurs with no assistance.

sprain A joint injury involving damage to supporting ligaments, and partial or temporary dislocation of bone ends.

stair chair A lightweight folding device that is used to carry a conscious, seated patient up or down stairs.

standard of care Written, accepted levels of emergency care expected by reason of training and profession; written by legal or professional organizations so that patients are not exposed to unreasonable risk or harm.

standing orders Written documents, signed by the EMS system's medical director, that outline specific directions, permissions, and sometimes prohibitions regarding patient care; also called protocols.

Star of Life The six-pointed star that identifies vehicles that meet federal specifications as licensed or certified ambulances.

status epilepticus The term used to describe a continuous seizure, or multiple seizures without a return to consciousness, for 30 minutes or more.

sternocleidomastoid muscles The muscles on either side of the neck that allow movement of the head.

sternum The breastbone.

sterilization A process, such as heating, that removes microbial contamination.

stimulant An agent that produces an excited state.

stoma Opening in the neck that connects the trachea directly to the skin.

strain Stretching or tearing of a muscle; also called a muscle pull.

strangulation Complete obstruction of blood circulation in a given organ as a result of compression or entrapment, an emergency situation causing death of tissue.

striated muscle Muscle that has characteristic stripes, or striations, under the microscope; voluntary, or skeletal, muscle.

stridor A harsh, high-pitched inspiratory sound that is often heard in acute laryngeal (upper airway) obstruction; may sound like crowing and be audible without a stethoscope.

stroke A loss of brain function in certain brain cells that do not get enough oxygen during a CVA. Usually caused by obstruction of the blood vessels in the brain that feed oxygen to those brain cells.

structure fire A fire in a house, apartment building, office, school, plant, warehouse, or other building.

stylet A plastic-coated wire that gives added rigidity and shape to the endotracheal tube.

subcutaneous emphysema A characteristic crackling sensation on palpation, caused by the presence of air in soft tissues.

subcutaneous (SC) injection Injection into the tissue between the skin and muscle; a medication delivery route.

subcutaneous tissue Tissue, largely fat, that lies directly under the dermis and serves as an insulator of the body.

sublingual (SL) Under the tongue; a medication delivery route.

substance abuse The knowing misuse of any substance to produce some desired effect.

sucking chest wound An open or penetrating chest wall wound through which air passes during inspiration and expiration, creating a sucking sound.

sudden infant death syndrome (SIDS) Death of an infant or young child that remains unexplained after a complete autopsy.

superficial Closer to or on the skin.

superficial burn A burn affecting only the epidermis, characterized by skin that is red but not blistered or actually burned through; traditionally called a first-degree burn.

superior The part of the body, or any body part, nearer to the head.

superior vena cava One of the two largest veins in the body; carries blood from the upper extremities, head, neck, and chest into the heart.

supine hypotensive syndrome A drop in blood pressure caused when the heavy uterus of a supine, third-trimester pregnant patient obstructs the vena cava, lowering blood return to the heart.

supine position The position in which the body is lying face up.

suspension A mixture of ground particles that are distributed evenly throughout a liquid but do not dissolve.

swathe A bandage that passes around the chest to secure an injured arm to the chest.

sweat glands The glands that secrete sweat.

symptom A subjective finding that the patient feels but that can be identified only by the patient.

syncope Fainting spell or transient loss of consciousness, often caused by an interruption of blood flow to the brain.

systole The contraction, or period of contraction, of the heart, especially that of the ventricles.

systolic pressure The increased pressure along an artery with each contraction (systole) of the ventricle.

tachycardia Rapid heart rhythm, more than 100 beats/min.

tachypnea Rapid respirations.

tactical situation A hostage, robbery, or other situation in which armed conflict is threatened or shots have been fired and the threat of violence remains.

technical rescue group A team of individuals from one or more departments in a region that is trained and on call for certain types of technical rescue.

technical rescue situation A rescue that requires special technical skills and equipment in one of many specialized rescue areas, such as technical rope rescue, cave rescue, and dive rescue.

telemetry A process in which electronic signals are converted into coded, audible signals; these signals can then be transmitted by radio or telephone to a receiver at the hospital with a decoder.

temporal regions The lateral portions on each side of the cranium.

temporomandibular joint The joint where the mandible meets with the temporal bone of the cranium just in front of each ear.

tendon A tough, ropelike cord of fibrous tissue that attaches a skeletal muscle to a bone.

tension pneumothorax An accumulation of air or gas in the pleural cavity that progressively increases the pressure in the chest with potentially fatal results.

testicle A male genital gland that contains specialized cells that produce hormones and sperm.

thoracic cage The chest or rib cage.

thoracic spine The 12 vertebrae that lie between the cervical vertebrae and the lumbar vertebrae. One pair of ribs is attached to each of the thoracic vertebrae.

thorax The chest cavity that contains the heart, lungs, esophagus, and great vessels (the aorta and the two venae cavae).

thrombosis Clotting of the cerebral arteries that may result in the interruption of cerebral blood flow and subsequent stroke.

thyroid cartilage A firm prominence of cartilage that forms the upper part of the larynx; the Adam's apple.

tibia The larger of the two lower leg bones responsible for supporting the major weight-bearing surface of the knee and the ankle; the shinbone.

tidal volume The amount of air that is delivered to the lungs and airways in one inhalation.

toddler The period following infancy until 3 years of age.

tolerance The need for increasing amounts of a drug to obtain the same effect.

tonic-clonic seizure A seizure that features rhythmic back-and-forth motion of an extremity and body stiffness.

tonsil tip A large, semirigid suction tip recommended for suctioning the pharynx; also called a Yankauer tip.

topical medications Lotions, creams, and ointments that are applied to the surface of the skin and affect only that area; a medication delivery route.

topographic anatomy The superficial landmarks of the body that serve as guides to the structures that lie beneath them.

torso The trunk without the head and limbs.

tourniquet The bleeding control method of last resort that occludes arterial flow; used only when all other methods have failed and the patient's life is in danger.

toxicity level A measure of the risk that a hazardous material poses to the health of an individual who comes into contact with it.

toxin A poison or harmful substance produced by bacteria, animals, or plants.

trachea The windpipe; the main trunk for air passing to and from the lungs.

tracheostomy tube A tube inserted into the trachea in children who cannot breathe on their own; passes through the neck directly into the major airways.

traction The act of exerting a pulling force on a structure.

trade name The brand name that a manufacturer gives a medication; capitalized.

tragus The small cartilaginous projection in front of the opening of the ear.

transcutaneous Through the skin; a medication delivery route.

transdermal medications Medications that are designed to be absorbed through the skin (transcutaneously).

transient ischemic attack (TIA) A disorder of the brain in which brain cells temporarily stop working because of insufficient oxygen, causing stroke-like symptoms that resolve completely within 24 hours of onset.

transmission The way in which an infectious agent is spread: contact, airborne, by vehicles, or by vectors.

transportation area   The area in a mass-casualty incident where ambulances and crews are organized to transport patients from the treatment area to receiving hospitals.

transportation officer   The individual in charge of the transportation sector in a mass-casualty incident, who assigns patients from the treatment area to awaiting ambulances in the transportation area.

treatment area   Location in a mass-casualty incident where patients are brought after being triaged and assigned a priority, where they are reassessed, treated, and monitored until transport to the hospital.

treatment officer   The individual, usually a physician, who is in charge of and directs EMS personnel at the treatment area in a mass-casualty incident.

Trendelenburg's position   The position in which the body is supine with the head lower than the feet.

triage   The process of sorting patients based on the severity of injury and medical need, to establish treatment and transportation priorities.

triage area   Designated area in a mass-casualty incident where the triage officer is located and patients are initially triaged before being taken to the treatment center.

triage officer   The individual in charge of the incident command triage sector, who directs the sorting of patients into triage categories in a mass-casualty incident.

triceps   The muscle in the back of the upper arm.

tripod position   An abnormal position to keep the airway open; it involves leaning forward onto two arms stretched forward.

tuberculosis   A chronic bacterial disease, caused by *Mycobacterium tuberculosis*, that usually affects the lungs but can also affect other organs such as the brain or kidneys.

turbinates   Layers of bone within the nasal cavity.

two- to three-word dyspnea   A severe breathing problem in which a patient can speak only two to three words at a time without pausing to take a breath.

tympanic membrane   The eardrum, which lies between the external and middle ear.

type I diabetes   The type of diabetic disease that usually starts in childhood and requires insulin for proper treatment and control.

type II diabetes   The type of diabetic disease that usually starts in later life and often can be controlled through diet and oral medications.

UHF (ultra-high frequency)   Radio frequencies between 300 and 3,000 MHz.

ulcer   Abrasion of the stomach or small intestine.

ulna   The bone on the small finger side of the forearm; most important for elbow function.

ulnar artery   One of the major arteries of the forearm; it can be palpated at the wrist on the ulnar side (at the base of the fifth finger).

umbilical cord   The conduit connecting mother to infant via the placenta; contains two arteries and one vein.

universal precautions   Protective measures that have traditionally been developed by the Centers for Disease Control and Prevention (CDC) for use in dealing with objects, blood, body fluids, or other potential exposure risks of communicable disease.

ureter   A small, hollow tube that carries urine from the kidneys to the bladder.

urethra   The canal that conveys urine from the bladder to outside the body.

urinary bladder   A sac behind the pubic symphysis made of smooth muscle that collects and stores urine.

urinary system   The organs that control the discharge of certain waste materials filtered from the blood and excreted as urine.

urticaria   Small spots of generalized itching and/or burning that appear as multiple raised areas on the skin; hives.

uterus   The muscular organ where the fetus grows, also called the womb; responsible for contractions during labor.

vagina   A muscular distensible tube that connects the uterus with the vulva (the external female genitalia); also called the birth canal.

vallecula   The space between the base of the tongue and the epiglottis; receives the tip of a curved laryngoscope blade during endotracheal intubation.

vasa deferentia (vas deferens)   The spermatic duct of the testicles; also called vas deferens.

vasoconstriction   Narrowing of a blood vessel.

vasodilation   Widening of a blood vessel.

vein   Any blood vessel that carries blood from the tissues to the heart.

ventral   The anterior surface of the body.

ventilation   Exchange of air between the lungs and the air of the environment, either spontaneously by the patient or with assistance from an EMT-B.

ventricle   One of two (right and left) lower chambers of the heart. The left ventricle receives blood from the left atrium (upper chamber) and delivers blood to the aorta. The right ventricle receives blood from the right atrium and pumps it into the pulmonary artery.

ventricular fibrillation   Disorganized, ineffective twitching of the ventricles, resulting in no blood flow and a state of cardiac arrest.

ventricular tachycardia   Rapid heart rhythm in which the electrical impulse begins in the ventricle (instead of the atrium), which may result in inadequate blood flow and eventually deteriorate into cardiac arrest.

vertebrae   The 33 bones that make up the spinal column.

VHF (very high frequency)   Radio frequencies between 30 and 300 MHz; the VHF spectrum is further divided into "high" and "low" bands.

virulence   The strength or ability of a pathogen to produce disease.

vital signs   The key signs that are used to evaluate the patient's overall condition, including respirations, pulse, blood pressure, level of consciousness, and skin characteristics.

voluntary activity   Actions that we consciously perform, in which sensory input determines the specific muscular activity.

voluntary muscle   Muscle that is under direct voluntary control of the brain and can be contracted or relaxed at will; skeletal, or striated, muscle.

vomitus   Vomited material.

weapons of mass destruction   Biological, chemical, and nuclear warfare mediums used for mass destruction, more prevalent in wartime and more closely associated with the military.

wheal   A raised, swollen, well-defined area on the skin resulting from an insect bite or allergic reaction.

wheeled ambulance stretcher   A specially designed stretcher that can be rolled along the ground. A collapsible undercarriage allows it to be loaded into the ambulance. Also called the cot or an ambulance cot.

wheeze   A high-pitched, whistling breath sound, characteristically heard on expiration in patients with asthma or COPD.

wheezing   A whistling breath sound caused by air traveling through narrowed air passages within the bronchioles; a sign of lower airway obstruction.

white blood cells   Blood cells that play a role in the body's immune defense mechanisms against infection; also called leukocytes.

xiphoid process   The narrow, cartilaginous lower tip of the sternum.

zygomas   The quadrangular bones of the cheek, articulating with the frontal bone, the maxillae, the zygomatic processes of the temporal bone, and the great wings of the sphenoid bone.

Index

Index

Student Resources

Student Workbook

ISBN: 0-7637-1943-9

This resource is designed to encourage critical thinking and aid comprehension of the course material through:

- case studies and corresponding questions
- figure labeling exercises
- crossword puzzles
- matching, fill-in-the-blank, short answer, and multiple-choice questions
- skill drill activities

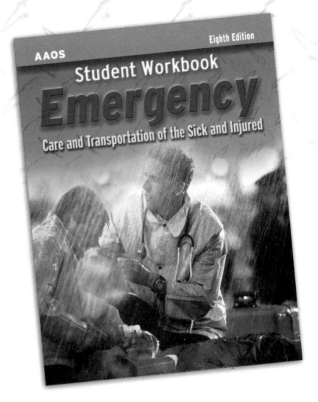

Review Manual

ISBN: 0-7637-1945-5 * Print

ISBN: 0-7637-1947-1 * CD-ROM

ISBN: 0-7637-1946-3 * Online at www.emtb.com

This Review Manual has been designed to prepare students to sit for exams by including the same type of scenario-based and multiple-choice questions that they are likely to see on classroom and national examinations. The manual is available in print, on CD-ROM, and Online. It provides answers to all questions with brief explanations and page references.

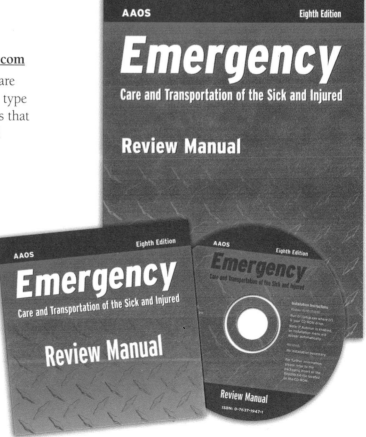